The Cleveland Clinic Intensive Review
of
Internal Medicine

The Cleveland Clinic Intensive Review
of
Internal Medicine

James K. Stoller, MD
Head, Section of Respiratory Therapy
Department of Pulmonary and Critical Care Medicine
The Cleveland Clinic Foundation
Professor of Medicine
The Cleveland Clinic Foundation Health Sciences Center of the Ohio State University
Cleveland, Ohio

Muzaffar Ahmad, MD
Chairman, Division of Internal Medicine
The Cleveland Clinic Foundation
Professor of Internal Medicine
The Cleveland Clinic Foundation Health Sciences Center of the Ohio State University
Cleveland, Ohio

David L. Longworth, MD
Chairman, Department of Infectious Disease
The Cleveland Clinic Foundation
Associate Professor of Medicine
The Cleveland Clinic Foundation Health Sciences Center of the Ohio State University
Cleveland, Ohio
Clinical Professor of Medicine
Pennsylvania State University
Hershey, Pennsylvania

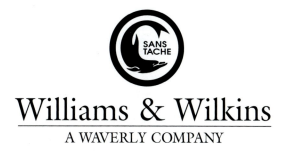

Williams & Wilkins
A WAVERLY COMPANY

BALTIMORE • PHILADELPHIA • LONDON • PARIS • BANGKOK
BUENOS AIRES • HONG KONG • MUNICH • SYDNEY • TOKYO • WROCLAW

Editor: Jonathan W. Pine, Jr
Managing Editor: Molly L. Mullen
Project Editor: Jeffrey S. Myers
Marketing Manager: Danielle Griffin
Designer: Mario Fernandez

Rose Tree Corporate Center
1400 North Providence Road
Building II, Suite 5025
Media, Pennsylvania 19063-2043 USA

Accurate indications, adverse reactions and dosage schedules for drugs are provided in this book, but it is possible that they may change. The reader is urged to review the package information data of the manufacturers of the medications mentioned.

Printed in the United States of America

Library of Congress Cataloging-in-Publication Data

The Cleveland Clinic intensive review of internal medicine / [edited
   by] Muzaffar Ahmad, David L. Longworth, James K. Stoller.
        p.   cm.
      Includes index.
      ISBN 0-683-30087-3
      1. Internal medicine.   2. Internal medicine—Examinations,
   questions, etc.   I. Ahmad, Muzaffar.   II. Longworth, David L.
   III. Stoller, James K.   IV. Cleveland Clinic Foundation.   V. Title:
   Intensive review of internal medicine.
      [DNLM: 1. Internal Medicine.   2. Internal Medicine—examination
   questions.   WB 115 C835 1998]
   RC46.C548   1998
   616'.0076—DC21
   DNLM/DLC   97-49226
   for Library of Congress   CIP

The publishers have made every effort to trace the copyright holders for borrowed material. If they have inadvertently overlooked any, they will be pleased to make the necessary arrangements at the first opportunity.

To purchase additional copies of this book, call our customer service department at **(800) 638-0672** or fax orders to **(800) 447-8438.** For other book services, including chapter reprints and large quantity sales, ask for the Special Sales department.

Canadian customers should call **(800) 665-1148,** or fax **(800) 665-0103.** For all other calls originating outside of the United States, please call **(410) 528-4223** or fax us at **(410) 528-8550.**

Visit Williams & Wilkins on the Internet: http://www.wwilkins.com or contact our customer service department at **custserv@wwilkins.com.** Williams & Wilkins customer service representatives are available from 8:30 am to 6:00 pm, EST, Monday through Friday, for telephone access.

98 99 00 01 02
2 3 4 5 6 7 8 9 10

Reprints of chapters may be purchased from Williams & Wilkins in quantities of 100 or more. Call Isabelle Wise in the Special Sales Department, (800) 358-3583.

Dedication

To our wives and families for their enduring love and support, and to our colleagues at The Cleveland Clinic Foundation for their passionate commitment to excellence in the practice of medicine.

J.K.S.
M.A.
D.L.L.

Preface

This book is the product of contributions by members of the Cleveland Clinic Foundation professional staff and by several other distinguished clinicians, and is born of a passion for excellence in the practice of medicine and of a commitment to education. These core values define the Cleveland Clinic Foundation as an institution and health care facility.

More specifically, this book has its roots in the Foundation's annual "Intensive Review of Internal Medicine Symposium," which celebrates its tenth anniversary this year under the co-direction of two of the editors (JKS, DLL). This course is designed to provide a comprehensive review of Internal Medicine for those preparing for Board Certification (or re-certification), as well as for those who simply wish to update their knowledge in the field. The course syllabus in years past has served as a nidus for this book, which is designed to provide a succinct, focused document that will help course participants follow the lectures and also provide a "stand-alone" study guide for later Board preparation. It also serves as a companion text for other educational offerings related to the course, including the CD-ROM, Videotapes and Self-Assessment Test. For some of these activities, CME credit is available; however, in each instance the book is meant to serve as a resource for the educational program, rather than as the basis for CME credit.

This book is not intended to be a comprehensive textbook of internal medicine, but rather attempts to highlight key points identified by clinician faculty. To enhance its utility as a study guide, ample use is made of bullet points. Case-based teaching has become the hallmark of the Course, as we believe that most practicing physicians learn best in a case-driven format. For this reason, case presentations are included in some chapters which pose specific diagnostic or management questions, along with discussions of those issues.

We are delighted to offer this book as a compilation of clinical wisdom from a distinguished roster of clinician-scholars. As editors, we take pride in this volume, no credit for its valuable content, but total responsibility for any of its short-comings. We hope that you will find the shortcomings to be few in number, and that this book enhances your knowledge and joy of clinical medicine, just as it has enhanced our own.

James K. Stoller, M.D.
Muzaffar Ahmad, M.D.
David L. Longworth, M.D.

The Cleveland Clinic Foundation,
Cleveland, Ohio
June 1998

Contributors

Karim A. Adal, M.D., M.S.
Department of Infectious Diseases
The Cleveland Clinic Foundation
Cleveland, Ohio

David J. Adelstein, M.D.
Vice-Chairman
Department of Hematology and Medical Oncology
The Cleveland Clinic Foundation
Cleveland, Ohio

Muzaffar Ahmad, MD
Chairman, Division of Medicine
The Cleveland Clinic Foundation

Steven W. Andresen, D.O.
Department of Hematology and Medical Oncology
The Cleveland Clinic Foundation
Cleveland, Ohio

Gerald B. Appel, M.D.
Professor of Clinical Medicine
Columbia University College of Physicians and Surgeons
Director of Clinical Nephrology
Columbia-Presbyterian Medical Center
New York, New York

Alejandro C. Arroliga, M.D.
Director, Fellowship Program
Department of Pulmonary and Critical Care Medicine
The Cleveland Clinic Foundation
Cleveland, Ohio

Gerald J. Beck, Ph.D.
Department of Biostatistics and Epidemiology
The Cleveland Clinic Foundation
Cleveland, Ohio

Brian J. Bolwell, M.D.
Director, Bone Marrow Transplant Program
Department of Hematology and Medical Oncology
The Cleveland Clinic Foundation
Cleveland, Ohio

David L. Bronson, M.D.
Chairman, Division of Regional Medical Practice
The Cleveland Clinic Foundation
Cleveland, Ohio

Aaron Brzezinski, M.D.
Inflammatory Bowel Disease Center
Department of Gastroenterology
The Cleveland Clinic Foundation
Cleveland, Ohio

Carol A. Burke, M.D.
Department of Gastroenterology
The Cleveland Clinic Foundation
Cleveland, Ohio

Leonard H. Calabrese, D.O.
Head, Section of Clinical Immunology
Vice-Chairman, Department of Rheumatic and
    Immunologic Disease
The Cleveland Clinic Foundation
Cleveland, Ohio

Darwin L. Conwell, M.D.
Assistant Staff
Department of Gastroenterology
The Cleveland Clinic Foundation
Cleveland, Ohio

Rossana D. Danese, M.D.
Department of Endocrinology
The Cleveland Clinic Foundation
Cleveland, Ohio

Charles Faiman, M.D.
Chairman, Department of Endocrinology
The Cleveland Clinic Foundation
Cleveland, Ohio

Gary W. Falk, M.D.
Staff Gastroenterologist
Department of Gastroenterology
The Cleveland Clinic Foundation
Cleveland, Ohio

Barri J. Fessler, M.D.
Staff Rheumatologist
Department of Rheumatic and Immunologic Diseases
The Cleveland Clinic Foundation
Cleveland, Ohio

Andrew Fishleder, M.D.
Chairman, Division of Education
The Cleveland Clinic Foundation
Cleveland, Ohio

Kevin R. Fox, M.D.
Associate Professor of Medicine
Department of Hematology/Oncology
University of Pennsylvania
Philadelphia, Pennsylvania

Kathleen N. Franco, M.D.
Head, Section of Consult/Liaison Psychiatry
Director, Residency Training Program
Department of Psychiatry and Psychology
The Cleveland Clinic Foundation
Cleveland, Ohio

Steven M. Gordon, M.D.
Hospital Epidemiologist
Department of Infectious Diseases
The Cleveland Clinic Foundation
Cleveland, Ohio

Brian P. Griffin, M.D.
Department of Cardiology
The Cleveland Clinic Foundation
Cleveland, Ohio

Richard A. Grimm, D.O.
Staff Cardiologist
Department of Cardiology
Section of Cardiac Imaging
The Cleveland Clinic Foundation
Cleveland, Ohio

Robert E. Hobbs, M.D.
Director, Heart Failure Clinical Trials
Department of Cardiology
The Cleveland Clinic Foundation
Cleveland, Ohio

Gary S. Hoffman, M.S., M.D.
Chairman, Professor of Medicine
Department of Rheumatic and Immunologic Diseases
The Cleveland Clinic Foundation
Cleveland, Ohio

Edward P. Horvath, Jr., M.D., M.P.H.
Director, Occupational Medicine
Department of General Internal Medicine
The Cleveland Clinic Foundation
Cleveland, Ohio
Volunteer Professor
Environmental Health
University of Cincinnati Medical Center
Cincinnati, Ohio

Carlos M. Isada, M.D.
Department of Infectious Diseases
The Cleveland Clinic Foundation
Cleveland, Ohio

George A. Kanoti, M.A., S.T.D.
F.J. O'Neill Bioethicist (RTD)
Department of Bioethics
The Cleveland Clinic Foundation
Cleveland, Ohio

Mani S. Kavuru, M.D.
Director, Pulmonary Function Laboratory
Department of Pulmonary and Critical Care Medicine
The Cleveland Clinic Foundation
Cleveland, Ohio

Thomas F. Keys, M.D.
Staff Physician
Department of Infectious Diseases
Director, Office of Quality Management
The Cleveland Clinic Foundation
Cleveland, Ohio

Richard S. Lang, M.D., M.P.H.
Head, Section of Preventive Medicine
Medical Director, Cleveland Clinic Telemedicine Center
Department of Internal Medicine
The Cleveland Clinic Foundation
Cleveland, Ohio

Julia Breyer Lewis, M.D.
Associate Professor of Medicine
Director, Renal Unit
Vanderbilt University Medical Center
Division of Nephrology
Nashville, Tennessee

Angelo A. Licata, M.D., Ph.D.
Head, Metabolic Bone and Calcium Disorders Section
Department of Endocrinology
The Cleveland Clinic Foundation
Cleveland, Ohio

Alan E. London, M.D.
Executive Director
Managed Care
The Cleveland Clinic Foundation
Cleveland, Ohio

David L. Longworth, M.D.
Chairman, Department of Infectious Diseases
The Cleveland Clinic Foundation
Cleveland, Ohio

Careen Y. Lowder, M.D., Ph.D.
Staff Physician
Department of Ophthalmology
The Cleveland Clinic Foundation
Cleveland, Ohio

Brian F. Mandell, M.D., Ph.D.
Education Program Director
Department of Rheumatic and Immunologic Disease
The Cleveland Clinic Foundation
Cleveland, Ohio

Maurie Markman, M.D.
Director, Cleveland Clinic Cancer Center
Chairman, Department of Hematology/Medical Oncology
The Cleveland Clinic Foundation
Cleveland, Ohio

Thomas H. Marwick, M.D.
Director of Cardiac Stress Imaging
Department of Cardiology
The Cleveland Clinic Foundation
Cleveland, Ohio

Arthur J. McCullough, M.D.
Associate Professor of Medicine
Case Western Reserve University School of Medicine
Director, Division of Gastroenterology
MetroHealth Medical Center
Cleveland, Ohio

Adi E. Mehta, M.D.
Department of Endocrinology
The Cleveland Clinic Foundation
Cleveland, Ohio

Atul C. Mehta, M.D., B.S.
Head, Section of Bronchology
Associate Professor of Medicine
Department of Pulmonary and Critical Care Medicine
The Cleveland Clinic Foundation
Cleveland, Ohio

Neil B. Mehta, M.D.
Department of General Internal Medicine
The Cleveland Clinic Foundation
Cleveland, Ohio

Douglas S. Moodie, M.D.
Chairman, Division of Pediatrics
Director, The Cleveland Clinic Children's Hospital
The Cleveland Clinic Foundation
Cleveland, Ohio

Kevin D. Mullen, M.D.
Associate Professor of Medicine
Case Western Reserve University School of Medicine
MetroHealth Medical Center
Department of Medicine
Division of Gastroenterology
Cleveland, Ohio

Joseph V. Nally, Jr., M.D.
Department of Nephrology and Hypertension
The Cleveland Clinic Foundation
Cleveland, Ohio

Jeffrey W. Olin, D.O.
Chairman, Department of Vascular Medicine
The Cleveland Clinic Foundation
Cleveland, Ohio

Beth A. Overmoyer, M.D.
Director, Breast Cancer Program
Department of Hematology/Medical Oncology
The Cleveland Clinic Foundation
Cleveland, Ohio

Robert M. Palmer, M.D., M.P.H.
Head, Section of Geriatric Medicine
Department of General Internal Medicine
The Cleveland Clinic Foundation
Cleveland, Ohio

Robert Pelley, M.D.
Department of Hematology and Medical Oncology
The Cleveland Clinic Foundation
Cleveland, Ohio

Elliot H. Philipson, M.D.
Department of Gynecology and Obstetrics
The Cleveland Clinic Foundation
Cleveland, Ohio

Marc A. Pohl, M.D.
Department of Nephrology and Hypertension
The Cleveland Clinic Foundation
Cleveland, Ohio

Brad L. Pohlman, M.D.
Staff Physician, Department of Hematology and Medical
    Oncology
The Cleveland Clinic Foundation
Cleveland, Ohio

Satti Sethu K. Reddy, M.D.
Program Director, Department of Endocrinology
The Cleveland Clinic Foundation
Cleveland, Ohio

Susan J. Rehm, M.D.
Staff Physician
Department of Infectious Diseases
Associate Director, Internal Medicine
Residency Training Program
The Cleveland Clinic Foundation
Cleveland, Ohio

Joel E. Richter, M.D.
Chairman, Department of Gastroenterology
Professor of Internal Medicine
The Cleveland Clinic Foundation Health Sciences Center
Ohio State University
Cleveland, Ohio

Curtis M. Rimmerman, M.D.
Staff Cardiologist
Department of Cardiology
The Cleveland Clinic Foundation
Cleveland, Ohio

Killian Robinson, M.D.
Associate Professor
Department of Cardiology
The Cleveland Clinic Foundation
Cleveland, Ohio

Raymond J. Scheetz, Jr., M.D.
Senior Staff Physician
Department of Rheumatic and Immunologic Disease
The Cleveland Clinic Foundation
Cleveland, Ohio

Steven K. Schmitt, M.D.
Staff Physician
Department of Infectious Diseases
The Cleveland Clinic Foundation
Cleveland, Ohio

Martin J. Schreiber, Jr., M.D.
Medical Director, Continuous Ambulatory Peritoneal
    Dialysis Unit
Department of Nephrology and Hypertension
The Cleveland Clinic Foundation
Cleveland, Ohio

Edy E. Soffer, M.D.
Staff Physician
Department of Gastroenterology
The Cleveland Clinic Foundation
Cleveland, Ohio

Glen D. Solomon, M.D.
Head, Section of Headache
General Internal Medicine
The Cleveland Clinic Foundation
Cleveland, Ohio
Clinical Professor of Medicine
Pennsylvania State University
Hershey, Pennsylvania

Dennis L. Sprecher, M.D.
Head, Section of Preventive Cardiology
Department of Cardiology
The Cleveland Clinic Foundation
Cleveland, Ohio

James K. Stoller, M.D.
Head, Section of Respiratory Therapy
Department of Pulmonary and Critical Care Medicine
The Cleveland Clinic Foundation
Cleveland, Ohio

Eugene J. Sullivan, M.D.
Department of Pulmonary and Critical Care Medicine
The Cleveland Clinic Foundation
Cleveland, Ohio

Holly L. Thacker, M.D., F.A.C.P.
Department of General Internal Medicine, Head, Section of
    Women's Health
Associate Program Director, Menopause Program
Department of Gynecology and Obstetrics
The Cleveland Clinic Foundation
The Cleveland Clinic Health Science Center
Ohio State University
Cleveland, Ohio

Kenneth J. Tomecki, M.D.
Staff Physician
Department of Dermatology
The Cleveland Clinic Foundation
Cleveland, Ohio

J. Walton Tomford, M.D.
Staff Physician
Department of Infectious Disease
The Cleveland Clinic Foundation
Cleveland, Ohio
Ohio State University College of Medicine
Columbus, Ohio
Associate Professor of Medicine
Pennsylvania State University
Hershey, Pennsylvania

Donald A. Underwood, M.D.
Head, Electrocardiography
Department of Cardiology
The Cleveland Clinic Foundation
Assistant Professor of Medicine
Ohio State University
Cleveland, Ohio
Clinical Professor of Medicine
Pennsylvania State University
Hershey, Pennsylvania

John J. Vargo, M.D.
Staff Physician
Department of Gastroenterology
The Cleveland Clinic Foundation
Cleveland, Ohio

Herbert P. Wiedemann, M.D.
Chairman, Department of Pulmonary and Critical Care
   Medicine
The Cleveland Clinic Foundation
Cleveland, Ohio

Contents

COLOR PLATES

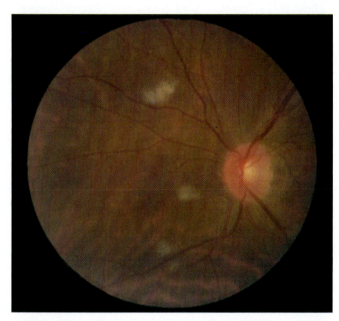

Figure 6.1.

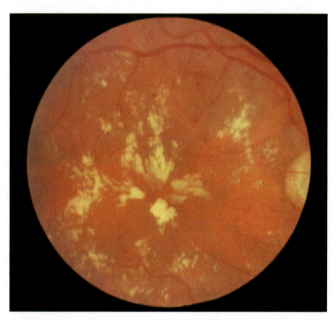

Figure 6.2.

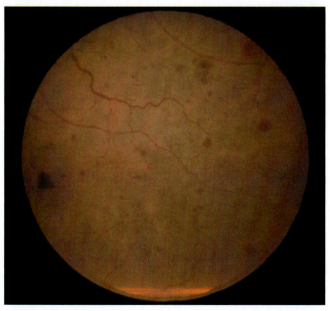

Figure 6.3.

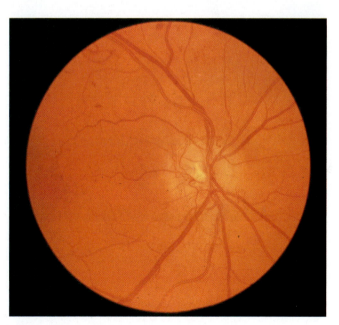

Figure 6.4.

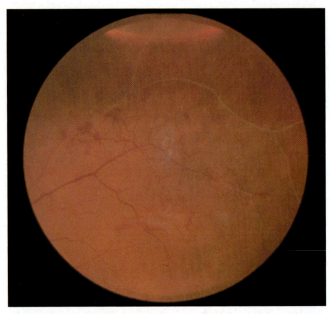

Figure 6.5.

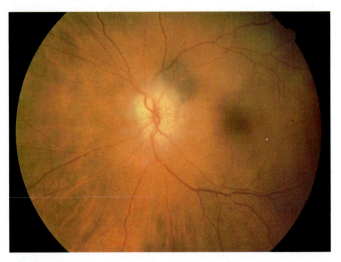

Figure 6.6.

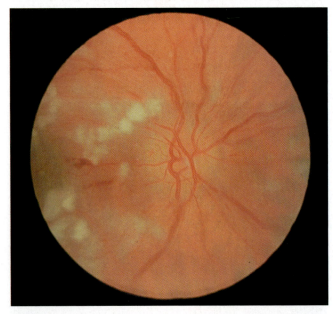

Figure 6.7.

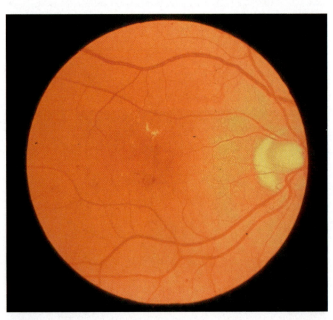

Figure 6.8.

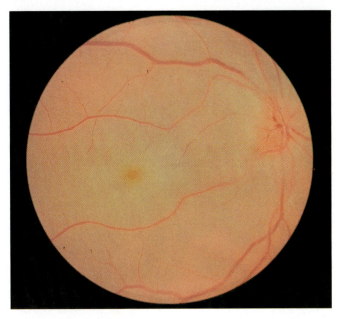

Figure 6.10.

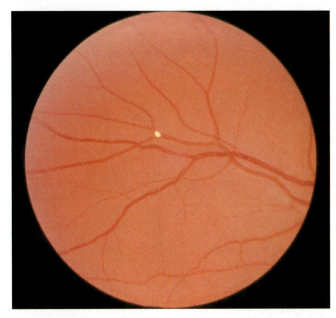

Figure 6.11.

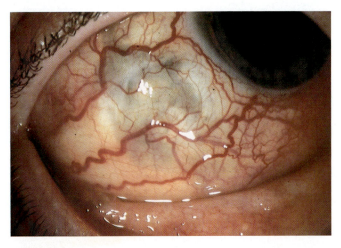

Figure 6.13.

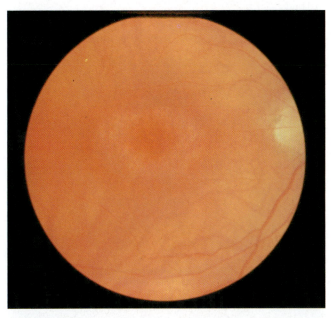

Figure 6.14.

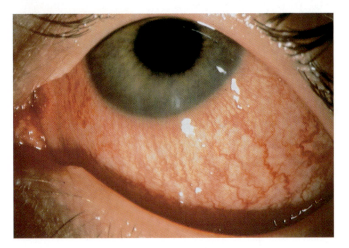

Figure 6.15.

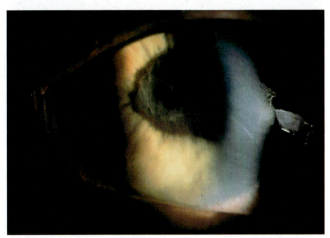

Figure 6.16.

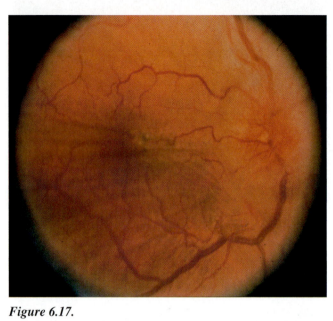

Figure 6.17.

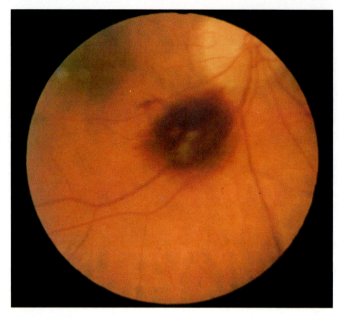

Figure 6.18.

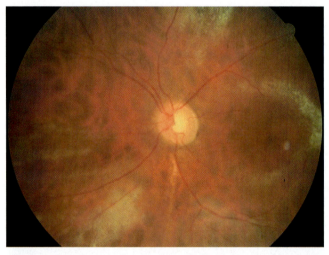

Figure 6.19.

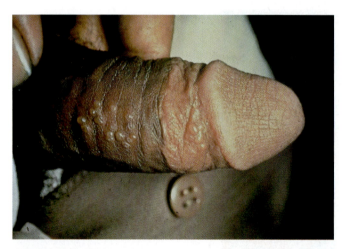

Figure 12.1.

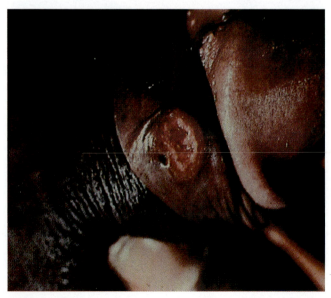

Figure 12.2.

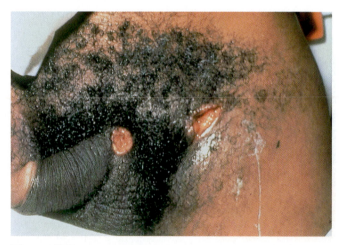

Figure 12.3.

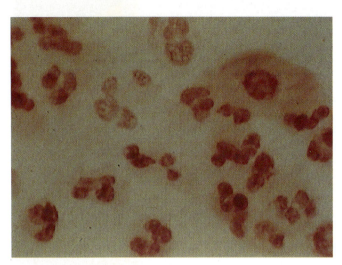

Figure 12.4.

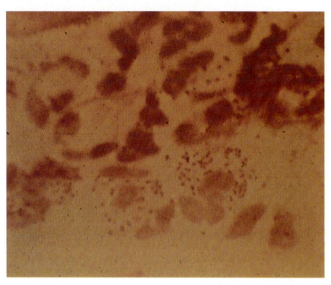

Figure 12.5.

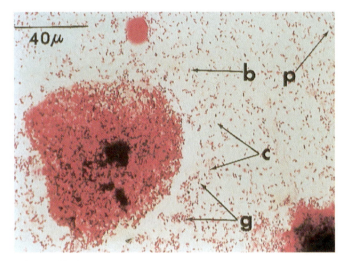

Figure 12.6.

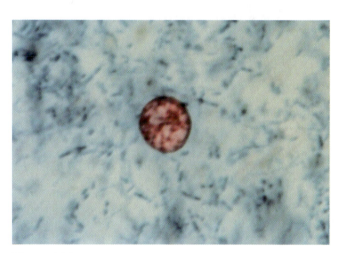

Figure 16.1.

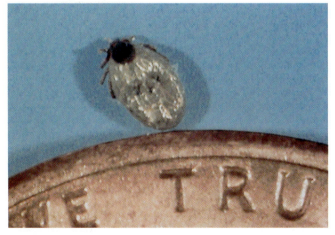

Figure 16.3.

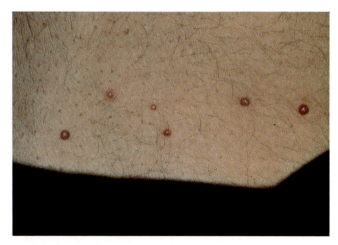

Figure 16.4.

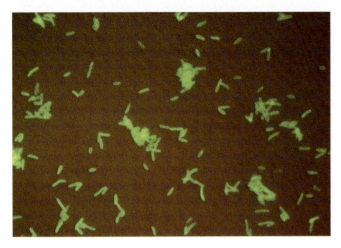

Figure 18.3.

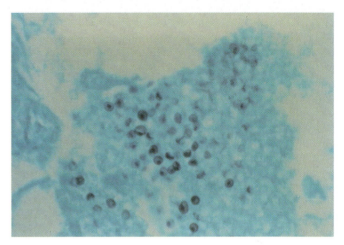

Figure 18.4.

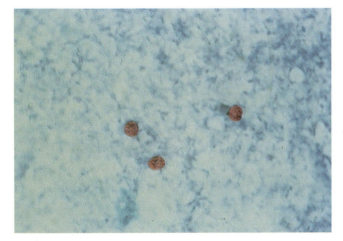

Figure 18.5.

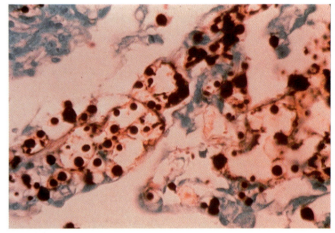

Figure 18.6.

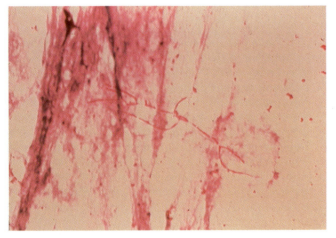

Figure 18.10.

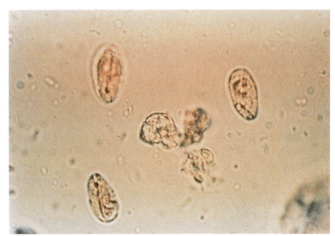

Figure 18.11.

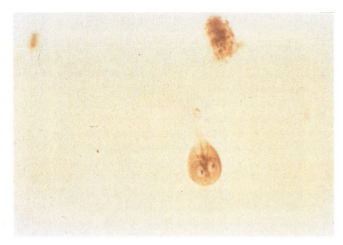

Figure 18.12.

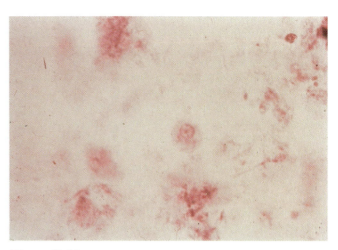

Figure 18.13.

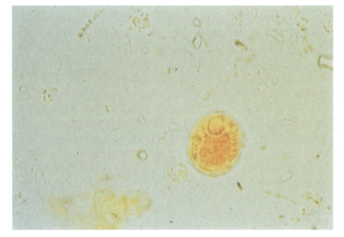

Figure 18.14.

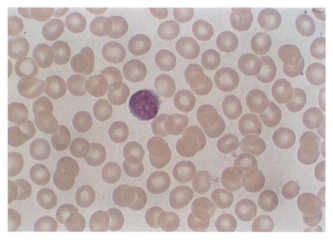

Figure 18.15.

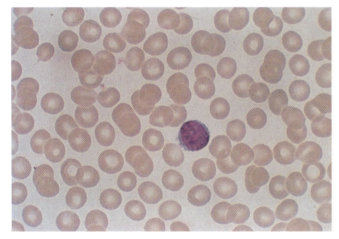

Figure 18.16.

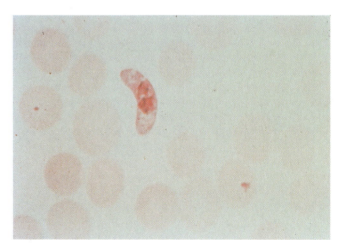

Figure 18.17.

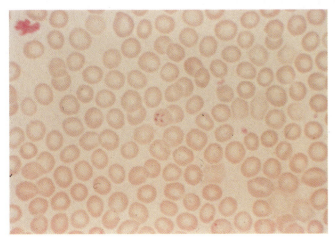

Figure 18.18.

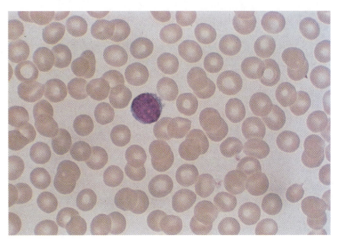

Figure 18.19.

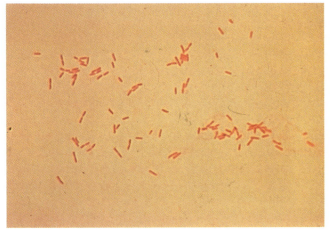

Figure 18.20.

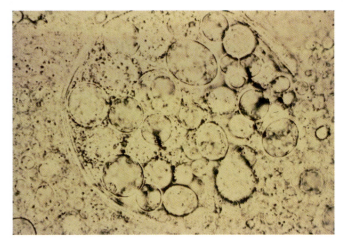

Figure 18.21.

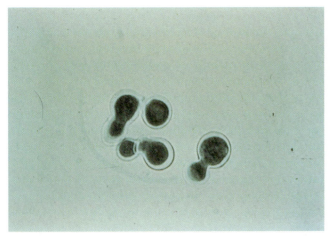

Figure 18.22.

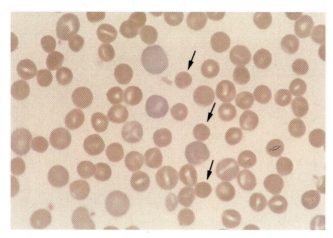

Figure 27.1.

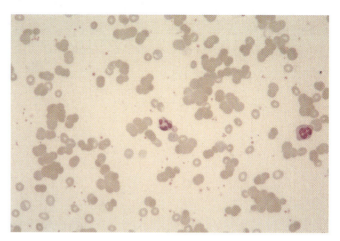

Figure 27.2.

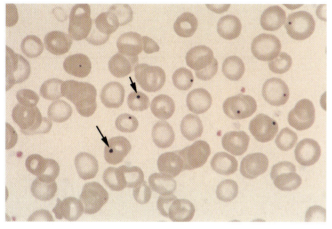

Figure 27.3.

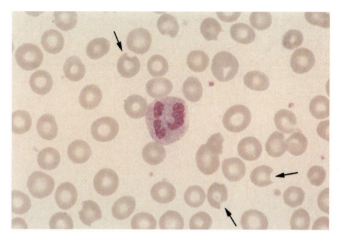

Figure 27.4.

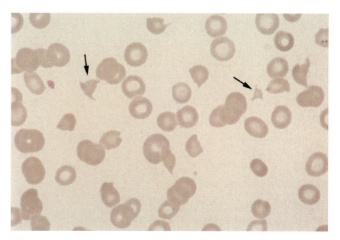

Figure 27.5.

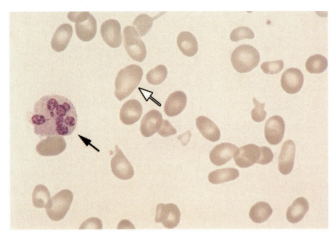

Figure 27.6.

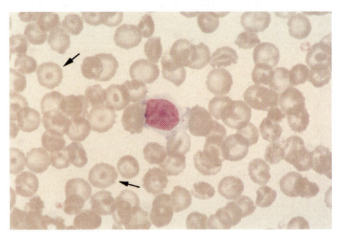

Figure 27.7.

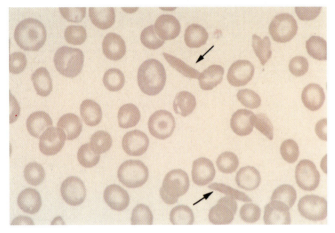

Figure 27.8.

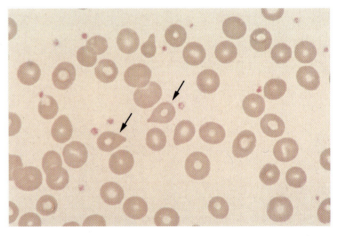

Figure 27.9.

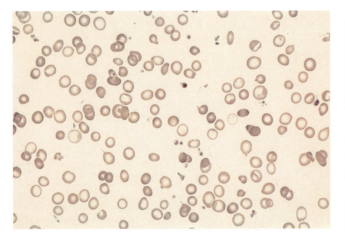

Figure 27.10.

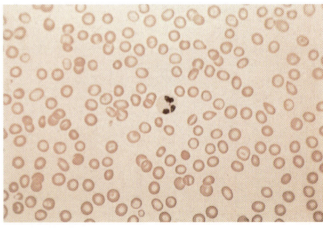

Figure 27.11.

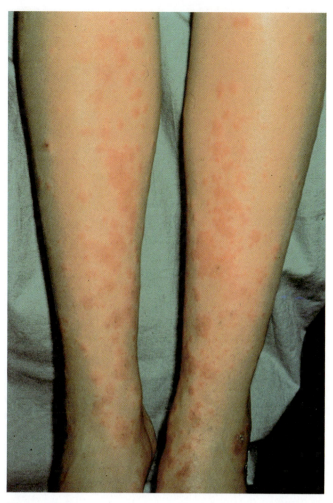

Figure 31.1.

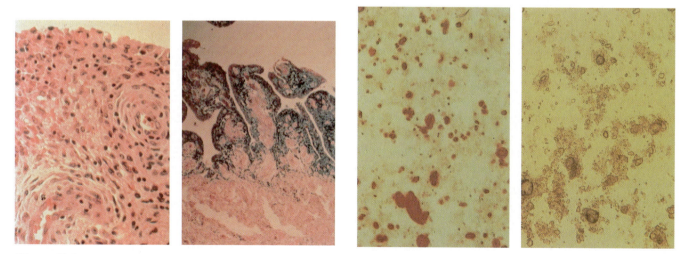

Figure 33.1.

Figure 33.2.

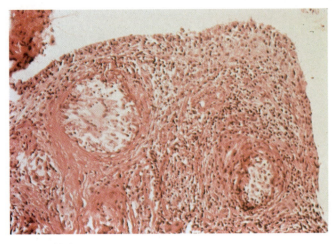

Figure 33.3.

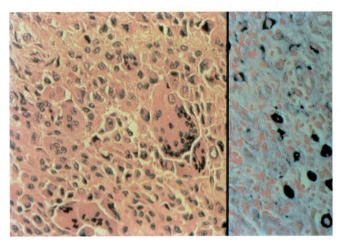

Figure 33.4.

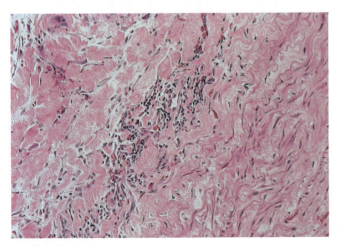

Figure 33.10.

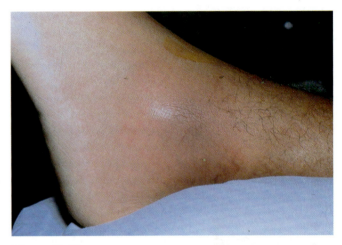

Figure 33.11.

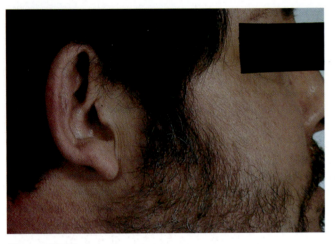

Figure 33.17.

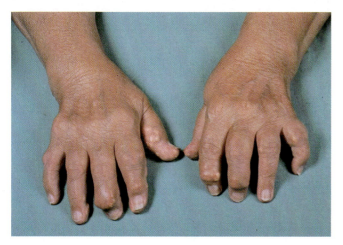

Figure 33.18.

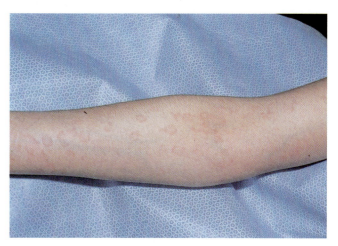

Figure 33.19.

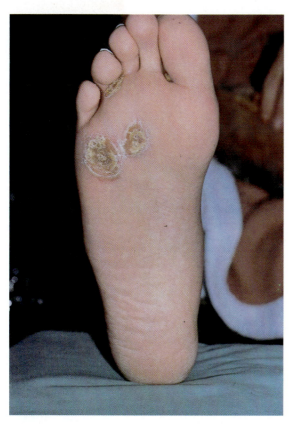

Figure 33.20.

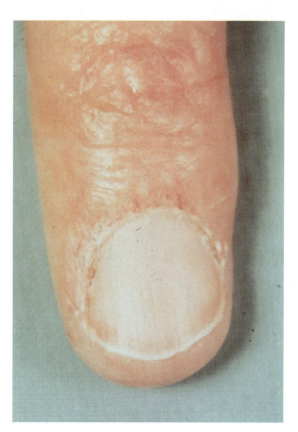

Figure 33.21.

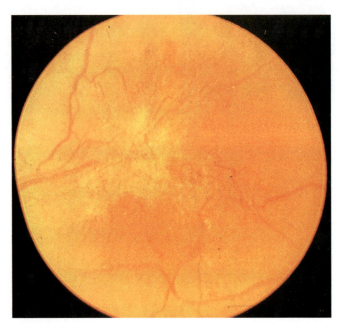

Figure 47.1.

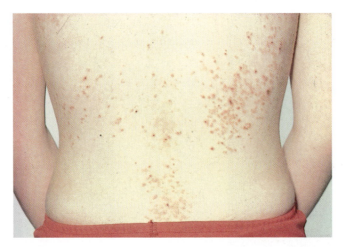

Figure 47.2.

S • E • C • T • I • O • N

I

Multidisciplinary Skills for the Internist

C·H·A·P·T·E·R

1

Health Screening and Immunization

Richard S. Lang

Conceptually, preventive medicine involves three tasks for the clinician: screening, counseling, and immunization and prophylaxis. Preventive interventions have been categorized as primary, secondary, and tertiary. *Primary prevention* is the reduction of risk factors before a disease or condition has occurred. Examples are immunization, use of safety equipment, dietary management, and smoking cessation. Primary prevention aims to reduce the incidence of a disease or condition. *Incidence* is the number of persons developing a condition or disease in a specific period of time. *Secondary prevention* is the detection of a condition or disease in order to reverse or slow the condition or disease and thereby improve prognosis. Examples of secondary prevention are mammography and Papanicolaou (Pap) smears. Secondary prevention ideally detects and intervenes in a condition before that condition is clinically apparent. Secondary prevention therefore aims to reduce the prevalence of a disease. *Prevalence* is the total number of individuals who have a condition or disease at a particular time. *Tertiary prevention* is the minimizing of future negative health effects of a disease or condition.

Considerations in screening for a disease or condition should include the following questions:

- Is the disease or condition an important problem? (What are the morbidity and mortality of the condition?)
- Is the disease or condition a common problem? (What are its prevalence and incidence?)
- Is the screening test accurate? (What are its sensitivity, specificity, and predictive value?)
- Does the screening determine prevalence or incidence?
- What is the cost of the screening procedure? (Consider both financial and health risks.)
- What are the available follow-up diagnostic procedures?
- What is the available treatment for the disease or condition?

- How acceptable to patients is the screening procedure?
- What are the circumstances for the screening? (What is the context—health maintenance, occupational, preoperative, screening, etc.?)
- What are the current recommendations for screening and the medical evidence to support these recommendations?

The ideal screening situation uses an inexpensive, noninvasive test with a high level of sensitivity and specificity to detect a common problem that can be treated but, if left untreated, leads to significant morbidity and mortality. Presently, medical practice and literature identify few such interventions.

Sensitivity is the ability of a test to correctly identify those who have a condition or disease. *Specificity* is the ability of a test to correctly identify those who do not have the disease or condition in question. *Predictive values* for a screening test are the proportions of people correctly labeled as having the condition or disease (*positive predictive value*) and those without the condition or disease (*negative predictive value*). Table 1.1 illustrates these terms. This "2×2" table is a common method for viewing the application of a screening test in a population.

LEADING CAUSES OF MORTALITY

The optimal use of screening requires a basic understanding of the common causes of mortality. Table 1.2 outlines the most common causes of mortality for adult age groups, and Table 1.3 shows the average life expectancy of males and females at different ages.

Accidents, homicide, and suicide are common causes of mortality in young adults. Motor vehicle injuries account for more than 35% of the deaths in persons aged 15–24. The use of seat belts can reduce crash mortality by as much as 50%. Homicide is the leading cause of death of black males in the

3

15–24-year-old age group. Counseling regarding hand gun safety is therefore an important intervention for this population. Suicide is another common cause of death in the young age group and is markedly more common in persons who have become HIV positive. Surveillance and counseling for suicide in this patient population are therefore important. HIV continues to rise as a cause of mortality, particularly in the age groups shown in Table 1.2. Preventive efforts related to sexual practices and the use of IV drugs are important interventions.

Heart disease and cancer are the leading causes of mortality in adults in the groups over age 35. Preventive efforts therefore should be directed to these conditions. Projections indicate that cancer will become the leading cause of adult mortality in the near future. Common cancer sites in women are the breast, lung, colon/rectum, uterus, and ovary. Leading cancer sites in males are the prostate, lung, colon/rectum, and bladder. Common causes of cancer death in women are lung, breast, colon/rectum, and ovary cancers; in men, lung, prostate, and colon/rectum cancers. Screening and prevention efforts are therefore targeted at those cancers that are the most common as well as the most common causes of cancer death: lung, colon/rectum, breast, and prostate cancers.

SCREENING TESTS BY ORGAN SYSTEM AND DISEASE

CARDIOVASCULAR SYSTEM

For preventive purposes, atherosclerotic heart disease, stroke, and peripheral vascular disease are grouped in terms of their similar risk factors. The risk factors include the following:

- Previous atherosclerotic vascular disease
- Family history of premature vascular disease
- Smoking
- Hypertension
- Diabetes
- Hyperlipidemia
- Age greater than 45 years in men and greater than 55 years in women
- Premature menopause in women without estrogen replacement therapy

An HDL cholesterol level greater than 60 mg/dL is thought to be a negative risk factor, or ''protective'' factor, for the development of coronary vascular disease. Most policy groups have recommended that total serum cholesterol level in a nonfasting state be measured in ''asymptomatic'' adults generally every 5 years. Presently, agreement has not been reached by authoritative groups on the use of lipoprotein subfractions.

Most authorities advise measurement of the blood pressure in normotensive persons at least every 2 years, particularly in persons with prior diastolic readings of 85–89 or those who are obese or who have a first-degree relative having hypertension. Lifestyle modifications should be made for mild to moderate hypertension. These modifications include optimizing weight, limiting alcohol, participating in regular aerobic exercise, reducing sodium intake, and maintaining adequate dietary potassium, calcium, and magnesium.

Low-dose aspirin therapy should be considered for primary prevention of ischemic heart disease in men over age 40 who are of high risk. The optimal preventive aspirin dosage is not clearly established, however. The side effects and potential complications of chronic aspirin usage should be considered carefully.

The electrocardiogram is not a sensitive screening test

Table 1.1. Predictive Value of Tests

	Disease	*No Disease*	*Total*
Test positive	True (+)	False (+)	All (+)
Test negative	False (−)	True (−)	All (−)
Total	All with disease	All without disease	Total patients

$$\text{Sensitivity} = \frac{\text{True } (+)}{\text{True } (+) + \text{False } (-)} = \text{how well the test correctly detects those with disease}$$

$$\text{Specificity} = \frac{\text{True } (-)}{\text{True } (-) + \text{False } (+)} = \text{how well the test identifies those without disease}$$

$$\text{Positive predictive value} = \frac{\text{True } (+)}{\text{True } (+) + \text{False } (+)} = \text{when a test is positive, the proportion of those with the disease}$$

$$\text{Negative predictive value} = \frac{\text{True } (-)}{\text{True } (-) + \text{False } (-)} = \text{when a test is negative, the proportion of those without the disease}$$

Table 1.2. Leading Causes of Death (1992)

Rank	Overall Population	Age 15–34	Age 35–54	Age 55–74	Age 75 & Over
1	Heart	Accidents	Cancer	Cancer	Heart
2	Cancer	Homicide	Heart	Heart	Cancer
3	Stroke	HIV	HIV	COPD	Stroke
4	COPD[a]	Suicide	Accidents	Stroke	Pneumonia/flu
5	Accidents	Cancer	Suicide	Diabetes	COPD
6	Pneumonia/flu	Heart	Cirrhosis of the liver	Accidents	Diabetes

[a] COPD, Chronic obstructive pulmonary disease

Table 1.3.   Average Life Expectancy

Gender	Years of Survival	Life Expectancy
Males		
65	15.1	80.1
70	12.3	82.3
75	9.8	84.8
Females		
65	19.9	84.9
70	16.3	86.3
75	13.0	88.0
85	6.2	91.2

for coronary artery disease in asymptomatic patients and therefore is not generally advised as a screening test. There is no consensus for the use of preoperative electrocardiograms. Considerations for the obtaining of a preoperative EKG include the patient's age, the procedure planned, the anesthesia to be used, the cardiovascular risk factors, and the presence of other systemic disease.

Exercise treadmill testing has limited sensitivity (approximately 65%) and specificity (approximately 75%) for detection of coronary artery disease. Stress testing is most useful when coronary artery disease is more likely. Therefore, treadmill testing is most effectively used for persons with multiple risk factors. Stress testing should also be considered for persons engaging in occupations that demand physical exertion or that may impact on public safety. Otherwise, exercise treadmill testing should not be used routinely.

Similarly, the use of noninvasive vascular evaluation of the carotid arteries should be reserved for patients in whom disease is suspected, based either on symptoms or the presence of carotid bruits. The prevalence of carotid bruits in the adult population is about 4–5%.

Overall, the risk factors for development of vascular disease should be assessed in all patients. Modifiable risk factors should be addressed. Blood pressure and cholesterol should be monitored and treated appropriately. Stress testing and assessment of carotid arteries are best used with patients in whom coronary artery disease or carotid atherosclerosis is most likely to be present.

LUNG CANCER

The numbers of new cancer cases and cancer deaths for specific types of cancers are shown in Figure 1.1. Lung cancer is the most common cause of cancer death in the United States.

Cigarette smoking is the most important risk factor for the development of lung cancer. Generally, smokers are 10 times more likely to die of lung cancer than nonsmokers. The risk for developing lung cancer depends on the number of cigarettes smoked, the age when smoking began, and the de-

gree of inhalation. The risk for lung cancer decreases after smoking is stopped, particularly after 5 years or more. Therefore, the most important preventive interventions for lung cancer are avoidance and cessation of smoking. Other risk factors for development of lung cancer are occupational exposures (asbestos, arsenic, chloromethyl ethers, chromium, polycyclic aromatic compounds, nickel, and vinyl chloride), chronic obstructive lung disease, previous lung cancer, previous head and neck cancer, and radon exposure.

Generally, screening for lung cancer in asymptomatic patients is not advised. Large-scale studies have not demonstrated a reduction in mortality when screening interventions such as serial chest x rays and frequent sputum cytology were applied to high-risk populations. Therefore, routine screening chest x rays should not be done unless clinical evidence suggests the presence of disease. Improved treatment and screening techniques may change the perspective for screening for lung cancer in the future.

BREAST CANCER

Risk factors for breast cancer include the following:

- Family history of breast cancer
- Menarche before age 12
- Late menopause (after age 50)
- Late first pregnancy (after age 35)
- Previous lobular carcinoma in-situ of the breast
- Previous breast cancer
- Previous cancer of the uterus, ovary, or salivary gland

A family history of breast cancer is a particularly important risk factor when diagnosed in a premenopausal first-degree relative or bilaterally in any first-degree relative. A woman with a premenopausal first-degree relative having had breast cancer has three times the risk for developing breast cancer. High socioeconomic status, nulliparity, and prior exposure to high-dose radiation also convey modestly increased risk.

Screening for breast cancer includes breast self-examination, clinical breast examination by a physician or nurse, and mammography. A large number of breast cancers are found by palpation. Breast self-examination has low sensitivity and unknown specificity. Appropriate teaching is required for effective breast self-examination. Although not of proven effectiveness, breast self-examination is recommended by some advisory groups. Annual clinical breast examination by a physician or health care professional is recommended by the major advisory panels for women over the age of 40. Mammography has a variable but good sensitivity for detecting breast cancer, in the range of 74–93%. Specificity is also relatively good at about 90–95%. The positive predictive value of an abnormal mammogram is about 10–20%. A normal mammogram has a negative predictive value of about 99%. All major authoritative groups recommend routine mammography screening after the age of 50. Studies have

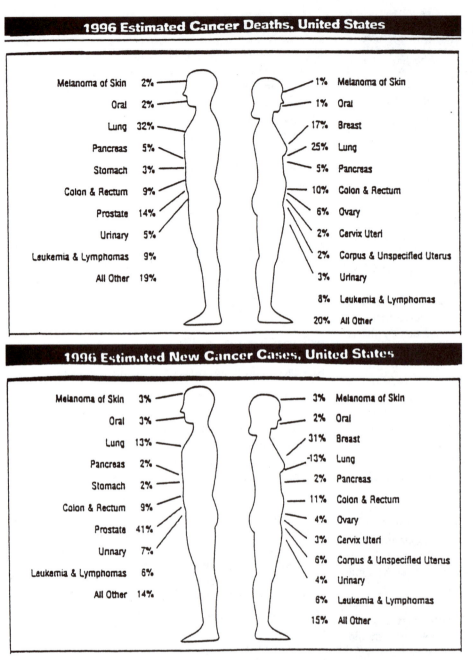

Figure 1.1. New cancer cases and cancer deaths for specific types of cancers.

shown that mammography screening in women of age 50–69 years leads to a reduction in breast cancer mortality of about 30%. The benefits of mammography for women of normal risk under the age of 50 have been uncertain, and most groups have therefore not recommended screening for this age group. More recent data suggest a positive benefit from screening in the age group of 40–50 years, leading some authorities to recommend mammography screening in these ages. Evidence is lacking as to the efficacy of screening mammography in women over the age of 70, but because of the high risk for breast cancer in this age group, many have recommended con-

tinuation of screening. Life expectancy of the individual woman is a major factor to consider for screening in this age group.

In general, then, clinical breast examinations should be instituted in women at around the age of 40, and mammography screening should be started at around the age of 40. Women with greatest risk should be considered for screening at an earlier age. Mammography frequency depends on the individual's risk factors. Less frequent screenings for low-risk women can be undertaken, but generally screening is done yearly. Screening should be continued into the later years until less-frequent screening in that age group is supported by clinical studies. Breast self-examination appears to be prudent but is of unproven efficacy.

COLON AND RECTAL CANCER

Risk factors for colon cancer include the following:

- Familial polyposis
- Ulcerative colitis
- Family history of colorectal cancer
- History of endometrial, ovarian, or breast cancer
- History of adenomatous polyps of the colon

The younger the age of a first-degree relative encountering colon cancer, the greater the risk to the patient. The primary prevention of colon cancer includes following a low-fat, high-fiber diet with a possible role for aspirin and/or other nonsteroidal anti-inflammatory drugs. Screening for colon cancer is best conducted by determining whether a patient has normal or high risk. The testing type and frequency can then be selected based on that risk stratification.

Fecal occult blood testing is a cheap screening test but often involves poor patient compliance, has a limited sensitivity of about 50–65% for colon cancer, and has a positive predictive value for cancer of about 10–15%. In persons of normal risk over the age of 50, yearly fecal occult blood testing has been advised by most authoritative groups.

Sigmoidoscopy has a relatively low sensitivity for detecting cancer of the colon: 40–60%. Sigmoidoscopy is limited by examiner technique and the length of colon examined. In persons of average risk, screening sigmoidoscopy is generally advised every 3–5 years beginning at about age 50.

In high-risk patients, most authoritative groups have advised screening starting at an earlier age, usually around 40. The advised type of screening varies. Some authorities recommend sigmoidoscopy combined with periodic colonoscopy. Others have suggested periodic colonoscopy without sigmoidoscopy at a frequency of about 5 years. Colonoscopy conveys a sensitivity for colon cancer of about 80–90%. An air-contrast barium enema also has a high sensitivity for colon cancer: about 90% or greater. The air-contrast barium enema is generally cheaper than a colonoscopy, has a lower complication rate, and can provide a better view of the cecum. In some patients, air-contrast barium enema is used because of patient preference.

In summary, the risk for future development of colon cancer should be assessed in each patient. In persons of low or average risk, screening should consist of fecal occult blood testing yearly and sigmoidoscopy done every 3–5 years after the age of 50. In high-risk groups, fecal occult blood testing and sigmoidoscopy can be initiated at around the age of 40, with colonoscopy done every 5 years after the age of 50.

PROSTATE CANCER

Risk factors for prostate cancer include the following:

- Advanced age
- African-American race
- Family history of prostate cancer
- Bladder outlet obstruction

Digital rectal examination has a sensitivity of about 33–70% and a specificity of 50–95% for detecting prostate cancer. Digital rectal examination has not been shown to decrease mortality from prostate cancer. Prostate specific antigen (PSA) has been used to screen for prostate cancer. A PSA level of greater than 4 ng/mL has sensitivity of about 71%, specificity of about 75%, positive predictive value of about 35–40%, and negative predictive value of about 90% for prostate cancer. PSA levels increase in both benign and malignant prostate disease. To date, no clear evidence has shown that early detection and treatment of prostate cancer decreases mortality. Screening for prostate cancer can lead to morbidity in persons who may never have been affected by the disease, and it is costly. The use of digital rectal examination and PSA to screen for prostate cancer is therefore controversial at this juncture and not advocated based on evidence. The American Cancer Society has recommended annual PSA testing in men over 50, screening in men under 50 who are in a high-risk group, and discontinuation of screening once the patient's life expectancy is less than 10 years. Other groups have not recommended the use of PSA as a screening test for prostate cancer. A transrectal prostate ultrasound is also unproven as a screening tool. Thirty percent of prostate cancers are isoechoic. Ultrasound is considered in patients found to have increased PSA levels.

CERVICAL CANCER

Risk factors for the development of cervical cancer include the following:

- First coitus at an early age
- Multiple sexual partners
- History of sexually transmitted disease (especially HPV and HIV)
- Smoking
- Low socioeconomic status

Use of the cervical Pap smear has been shown to decrease mortality from invasive cervical cancer. The positive benefit of cervical Pap smear screening occurs because the natural history of the disease is known, the disease progresses relatively slowly, and screening via Pap smear is relatively accurate, inexpensive, and safe. A Pap smear has a low sensitivity of about 30–40% but a high specificity greater than 90%. Most advisory groups suggest Pap screening be initiated with the onset of sexual activity or at age 18, whichever occurs first. Thereafter, organizations advise various intervals for screening from 1–5 years. Most groups suggest at least two initial screens 1 year apart in order to provide diagnostic accuracy. Thereafter, the screening interval usually depends on individual risk factors. In years beyond age 65, screening should be continued based on risk; in women who have been adequately screened in earlier ages whose tests have been consistently negative, screening may be discontinued.

GENERAL PHYSICAL EXAMINATION

The use of the general physical examination as a screening tool has changed much over time. The general physical examination is now usually employed to establish a data base. Thereafter, only blood pressure, weight, breast examination, and pelvic examination are advised by most advocacy groups for screening asymptomatic adults. The intervals to perform these are not generally agreed upon. Other components of the physical examination are not generally advised in truly "asymptomatic" persons. It is more cost effective to counsel patients about the following:

- Smoking
- Diet
- Exercise
- Mental health
- Sexual practices
- Alcohol use
- Drug abuse
- Use of seat belts

OTHER TESTS

Hearing testing is advised in all adults when hearing loss is suspected. In patients exposed on a regular basis to excess noise, audiograms should be done periodically.

There is no general consensus for visual acuity testing. Some authorities have recommended screening in adults over the age of 65.

Tonometry is generally not recommended because of the lack of a good screening test. Schiotz tonometry has a specificity of 10–30% and a sensitivity of 50–70%. Patients at high risk for glaucoma should be referred to an ophthalmologist for evaluation. Glaucoma prevalence is significantly higher in African-Americans; the risk steadily increases with age.

Neither hematocrit/hemoglobin or leukocyte determinations have been shown to be useful in screening asymptomatic patients. Chemistry profile panels are also generally not recommended for screening asymptomatic healthy adults. Fasting plasma glucose levels should be measured in patients at a high risk for diabetes because of a family history of diabetes; in persons over age 40 with obesity; and in women with a personal history of gestational diabetes. Native Americans, Hispanics, and African-Americans have a higher risk for the development of diabetes mellitus. Urinalysis also is generally not advised for screening asymptomatic patients. Population-based studies have shown low rates of detecting serious and treatable urinary tract disorders in asymptomatic adults with either hemoglobin or protein present on dipstick urinalysis. All major authorities do recommend screening urinalysis in the prenatal care for pregnant women. Urinalysis for asymptomatic bacteriuria has been advised by some groups in diabetic patients and elderly patients over the age of 65.

Generally, laboratory tests such as chemistry profiles, blood count, urinalysis, and other similar tests should be used for targeted select patients based on their risk and the likelihood of disease. Routine screening of asymptomatic healthy adults via these methods is not advised or supported by the current medical literature.

ADULT IMMUNIZATIONS

INFLUENZA

Influenza vaccine is made from an inactivated virus grown in eggs. The vaccine is given yearly in the fall, optimally in November. It is 65–80% effective. Side effects include local skin reaction, fever, myalgia, and malaise. Hypersensitivity reactions are rare. The vaccine should be avoided in persons with a history of hypersensitivity reactions to eggs or persons with a febrile illness. The vaccination can be given safely in pregnant women. Recommended recipients of the vaccine include the following:

- People over age 65
- Nursing home patients
- Medical personnel
- Persons infected with HIV or having other immunocompromise
- Persons under age 18 on long-term aspirin therapy (to prevent Reye's syndrome)
- Persons frequently exposed to or living with persons of high risk
- Persons who perform essential community service

The vaccine, particularly in the elderly, is less protective for the recipient contracting the illness but does reduce the severity of the illness. The greatest percentage of deaths due to influenza occurs in persons over the age of 65. Consequently, vaccination in this age group is particularly important.

PNEUMOCOCCAL VACCINATION

The current 23 valent vaccine was established in 1983. The vaccine is about 60% effective for establishing immunity and covers about 88% of bloodstream isolates of pneumococcal infections in the United States. High-risk patients include those with the following conditions:

- Chronic cardiac or pulmonary conditions
- Anatomic or functional asplenia
- Chronic liver disease
- Alcoholism
- Diabetes
- Immunocompromise

Patients with chronic renal disease, Hodgkin's disease, multiple myeloma, or organ transplantation and those receiving hemodialysis or chemotherapy for cancer may have a diminished response to the vaccine. Adverse reactions to the vaccine are rare. Minor local side effects such as pain and redness are common. Revaccination is recommended for persons who received the 14 valent pneumococcal vaccine prior to 1983 and for those adults who are most at risk for serious pneumococcal infection who received the 23 valent vaccine 6 or more years previously. This is particularly important in patients with functional or anatomic asplenia. Persons who are likely to have diminishing antibody levels (e.g., patients on dialysis, those with nephrotic syndrome, or those having had organ transplantation) should receive a booster vaccination every 6 years. Revaccination for healthy adults including the elderly is presently not advised.

HEPATITIS B VACCINATION

Hepatitis B vaccination is a three-part vaccination presently given at 0, 1, and 6 months. The vaccination is 85–95% effective and is administered in the deltoid muscle. A decreased antibody response is seen in the presence of renal failure, diabetes, chronic liver disease, HIV infection, smoking, and advanced age. The vaccination series is advised for persons at high risk, including the following:

- Health care workers
- Dentists
- Hemodialysis patients
- IV drug users
- Institutionalized persons
- Homosexuals and bisexuals

Vaccination also is recommended for contacts of hepatitis B virus carriers, heterosexuals with multiple partners, and persons with recent sexually transmitted disease. The vaccine is contraindicated for those with yeast hypersensitivity or pregnancy. The vaccine is safe, producing in some patients only mild soreness at the injection site that may last 1–2 days. Rarely, constitutional symptoms have been experienced. Postvaccination serological testing to demonstrate immunity is advised. When antibodies to the hepatitis B surface antigen are not present, up to three additional doses of the vaccine at 1–2-month intervals should be undertaken. After one dose, 20% of nonresponders will produce antibodies. Between 30% and 50% will respond after three additional doses. After six doses, further attempts to immunize the patient are not likely to be fruitful. The need for booster vaccinations to provide clinical protection is unresolved at this time. In patients receiving hemodialysis whose immunity declines rapidly, annual serologic testing is recommended and booster vaccination administered to those whose antibody level falls below 10 mIU/mL.

TETANUS/DIPHTHERIA VACCINATION

The primary tetanus/diphtheria toxoid vaccination should be given to all adults who have not received the primary series previously. The general recommendation for booster dosing has been every 10 years throughout life. The Task Force on Adult Immunization recommends an alternative strategy of a single adult booster vaccination at age 50. Local reactions of tenderness and erythema are common following tetanus/diphtheria injections. Severe reactions to the vaccine are rare. Hypersensitivity occurs most commonly in persons receiving multiple booster vaccinations; therefore, persons who have received the vaccination within 5 years should not be revaccinated.

RUBELLA VACCINATION

The rubella vaccine is a live attenuated virus vaccine. It is available alone or in combination with measles and mumps (MMR). Rubella vaccine is recommended for all adults, particularly women. Susceptible women of childbearing age who have not received a previous vaccine should be vaccinated. In this situation, serologic testing is not advised because such a strategy is expensive and has been ineffective because of low rates of follow-up immunization. Women of childbearing age should receive the vaccine only if they say they are not pregnant. They should be counseled not to become pregnant for 3 months after receiving the vaccination. Adverse reactions occur only in susceptible persons. Those already immune to rubella who are receiving a second vaccination are not at risk for developing side effects. Side effects have included joint pain and inflammation, which in some persons have been persistent. Hospital workers who have the potential to transmit rubella to pregnant females should have their immunity checked and be vaccinated appropriately.

MEASLES VACCINATION

Measles vaccine is a live attenuated vaccine. Persons born prior to 1956 are likely to have had the virus and need not be vaccinated. Persons vaccinated in the years 1963 to 1967 with an inactivated virus should be revaccinated with the live virus vaccine. Reactions to the vaccine are local redness, sometimes accompanied by a low-grade fever. Higher fevers developing 5–12 days after the vaccination and lasting 1–2 days occurs in 5–15% of recipients.

MUMPS VACCINATION

Mumps vaccine should be administered to adolescent males who previously have not had mumps or been given the vaccine. The vaccine should be avoided when hypersensitivity to eggs is present. Contraindications include pregnancy, anaphylaxis to neomycin, and the presence of immunosuppressive conditions. Asymptomatic HIV-positive patients can receive the vaccine. Side effects include fever and rash 5–14 days after the vaccination, arthralgia or arthritis when given with the rubella vaccine, and local pain.

HEPATITIS A VACCINE

Preexposure immunization with the hepatitis A vaccine is advised for the following groups:

- Adults traveling to or working in countries in which hepatitis A is endemic
- Homosexual men
- Users of elicit drugs
- Persons with chronic liver disease
- Persons with an occupational risk for developing the disease

The intramuscular injection is given as a primary vaccination followed in 6–12 months by a booster vaccination. Postexposure management of hepatitis A should employ immune globulin. Side effects of the vaccine include soreness at the injection site, headache, and malaise. Generally, the vaccine has a very good safety profile.

VARICELLA VACCINE

Persons with a history of having varicella are assumed to be immune and do not need to be considered for vaccination.

Many other adults without a reliable history of varicella infection often carry immunity to varicella. Therefore, serologic testing before vaccination should be considered. Persons for whom the varicella vaccination should be considered include the following groups:

- Health care workers
- Household contacts of immunocompromised patients
- Persons living or working in high-risk environments for varicella transmission, such as schools and day-care centers
- College students
- Military personnel
- Nonpregnant women of childbearing age
- International travelers
- Persons without a history of the disease

The vaccine is given subcutaneously in two doses 4–8 weeks apart. The vaccine is of the live attenuated virus type and therefore is contraindicated in immunocompromised individuals. The vaccine is also contraindicated in persons who have anaphylaxis to neomycin, untreated active tuberculosis, or pregnancy. Side effects may include pain and erythema at the injection site or a varicella-like rash.

REVIEW EXERCISES

QUESTIONS

1. All of the following should receive yearly influenza vaccination *except*

   a. A radiology technician
   b. An adult on long-term aspirin therapy
   c. The parents of a 12-year-old son who has cystic fibrosis
   d. A pregnant woman with steroid-dependent asthma
   e. A 35-year-old healthy office worker requesting a flu vaccination

2. A 58-year-old patient with progressive nephrotic syndrome should

   a. Not need antibody titres assessed after the hepatitis B vaccination series
   b. Undergo pneumococcal vaccination once as a single lifetime vaccination
   c. Avoid revaccination for pneumococcal infection because of having received vaccination in 1975
   d. Undergo pneumococcal vaccination every 6 years
   e. Avoid taking the influenza vaccination

3. The optimal timing for administration of the pneumococcal vaccination includes all of the following *except*

   a. Prior to a planned splenectomy
   b. Every 6 years in a patient with chronic renal failure
   c. Prior to administration of chemotherapy in a patient with lymphoma
   d. When clinical AIDS develops in an HIV-infected patient
   e. Prior to immunosuppressive therapy in a patient undergoing organ transplantation

4. All of the following statements regarding influenza flu vaccination are true *except*

   a. It can be given at the same time as the pneumococcal vaccination
   b. It is 60% to 70% effective
   c. It often causes an influenza-like illness
   d. It is contraindicated in the presence of allergy to eggs
   e. It should be postponed in the setting of a febrile illness

Answers

1. b

   A radiology technician is a health care worker and should receive the influenza vaccination. An adult on long-term aspirin therapy is not specifically in a high-risk group advised to undergo the influenza vaccination, whereas a child or young adult on aspirin therapy should receive the vaccination because of the possibility of aspirin therapy and influenza in this age group leading to Reye's syndrome. The correct answer is therefore B. The parents of a young child with cystic fibrosis should receive the vaccination so that they do not potentially expose their child to this illness. A pregnant woman with steroid-dependent asthma is in a high-risk group for influenza infection and therefore should receive the vaccination even though she is pregnant. The vaccine is not contraindicated in pregnancy. Last, healthy adults who wish to receive the vaccination may safely be given it.

2. d

   A person with progressive nephrotic syndrome is in a high-risk group for hepatitis B and pneumococcal and influenza infections. Therefore, these vaccinations should all be administered in this situation. In progressive nephrotic syndrome, antibody response to these vaccinations wanes. Therefore, antibody titers should be obtained after patients receive the hepatitis B series. These patients likewise should receive the pneumococcal vaccination every 6 years. Thus,

the answer is D. This person should be given the influenza vaccination, and if he or she had received only the early 14 valent pneumococcal vaccination, a repeat updated pneumococcal vaccination should be administered.

3. d

   Generally, the pneumococcal vaccination should be given to immunosuppressed patients before their immunosuppression occurs or becomes advanced. Therefore, the vaccination should be given prior to a planned splenectomy, the administration of chemotherapy, or immunosuppressant therapy, and when HIV infection is first detected. The correct answer therefore is D. Because of waning immunity, the vaccination should be given every 6 years in patients with chronic renal failure.

4. c

   A common misconception among patients is that the influenza vaccination causes an influenza-like illness. The vaccine may cause local skin reaction, fever, myalgia, and malaise but does not cause an influenza-like illness. The vaccine is contraindicated in those allergic to eggs because the vaccine is made from inactivated virus grown in eggs. It should be postponed in those with a febrile illness. It is 60–70% effective and can safely be given at the same time as the pneumococcal vaccination. The correct answer is therefore C.

SUGGESTED READINGS

GENERAL

Matzen RN, Lang RS, eds. Clinical Preventive Medicine. Mosby Year Book Company, 1993.

U.S. Department of Health and Human Services. Put prevention into practice: clinicians handbook of preventive services. U.S. Department of Health and Human Services, Public Health Service, Office of Disease Prevention and Health Promotion, 1994.

U.S. Preventive Services Task Force. Report. Guide to clinical prevention services, 2nd ed. International Medical Publishing, 1996.

SCREENING

American Cancer Society. Guidelines for the cancer-related check-up. Recommendations and rationale. CA 1980;30L: 194–240. Also yearly updates.

American College of Physicians. Guidelines for using cholesterol, HDL cholesterol, and triglyceride levels as screening tests for preventing coronary artery disease in adults. Ann Int Med 1996;124:515–517.

Berlin NI et al. The National Cancer Institute Cooperative Early Lung Cancer Detection Program. (Prevalence reports from Mayo, Johns Hopkins, and Memorial Sloan-Kettering Studies). Am Rev Respir Dis 1984;130:545, 549, 555, 561–565.

Canadian Task Force on the Periodic Health Examination. Spitzer W et al. The periodic health examination. Can Med Assoc J 1979;121:1193. 1984;130:1276. 1986;134:721. Also yearly updates.

Carter HB et al. Longitudinal evaluation of prostate specific antigen levels in men with and without prostate disease. JAMA 1992;267:2215–2220.

Dorr VJ et al. An evaluation of prostate specific antigen as a screening test for prostate cancer. Arch Int Med 1993;153: 2529–2537.

Garber AM, Browner WS, Halley SB. Cholesterol screening in asymptomatic adults, revisited. Ann Int Med 1996;124: 518–531.

Harris R, Leininger L. Clinical strategies for breast cancer screening: weighing and using the evidence. Ann Intern Med 1995;122:539–547.

IARC Working Group on Evaluation of Cervical Cancer Screening Programmes. Screening for squamous cervical cancer: duration of low risk after negative results of cervical cytology and its implication for screening policies. Br Med J 1986;293:659–664.

Oboler SK, La Force FM. The periodic physical examination in asymptomatic adults. Ann Int Med 1989;110:214–226.

Oesterling JE. Prostate specific antigen improving its ability to diagnose early prostate cancer. JAMA 1992;267:2536–2538.

Report of the Joint American College of Cardiology & American Heart Association Task Force on Assessment of Cardiovascular Procedure. Schlant RC et al. Guidelines for exercise testing. Circulation 1986;74:653A–667A.

Ruckle HC et al. Prostate specific antigen: critical issues for the practicing physician. Mayo Clinic Proc 1994;69:59–68.

Sickles EA, Kopans DB. Mammographic screening for women aged 40 to 49 years: the primary practitioner's dilemma. Ann Int Med 1995;122:534–538.

Sox HC. Preventive health services in adults. NEJM 1994; 330:1589–1595.

Toribara NW, Sleisinger MH. Screening for colorectal cancer. NEJM 1995;332:861–867.

IMMUNIZATIONS

ACP Task Force on Adult Immunization and Infectious Diseases Society of America. Guide for adult immunization. 1994.

Gardner P, Schaffner W. Immunization of adults. NEJM 1993; 328:1252–1258.

Gardner P et al. Adult immunizations. Ann Int Med 1996; 124:35–40.

Women's Hormonal Health Issues: Menopause, Hormone Replacement Therapy, and Hormonal Contraception

Holly L. Thacker

The American Board of Internal Medicine has asserted that internists should be proficient in providing comprehensive women's health care. By understanding the hypothalamic/pituitary/ovarian/endometrial axis, the internist can understand menstrual abnormalities, menopause, and hormonal contraception (Fig. 2.1). Most women live long enough to become menopausal. The average age of menopausal onset has not changed much in the last century; however, the average life span of a woman is increasingly lengthening. Therefore, the amount of time that a woman spends in a potential estrogen-deficient and progesterone-deficient state is increasing with certain physiologic and metabolic consequences. The onset of menopause is an excellent time for the internist to assess a woman's overall health. *For most menopausal women, the benefits of hormone replacement therapy (HRT) outweigh the risks.*

ANATOMY AND PHYSIOLOGY OF THE FEMALE REPRODUCTIVE ORGANS

MENSTRUAL CYCLE

Between menarche (approximate age, 12 years) and natural menopause (approximate age, 51 years), the hypothalamic/pituitary/ovarian/endometrial axis directs the reproductive organs in the menstrual cycle. The menstrual cycle can be divided into three distinct phases: follicular, ovulation, and luteal.

The usual menstrual cycle length is 28 days; normal ovulatory menstrual cycles, however, may range from 3 to 6 weeks in cycle length. Menstrual cycles are the most variable in length in the years immediately following menarche and in the perimenopausal years, largely owing to a higher incidence of anovulatory cycles. Other causes of change in the menstrual cycle length may be due to abrupt changes in the body mass index, a change in exercise pattern, significant psychosocial distress, and parturition. The age of menopause is lowered by smoking. Menopause may be a potent biological marker of aging.

The follicular phase—an estrogen-dominant phase with proliferation of the endometrium—begins with the first day of the menstrual period. The oocyte is released from a mature follicle after the onset of the preovulatory surge of luteinizing hormone (LH) by the pituitary gland. (At the time of ovulation, some women experience dull pelvic pain, which is termed "mittelschmerz.") As peak LH levels are reached, estradiol (E2) levels drop, while progesterone levels continue to increase. The luteal phase, which is more consistent in duration than the follicular phase, is approximately 2 weeks long and ends with the onset of the menses. The luteal/secretory phase results from the corpus luteum, which secretes progesterone. Progesterone causes the endometrium to become secretory in nature.

The ovaries synthesize estrogens, androgens, progesterone, and peptides, including inhibin (folliculostatin), a hormone that specifically inhibits the release of follicle-stimulating hormone. (See Fig. 2.1.) Inhibin, like estradiol, is produced by ovarian granulosa cells, the major cell type of the ovarian follicle. Inhibin is not measurable in the postmenopausal woman.

Progesterone, the name of the class, is the sole naturally occurring progesterone. Produced by the corpus luteum, it prepares the endometrium to be secretory in preparation for a fertilized ovum. Progesterone opposes the action of estrogen in various tissues, most notably the endometrium. Progesterone deficiency may occur during the perimenopausal time because of defects in the luteal phase. This can result in dysfunctional uterine bleeding caused by a proliferative endometrium. Progestins are synthetic substances that are manufactured by chemically altering naturally occurring pro-

Hypothalamic-Pituitary-Ovarian-Endometrial Axis

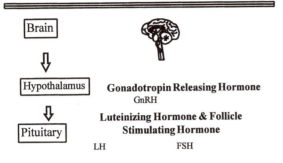

Pituitary-Ovarian-Endometrial Axis (cont.)

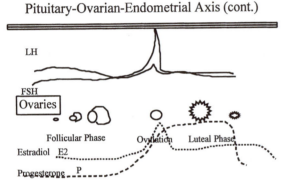

Ovarian-Endometrial Axis (cont.)

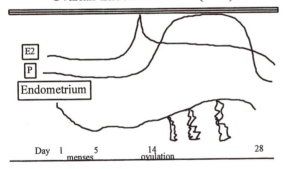

Figure 2.1. Hypothalamic-pituitary-ovarian-endometrial axis

gesterone (derived primarily from plant sources). Clinically, progestins are used solely to oppose estrogenic effects on the endometrium.

The premenopausal adult ovary consists of germ cells and stroma. The germ cells are eliminated from the ovaries by ovulation and by atresia. The latter accounts for the elimi-

nation of over 99% of all germ cells. After approximately 400 menstrual cycles, the reproductive capacity of the ovaries is exhausted. The numbers of ovarian follicles present in the ovary are the initial determinants of the age at menopause. The ovarian follicle granulosa cells produce estradiol, which is the most potent naturally occurring estrogen. The three estrogens that occur naturally are estrone (E1), estradiol (E2), and estriol (E3). Estradiol and estrone are mutually interconvertable by a redux reaction in the liver. Estrone, the dominant menopausal estrogen, is formed by the peripheral conversion of androstenedione into estrone in the adipose tissue. The premenopausal and postmenopausal ovary produces androgens from ovarian stroma. However, in some women, the ovarian stroma becomes fibrotic and does not produce postmenopausal androgens.

MENOPAUSE

The term natural menopause is defined as the permanent cessation of menstruation resulting from the loss of ovarian follicular activity. Natural menopause is a retrospective diagnosis made after 12 consecutive months of amenorrhea from the final menstrual period. Perimenopause includes the period prior to menopause. Perimenopause begins with a transition phase of declining ovarian function that may occur five to seven years before the final menstrual period. The decline of ovarian function is gradual and begins in the 30s, corresponding to a decrease in fertility. The term ''premenopausal'' encompasses the entire reproductive period up to the final menstrual period. Postmenopause is defined as dating from the final menstrual period, regardless of whether the menopause was natural or induced. Induced menopause is defined as the absence of menstruation, which follows either surgical removal of both ovaries (castration with or without a hysterectomy) or iatrogenic ablation of ovarian function (which may follow either chemotherapy or radiation treatment). Premature menopause is defined as occurring before the age of 40, although the usual range for menopause is between the ages of 45 and 55.

In both natural and induced menopause, there is no longer production of estradiol because follicular development has ceased. In naturally menopausal women, however, the ovarian stroma usually continues to produce some androgens, which can be converted to estrone peripherally. Constitutional, genetic, and environmental factors account for the differing effects of menopause in individual women. Women who have induced menopause abruptly lose all production of estradiol and approximately half of the production of androgens (as the remaining androgens are produced in the adrenal gland). The adrenal androgen, dehydroepiandrosterone-sulfate (DHEA-s) decreases linearly with age and is not specifically decreased by the menopause.

PATHOPHYSIOLOGY OF SEX HORMONE DEFICIENCY AND EXCESS

Estrogen deficiency is associated with osteoporosis, genitourinary atrophy, and an increased risk of atherosclerosis. Andro-

Table 2.1. Oral Estrogen						
Drug	*Dosages*	*Standard Dose*				
Premarin (CEE)	0.3 mg	0.625 mg po q d	0.9 mg	1.25 mg		2.5 mg
Estrace (micronized estradiol)	0.5 mg	1.0 mg po q d		2.00 mg		
Ogen (estrone)		0.625 mg po q d		1.25 mg		
Ortho-Est (estrone)		0.625 mg po q d		1.25 mg		

gen deficiency in women usually is the result of castration or surgical procedures that affect ovarian blood supply or spontaneous fibrosis of the stroma of the postmenopausal ovary. Androgen deficiency is associated with a decreased libido and a decreased sense of well being. Progesterone deficiency in the perimenopause from defective corpus luteum production can result in dysfunctional uterine bleeding, which is manifested by heavy and/or irregular menstrual bleeding.

Chronic anovulation may lead to irregular and heavy menstrual cycles and an increased risk of endometrial hyperplasia and cancer (due to unopposed estrogen) (Table 2.1). The causes of chronic anovulation include:

- Chronic anovulation due to inappropriate pituitary feedback (such as in polycystic ovary syndrome)
  - Excessive extra-glandular estrogen (as in obesity)
  - Functional androgen excess from adrenal or ovarian cause
  - Neoplasms that produce either androgens or estrogens
  - Neoplasms that produce chorionic gonadotropin
  - Abnormal sex hormone binding globulin (including liver disease)
- Chronic anovulation due to endocrine or metabolic disorders
  - Thyroid dysfunction
    - Hyperthyroidism
    - Hypothyroidism
  - Prolactin and/or growth hormone excess
    - Pituitary microadenomas or macroadenomas
    - Hypothalamic dysfunction
    - Drug-induced hyperprolactinemia
  - Malnutrition
  - Adrenal hyperfunction (Cushing's disease)
  - Congenital adrenal hyperplasia
- Chronic anovulation of hypothalamic pituitary origin
  - Hypothalamic chronic anovulation
    - Psychogenic
    - Exercise induced
    - Associated with malnutrition, weight loss, or systemic illness
    - Eating disorders, including anorexia nervosa and bulimia
  - Isolated gonadotropin deficiency (Kallmann's syndrome)
  - Hypothalamic pituitary damage

- Following surgery, trauma, radiation, or infection
- Empty sella syndrome
- Following infarction (post delivery Sheehan's syndrome)
- Pituitary and parapituitary tumors
- Idiopathic hypopituitarism

CLINICAL PRESENTATION OF MENOPAUSE

Menopause can be viewed medically as an adult-onset, potential primary hypogonadism with various target tissues affected. The primary areas affected (as discussed in the following sections) are the:

- Integument
- Genitourinary system
- Neuroendocrine system
- Skeleton
- Cardiovascular system

Menopausal changes may affect women differently and may occur over a variable time span. Constitutional factors, genetic predisposition, diet, and the level of endogenous estrogen and androgen production all play a role in this variability.

INTEGUMENT

Estrogen-deficiency skin changes include loss of elasticity and decreased production of collagen. Dryness of mucosal surfaces may be manifested as dryness of the eyes, nose, mouth, and vagina. Many postmenopausal women have relative androgen excess as the ovarian stroma continues to produce androgens. Skin manifestations of androgen excess include minimal facial hirsutism, acne, and male-patterned androgenic hair loss.

GENITOURINARY SYSTEM

Genitourinary atrophy from estrogen deficiency can be manifested by dyspareunia, blood-tinged vaginal discharge from an atrophic vagina, urethral caruncle, irritable bladder with both urinary frequency and urgency, and an exacerbation of stress incontinence.

Urinary incontinence is a significant problem for many older women. The types of incontinence are:

- Stress
- Urge
- Overflow
- Functional

There may be a combination of these types of incontinence present in the postmenopausal woman. Stress urinary incontinence occurs primarily in women during pelvic-stress maneuvers, such as coughing, sneezing, exercise, and any Valsalva maneuver. Risk factors for stress urinary incontinence include estrogen deficiency, chronic cough, obstetrical trauma, and weak pelvic-floor muscles.

Pelvic-floor exercises, which are done to strengthen the voluntary muscles of the urinary sphincter and pelvic-floor muscles, may be helpful in the treatment of mild stress urinary incontinence. Estrogen-replacement therapy (ERT), either topically or systemically, may improve stress urinary incontinence symptoms by improving the formation of collagen and the integrity of the vagina and urethra. Bladder training, behavioral modification, pelvic-floor biofeedback, and pelvic-floor muscle strengthening with various vaginal cones may be beneficial. Pelvic-floor muscle relaxation may lead to incontinence, cystocele, rectocele, enterocele, or frank prolapse of the uterus at the introitus.

Urge incontinence occurs when an uninhibited bladder contraction is of significant strength to overcome the baseline urethral sphincter tone. This may be associated with pelvic floor relaxation and often coexists with genuine stress urinary incontinence. Bladder irritability that leads to the sensation of urgency may be increased when there is atrophy of the estrogen-sensitive trigone of the bladder. Certain substances in the diet, including caffeine and spices, may also irritate the bladder.

NEUROENDOCRINE CHANGES

Neuroendocrine changes in the perimenopausal and postmenopausal woman include the vasomotor symptoms of the hot flash (a sensation of warmth) or hot flush (a sensation of warmth coupled with an erythematous appearance of the head and neck), which can range from a minor inconvenience in some women to debilitating symptoms in others. Vasomotor symptoms may be accompanied by diaphoresis. This phenomenon is more likely to occur at night, in warm environments, after the ingestion of caffeine or alcohol, and during periods of stress. If hot flashes occur at night, it can lead to a sleep disturbance with consequent fatigue and depression. The physiology of the hot flash/flush is not defined clearly; however, it is thought to involve the hypothalamus with pulses of gonadotropin-releasing factors that affect the autonomic nervous system. Untreated hot flashes may last for a few years;

in some women, however, the flashes may continue for decades.

Contrary to common belief, hot flashes are not linked directly with estradiol levels and do not always occur in induced menopause; however, induced menopausal women may have the most intense hot flashes if they experience them. The amount of estrogen receptors in the hypothalamus and other constitutional factors probably account for the varying intensity of hot flashes. Vasomotor instability may also be manifested as palpitations, which are common in both perimenopausal and postmenopausal women.

Psychiatric disease is not increased in menopausal women; however, women with preexisting psychiatric disturbances can have exacerbations if they are having significant menopausal symptoms as well. Preexisting major depression and panic disorder can be exacerbated by vasomotor symptoms in menopause. Estrogens, progesterone, and androgens all have effects on the CNS and the neurotransmitter system. Hormone replacement or hormone supplementation is not a method of treatment for neurotransmitter imbalance, although many minor mood disturbances can certainly be improved in menopausal women with hormone replacement regimens.

SKELETON

Peak bone mass is reached by age 30, with a gradual loss occurring thereafter and rapid bone loss occurring at the time of menopause. Estrogen acts as an antiresorptive agent and inhibits bone loss. Progesterone may stimulate bone growth by stimulating osteoblasts. Postmenopausal use of estrogen and other indicators of estrogen status have been strongly correlated with a higher bone mineral density. Estrogen used many years after menopause is beneficial to the skeleton. Although estrogen and bisphosphates, such as alendronate, can treat osteoporosis, estrogen is the best studied.

Routine testing of bone mineral density for all menopausal women is not indicated. However, women who have evidence of vertebral deformity or a history of fractures should have bone density tested. Women with premature menopause, women with any risks for osteoporosis, and women who decide to take HRT if they were found to have low bone density should be offered screening.

CARDIOVASCULAR SYSTEM

Cardiovascular disease is the leading cause of death and disability in American women. Gender-specific risk factors for cardiovascular disease in women include diabetes mellitus, low levels of high-density-lipoprotein (HDL) cholesterol, hypertriglyceridemia, and hormonal status.

The risk of a 50-year-old Caucasian woman dying of cardiovascular disease is 10 times greater than her combined risk of dying as the result of a hip fracture or of breast cancer.

Hispanic and African-American women have an even greater risk of cardiovascular disease. Induced menopause and premature menopause without the benefit of ERT are significant risk factors for coronary artery disease. Natural menopause also may be a risk factor for coronary artery disease. Epidemiologic studies strongly suggest that ERT reduces the incidence of cardiovascular death.

Oral conjugated estrogen decrease total cholesterol and low-density-lipoprotein (LDL) cholesterol and increase HDL cholesterol. Transdermal estradiol decreases both total cholesterol and LDL cholesterol and, unlike oral estrogens in some predisposed women, does not elevate triglycerides. The favorable lipid effects associated with ERT are only a small part of the cardiovascular benefit derived. Estradiol relaxes smooth muscle tone and has a direct beneficial effect on vessel wall physiology and endothelial function. Menopausal progestins do not appear to attenuate the beneficial effects of estrogen on the lipoprotein moieties. However, preliminary research indicates that natural progesterone may be preferable to synthetic progestins in women with existing coronary artery disease and myocardial ischemia.

DIAGNOSIS OF MENOPAUSE

The diagnosis of menopause is usually straightforward. The absence of menstruation in a woman with characteristic menopausal symptoms does not require any specific laboratory testing. However, pregnancy should always be considered in the differential of secondary amenorrhea. Causes of secondary amenorrhea include:

- Pregnancy
- Ovarian failure (menopause)
- Chronic anovulation
- Traumatic amenorrhea (Asherman's syndrome)
- Adrenal and/or thyroid dysfunction
- Endometrial atrophy (e.g., from continuous progestin use)
- Pituitary prolactinoma
- Gestational trophic disease

HISTORY AND PHYSICAL EXAMINATION

The history and physical examination in the menopausal woman should focus on the areas affected by menopause:

- Cardiovascular system
- Skeleton
- Genitourinary system
- Neuroendocrine system
- Integument

The examiner should ask specifically about:

- Symptoms of estrogen deficiency
  - Hot flashes
  - Sleep disturbance
  - Palpitations
  - Dry skin
  - Irritable bladder
  - Dyspareunia
- Symptoms of androgen deficiency
  - Decreased libido
  - Decreased ability to reach sexual climax
- Symptoms of progesterone deficiency (may be manifested as heavy irregular menses)

The height, weight, and blood pressure should be recorded during the physical examination. Thyroid examination, breast examination, cardiovascular examination, and pelvic and rectal examinations should be performed. Signs of genitourinary atrophy include a thin, pale, atrophic vaginal mucosa, either diffuse or in patches. The periurethral tissue is the most estrogen-sensitive and usually shows signs of estrogen deficiency first. Severe cases of vaginal estrogen deficiency include a stenotic introitus, a urethral caruncle, and a small cervix with a stenotic cervical os. In severe cases, the cervix may be flush with the vaginal wall. A screening Papanicolaou (Pap) smear should be obtained of the exocervix and endocervix using a spatula and cytobrush to screen for cervical cancer.

LABORATORY STUDIES

Follicle-stimulating hormone (FSH) and estradiol levels are usually not needed to diagnose the menopausal state. Knowing these levels, however, can occasionally be helpful, such as when deciding whether to institute ERT in a woman who has had a simple hysterectomy (i.e., one in which at least one ovary is conserved). Ovarian function may or may not persist for a variable period after a simple hysterectomy.

Measuring hormone levels also may be helpful with a healthy, nonsmoking woman who continues to take oral contraceptives up through the menopause, and in whom it may be difficult to determine when menopause has occurred. In such women, the FSH level is usually measured on day 5 of the pill-free week. An assay-specific, FSH level greater than 20 IU/L (and particularly greater than 40 IU/L), with an estradiol level less than 20–40 pg/mL, usually confirms primary gonadal failure. Perimenopausal women may have similar values that may fluctuate widely in the perimenopause; therefore, the diagnosis of menopause is always retrospective. The differential diagnosis of hypergonadotrophic hypogonadism (FSH > 20–40 IU/L) include:

- Natural menopause
- Physical causes
  - Surgical removal (castration)
  - Gonadal irradiation
  - Chemotherapy (especially alkylating agents)
- Autoimmune disorders
  - Polyglandular failure involving the ovaries
  - Isolated ovarian failure associated with ovarian antibodies

- Chromosomal abnormalities
- Inherited tendencies producing premature ovarian failure
  - Genetically reduced cell endowment
  - Accelerated atresia
- Gonadotropin receptor and/or postreceptor defects causing the resistant ovary syndrome

A thyroid-stimulating hormone (TSH) can help detect possible overreplacement in women receiving thyroxine who may be at increased risk for bone loss. Such women can be clinically euthyroid but biochemically hyperthyroid, as evidenced by suppressed TSH level. In addition, any perimenopausal women with nonspecific symptoms and/or a menstrual disorder should have TSH done, as symptoms of the perimenopause may overlap with symptoms of thyroid dysfunction. A screening mammogram should be obtained yearly in perimenopausal and postmenopausal women. Approximately 10–20% of women on HRT will have an increased density in their breast after beginning HRT, which may make detection of breast cancer more difficult.

Bone densitometry with dual energy x-ray absorptiometry of the hip and spine as a baseline in healthy menopausal women should generally be reserved for those in whom its results would affect the decision to institute HRT (Fig. 2.2).

Total and HDL cholesterol should be measured to help ascertain cardiovascular risk in the menopausal woman. If the total cholesterol concentration is elevated or the HDL-cholesterol concentration is low, a 12-hour fasting lipid profile (including triglycerides) is needed. Marked hypertriglyceridemia is an independent risk factor for coronary artery disease in women.

TREATMENT OF MENOPAUSE

HORMONE TREATMENT OF MENOPAUSE

Figure 2.2 can help guide the institution of HRT, but treatment plans must be tailored for the individual woman. The goal of HRT is not to normalize the FSH value (which would be difficult to do in the absence of inhibin), but rather to use the minimum effective dosage to suppress vasomotor symptoms, treat genitourinary atrophy, prevent bone loss, and reduce cardiovascular risk. Benefits and risks include the following:

- Benefits
  - Cardiovascular risk reduction
  - Prevention of postmenopausal osteoporosis, fractures, and dental loss
  - Relief of vasomotor symptoms
  - Curing genitourinary atrophy
  - Possible improvement in mood, energy, and recent memory
  - Possible reduction in the prevalence of senile dementia of the Alzheimer's type
- Risks

- Growth acceleration of an already preformed breast cancer
- Five-to-ten-fold increase of endometrial cancer risk if estrogen is unopposed
- Premenstrual syndrome-like side effects on progestin-estrogen program
- Increased incidence of gallbladder disease
- Nuisance of withdrawal menstrual bleeding on cycled program

Women who have had a simple hysterectomy can take estrogen alone. However, if the uterus and/or endometrial lining is present, an estrogen-only regimen can lead to endometrial hyperplasia and an increased incidence of uterine cancer. Therefore, women with a uterus need combined progestin estrogen replacement (PERT). Women practicing contraception before menopause should continue to do so for 1 year, as PERT does not provide contraceptive levels of these hormones, and, therefore, an occasional ovulation may occur prior to the final menstrual period.

Estrogen and the Breast

Estrogen is a trophic growth hormone and therefore may theoretically promote the growth of a preexisting breast cancer; however, estrogen is not carcinogenic per se. Moreover, the use of synthetic oral contraceptives has not been associated with an increased risk of breast cancer. A meta-analysis of the major breast cancer studies did not show an increased risk of breast cancer in women who had ever received ERT compared with those who had not. Women with premenopausal breast cancer are no longer treated with induced menopause. There are no prospective controlled trials showing a worsening of prognosis of women with breast cancer on HRT, and women who have received HRT and have breast cancer may have a better outcome. There has been much discussion in the recent literature about re-evaluating the dogmatic stance of precluding HRT in women with a history of breast cancer.

Because of the documented benefits of ERT, one must be circumspect in denying HRT for the symptomatic menopausal woman requesting a trial, regardless of her breast status. The benefit of HRT in reducing the risk of developing cardiovascular disease appears to outweigh the risk of breast cancer in virtually all women in whom this therapy might be considered. A recent decision analysis supports the broader use of HRT in postmenopausal women.

Estrogen Therapies

Conjugated Equine Estrogens   Of the oral estrogen preparations, the conjugated estrogen preparation Premarin (a complex blend of multiple estrogens) has been available the longest (see Table 2.1). Consequently, Premarin has been studied the most. It is the preferred estrogen preparation with regard to cardiac protection. Esterified estrogen preparations (Estratab and Menest) principally contain estrone and equiva-

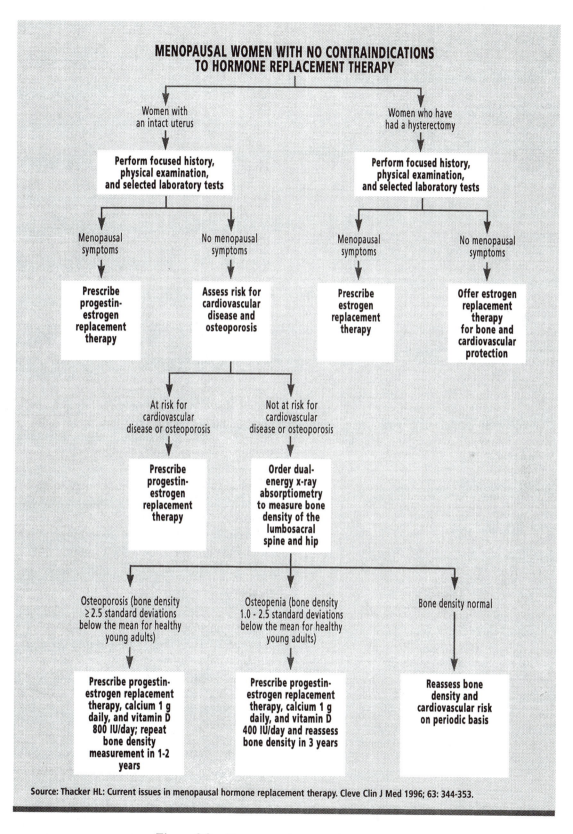

Figure 2.2.   Hormone replacement therapy algorithm

Table 2.2.	Estradiol Patches				
Drug	*Dosages*	*Standard Dose*			*Change Patch*
Estraderm		0.05 mg		0.10 mg	Every 3½ days
Vivelle	0.0375 mg	0.05 mg	0.075 mg	0.10 mg	Every 3½ days
Climara		0.05 mg		0.10 mg	Weekly
Alora		0.05 mg	0.075 mg	0.10 mg	Every 3½ days
Fempatch	0.025 mg				Weekly

lent sulfate but are not biochemical equivalents to conjugated equine estrogens.

Estradiol is the principal estrogen secreted by the premenopausal ovary. Given orally, micronized 17-beta estradiol (Estrace) is converted and metabolized by the liver to estrone. It increases sex-binding globulin protein levels and may be beneficial for women with skin and hair problems related to androgen excess. Oral estradiol is rapidly absorbed from the gut and has a short half life. Therefore, the total daily dose needs to be split in a twice-a-day regimen.

Estropipate (estrone) (Ogen, Ortho-Est) contains purified estropipate without any equine estrogen. Physiologically, these formulations are weaker than the conjugated or esterified estrogens at comparable dosages because they contain only the weakest estrogen, estrone.

The estradiol patch avoids enterohepatic metabolism (Table 2.2). The transdermal estradiol does not affect hepatic coagulation proteins. The patch may be preferable in a woman who has:

- Nausea on oral preparations
- Drug-induced hypertension while taking an oral estrogen-replacement formulation (a rare occurrence)
- A history of thromboembolism

Side effects occur much less frequently during ERT than with oral contraceptive use because the estrogenic dosages are approximately four to five times lower than with low-dose oral contraceptives.

As shown in Table 2.1, the lowest effective estrogen dose for most menopausal women is 0.625 mg daily of conjugated equine estrogens (CEE) or an equivalent. The estrogen dose can be increased if needed to control vasomotor symptoms, but should not be decreased to less than the recommended starting dose if the prevention of osteoporosis and heart disease is the treatment goal. Women without vasomotor symptoms who cannot tolerate higher dosages of estrogen because of mastalgia or fluid retention, however, can receive a lower dose (e.g., conjugated estrogens 0.3 mg; micronized estradiol 0.5 mg; or estradiol patch 0.0375 mg or the lowest dose patch 0.025 mg).

Vaginal preparations, such as Estrace vaginal cream (2 g daily for 2 weeks, then 1 g 1–3 times per week), are good options for women who still have mild residual genitourinary atrophy while taking the standard doses of systemic estrogens. There may be some initial systemic absorption of vaginal estrogen through the thin atrophic vaginal mucosa; however, once mucosal integrity is restored with local therapy, systemic absorption of estradiol is generally not a concern. Therefore, vaginal estrogen alone is an option for women who only need treatment of genitourinary atrophy. A new vaginal estrogen ring (Estring), changed every 3 months by the patient or the physician, is available to treat genitourinary atrophy and is not associated with systemic absorption. This is optimal treatment for the woman who cannot or will not tolerate any systemic absorption of estrogen.

Younger women and women who have undergone induced menopause may need at least twice the minimum estrogen dose to suppress vasomotor symptoms (e.g., conjugated estrogen 1.25–2.5 mg daily; transdermal estradiol 0.10 patch; or oral estradiol 2 mg). Estratest or Estratest HS is indicated for women with low levels of free testosterone (e.g., esterified estrogen 1.25 mg or 0.625 mg and methyltestosterone 2.5 mg or 1.25 mg). Oral androgens may be associated with abnormal liver enzyme tests and, in high doses, potential liver damage. Therefore, periodic monitoring of liver function is recommended for women who take oral androgens. Very rarely, a woman taking menopausal estrogen-testosterone preparations may experience acne, hirsutism, or other virilizing effects. It can be helpful to measure blood estradiol and free testosterone levels during treatment. The minimum target level is approximately 60 pg/mL of estradiol and 1–9 pg/mL of free testosterone.

Progestins

A woman taking estrogen who has a uterus (and therefore an endometrial lining) needs a progestin to prevent endometrial hyperplasia associated with unopposed estrogen therapy. In general, progestins are not recommended after hysterectomy unless residual endometriosis is of concern. Progestins may have androgenic effects depending on the agent, dose, and route of administration. In combination with estrogen, progestins can cause premenstrual-like symptoms, the most common limiting side effect. Current epidemiologic studies do not support adding synthetic progestins to estrogen to protect the bones or the breast.

Progestins can either be taken for the first 12 days of every calendar month (a cycled regimen usually associated with withdrawal bleeding), or every day with a lower dosage (the continuous regimen, which usually induces amenorrhea in women within 6 to 9 months).

Table 2.3. Medroxyprogesterone Acetate (MPA) Regimens

Brand Name	Dosage
Provera	MPA 5–10 mg on days 1–12, or 2.5 mg daily
Cycrin	MPA 5–10 mg on days 1–12, or 2.5 mg daily
Amen	MPA 10 mg on days 1–12 (the tablet is scored)
PremPro	MPA 2.5 mg daily in conjugated equine estrogens 0.625 mg daily (28-day pill pack)
Premphase	MPA 5 mg/day for 14 days with conjugated equine estrogens 0.625 mg daily (28-day pill pack)

As shown in Table 2.3, the standard cycled progestin dosage is medroxyprogesterone acetate (MPA, available as Provera, Cycrin, Amen) available in 5–10 mg on days 1 through 12 of every calendar month.

During cycled treatment, mild-to-moderate uterine bleeding generally occurs mid month, usually between days 10 and 15. If the cervical os is not occluded or stenosed, the absence of withdrawal menstrual bleeding indicates there is no endometrial lining to be shed. Any abnormal uterine bleeding needs to be investigated. Cycling the estrogen alone does not protect against endometrial hyperplasia and is not routinely advocated when cardiovascular and osteoporosis prevention are the intended treatment goals.

If the goal of HRT is solely to relieve menopausal symptoms, the treatment duration is generally 2–3 years with a gradual tapering off of the medication. If the goal is to provide cardiac protection and prevent osteoporosis, long-term, possible lifetime treatment is needed. HRT should increase life expectancy for nearly all postmenopausal women, with some gains exceeding 3 years depending on the women's individual risk factors for coronary artery disease and breast cancer. Overall, the benefits of HRT outweigh the risks for many menopausal women.

Contraindications to HRT

Undiagnosed vaginal bleeding is an absolute contraindication to ERT. Postmenopausal bleeding must always be evaluated because 5–10% of women with spontaneous, unexplained postmenopausal bleeding will be diagnosed with abnormalities such as atypical hyperplasia, adenomatous hyperplasia, or endometrial cancer. The remainder of women with postmenopausal bleeding have a proliferative endometrium due to lack of progesterone, endometrial polyps, cervical or vulvar lesions, submucosal fibroids, or simply an atrophic vagina or atrophic endometrium.

A history of uterine cancer (estrogen-dependent cancer) is not necessarily a contraindication for ERT, provided that the uterine cancer is considered to be cured, either by surgical excision of a low-grade, early-stage cancer or by lack of evidence of recurrence after 5 years from the initial surgical treatment. When a progestin is prescribed to a woman with an intact uterus, the increase in endometrial cancer associated with ERT alone can be prevented. Ovarian cancers generally are thought not to be estrogen dependent and therefore do not constitute a contraindication to HRT.

Uterine leiomyomata (fibroids) are not an absolute contraindication to ERT. Fibroids generally shrink in the menopause because of estrogen deficiency. The low doses of ERT used for menopause do not generally cause fibroid enlargement.

A remote history of deep venous thrombosis is not a contraindication to HRT. However, one may want to consider the use of transdermal estradiol, as it does not affect hepatic coagulation proteins. Migraineurs may enjoy relief of headaches at the onset of menopause; conversely, they may have worsening of migraines. Avoiding cyclic variation in hormone levels may be beneficial to the patient with migraines.

HRT is associated with lowering of the mean diastolic and systolic blood pressure; however, an occasional woman will have idiosyncratic elevation of the blood pressure on oral estrogen replacement. The blood pressure, therefore, should be checked after instituting HRT. In women with existing hepatic or gallbladder disease, one may want to consider transdermal estradiol. Transdermal progestin is not yet available in the United States, but it is under investigation.

ALTERNATIVE TREATMENTS OF MENOPAUSAL SYMPTOMS

There are a variety of over-the-counter, nonhormone lubricants that help with vaginal dryness, but they do not restore the integrity of the vaginal mucosa. For the treatment of hot flashes, Clonidine and methyldopa have shown some efficacy. Megace (megestrol acetate) has been used in women with breast cancer for the treatment of hot flashes. Some women may turn to "natural remedies," such as herbs and other plant substances. Black Cohosh, an herb with possible estrogen-like effects, may be effective in reducing hot flashes. Many of these "natural remedies" have potent estrogenic and progestogenic actions. Although they may provide relief from symptoms, however, they have not yet been studied in controlled, prospective trials; the risk-benefit equation is not defined nearly as well as it is for the standard medical regimen of progestin/estrogen therapy.

MANAGEMENT OF THE PERIMENOPAUSAL WOMAN

Some perimenopausal women begin to experience vasomotor symptoms while they are still menstruating regularly. Low-dose estrogen therapy, such as Premarin 0.3 mg daily or Vivelle 0.0375 mg patch, may be helpful. Alternatively, the perimenopausal woman may experience periods of estradiol excess as the failing ovary temporarily responds to the elevated level of stimulating gonadotropins with estrogen-production surges. Periodic monitoring of the endometrium is mandatory for any woman exposed to unopposed estrogen, either endogenously from chronic anovulation or exogenously from ERT.

Some perimenopausal women who produce adequate estrogen (from ovarian and adrenal production) may have progesterone deficiency from a defective corpus luteum. This may be manifested by mood changes and menstrual disturbances, particularly heavy bleeding. The use of natural progesterone or synthetic progestins can regulate menstrual flow. Natural progesterone is not commercially available from a pharmaceutical company but can be compounded to oral formulations by some compounding pharmacists.

Low-dose oral contraceptives (30–35 mcg of ethinyl estradiol) have minimal impact on carbohydrate metabolism and appear to have no effect on the long-term development of diabetes. Large epidemiologic studies have shown no increased risk of diabetes among women using oral contraceptives even for a long period of time. There does not seem to be any increased risk of breast cancer with long-term oral contraceptive use. All oral contraceptives suppress androgen production both from the ovaries and in part from the adrenal glands. This suppression probably outweighs the androgenic properties of any progestational compound contained in oral contraceptives.

CONTRACEPTION

Oral Contraceptives

A nonsmoking, healthy, perimenopausal woman up to the age of 50 can continue on oral contraceptives. Oral contraceptives will suppress vasomotor menopausal symptoms, provide menstrual-cycle regularity, and may have a protective effect on bone density. Thus, the low-dose oral contraceptive pills are a good therapeutic option for the symptomatic perimenopausal woman with oligomenorrhea because they provide cycle control, birth control, and vasomotor symptom control. The newer low-dose oral contraceptives are four-to-five times the amount of estrogen needed for postmenopausal replacement purposes; therefore, changing to PERT is recommended when the woman becomes menopausal.

Very-low-dose oral contraceptives containing 20 mcg of ethynodiol estradiol should preserve bone-marrow density, alleviate dysmenorrhea, and reduce iron deficiency anemia; however, they are not as likely to prevent ovarian cyst formation. The strength of the inhibition of the formation of ovarian cysts is attenuated with the newer low-dose pills.

Oral contraceptives raise sex-hormone-binding globulin levels to varying degrees; however, they reduce absolute free testosterone values and hence the propensity to acne. Oral contraceptives exert a significant effect on androgen secretion via the suppression of ovarian steroidogenesis. Suppressing ovarian and some adrenal androgen production has a substantial effect on preventing acne.

Cardiovascular complications in women using oral contraceptives are not atherogenic in origin. The latest data from the Nurses Health Study indicate that there is no increased risk for coronary heart disease, stroke, or other heart disease among former oral contraceptive users. The concern about cardiovascular complications in oral contraceptive users is primarily in older women over age 35 who continue to smoke while using the birth control pill; they are at increased risk for thrombotic coronary disease.

Women at low cardiovascular risk—that is, nonsmoking, normotensive women with relatively normal cholesterol values—can be safely continued on low-dose oral contraceptives past the age of 35. In addition to providing contraceptive efficacy, noncontraceptive health benefits of the pill include:

- A decreased risk of ovarian cancer (the most important benefit) and endometrial cancer
- Menstrual cycle regularity
- A reduced incidence of vasomotor hot flashes
- Stabilization of bone-mineral density
- A decrease in dysmenorrhea
- A decrease in iron deficiency anemia due to lighter menses

Other benefits of the oral contraceptive pill include:

- A reduced risk of benign breast disease
- Fewer uterine fibroids
- A decreased incidence in salpingitis/pelvic inflammatory disease
- A probable decrease in the incidence of endometriosis
- A possible reduction in the incidence of rheumatoid arthritis

Progestins, especially in higher doses, can cause some undesirable changes in glucose tolerance and serum lipid values. As a consequence, there is interest in designing new progestins with less androgenic metabolic effects. Desogestrel is a newer progestin synthesized from a precursor extracted from Mexican yams that appears to have fewer androgenic-related adverse effects. Desogen and Ortho-Cept contain this newer progestin. Ortho-Cyclen is a newer contraceptive containing norgestimate that is also considered a less androgenic progestin.

Recently, concern has risen about a possible increased risk of thromboembolism with the newer progestins of desogestrel and gestodene (the latter available only in Europe). This concern about a possible risk of venous thrombosis is based on three case-controlled studies that indicate an increased risk in thromboembolism when contraceptives containing desogestrel or gestodene were compared to products with other progestins (such as the older norethindrone and levonorgestrel). It is probably too premature to conclude that the newer oral contraceptives have a different risk for venothrombosis. It has been conventional wisdom that venous thrombosis is a synthetic estrogen dose-related complication and not a progestin effect; however, women at risk for venous thromboembolism (including those with obesity, varicose veins, and a history of thrombosis from any cause) should avoid oral contraceptives containing desogestrel or gestodene.

One oral contraceptive has been recently approved for the treatment of acne vulgaris. The FDA approved the triphasic oral contraceptive, orthotricyclen, containing 35 mcg of ethinyl estradiol and norgestimate.

DepoProvera

DepoProvera, a sterile medroxyprogesterone acetate suspension available as an injectable contraceptive, inhibits the secretions of gonadotropins. This in turn prevents follicular maturation and ovulation, resulting in endometrial atrophy. The contraceptive action of DepoProvera is effective for 14 weeks. Current recommendation is to give an intramuscular injection of DepoProvera 150 mg every 3 months. Women with medical contraindications to synthetic estrogen progestin oral contraceptives can use DepoProvera.

Medical conditions that make use of DepoProvera more desirable over oral contraceptives include:

- The postpartum state in lactating mothers
- Hypertension
- Renal disease
- Hepatic disease
- Vascular disease
- Prior thromboembolism
- Valvular heart disease
- Hemoglobinopathies
- Seizure disorder
- Cognitive problems that interfere with pill adherence
- Leiomyoma uteri

DepoProvera is over 99% effective, with a failure rate of only 0.3%. Contraindications to DepoProvera include:

- Pregnancy

- Undiagnosed vaginal bleeding
- Known or suspected malignancy of the breast
- Active thrombophlebitis
- Active liver disease
- Known hypersensitivity to MPA

The most common side effects of DepoProvera are menstrual irregularities, which occur in the majority of women. This menstrual irregularity has to be investigated in the perimenopausal woman, thus making DepoProvera somewhat less appealing in this age group. The incidence of amenorrhea due to endometrial atrophy increases over time and is certainly the most commonly reported side effect. DepoProvera causes a tendency toward weight gain, with an average weight gain of 2 kg in the first year of use. The use of progestins is associated with a reduced risk of endometrial cancer. Long-term use of only progestins may theoretically increase the risk for osteoporosis due to a low estrogen state.

Other contraceptive agents available to women include the female reality condom, standard spermicides (including non-oxyl 9), male condoms, and the latex diaphragm. Any of these latex products would be contraindicated in a person with a history of latex allergy. The most popular form of contraception includes permanent sterilization with tubal ligation and vasectomy, which are considered irreversible procedures. The vaginal sponge has been taken off the U.S. market. The two IUD's that remain on the market are an excellent option for a parous, monogamous woman.

CONCLUSION

Understanding the hypothalamic/pituitary/ovarian/endometrial axis allows the internist to understand, evaluate, and manage menstrual disorders, menopause, and hormonal contraception. Oral contraceptives have many noncontraceptive health benefits. HRT is safe and effective and is indicated for the majority of postmenopausal women. The 1996 United States Preventive Health Task Force recommends the counseling of all perimenopausal and postmenopausal women about the benefits and risks of HRT.

REVIEW QUESTIONS

QUESTIONS

1. The following are cardiovascular disease risk factors that are more important in women compared to men except:

    a. HDL cholesterol levels
    b. Triglycerides levels
    c. Smoking
    d. Diabetes mellitus

2. A 58-year-old woman with diabetes mellitus and type II hypercholesterolemia is status post a simple hysterectomy for fibroids. She has no menopausal symptoms, yet despite intensive hygienic measures, she still has an abnormal lipid profile (total cholesterol of 248, LDL cholesterol of 185, and an HDL cholesterol of 44). Your recommendation is to:

    a. Start a statin drug to lower the LDL cholesterol
    b. Start conjugated equine estrogens 0.625 mg to reduce the LDL cholesterol and increase the HDL cholesterol
    c. Start her on low-dose oral contraceptives
    d. Start conjugated equine estrogens 0.625 mg daily along with MPA 2.5 mg daily

3. A 70-year-old woman with natural menopause at age 52 has not been on any HRT. She has frequent urinary tract infections, bladder irritability, dyspareunia, and vaginal spotting after intercourse due to severe atrophic vaginitis. She has two first-degree relatives with breast cancer, and the patient is afraid of using any systemic HRT. You recommend:

    a. The use of over-the-counter nonhormonal vaginal lubricants
    b. The use of synthetic progestins such as Megace
    c. The use of Estring, the vaginal estrogen ring
    d. The use of the menopausal pill

4. A 45-year-old woman has menstrual cycles ranging from every 21 to every 42 days and flowing for 3 days. She is having significant vasomotor symptoms with hot flashes that are interfering with sleep. She is a smoker and wants HRT. You recommend:

    a. Starting on low-dose birth control pills such as Loestrin
    b. Starting on transdermal estradiol patch at 0.0375 dose
    c. Starting on standard HRT
    d. Avoiding all hormones until she is menopausal and has cessation of menses

Answers

1. c

    The gender-specific risk factors for women are the hormonal status of the woman; the specific lipid values of the HDL cholesterol and triglycerides; and diabetes mellitus (which confers a markedly increased risk for cardiovascular events in diabetic women as compared to diabetic men). Smoking is a modifiable cardiovascular risk that is equally important in males and females.

2. b

    The National Cholesterol Education Panel recommends considering the use of estrogen as first-line treatment for postmenopausal women with persistent hypercholesterolemia. MPA, a progestin, is not needed as the patient has had a hysterectomy. Statins will not significantly improve HDL and do not have the other benefits on the integument, bone, and genitourinary system that estrogen replacement has.

3. c

    The use of vaginal Estring, a vaginal estrogen ring, will deliver local estradiol to the genitourinary tissue without any systemic absorption. Local estradiol will treat the symptoms of genitourinary atrophy.

4. b

    The patient is perimenopausal. She is not yet menopausal and therefore would not be offered standard HRT at this time. Because she is a smoker of advanced age, she is not a candidate for oral contraceptives. In terms of hormonal therapy to control her perimenopausal symptoms of hot flashes, transdermal estradiol like Vivelle 0.0375 mg changed every 3½ days could be offered. When she has cessation of menstrual bleeding (indicating menopause) or menstrual bleeding that becomes heavier (indicating progesterone deficiency), she will need the addition of a cycled progestin such as 5 mg of MPA, as long-term unopposed estrogen is not recommended owing to the increased risk of endometrial cancer.

5. A 48-year-old women has had irregular menstrual cycles for the last year. She has been bleeding every 18 to 21 days and flowing for 10 days with heavy clots. She is not having any hot flashes. On examination, she is obese but otherwise has an unremarkable examination. She is otherwise asymptomatic and has a hematocrit of 30%. You recommend:

a. Starting on low-dose oral contraceptives
b. Starting on standard HRT regimen
c. Performing an endometrial biopsy and then a cycled progestin
d. Performing a bowel evaluation and, if negative, recommending iron supplementation

6. A 40-year-old women is status post induced menopause at age 38 with a TAH BSO for benign reasons. She is on ERT with an adequate serum beta-estradiol level at 100 pg/mL. She complains of sexual dysfunction with decreased libido and decreased ability to climax. You recommend:

a. The addition of a cycled progestin such as MPA 5 mg
b. The addition of androgen replacement with Estratest HS
c. The addition of vaginal estrogen
d. Referral to a sex therapist

7. A 65-year-old woman is status post a simple hysterectomy. She has been on oral estrogen and has elevated triglycerides at 400 mg/dL. You recommend:

a. A change to transdermal estradiol and a recheck of the triglycerides
b. Addition of a progestin
c. Addition of a statin drug
d. An increase in the oral estrogen dosage

8. A 70-year-old woman with natural menopause at age 51 is slender and physically active. Her bone density is greater than 2.5 SD below young normal. She has lost over 2 inches in height in the last 2 years. She had refused HRT because of menstrual bleeding. She has tried alendronate (Fosamax) but has been unable to tolerate the medication because of the gastrointestinal side effects. You recommend:

a. The use of sodium fluoride
b. Vaginal estrogen cream
c. Cycled HRT with Premphase
d. Continuous combined hormone replacement with PremPro

Answers

5. c

The patient is perimenopausal. She is progesterone-deficient but not estrogen-deficient. Because of her age, obesity, and irregular menses, she has an increased risk for endometrial hyperplasia or cancer and, therefore, should have an endometrial biopsy. Thyroid-function tests should be considered because hypothyroidism can cause menorrhagia. After an endometrial biopsy is done to exclude malignancy, the patient should be offered a cycled progestin, such as 10 mg of MPA for 12 days of every month, to control her menstrual bleeding, iron supplementation, and a hemoccult (as well as a history to exclude concurrent gastrointestinal (GI) bleeding as a cause for her low hematocrit).

6. b

Induced menopause with adequate estrogen replacement but persistent sexual dysfunction (usually a result of a lack of testosterone) indicates the need for androgen replacement. Currently there is no ideal method of androgen replacement in women; however, low doses of oral androgens in Estratest half strength (1.25 mg of Methyltestosterone with 0.625 mg of esterified estrogens) can be used. Baseline liver functions and a free testosterone level should be done, and the patient should have liver functions followed on oral androgen replacement.

7. a

A patient with baseline elevated triglycerides (TG) may have a worsening of TG on oral estrogens. The patient should be offered transdermal estradiol such as Vivelle 0.05, Climara 0.05, or Estraderm 0.05 with a recheck of the triglycerides along with weight loss, dietary changes, and an investigation into the possibility of diabetes or other medical conditions that can cause hypertriglyceridemia.

8. d

Continuous combined HRT has the advantage of inducing amenorrhea within 6–9 months in the majority of postmenopausal women. The patient should be counseled on adequate calcium and vitamin D supplementation. HRT is the preferred pharmacologic treatment for the prevention of osteoporosis as well as the treatment of established osteoporosis. Sodium fluoride remains investigational. Vaginal estrogen does not provide reliable systemic absorption, which is needed for the prevention/treatment of osteoporosis.

9. All of the following are reasons why oral contraceptives (OCs) are generally beneficial for acne vulgaris except that they:

a. Suppress androgen production from the ovary
b. Suppress androgen production from the adrenal gland
c. Lower the sex hormone, binding globulin levels
d. Reduce free testosterone levels

10. One of the health benefits of OCs that may be lessened when using OCs with 20 mcg of ethinyl estradiol is:

a. Alleviation of dysmenorrhea
b. Prevention of ovarian cyst formation
c. Reduction of iron deficiency anemia
d. Prevention of endometrial cancer

Answers

9. c

OCs are beneficial in the treatment of acne because they suppress ovarian androgen production and some adrenal androgen production. OCs do not lower SHBG levels, but may raise SHBG levels to varying degrees. OCs reduce absolute free testosterone levels and are, therefore, beneficial in women with androgenic problems such as acne vulgaris and/or hiruitism.

10. b

There is nearly complete ovarian suppression with the older high-dose birth control pills of 50 mcg of ethinyl estradiol. The standard 30–35 mcg of ethinyl estradiol suppresses the majority of corpus luteum cysts; however, the lowest dose ethinyl estradiol pills of 20 mcg do not inhibit ovarian cyst formation as much as the higher dose pills.

SUGGESTED READINGS

Col NF, Eckman MH, Karas RH, et al. Patient-specific decisions about hormone replacement therapy in postmenopausal women. JAMA 1997;277:1140–1147. (A decision analysis examining the effect of hormone replacement therapy on life expectancy in postmenopausal women with different risk profiles for heart disease, breast cancer, and hip fracture.)

Thacker HL. Current issues in menopausal hormone replacement therapy. CCF J Med 1996;63:344–353. (A recent review of current drug therapy hormone replacement therapy and a review of endometrial biopsy.)

U.S. Preventive Health Task Force: Guide to Clinical Preventive Services, 2nd ed. Baltimore: Williams & Wilkins, 1996: 829.

W.H.O. Scientific group on research on the menopause in the 1990s. WHO technical report series. Geneva, Switzerland, 1996:886. (The latest WHO Scientific Group on research on menopause which summarizes current knowledge and recommendations regarding menopause and its management.)

3

Medical Complications of Pregnancy

Elliot H. Philipson

The medical complications of pregnancy are complex and extensive. This chapter does not address all the medical complications of pregnancy but reviews and summarizes some of the major medical diseases and their impact in obstetrics.

Maternal mortality is the number of maternal deaths per 100,000 live births, although most other obstetrical statistics use 1,000 live births as a denominator. In the United States, maternal mortality is approximately 7.8 per 100,000 live births. Although the difference in rates has decreased in recent decades, maternal mortality remains higher in black women than in white women. The most common causes of maternal mortality in the United States are embolism, hypertension, and infection. In some undeveloped countries, infection and hemorrhage are the most common causes of maternal mortality.

Perinatal mortality is the number of stillbirths plus neonatal deaths per 1,000 live births. Stillbirth is defined as the delivery of a nonliving fetus after 20 weeks of gestation. A neonatal death is one that occurs between birth and the 28th day of life. Neonatal death is sometimes also reported as that occurring within the first 7 days of life. In the United States, perinatal mortality has also dropped significantly over the last several decades and is now about 7.3 per 1,000.

THROMBOEMBOLISM

Pregnancy is a hypercoagulable state. Deep venous thrombosis and pulmonary embolism fortunately do not occur commonly in pregnancy, but when they do occur, maternal mortality is high. Deep venous thrombosis often can be difficult to diagnose because the large pregnant uterus compresses the major vessels of the extremities. Impedance plethysmography and ultrasound can be helpful. Chest x rays, ventilation-perfusion lung scans, and pulmonary angiography are sometimes necessary to confirm the diagnosis of pulmonary embolism. With a high index of suspicion, it may be necessary to start heparin therapy before these tests are obtained to make a definitive diagnosis. The oral anticoagulant Coumadin (warfarin) is contraindicated in pregnancy. A warfarin embryopathy has been described, the features of which include mental deficiencies, seizures, mild facial hypoplasia, stippling in uncalcified epiphyseal regions, and growth restriction. However, the risks of Coumadin use in pregnancy have recently been challenged, although the drug remains contraindicated in pregnancy. Heparin or low-molecular-weight heparin can be used if anticoagulation is necessary.

ASTHMA

Asthma, a chronic medical condition, generally follows the "rule of thirds:" a third of the time it gets better during pregnancy, a third of the time it gets worse, and a third of the time it is unchanged. Asthma complicates pregnancy by causing frequent emergency room visits and hospitalizations. The two major complications associated with asthma are preterm labor and delivery and intrauterine growth restriction (IUGR). Treatment is based on the same pathophysiologic principles as in nonpregnant patients, using early intervention and pharmacotherapy to reduce the severity of the attacks. Well-controlled and treated asthma can allow a normal pregnancy to proceed with little increased risk. The asthma medications required to achieve control in pregnant patients are the same as in nonpregnant patients. Although good studies of asthma medications in human pregnancy are limited, these medications do not appear to be detrimental in pregnancy. The risks of the medications used for asthma in pregnancy are probably less than the risks of a pregnant woman not maintaining normal oxygenation and air exchange.

CARDIAC DISEASE

For cardiac disease that complicates pregnancy, the New York Heart Association Classification system has been widely used for prognosis. Class I patients are asymptomatic; Class II patients have symptoms with normal activity; Class III patients have symptoms at rest; and Class IV patients are the more-severe cases and therefore have the highest risks. More recently, cardiac disease has been classified by the risk of maternal death. Conditions associated with a maternal mortality lower than 1% are atrial septal defect (ASD), ventricular septal defect (VSD), patent ductus arteriosis (PDA), mild mitral stenosis, and corrected tetralogy of Fallot. A maternal mortality of 5–15% has been found with mitral stenosis, aortic stenosis, uncorrected tetralogy of Fallot, previous myocardial infarction, and Marfan's syndrome with a normal aorta. The highest risk group of patients, with a 25–55% mortality, have primary or pulmonary hypertension, coarctation of the aorta, or Marfan's syndrome within aortic root dilation. An important contraindication to pregnancy is any condition associated with pulmonary hypertension.

Various cardiac problems involve different specific considerations. One tenet of the management of cardiac disease in pregnancy is maintaining cardiac output. Mitral stenosis can result in an obstruction to left ventricular diastolic filling. With a drop in diastolic filling, the cardiac output also may drop. Therefore, hydration and blood pressure control can be critical. For example, in a patient with severe mitral stenosis, it is critical that fluids be used to maintain the cardiac output, but too much fluid may result in pulmonary edema. Pulmonary artery catheter monitoring can be used to optimize the cardiac output. A pulmonary capillary wedge pressure between 12 and 14 mmHg would allow maintenance of cardiac output. With an increase in maternal pulse, medication may be necessary.

Patients at risk for subacute bacterial endocarditis should receive appropriate antibiotics before delivery in accordance with American Heart Association guidelines.

The mode of delivery depends on obstetric indications, and vaginal births are not contraindicated in most cases. Epidural anesthesia also is not contraindicated. The second stage of labor, the time from complete cervical dilatation to delivery, can be shortened with the use of forceps or vacuum.

Aortic stenosis, most commonly rheumatic in origin, is a lesion in which the cardiac output is fairly well maintained. When severe, pulmonary artery catheter monitoring may be necessary. Aortic stenosis leading to ischemic heart disease, myocardial infarction, or death is rare.

Atrial septal defect, a more common condition, does not usually complicate the antenatal or intrapartum period.

Atrial fibrillation, although not common, can be treated with either digoxin or heparin in a manner similar to that used with nonpregnant patients.

Patients with prosthetic valves may need special attention. If a patient has a mechanical valve, anticoagulation is necessary. Traditionally, heparin has been recommended, par-

ticularly in the first and third trimesters of pregnancy. As stated previously, Coumadin or warfarin has been associated with embryopathy and therefore is not recommended for use. Some older literature has recommended its use after embryogenesis (in the second trimester). Coumadin could be discontinued in the third trimester, when heparin would be reinitiated. In this way, heparin can be reversed with Protamine to avoid excessive bleeding at delivery. More recently, low-molecular-weight heparin has been used during pregnancy without problems. It is well tolerated during pregnancy, but currently is quite expensive. If a patient has a tissue valve, anticoagulation is not necessary.

Eisenmenger syndrome is an unusual syndrome characterized by pulmonary hypertension. Any condition with pulmonary hypertension markedly increases maternal mortality and is generally a contraindication to pregnancy.

Epstein's anomaly is characterized by a downward displacement of the tricuspid valve, leading to tricuspid regurgitation and an enlarged right atrium. It is important because it has been associated with the use of lithium.

Marfan's syndrome, an autosomal dominant condition, will affect 50% of the offspring. Flo Heyman, a U.S. athlete with Marfan's syndrome, suffered a ruptured aortic aneurysm with sudden death several years ago. The cardiovascular system is affected as well as the ophthalmologic and skeletal systems. In pregnancy, an aortic root measuring greater than 4 cm has been associated with a worse prognosis. The risk of aortic rupture is high.

Cardiomyopathies generally occur in the third trimester of pregnancy or during the intrapartum period. Postpartum cardiomyopathy can occur up to 6 months postpartum. Signs and symptoms are characteristic of ventricular failure, with orthopnea, dyspnea, fatigue, and edema occurring. The diagnosis needs to be made in the absence of hypertension or any obvious signs of infection, valvular disease, or metabolic process. Some believe that these cardiomyopathies may be related to viral infections. Maternal mortality is high in these patients, and early, aggressive therapy is indicated. Finally, there is a high risk of recurrence if the patient has had a previous cardiomyopathy.

DIABETES MELLITUS

All patients should be screened for diabetes mellitus in pregnancy. Recently, some have argued against testing all patients and have advocated screening only for those with specific risk factors. Pregnancy is a diabetogenic state, however. The 1-hour glucose test is a screening test; the 3-hour 100-g glucose tolerance test is the definitive test. If the oral glucose tolerance test result was abnormal, a nutritional consult and meal plan should be started. The 1-hour glucose test should not be repeated unless there was something unusual about the test; e.g., the patient was chewing gum or candy or taking a medication that may alter the glucose level. Approximately 2–3% of patients will have an abnormal glucose tolerance test result as determined by any two or more of the glucose values being met or exceeded. These patients are gestationally diabetic and require a meal plan and dietary consultation. Euglycemia is the goal. If fingerstick glucose testing of fasting and postprandial glucose levels indicates hyperglycemia, insulin therapy becomes necessary. Insulin therapy generally would not be started based on the results of the 1-hour test.

There is a correlation between mean maternal glucose levels and infant mortality. As the mean glucose level decreases, infant mortality decreases. Therefore, treatment should attempt to achieve euglycemia, which may be lower than traditionally taught. A normal fasting glucose level would be less than 100 mg/dL, and a normal postprandial glucose level would be less than 120 mg/dL. The normal fasting glucose level in nonpregnant women is 78–80 mg/dL. In early pregnancy, there is a marked drop in the fasting glucose level that continues to decrease until the third trimester of pregnancy, when a normal fasting glucose is 65–70 mg/dL. This phenomenon in pregnancy is referred to as "accelerated starvation." The postprandial glucose response is altered in pregnancy, with a higher glucose response to the same meal than occurs in nonpregnant women. In contrast to women with gestational diabetes, insulin-dependent diabetic women have an increased risk for offspring with congenital anomalies. This risk has been associated with insulin-dependent diabetes and not with gestational diabetes.

The Pederson hypothesis relates to the maternal hyperglycemia that leads to fetal hyperglycemia. Fetal hyperglycemia results in fetal hyperinsulinemia, because the maternal insulin does not cross the placenta. The fetus makes its own insulin, with high insulin levels at delivery resulting in neonatal hypoglycemia. Figure 3.1 shows a newborn from a mother with undetected gestational diabetes. This baby weighed 11.5 pounds. A large size does not necessarily indicate health, however, as this baby's face is bruised, and the baby is intubated and on a respirator. Excessive birth weight can result in birth

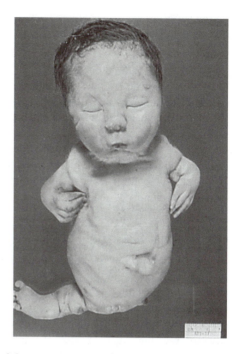

Figure 3.2.   A newborn with caudal regression syndrome, a congenital anomaly considered pathognomonic for diabetes mellitus.

trauma. The management plan consists of a meal plan and added insulin as needed. Usually, regular insulin with long-acting insulins are used to maintain euglycemia. Hemoglobin A1C can be helpful for preconceptional counseling. In patients with insulin-dependent diabetes, a congenital anomaly is less likely if the maternal glucose is well controlled in the periconceptional period. Figure 3.2 shows a newborn with caudal regression syndrome, often thought of as a congenital anomaly that is pathognomonic for diabetes mellitus. Generally speaking, the caudal regression syndrome is characterized by the absence of the lower portion of the spine and sacrum.

PREGNANCY-INDUCED HYPERTENSION

Pregnancy-induced hypertension is the correct term for eclampsia or pre-eclampsia. It encompasses both conditions plus chronic hypertension, chronic hypertension with superimposed pregnancy-induced hypertension, transient hypertension during pregnancy, and the HELP (hemolysis-elevated liver enzymes, low platelet) syndrome. The cause of pregnancy-induced hypertension is unknown. Often there is a strong family history of hypertension. The underlying pathophysiologic process in pregnancy-induced hypertension is vasoconstriction and vasospasm. There is an increase in peripheral vascular resistance, sensitivity to angiotensin, and decreased uterine placental blood flow. Vasospasm and vasoconstriction can also affect other organs, including the kidney, liver, and central nervous system. Endothelial damage, hemolytic anemia, platelet consumption, thrombocytopenia, red blood cell destruction, congestion, and renal or

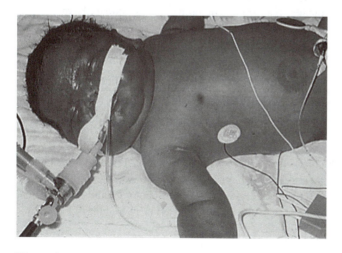

Figure 3.1.   The newborn of a mother with undetected gestational diabetes.

glomerular damage can all become key features of this condition. Magnesium sulfate is used to stabilize the mother and prevent seizures. Vaginal delivery is not contraindicated, but a cesarean section may be required if labor cannot be achieved or if the patient's condition deteriorates. In obstetrics, the real treatment of pregnancy-induced hypertension does not occur until after the placenta is delivered. The HELP syndrome can be thought of as a variant of pre-eclampsia or pregnancy-induced hypertension. Often, the diagnosis is made late in a patient with mild or unrecognized symptoms when thrombocytopenia is incidentally found. These patients should be managed aggressively, hospitalized, and delivered.

CHRONIC HYPERTENSION

Chronic hypertension with an increased risk of abruptio placenta, prematurity, and intrauterine growth restriction (IUGR) may also require hospitalization or early delivery. Methyldopa is the drug of choice for most obstetricians because this drug has been used for many years with good experience. Diuretics are generally not recommended, because the intracellular blood volume may be additionally depleted. If the patient was on diuretics before her pregnancy, the diuretic may be continued. The use of the angiotensin-converting enzyme inhibitors is contraindicated in pregnancy.

SYSTEMIC LUPUS ERYTHEMATOSUS

Systemic lupus erythematosus (SLE) is associated with an increased risk of pregnancy loss, spontaneous miscarriage, preterm delivery, IUGR, and fetal demise late in pregnancy. The prognosis for patients with SLE appears to depend on the degree of activity of the condition at the time of conception. If a pregnant patient presents with SLE and the SLE is in remission, the prognosis is generally good. If the SSA or RO antibodies are present, there is a greater risk of congenital heart block in the fetus. Frequent office visits or hospitalization may be necessary with fetal monitoring in the second or third trimester of pregnancy. A patient who has an acute flare-up or active disease is at greater risk for the problems listed above.

"Lupus anticoagulant" is a common term in the obstetric literature. It is a misnomer and is not related to lupus. It is an antibody to the phospholipid and is associated with recurrent, spontaneous miscarriage and thrombosis. The therapy consists of aspirin with heparin if the levels are very elevated. Steroid therapy may not be helpful.

TERATOGENS

A teratogen is any agent or factor that can produce a permanent alteration in the form or function of the offspring following exposure. The most crucial period is the embryonic period, from the second to the eighth week of pregnancy, when an early insult or event in the pregnancy may result in the "all or none phenomenon." The fetus and pregnancy may be very abnormal, or nothing at all may happen. A few of the most commonly known teratogens are as follows, along with some of the associated conditions:

- Alcohol, with mid-facial defects, IUGR, and central nervous system abnormalities
- Coumadin, with the warfarin embryopathy
- Anticonvulsants, with the fetal hydantoin syndrome (this syndrome may be associated with other antiepileptics, and not necessarily phenytoin)
- Methimazole, with hypothyroid and aplasia cutis
- Isoretinoids, with facial, central nervous system, and cardiac defects
- Tetracycline, with staining and bone growth
- Thalidomide, with limb defects

Medication risk factors include the categories A, B, C, D, and X. These categories have been assigned to all drugs by most manufacturers. Some authorities have assigned categories different from the manufacturer's. Generally speaking, A, B, and C categories are for medications that are used frequently in pregnancy with little risk. Category A includes drugs with well-controlled studies performed in human pregnancy without demonstrating any risk to the fetus. Few drugs, unfortunately, fall into Category A. Category B is for drugs for which animal reproduction studies have not demonstrated a fetal risk but for which there are really no controlled studies. Category C is for drugs that should be given if the potential benefit justifies the potential risk to the fetus. Early studies may have revealed an adverse effect, but there are no controlled studies in human pregnancy. There may have been some studies in animals, or there are no available studies. With Category D drugs, there is positive evidence of fetal risk in human pregnancy, but the benefits for use in pregnancy may be acceptable even though there is a risk. Category X indicates that animal or human being studies have demonstrated a definite fetal risk, and these medications should be avoided in pregnancy.

HIV IN PREGNANCY

The best study of HIV in pregnancy justifies the use of AZT in pregnancy. The risk of perinatal transmission of HIV can be markedly reduced with the use of AZT. Newer medications may also reduce the risk of perinatal transmission. The American College of Obstetrics and Gynecology publishes technical bulletins helpful for managing HIV in pregnancy.

REVIEW EXERCISES

QUESTIONS

1. A 28-year-old gravida 3, para 2 was tested for diabetes in this pregnancy at 26 weeks' gestation. Her glucose after a 1-hour 50-g glucose test was 150 mg/dL. The next step should be:

    a. Insulin therapy
    b. To perform a 3-hour glucose tolerance test
    c. To obtain a nutrition consult and start a diet
    d. To repeat the 1-hour glucose test
    e. To call an endocrinologist

2. A 16-year-old female presents to the emergency room with seizures. A friend with her states that she is almost due but that she has never been examined by a doctor. On cursory examination, her abdomen is enlarged and soft with no vaginal bleeding. The most likely diagnosis is:

    a. Epilepsy
    b. Hypertensive crisis
    c. Renal failure
    d. Eclampsia
    e. Cocaine abuse

3. The same patient is now postictal, and her blood pressure is 150/90, her pulse is 90, and her respirations are 24 per minute. Her abdomen measures 40 cm in height, and the fetal heart rate is found to be 150 beats per minute. The most appropriate next step would be to:

    a. Perform an emergency cesarean section
    b. Start phenytoin
    c. Start magnesium sulfate
    d. Start antihypertensive therapy
    e. Call the obstetrician to come in from home

Answers

1. b

    The 3-hour glucose tolerance test is the definitive test. Insulin therapy would not normally be started based on the results of the 1-hour test. The 1-hour test should not be repeated unless there was something unusual about the circumstances.

2. d

    There might be some controversy about the correct answer to this question, but in the context of obstetrics, the correct answer is eclampsia, which is the most likely diagnosis in this setting. When a young patient who is pregnant for the first time and who has had little or no prenatal care presents with the described characteristics, the diagnosis should be considered eclampsia until proven otherwise.

3. c

    This situation might also raise some controversy, but not among obstetricians. This patient has stable vital signs, and the fetal heart rate is normal (normal is 120–160 beats per minute). An emergency cesarean section is not indicated; general anesthesia and the possibility of aspiration should be considered. In the absence of fetal distress, this stable patient should be treated with magnesium sulfate to prevent additional seizures. Phenytoin therapy, Valium, or other antiepileptic medications may be suggested by some, but most obstetricians in North America use magnesium sulfate to prevent seizure disorder. It is usually given as a 2–4-g intravenous bolus followed by a continuous 1-, 2-, or 3-g/hour intravenous infusion. Antihypertensive therapy can be considered, but any antihypertensive therapy may also lower the blood pressure in the uteroplacental bed, resulting in hypoperfusion and fetal distress.

SUGGESTED READINGS

American College of Obstetricians and Gynecologists Educational Bulletins

1. Cardiac Disease in Pregnancy, 168 (June 1992)
2. Hepatitis in Pregnancy, 174 (November 1992)
3. Thyroid Disease in Pregnancy, 181 (June 1993)
4. Diabetes and Pregnancy, 200 (December 1994)
5. Hypertension in Pregnancy, 219 (January 1996)
6. Hemoglobinopathies in Pregnancy, 220 (February 1996)
7. Pulmonary Disease in Pregnancy, 224 (June 1996)
8. Seizure Disorders in Pregnancy, 231 (December 1996)
9. Human Immunodeficiency Virus Infections in Pregnancy, 232 (January 1997)
10. Thromboembolism in Pregnancy, 234 (March 1997)
11. Teratology, 236 (April 1997)
12. Antiphospholipid Syndrome, 244 (February 1998)

Ashmead GG, Reed GB, eds. Essentials of Maternal-Fetal Medicine. New York: Chapman & Hall, 1997.

Briggs GG, Freeman RK, Yaffe SJ, eds. Drugs in Pregnancy and Lactation. Baltimore, Williams & Wilkins, 1994.

Creasy RK, Resnik R. Maternal-Fetal Medicine Principles and Practice, 3rd ed. Philadelphia: W.B. Saunders, 1994.

Cunningham FG, MacDonald PC, Grant NF, et al, eds. Williams Obstetrics, 20th ed. Stamford, CT: Appleton & Lange, 1997.

Biostatistics in Clinical Medicine: Diagnostic Tests

Gerald J. Beck

When determining the presence of disease in a patient, physicians use the results of diagnostic tests (e.g., laboratory, radiologic, and/or physical symptoms) to modify their pretest impressions on the likelihood of the presence of the disease. Therefore, it is important that clinicians understand how diagnostic tests are useful in reaching clinical decisions and how the accuracy of diagnostic tests can impact the conclusions.

This chapter defines and illustrates the concepts of sensitivity, specificity, and predictive value of diagnostic tests. (For a good general reference to the interpretation and use of diagnostic tests, see Griner et al. [3].)

QUANTIFYING DIAGNOSTIC TESTS

Diagnostic tests are used as decision-making tools because the test results are used to predict whether a disease is present or absent. The relationship between a dichotomous test result (i.e., positive or negative) and the true diagnosis of disease appears in Figure 4.1. As illustrated, tests may provide the correct answer (true positive [A] or true negative [D]) or the wrong conclusion (false positive [B] or false negative [C]).

SENSITIVITY AND SPECIFICITY OF DIAGNOSTIC TESTS

To quantify the accuracy of a test used in making a decision, several diagnostic summary values can be calculated. Figure 4.2 presents hypothetical data on the relationship of a screening test using prostate-specific antigen (PSA) in diagnosing prostate cancer. In the group of 400 men, all of whom were given both the PSA test and the definitive (i.e., gold standard test) biopsy, 160 men were correctly identified as having prostate cancer and 120 were correctly identified as not having prostate cancer. However, there were 120 men who were misdiagnosed as either false positives

(80) or false negatives (40). The accuracy of the PSA test can be summarized by the following:

*   The proportion of truly diseased patients who test positive (called the sensitivity of the test) = 160/200 = 0.80 (80%)
*   The proportion of truly nondiseased patients who test negative (called the specificity of the test) = 120/200 = 0.60 (60%)

Accordingly, the false positive rate would be 80/200 or 40% (100% minus the specificity) and the false negative rate would be 40/200 or 20% (100% minus the sensitivity) .

In general, the sensitivity and specificity of a diagnostic test can be determined when the test result and the true disease status are known for a group of patients. As shown in Figure 4.1, cells A, B, C, and D represent the frequencies of various combinations of test and disease status. The sensitivity of the diagnostic test is A/(A + C), and the specificity is B/(B + D).

CUT POINT OF DIAGNOSTIC TESTS

Many diagnostic tests are based on a continuous measurement. The accuracy of these tests is specific to the "cut point" value of the test that distinguishes between a positive and negative test. As shown in Figure 4.3, the choice of the cut point affects the sensitivity and specificity and in turn the false-positive and false-negative rates. The two curves represent the frequency distribution of the test value in the "disease absent" and "disease present" populations. (These curves usually overlap because no test perfectly discriminates between the "disease absent" and "disease present" groups.) The different areas under the curves give the proportions of persons that are correctly or incorrectly classified in the "disease absent" and "disease present" groups.

Figure 4.1. The relationship between a dichotomous diagnostic test result and the occurrence of
disease.

True Disease Status

	Disease Present	Disease Absent	Total
Positive	True Positive (A)	False Positive (B)	A+B
Negative	False Negative (C)	True Negative (D)	C+D
Total	A+C	B+D	

Test Result

Figure 4.2. The relationship between the PSA test
and the occurrence of prostate cancer (hypothetical
data)

True Disease Status

PSA Test	Prostate Cancer	No Prostate Cancer	Total
Positive (≥ 4 mg/L)	160	80	240
Negative (< 4 mg/L)	40	120	160
Total	200	200	400

Moving the cut point affects all areas under the curves. For example, moving the cut point to the left (lower test value) increases the sensitivity but decreases the specificity (assuming that a larger test value indicates the presence of disease). Hence, changing the cut point cannot simultaneously increase both the sensitivity and specificity or simultaneously decrease the false-positive and false-negative rates.

The choice of an optimal cut point—a discussion of which is beyond the scope of this chapter—can be determined using receiver operating characteristic (ROC) curves (4). The cut point choice also depends on the purpose of the diagnostic test. For example, when screening donated blood for HIV, one should choose a cut point that would reduce the false-negative rate as much as possible. However, if one uses the HIV blood test to identify infected individuals, one should reduce the false-positive rate as much as possible in order to avoid falsely alarming individuals about the presence of disease. In practice, to confirm the diagnosis, tests are often repeated or other types of tests are performed.

PREDICTIVE VALUES OF DIAGNOSTIC TESTS

The probability of actually having a disease when the test result is positive is of considerable interest to physicians and patients. As shown in the PSA example in Figure 4.2, of the 240 men with a positive test, 160 have prostate cancer. That is, the test gave the correct diagnosis 0.667 or 66.7% of the time (the number of times the test was positive and the disease was present out of the total number of positive tests). This quantity, called the positive predictive value, is calculated by A/(A + B) using the general frequencies in Figure 4.1.

Similarly, the negative predictive value is the proportion of patients who have a negative test and actually have no disease out of the total number with a negative test. In the example, this is 120/160 = 0.75 or 75%, or, in general, D/(C + D). In practice, the clinician, who only knows the result of the diagnostic test, must try to determine the true disease status of the patient without having knowledge of the frequencies in Table 4.1. A technique, described below, is available to accomplish this.

The pretest probability of disease in a given individual is based upon the physician's personal experience with patients who have characteristics similar to the patient being diagnosed and/or on the prevalence of the disease in such patients as given in the published literature. The key point is that the pretest probability is modified to the posttest probability (the positive predictive value) by incorporating the information on the accuracy of the test. In the PSA example, the pretest probability of disease was 0.50 because 200 of the 400 men represented in Figure 4.2 had prostate cancer, but this is not likely in practice. Therefore, a general way of calculating the positive and negative predictive values is needed.

In general, the positive and negative predictive values are calculated using the two equations below (derived from Bayes' Theorem):

Positive predictive value

$$= \frac{(Prevalence)(Sensitivity)}{(Prevalence)(Sensitivity) + (1 - Prevalence)(1 - Specificity)}$$

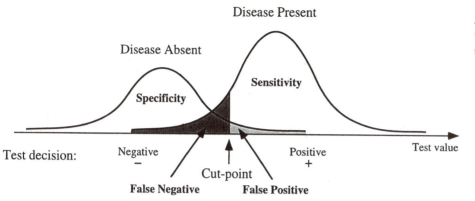

Figure 4.3. Diagnostic test terms when there is a continuous outcome for the test.

Table 4.1. The Influence of the Prevalence of Disease on the Positive and Negative Predictive Probabilities (Hypothetical Data, Assuming 80% Sensitivity and 60% Specificity)

Prevalence	Positive Predictive Value	Negative Predictive Value
0.10	0.182	0.964
0.30	0.462	0.875
0.50	0.667	0.750
0.70	0.926	0.562
0.90	0.947	0.250

Negative predictive value

$$= \frac{(1 - Prevalence)(Specificity)}{(1 - Prevalence)(Specificity) + (Prevalence)(1 - Sensitivity)}$$

In the PSA example, the sensitivity is 0.80, the specificity is 0.60, and the prevalence (as assumed above) is 0.5. Accordingly,

Positive predictive value =

(0.5)(0.80)/[(0.5)(0.80) + [(1 − 0.5)(1 − 0.60)] = 0.667

Note that this answer is the same (160/240) as previously determined from Figure 4.2. Likewise:

Negative predictive value =

(1 − 0.5)(0.60)/[(1 − .05)(0.60) + (0.5)(1 − 0.80)] = 0.75

Again, this answer matches the answer (120/160) from Figure 4.2.

Suppose now that the prevalence (pretest probability) is 0.1 instead of 0.5. Applying the above equations would give a positive predictive value of 0.182 and a negative predictive value of 0.964, quite a bit different from the values when the prevalence was 0.5 (Table 4.1). Table 4.1 shows that the positive and negative predictive values are dependent upon the prevalence of the disease and that, as the prevalence in-

creases, the positive predictive value increases while the negative predictive value decreases. This will occur even if the diagnostic test has very high sensitivity and specificity.

The equations above demonstrate that the positive predictive value can be increased by increasing the specificity of the test, and the negative predictive value can be increased by increasing the sensitivity of the test.

Clinicians must understand these interrelationships when interpreting diagnostic tests or beginning a screening program. For example, if the general population with low prevalence of HIV infection is screened for HIV, the positive predictive value may be very low in spite of a very high sensitivity and specificity of the test, a situation that could lead to many more false-positive results than the number of true cases identified (5).

Also, it is important to understand how diagnostic test results can modify pretest probability (prevalence) values into posttest probabilities. That is, a positive test will give a posttest probability (the positive predictive value) larger than the pretest probability, whereas a negative test will give a posttest probability (equal to 1 minus the negative predictive probability) smaller than the pretest probability. For example, as Table 4.1 shows, with a pretest probability of disease equal to 0.1, if the diagnostic test is positive, the posttest probability of disease is increased to 0.182 while if the test is negative, the probability of disease is decreased to 1 − 0.964, or 0.036.

NOMOGRAM OF FAGAN

Instead of using the equations based on Bayes' theorem for determining the positive and negative predictive probabilities from the sensitivity, specificity, and prevalence of the disease (in a group similar to the individual being treated), clinicians can use the simple nomogram of Fagan (2) to go from the pretest to the posttest probability (Fig. 4.4). This nomogram uses the ratio of the sensitivity and the false positive rate (or 1 − specificity) as a way of incorporating both the sensitivity and specificity. Also called the likelihood ratio, it is the ratio of obtaining a positive test result given the disease is present versus given when the disease is absent.

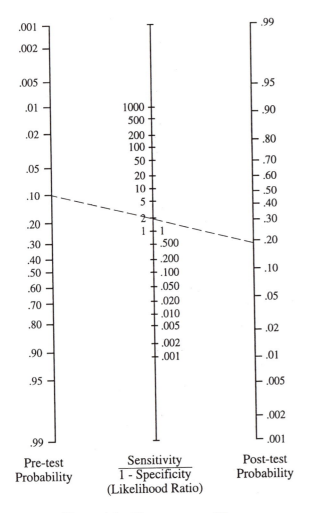

Figure 4.4.   The nomogram of Fagan.

As in the PSA example, if the sensitivity is 80% and the specificity is 60%:

The likelihood ratio = 0.80/(1 − 0.60) = 2.0

If the pretest probability is 0.10, the posttest probability can be obtained using the nomogram in Figure 4.4 by drawing a straight line between the pretest value and the likelihood ratio and extending it to the posttest probability scale to give a value (in this example, about 0.18, close to the exact value of 0.182 previously calculated). As expected, selecting other pretest probabilities will yield different posttest probabilities, and changing the sensitivity and/or specificity of the test will give different results. If the likelihood ratio is above (below) one, the posttest probability will be larger (smaller) than the pretest probability.

CONCLUSION

Understanding the interpretation of diagnostic tests is important in the practice of medicine. Clinicians should know the concepts of sensitivity, specificity, and positive and negative predictive value, their relationships, and the influence of the setting in which the test is applied (that is, the prevalence, or pretest probability, of the disease).

For a more in-depth understanding of this topic, physicians should study other biases that can occur when using diagnostic tests that have not been covered (1). These biases include referral or verification bias, the use of an imperfect gold standard, how to handle uninterpretable results, and the influence of the case-mix or spectrum of the patients to which the test is being applied.

REVIEW EXERCISE

Evaluate "X-ometry," a new test for Disease X, after testing 100 patients in your office. Given:

- the population prevalence of disease X is 20%—that is, 20% of patients truly have Disease X.

- 40 of 100 patients tested positive for disease X
- the specificity of X-ometry equals 60%

What is the positive predictive value of the X-ometry test?

Answer

Step 1: With a population prevalence of disease X of 20%, 20 of 100 patients are expected to have Disease X (i.e., cells A + C in Figure 4.1 equal 20) (Fig. 4.5).

Step 2: The test results show that 40 of the 100 patients tested have a positive test, thus cells A + B equal 40 (Fig. 4.6). Other marginal values can be determined by subtracting the known values from 100, the total number of patients examined in this example.

Step 3: With a test specificity of 60%, 60% of the 80 patients without Disease X in this example have a negative X-ometry test (Fig. 4.7). Cell D is thus 60% of 80, or 48. The contents of the other cells in this table can then be specified.

Once all the cells are filled in, it is possible to calculate the value of the positive predictive value:

Positive   predictive   value $= A/(A+B) = 8/(8+32) = 8/40 = 20\%$

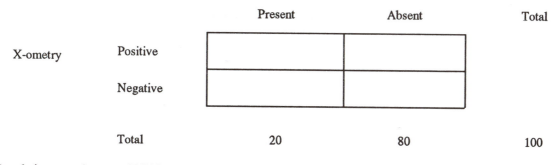

Population prevalence = 20/100 (20%)

Figure 4.5.   Determining the positive predictive value of X-ometry (Step 1).

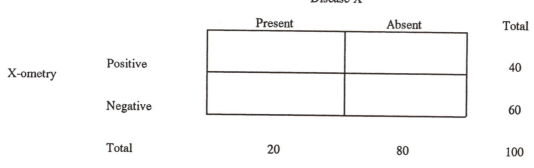

Population prevalence = 20%
Positive X-ometry rate = 40/100 (40%)

Figure 4.6.   Determining the positive predictive value of X-ometry (Step 2).

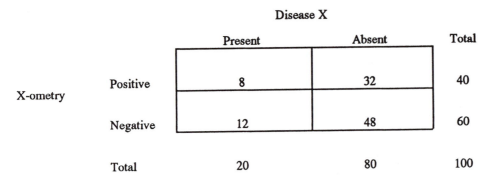

Figure 4.7. Determining the positive predictive value of X-ometry (Step 3).

Population prevalence = 20%
Positive X-ometry rate = 40%
Specificity X-ometry = 60%

REFERENCES

1. Begg CB. Biases in the assessment of diagnostic tests. Stat Med 1987;6:411–423.
2. Fagan TJ. Nomogram for Bayes's theorem (letter). N Engl J Med 1975;293:257.
3. Griner PF, Mayewski RJ, Mushlin AI, Greenland P. Selection and interpretation of diagnostic tests and procedures: principles and applications. Ann Intern Med 1981;94:553–600.
4. Metz CE. Basic principles of ROC analysis. Semin Nucl Med 1978;8:283–298.
5. Meyer KB, Pauker SG. Screening for HIV: can we afford the false positive rate? N Engl J Med 1987;317:238–241.

Headache

Glen D. Solomon

Headache is the most common pain complaint of humankind. Common headache disorders include migraine; cluster; tension-type; substance-withdrawal; and post-traumatic headaches. The vast number of different types of headache and their associated causes, signs, symptoms, natural history, and treatments can make headache difficult to diagnose and treat, especially in primary-care settings, where some headache disorders may be seen only rarely. Nevertheless, the vast majority of headaches can be treated effectively once the diagnosis has been made.

EPIDEMIOLOGY OF HEADACHE

Headache is the seventh most common presenting complaint for ambulatory care encounters in the United States. The problem of headache generates 18.3 million outpatient physician visits in the United States per year.

A new understanding of the epidemiology of headache emerged in the early 1990s with the advent of sophisticated epidemiologic methodology and the widespread acceptance of the International Headache Society's (IHS) criteria for the diagnosis of headache disorders. To determine the overall prevalence of headache in the general population, Rasmussen and colleagues examined 740 people aged 25–64 who had been randomly chosen to constitute a representative sample of the population of Copenhagen, Denmark. The study group was representative of the Danish population with regard to gender, age distribution, and marital status. Subjects underwent a structured interview, examination by a neurologist, and laboratory evaluation. Headache disorders were classified according to the IHS criteria. Although this in-depth evaluation offered the highest likelihood of differentiating among headache disorders and recognizing tension-type headache and migraine, the size of the population studied was, of necessity, limited. Results of the Rasmussen study included:

- A lifetime prevalence of headache of 96%
- Prevalence significantly higher among women (99%) than among men (93%)
- Headache at the time of examination (point-prevalence rate) was twice as common in women as in men
- Men aged 55–64 had the lowest lifetime and last-year prevalence of headache
- One case of cluster headache

Migraine-related results included:

- An overall lifetime prevalence of migraine of 16%
- A male:female ratio of about 1:3 (8% among men and 25% among women)
- 4% of the patients reported a migraine during the last month
- No significant differences in migraine prevalence rates according to age
- Of migraine sufferers, 15% had migraine 8–14 days per year and 9% had it more than 14 days per year.
- 85% of migraine sufferers reported severe pain intensity.

A summary of the epidemiology of the migraine headache is as follows:

- Prevalence: 6–8% men, 18–25% women
- Age of onset: childhood to twenties
- Peak prevalence: age 40; ages 25–55

Tension-type headache results included:

- A lifetime prevalence of tension-type headache is 78% (97% episodic, 3% chronic)
- A male:female ratio of 4:5 (69% among men and 88% among women)
- 48% of subjects had a tension-type headache in the previous month

- Men aged 55–64 had the lowest lifetime prevalence of tension-type headache
- Among women, there was a significant decrease in the prevalence of tension-type headache with increasing age
- 23% had headache 8–14 days per year and 36% had it several times per month
- Chronic tension-type headache (tension-type headache occurring > 180 days/year) was noted by 3% of the population
- Only 1% of tension-type headache patients reported severe pain intensity, whereas moderate pain was noted by 58%, and mild pain by 41%
- Age of onset: teens to thirties

DIAGNOSIS OF HEADACHE

Headache may be categorized as benign (primary headache disorder) or organic (secondary headache disorder). Benign headaches are further classified by temporal patterns and symptoms, including migraine headache and cluster headache.

Organic headaches present as a symptom of an underlying disease, including:

- Giant-cell arteritis
- Subarachnoid hemorrhage
- Meningitis
- Intracranial mass lesion
- Temporal arteritis
- Arterial dissection
- Stroke

SCREENING

The appropriate screening for the outpatient with recurrent headaches includes:

- A complete headache history
- Both a physical and a neurologic examination
- Laboratory tests (if indicated by the history and physical)
- Computed tomography (CT) or magnetic resonance imaging (MRI) studies if the headaches are:
  - Of recent onset
  - Indicated by troubling neurologic symptoms in the patient's headache history
  - Associated with abnormalities on the neurologic examination

HISTORY OF HEADACHE

The first step in evaluating any patient with headache is to obtain a thorough headache history. This should include the:

- Duration of the headache disorder
- Age of onset
- Temporal pattern

- Quality of pain
- Location of pain
- Trigger factors
- Associated symptoms

The headache history is the key to determining whether a headache is benign or organic. Most often, a careful and complete history will provide a presumptive diagnosis, which can then be confirmed by physical examination and laboratory or radiographic studies.

Evaluating factors such as age of onset, temporal pattern, quality and location of pain, and headache triggers usually allows the physician to diagnose the headache and to initiate therapy. Temporal-pattern characteristics include:

- Constant
  - Chronic tension-type
- Daily
  - Chronic tension-type
  - Analgesic rebound
  - Chronic cluster
- Cyclic
  - Episodic cluster
- Intermittent
  - Migraine
  - Episodic tension-type

The duration of the headache problem is often a key indicator of its probable cause:

- Sudden onset
  - Hemorrhage
  - Meningitis
- Chronic
  - Migraine
  - Tension-type
  - Cluster
- Developing over weeks to months
  - Sinusitis
  - Subdural hematoma
  - Mass lesion
  - Hydrocephalus
  - Giant-cell arteritis
  - Ocular disease

Severe headache of sudden onset, especially if associated with focal neurologic signs or changes in the level of consciousness, suggests serious illness such as intracerebral hemorrhage or meningitis (which must be immediately ruled out by physical examination and laboratory evaluation). Recurrent episodic headaches dating back many years, on the other hand, are more likely a type of vascular headache, such as migraine or cluster headaches. A long history of daily headaches without associated symptoms suggests a chronic tension-type headache. An initial migraine headache, unless preceded by a characteristic aura, may be confused with serious neurologic problems such as meningitis or intracerebral hemorrhage.

Among the most difficult headaches to interpret are those

that develop over weeks or months. These headaches may be benign or arise from conditions as diverse as sinusitis, ocular disease, subdural hematoma, mass lesion, hydrocephalus, or—in the patient over age 60—giant-cell arteritis.

In addition to the frequency and duration, the timing of the headache with respect to other physiological events can be crucial to a correct diagnosis.

- Childhood
  - Migraine
  - Tension-type
- Puberty
  - Migraine
- Twenties
  - Tension-type
  - Migraine
  - Cluster
- After age 50
  - Giant-cell arteritis
  - Tension-type/cervical osteoarthritis
  - Organic

One should determine the time of day the headache occurs as well as its relationship to puberty, menses, pregnancy, menopause, or the use of hormones.

Migraine headaches often initially occur during puberty and for women may resolve after menopause. Migraine headaches may occur irregularly for months to years or, for women, may occur with menses. An acute migraine attack can last 4–72 hours, with headache-free intervals between attacks.

Episodic cluster headache follows a cyclical pattern of attacks, lasting from 2 weeks to several months, often in the spring and fall. These bouts are separated by quiescent periods lasting from months to years. During these bouts, severe headaches, lasting from 15 minutes to 3 hours, may occur from one to four times a day, often awakening the patient from sleep at night. The duration of the cluster headache attack distinguishes it from trigeminal neuralgia, which presents with recurrent jabs of pain lasting less than a minute. The duration of the cluster headache can categorize it as follows:

- Seconds
  - Trigeminal neuralgia
  - Idiopathic stabbing
- Minutes
  - Cluster/chronic paroxysmal hemicrania (CPH)
- Hours
  - Migraine
  - Episodic tension-type
- Days
  - Migraine
  - Chronic tension-type
- Constant
  - Chronic tension-type

Cluster-variant headaches, such as CPH, show a pain pattern similar to cluster headache, but the attacks are more frequent and occur predominantly during the day. Chronic tension-type headaches show no periodicity and have few headache-free intervals: the patient typically describes a daily, unrelenting headache. The mixed headache syndrome is characterized by intermittent paroxysms of severe, throbbing, "sick" (migraine) headache superimposed on a constant daily headache.

The location of the pain can sometimes aid in diagnosis, such as in cluster headache or trigeminal neuralgia, but it also may be misleading.

- Unilateral
  - Cluster
  - Trigeminal neuralgia
  - Migraine (two out of three)
  - Local disease of eye, nose, or sinus
- Bilateral
  - Tension-type
  - Hemorrhage/mass lesion (may begin unilaterally)
  - Migraine (one out of three)

Chronic tension-type headache is usually bilateral but may be unilateral. Headaches arising from hemorrhage or space-occupying lesions may begin unilaterally but usually become bilateral. Migraine usually alternates sides with different attacks, but it may be predominantly unilateral throughout life. Cluster headache is invariably unilateral and affects only one side during a series of attacks.

The patient's description of the quality of the pain can be valuable:

- Throbbing
  - Migraine
- Pressure/ache
  - Tension-type
- Boring
  - Cluster
- Shock-like
  - Trigeminal neuralgia

Migraine is usually throbbing or pulsatile, whereas a constant ache suggests tension-type headache, and deep, boring, intense pain points to cluster headache. Trigeminal neuralgia is marked by short, intense, shock-like jabs. The intensity of pain in cluster headache and trigeminal neuralgia is invariably described as so severe that the cluster headache patient usually cannot remain still. The migraine sufferer, by contrast, often seeks to rest in the stillness of a darkened room.

If the patient tells of an aura or warning signs, this generally means migraine with aura (classic migraine), the only type of headache with a recognizable prodrome. Visual or neurologic symptoms commonly precede the headache by 10–60 minutes (usually 20 minutes). Premonitory symptoms, which can include euphoria, fatigue, yawning, and craving for sweets, may occur 12–24 hours before an attack. In addition to focal neurologic signs, associated symptoms that may accompany migraine include:

- Aura
- Premonitory symptoms

- Photophobia/phonophobia
- Anorexia/nausea/vomiting
- Exacerbation with exertion
- Lacrimation/rhinorrhea/Horner's syndrome
- Dysthymia/depression

Conditions associated with cluster headache include:

- Horner's syndrome
- Constricted pupils
- Injected conjunctiva
- Unilateral lacrimation and rhinorrhea

Rhinorrhea and nasal congestion are also common in sinusitis.

Neck stiffness or other signs of meningeal irritation can signal meningitis, encephalitis, or intracerebral hemorrhage. A mass lesion, hydrocephalus, or encephalitis may be suggested by decreased consciousness or obtundation. Seizures can reflect cortical irritation resulting from a mass lesion or arteriovenous malformation. Fever and sweating may suggest an infectious process.

One also should consider precipitating factors or "triggers" such as:

- Hormonal changes/menses
- Changes in sleep
- Stress/post-stress
- Foods/alcohol
- Missing meals
- Weather changes

Fatigue, particularly loss of sleep, may cause either migraine or tension-type headache. Stress may exacerbate tension-type headache, whereas migraine may occur after a period of stress, often on weekends or vacations. Migraine sufferers may associate their headaches with menses, missing meals, or imbibing foods rich in tyramine, such as red wine or aged cheese. Alcohol may trigger a cluster attack during a cluster cycle, but will have no effect during a quiescent period. Weather changes can be associated with migraine or exacerbation of sinusitis. Symptoms of depression, such as sleep and appetite disturbances, are commonly associated with chronic tension-type headache.

One also should assess possible exposure to occupational toxins, chemicals, or infectious agents. Carbon monoxide poisoning, for example, often manifests as headache. Certain chemicals, such as nitrates, induce withdrawal and reintroduction headache. Exposure to infectious agents in immunosuppressed or AIDS patients also may induce encephalitis or meningitis, unaccompanied by the classic fever and stiff neck.

Reviewing the patient's family history may prove rewarding. Migraine is a familial disorder, with a positive family history in two-thirds of cases. Cluster headache is familial in only about 3% of patients. In tension-type headache, a family history of depression or alcohol abuse is common.

The patient's medical-surgical history and medication history can aid in diagnosis. Head trauma, for instance, may suggest subdural hematoma or skull fracture. Certain medications can trigger the onset of headache or exacerbate headache in patients with an underlying headache disorder. Medication-induced headache has been commonly reported for:

- Indomethacin (Indocin)
- Nifedipine (Procardia, Adalat)
- Cimetidine (Tagamet)
- Atenolol (Tenormin)
- Trimethoprim-sulfamethoxazole (Bactrim, Septra)
- Nitroglycerin
- Isosorbide dinitrate (Isordil)
- Ranitidine (Zantac)
- Isotretinoin (Retin-A)
- Captopril (Capoten)
- Piroxicam (Feldene)
- Granisetron (Kytril)
- Erythropoetin (Epogen)
- Metoprolol (Lopressor, Toprol)
- Diclofenac (Voltaren)

Medications that may aggravate existing migraine include:

- Vitamin A and its retinoic acid derivatives
- Hormone therapy
  - Oral contraceptives
  - Clomiphene
  - Postmenopausal estrogens

Migraine and cluster headaches may be exacerbated by vasodilators, such as:

- Nitrates
- Hydralazine (Apresoline)
- Minoxidil (Loniten)
- Nifedipine (Procardia, Adalat)
- Prazocin (Minipress)

Reserpine, a serotonin antagonist, can cause depression, migraine, and tension-type headaches. Indomethacin, although useful in treating cluster variant headaches, can cause generalized headache. Frequent or chronic use of some prescription and over-the-counter medications used to treat headache, including opioids, barbiturates, caffeine, and ergots, can lead to rebound or withdrawal headaches.

The following symptoms strongly suggest headache of organic etiology:

- Newly developed, massive, or gradually increasing headache
- Alterations in personality
- Constant headache that worsens when lying down
- Headache in the late night or morning
- Headaches precipitated by coughing
- Headache with exertion
  - Physical exertion
  - Coitus and orgasm
- Epileptic attacks

- Diplopia
- Headache following head trauma
- The presence of other symptoms
  - Fever
  - Nausea and/or vomiting
  - Generalized or focal neurologic symptoms
  - Cerebrospinal rhinorrhea
- The start of headaches after age 50

PHYSICAL EXAMINATION

After evaluating the headache history, the physician should perform a targeted physical examination of:

- Fever and other vital signs
- Skull examination
- Papilledema
- Neck stiffness
- Generalized neurologic signs
- A decreased level of consciousness
- Abnormal behavior
- Focal neurologic signs

This examination should include:

- Mental status (often performed as part of obtaining the history)
- Blood pressure
- Pulse measurement
- Cranial nerves
- Funduscopic examination
- Palpation of the head and neck
- Auscultation of the carotid arteries and heart
- Evaluation of motor nerves and balance
- Palpation of peripheral pulses (particularly if vasoconstrictor medications are to be prescribed).

The following signs strongly suggest headaches of organic cause:

- Fever plus rigidity of the neck
- Papilledema
- Tender temporal arteries
- Loss of local neurologic function, including loss of sight

Diagnostic tests for the headache patient should be chosen on the basis of the results of the history and physical examination. In a patient with a typical headache history of several years' duration and a normal neurologic examination, no further evaluation may be needed.

IMAGING STUDIES

Several commonly ordered tests have little or no value in evaluating headache. Electroencephalograms (EEG) may be abnormal in some migraine patients, but EEG changes are neither specific for nor diagnostic of migraine. As a screening test to localize organic lesions, EEG has been supplanted by more specific imaging (CT and MRI). Evoked potentials (visual, auditory, and somatosensory) fail to show specific findings in migraine. Like EEG, evoked potentials have no utility as a screening test for headache. The medical literature does not support the use of thermography in generating a diagnosis, in guiding therapy, or in determining a prognosis for headache disorders. Radiographs of the cervical spine are rarely useful in the diagnosis and management of headache.

Neuroradiology has little role in the diagnosis of headache, beyond ruling out occult lesions such as neoplasm, hemorrhage, vascular malformations, brain abscesses, hydrocephalus, or congenital malformations (i.e., Arnold-Chiari malformations). MRI and CT will not identify other organic causes of headache, such as idiopathic intracranial hypertension (pseudotumor cerebri), meningitis or other infections, glaucoma or eye disease, or metabolic or toxic causes of headache. The physician must obtain a complete history and examination and not rely solely on the MRI or CT to eliminate organic causes of headache.

Most patients suffering from acute severe headaches should undergo imaging with CT or MRI to rule out the organic causes listed above. Because organic causes of headache are rare (estimated to be less than 1% in headache clinics), these tests will generally be unrevealing. The benefits of a normal CT or MRI in reassuring the patient and doctor should not be overlooked, however. Some patients (and physicians) may be unwilling to embark on a course of therapy for a benign headache disorder without the reassurance of a normal scan.

LABORATORY STUDIES

All patients older than 60 years with new-onset headache or a change in their headache pattern should have their sedimentation rate or C-reactive protein levels measured to evaluate for giant-cell arteritis. If either measurement is elevated, a temporal artery biopsy should be obtained to confirm the diagnosis.

Routine laboratory screening with a complete blood count, urinalysis, and a chemistry profile adds little diagnostic information. However, these studies may rule out the diseases that typically present with headache.

DIFFERENTIAL DIAGNOSIS

In medical practice, most headaches are not caused by underlying disease. It is important to recognize, however, that headache can be the presenting symptom of several diseases. Fever, regardless of cause, is probably the most common medical problem that causes headache. Less common causes include:

- Pheochromocytoma
- Chronic renal failure
- Hyperthyroidism

- Organ transplantation
- Malignant hypertension

Pheochromocytoma may present with a pounding headache associated with hypertension, diaphoresis, tachycardia, and palpitations.

Rheumatologic diseases may have headache as an early manifestation. Headache is common in systemic lupus erythematosus, polyarteritis nodosa, and giant-cell arteritis. About two-thirds of patients with either fibromyalgia or chronic fatigue syndrome report headache, usually tension-type headache. Many types of vasculitis can also present with headache.

Headache on awakening may be the initial symptom of sleep-apnea syndrome. The headache often will improve as the day progresses. Sleep apnea is most commonly observed in obese, middle-aged males. Associated symptoms include snoring, daytime somnolence, hypertension, and arrhythmias.

SPECIFIC HEADACHES

MIGRAINE HEADACHE

Pathophysiology of Migraine Headache

The pathophysiology of migraine is still uncertain. The initiating event in migraine is still unknown; however, it is believed that either an ischemic or a neurochemical noxious trigger stimulates the trigeminal nerve. Through antidromic conduction in the trigeminal nerve, substance P and CGRP are released from small-diameter sensory afferents. These neuropeptides, possibly acting through nitric oxide, initiate a sterile inflammatory response in the cerebral blood vessels. It is likely that local inflammation and sensitization of polymodal nociceptors by substance P cause the pain of migraine.

Clinical Presentation of Migraine Headache

Migraine is a syndrome of intermittent, moderate-to-severe intensity headaches, lasting 4–72 hours. The headaches are typically unilateral, throbbing, associated with nausea or vomiting, and aggravated by light, noise, or both. Clinical features are summarized as follows:

- Frequency: intermittent, 1–4/month
- Location: unilateral
- Character: throbbing
- Intensity: moderate to severe; increases with exertion
- Duration: 4–72 hours
- Associated symptoms: photophobia, phonophobia, anorexia, nausea, and vomiting

Aura, usually scintillating scotomata or fortification spectra, precede the headache in about 15% of patients.

- Without aura (common): 80%
- With aura (classic): 20%
  - Symptoms of focal brain dysfunction

- Gradual onset over 4 minutes or more
- Duration under 60 minutes
- Headache follows in under 60 minutes
- Varients
- Basilar migraine
- Retinal migraine
- Ophthalmoplegic migraine
- Migraine with complicated aura
- Migrainous stroke
- Migraine aura without headache

The prevalence of migraine in the U.S. is 6–8% in men and 18–25% in women.

Most migraines are precipitated only when several triggers occur at about the same time, usually in the 12 hours preceding onset:

- Stress letdown
- Sleep changes
- Fasting
- Diet
- Hormones
- Weather changes

The simultaneous elimination of multiple headache triggers has an additive effect in decreasing the probability that migraine will occur. Migraines are rarely induced every time by exposure to individual triggers.

The most common migraine triggers are alcohol and four food substances:

- Tyramine (found in aged cheese and fermented foods)
- Aspartame (found in many diet soft drinks)
- Monosodium glutamate (MSG, found in Chinese restaurant food and flavor enhancers)
- Phenylethylamine (found in chocolate)

Additional common triggers include:

- Hormonal changes (menses, climacteric)
- Alterations in sleep patterns (shift changes, jet lag, sleeping late on weekends)
- Fasting
- Weather changes
- ''Let down'' periods (weekends, vacations) after stressful periods

Treatment of Migraine Headache

Pharmacologic Treatment of Migraine—Prophylactic A variety of medications have been used to prevent migraine:

- Methysergide (Sansert)
- Cyproheptadine (Periactin)
- Beta blockers
- Calcium channel blockers
- Nonsteroidal anti-inflammatory drugs (NSAIDs)
- Tricyclic antidepressants
- Divalproex (Depakote)
- Valporic acid

Methysergide (Sansert) is less commonly used today for migraine prophylaxis because of the risk of serious complications, such as retroperitoneal fibrosis. Cyproheptadine (Periactin) is generally used for migraine prophylaxis in children. Adults often find the side effects of fatigue and weight gain from this antihistamine-antiserotonin drug to be intolerable.

Beta blockers, calcium channel blockers, and NSAIDs are first-line drugs for preventing migraine. Several beta blockers are effective:

- Propranolol (Inderal), 60–160 mg/day
- Timolol (Blockadren), 10–40 mg/day
- Nadolol (Corgard), 20–160 mg/day
- Metoprolol (Lopressor, Toprol), 50–200 mg/day
- Atenolol (Tenormin), 25–100 mg/day

Propranolol and timolol are the only beta blockers currently approved by the U.S. Food and Drug Administration for migraine prophylaxis. Beta blockers with intrinsic sympathomimetic activity, such as pindolol (Visken) and acebutolol (Sectral), are not useful in migraine prophylaxis. Although generally well tolerated, beta blockers are contraindicated in patients with congestive heart failure, bronchospastic disease (i.e., asthma, emphysema, chronic bronchitis), diabetes mellitus, and Wolff-Parkinson-White syndrome. Beta blockers also may exacerbate Raynaud's phenomenon, a condition found more commonly in migraine sufferers. Side effects of beta blockers include depression, fatigue, and sleep disorders. Depression is more commonly reported with propranolol (Inderal) than with other beta blockers.

Calcium entry blockers useful in preventing migraine and cluster headache include:

- Verapamil (Isoptin, Calan, Verelan), 120–480 mg/day
- Diltiazem (Cardizem), 90–360 mg/day
- Flunarizine, 5–10 mg/day
- Nimodipine (Nimotop), 60–120 mg/day
- Nicardipine (Cardene), 40–90 mg/day

Nifedipine (Procardia, Adalat) is either weakly effective or ineffective for migraine prophylaxis and can exacerbate migraine in some patients because of profound vasodilation. In the United States, verapamil (Isoptin, Calan, Verelan) is considered the calcium channel blocker of choice for migraine and cluster prophylaxis.

The calcium entry blockers are a diverse group of drugs with varying effects on the heart and peripheral vasculature. Verapamil (Isoptin, Calan, Verelan) and diltiazem (Cardizem) have negative inotropic effects and slow conduction through the AV node. Therefore, these agents should be avoided in patients with congestive heart failure, advanced heart block, or sick sinus syndrome. The dihydropyradine calcium entry blockers, nifedipine (Procardia, Adalat), nicardipine (Cardene), and nimodipine (Nimotop), have no effect on cardiac conduction but can cause marked vasodilation.

Adverse effects with calcium entry blockers include:

- Verapamil (Isoptin, Calan, Verelan): constipation
- Flunarizine: sedation, weight gain, and Parkinsonism
- Nifedipine (Procardia, Adalat): flushing and edema
- Diltiazem (Cardizem): gastrointestinal upset and Parkinsonism

NSAIDs are valuable both in preventing migraine and as adjunctive therapy for tension-type headache. This dual effect on migraine and tension-type headache allows NSAIDs to be used as single-drug therapy in some patients with the mixed headache syndrome. Several NSAIDs have been reported to prevent migraine:

- Aspirin, 325 mg qd
- Naproxen (Naprosyn), 250–500 mg bid
- Flurbiprofen (Ansaid), 100 mg bid
- Ketoprofen (Orudis), 75 mg tid
- Fenoprofen (Nalfon), 600 mg tid

Adverse effects from NSAIDs are relatively common and may include gastrointestinal symptoms, such as dyspepsia, heartburn, nausea, vomiting, diarrhea, constipation, and generalized abdominal pain. Most NSAIDs can cause bleeding of the upper gastrointestinal tract. Renal effects of NSAIDs may include decreased glomerular filtration rate (GFR) with sodium, chloride, and water retention. Renal problems are most likely to occur in patients who are elderly, hypertensive, have renovascular or advanced atherosclerotic disease, or who take diuretics. Indomethacin (Indocin) and fenoprofen (Nalfon) appear to be more nephrotoxic than other NSAIDs. Analgesic nephropathy, the most common cause of drug-induced renal failure, has been associated with excessive use of NSAIDs in conjunction with phenacetin or acetaminophen (Tylenol).

For patients who do not respond to first-line therapies, alternatives include the monamine oxidase inhibitor phenelzine (Nardil) or divalproex (Depakote). Because of their potential for serious toxicity, these agents should be prescribed only by physicians experienced in their use.

Several complementary (alternative) medicine approaches have been used to prevent migraine. The following have been evaluated in randomized clinical trials and shown to be effective:
- The medicinal herb feverfew
- Magnesium
- High-dose vitamin B_2 (riboflavin)

Pharmacologic Treatment of Migraine—Abortive Migraine headache abortive therapies include:

- Serotonin agonists
- Isometheptene/mucate combination
- NSAIDs
- Antiemetics
- Lidocaine
- Corticosteroids
- Analgesics

Treatment of Migraine Headache With Moderate Disability
For the management of migraine attacks of moderate disability, the following are prescribed:

- NSAIDs
- Isometheptene mucate
- Sumatriptan PO
- Ergotamine tartrate (PO, PR)
- Analgesic (if infrequent)

Usually an NSAID or isometheptene compound (Midrin) is prescribed initially for the abortive (acute) treatment of migraine headaches
The most effective NSAIDs to abort migraine attacks are:

- Naproxen sodium (Anaprox, Aleve), 550 mg/550 mg
- Flurbiprofen (Ansaid), 100 mg/100 mg
- Meclofenamate (Meclomen), 200 mg/200 mg

Generally, a dose is given at the onset of the headache, then repeated in one hour if the headache is still present. Ketorolac (60 mg 1M) also is prescribed.

An isometheptene compound (Midrin) is prescribed as two capsules initially, followed by one capsule every hour, as needed, with a limit of five per day and 15 per week. Characteristics of isometheptene mucate (Midrin) include:

- Isometheptene mucate: sympathetic amine with vasoconstrictor effects
- Dichloralphenazone: mild sedative
- Acetaminophen: analgesic
- Contraindications: Coronary +/or peripheral vascular disease, hypertension, monoamine oxidase inhibitors (MAOIs)

Treatment of Migraine Headache With Significant Disability   Management of migraine attacks of significant disability includes:

- Sumatriptan PO, SC
- Dihydroergotamine SC, IM, IV
- Dihydroergotamine + metoclopramide IV
- Prochlorperazine 10 mg IV

Migraine abortives include:

- Antiemetics
  - Prochlorperazine (10 mg)
  - Metoclopramide (10 mg)
- Corticosteroids
  - Dexamethasone (1.5 mg bid × 2 days)
    - Limit usage to one attack per month
- Lidocaine
  - 4% topical solution
    - 0.5 mL in ipsilateral nostril over 30 seconds

When initial therapy is ineffective, or when the migraine is associated with marked disability, serotonin agonists should be considered. Oral sumatriptan (Imitrex), a serotonin 1-D agonist, is effective in about 60% of migraine attacks; subcutaneous administration is effective in about 80%. When given subcutaneously (6 mg), it acts rapidly, often within 20 minutes. Both subcutaneous and oral (25–100 mg) formulations are generally well tolerated, with chest pressure and sensations

of heaviness being common adverse reactions. Limitations to its use include expense and the problem of recurrent headache in up to 40% of patients. The characteristics of sumatriptan include the following:

- Clinical experience
  - Effective in about 80% of migraine attacks
  - Recurrence of headache in about 40% of attacks
  - Cost: $30–35 per injection; $9–15 per tablet
  - Rapid onset of action: 20–30 min SQ, 30–120 min PO
- Adverse effects
  - Atypical sensations: tingling, warm/hot sensation, heaviness
  - Tightness in chest
  - Flushing
  - Dizziness
  - Injection-site reaction
- Oral Sumatriptan
  - Dosages: 25 mg and 50 mg in U.S.; 100 mg worldwide
  - Response: 50–70% at 2 hours
  - Recurrence rate: 30–48%
  - Efficacy: greater than placebo
    - greater than ergotamine 2 mg + caffeine 200 mg
    - equals aspirin 900 mg + metoclopramide 10 mg

Newer serotonin 1-D agonists, including naratriptan, zolmetriptan, rizatriptan, alniditan, eletriptan, and VML 251, have efficacy similar to sumatriptan. Preliminary research suggests that they may have lower recurrence rates. Dihydroergotamine (DHE-45) can be given intramuscularly (1 mg), subcutaneously (1 mg), or intranasally (2 mg). Repetitive doses of intravenous DHE may be given to abort prolonged (status) migraine. Parenteral DHE will usually induce nausea; pretreatment with an antiemetic is recommended. Several other serotonin agonist drugs are under development for the acute treatment of migraine.

Ergotamine tartrate (Wigraine, Cafergot) is often effective for the acute treatment of migraine. Because of the problem of ergotamine rebound with frequent use, ergot alkaloids are used only when other medications are ineffective. The usual oral dose is 2 mg initially, followed by 1 mg every 30 minutes, as needed, with a maximum of 6 mg daily and 10 mg/week. Rectal absorption of ergotamine is greater than oral absorption. To reduce the likelihood of nausea, a 2-mg rectal suppository should be cut into thirds, with one-third given as the initial dose and additional thirds given every hour as needed, up to the maximum of 6 mg/day. When ergotamine is prescribed, it should be given no more often than every 4 days to prevent rebound headaches. Vasoconstrictors, such as ergotamine preparations, sumatriptan, and isometheptene products, should be avoided in patients with coronary artery disease, peripheral vascular disease, or poorly controlled hypertension.

CHRONIC TENSION-TYPE HEADACHE

Etiology of Chronic Tension-Type Headache

The tension-type headache is the most common form of headache, at least in Western populations. Previously used names for tension-type headache included muscle contraction headache, psychogenic headache, and chronic daily headache. The term ''muscle-contraction headache'' was abandoned because electromyographic (EMG) evidence failed to show consistent changes in muscle tone in patients with tension-type headache. Further, it suggested a pathophysiologic mechanism for the headache that has yet to be proven.

The concept that tension-type headache is a ''psychogenic'' headache has also been questioned. Patients with chronic tension-type headache, like patients with other chronic pain disorders, have about a 25% likelihood of developing secondary depression. Half of these patients develop depression simultaneously with the pain, whereas the development of depression is more insidious in the other half of the patients. Tension-type headache may be present in almost all psychiatric disturbances. This should not suggest, however, that most tension-type headaches are associated with psychiatric or psychological disorders.

The term ''chronic daily headache'' usually refers to patients with headaches that meet IHS criteria for both tension-type headache and migraine (usually without aura). This group often includes patients with analgesic-abuse or ergotamine-rebound headaches. Other well-defined primary headaches can occur on a daily basis (i.e., cluster headache, CPH, hemicrania continua, idiopathic stabbing headache), but are not considered as ''chronic daily headache.''

Most people with tension-type headache have it once a month or less, but about 40% have it several times per month. Headache occurring at least 180 days per year (half the days of the year) is reported by 4% of people. The severity of tension-type headache increases significantly with its frequency. In 59% of people with tension-type headache, their daily activities were impaired because of the headache.

Because of the large number of sufferers in the general population, the economic impact of tension-type headache is enormous. On average, 5% of the total employed population between the ages of 25 and 64 were absent for 4 days; 2% were absent for 11 days, and 2% were absent about 20 days per year. The number of days lost from work that was attributable to tension-type headache was 820 workdays per 1000 employed persons per year.

Pathophysiology of Chronic Tension-Type Headache

The pathophysiology of tension-type headache is poorly understood. Probably, episodic tension-type headache is predominantly a disorder of peripheral mechanisms, whereas chronic tension-type headache reflects a central pain disturbance.

Episodic tension-type headache is thought to be caused by either increased nociception from strained muscles, as occurs with inadequate rest or poor posture, or increased muscle tension, as occurs with stress. Increased pain impulses may cause an increased sensitivity of neurons of the trigeminal tract and then pain may propagate itself to some extent. Recurrent bouts of tension-type headache may lower the threshold for new episodes by altering the myofascial tissues, potentiating nociceptive neurons, or decreasing the activity of the anti-nociceptive system.

Chronic tension-type headache appears to be one of a group of disorders marked by low levels of brain serotonin. Like other chronic pain disorders, chronic tension-type headache is also associated with hypofunction of the central opioid system. Patients with chronic tension-type headache commonly report symptoms of constant headache, generalized myalgias and arthralgias, difficulty in initiating and maintaining sleep, chronic fatigue, carbohydrate craving, decreased libido, irritability, and disturbed memory and concentration. This disorder is similar to the disease depression; however, in chronic tension-type headache, anhedonia is not present, the mood disturbance is less marked or may even be absent, and the primary symptom is headache pain. It also resembles the disease fibromyalgia, characterized by generalized myofascial pain and sleep disturbance.

Clinical Presentation of Chronic Tension-Type Headache

Chronic tension-type headache typically is described as a band-like pressure headache without associated symptoms. The IHS defines tension-type headache as a bilateral headache having a pressing or tightening quality of mild-to-moderate severity. Unlike migraine, it is neither aggravated by physical activity nor associated with vomiting. Phonophobia or photophobia may be present, but not both. In chronic tension-type headache—but not in episodic tension-type headache—patients may experience nausea. By definition, chronic tension-type headache occurs at least 15 days per month for at least 6 months, although in clinical practice, it is usually a daily or almost daily headache. To summarize clinical features:

- Frequency: daily or nearly daily
- Location: frontal, bitemporal, occipital, holocephalic
- Character: pressure, vise-like, weight-like
- Intensity: mild to moderate
- Duration: constant, daily
- Associated symptoms: none
- Neurovegetative symptoms
  - Mood lability
  - Appetite or weight change
  - Fatigue
  - Sleep disturbance
  - Memory and concentration difficulties

Treatment of Chronic Tension-Type Headache

Pharmacologic Treatment of Chronic Tension-Type Headache Despite its frequency in the population and its societal impact, there are very few well-controlled studies of treatment of tension-type headache. Many earlier trials included patients with combined tension-type headache and migraine without aura and patients with medication-overuse headache.

Given the chronic nature of the disorder and the risk of medication-overuse headache in patients with frequent headaches, prophylactic therapy is warranted for most patients with chronic tension-type headache:

- NSAIDs
- Antidepressants
- Muscle relaxants

Antidepressants are the drugs of choice for chronic tension-type headache; several are also effective in preventing migraine. Of the antidepressants, the tricyclic drugs and the newer serotonin reuptake inhibitors are usually the first choice because the incidence of side effects and the seriousness of drug interactions are lower than those of the monamine oxidase inhibitors (MAOIs).

The selection of a specific antidepressant drug should be based primarily on whether the patient has a sleep disturbance. Patients who initiate and maintain sleep easily generally tolerate nonsedating drugs better than sedating agents. Those patients who have difficulty initiating or maintaining sleep respond better to sedating drugs. Patients often note improvement in headaches within 1 or 2 weeks after their sleep disturbance is corrected.

The nonsedating antidepressants include:

- Fluoxetine (Prozac)
- Sertraline (Zoloft)
- Bupropion (Wellbutrin)
- Paroxetine (Paxil)
- Nefazadone (Serzone)
- Venlafaxine (Effexor)
- Protriptyline (Vivactil)
- Desipramine (Norpramin)

The MAOIs are nonsedating and may induce insomnia. The sedating antidepressants include:

- Amitriptyline (Elavil, Endep)
- Doxepin (Sinequan)
- Nortriptyline (Pamelor)
- Imipramine (Tofranil)
- Trimipramine (Surmontil)
- Trazodone (Desyrel)

Of these drugs, nortriptyline (Pamelor) appears to cause the least amount of morning sedation.

The second consideration after the drug's effect on sleep is whether the patient is likely to tolerate anticholinergic side effects. The common anticholinergic side effects of the tricyclic antidepressants are urinary retention (primarily in men with prostatic hypertrophy), dry mouth, blurred vision, and constipation.

All tricyclic antidepressants have anticholinergic side effects. Of the tricyclics, doxepin (Sinequan) appears to cause the fewest such side effects. Serotonin reuptake inhibitors and

the newer antidepressants, such as fluoxetine (Prozac), sertraline (Zoloft), bupropion (Wellbutrin), paroxetine (Paxil), nefazadone (Serzone), and venlafaxine (Effexor), are generally free of anticholinergic effects.

Treatment of the daily, tension-type headache with abortive medications is difficult. Abortive therapies include:

- NSAIDs
- Muscle relaxants
  - Metaxalone, 800 mg tid-qid prn
  - Orphenadrine, 50 mg bid-tid prn
  - Chlorzoxazone, 500 mg qid prn
  - Carisoprodal, 200 mg tid prn
  - Methocarbamol, 500–1,000 mg qid prn
  - Cyclobenzaprine, 10 mg qid-tid prn

Muscle relaxants, such as chlorzoxazone (Parafon forte), orphenadrine citrate (Norflex), carisoprodol (Soma), and metaxalone (Skelaxin), either alone or in combinations with aspirin, acetaminophen, caffeine, or all three, are generally helpful. NSAIDs are also useful as analgesics for daily headache. Benzodiazepines, butalbital combinations (Fiorinal, Fioricet, Esgic, Axotal, Phrenelin), and narcotics should be avoided, or their use carefully controlled, because of the risk of habituation and rebound headache.

Nonpharmacologic Treatment of Chronic-Tension-Type Headache   Nonpharmacologic therapy is also important in the management of chronic headache syndromes. Biofeedback can help patients to change vasomotor tone and to relax tight muscles. Physical therapy is used to train patients to strengthen neck muscles, improve mobility, and correct poor posture. Physical therapy should not be limited to heat and massage. Although heat and massage provide short-term pain relief, only strengthening exercises provide long-term benefit.

CLUSTER HEADACHE

Etiology of Cluster Headache

Cluster headache is an uncommon headache disorder with a prevalence of about 1 in 1000, with a male-to-female ratio of 6 : 1. Cluster headache is marked by cycles of headache lasting 1–4 months, separated by remissions of 6 to 24 months. Ten to 15% of these patients suffer from chronic cluster headache that lasts greater than one year without remission. The epidemiological features of the cluster headache include:

- Age of onset: age 25; twenties to fifties
- Prevalence: 1 per 1000 males
- Six times more common in males
- Typical patient: Tall, slender smoker with ''lionine'' facies and hazel eyes

Clinical Presentation of Cluster Headache

The cluster headache attacks are always unilateral and are located around the eye, temple, or upper jaw. Associated symptoms include reddening and tearing of the eye, drooping of the eyelid, nasal stuffiness, and rhinorrhea. The attacks generally last from 15 minutes to 2 hours, occur one to four times daily, and often awaken the patient after 90 to 120 minutes of sleep. The pain is excruciating, and the patient commonly will pace the floor during an attack. The clinical features of the cluster headache are summarized as follows:

- Frequency: 1–4 attacks per day
- Location: unilateral/periorbital
- Character: boring, stabbing
- Intensity: severe
- Duration: 15–120 minutes
- Associated symptoms:
  - Ipsilateral lacrimation and nasal congestion
  - Scleral injection
  - Partial Horner's syndrome
- Periodicity of clusters of headache
  - 4–16 weeks in duration
  - Remission 6–12 months; can be years between cycles
  - Seasonal—spring and autumn most likely
- Periodicity within a cluster of headaches
  - 90–120 minutes after sleep onset

Treatment of Cluster Headache

Medications used to prevent cluster headache include:

- Ergotamine
- Glucocorticoids
- Methysergide (Sansert)
- Verapamil (Isoptin, Calan, Verelan)
- Lithium carbonate (Eskalith, Lithobid)

Verapamil, 240–480 mg daily, is useful in both episodic and chronic cluster headache and generally is considered the drug of choice for cluster prophylaxis. Prednisone (Deltasone)—40 mg every morning for 1 week, tapering by 10 mg every week—or methysergide (Sansert) are used only in episodic cluster headache because of potential adverse effects with long-term use. Verapamil may be combined with either prednisone or ergotamine tartrate (Wigraine, Cafergot), 1 mg at bedtime, if it is ineffective as monotherapy. Lithium carbonate (Eskalth, Lithobid), 300 mg three times daily, is generally reserved for patients with chronic cluster headache because of its slow onset of action. Corticosteroids (such as prednisone, 40 mg qd × 1 week, tapering by 10 mg/wk) also are prescribed.

For the acute treatment of cluster headache, the drug of choice is oxygen—8–10 L/min by mask for 10 minutes. Other useful abortive medications include:

- Ergotamine (Wigraine, Cafergot)
  - Sublingual
  - Parenteral
- Dihydroergotamine (DHE-45)
- Sumatriptan (Imitrex), 6 mg

- Lidocaine (Xylocaine)
  - Nosedrops
  - Topical, 4% solution

GIANT-CELL ARTERITIS

Giant-cell arteritis should be considered in any patient older than 55 who presents with a new-onset headache. Symptoms may include:

- Subacute headache
  - Stable location
  - Steady worsening
- Constitutional symptoms
- Shoulder and hip girdle aches
- Neck or ear pain
- Jaw claudication
- Swollen and tender (or pulseless) scalp artery
- Elevated sedimentation rate (elevated WSR and/or C-RP)
- Myalgias
- Visual obscurations

Because giant-cell arteritis can affect the ophthalmic arteries (leading to partial or complete blindness as a result of retinal ischemia), treatment should begin as early as possible. Treatment is with glucocorticoids, often given over a period of months to years. The headache will invariably disappear within 48 hours of glucocorticoid therapy.

DRUG-HABITUATION AND DETOXIFICATION HEADACHE

Because drug habituation commonly accompanies many chronic headache syndromes, it is often the first issue that must be considered in patient management. Substances known to cause headaches include:

- Caffeine
  - Beverages
  - Combination preparations
- Analgesics
  - Narcotic
  - Opioid
  - Butalbital containing compounds
- Benzodiazepines
- Ergotamines

Medications that are known to cause habituation and rebound headaches include:

- Opioids
- Barbiturates (Fiorinal, Fioricet, Esgic, Axotal, Phrenelin)
- Ergotamine tartrate compounds (Cafergot, Wigraine)
- Benzodiazepines
- Caffeine-containing analgesic preparations (Anacin,

Excedrin, Vanquish, and others). There is no evidence that simple analgesics, such as aspirin, acetaminophen, or NSAIDs, cause rebound headaches with daily use.

Detoxification from habituating drugs is the initial step in the treatment of patients who are taking excessive pain medications (i.e., using daily or almost daily habituating pain medication, or taking ergotamine more than twice weekly). Prophylactic medication is ineffective in patients suffering from rebound or withdrawal headaches. Frequently, patients say that they ''would stop taking pain medication if only the preventative medication prevented the headaches.'' Patients must be instructed that the ''pain medication'' itself is part of the cause of the headaches, and that headache therapy is futile until the rebound-habituation cycle is resolved.

Management of the habituated patient can be difficult, and the medical literature offers little insight into proper techniques of detoxification. Patients who are habituated to opioids can benefit from clonidine (Catapres) to prevent phys-

ical signs and symptoms of withdrawal. Glucocorticoids and phenothiazines may be prescribed for outpatient detoxification from butalbital, ergotamine, or low doses of opioids. Generally, a 6–14 day tapered course of glucocorticoid is given, with chlorpromazine (Thorazine) suppositories prescribed for severe withdrawal headaches associated with vomiting. For patients with concomitant medical problems, a history of seizures, or unsuccessful outpatient detoxification, inpatient detoxification is often required.

CONCLUSION

The management of chronic headache disorders requires close follow-up and frequent physician visits until therapy is successful with a minimum of adverse effects. Although this approach takes commitment on the part of both the practitioner and the patient, good results should be expected in the vast majority of cases.

REVIEW EXERCISES

QUESTIONS

1. A 25-year-old woman presents with a 6-year history of monthly, unilateral headaches, always occurring 2 days before her menses. The headaches can occur on either side of the head and are associated with nausea and photophobia. Her physical and neurologic examinations are normal. Appropriate work-up for this patient includes:

   a. CT with contrast
   b. MRI without gadolinium
   c. Sed rate and TSH
   d. No further workup

2. A 35-year-old man presents with daily headaches for the past 2 weeks. He describes them as severe, always behind the right eye, and associated with runny nose and tearing of the eye. They occur twice a day, usually in the evening and at night. Two years ago he had a similar episode, resolved after 6 weeks with antibiotics. Appropriate therapy for this patient includes:

   a. Augmentin
   b. Propranolol
   c. Amitriptyline
   d. Verapamil

3. A 34-year-old female has had headaches almost daily for the past 5 years. The headaches are band-like pressure, without associated symptoms. They are generally well controlled with over-the-counter analgesics. She wants to become pregnant in the next few months and seeks your advice on headache management. You advise:

   a. Biofeedback training
   b. Relaxation techniques such as guided imagery
   c. It is OK to continue OTC analgesics; suggest she use acetaminophen
   d. All of the above
   e. Headache is a hereditary disorder; pregnancy is not advised

Answers

1. d
   This patient has had typical migraine headaches for several years. She has no "warning signs" of organic disease on history or examination. No further work-up is needed before initiating treatment.

2. d
   This case is episodic cluster headache. Cluster headaches are daily, unilateral and around the orbit, with associated rhinorrhea, lacrimation, Horner's syndrome, and conjunctival injection. The headaches usually are nocturnal or occur at rest. Cycles last 4–16 weeks. It is often misdiagnosed as sinusitis.

3. d
   When a headache patient wants to become pregnant, the ideal therapy should be nonpharmacologic. Biofeedback and relaxation are both useful in treating tension-type headache. Many patients still will require pain medication. Acetaminophen is the drug of choice in pregnancy. If her tension-type headaches are not manageable, fluoxetine could be prescribed.

SUGGESTED READING

Cady R, Wendt J, Kirchner J, et al. Treatment of acute migraine with subcutaneous sumatriptan. JAMA 1991;265: 2831–2835.

Goadsby P, Zagami A, Donnan G, et al. Oral sumatriptan in acute migraine. Lancet 1991;338:782–783.

Health and Public Policy Committee, American College of Physicians. Biofeedback for headaches. Ann Int Med 1985; 102:128–131.

Olesen J, Tfelt-Hansen P, Welch KMA, eds. The headaches. New York: Raven Press, 1993.

Pradalier A, Clapin A, Dry J. Treatment review: nonsteroid anti-inflammatory drugs in the treatment and long-term prevention of migraine attacks. Headache 1988;28:550–557.

Raskin N. Repetitive intravenous dihydroergotamine as therapy for intractable migraine. Neurology 1986;36:995–997.

Rasmussen, BK, et al. Epidemiology of headache in a general population: a prevalence study. J Clin Epidemiol 1991;44: 1147–1157.

Solomon GD. Headache. In: Rakel RE, ed. Conn's current therapy. Philadelphia: WB Saunders, 1997.

Subcutaneous Sumatriptan International Study Group. Treatment of migraine attacks with sumatriptan. N Engl J Med 1991;325:316–321.

Tollison CD, Kunkel RS, eds. Headache. Diagnosis and treatment. Baltimore: Williams & Wilkins, 1993.

C•H•A•P•T•E•R

6

Ocular Manifestations of Systemic Disease

Careen Y. Lowder

The ability of the physician to directly visualize ocular structures is unique to the eye as an organ system. The physician is able to make an immediate assessment of many systemic diseases with ocular manifestations such as diabetes and hypertension. In systemic diseases with ocular manifestations, close collaboration between the ophthalmologist and the internist is required in order to provide the best medical care to the patient.

EYE EXAMINATION

The internist can obtain valuable information by using a systematic approach in the examination of the eye, performing each of the following eight steps:

1. Vision
2. External examination
3. Pupils
4. Extraocular muscles
5. Anterior segment (conjunctiva, sclera, cornea, anterior chamber, iris, and lens)
6. Fundus ophthalmoscopy
7. Confrontation visual fields
8. Intraocular pressure

A significant number of pathologic conditions may be detected by careful examination and with a handheld ophthalmoscope. For example, the external examination may reveal exophthalmos, lid lesions, and edema. A pupil check may demonstrate relative afferent pupillary defects and Argyll-Robertson pupils. Evaluation of ocular movements may reveal palsies. Conjunctival and scleral examination will give clues to systemic diseases by noticing signs such as jaundice, paleness of the tarsal conjunctiva in anemic patients, subconjunctival hemorrhages in patients with bleeding tendencies, or blood sludging in the conjunctival vessels in patients with hyperviscosity syndromes. Congestion of the conjunctival vessels is seen in conjunctivitis, conjunctival chemosis or edema in allergies, and characteristic changes in conjunctival vessels in patients with sickle cell anemia, diabetes, and acquired immunodeficiency syndrome (AIDS). Gross corneal examination may reveal crystalline deposits such as calcium or copper. The clarity of the lens and vitreous cavity can be assessed through an undilated pupil. Important structures of the posterior segment such as the optic nerve, macula, and the major arcades and some of their branches are easily visualized using a handheld ophthalmoscope.

Narrowing and tortuosity of the arteries, arteriolar sclerosis, congestion and tortuosity of the veins, and arterial-venous (AV) crossing changes reflect disease processes such as hypertension, anemia, diabetes, and vasculopathies, among others. Most of the findings detectable on fundoscopic examination are nonspecific, as the tissues of the eye can only react in a small number of ways. It is the pattern of the findings, specific for various diseases, that provide clues to different systemic conditions.

NONSPECIFIC SIGNS

Cotton-wool spots, hard exudates, and intraretinal hemorrhages are the most common nonspecific manifestations of retinopathy. All of these findings can be seen in disease processes such as diabetes, hypertension, venous stasis, and collagenoses.

Cotton-wool spots result from swelling of nerve fibers in areas of microinfarcts owing to obstructed precapillary arterioles. They appear as small fluffy white lesions that may obscure the retinal blood vessels (Fig. 6.1).

Hard exudates are visualized as punctate yellowish spots resulting from conditions that produce leaky blood vessels (Fig. 6.2).

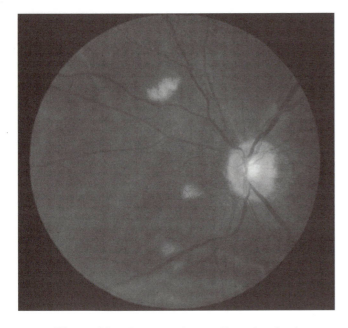

Figure 6.1.   Cotton-wool spots. (See color plate.)

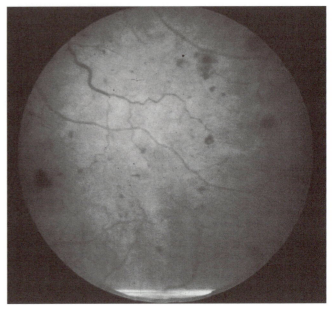

Figure 6.3.   Intraretinal hemorrhages. (See color plate.)

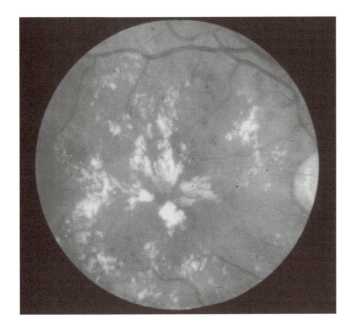

Figure 6.2.   Hard exudates. (See color plate.)

Figure 6.4.   Neovascularization of the disc (NVD). (See color plate.)

Hemorrhages may be intraretinal or extraretinal extravasation of blood. Intraretinal hemorrhages may be flame shaped when present in the nerve fiber layer or dot shaped if in the outer plexiform layer (Fig. 6.3).

Abnormal blood vessels proliferate into the vitreous cavity in those disorders such as diabetes that lead to retinal ischemia. The vascular proliferation in diabetes is typically on the optic nerve head (neovascularization of the disc, or NVD, Fig. 6.4) or may be present elsewhere (neovascularization elsewhere, NVE, Fig. 6.5) but is usually along blood vessels in the posterior pole. These new vessels tend to leak serum and blood elements.

Papilledema refers to swelling of the optic nerve head in patients with increased intracranial pressure; it is associated with stasis rather than inflammation. Swelling of the optic nerve associated with inflammation is called papillitis and is differentiated from papilledema by a reduction in vision.

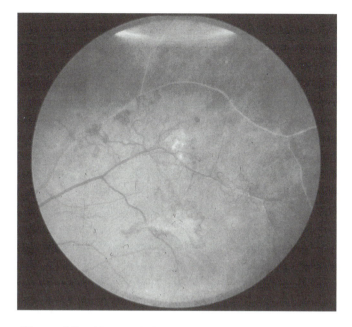

Figure 6.5. Neovascularization elsewhere (NVE). (See color plate.)

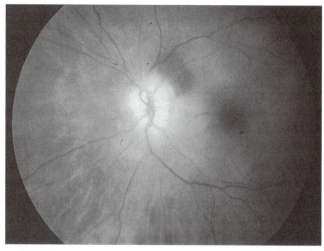

Figure 6.6. Pallid optic nerve edema in giant cell arteritis. (See color plate.)

Papilledema does not cause reduction in vision unless it has been longstanding.

OCULAR SIGNS OF SPECIFIC CONDITIONS

GIANT CELL ARTERITIS

Giant cell arteritis (GCA) is a systemic vasculitis that affects people over 60 years of age with increasing prevalence in each subsequent decade. The arteritis consists of cellular infiltration by multinucleated giant cells and a breakdown of the internal elastic lamina; at a minimum, the demonstration of epithelioid cells and a ruptured elastica are needed for diagnosis of GCA.

GCA may present with sudden loss of vision or diplopia. Patients may have systemic symptoms such as headache, arthralgias, myalgias, fever, weight loss, anemia, and depression prior to loss of vision. Sudden loss of vision is attributed to the involvement of the posterior ciliary blood vessel supply to the optic nerve leading to an anterior ischemic optic neuropathy. Ophthalmoscopy will disclose typical pallid edema of the optic nerve head (Fig. 6.6).

Oral corticosteroid should be started immediately, prednisone 60–100 mg daily, as soon as the patient is suspected of having GCA. A biopsy should be scheduled within the next few days. Several studies have demonstrated that the biopsy remains positive for at least 3 weeks even with appropriate corticosteroid treatment. Therapy is started immediately to prevent further vascular occlusions such as loss of vision in the other eye. Response to therapy and tapering of corticosteroids are guided by the erythrocyte sedimentation rate, which should be kept below 30 mm.

HYPERTENSION

Hypertensive retinopathy may develop through several stages, but in severe hypertension these stages may not be detected because of the accelerated nature of the hypertensive retinopathy. Following are the stages of hypertensive retinopathy:

1. Vasoconstrictive phase
2. Sclerotic phase
3. Exudative phase
4. Complications of the sclerotic phase

In the vasoconstrictive phase, the elevated blood pressure causes the retinal arteries to increase their tone by autoregulation. The arteries may be narrowed and irregular. The primary site of vasoconstriction is the precapillary arteriole, and vasoconstriction is most prominent in the second-order and third-order arteries. Persistent elevation in blood pressure leads to hyalinization of the blood vessels, leading to a change in the light reflex of the vessel wall; arterial-venous crossing changes develop, and the arteries become more tortuous. In the exudative phase, flame-shaped hemorrhages develop from damaged blood vessel walls; cotton-wool spots or microinfarcts develop from closure of the precapillary arterioles.

MALIGNANT HYPERTENSION

Malignant hypertension is characterized by papilledema and large numbers of flame-shaped hemorrhages and cotton-wool spots in the peripapillary area and posterior pole (Fig. 6.7). Malignant hypertension is a medical emergency, but care must

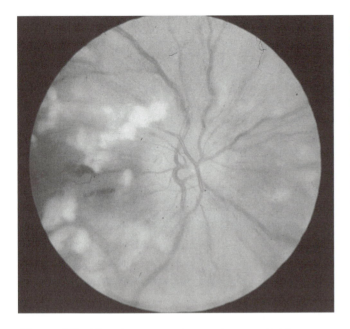

Figure 6.7.   The edematous optic nerve is surrounded by cotton-wool spots and intraretinal hemorrhages in malignant hypertension. (See color plate.)

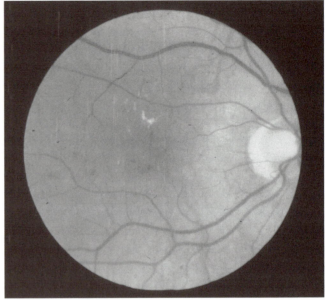

Figure 6.8.   Background diabetic retinopathy consisting of dot hemorrhages and hard exudates. (See color plate.)

be taken not to decrease the systemic blood pressure too rapidly, as this may lead to infarction of the optic nerve.

DIABETIC RETINOPATHY

Diabetic retinopathy is the leading cause of blindness in patients under 65 years of age. The onset of diabetic retinopathy varies with the type of diabetes. In Type I diabetes, there is a delay of approximately 5 years between the diagnosis of diabetes and the onset of retinopathy. In Type II diabetes, the retinopathy may be present at the time of diagnosis. Patients with diabetes should be referred to an ophthalmologist for proper detection and care.

Retinal hemorrhages and hard exudates are not peculiar to diabetes, but their distribution and relative proportions lead to the highly characteristic and essentially pathognomonic appearance in patients with diabetes. The hemorrhages and exudates are usually confined to the posterior pole, bounded by the superior and inferior temporal vessels (Fig. 6.8).

Fluorescein angiography is necessary to identify areas of precapillary closure and capillary nonperfusion (Fig. 6.9). Clinically, areas of capillary nonperfusion may have overlying cotton-wool spots. Patients with extensive capillary closure are at high risk for development of proliferative diabetic retinopathy. Diabetic patients who are noted to have cotton-wool spots should be monitored closely for the development of neovascularization or proliferative diabetic retinopathy. Neovascularization of the disc or of blood vessels elsewhere in the posterior pole characterize the proliferative stage. Panretinal laser photocoagulation is indicated in these patients.

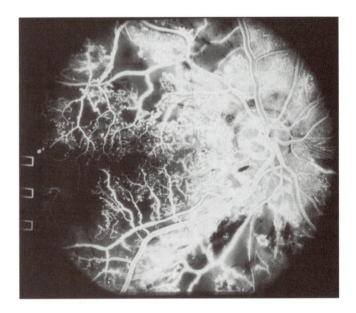

Figure 6.9.   Fluorescein angiogram reveals areas of capillary nonperfusion.

RETINAL ARTERY OCCLUSION

Patients with central retinal artery occlusion have sudden loss of vision. Examination will reveal markedly narrow arteries with box-car segmentation. The retina is opacified with a cherry-red spot in the macular area (Fig. 6.10). Central retinal artery occlusion is a true medical emergency, and prompt intervention is necessary to restore blood flow. The usual site of obstruction is at the lamina cribrosa, the sieve-like membrane at the optic nerve head. This is the location where the

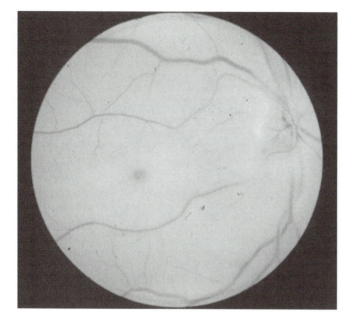

Figure 6.10. The retina is edematous and there is a cherry-red spot in the macula of a patient with central retinal artery occlusion. (See color plate.)

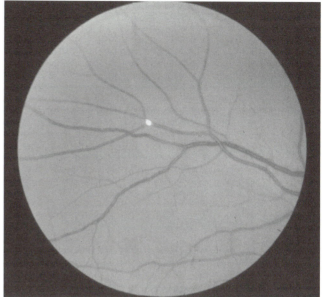

Figure 6.11. Hollenhorst plaque. (See color plate.)

periarterial fibrous membrane becomes a mechanical barrier to expansion of the artery. Digital massage over closed lids after instillation of antihypertensive drops such as a beta blocker (timolol 0.5%) or an alpha-adrenergic agonist (alphagan) should be performed immediately to decrease the intraocular pressure. Systemic medications such as a carbonic anhydrase inhibitor may also be given to the patient. Lowering the intraocular pressure may dislodge emboli and improve circulation. Visual loss is permanent if the circulation is not restored within 90 minutes.

Atheromata and emboli are the most common causes of artery obstruction. The emboli may consist of calcific vegetations that originate from valvular disease of the heart, or they may be particles from atheromatous plaques found in the carotid artery or aorta. Calcific emboli are mat white and non-scintillating, in contrast to lipid emboli, which appear yellowish and scintillating (Fig. 6.11). Lipid emboli usually originate in an atheroma of a stenotic carotid artery. Usually multiple lipid emboli may be seen clinically, and they tend to lodge at the bifurcations of the retinal arteries. These emboli are responsible for transient ischemic attacks. Platelet-fibrin emboli cause transient blindness and usually occur after myocardial infarction. Platelet-fibrin emboli are abolished with aspirin intake.

WEGENER'S GRANULOMATOSIS

Wegener's granulomatosis is a necrotizing vasculitis of small arteries and veins associated with granuloma formation. About 95% of patients have respiratory tract disease; 85%

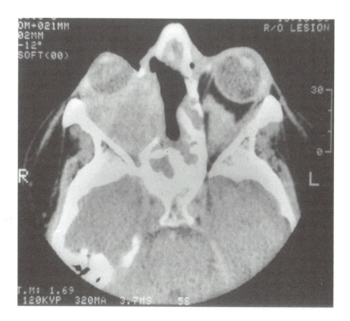

Figure 6.12. Computed tomography reveals involvement of the paranasal sinuses and orbits in a patient with Wegener's granulomatosis.

may have renal disease. Eye, adnexal, and orbital involvement are present in 50% of patients. Virtually any vascularized part of the eye may be involved. Orbital disease is the most common ophthalmic manifestation of Wegener's granulomatosis and is usually secondary to nasal or paranasal sinus disease (Fig. 6.12). Orbital disease presents with pain, tenderness, limited extraocular movement, and proptosis. Optic nerve compression is the usual cause of blindness.

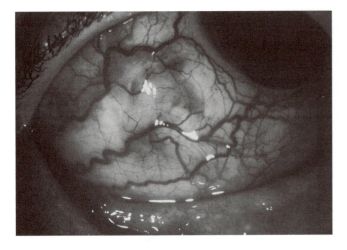

Figure 6.13. Avascularity of the sclera leads to scleromalacia in a patient with rheumatoid arthritis. (See color plate.)

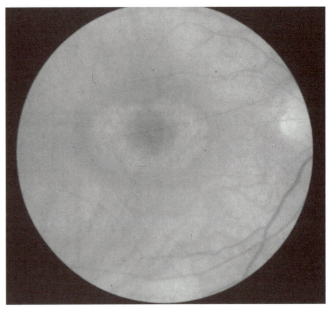

Figure 6.14. Bull's eye of hydroxychloroquine pigmentary maculopathy. (See color plate.)

RHEUMATOID ARTHRITIS

The most common ocular problem in patients with rheumatoid arthritis is keratoconjunctivitis sicca or secondary Sjogren's syndrome associated with connective tissue disease. Dry eyes occur in 11–13% of patients. The lacrimal and salivary glands are infiltrated by lymphocytes, leading to glandular destruction with loss of tear and saliva production. Dry eyes should be treated with frequent instillation of tears or bland ointment to prevent corneal opacification and melting.

Scleritis is the second most common ocular finding, occurring in 1–6% of patients with rheumatoid arthritis. The scleritis may be anterior, posterior, or necrotizing. Necrotizing scleritis has poor prognosis because it is usually associated with systemic vasculitis (Fig. 6.13). Scleritis requires systemic treatment with nonsteroidal antiinflammatory agents in addition to topical corticosteroids. In severe cases, systemic corticosteroids and immunosuppressive drugs may be necessary.

Posterior segment lesions due to rheumatoid arthritis are rare. Probably the most common reason for a dilated eye examination in patients with rheumatoid arthritis is to screen for antimalarial drug toxicity. Hydroxychloroquine is accumulated in pigmented tissues such as the retinal pigment epithelium and may cause a bull's eye pigmentary maculopathy (Fig. 6.14). The retinopathy may be reversible if discovered early but is irreversible and even progressive despite discontinuation of the drug if not detected early. The frequency of retinopathy is less than 5% when dosages of less than 6.5 mg/kg/day of hydroxychloroquine are used (less than 400 mg/day).

HLA-B27-ASSOCIATED UVEITIS

Over 50% of acute anterior uveitis (iritis or iridocyclitis) is associated with the HLA-B27 antigen. In patients who have

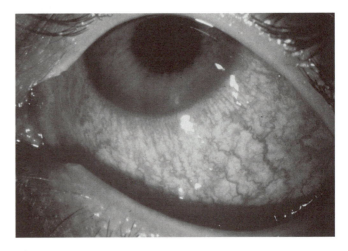

Figure 6.15. Marked conjunctival injection and ciliary flush in acute iritis. (See color plate.)

recurrent, unilateral, or acute attacks of iritis that alternate between the eyes, almost 90% of patients have the HLA-B27 antigen. The iritis is characterized by severe pain, redness, and photophobia. Clinically, there is marked conjunctival injection and ciliary flush (Fig. 6.15). The cornea may be hazy, and fibrinous exudates or a hypopyon may be present. The anterior lens surface may be obscured by fibrin (Fig. 6.16). All of the findings may be visualized using a direct ophthalmoscope. Both men and women may be affected, and approximately 50% of patients have an associated seronegative spondyloarthropathy. The most commonly associated sys-

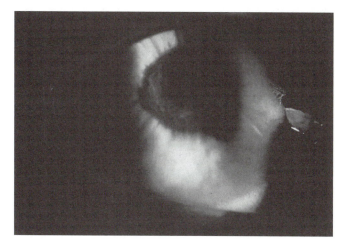

Figure 6.16. The anterior lens capsule is covered by a fibrinous exudate in a patient with HLA-B27-associated acute iritis. (See color plate.)

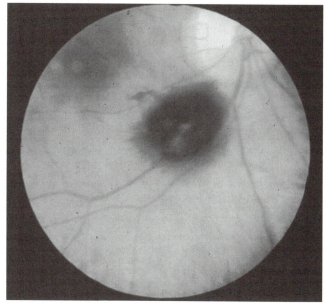

Figure 6.18. Leukemic retinopathy characterized by intraretinal and preretinal hemorrhages. (See color plate.)

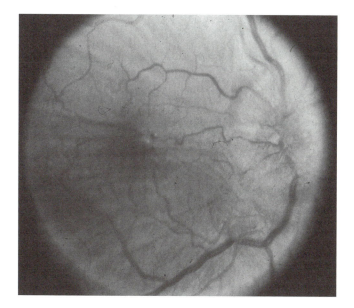

Figure 6.17. Fundus photographs show a swollen optic nerve and choroidal folds secondary to compression by enlarged muscles in a patient with thyroid optic neuropathy. (See color plate.)

temic diseases are ankylosing spondylitis, Reiter's syndrome, psoriatic arthritis, and inflammatory bowel disease.

THYROID EYE DISEASE

Thyroid-related immune orbitopathy (Graves' orbitopathy, dysthyroid ophthalmopathy, thyroid eye disease) is the most common cause of unilateral or bilateral proptosis in adults. Thyroid eye disease usually occurs between the ages of 25 and 50. Findings include proptosis, eyelid retraction and lagophthalmos, and restriction of extraocular muscles resulting

in diplopia. The signs may occur alone or all at the same time. Compression of the optic nerve as a result of extraocular muscle enlargement is sight threatening and should be looked for in every thyroid patient (Fig. 6.17). Formal visual field tests will reveal scotomas in patients with thyroid optic neuropathy.

The clinical course of thyroid eye disease does not usually follow a linear progression in severity. Patients may have acute episodes characterized by edema and swelling of the tissues, followed by resolution and scarring. Swelling of the extraocular muscles causes diplopia. The patient, however, should not have corrective strabismus surgery until the inflammatory process has subsided and stabilized with the development of scarring.

LEUKEMIA

Ocular involvement in leukemia varies in different series from a prevalence of 28–82% in an autopsy series. Leukemic infiltrates may be seen in the iris, retina, choroid, and optic nerve. Leukemic cells invading the anterior chamber mimic iritis, and in the vitreous, vitreitis.

Leukemic retinopathy refers to the ocular findings in patients with leukemia who are suffering with anemia, thrombocytopenia, or increased blood viscosity. Hemorrhages may present as blots, dots, and flame shapes with or without white centers. The hemorrhage may spill into the vitreous. Cotton-wool spots also are commonly seen. Hyperviscosity of the blood may lead to vein occlusions, microaneurysms, retinal hemorrhages, and neovascularization (Fig. 6.18).

ACQUIRED IMMUNODEFICENCY SYNDROME (AIDS)

The most common ocular manifestation in AIDS is the cotton-wool spot, a nonspecific finding seen in many other diseases. Infections of every ocular structure by unusual organisms have been reported in patients with AIDS. The most common and sight-threatening ocular infection is cytomegalovirus (CMV) retinitis (Fig. 6.19), which affects 20–35% of patients with AIDS and 30–40% of patients with a CD4 + cell count under 50/uL. Treatment of CMV retinitis with currently available antiviral agents such as ganciclovir, foscarnet, and cidofovir requires close collaboration between the ophthalmologist and the internist.

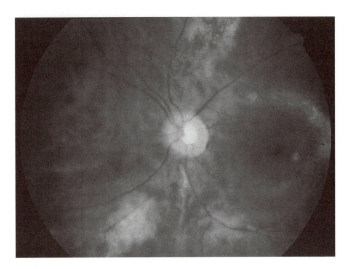

Figure 6.19. Cytomegalovirus retinitis in a patient with AIDS. (See color plate.)

SUGGESTED READINGS

Boskovich SA, Lowder CY, Meisler DM, Gutman FA. Systemic diseases associated with intermediate uveitis. Cleve Clin J Med 1993;60:460–465.

Diabetes Control and Complications Trial Research Group. Progression of retinopathy with intensive versus conventional treatment in the diabetes control and complications trial. Ophthalmology 1995;102:647–661.

Diabetes Control and Complications Trial Research Group. The effect of intensive diabetes treatment on the progression of diabetic retinopathy in insulin-dependent diabetes mellitus. Arch Ophthalmol 1995;113:36–51.

Ernst BB, Lowder CY, Meisler DM, Gutman FA. Posterior segment manifestations of inflammatory bowel disease. Ophthalmology 1991;98:1272–1280.

Fauci AS, Haynes BF, Katz P, Wolff SM. Wegener's granulomatosis: prospective clinical and therapeutic experience with 85 patients for 21 years. Ann Intern Med 1983;98:76–85.

Foster RE, Lowder CY, Meisler DM, Huang S, Longworth DL. *Pneumocystis carinii* choroiditis. Ophthalmology 1991; 98:1360–1365.

Freeman WR, et al. Risks factors for development of rhegmatogenous retinal detachment in patients with CMV retinitis. Am J Ophthalmol 1993;116:713–720.

Holland GN, Levinson RD, Jacobson MA, AIDS Clinical Trials Group. Dose-related difference in progression rates of CMV retinopathy during foscarnet maintenance therapy. Am J Ophthalmol 1995;119:576–86.

Holland GN, et al. Ocular toxoplasmosis in patients with AIDS. Am J Ophthalmol 1988;106:653–657.

Pepose J, Wilhelmus K, Holland GN, eds. Ocular Infection and Immunity. St Louis: Mosby-Yearbook, 1995.

Johnson MW, Vine AK. Hydroxychloroquine therapy in massive total doses without retinal toxicity. Am J Ophthalmol 1987;104:139–144.

Keltner JL. Giant cell arteritis; signs and symptoms. Ophthalmology 1982;89:1101–1110.

Kishi S, Tso MO, Hayreh SS. Fundus lesions in malignant hypertension. Arch Ophthalmol 1985;103:1198–1206.

Laties AM. Central retinal artery innervation; absence of adrenergic innervation to the intraocular branches. Arch Ophthalmol 1967;77:405–409.

Lowder CY, Meisler DM, McMahon JT, Longworth DL, Rutherford I. *Microsporidia* infection of the cornea in a man seropositive for human immunodeficiency virus. Am J Ophthalmol 1990;109:242–244.

Lowder CY, Butler CP, Dodds EM, Secic M, Recillas-Gispert C. CD8 + T-lymphocytes and CMV retinitis in patients with AIDS. Am J Ophthalmol 1995;120:283–290.

Margolis TP, Lowder CY, Holland G, Spaide RF, Logan AG, Weissman SS, Irvine AR, Josephberg R, Meisler DM, O'Donnell JJ. Varicella zoster virus retinitis in patients with the acquired immunodeficiency syndrome. Am J Ophthalmol 1991; 112:119–131.

Mizen TR. Giant cell arteritis: diagnostic and therapeutic considerations. Ophthalmol Clin North Am 1991;4:547–556.

Moss SE, et al. Ocular factors in the incidence and progression of diabetic retinopathy. Ophthalmology 1994;101:77–83.

Studies of the Ocular Complications of AIDS Group. Foscarnet-ganciclovir cytomegalovirus retinitis trial: 4. Visual outcomes. Ophthalmology 1994;101:1250–1261.

Tay-Kearney ML, Schwam BL, Lowder C, Dunn JP, Meisler DM, Vitale S, Jabs DA. Clinical features and associated systemic diseases of HLA-B27 uveitis. Am J Ophthalmol 1996; 121:47–56.

Tso MO, Jampol LM. Pathophysiology of hypertensive retinopathy. Ophthalmology 1982;89:1132–1145.

Tso MO, Kurosawa A, Benhamou E, et al. Microangiopathic retinopathy in experimental diabetic monkeys. Trans Am Ophthalmol Soc 1988;86:389–421.

Preoperative Evaluation and Management Before Major Noncardiac Surgery

David L. Bronson

Each year more than 28 million adults undergo noncardiac surgical procedures, of whom 1 million have known coronary artery disease, 2–3 million have known cardiac risk factors, and more than 4 million are 65 or more years old. Of the 1 million patients with cardiac complications associated with surgery, more than 80% are in these groups, with a similar number of pulmonary complications. In addition to the assessment of cardiac risk, the internist must assess all risks and intervene or recommend actions to reduce the potential medical complications of anesthesia and surgery. Effective preoperative internal medicine consultation depends on the internist understanding the issues faced by anesthesiologists and surgeons in planning and performing a surgical procedure and on communicating clear strategies to maximize the patient's medical status.

Perioperative risks the internist can help reduce fall into three major categories: patient-specific, procedure-specific, and anesthesia-specific risks. Patient-specific risks refer to the many interdependent variables that define the patient and the patient's surgical indications and comorbid diseases. These factors include age, race, gender, nutritional status, level of fitness, and comorbid diseases. The American Society of Anesthesiologists (ASA) Physical Status Scale (Table 7.1) roughly classifies patients into groups correlated with overall and anesthesia specific risk. It is a useful tool to quickly define a patient's risk, but it does not consider procedure-specific issues. The death rate from anesthesia in healthy patients in class I and class II is 1 in 200,000. In emergency surgery, anesthetic and surgical mortality double for classes I, II, and III.

The risk of a specific procedure is proportional to the physiological stress associated with the procedure. Procedures associated with higher levels of risk include the following:

• Thoracic surgery

• Major joint replacement
• Craniotomy
• Cardiac procedures
• Large bowel surgery
• Exploratory laparotomies

Low levels of risk are associated with plastic surgical procedures, tubal ligation, D & C, hysterectomy, eye and oral surgery, and herniorrhaphy.

Anesthesia-specific risks involve the direct and indirect effects of anesthetic agents and the physiologic responses to surgical-induced hypotension, blood loss, anemia, and postoperative pain. During anesthesia induction, tachycardia and hypertension occur in response to anxiety and the mechanical effects of tracheal manipulation with intubation. Ten percent of cardiac events occur during this time. Later, hypotension may occur as a result of vasodilation and myocardial depression associated with anesthetic agents, intermittent positive pressure ventilation, hemorrhage, or infection. Balanced anesthetic techniques using opiates, sedative hypnotics, neuromuscular blockers, and inhalation agents cause fewer cardiovascular effects than with inhalation agents alone. Newer inhalation agents such as isoflurane produce less myocardial depression than older agents. Most anesthetic deaths are due to failure to ventilate adequately, unsuspected hypoxia, or anesthetic agent overdose. The risk of anesthesia has lessened dramatically in recent years. It has not yet been established that any one method of anesthesia is safer than another when used properly, and the skill of modern practicing anesthesiologists is generally excellent in managing these issues. It is a common misconception that spinal anesthesia is safer than general anesthetic agents. From a cardiac perspective, spinal anesthesia is associated with wider variations in blood pressure with more difficult physiologic management and lack of airway or ventilatory control.

Table 7.1. ASA Physical Status Scale

ASA Class	Definition	7-day Mortality
Class I	No organic or psychiatric disease	0.07%
Class II	Mild to moderate systemic disturbance	0.20%
Class III	Severe systemic disturbance, but not necessarily life-threatening	1.15%
Class IV	Severe systemic disturbance; life-threatening	7.66%
Class V	Moribund with little chance of survival	33.58%

CARDIOVASCULAR COMPLICATIONS

Cardiac events are among the most important complications of noncardiac surgery. The most common cardiovascular complications are the following:

- Perioperative acute ischemia and myocardial infarction (MI)
- Congestive heart failure
- Arrhythmias
- Hypotension
- Hypertension

In the early postoperative period, pain, hypertension, and increased catecholamines with associated tachycardia may lead to cardiovascular stress by increasing myocardial oxygen demand and coronary vascular tone. The catecholamine effects may also increase plaque instability and, with enhanced platelet aggregation and hypercoagulability owing to tissue injury, elevate the risk of coronary thrombosis. Limited cardiovascular reserve, particularly in the elderly, increases the risk of a cardiac event. The incidence of myocardial infarctions peaks on the third postoperative day, and increased risk persists for up to 6 months following the surgery. The greatest risk for acute pulmonary edema is in those patients with known congestive heart failure; this risk occurs especially in the first few hours after anesthesia when anesthesia-induced hypotension abates and fluid resorption is most vigorous.

The major predictors of cardiac events are active ischemic disease and left ventricular function. The Goldman index of cardiac risk assessment (Table 7.2) is a useful instrument for assessing cardiac risk in a multivariate model, primarily because of its ease of use and relative weighting of risk factors. However, it has several limitations. First, it was developed from a data set in the mid 1970s and therefore does not reflect more recent practices in anesthesia, medicine, or surgery. Second, it may not fairly represent the pretest probabilities of events for other institutions, other surgical teams at the same

Table 7.2. Goldman Index of Cardiac Risk Assessment

Goldman Multifactorial Index	Points
History	
MI within 6 mos	10
Age > 70 yrs	5
Physical Exam	
S-3 or JVD	11
Important AS	3
Electrocardiogram	
Rhythm other than sinus or sinus & APCs on last preop ECG	7
>5 PVCs/min anytime preop	7
Poor general medical status[a]	3
Intraperitoneal, intrathoracic or aortic surgery	3
Emergency Operation	4

[a] $pO_2 < 60$ mm Hg; $pCO_2 > 50$ mm Hg; K < 3.0 meq/L; $HCO_3 < 20$ meq/L; BUN > 50, Cr > 3.0; abnormal SGOT; signs of chronic liver disease; bedridden from noncardiac causes.

	Cardiac Risk Index	
Class (Points)	Life-threatening Complications	Cardiac Deaths
I (0–5)	0.7%	0.2%
II (6–12)	5%	2%
III (13–25)	11%	2%
IV (26 or higher)	22%	56%

Reprinted with permission from Goldman L, Caldera DL, Nussbaum SR, Southwick FS, Krogstad D, Murray B, Burke CH, Nolan J, Carabello B, Slater EF. Multifactorial index of cardiac risk in noncardiac surgical procedures. N Engl J Med 1977;297:845–850.

institution, or specific surgical procedures. Third, the level of risk for patients in class IV is higher than has been found at most institutions. Fourth, the data set included relatively few vascular surgical patients, who have been shown to have a higher event rate in classes I to III. Finally, although this index is useful in predicting risk, its sensitivity is relatively low, and important disease can be missed. The performance of the Multifactorial Cardiac Risk Index is shown in Table 7.3.

The major concern for perioperative management of the patient with a history of ischemic heart disease is cardiovascular instability, particularly intraoperative hypotension and/or congestive heart failure (CHF). These events predispose the patient to perioperative myocardial infarction or other significant cardiac events. More recently, coronary plaque instability owing to perioperative catecholamine release has been postulated as a mechanism of perioperative ischemic events. Arrhythmias are of concern if they are new in onset or otherwise likely to cause or contribute to hypotension.

An MI within 6 months preceding surgery carries a signif-

Table 7.3. Multifactorial Cardiac Risk Index Death and Major Complication Rate

Patient	Class I	Class II	Class III	Class IV
Goldman (1977) > 40 yrs	5/537 (1%)	21/316 (7%)	18/130 (14%)	14/18 (78%)
Zeldin (1984) > 40 yrs	4/590 (1%)	13/453 (3%)	11/74 (15%)	7/23 (30%)
Detsky (1986) Preop consults	8/134 (6%)	6/85 (7%)	9/45 (20%)	4/4 (100%)
Pooled Data —	17/1265 (1.3%)	40/854 (4.7%)	38/249 (15.2%)	24/45 (56%)

icant risk of perioperative infarction, although contemporary anesthetic technique emphasizing careful monitoring and hemodynamic intervention have lowered this risk considerably. For elective procedures, there is a 5.8% rate of MI for 0–3 months after surgery, a rate of 2.3% after 3–6 months, and a rate of 1.3% after 6 months or more (Rao 1983) For urgent and emergency procedures, there is a 16.7% rate of MI or cardiac death for 0–3 months after surgery (Shah 1990) However, these risk assessments were prior to the era of assessment of residual ischemia risk after an MI and may not apply to patients who have no evidence of active ischemia on noninvasive testing 6 weeks after an MI. Nonetheless, elective procedures should usually be delayed, or if they are essential, preoperative thallium or echocardiographic stress testing should be undertaken. Invasive monitoring should be considered to minimize cardiovascular instability, depending on the planned procedure and the individual's risk. A poorly functioning left ventricle (LVEF below 30%) necessitates monitoring for most procedures associated with significant physiologic stress.

In a study of consecutive noncardiac surgical procedures in 1,487 men over 40 years old scheduled for major elective or urgent noncardiac surgery, Ashton and colleagues found that risk could be stratified by the history, physical examination, and baseline electrocardiogram (ECG)(2). High-risk patients were those with known coronary disease (i.e., history of MI, old MI by ECG, typical angina, coronary artery bypass graft [CABG], or angiographic coronary artery disease [CAD] with greater than 70% stenosis) and had a 4.1% rate of MI and a 2.3% rate of cardiac death. Intermediate-risk patients had other vascular disease without known CAD or had atypical chest pain syndromes. These patients had a 0.8% rate of MI and 0.4% rate of cardiac death. The low-risk group had no known atherosclerosis but were older than 75 years or were classified as high risk per the Framingham instrument (greater than 15% event rate in 6 years). None had MIs, and there was only a 0.4% cardiac death rate. In the negligible-risk group, there was no atherosclerosis, a low-risk profile, and no cardiac deaths. It is apparent from the above data that even in the high-risk group, the event rate is low. This is further supported by the findings of the CASS study, which showed that medically managed post-MI patients with mild or no symptoms

undergoing elective noncardiac surgery had a cardiac mortality rate of only 1.3%. Chronic stable angina can be managed medically in the perioperative period, but unstable angina requires intervention prior to surgery. Climbing two flights of stairs without angina or significant dyspnea implies adequate cardiopulmonary reserve. Patients in Canadian Cardiovascular Society Angina class I or II generally require no further intervention, whereas patients with higher levels of angina should receive consideration for surgical intervention or PTCA, independent of the planned surgical procedure and prior to it. Those patients less than 70 years old, without a history of MI or angina, significant Q waves on ECG, ventricular arrhythmias, or an S_3 or other evidence of CHF are at low risk and need no additional testing.

The use of noninvasive cardiac testing has exploded in recent years. The role of testing in those with multiple risk factors but no evidence of disease remains uncertain, and recent studies by Mangano, Baron, Seeger, and Fleisher question the value of dipyridamole-thallium stress testing in improving outcomes (3, 10, 16, 21). Like many interventions, the initial enthusiasm has been tempered by the reality that in usual clinical settings, the testing performs less well than first reported. In Seeger's study, those patients having preoperative stress thallium testing and coronary intervention had an 11.6% rate of serious cardiac events, compared to an 11.1% rate in a comparable group having preoperative clinical evaluation only (21). The performance of dipyridamole-thallium stress testing in several studies is shown in Table 7.4.

When needed, the selection of a noninvasive testing approach largely depends on local experience and availability. Dobutamine stress ECG has some advantages over other techniques. First, it measures both left ventricular function and the potential for ischemia, the major determinants of cardiac risk. Second, it is physiologic in reproducing the increased myocardial oxygen demand of perioperative ischemia. Additionally, it can detect unsuspected or underappreciated valvular heart disease. However, it is not available in all centers, and its interpretation can be rather subjective. The predictive value of stress echocardiography from several studies is shown in Table 7.5. Still, the presence of preoperative ischemia on holter, dipyridamole-thallium, or stress ECG seems to define a risk for serious cardiac events of 9–38% and a

Table 7.4.   Dipyridamole Thallium Stress Testing in Vascular Surgery Patients Predictive Value of Known Cardiac Events

Study	No. of Patients	PV +	PV − (normal test)
Boucher 1985	48	8/16 (50%)	32/32 (100%)
Eagle 1989	200	25/82 (30%)	113/118 (96%)
Lette 1989	66	9/27 (33%)	39/39 (100%)
Youris 1990	111	6/50 (12%)	41/41 (100%)
Mangano 1991	60	6/22 (27%)	17/20 (85%)
Baron 1994	457	31/160 (19%)	171/203 (84%)
Elliott 1991	126	9/18 (50%)	53/54 (96%)
Fleisher 1995	172	10/65 (15%)	101/107 (94%)
Pooled Data	1477	175/550 (23%)	664/713 (93%)

Table 7.5.   Pharmacologic Stress Echocardiography in Vascular Surgery Patients; Predictive Values of Serious Cardiac Events

Study	n	Stress	PV+	PV−
Tischler	109	DP	7/9 (78%)	99/100 (99%)
Marwick	67	DP	12/18 (67%)	46/49 (94%)
Lane	57	Db	4/19 (21%)	19/19 (100%)
Lalka	60	Db	10/30 (33%)	28/30 (93%)
Davila-Roman	91	Db + At	17/23 (74%)	68/68 (100%)
Poldermans	131	Db + At	15/35 (43%)	96/96 (100%)
Langan	81	Db	3/16 (19%)	31/31 (100%)
Pooled	596		68/150 (45%)	387/393 (98%)

DP, Dipyridamole; Db, Dobutamine; At, Atropine; PV +, Predictive Value Positive; PV −, Predicted Value Negative

risk of death of 1–7%, with the lower numbers reported in the last few years. Those patients at very high risk may be referred directly for coronary angiography and intervention prior to the desired procedure if the risk of the planned procedure is greater than the risk of a staged intervention (catheterization, CABG, or angioplasty) and the planned procedure. However, this is a rare event.

There is a growing shift of emphasis in the evaluation and management of the higher-risk patient. Mangano and colleagues recently reported a randomized controlled trial of the use of atenolol in patients with known CAD or at high risk for CAD prior to major noncardiac surgery (17). They found that the use of atenolol was associated with a markedly reduced 6-month mortality rate of 1% compared to 9% in the control group. This is the first report of a broad intervention to reduce adverse outcomes, and the literature should be followed carefully to see if this approach is generalizable.

For those patients with chronic stable angina, therapy should be intensified and further testing considered for those with low threshold symptoms. Those who clearly are at high risk, such as patients with known coronary disease evidenced

by a MI 6 months ago, or those patients at risk who cannot exercise to a level consistent with American Heart Association (AHA) functional class I or II because of dyspnea or chest discomfort, would have a high pretest probability of CAD and should be evaluated or intensively medically managed.

CHF represents a significant risk for adverse events. The presence of an S_3 or jugular venous distention denotes a severity of failure indicating added risk for cardiac death or complications. Patients with CHF have an increased risk of both pulmonary edema and acute ischemia, with events occurring in up to 25% of patients. Careful preoperative management to optimal hemodynamics decreases risk. Perioperative hemodynamic monitoring and management may lead to improved outcomes in patients with more severely impaired left ventricular function (LVEF below 30%) and higher levels of hemodynamic stress. In all circumstances, the anesthesiologist needs to be aware of left ventricular function to manage fluids and anesthetic choice appropriately. Preoperative ECG has not been found useful in managing CHF risk.

Valvular aortic stenosis is associated with an increased risk of cardiac events. When severe, aortic stenosis leads to

Table 7.6.   Guidelines for Cardiac Testing Prior to Major Noncardiac Surgery

Category	Risk for Cardiac Complications	Guidelines for Testing
No known CAD		
Men < 45 years, women < 55 years	Negligible	No further testing
Men > 45 years, women > 55 years	Negligible	Resting ECG
Known CAD		
MI < 6 months ago	High	Postpone surgery if possible; stress test; cardiac catheterization if positive
MI > 6 months ago; now asymptomatic	Low	Resting ECG
Unstable angina	High	Postpone surgery if possible; cardiac catheterization
Stable angina (moderate-to-high exercise threshold)	Low	Resting ECG and maximize therapy
Stable angina (low exercise threshold)	Medium/high	Stress test and maximize therapy
History of revascularization (now asymptomatic)	Low	Resting ECG, stress test if patient has multiple risk factors
Hypertension (BP > 110 mgHg diastolic)	High	Lower BP prior to surgery
Multiple risk factors	Medium/high	Consider stress test—medical intervention or cardiac catheterization if positive
Vascular surgery patient		
No clinical variables[a]	Low	Resting ECG
> 1 clinical variable[a]	Medium/high	Stress test—medical intervention or cardiac catheterization if positive

CAD, coronary artery disease; ECG, electrocardiogram; MI, myocardial infarction; BP, blood pressure.

[a] Eagle criteria: age > 70 yrs., Q-waves, congestive heart failure, arrhythmias requiring treatment, diabetes requiring treatment

a limited cardiac output and an inability to respond to anesthesia-induced hypotension. A Mayo Clinic series found, when this is recognized and managed carefully, a 10% incidence of intraoperative hypotension but a low risk of cardiac events. However, significant aortic stenosis requires careful assessment and often aortic valve replacement. Patients with mitral regurgitation usually tolerate anesthesia-induced hypotension well. In both disorders, antimicrobial prophylaxis is essential for most major procedures.

Hypertension can be safely managed in most circumstances. Poorly controlled blood pressure results in greater perioperative blood pressure lability, and a diastolic blood pressure over 110 mmHg indicates a higher risk of complications. Chronic antihypertensive medications can be continued in the perioperative period. Beta blockers reduce the incidence of perioperative arrhythmias. Limits of 110 mmHg for diastolic blood pressure and 180 mmHg for systolic blood pressure are appropriate points to intervene preoperatively to lower the risk, although there are many other reasons to intervene for long-term care.

Table 7.6 outlines a suggested approach to the preoperative evaluation of patients at risk for cardiovascular events.

PULMONARY COMPLICATIONS

Pulmonary complications occur in about one-third of patients in the postoperative period. Those patients with chronic ob-structive pulmonary disease (COPD), active asthma, and a current infection have the greatest risk. Upper abdominal and thoracic surgery carry the highest procedural risk. Pulmonary function testing is indicated for lung resections but is not necessary for other procedures in patients who are free of pulmonary symptoms.

The clinical history is the best screening tool, with significant dyspnea on climbing two flights of stairs deserving further testing. Patients with asthma should be free of wheezing prior to surgery. Symptomatic patients with chronic pulmonary disease should have further testing prior to most major surgical procedures, and the FEV_1 remains a good indicator of surgical risk. If the FEV_1 is greater than 2 liters, the risk of complications is low. An FEV_1 less than 1 liter is associated with a high risk of pulmonary complications and/or prolonged ventilation, whereas those patients with an FEV_1 between 1 and 2 liters have a moderately elevated risk that must be weighed against the need for the procedure. Carbon dioxide retention with pCO_2 above 45 mmHg and an FEV_1 below 500 mL are relative contraindications to most elective surgery.

Stopping smoking at least 2 months prior to surgery significantly decreases the risk of pulmonary complications from 33% to 14.5% (Warner 1989). However, stopping for as little as 24 hours will significantly reduce carbon monoxide levels and improve myocardial oxygen delivery (Pearce 1984).

Following are the American College of Physicians guidelines for situations in which preoperative spirometry is indicated (1):

1. Lung resection
2. Coronary artery bypass surgery and smoking history or dyspnea
3. Upper abdominal surgery and smoking history or dyspnea
4. Lower abdominal surgery and uncharacterized pulmonary disease, particularly if the surgery will be prolonged or extensive
5. Other surgery and uncharacterized pulmonary disease, particularly in those who might require strenuous postoperative rehabilitation programs

ENDOCRINE COMPLICATIONS

Diabetes mellitus is associated with higher levels of perioperative risk. Preoperative glucose levels greater than 300 mg% cause an osmotic diuresis, complicating volume management. Therefore, surgery usually should be delayed until the fasting glucose is less than 250 mg%. Patients with diabetes mellitus also have an 11% noncardiac and 7% cardiac complication rate. The presence of end-organ complications (nephropathy, neuropathy, or retinopathy), CHF or valvular heart disease, or peripheral vascular disease accompanied by infection predicts a higher noncardiac complication rate. In insulin-dependent diabetes mellitus, the insulin doses are generally reduced to one-third or one-half the usual morning dose prior to surgery, and the anesthesiologist will monitor glucose control intraoperatively. Oral hypoglycemic agents generally can be managed safely by holding on the day of the procedure, but chlorpropamide use risks hypoglycemia because of its unusually long half-life.

Patients who have used corticosteroids in the last 6 months may have impaired adrenal reserve and hence increased risk of adrenal insufficiency. If the patient has received a 2-week course of systemic steroids in the last 6 months, stress doses of steroids should be added to the perioperative care regimen.

OTHER COMPLICATIONS

Cirrhosis of the liver is associated with a 60% major morbidity rate and a 30% mortality rate for abdominal surgery. The presence of a coagulopathy, a higher Childs class, and infection predicts complications.

Surgery can be performed safely in most patients with renal disease, although a preoperative creatinine greater than 4.0 mg% is associated with increased morbidity in patients undergoing abdominal aortic aneurysm repair.

Delirium is a common postoperative complication associated with both higher mortality and poor functional recovery. The costs of care increase substantially when an acute confusional state complicates postoperative recovery. A recent study by Marcantonio and colleagues developed and validated a clinical prediction rule for the postoperative development of delirium (18). Independent correlates included an age over 70 years, self-reported alcohol use, poor cognitive status, poor functional status, markedly abnormal serum sodium, potassium, or glucose level, noncardiac chest surgery, and aortic abdominal surgery. The tool allows for preoperative risk stratification and potentially for interventions to reduce delirium risk. In addition to correcting preoperative metabolic abnormalities, the best intervention is to avoid psychotropic drug use and hypoxia perioperatively.

PREOPERATIVE LABORATORY STUDIES

In recent years, ample literature has shown the lack of value of most preoperative laboratory testing in otherwise healthy patients undergoing elective noncardiac surgery. In general, laboratory testing should be done only for specific indications associated with known clinical conditions or specific risks. Baseline ECGs are often useful in patients over the age of 50 years, because most cardiac events occur in this age group. Baseline chest x rays are seldom indicated in the absence of pulmonary disease or symptoms. In patients over the age of 70 years, a baseline chest x-ray may be useful for postoperative comparison purposes, again because of a higher incidence of events.

CONCLUSION

There are many medical considerations in the perioperative evaluation and management of patients having major noncardiac surgery. Careful attention to detail and optimization of the preoperative medical condition will assist the anesthesiologist and surgeon in delivering the best care. Much further work is needed to better understand the roles of noninvasive cardiac testing and prophylactic management for achieving the best outcomes.

REVIEW EXERCISES

QUESTIONS

1. A 57-year-old man presented with new-onset angina pectoris 6 months ago. He underwent coronary angiography that revealed significant stenoses of the LAD and circumflex arteries and subsequently underwent CABG surgery without complications. Since then he has completed a cardiac rehabilitation program and returned to work. He presents now for preoperative evaluation prior to elective right hemicolectomy for a newly found cancer. You recommend the following cardiac evaluation:

   a. No further testing
   b. A resting EKG
   c. A thallium stress test
   d. Cardiac catheterization

2. The peak perioperative period for ischemic cardiac events is:

   a. During anesthesia induction
   b. During the surgical procedure
   c. During anesthetic recovery
   d. During the first 3 postoperative days

3. A 60-year-old man with longstanding COPD presents for preoperative evaluation before an elective total hip replacement. He quit smoking 5 years ago. He walks 1 mile daily for exercise and can climb two flights of stairs without difficulty. His physical examination reveals mild wheezing in forced expiration but is otherwise normal. His chest x-ray shows diaphragmatic flattening. Preoperative pulmonary evaluation should include:

   a. Spirometry
   b. Pulse oximetry with exercise
   c. Arterial blood gases
   d. No further testing

4. Which risk factor is not a major contributor to postoperative pulmonary complications?

   a. Upper abdominal surgery
   b. Anesthetic time longer than 4 hours
   c. Morbid obesity
   d. Laparoscopic surgery
   e. Cigarette use over 20 packs a year

Answers

1. b

   The CASS study showed that patients who have had successful coronary revascularization return to a low baseline level of risk. This patient's risk is low, similar to noncoronary disease populations. The resting ECG to assess for interval change is the only requirement.

2. d

   The peak perioperative period for ischemic cardiac events is during the 3 postoperative days. This is primarily related to changes in coronary vascular tone, plaque rupture, and hypercoagulability. After 3 days, the level of risk drops significantly.

3. d

   This patient displays an excellent level of physical capacity. The ability to climb two flights of stairs without difficulty indicates a low level of pulmonary risk. No further testing is required.

4. d

   This answer seems obvious. The other answers are associated with impairment of diaphragmatic motion secondary to upper abdominal incisional pain or morbid obesity or are associated with the impairment of mucociliary function. Laparoscopic surgery is not totally without risk. Often, there is some level of incisional or diaphragmatic pain, although the levels of risk are relatively low compared to the other answers.

SUGGESTED READINGS

1. American College of Physicians. Preoperative pulmonary function testing. Ann Intern Med 1990;112(10):793–794.

2. Ashton CM, Petersen NJ, Wray NP, Kiefe CI, Dunn JK, Wu L, Thomas JM. The incidence of perioperative myocardial infarction in men undergoing noncardiac surgery. Ann Intern Med 1993;118:504–510.

3. Baron J, Mundler O, Bertyrand M, Vicaut E, Barre E, Godet G, Samama C, Coriat P, Kieffer E, Viars P. Dipyridamole-thallium scintigraphy and gated radionuclide angiography to assess cardiac risk before abdominal aortic surgery. N Engl J Med 1994;330:663–669.

4. Boucher CA, Brewster DC, Darling RC, Okada RD, Strauss HW, Pohost GM. Determination of cardiac risk by dipyridamole-thallium imaging before peripheral vascular surgery. N Engl J Med Feb 14, 1985;312(7):389–394.

5. Coley CM, Eagle KA. Preoperative assessment and perioperative management of cardiac ischemic risk in noncardiac surgery. Curr Probl Cardiol 1996;26:291–382.

6. Davila-Roman VG, Waggoner AD, Sicard GA, et al. Dobutamine stress echocardiography predicts surgical outcome in patients with an aortic aneurysm and peripheral vascular disease. J Am Coll Cardiol 1993;21:957.

7. Detsky AS, Abrams HB, McLaughlin JR, Drucker DJ, Sason Z, Johnston N, Scott JG, Forbath N, Hilliard JR. Predicting cardiac complications in patients undergoing noncardiac surgery. J Gen Intern Med 1986;1:211–219.

8. Eagle KA, Coley CM, Newell JB, Brewster DC, Darling RC, Strauss HW, Guiney TE, Boucher CA. Combining clinical and thallium data optimizes preoperative assessment of cardiac risk before major vascular surgery. Ann Int Med Jun 1, 1989;110(11):859–866.

9. Elliott BM, Robison JG, Zellner JL, Hendrix GH. Dobutamine-201Tl imaging. Assessing cardiac risks associated with vascular surgery. Circulation Nov 1991;84(5 Suppl):11154060.

10. Fleisher LA, Rosenbaum SH, Nelson AH, Jain D, Wackers FJ, Zaret BL. Preoperative dipyridamole thallium imaging and ambulatory electrocardiographic monitoring as a predictor of perioperative cardiac events and long-term outcome. Anesthesiology 1995;83:906–917.

11. Goldman L, Caldera DL, Nussbaum SR, Southwick FS, Krogstad D, Murray B, Burke CH, Nolan J, Carabello B, Slater EF. Multifactorial index of cardiac risk in noncardiac surgical procedures. N Engl J Med 1977;297:845–850.

12. Lalka SG, Sawada SG, Dalsiing MC, et al. Dobutamine stress echocardiography as a predictor of cardiac events associated with aortic surgery. J Vasc Surg 1992;15:831; discussion 841.

13. Lane RT, Sawada SG, Segar DS, et al. Dobutamine stress echocardiography for assessment of cardiac risk before noncardiac surgery. Am J Cardiol 1991;68:976.

14. Langan EM, Youkey JR, Franklin DP, et al. Dobutamine stress echocardiography for cardiac risk assessment before aortic surgery. J Vasc Surg 1993;18:905; discussion 912.

15. Lette J, Waters D, LaPointe J, et al. Usefulness of the severity and extent of reversible perfusion defects during thallium dipyridamole imaging for cardiac risk assessment before noncardiac surgery. Am J Cardiol 1989;64(5):276.

16. Mangano DT, London MJ, Tubau JF, Browner WS, Hollenberg M, Krupski W, Layug EL, Massie B. Dipyridamole thallium-201 scintigraphy as a preoperative screening test. A reexamination of its predictive potential. Study of Perioperative Ischemia Research Group (see comments). Circulation Aug 1991;84(2):493–502.

17. Mangano DT, Layug EL, Wallace A, Tateo T. Effect of atenolol on mortality and cardiovascular morbidity after noncardiac surgery. N Engl J Med 1996;335:1713–1720.

18. Marcantonio E, Goldman L, Mangione C, Ludwig L, Muraca B, Haslauer C, Donaldson C, Whittemore A, Sugarbaker D, Poss R, Haas S, Cook E, Orav J, Lee T. A clinical prediction rule for delirium after elective noncardiac surgery. JAMA 1994;271:134–139.

19. Marwick TM, Vincent M, D'Ondt AM. Predictions of perioperative events. Circulation 1992;86:I-790.

20. Poldermans MD, Paolo M, Fioretti MD, et al. Dobutamine stress echocardiography for assessment of perioperative cardiac risk in patients undergoing major vascular surgery. Circulation 1993;87:1506.

21. Seeger JM, Rosenthal GR, Self SB, et al. Does routine stress-thallium cardiac scanning reduce postoperative cardiac complications? Ann Surg 1994;219:654–663.

22. Tishler MD, Lee TH, Hirsch AT, et al. Prediction of major cardiac events after peripheral vascular surgery using dipyridamole echocardiography. Am J Cardiol 1991;68:593.

23. Younis LT, Aguirre F, Byers S, Dowell S, Barth G, Walker H, Carrachi B, Peterson G, Chaitman BR. Perioperative and long-term prognostic value of intravenous dipyridamole thallium scintigraphy in patients with peripheral vascular disease. Am Heart J June 1990;119(6):1287–1292.

24. Zeldin RA. Assessing cardiac risk in patients who undergo noncardiac surgical procedures. Can J Surg 1984;27:402.

Geriatric Medicine

Robert M. Palmer

The aging process predisposes elderly patients to homeostatic failure, chronic disease, and functional decline (a loss of independence in performing daily activities). Illness often manifests as a "geriatric syndrome," a clinical problem with a wide array of etiologies and complex pathophysiology. Included among these geriatric syndromes are:

- Cognitive dysfunction (altered mental status)
- Falls
- Urinary incontinence

These syndromes, which increase in frequency and importance in advanced age (over age 75 years), are frequently encountered by internists in ambulatory, hospital, and long-term care settings. Recent studies highlight the potential to accurately detect and effectively manage these common problems of old age.

COGNITIVE DYSFUNCTION: DELIRIUM

Common causes of cognitive dysfunction in elderly patients are dementia, delirium, and depression. (Dementia and depression are discussed elsewhere, but key points are included here). Delirium (acute confusion) is an organic mental syndrome characterized by:

- A reduced ability to maintain or shift attention
- Disorganized thinking
- An altered level of consciousness
- Perceptual disturbances
- Increased or decreased psychomotor activity
- Disturbances of the sleep-wake cycle
- Disorientation to time, place, or person
- Memory impairments

Typically, the disturbance in cognition develops over a short period of time (hours to days) and fluctuates throughout the day. Delirium occurring in hospitalized elderly patients often goes undetected or is misdiagnosed as dementia, depression, functional psychosis, or personality disorder. The sequelae of delirium include prolonged length of hospitalization, higher costs of care, and greater risk of institutionalization—underscoring the importance of early detection, a search for likely etiologies, and appropriate therapeutic interventions designed to prevent or rapidly resolve the syndrome of delirium.

ETIOLOGY OF DELIRIUM

Virtually any acute physical stress can precipitate delirium in vulnerable patients. Delirium is most commonly associated with:

- Infection (e.g., urosepsis or pneumonia)
- Hypoxemia
- Hypotension
- Psychoactive medications (e.g., narcotics or benzodiazepines)
- Anticholinergic medications

Other causes of delirium include:

- Alcohol withdrawal or intoxication
- Partial-complex seizures
- Stroke
- Uremia
- Electrolyte disorders (e.g., hyponatremia)

Drugs are common, but preventable, causes of delirium. Many antiarrhythmics, tricyclic antidepressants, neuroleptics, analgesics, and gastrointestinal medications can induce delirium in elderly patients. One common characteristic of many of these agents is their central anticholinergic effect.

EPIDEMIOLOGY OF DELIRIUM

Delirium occurs primarily in patients who are acutely ill or hospitalized. Among medically ill hospitalized elderly patients, the prevalence of delirium at admission is 10–15%, whereas the incidence is 5–10% during hospitalization. Postoperative delirium occurs in 10–15% of general surgical patients and in 30–50% of patients admitted to the hospital with hip fractures or to undergo knee surgery.

The risk factors for delirium have been recently elucidated in prospective cohort studies. Independent risk factors for prevalent delirium in elderly patients admitted to the hospital include:

- Dementia
- Fever
- The use of psychoactive drugs
- Azotemia
- Fracture
- Abnormal serum sodium

Dementia is the major risk factor for delirium, increasing the risk nearly threefold. Other medical conditions that are often associated with delirium include:

- Prolonged sleep deprivation
- Sensory impairments (vision and hearing)
- Changes in environment

Risk factors for incident delirium (i.e., occurring in hospitalized patients without evidence of delirium at admission) include:

- Severe illness
- Cognitive impairment (dementia)
- Visual impairment
- High blood urea nitrogen-to-creatinine ratio (implying dehydration)

Delirium that occurs in the hospital in high-risk patients is precipitated by factors that are potentially amenable to medical interventions or change in therapies. In one study, five independent precipitating or antecedent factors for delirium in the hospital were identified:

- The use of physical restraints
- Malnutrition
- More than three added medications
- The use of a bladder catheter
- Any iatrogenic event (e.g., unintentional injury or pressure ulcer)

PATHOPHYSIOLOGY OF DELIRIUM

The pathophysiology of delirium remains poorly understood. Patients with risk factors for delirium are regarded as vulnera-

ble based on the hypothetic assumption of limited homeostatic (brain) reserves. The most important unifying hypothesis is that of neurotransmitter disturbances, especially cholinergic failure; acetylcholine transmission (e.g., secondary to anticholinergic drugs with central effects) can disturb normal cognition as well. This hypothesis is supported by animal and human studies and "models" of cholinergic failure (such as Alzheimer's disease). In these cases, patients are clearly "sensitive" to the central anticholinergic effects of various drugs and may show improved cognition with acetylcholinesterase inhibitors (e.g., tacrine), which potentiate central cholinergic transmission. In some conditions, such as hepatic encephalopathy, the presence of delirium correlates with the accumulation of toxic metabolites (e.g., ammonia). Abnormalities in lymphokine elaboration, especially interleukin-1 and interleukin-2, are associated with delirium.

CLINICAL PRESENTATION OF DELIRIUM

An acute change in mental status with disturbed consciousness, impaired cognition, and fluctuating course is characteristic of delirium. A reduced ability to focus, sustain, or shift attention is evident and accounts for behavioral manifestations of incoherent or tangential speech and disorganized or erratic thought processes. Perceptual disturbances (misperceptions), illusions, or delusions and hallucinations are common, particularly in patients with increased psychomotor activity. Most often, delirium presents as a "quiet confusion" in acutely ill patients, although extremes in behavior and cognition may occur throughout the day. Delirium is often the initial symptom or a common presentation of many acute illnesses.

DIAGNOSIS OF DELIRIUM

The diagnostic evaluation of a patient with detected delirium is driven by a search for the most probable etiologies and the need to exclude life-threatening diseases. In many cases, the etiology will be obvious (e.g., urosepsis), but vigilance is needed to exclude other possible causes (e.g., hypoxemia) that may contribute to the delirium. Rarely is an extensive laboratory evaluation needed.

Because infection is so frequently the precipitant of delirium, a complete blood count and blood chemistry panel should be obtained when the etiology is uncertain. In select cases (e.g., fever, hypotension), blood and urine cultures will be warranted; likewise chest films, an electrocardiogram, arterial blood gases, lumbar puncture, head neuroimaging, or an electroencephalogram may be useful.

Screening

Even subtle cases of delirium can be detected through careful observation of the patient (change in cognition, reasoning, alertness), and the use of screening instruments such as the

Table 8.1.   Delirium Versus Dementia

Feature	Delirium	Dementia
Onset	Rapid, often at night	Usually insidious, as in Alzheimer's disease
Duration	Hours to weeks (usually transient)	Months to years (persistent)
Consciousness	Depressed	Normal
Awareness	Always impaired	Usually normal
Alertness	Reduced or increased (fluctuates)	Usually normal
Attention span	Decreased (less than 4 digits)	Usually normal (in mild to moderate states)

digit span test and the confusion assessment method (CAM). With the CAM, a diagnosis of delirium can be achieved with greater than 90% sensitivity and specificity by requiring evidence of inattention, an acute onset and a fluctuating course and either or both disorganized thinking or an altered level of consciousness.

Differential Diagnoses

Delirium should be distinguished from functional psychosis, depression, and dementia as follows:

- Functional psychosis (e.g., late-onset schizophrenia) is not characterized by impaired attention or fluctuating mental status.
- Depression is suspected in patients who give variable responses or many ''I don't know'' answers to questions during a mental status examination. A dysphoric mood, irritability, and a withdrawn appearance further suggest the diagnosis. Depressed patients are alert and attentive, although their ability to concentrate may be limited, especially in anxious or agitated patients.
- Although delirium occurs more often in demented patients, clinical features help to distinguish these conditions (Table 8.1).

TREATMENT OF DELIRIUM

The management of delirium begins with treatment of the underlying etiologies. Effective nursing and environmental interventions include:

- Continuity of nursing care
- Alternatives to physical restraints (which can paradoxically increase patient agitation)
- Correction of sensory impairments (visual and hearing)

- Placement of the patient in a room near the nurses' station for closer observation and greater socialization
- Social visits with a family member, caregiver, or hired sitter
- The promotion of normal sleep cycles through noise control, dim lighting at night, and reality orientation

Pharmacologic Treatment of Delirium

Medications are warranted for treatment of symptoms that disturb the patient or behaviors that threaten to disrupt life-maintaining therapies. For treatment of hallucinations, delusions, or frightening illusions, antipsychotic agents may be useful. Haloperidol 0.5 mg to 1.0 mg can be given orally or intramuscularly. Patients with anxiety, agitation, insomnia, or drug or alcohol withdrawal may benefit from treatment with lorazepam 0.5 mg to 1.0 mg given orally or parenterally. Delirious patients in severe pain can be treated with morphine sulfate 4–6 mg (lower doses in very old or frail patients). Repeated doses of meperidine should be avoided because of the neurotoxic effect of its metabolite.

PROGNOSIS OF DELIRIUM

Most episodes of delirium improve rapidly, usually within days of appropriate therapy. Recent studies, however, suggest that functional and cognitive deficits often persist after discharge. This is probably related to the underlying etiology or risk factors, especially dementia.

FALLS

Unintentional injury, most often attributed to falls, is the sixth leading cause of death in elderly persons. Accidental falls (unintentionally coming to rest on the ground, floor, or other lower level) occur in about one third of community-residing persons over age 65 years and account for many serious injuries, including hip fractures and soft tissue trauma. A loss of mobility or fear of falling are common consequences of a fall and contribute to the patient's inability to live independently. Recent studies have identified risk factors for falls and interventions that reduce the risk of recurrent falls.

ETIOLOGY OF FALLS

Epidemiology of Falls

The incidence of falls and related injuries increases with advancing age. About 50% of persons 80 years and older fall each year, and multiple episodes of falls are common. About 5% of falls by community-residing elderly persons result in a fracture. Falling increases the probability of hospitalization, nursing home placement, and death. About 90% of hip fractures in elderly people result from falls.

Risk factors for falling include:

- Disturbances of balance and gait
- Medications (psychoactive, cardiovascular)
- Environmental factors (e.g., poor lighting, cords, frayed rugs)
- Cognitive dysfunction

In retrospective studies, risk factors for hip fractures resulting from falls included:

- Low bone-mineral density
- Use of long-acting benzodiazepines (e.g., diazepam)
- Visual impairment
- Reduced mobility and physical independence
- Cognitive dysfunction

In a recent prospective study, independent predictors of hip fracture related to falls in very old women included lower gait speed, difficulty performing tandem gait, reduced visual acuity, and small calf circumference.

Clinical Causes of Falls

Accidents, usually associated with environmental hazards, are the most common cause of falls. Lower extremity weakness from deconditioning, stroke, and chronic diseases is the second most common cause of gait impairment leading to falls. Syncope accounts for less than 3% of falls. Dizziness, vertigo, delirium, postural hypotension, and visual disorders are less frequent causes of falls.

PATHOPHYSIOLOGY OF FALLS

The maintenance of normal balance and gait requires the successful integration of sensory (afferent), central (brain and spinal cord), and musculoskeletal systems. A disturbance in sensory input (e.g., peripheral neuropathy), central nervous system functioning (e.g., dementia), or motor function (e.g., arthritis, muscle weakness) will predispose elderly patients to falls. The aging process may predispose patients to falls by increasing postural sway and reducing adaptive reflexes.

DIAGNOSIS OF FALLS

Patients at risk for falls can be identified through:

- Medical history
- Physical examination
- Laboratory studies

A review of risk factors, medications (vasodilators, adrenergic blockers, psychotropic agents) and screening instruments (vision, mental status, balance, and gait) help to identify patients at risk. Observation of the patient is most useful as the patient stands from a chair, walks 10 feet, turns around, and returns to sit in the chair. Postural instability, weakness, poor steppage, asymmetry of gait, and unsteadiness will identify the patient in need of further evaluation.

The further diagnostic evaluation of a patient who has fallen is based on the circumstances surrounding the fall. An ambulatory cardiac monitor, for example, is indicated for the patient with syncope, unexplained lightheadedness, or palpitations preceding the fall.

TREATMENT OF FALLS

Obvious causes of falls are quickly treatable (e.g., syncope owing to complete heart block). More often, the intervention to reduce the risk of fall is multifactorial, directed at optimizing the patient's sensory, central, and musculoskeletal systems (Table 8.2).

Recent clinical trials support the effectiveness of multifactorial interventions. In a trial involving community-residing persons aged 70 and older who had risk factors for falling, an intervention that included an adjustment of medications, behavioral instructions, and an exercise program (balance exercises, gait training, low-impact resistive exercises) led to a significant reduction in the numbers of falls in the subsequent year compared to controls. Tai Chi exercises to enhance balance and body awareness when combined with balance training may also reduce the rate of falls.

The risk for falls may even be reduced in frail, nursing-home residents. In a clinical trial with nursing home residents with a mean age of over 85 years, an intervention that included progressive resistance exercise training led to a significant increase in muscle strength in the legs and increase in gait velocity. These studies support the effectiveness of measures directed at reducing the frailty of very old patients.

Table 8.2. Intervention to Decrease the Risk of Falls

Risk Factor	Intervention
Polypharmacy	Medication review: reduce or discontinue doses of psychotropic agents, vasodilators, and adrenergic blockers
Lower extremity weakness, deconditioning	Low-impact resistive exercises, high-impact-resistance exercises under therapist supervision, Tai Chi exercises, water-walking exercises, and assistive devices (e.g., cane, walker)
Hearing and visual impairment	Hearing aid and corrective lenses
Postural hypotension	Reconditioning exercises, graded compression stockings, salt repletion, and medication changes (diuretics, vasodilators)

URINARY INCONTINENCE

Urinary incontinence is the involuntary loss of urine of sufficient severity to be a social or health problem. Incontinence is a source of social embarrassment for older patients and a risk factor for institutionalization. Never a consequence of normal aging, urinary incontinence is always treatable and often curable.

EPIDEMIOLOGY OF URINARY INCONTINENCE

The prevalence of urinary incontinence in community-residing elderly increases with advancing age from 5–15% in women aged 65 years to more than 25% in men and women age 85 years and older. The prevalence of incontinence approaches 50% in nursing home residents. Urinary incontinence is strongly associated with impaired cognition and physical function. The economic costs of treating urinary incontinence and its complications exceeds $10 billion annually in the United States.

PATHOPHYSIOLOGY OF URINARY INCONTINENCE

Urinary incontinence results from neurologic or anatomic defects that interfere with normal urinary micturition. The urinary bladder is responsible for storage and emptying of urine. Lesions that interfere with bladder contraction and emptying (e.g., sensory neuropathy) predispose patients to incontinence. Parasympathetic stimulation by the sacral nerves (S2–S4) produces detrusor muscle contractions; disruption of these nerves results in an acontractile bladder. As the bladder fills, the parasympathetic system is inhibited. When intravesical pres-

sure increases (typically with bladder volumes of greater than 250 mL), inhibitory pathways from the frontal lobe are overcome and detrusor contraction is able to exceed urethral resistance to allow urinary flow from the bladder.

Contraction of the detrusor muscle at low bladder filling volumes (detrusor instability or overactivity) occurs in patients with central nervous system disease (e.g., stroke) or increased sensory stimulation from the bladder (e.g., urinary tract infection, prostatic hyperplasia). Loss of detrusor contractility or bladder outlet obstruction results in a distended bladder; intravesical pressure exceeds urethral resistance, resulting in incontinence. Incompetence of the internal urethral sphincter (e.g., secondary to pelvic relaxation) allows urine to leak from the bladder during increases in intraabdominal pressure).

CLINICAL PRESENTATIONS OF URINARY INCONTINENCE

Four basic types of urinary incontinence occur in elderly patients (Table 8.3):

- Stress incontinence
- Urge incontinence
- Overflow incontinence
- Functional incontinence

Stress incontinence is the most common type in women less than age 75 years, whereas urge incontinence is the most common type in patients older than 75 years. Stress incontinence results from sphincteric incompetence; urge incontinence results from detrusor overactivity. Overflow incontinence is seen in patients with an acontractile bladder or bladder outlet obstruction. Functional incontinence occurs

Table 8.3.   Types, Characteristics, and Treatment of Urinary Incontinence

Type	*Characteristics*	*Cause*	*Treatments*
Stress	Urinary leakage with an increase in intraabdominal pressure (cough, sneeze, physical exertion)	Sphincteric incompetence	Medical: pelvic-muscle exercises, scheduled toileting, alpha-adrenergic agonists, estrogen Surgical: bladder-neck suspension and periurethral injections
Urge	Urinary urgency and frequency, usually with small-to-moderate volume of urine	Detrusor overactivity	Bladder retraining (scheduled or prompted voiding) and anticholinergics/bladder relaxants (e.g., oxybutynin)
Overflow	Incomplete or unsuccessful voiding or continuous dribbling	Outlet obstruction or inability to toilet	Acontractile bladder: intermittent or chronic catheter drainage Obstructed outlet: surgical relief of obstruction
Functional	Inability or unwillingness to get to toilet	Physical or cognitive disability	Change treatments (e.g., loop diuretics, restraints); bedside commode or urinal, prompted voiding, and absorbent pads and garments

as a consequence of cognitive, physical, psychologic, or environmental barriers to urination (e.g., delirious patient in physical restraint). Often two or more mechanisms are operative in frail elderly patients. Patients with polyuric states (e.g., uncontrolled diabetes), gait impairments, and cognitive impairments are particularly likely to have a functional component of incontinence.

DIAGNOSIS OF URINARY INCONTINENCE

The clinical type and most likely cause of urinary incontinence can usually be determined by a careful medical history, a brief physical examination (genitourinary), and a few laboratory studies (urinalysis, blood chemistries). On occasion, urodynamic studies (e.g., cystometry) are needed to determine the diagnosis. The medical history is key to the diagnosis (see Table 8.3). A postvoid residual obtained by straight catheterization of the bladder is useful in excluding urinary retention (e.g., due to an acontractile bladder). A residual of greater than 150 mL is abnormal and indicates the need for further urologic evaluation.

TREATMENT OF URINARY INCONTINENCE

Detrusor instability often responds to behavioral therapies such as scheduled toileting and bladder retraining. Cognitively impaired patients also benefit from scheduled toileting (e.g., every 2 hours) or prompted voiding. Anticholinergic medications (e.g., oxybutynin) can suppress detrusor contractions, but side effects (e.g., constipation, dry mouth) are common.

Women with stress incontinence may benefit from pelvic muscle exercises, scheduled toileting, and pharmacologic therapies (vaginal or oral estrogens or alpha-adrenergic agonists). Surgical options include bladder-neck suspension or periurethral injections of collagen. Patients with acontractile bladders require intermittent or chronic indwelling catheterization. Bladder-outlet obstructions are usually treated surgically (e.g., transurethral prostatectomy). Functional incontinence responds to improved care giving, frequent toileting, and treatment of underlying causes. When incontinence is incurable, incontinence aids such as absorbent pads or external catheters are useful.

REVIEW EXERCISES

1. A previously well 78-year-old man is admitted to the hospital for treatment of community-acquired pneumonia. The nurses report that he is sometimes hard to arouse, quiet and withdrawn, and other times agitated, disoriented, accusatory, and inappropriate in behavior. Physical examination is unremarkable except for findings of pneumonia. The most likely cause of his change in mental status is:

   a. Alzheimer's Disease
   b. Vascular dementia
   c. Delirium
   d. Major depressive episode
   e. Late-onset schizophrenia

2. An 82-year-old woman presents with a history of urinary frequency and urgency, with leakage of moderate amounts of urine, which began after a stroke 3 months earlier. Physical examination is now normal. A postvoid residual urine is 35 mL. A chemistry panel and urinalysis are normal. The treatment most likely to improve this patient's symptoms is:

   a. Anticholinergic drug (oxybutynin)
   b. Vaginal estrogen
   c. Intermittent catheterization
   d. Bladder-neck suspension
   e. Periurethral injections

Answers

1. c

   The acute onset of change in mental status, the fluctuating course and altered level of consciousness are diagnostic of delirium. Although cognitive dysfunction is seen in Alzheimer and vascular dementias, the symptoms usually progress over a duration of months to years, and attention and level of consciousness are normal. Major depression is often accompanied by cognitive impairment, but patients are alert and attentive. Likewise, patients with late-onset schizophrenia are alert and usually have normal cognition.

2. a

   Urinary frequency and urgency with leakage of urine and small residual volumes is characteristic of urge incontinence resulting from detrusor instability. Stroke is a common cause of urge incontinence. Anticholinergic agents/bladder relaxants, including oxybutynin, may lessen the intensity of uninhibited contractions and relieve the symptoms of urge incontinence. Vaginal estrogen, bladder-neck suspension, and periurethral injections can lessen or eliminate the symptoms of stress incontinence but have less or no effect on urge incontinence. Intermittent catheterization is reserved for patients with overflow incontinence, usually due to either an acontractile bladder or bladder outlet obstruction.

SUGGESTED READINGS

Fiatarone MA, O'Neill EG, Ryan ND, et al. Exercise training and nutritional supplementation for physical frailty. N Engl J Med 1994;330:1769–1775. (*High-intensity resistance exercise training increases muscle strength and gait velocity in very elderly people.*)

Dargent-Molina P, Favier F, Grandjean H, et al. Fall-related factors and risk of hip fracture: the EPIDOS prospective study. Lancet 1996;348:145–149. (*Neuromuscular and visual impairments, and low bone-mineral density are independent predictors of hip fracture in elderly women.*)

Inouye SK, Viscoli CM, Horwitz RI, Hurst LD, Tinetti ME. A predictive model for delirium based on admission characteristics. Ann Intern Med 1993;119:474–481. (*Risk factors for incident delirium in hospital are severe illness, cognitive impairment, visual impairment, and a high BUN/creatinine ratio.*)

Inouye SK, Charpentier PA. Precipitating factors for delirium in hospitalized elderly persons. JAMA 1996;275:852–857. (*Factors preceding the onset of delirium in the hospital include use of physical restraints, more than three medications added, use of bladder catheter, malnutrition, and any iatrogenic event.*)

Ouslander JG, Schnille JF. Incontinence in the nursing home. Ann Intern Med 1995;122:438–449. (*A comprehensive review of the evaluation and management of urinary incontinence*)

Schor JD, Levkoff SE, Lipsitz LA, et al. Risk factors for delirium in hospitalized elderly. JAMA 1992;267:827–831. (*Delirium is most closely associated with factors present on admission such as prior cognitive impairment, advanced age, and fracture.*)

Tinetti ME, Baker DI, McAvay G, et al. A multifactorial intervention to reduce the risk of falling among elderly people living in the community. N Engl J Med 1994;331:821–827. (*The risk of falling is reduced by an intervention that includes decreased use of medications, behavioral instructions, and exercise programs.*)

Skin Signs of Systemic Disease

Kenneth J. Tomecki

SKIN DISEASE AND CANCER

CUTANEOUS METASTASES

Cutaneous metastases (Fig. 9.1) occur in 3–5% of patients with cancer; they most commonly occur on the head, neck, and trunk, often in close proximity to the underlying tumor. Metastases typically reflect the more common types of cancer in the general population, e.g., cancers of the breast, lung, or gastrointestinal tract.

GLUCAGONOMA SYNDROME

The glucagonoma syndrome (Fig. 9.2), characterized by a distinctive necrolytic migratory erythema (erosive, crusted plaques on the perineum, sometimes on the face and trunk), invariably represents an islet cell tumor of the pancreas, or occasionally malabsorption, e.g., zinc deficiency. Affected patients usually have weight loss, diarrhea, stomatitis, glossitis, and anemia. An elevated serum glucagon level confirms the diagnosis.

PAGET'S DISEASE OF THE BREAST

Paget's disease of the breast (Fig. 9.3), a unilateral, eczematous plaque of the nipple and areola, invariably implies an underlying intraductal carcinoma of the breast. Extramammary Paget's disease (Fig. 9.4), typically a persistent, eczematous plaque on the perineum, often indicates the presence of an underlying adnexal (apocrine) carcinoma or an underlying cancer of the genitourinary tract or distal gastrointestinal tract; such cancers occur in approximately 50% of affected patients.

SWEET'S SYNDROME

Sweet's syndrome (Fig. 9.5), or acute febrile neutrophilic dermatosis, is characterized by the presence of painful, reddened plaques on the face, extremities, and trunk. The syndrome has a strong association with acute leukemia, either myelocytic or myelomonocytic. Often preceded by a flu-like illness and accompanied by arthralgias, the syndrome primarily affects women.

ACANTHOSIS NIGRICANS

Acanthosis nigricans (Fig. 9.6)—smooth, velvet-like, hyperkeratotic plaques of intertriginous areas (i.e., the groin, axillae, neck)—may indicate an underlying adenocarcinoma of the gastrointestinal tract, usually the stomach. Other causes of acanthosis nigricans are obesity, insulin-resistant diabetes, and certain medications, e.g., systemic corticosteroids, nicotinic acid, diethylstibesterol, and INH (isoniazid).

DERMATOMYOSITIS

Dermatomyositis (Fig. 9.7) is a photosensitive skin disease characterized by symmetric proximal muscle weakness (myositis); papules and plaques on the hands, elbows, and knees (Gottron's papules); and periorbital edema with a violaceous hue (heliotrope). Other features include poikiloderma-like changes (scaly, telangiectatic macules and papules) on the face, neck, trunk, and extremities; malar erythema; and nail abnormalities (periungual telangiectasiae and cuticular hypertrophy). Accurate diagnosis requires a muscle biopsy, electromyogram (EMG), and muscle enzyme tests. Adult dermatomyositis has a strong association with malignant dis-

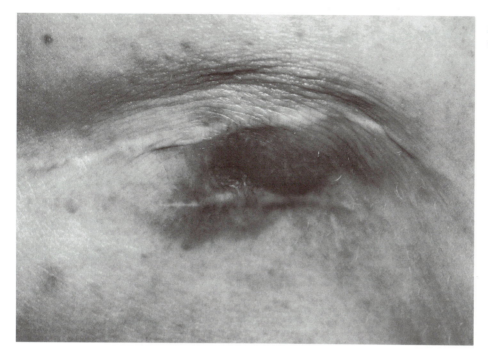

Figure 9.1. Metastatic breast cancer: thoracic nodule.

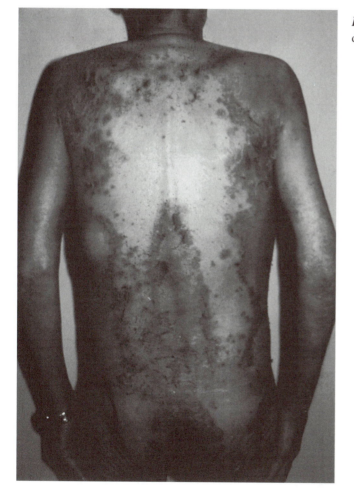

Figure 9.2. Necrolytic migratory erythema (glucagonoma syndrome): erosive, necrolytic plaques.

Figure 9.3. Paget's disease: unilateral eczematous plaque on areola.

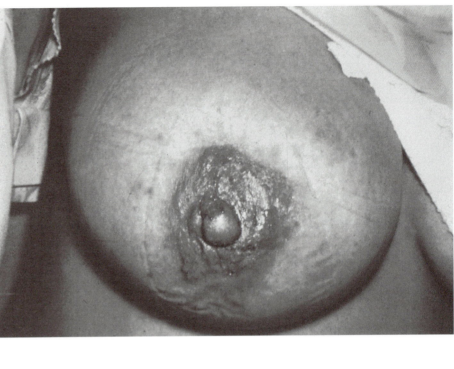

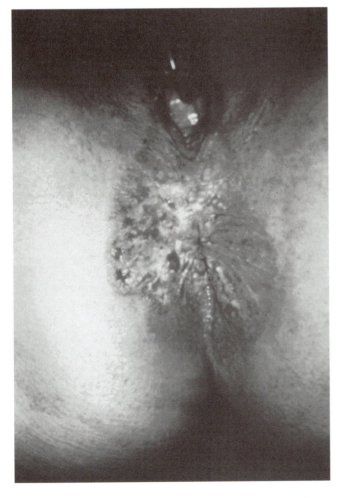

Figure 9.4. Extramammary Paget's disease: eczematous plaque on perineum.

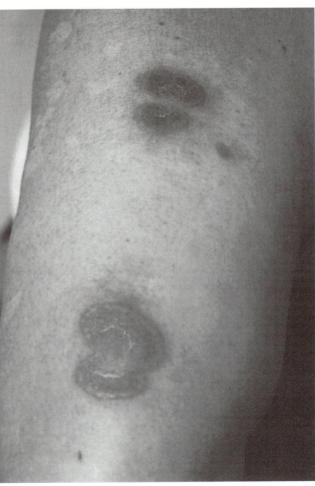

Figure 9.5. Sweet's syndrome: juicy, reddened plaques.

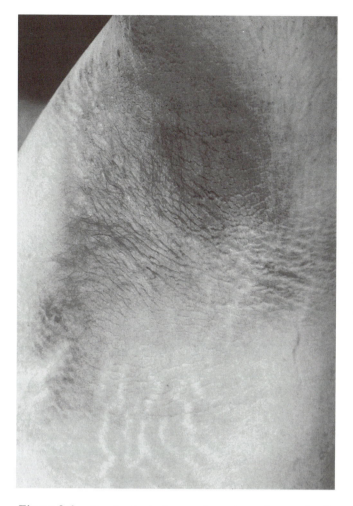

Figure 9.6. Acanthosis nigricans: velvety, hyperpigmented axillary plaques.

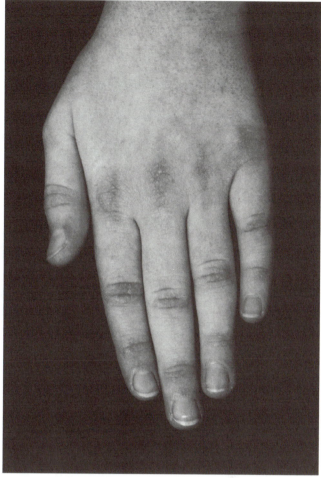

Figure 9.7. Dermatomyositis: Gottron's papules and plaques.

ease, usually an adenocarcinoma of the breast, gastrointestinal tract, or lung.

ACQUIRED ICHTHYOSIS

Acquired ichthyosis (Fig. 9.8), a scaly, plate-like thickening of the skin, is a relatively specific marker for lymphoma when it appears *de novo* in an adult.

HIRSUTISM

Hirsutism (Fig. 9.9), the presence of coarse, male-type hair in a woman, may indicate androgen excess, with or without an adrenal or ovarian tumor.

HYPERTRICHOSIS

Hypertrichosis, the presence of increased hair growth (usually fine, lanugo type hair growth) without androgen excess, can

occur with carcinoid tumor, adenocarcinoma of the breast or gastrointestinal tract, and other cancers.

AMYLOIDOSIS OF THE SKIN

Amyloidosis of the skin, typically expressed as waxy papules of the orbits and mid-face that become purpuric with pressure or rubbing, may be a sign of multiple myeloma. Other features of primary amyloidosis include macroglossia, ''pinch-purpura'' after trauma, and alopecia.

AUTOIMMUNE BULLOUS DISEASES

Autoimmune bullous diseases, characterized by the deposition of immunoglobulin within the epidermis (pemphigus) or at the dermal-epidermal junction (dermatitis herpetiformis, bullous pemphigoid, epidermolysis bullosa), may have a link with malignancy. Paraneoplastic pemphigus has clinical and histologic features of pemphigus, lichen planus, and erythema multiforme; the disease has a strong association with leukemia and lymphoma. Pemphigus may occur with thymoma, either

Figure 9.8. Acquired ichthyosis: plate-like, scaly plaques.

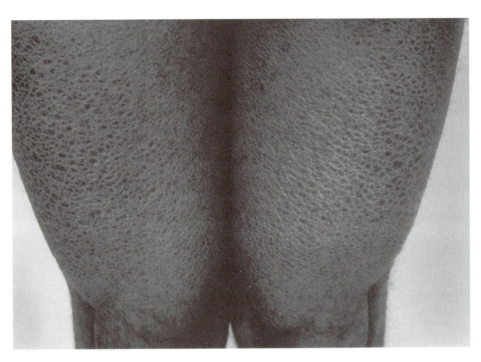

Figure 9.9. Hirsutism: coarse, male-type hair.

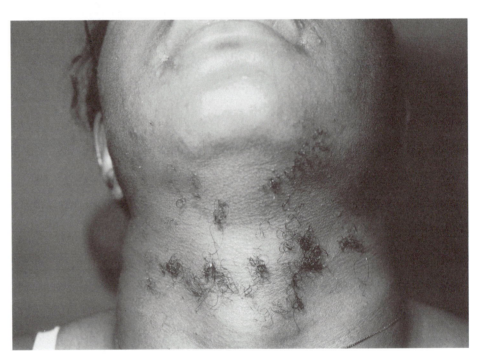

with or without myasthenia gravis. Although rare, dermatitis herpetiformis may precede an intestinal lymphoma. Epidermolysis bullosa acquisita has a weak association with multiple myeloma.

ERYTHEMA GYRATUM REPENS

Erythema gyratum repens, a rare but distinctive skin disease characterized by reddened concentric bands in a whorled pattern, has a strong association with breast cancer.

SEBORRHEIC KERATOSES

Seborrheic keratoses—warty, age-related plaques of the skin—may indicate an underlying adenocarcinoma of the gastrointestinal tract if they appear suddenly in great numbers (sign of Leser-Trélat).

GENERALIZED PRURITUS

Generalized pruritus, a common occurrence with or without skin disease, may be an early symptom of lymphoma.

SKIN DISEASE AND CARDIOVASCULAR DISEASE

EHLERS-DANLOS SYNDROME

Ehlers-Danlos syndrome, characterized by hyperextensibilty, hypermobility, fragile skin, and ''fish mouth'' scars, represents an abnormality in collagen biosynthesis. Associated features include hernias, angina, gastrointestinal bleeding (perforation), and peripheral vascular disease.

PSEUDOXANTHOMA ELASTICUM

Pseudoxanthoma elasticum (Fig. 9.10)—an inherited disease (either autosomal dominant or recessive) characterized by yellowed, pebbled skin on the neck, abdomen, and intertriginous areas (e.g., axillae, groin)—represents a defect in elastic fibers, which become brittle and calcified. Associated features include hypertension, peripheral vascular and coronary artery disease, and retinal and gastrointestinal hemorrhage. Fundos-

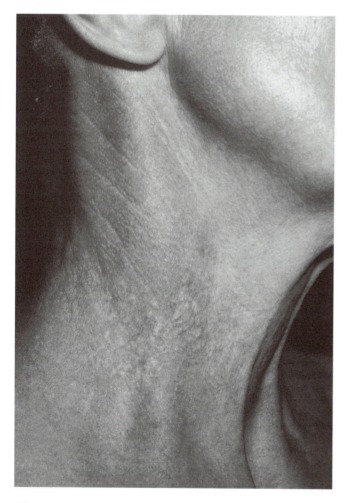

Figure 9.10. Pseudoxanthoma elasticum: pebbled skin on the neck.

copic examination reveals angioid streaks in Bruch's membrane.

MULTIPLE LENTIGINES

Multiple lentigines occur with cardiac abnormalities, namely LEOPARD syndrome (also known as Moynanan's syndrome), a mnemonic for **L**entigines, **E**lectrocardiographic (ECG) changes, **O**cular telorism, **P**ulmonary stenosis, **A**bnormal genitalia, **R**etarded growth, and **D**eafness. Variants of LEOPARD syndrome include LAMB syndrome (**L**entigines, **A**trial myxoma, **M**ucocutaneous myxomas, and **B**lue nevi) and NAME syndrome (**N**evi, **A**trial myxoma, **M**yxoid neurofibromas, and **E**phelides).

SKIN DISEASE AND ENDOCRINE OR METABOLIC DISEASE

SKIN DISEASE WITH DIABETES

Skin disease may occur with diabetes, e.g., necrobiosis lipoidica diaticorum, shin spots, eruptive xanthoma, scleredema, stiff hand syndrome, or granuloma annulare. Necrobiosis lipoidica diabeticorum (NLD) (Fig. 9.11) exhibits thin, yellowed, atrophic plaques of the skin, which may ulcerate; most patients with NLD have diabetes. Shin spots (diabetic dermopathy) are small, discrete scar-like plaques on the legs; they are common with diabetes. Eruptive xanthoma—a result of hyperlipidemia (elevated triglycerides) and characterized by discrete, yellow papules with a predilection for the extremities and buttocks—invariably represent uncontrolled diabetes; with control of the lipids and the diabetes, the xanthoma resolve. Scleredema is a chronic thickening of the skin on the upper back, usually in men with long-standing, uncontrolled diabetes. Stiff hand syndrome, a waxy thickening of the skin combined with restricted mobility, occurs with insulin-dependent juvenile diabetes; renal and retinal vascular disease often follows the syndrome. Granuloma annulare, characterized by reddened, annular papules and plaques, usually on the hands and feet, may occur with or without diabetes.

PORPHYRIAS

Porphyrias are a group of disorders resulting from abnormalities of heme biosynthesis. Porphyrias may be erythropoietic, hepatic, or mixed in nature; each type, whether inherited or acquired, has a specific enzyme defect. Porphyria cutanea tarda (PCT) (Fig. 9.12), the most common porphyria, is a hepatic porphyria that may be inherited or acquired. Affected patients lack uroporphyrinogen decarboxylase, which converts uroporphyrin to coproporphyrin; as such, uroporphyrins accumulate in the urine. Precipitating factors include alcohol ingestion, estrogen, and certain toxins. Skin disease typically includes photosensitivity, skin fragility, dermatitis (vesicles,

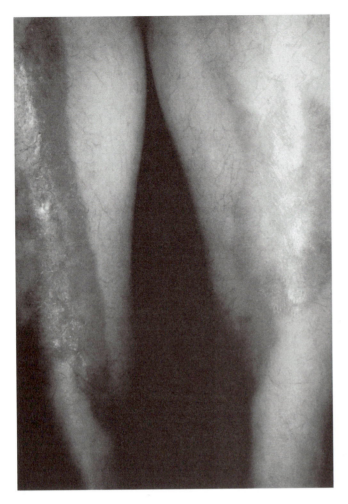

Figure 9.11. Necrobiosis lipoidica diabeticorum: shiny atrophic plaques.

Figure 9.12. Porphyria cutanea tarda: vesicles and erosions.

bullae, erosions), especially on the hands and often with hyperpigmentation and hypertrichosis (excess hair growth).

SKIN DISEASE AND GASTROINTESTINAL DISEASE

APHTHAE

Aphthae, painful, superficial ulcerations of the mucosae, may occur with Crohn's disease and gluten-sensitive enteropathy.

ACRODERMATITIS ENTEROPATHICA

Acrodermatitis enteropathica is an inflammatory disease, either inherited or acquired, that is characterized by a deficiency of zinc. Clinical features are diarrhea, alopecia, and erosive plaques in the perineum and on the face, hands, and feet.

DERMATITIS HERPETIFORMIS

Dermatitis herpetiformis (Fig. 9.13) is an intensely pruritic, vesicular-bullous disease, characterized by the deposition of IgA at the dermal-epidermal junction. Skin disease has a predilection for the elbows, knees, scalp, and buttocks. Most affected patients have an asymptomatic gluten-sensitive enteropathy; some patients have thyroid disease.

HEREDITARY HEMORRHAGIC TELANGIECTASIA

Hereditary hemorrhagic telangiectasia (Osler-Weber-Rendu syndrome) (Fig. 9.14) is an autosomal dominant disease char-

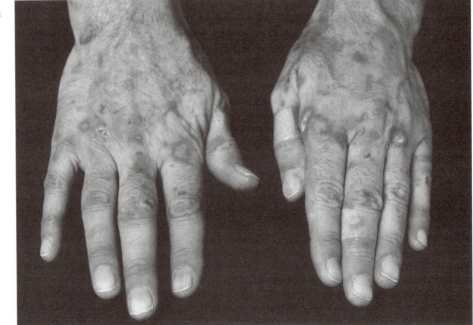

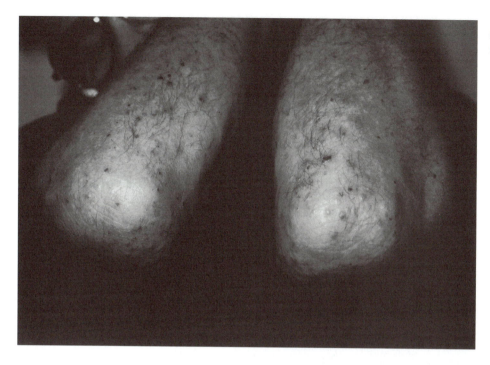

Figure 9.13. Dermatitis herpetiformis: excoriated papules and vesicles.

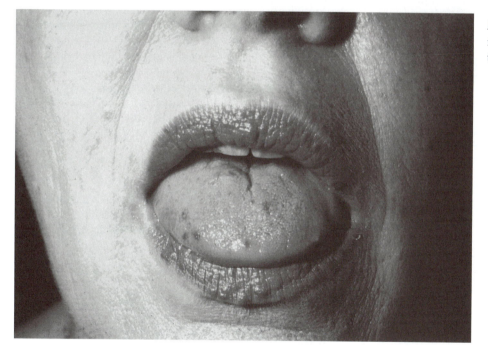

Figure 9.14. Hereditary hemorrhagic telangiectasia: telangiectasiae of the skin and mucosa.

acterized by cutaneous (typically on the palms, but elsewhere as well) and mucosal (lips, nose, and tongue) telangiectasiae that may bleed. Affected patients typically have frequent nosebleeds (epistaxis) and occasionally gastrointestinal bleeding (melena). Pulmonary arteriovenous fistulae and CNS vascular malformations may occur; aortic aneurysms are rare.

PEUTZ-JEGHERS SYNDROME

Peutz-Jeghers syndrome (Fig. 9.15) is an autosomal dominant disease characterized by perioral and mucosal lentigines and

gastrointestinal polyps, usually hamartomas in the small intestine. The malignant potential of the polyps is low, but affected patients have a higher risk of colon cancer than the general population.

PYODERMA GANGRENOSUM

Pyoderma gangrenosum (Fig. 9.16) is an inflammatory ulcerative disease of the legs with a distinctive morphology: inflammatory ulcers with undermined edges and a border of grey or

Figure 9.15. Peutz-Jeghers syndrome: hyperpigmented macules (lentigines) on the skin and mucosa.

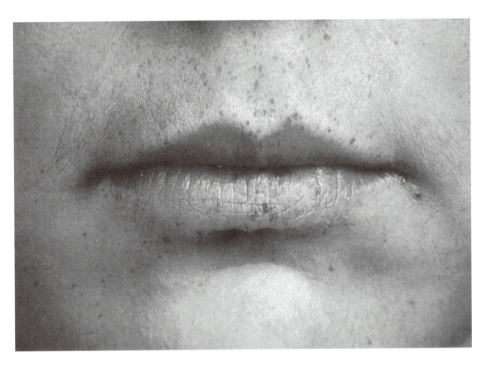

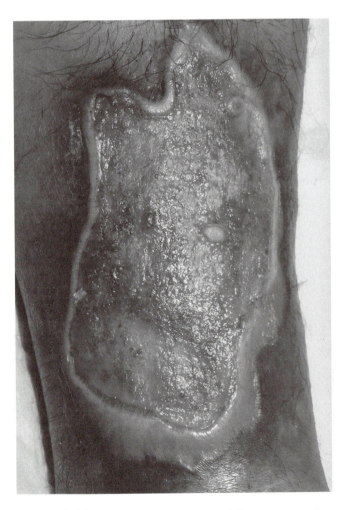

Figure 9.16. Pyoderma gangrenosum: inflammatory, undermined ulcer.

purple pigmentation. Skin disease and ulcers typically follow trauma. Most patients have inflammatory bowel disease (usually ulcerative colitis), rheumatoid arthritis, or a paraproteinemia, usually an IgA gammopathy. A bullous variant of pyoderma gangrenosum occurs with leukemia.

SKIN DISEASE AND PULMONARY DISEASE

SARCOIDOSIS

Sarcoidosis (Fig. 9.17) is a chronic, often multisystem, granulomatous disease with a variety of presentations on the skin, including nasal edema (lupus pernio), midfacial papules, annular plaques, and plaques or nodules. Skin disease occurs in approximately one-third of patients with sarcoidosis. Erythema nodosum, an acute, painful panniculitis that commonly affects the shins, may accompany acute sarcoidosis.

SKIN DISEASE AND RHEUMATIC DISEASE

PSORIASIS

Psoriasis (Fig. 9.18) is a common disease that affects 1–2% of the population. Psoriatic arthritis, which affects approximately 5% of patients with psoriasis, is an asymmetric, fusiform swelling of the distal and proximal interphalangeal joints that may resemble rheumatoid arthritis.

REITER'S SYNDROME

Reiter's syndrome (Fig. 9.19) is an inflammatory disorder with three features: urethritis, conjunctivitis, and arthritis. It

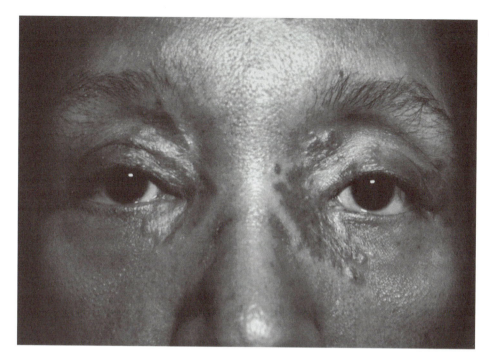

Figure 9.17. Cutaneous sarcoidosis: annular facial plaques.

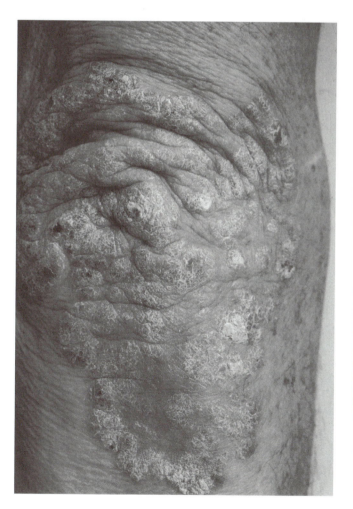

Figure 9.18. Psoriasis: scaly plaques.

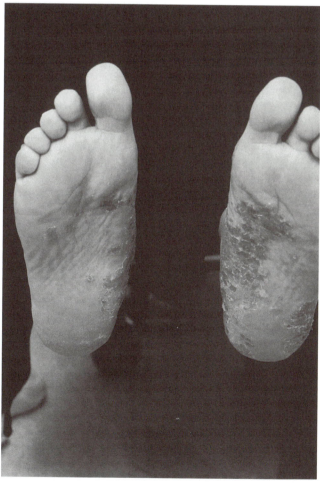

Figure 9.19. Reiter's syndrome: psoriasiform plaques of the feet (keratoderma blenorrhagicum).

Figure 9.20. Acrosclerosis: thickened, sclerotic digits.

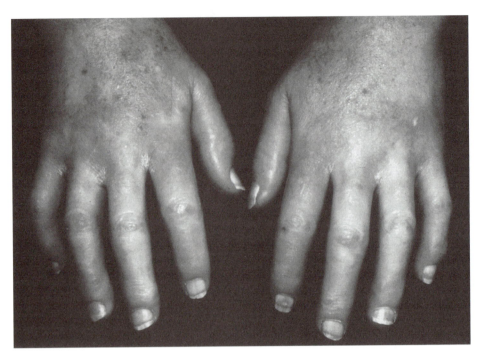

invariably affects young men. Most patients have skin disease that resembles psoriasis: psoriatic plaques on the penis (circinate balanitis) and palms and soles (keratoderma blenorrhagicum). Most patients have the HLA-B27 antigen.

ACROSCLEROSIS

Acrosclerosis (Fig. 9.20), a thickened tapering of the skin, often with secondary ulceration, may occur with angiitis, chilblains, cryopathies, and scleroderma, or it may follow exposure to polyvinyl chlorides.

ERYTHEMA CHRONICUM MIGRANS

Erythema chronicum migrans (Fig. 9.21), an annular, reddened plaque that follows and surrounds a tick bite, is the cutaneous manifestation of Lyme disease, a multisystem disease that usually includes fever, arthralgia, and myalgia and may include meningoencephalitis, myocarditis, and peripheral neuropathy. The usual causative agent in the United States is *Ixodes dammini,* or *I. pacificus* in the Pacific Northwest. In Europe, the causative agent is *I. ricinus.* The plaques are usually solitary (75% of patients), but may be multiple.

SKIN DISEASE AND HIV INFECTION

Skin disease is common with HIV infection. Epidemic Kaposi's sarcoma, now thought to be an infectious disease (HHV-8), is common with HIV infection. Unlike the classic Kaposi's sarcoma seen in elderly patients, this disease affects the mucosa, face, and trunk. Infectious skin disease is ex-

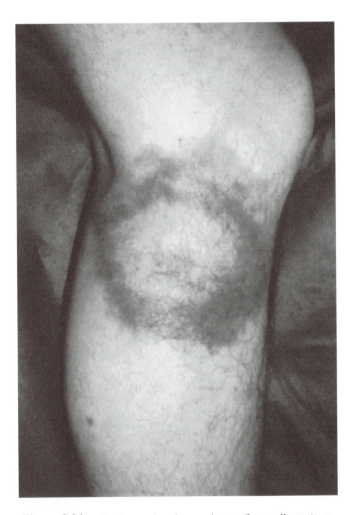

Figure 9.21. Erythema chronicum migrans (Lyme disease): annular, reddened plaque.

tremely common and may be the first sign of HIV disease. The more common bacterial infections include:

- Bacillary angiomatosis (BA), a newly described disease caused by *Bartonella henselae,* which is somewhat specific for HIV infection. BA exhibits vascular, friable papules and nodules that are often painful and numerous.
- Staphylococcal skin disease, e.g., impetigo, ecthyma, folliculitis, and abscesses, which may assume unusual patterns and be refractory to treatment

The more common viral infections include:

- HSV disease, often persistent with advanced HIV infection
- VZV disease (varicella), which may have a benign course, although complications are common, and herpes zoster, a common occurrence with its attendant painful ulcerations, postherpetic neuralgia, and, occasionally, dissemination

- Molluscum contagiosum, markers for advanced human immunodeficiency virus (HIV) infection
- Oral hairy leukoplakia, usually present with advanced disease

The three most common fungal infections are cryptococcosis, coccidioidomycosis, and histoplasmosis, each of which has cutaneous manifestations, particularly cryptococcal skin disease, which may resemble molluscum.

OTHER CONDITIONS
ERYTHEMA MULTIFORME

Erythema multiforme (Fig. 9.22) is a hypersensitivity reaction of the skin and mucosal surfaces, characterized by macules, papules, plaques, vesicles, or bullae, often with a targetoid or iris appearance. The most common cause is herpetic (HSV) infection; less common causes are drugs such as sulfonamides, barbiturates, or antibiotics.

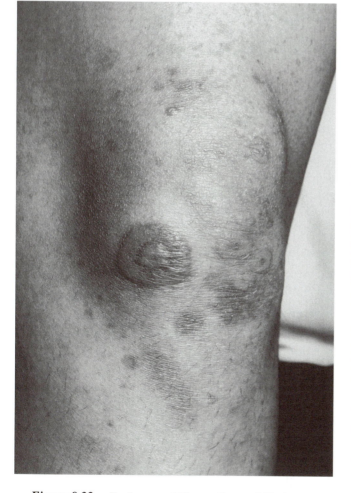

Figure 9.22. Erythema multiforme: ''targetoid'' plaques.

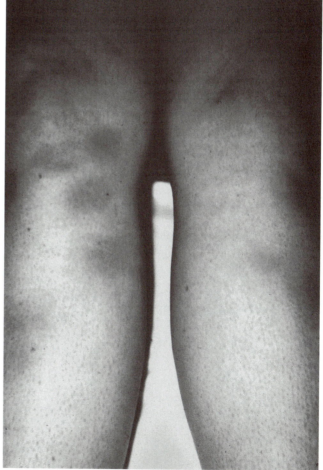

Figure 9.23. Erythema nodosum: reddened nodules on the shins.

Figure 9.24. Exfoliative dermatitis: eczematous, scaly plaques.

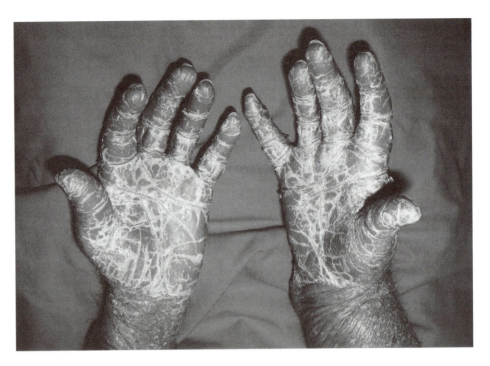

ERYTHEMA NODOSUM

Erythema nodosum (Fig. 9.23) is a hypersensitivity reaction—a panniculitis, characterized by painful, reddened nodules on the shins. The most common cause of erythema nodosum is a streptococcal pharyngitis; other causes include drug sensitivity (e.g., to sulfonamides, oral contraceptives) and a variety of illnesses, including inflammatory bowel disease and sarcoidosis.

EXFOLIATIVE DERMATITIS

Exfoliative dermatitis (Fig. 9.24) is an itchy, eczematous disease that is usually generalized and insidious in nature. The most common causes are a preexisting skin disease (e.g., psoriasis, atopic eczema) and drug hypersensitivity (drug rash); a less common but important etiology is a cutaneous lymphoma (T-cell type).

SUGGESTED READINGS

Gregory B, Ho VC. Cutaneous manifestations of gastrointestinal disorders. Am Acad Dermatol 1992;26:153, 371.

Helm KF, Peters MS. Imuunodermatology update: the immunologically mediated vesiculobullous diseases. Mayo Clin Proc 1991;66:187.

Heyman WR. Cutaneous manifestations of thyroid disease. J Am Acad Dermatol 1992;26:885.

Loucas E, Russo G, Millikan LE. Genetic and acquired cutaneous disorders associated with internal malignancy. Int J Dermatol 1995;34:749.

Perez MI, Kohn SR. Cutaneous manifestations of diabetes mellitus. J Am Acad Dermatol 1994;30:519.

Poole S, Fenske NF. Cutaneous markers of internal malignancy I & II. J Am Acad Dermatol 1993;28:1, 147.

Roe DA. Cutaneous manifestations of nutritional diseases. Semin Dermatol 1991;10:269.

Schwartz RA. Cutaneous metastatic disease. J Am Acad Dermatol 1995;33:161.

Tschachler E, Bergstresser PR, et al. HIV-related skin diseases. Lancet 1996;348:659.

Von den Driesch P. Sweet's syndrome (acute febrile neutrophilic dermatosis). J Am Acad Dermatol 1994;31:535.

Zalla MJ, Su WPD, et al. Dermaologic manifestations of human immunodeficiency virus infection. Mayo Clin Proc 1992;67:1089.

C·H·A·P·T·E·R

10

Occupational Medicine

Edward P. Horvath, Jr.

LEAD

Lead has been used extensively since antiquity. Considerable information regarding the cause, clinical effects, prevention, and treatment of lead poisoning has been compiled. However, despite a reduction in clinical cases arising in industrialized settings, lead poisoning continues to occur in both occupational and nonoccupational environments, providing a challenge to both internists and pediatricians.

OCCUPATIONAL EXPOSURE TO LEAD

Although many industrial workers still regularly come in contact with lead-containing compounds, modern control measures, such as those found in the Occupational Safety and Health Administration's (OSHA) lead standard, have reduced the incidence of overt cases of clinical poisoning in high-risk operations such as battery manufacturing, brass and bronze foundry work, and lead smelting/refining. However, cases continue to be reported in occupations in which lead exposure is less well appreciated. Bridge reconstruction workers are exposed to airborne lead arising from lead-painted surfaces that are subjected to abrasive blasting or oxyacetylene torch cutting or welding. Avid marksmen, particularly those frequently engaged in shooting competitions, may develop symptoms from exposures in inadequately ventilated indoor firing ranges. The risk of clinical toxicity is generally low in occupations such as soldering and lead glass manufacturing.

ENVIRONMENTAL EXPOSURE TO LEAD

Exposure to leaded paint continues to be a serious hazard to both children and adults. Youngsters, particularly those in inner cities, regularly ingest paint chips from deteriorating interior surfaces. Adults are exposed to lead-containing dust generated by the abrasion of painted surfaces during building renovation. Although lead water pipes and storage tanks are no longer used in homes, some pipes may still contain lead solder. Lead can enter domestic water supplies under certain conditions, particularly if the water is slightly acidic and has been in contact with a leaded surface for a prolonged time. The declining use of alkyl lead compounds as antiknock agents in gasoline has decreased the risk from this source of exposure. Improperly manufactured lead-glazed earthenware can be an unusual source of lead poisoning, particularly with acidic foods and beverages, which may dissolve lead from the glaze. The risk is low with commercially manufactured stoneware, which was fired at a sufficiently high temperature. Although improvements in canning technology have substantially decreased the lead content of canned foods, folk remedies and "health foods" are generally unregulated, and may be a source of unsuspected exposure.

CLINICAL EFFECTS OF LEAD POISONING

Inorganic lead can enter the body by inhalation or ingestion. The former is more common in occupational exposures and the latter in environmental settings. Following absorption, it is distributed to the erythrocytes, liver, and kidneys. Over time, lead is redistributed to the bones, following a metabolic pathway similar to that of calcium. Through its ability to interact with sulfhydryl groups, lead exerts toxic effects on a number of organ systems, resulting in a wide range of clinical effects.

Classic lead colic, which is due to spasmodic contraction of intestinal smooth muscle, is now encountered only rarely. More common are insidious gastrointestinal symptoms, including vague abdominal discomfort, anorexia, and constipa-

91

tion. Because lead interferes with hemoglobin synthesis, anemia is a frequent clinical finding. This has been variously described as microcytic, hypochromic and normocytic, normochromic. Lead also shortens erythrocyte lifespan by a poorly understood mechanism. The resulting increased erythropoiesis in the bone marrow leads to the additional findings of reticulocytosis and basophilic stippling of red cells. Heavy, persistent exposure lasting 10 years or more may result in lead nephropathy characterized by progressive renal impairment and hypertension. Tubular dysfunction may be sufficiently severe as to result in a Fanconi-like syndrome with aminoaciduria, glucosuria, and hyperphosphaturia. Lead interferes with the excretion of urates. The resulting hyperuricemia can lead to a form of gout referred to as saturnine, an old term for lead poisoning.

Severe involvement of the peripheral nervous system, leading to paralysis of the extensor muscles of the wrist (wrist drop) or ankles (foot drop), is now uncommon. Likewise, occupationally induced lead encephalopathy is rare. However, acute encephalopathy remains a regrettably frequent and serious complication of childhood lead poisoning. Although chelation treatment has substantially reduced the mortality, approximately 25% of survivors exhibit permanent brain damage. Some cases of mild poisoning in adults may present with vague neuropsychiatric complaints such as headache, poor concentration, and memory loss. Because these symptoms are relatively common nonspecific complaints in clinical practice, the diagnosis of lead poisoning may not be suspected without obtaining a thorough occupational history. Reproductive effects in both males and females have been described, including increased rates of miscarriages and stillbirths, prematurity, reduced birth weight, and decreased sperm counts and motility.

LABORATORY STUDIES FOR LEAD POISONING

The diagnosis of lead poisoning, like that of all occupational and environmental disorders, is an exercise in clinical judgment requiring full consideration of the medical and occupational history, the physical examination, and relevant laboratory studies. Measurement of blood lead is the single most useful diagnostic test. It is also the preferred test for biological monitoring of exposed workers. It reflects recent exposure and is less variable than urinary lead measurements. However, the mere elevation of blood lead slightly above the upper limits of laboratory ''normal'' should not necessarily lead to a diagnosis of lead poisoning. Clinical symptoms (e.g., abdominal complaints) and/or organ system effects (e.g., anemia) should be present before the diagnosis is made. Concentrations greater than 40 μg/dL, but less than 60 μp/dL, indicate increased absorption, but may or may not be accompanied by clinical symptoms. Patients with blood lead levels greater than 80 μg/dL usually have clinical manifestations of lead toxicity and detectable anemia. Although an approximate dose-response relationship exists between blood lead levels and clinical effects, there are differences in individual susceptibility and in interpretation of test results.

Measurement of free erythrocyte protoporphyrin (FEP) or zinc protoporphyrin (ZZP) relate to lead's effect on heme synthetase. FEP and ZZP levels begin to increase when the blood lead level exceeds 40 μg/dL. They stay elevated longer than blood lead and are therefore better indicators of chronic intoxication. However, they are less specific than blood lead and may also be elevated in patients with iron deficiency anemia. Other laboratory studies that should be ordered in the initial assessment of any lead-exposed patient include a complete blood count with peripheral smear, blood urea nitrogen (BUN) creatinine, and urinalysis.

The assessment of a causal role for remote lead exposure in a chronic disorder, such as nephropathy, can be difficult. The usual measures of recent exposure, such as the blood lead level, are generally normal. Over time, most of the body burden is redistributed to the kidneys, liver, and especially bone. A lead-mobilization test utilizing edetate calcium disodium (Ca EDTA) has been advocated. A newer technique utilizing x-ray fluorescence and bone densitometry can also measure accumulated lead.

TREATMENT FOR LEAD POISONING

The initial treatment of lead poisoning is removal from further exposure. In adults with mild symptoms and only slight anemia, this may be all that is necessary. In patients with higher blood levels, more striking clinical symptoms, and significant anemia, chelation therapy is indicated. Ca EDTA is the parenteral agent of choice and is usually given in cases of acute or severe poisoning. An orally administered agent, 2,3 dimercaptosuccinic acid (Succimer) has gained acceptance for lead poisoning in both children and adults. The prophylactic use of chelating agents to prevent elevated blood lead levels in workers occupationally exposed is expressly prohibited by OSHA's lead standard.

ORGANOPHOSPHATE INSECTICIDES

Internists occasionally encounter patients either acutely poisoned by pesticides or fearful of potential long-term effects from past exposure. Although a large number of different pesticides are in commercial use, physicians are most likely to encounter clinical problems caused by the organophosphate insecticides. This group of compounds is classified according to its common mode of action, the inhibition of the enzyme acetylcholinesterase. The toxicity of organophosphate insecticides varies widely. One of the least toxic, malathion, commonly results in home-use exposures. Poisoning from more toxic agents, such as parathion, is rare except in agricultural regions or in a pesticide manufacturing or formulating facility.

OCCUPATIONAL EXPOSURE TO ORGANOPHOSPHATES

In occupational settings, exposures occur during the manufacturing, formulation, transportation, and application of pesticides. Firefighters and hazardous waste workers may also encounter these substances in their work. Organophosphate insecticides are readily absorbed by inhalation, through intact skin, and by ingestion.

ENVIRONMENTAL EXPOSURE TO ORGANOPHOSPHATES

Exposures may occur among families of field workers or farmers who come in contact with contaminated clothing. Haphazard aerial spraying can also result in exposure in rural families. The general public often expresses concern about pesticide contamination of food or water, although actual clinical toxicity in such circumstances is rare. Organophosphate poisoning from accidental ingestion by children remains regrettably common, particularly when unused pesticide is stored in an inappropriate container such as a pop bottle or can.

CLINICAL EFFECTS OF ORGANOPHOSPHATE POISONING

Anticholinesterase compounds produce their clinical effects through phosphorylation of acetylcholinesterase enzyme (AChE) at nerve endings. The resultant accumulation of the neurotransmitter, acetylcholine, at these nerve endings produces overstimulation and then paralysis of nerve transmission. Both nicotinic (ganglionic and neuromuscular) and muscarinic (parasympathetic) effects are observed. Various mnemonics have been devised to assist clinicians in remembering the clinical signs and symptoms of cholinesterase inhibition. A common one, DUMBELS, stands for Diarrhea, Urination, Miosis, Bronchospasm, Emesis, Lacrimation, and Salivation. The developmental sequence of systemic effects and the time of onset after exposure can vary. Acute toxicity is usually rapid in onset, although symptoms may be delayed up to 12 hours after exposure. In cases of inhalation, respiratory and ocular symptoms may appear first. In cases of ingestion, gastrointestinal effects may be the initial manifestations. Occupational exposures insufficient to produce symptoms following a single event can result in symptoms after continued daily exposure. Depending on treatment, complete symptomatic recovery usually occurs within a week. However, increased susceptibility to the effects of anticholinesterase agents may persist for several weeks after a single exposure.

A delayed peripheral neuropathy has been reported after poisoning by some organophosphates. This condition, organophosphate-induced delayed neuropathy (OPIDN), is thought to be due to phosphorylation and inhibition of the enzyme neurotoxic esterase (NTE) followed by degradation of the phosphoryl-enzyme complex. This predominantly motor polyneuropathy occurs 2–3 weeks after acute poisoning, usually by intentional ingestion. An "intermediate syndrome" following acute poisoning has also been reported. This consists of a paralytic syndrome, involving primarily proximal limb muscles, neck flexors, certain cranial motor nerves, and the muscles of respiration, that occurs 24–96 hours after heavy exposure. Neuropsychiatric or cognitive complaints, such as irritability, depression, anxiety, fatigue, difficulty in concentration, and short-term memory impairment, are commonly reported after acute exposures. However, in the assessment of individual cases, it is often difficult to distinguish organically based neurobehavioral symptoms from the psychologic reactions likely to occur after exposure events.

LABORATORY STUDIES FOR ORGANOPHOSPHATE POISONING

The diagnosis of organophosphate poisoning depends on a history of exposure, the presence of typical signs and symptoms, and laboratory documentation of cholinesterase inhibition. Two types of cholinesterase levels can be measured: plasma cholinesterase (pseudocholinesterase) and red cell cholinesterase (true acetylcholinesterase). Plasma cholinesterase, which is synthesized by the liver, declines sooner but regenerates faster than red cell cholinesterase. Typical regeneration time is days to a few weeks. Depressed plasma cholinesterase levels also are seen in genetic pseudocholinesterase deficiency and in chronic liver disease. Red cell cholinesterase more accurately reflects the degree of actual enzyme inactivation at neuroeffector sites. However, it is depressed more slowly and for longer periods of time than plasma cholinesterase. Typical regeneration time is 1–3 months. Cholinesterase levels are of greater clinical utility when they can be compared to a preexposure baseline. Unfortunately, such data are rarely available except in pesticide-exposed workers in whom prior medical surveillance testing has been conducted. A cholinesterase depression of 25% or more, compared to the preexposure baseline, is regarded as evidence of excessive absorption. A reduction of greater than 50% is usually seen with frank poisoning.

TREATMENT FOR ORGANOPHOSPHATE POISONING

For relatively mild cases, treatment may consist only of removal from further exposure and decontamination of clothing and skin. Healthcare personnel need to avoid direct cutaneous contact with obviously contaminated clothing inasmuch as organophosphate compounds are readily absorbed through intact skin. Gastric lavage is indicated in cases of pesticide ingestion. Anticonvulsant medication may be necessary. In severe cases, a patent airway needs to be established, both for removal of excess secretions and to institute ventilatory support. In the absence of cyanosis, atropine sulphate should be administered intravenously in high doses, typically 1–4 mg. This is repeated every 15 minutes until signs of atropinization appear: a dry, flushed skin; tachycardia as high as 140 beats per minute; and a pupillary dilatation. A mild degree of atropinization should be maintained at least 24 hours. Pralidoxime chloride (Protopam) reactivates the enzyme cholinesterase by breaking the acetylcholinesterase-phosphate complex. One to 2 grams are given as an intravenous infusion and can be repeated 1–2 hours later if muscle weakness has not improved. Additional doses can be given at 10–12 hour intervals. Treatment with pralidoxime chloride is most effective if initiated within 24 hours after exposure. In addition to assessment of clinical response, red cell cholinesterase levels should be monitored.

CARBON MONOXIDE

Carbon monoxide poisoning is one of the most common forms of poisoning in both occupational and nonoccupational settings. As a biproduct of incomplete combustion, it is present in virtually every workplace and home environment, particularly during the heating season. As an odorless, colorless, and tasteless gas, it gives no warning of its presence. Additionally, its typical early symptoms of nausea, headache, and dizziness occur frequently with common disorders such as viral illness. Practicing physicians must be aware of the possibility of carbon monoxide poisoning, particularly among certain workers and during the heating season. Measurement of blood carboxyhemoglobin should always be obtained in such circumstances.

OCCUPATIONAL EXPOSURE TO CARBON MONOXIDE

Certain employees are recognized as being at particular risk for carbon monoxide poisoning. These include firefighters, coal miners, coke oven and smelter workers, mechanics, and drivers. Exhaust from the operation of vehicles indoors, such as propane-powered forklift trucks, is a frequently overlooked source of exposure. Overexposure is particularly likely to occur during winter months when ventilation of the work environment may be decreased to lower costs of heating. Methylene chloride, a solvent widely used as a paint stripper, produces a unique form of carbon monoxide poisoning by being metabolized to carbon monoxide in the body.

ENVIRONMENTAL EXPOSURE TO CARBON MONOXIDE

Carbon monoxide is also a significant cause of poisoning in the nonoccupational environments. Despite widespread recognition of this hazard, fatalities occur each year from prolonged exposure to automobile exhaust in enclosed spaces. Deaths of entire families from carbon monoxide poisoning caused by a malfunctioning furnace or space heater are disturbingly common. Deliberate personal exposure from cigarette or cigar smoke can produce blood carboxyhemoglobin levels from 2–10%, sometimes as high as 18%. (Nonexposed individuals have an average level of 1% or less from endogenous hemoglobin metabolism.)

CLINICAL EFFECTS OF CARBON MONOXIDE POISONING

Carbon monoxide has an affinity for hemoglobin approximately 200–300 times that of oxygen. However, the formation of carboxyhemoglobin is not the only way in which carbon monoxide exerts adverse physiologic effects. It also shifts the oxygen-hemoglobin dissociation curve and binds to both myoglobin and cytochrome oxidase. The central nervous system and myocardium are sensitive to tissue hypoxia produced by carbon monoxide. Clinical effects in a given patient depend on the intensity and duration of clinical exposure and the presence of any preexisting conditions such as atherosclerosis. Blood carboxyhemoglobin levels of 10% or less rarely produce symptoms. At levels of 10–30%, patients may complain of headache, nausea, weakness, and dizziness. Mentation begins to be impaired at 30–35%, and levels of 35–40% may result in coma. Death can occur with levels greater than 50%. As with many chemical exposures, there is considerable individual variation. Death has occurred from blood levels of 36–38% in circumstances of prolonged exposure, presumably from the longer period of time available for the cytochromes to be inhibited. Whereas many patients with carbon monoxide poisoning recover completely, others exhibit delayed neurologic and neuropsychiatric manifestations thought to be due to diffuse demyelination. These complications can include a Parkinsonian movement disorder, cranial nerve dysfunction, peripheral motor or sensory loss, and disorders of cognition and affect.

LABORATORY STUDIES FOR CARBON MONOXIDE POISONING

A person who has been overcome by carbon monoxide and brought to the emergency room from a typical exposure environment (e.g., a running vehicle in a closed garage), seldom poses a diagnostic problem. However, in some instances, exposure to carbon monoxide may not be readily apparent, and the patient's symptoms may be nonspecific. Physicians should maintain a high index of suspicion and obtain a blood carboxyhemoglobin level. For more severely affected individuals, the physician should obtain arterial blood gases to check for metabolic acidosis. The pO_2 is usually normal, although oxygen saturation is decreased (as measured by direct CO-oximetry). Electrolytes may show hypokalemia. In the presence of tissue damage, creatinine kinase (CK) and lactate dehydrogenase (LDH) will be elevated. The electrocardiogram may show ischemic changes.

TREATMENT FOR CARBON MONOXIDE POISONING

The objectives of treatment are to increase tissue oxygenation and speed the elimination of carbon monoxide. Administration of 100% oxygen by tightly fitting face mask reduces the half-life from 5½ hours to approximately 1½ hours. Assisted ventilation is required for patients in respiratory distress. In addition, hospitalization should be considered if there is evidence of end-organ dysfunction (e.g., an abnormal electrocardiogram or neurologic findings) or carbon monoxide levels greater than 25%. Treatment with hyperbaric oxygen at two to three atmospheres should be considered for severely affected patients with coma or seizures, or for those in whom neurologic and cardiovascular dysfunction does not resolve with other forms of oxygen therapy. Oxygen at three atmospheres not only reduces the half-time for carbon monoxide elimination to 23 minutes, but also results in enough available oxygen dissolved in the plasma to support metabolism even in the absence of functioning hemoglobin. The prompt use of hyperbaric oxygen may also reduce the risk of delayed neurologic symptoms.

REVIEW EXERCISES

QUESTIONS

1. A 56-year-old bridge reconstruction worker who has been engaged in abrasive blasting of painted surfaces presents with a 2-month history of vague abdominal discomfort, constipation, fatigue, arthralgia, and headache. Based on the exposure history and symptoms, initial diagnostic studies should include:

   a. Blood lead, zinc protoporphyrin (ZPP)
   b. Complete blood count (CBC) with peripheral smear
   c. Blood urea nitrogen (BUN), serum creatinine (Cr)
   d. Blood lead only
   e. A, B, and C above

2. In the proper medical management of lead toxicity, all of the following are true except:

   a. Removal from exposure is mandatory.
   b. Symptomatic patients with high lead levels should undergo chelation therapy.
   c. All patients with elevated blood lead levels should be chelated even if asymptomatic.
   d. Edetate calcium disodium (CaEDTA) is the preferred parenteral agent.
   e. 2,3-dimercaptosuccinic acid (Succimer) is the oral agent of choice.

3. The appropriate management of a patient poisoned by organophosphate cholinesterase-inhibiting agents includes all of the following except:

   a. Atropine
   b. Sodium nitrite
   c. Pralidoxime chloride (Protopam)
   d. Maintenance of airway
   e. Decontamination

4. A 62-year-old warehouse worker is seen in an industrial clinic complaining of headache, nausea, lightheadedness, and chest discomfort that developed toward the end of his work shift. He had noticed similar symptoms in the past when ventilation of the building was poor. His physical examination is unremarkable. The proper initial management should include all of the following except:

   a. Blood carboxyhemoglobin level, arterial blood gases
   b. Creatine phosphokinase (CPK), lactate dehydrogenase (LDH)
   c. Electrocardiogram (ECG)
   d. 100% oxygen by face mask
   e. Hyperbaric oxygen

5. The most likely source of carbon monoxide poisoning in a warehouse operation is:

   a. Malfunctioning central heating unit
   b. Indoor vehicular exhaust
   c. Employee smoking
   d. Ambient (outside) air pollution
   e. Methylene chloride

Answers

1. e
2. c
3. b
4. e
5. b

SUGGESTED READINGS

Agency for Toxic Substances and Disease Registry (ATSDR). Case studies in environmental medicine. Washington, D.C.: U.S. Department of Health and Human Services, 1990–1993.

Brooks SM, Gochfeld M, Herzstein J, Jackson RJ, Schenker MB, eds. Environmental medicine. St. Louis: Mosby-Yearbook, Inc., 1995.

McCunney RH, ed. Handbook of occupational medicine. Boston: Little, Brown & Co., 1988.

LaDou J, ed. Occupational and environmental medicine, 2nd ed. Stamford, CT: Appleton & Lange, 1997.

Proctor NH, Hughes JP, Fishman ML. Chemical hazards of the workplace, 2nd ed. Philadelphia: JB Lippincott, 1988.

Rom WN. Environmental and occupational medicine, 2nd ed. Boston: Little, Brown & Co., 1992.

Rosenstock L, Cullen MR, eds. Textbook of clinical occupational and environmental medicine. Philadelphia: WB Saunders, 1994.

Sullivan JB, Krieger GR. Hazardous materials toxicology: clinical principles of environmental health. Baltimore: Williams & Wilkins, 1992.

Waldron HA. Lecture notes in occupational medicine. Oxford, United Kingdom: Blackwell Scientific Publications, 1990.

Zenz C, Dickerson OB, Horvath EP, eds. Occupational medicine, 3rd ed. St. Louis: Mosby-Yearbook, Inc., 1994.

Board Simulation: Psychiatric Disorders in Medical Practice

Kathleen Franco-Bronson

Internists frequently find themselves treating a variety of psychiatric patients, some of whom present particular challenges to diagnose or treat. Following are a few real-life cases of patients.

CASE 1

Patient Information

A 45-year-old female presents to your office complaining of intermittent chest pain for the past month. She initially noticed it walking up the stairs from her basement with a basket of laundry. Since then she has been aware of the pain on several occasions: once at the office while working on a complex project for her boss, another time when rushing to the school performance of their youngest child and, most recently, during a phone call with her mother. She believes the pain is growing in intensity and is taking longer before it passes.

QUESTION

1. Should your first step be:

   a. Reassure her and have her call back if the pain continues to occur over the next 2 weeks
   b. Schedule her for a stress-echocardiogram
   c. Gather additional personal and family history
   d. Prescribe an anxiolytic, such as Xanax (alprazolam)
   e. Prescribe a selective serotonin inhibitor such as Zoloft (sertraline)

Discussion and Answer Explanation

The information provided in Case 1 suggests that some or all of these episodes occur when the patient is fatigued or potentially under duress. Rather than jumping in to order costly tests or prescribe unnecessarily, the optimal choice is first to gather further history.

The patient confirms that her demands at work are increasing and it is hard to get everything done on time, both at work and at home. The history from the patient includes irregular menses, double vision, pelvic pain, fatigue, headaches, nausea/vomiting, joint symptoms, insomnia, bouts of diarrhea, and frequent upper respiratory infections (URIs) and urinary tract infections (UTIs), among a variety of other symptoms. As you flip through the archival record, you notice your predecessor has worked up the patient extensively on a variety of occasions and found little. As you talk further with her, she tells you that her 75-year-old father died of a myocardial infarction several months ago. She describes her mother as one who frequently requests others to take her to the doctor for a variety of concerns. Her mother is now quite distraught and needs or requests more visits with her doctors and more time from her daughter. The rest of the family history is unremarkable. Sleeping and eating patterns, concentration, and general interest level are all good at this time. The physical examination on the patient is completely normal.

Diagnostic Criteria for Somatoform Disorder (DSM-IV)

A history of many physical complaints beginning before age 30 years that occur over a period of several years and result in treatment being sought or significant impairment in social, occupational, or other area of functioning suggests a diagnosis of somatoform disorder. Following are the criteria:

- Four pain symptoms: different sites or functions
- Two gastrointestinal symptoms other than pain
- One sexual symptom

- One pseudoneurologic symptom
- After appropriate investigation, symptoms cannot be fully explained by a known medical condition or effects of a substance
- When there is a related general medical condition, the physical complaints or resulting social or occupational impairment are in excess of what would be expected

You watch closely the patient's affect and behavior while questioning about how easy or difficult daily life has been and how upsetting recent social changes have been. These responses can add clues for a psychosocial connection when there is a lack of support from physical findings. Reviewing medical records and emergency room visits is also a must.

Evaluating for Somatoform Disorders

Evaluate the following patient issues:

- Ease or difficulty with daily life
- Recent stressors
- Anniversary responses to past loss
- Time connection with physical symptom(s)
- Could symptom(s) serve to distract from emotional conflict?
- Are there any gains or benefits from the symptom(s)?

Treating the patient with short but regularly scheduled visits, reassurance, referral to a psychoeducational group (if available) to enhance optimal health, ordering only necessary testing, and treating comorbid psychiatric disorders such as depression if it arises are cornerstones of managing these cases.

Somatoform disorders respond better when intervention is early, without reinforcement by excessive ordering of tests and evaluations, and when patients are told the symptoms are ''real'' but not life-threatening, and you will want to see them again for a scheduled return visit.

CASE 2

Patient Information

A 76-year-old female has complained about epigastric pain, constipation, and a secondary loss of appetite for over 1 month. The pain wakes her at night, she believes causing daytime fatigue. Various gastrointestinal (GI) medications have been tried without success. Upper and lower GI series ordered by your partner for this patient yield normal results. Although the chart indicated her husband died 3½ months ago, she states she does not feel that is holding her back and would not describe herself as depressed. She has been devoted to her church throughout her life, but feels her physical symptoms have kept her from going to services the past few months. She moved out of her home a month ago and into a seniors

apartment to live near a female friend. Her friend was admitted to the hospital 2 weeks earlier and has been diagnosed with cancer.

The patient has never been treated for a psychiatric disorder and there is no family history for this. The patient has a 10-pound weight loss since her last visit 6 weeks ago. She has a history of partially controlled hypertension. Heart rate is 82, PR 120, QRS 100, QT 430/465. She has a 15-mm orthostatic BP drop, but does not complain of dizziness. Her electrolytes, blood urea nitrogen (BUN), creatinine, and physical examination indicate dehydration. Her total protein is slightly low, as well as her hemoglobin and hematocrit. Her liver function tests and urine analysis are normal. Her physical examination and x ray do not turn up any additional information.

QUESTION

1. What is your plan?

   a. Let this probably normal grief response run its course.
   b. Admit her to the hospital for a full work-up.
   c. Prescribe alprazolam (Xanax) for 2 weeks and have her return for a follow-up visit.
   d. Order a laboratory study for thyroid-stimulating hormone (TSH); call the patient's daughter for additional information; consider prescribing a selective serotonin reuptake inhibitor.
   e. Refer her to a gastroenterologist.

Discussion and Answer Explanation

Bereavement generally occurs within the first 2–3 months after the loss of a close loved one. Subjects with depression at 2 months are much more likely to be depressed at 2 years. They are less likely to engage in new relationships and more likely to experience worse generalized health than prior to their loss. Admitting the patient to the hospital does not seem necessary at this stage, although we would want to do some basic laboratory studies, including a TSH. It would be unlikely that referral to a gastroenterologist is necessary with two normal GI series. The weight loss, insomnia, fatigue, and discontinuation of her normal activities are possibly symptoms of depression. Starting an anxiolytic is not advisable and would likely slow recognition and treatment of major depression. Additional information and observations by family are always helpful.

As you talk to her longer, you learn that she believes she must have done something wrong for her husband to die and now she is losing her best friend. She talks about her daughters, one who is a nun and has much responsibility, and the other who lives in a distant state with her husband and the patient's only grandchildren. She admits to withdrawal from others. ''I should be stronger. My daughters have important things to do. As for other friends, if I get close, they'll just be taken away from me.'' The patient acknowledges she thinks of this a great deal. She also wonders if her body is developing cancer. She does not drink alcohol or smoke cigarettes, and she has no suicidal thoughts.

Patients may not identify themselves as depressed and stoically continue on despite their losses. It may take some additional questions to find the psychologic aspects of their condition. Ruminating on negative thoughts, excessive guilt, or belief of punishment and a lack of interest and pleasure in former activities are key symptoms. Physical symptoms of weight loss and insomnia may be associated with a variety of conditions and can be further explored, but depression should be treated when the criteria exist.

Sixty to 80% of the general public have a physical complaint during any given week, and physicians may be unable to identify organic cause in 20–80% of patients bringing these symptoms to the office visit. Patients with a diagnosis of major depression more often present with physical symptoms to their primary care physician.

Treat patients who meet criteria for major depression whether or not there is a comorbid physical illness or any "good reason to be depressed."

Signs and symptoms of depression in a medically ill patient include:

S⇕	sleep	W↑	withdrawal from others
I↓	interest	A↑	anhedonia
G↑	guilt	R↑	ruminating thoughts
E↓	energy	T↑	tearfulness
C↓	concentration		
A⇕	appetite		
P⇕	psychomotor		
S↑	suicidal thoughts or thoughts of death		

QUESTION

2. What do you think most closely identifies her condition?

   a. Generalized anxiety disorder
   b. Occult affective disorder (major depression without psychosis; single episode)
   c. Hypochondriasis
   d. Psychotic delusional disorder
   e. Posttraumatic stress disorder

Discussion and Answer Explanation

The patient does have many of the criteria for major depressive disorder and few of those for the other diagnoses.

Criteria for Major Depressive Episode (DSM-IV)

For a major depressive disorder, five (or more) of the following symptoms have been present during the same 2-week period and represent a change from previously functioning; at least one of the symptoms is either (1) depressed mood or (2) loss of interest or pleasure:

- Depressed mood most of the day or observation by others of depression
- Markedly diminished interest or pleasure; subjective account or observation made by others
- Significant weight loss when not dieting or weight gain, or decrease/increase in appetite nearly every day
- Insomnia or hypersomnia
- Psychomotor agitation or retardation
- Fatigue or loss of energy
- Feelings of worthlessness or excessive or inappropriate guilt
- Diminished ability to think or concentrate, or indecisiveness
- Recurrent thoughts of death or suicidal ideation

QUESTION

3. An effective, appropriate, and safe treatment to begin today is:

   a. Sertraline 50 mg qd
   b. Electroconvulsive therapy (ECT)
   c. Amitriptyline 75 mg bid
   d. Doxepin 150 mg qhs
   e. Psychoanalytic psychotherapy

Discussion and Answer Explanation

In this case, avoiding additional orthostasis, cardiac conduction delay (quinidine-like), and anticholinergic effects would recommend against a tricyclic. A rapid, safe first line choice would be a selective serotonin reuptake inhibitor, such as sertraline. Psychoanalytic psychotherapy is very lengthy and would not be recommended alone in this case. ECT would be a later option if two or more antidepressants were not effective or if the patient was acutely suicidal.

CASE 3

Patient Information

A 20-year-old male presents to the office. He tells you that last week, during his examination at the university, he had two episodes of choking. They came on unexpectedly and made it very difficult for him to finish the test. On another occasion he was just watching television in his room. The patient is concerned that these episodes will return and is fearful of going anywhere alone that would make it difficult for him to get to medical care. As you begin to question him further, he answers that he did feel short of breath and as though he might pass out after some minutes. He does not recall chest pain, headache, or abdominal pain. The patient takes Seldane for an allergy and has not been bothered by his symptoms.

The patient describes that he remembers feeling dizzy and sweaty toward the end of the episode. Family history indicates some complaints of dizziness 2 years earlier that did not occur on more than a few occasions and then disappeared. He stated he was told once he might have mitral valve prolapse. Although he states that he never visited a mental health professional, his parents had planned to take him to one during elementary school because he did not want to leave them to attend class. In addition, a 35-year-old aunt used to have chest pain and a rapid heart rate off and on and has been on Prozac for several years.

PANIC ATTACK AND PANIC DISORDER

Criteria for Panic Attack (DSM-IV)

Panic attack is diagnosed as a discrete period of intense fear or discomfort, in which four (or more) of the following symptoms developed abruptly and reached a peak within 10 minutes.

- Palpitations, pounding heart, or accelerated heart rate
- Sweating
- Trembling or shaking
- Sensations of shortness of breath or smothering
- Feeling of choking
- Chest pain or discomfort
- Nausea or abdominal distress
- Feeling dizzy, unsteady, lightheaded, faint
- Derealization (feelings of unreality) or depersonalization (being detached from oneself)
- Fear of losing control or going crazy
- Fear of dying
- Paresthesias (numbness or tingling sensation)
- Chills or hot flashes

Criteria for Panic Disorder (DSM-IV)

The patient must have recurrent unexpected panic attacks *and*

- At least one of the attacks has been followed by 1 month (or more) of one (or more) of the following:
  - persistent concern about having additional attacks
  - worry about the implications of the attack or its consequences
  - a significant change in behavior related to attacks
  - The diagnosis should also include *with* or *without* agoraphobia.
- The panic attacks are not due to the direct physiologic effects of a substance (e.g., a drug of abuse, a medication) or a general medical condition (e.g., hyperthyroidism).

QUESTION

1. Your impression is that he:

   a. Probably plans to request a medical note to allow him to drop two classes

   b. May have panic disorder and requires further assessment

   c. Should be referred to your ear, nose, and throat (ENT) colleague

   d. Needs a bronchoscopy

   e. Should take a semester off and he'll be fine

Discussion and Answer Explanation

The patient has had panic attacks and now has increased concern about future ones. He is also at risk for agoraphobia, considering he is starting to alter where he will go for fear of an attack. Any medical concerns and substance issues should be explored.

It is reported that patients with panic disorder have often had six medical visits or more before the diagnosis is entertained. Past history of separation anxiety or school phobia during childhood may be an important clue, as well as a positive family history. After basic laboratory studies, a chest film, and ECG are normal, the patient can be reassured and educated about panic disorder.

A wide range of therapeutic options are available, including antidepressants, anxiolytics, and cognitive/behavioral therapy. A frequently chosen option is low-dose antidepressants to avoid frequent side effects that panic patients experience, and a small amount of benzodiazepine as required, usually at night. Panic patients require tiny increments of antidepressant until they are able to tolerate a therapeutic amount with good control of symptoms.

CASE 4

Patient Information

A 51-year-old male patient in the intensive care unit (ICU) presents with acute onset of confusion 36 hours postoperatively, after a successful CABG. The patient is on a number of medications, including insulin, atenolol, promethazine, metoclopramide, and synthroid. The patient has no respiratory distress and has good arterial blood gases (ABGs). His electrolytes, blood sugar, ECG, creatinine, and liver function tests are within normal range at present. A TSH is ordered and oral haloperidol (5 mg) is given to reduce symptoms of delirium. The patient does not improve, and, in fact, the nurses report that his behavior has further deteriorated and his arms and legs have become somewhat rigid.

QUESTION

1. Your plan is to:

   a. Reconfirm that the patient has not used alcohol or benzodiazepines daily

   b. Consider the possibility of anticholinergic activity causing his agitation and other symptoms

   c. Try a dose of lorazepam (1–2 mg)

d. Monitor vital signs and cogwheeling and hold the haloperidol; consider checking creatine phosphokinase (CPK), iron (Fe), and white blood cells (WBC) if his temperature increases or stiffness occurs
e. All of the above

Discussion and Answer Explanation

The correct answer to this question is "all of the above."

Drug-to-drug interactions are frequent delirium inducers. It is wise to avoid multiple anticholinergic drugs that may cause delirium:

*   Antipsychotic agents
*   Antiemetic agents
*   Antiparkinsonian agents
*   Tricyclic antidepressants
*   Antihistamines

Using multiple agents that block dopamine (i.e., haloperidol, promethazine, metoclopramide) may affect multiple dopamine receptors, producing a paradoxical response and severe hypotension. Use a nondopaminergic pressor agent to treat if this occurs.

Avoid multiple drugs that prolong conduction on ECG (QTc)

*   Tricyclic antidepressant
*   Carbamazepine
*   Antipsychotics including pimozide
*   Antiarrhythmics including lidocaine, propafenone, and quinidine
*   Even haloperidol in patients with a history of Torsades de Pointes or alcohol cardiomyopathy

Prolonged metabolism of some QTc-increasing drugs can occur with fluoxetine, fluvoxamine, grapefruit juice, sertraline, nefazodone, ketoconazole, and hismanol via P450-34A isoenzyme.

Multiple reasons may exist for this patient's acute confusional state. Ruling out medication-induced delirium (anticholinergic), thyroid, alcohol or benzodiazepine withdrawal, should suggest other possible causes. It is less likely, but a possibility, that he is developing neuroleptic malignant syndrome. It is more likely that the metoclopramide and oral haloperidol may have increased the extrapyramidal side effects. Close monitoring of vital signs, laboratory studies, and patient responses will further direct treatment.

CASE 5

Patient Information

A 32-year-old female reports frequent headaches that extend from both temples to the back of her head and down her neck. As you further explore the history and complete your physical examination, you find there are adequate criteria to merit a diagnosis of major depressive disorder, recurrent. Although she is willing to try an antidepressant medication, because her symptoms responded in the past, she admits she discontinued it early because she experienced side effects.

QUESTIONS

1. Patients on which antidepressant are more likely to complain of sexual dysfunction?

    a. Nefazodone (Serzone)
    b. Buproprion (Wellbutrin)
    c. Paroxetine (Paxil)
    d. Lithium
    e. Mirtazapine (Remeron)

2. The antidepressant more likely to lead to weight gain is

    a. Mirtazapine (Remeron)
    b. Fluoxetine (Prozac)
    c. Venlafaxine (Effexor)
    d. Nefazodone (Serzone)
    e. Sertraline (Zoloft)

3. Akasthesia is more common with

    a. Venlafaxine (Effexor)
    b. Nefazodone (Serzone)
    c. Mirtazapine (Remeron)
    d. Fluoxetine (Prozac)
    e. Trazadone (Desyrel)

4. Insomnia could more likely be a side effect of which antidepressant?

    a. Imipramine (Tofranil)
    b. Sertraline (Zoloft)
    c. Nefazodone (Serzone)
    d. Trazadone (Desyrel)
    e. Mirtazapine (Remeron)

Discussion and Answer Explanations

1. Patients taking selective serotonin reuptake inhibitors (SSRIs) (fluoxetine, sertraline, paroxetine, fluvoxamine) are more likely to report sexual dysfunction than the other agents listed.
2. Although there are many cases in which it has great benefit, the agent mirtazapine is associated with weight gain.
3. Again, the traditional SSRIs (i.e., fluoxetine) are more likely to induce this side effect than the other options given.
4. Although only a minority of patients will report insomnia, this side effect is more prominent in patients taking SSRIs (i.e., sertraline).

SUGGESTED READINGS

Barsky AJ. Amplification, somatization, and the somatoform disorders. Psychosomatics 1992;33:28–34.

Barsky AJ, Syshak G, Klerman GL. Hypochondriasis. Arch Gen Psychiatry 1986;43:493–500.

Bezchlibnyk-Butler KZ, Jeffries JJ, Martin BA. Clinical handbook of psychotropic drugs, 5th ed. Seattle: Hogrefe and Huber Publishers, 1995.

Bowen RC, D'Arcy C, Orchard RC. The prevalence of anxiety disorders among patients with mitral valve prolapse syndrome and chest pain. Psychosomatics 1991;32:400–406.

Cassem NH, Barsky AJ. Functional somatic symptoms and somatoform disorders. In: Casem NH. The Massachusetts General Hospital handbook of general hospital psychiatry, 3rd ed. St. Louis: Mosby-Yearbook, 1991:131–157.

DeVane CL. Pharmacogenetics and drug metabolism of newer antidepressant agents. J Clin Psychiatry 1994;55(12):38–45.

Franco-Bronson KN. Emotional and psychiatric problems in patients with cancer. In: Skeel RT, Larchant NA, eds. Handbook of cancer chemotherapy, 4th ed. Boston: Little, Brown & Co., 1995:653–669.

Hollander E, Simeon D, Gorman J. Anxiety disorders. In: Hales R, Yudofsky S, Talbott J. Textbook of psychiatry, 2nd ed. Washington, D.C.: American Psychiatric Press, 1994: 495–563.

Kashner TM, Rost, K, Cohens B, et al. Enhancing the health of somatization disorder patients. Psychosomatics 1995;36(5): 462–470.

Leonard B. The comparative pharmacology of new antidepressants. J Clin Psychiatry 1993;54(8):3–15.

Lipowski ZJ. Somatization and depression. Psychosomatics 1990;31:15.

Merikangas JR. Headache syndromes. In: Stoudemire A, Fogel B. Medical Psychiatric Practice Washington, D.C.: American Psychiatric Press, 1991:393–424.

Preskorn SH. Comparison of the tolerability of buproprion, fluoxetine, imipramine, nefazodone, paroxetine, sertraline, venlafaxine. J Clin Psychiatry 1995;56(6):12–21.

Smith GR Jr., Monson RA, Ray DC. Psychiatric consultation in somatization disorder: a randomized, controlled study. N Engl J Med 1986;341:1407–1413.

Stoudemire A. Expanding psychopharmacologic treatment options for the depressed medical patient. Psychosomatics 1995;36:S19–S26.

Wise MG, Rundell JR. Physical symptoms and somatoform disorders. In: Wise MG, Rundell JR. Consultation psychiatry, 2nd ed. Washington, D.C.: American Psychiatric Press, 1994: 91–110.

Infectious Disease

Sexually Transmitted Diseases

Karim A. Adal

Sexually transmitted diseases (STDs) remain a diagnostic and therapeutic challenge for the general internist. This review focuses on the clinical manifestations, diagnosis, and treatment of the more classic STDs:

- Genital ulcers with regional adenopathy
- Urethritis
- Mucopurulent cervicitis (MPC)
- *Chlamydia trachomatis* infections
- Gonococcal infections
- Vaginal infections

This chapter discusses common clinical syndromes relevant to the internist. Treatment recommendations are based on the 1993 recommendations from the Centers for Disease Control and Prevention (MMWR 1993;42(RR-14):1–102).

GENITAL ULCERS WITH REGIONAL ADENOPATHY

Most commonly, genital ulcers are a manifestation of one or more sexually transmitted disease. Inguinal lymphadenopathy commonly accompanies the genital ulceration and can be a useful clue in diagnosis. Genital ulceration with regional adenopathy is characteristic of five of the six "classic" sexually transmitted diseases:

- Primary genital herpes simplex virus
- Primary syphilis
- Chancroid
- Lymphogranuloma venereum
- Granuloma inguinale

An increased risk of HIV infection is associated with each of these causes. Of note, gonorrhea is not a cause of this syndrome. Genital ulcers are frequently misdiagnosed when

history and physical examination are used alone; thus, laboratory tests are important to confirm the clinical suspicion.

In the U.S., genital herpes simplex infection is the most common cause of the syndrome of genital ulceration with regional adenopathy. The second most common cause of this syndrome in the U.S. is primary syphilis. The other infectious causes (the "minor venereal diseases") are relatively uncommon, although outbreaks have been reported. In 1984, the Centers for Disease Control gave the following estimates of new cases that year:

- Primary genital herpes simplex virus: 250,000–500,000
- Primary syphilis: 29,000
- Chancroid: 665
- Lymphogranuloma venereum: 170
- Granuloma inguinale: 30

Table 12.1 summarizes the clinical presentation of genital lesions and inguinal adenopathy for genital ulcers with regional adenopathy.

PRIMARY GENITAL HERPES SIMPLEX VIRUS (CAUSATIVE AGENT: HERPES SIMPLEX VIRUS 2 OR 1)

CLINICAL PRESENTATION OF PRIMARY GENITAL HERPES SIMPLEX VIRUS

Genital Lesion

The incubation period for primary genital herpes simplex virus (HSV) is 1–26 days following exposure, with an average of 1 week. Prior to lesions appearing, the patient may complain of burning or pruritus. The initial lesions are grouped papules

Table 12.1. Clinical Presentation of Genital Ulcers with Regional Adenopathy

	Clinical Presentation of Genital Lesions				
	Incubation	*Type*	*Pain*	*Number*	*Duration*
Primary syphilis	3–90 days	Clean ulcer; raised	no	Usually single	3–6 weeks
Primary HSV	1–26 days	Grouped papules, vesicles, pustules, ulcers	yes	Often multiple	1–3 weeks
Chancroid	1–21 days	Purulent ulcer, shaggy border	yes	Single in men, multiple in women	Progressive
LGV	3–21 days	Papule, vesicle, ulcer	no	Usually single	Few days
Granuloma inguinale	8–80 days	Nodules, coalescing granulomatous ulcers	no	Single/multiple	Progressive

	Clinical Presentation of Inguinal Adenopathy				
	Onset	*Pain*	*Type*	*Frequency*	*Symptoms*
Primary syphilis	Same time	no	Firm	80%, 70% bilateral	Absent
Primary HSV	Same time	yes	Firm	80%, usually bilateral	Common
Chancroid	Same time	yes	Fluctuant; may fistulize	50–65%, usually unilateral	Uncommon
LGV	2–6 wks later	yes	Indurated; fluctuant; may fistulize	$\frac{2}{3}$ unilateral, $\frac{1}{3}$ bilateral	Common
Granuloma inguinale	Variable	+/−	Suppurating pseudobubo	10%	1–5%

that often are painful. The lesions go on to vesiculate, pustulate, and then form small ulcerations that are clean-based.

The diagnostic evaluation of patients with genital ulceration and regional adenopathy includes:

- Serologic test for syphilis
- Dark-field examination or direct immunofluorescence test for *T. pallidum*
- Culture or antigen test for HSV
- Select cases
  - Culture for *H. ducreyi*
  - LGV titers
  - Biopsy for Donovan bodies

In most parts of the U.S., genital herpes and syphilis represent the primary differential diagnostic concerns. Select individuals, however, may require culture for *Haemophilus ducreyi,* biopsy for Donovan bodies, or LGV titers if these less-common entities are suspected.

Lymphadenopathy

Inguinal lymphadenopathy is apparent at the same time as the genital lesions in about 80% of cases. Adenopathy is usually bilateral. The nodes are firm and painful.

Constitutional Symptoms

It is important to note that primary genital HSV is often a systemic illness, with patients complaining of low-grade fever, malaise, headache, and fatigue. In severe cases, patients with primary genital HSV may present with aseptic meningitis, pelvic radiculomyelitis, flank pain—simulating pyelonephritis, or abdominal pain—resembling a surgical abdomen.

DIAGNOSIS OF PRIMARY GENITAL HERPES SIMPLEX VIRUS

Although the presence of grouped vesicles in the genital region is nearly pathognomonic for HSV, many patients present later in the course of the infection when vesicles have already ulcerated. Thus, laboratory confirmation is important in many instances. Several methods are available for confirming the presence of HSV in genital ulcerations:

- The *Tzanck smear* is an established, rapid, and reasonably accurate method for presumptively diagnosing HSV.
- The definitive diagnosis is still isolation of HSV in *tissue culture,* a technique available in most laboratories. In most cases, the turnaround time to isolation of the virus is short (relative to other viruses such as Varicella zoster or cytomegalovirus) because HSV grows rapidly and well in tissue culture systems.
- The recent introduction of the *shell vial* for primary viral isolation has further shortened the time for identification of HSV to 48 hours in many cases.

- Newer methods for HSV detection include several *enzyme immunoassays,* which identify HSV 1 and 2 antigen directly from clinical specimens.
- HSV can also be detected using the *polymerase chain reaction (PCR),* but this technique remains experimental.
- *Serologic studies* may be useful in certain cases of culture-negative primary infections, with the detection of specific HSV IgM strongly suggestive of recent infection. IgM antibody may also be detectable in some individuals during recurrent episodes of genital HSV. A fourfold rise in HSV IgG between the acute and convalescent period is also diagnostic of a primary HSV episode.

TREATMENT OF PRIMARY GENITAL HERPES SIMPLEX VIRUS

First Episode of Primary Genital Herpes Simplex Virus

Treat the first episode of primary genital HSV with acyclovir 200 mg PO 5 times qd for 7–10 days. Patients with severe disease or with complications of primary genital HSV (e.g., pneumonitis, encephalitis, or hepatitis) may be treated with acyclovir 5 mg/kg IV q8h for 5–7 days. Acyclovir affords only partial control of the symptoms of HSV, with documented accelerated healing, but does not impact on the subsequent rate of recurrences. The drug is active only against replicating virus and does not target latent HSV. Topical acyclovir is even less effective than acyclovir given orally.

The safety of acyclovir in pregnancy has not been definitively established. The U.S. Public Health Service recommends that pregnant women should be treated only if there is life-threatening maternal primary genital HSV.

Recurrent Genital Herpes Simplex Virus

Recurrences of genital HSV are common and problematic. Recurrent attacks are less frequently associated with regional adenopathy and constitutional symptoms than primary genital HSV infection; in addition, the genital lesions heal more quickly than with primary genital HSV. The optimal therapy of recurrent attacks remains controversial. Data from large studies suggest that acyclovir is of limited benefit when recurrent episodes are treated individually, shortening the duration of viral shedding and the time to crusting of lesions by less than 1 day. There is no beneficial effect on the rate of recurrences. In severe recurrent disease, some individuals start acyclovir at the start of the prodrome and continue therapy for 5 to 7 days. Possible regimens include:

- Acyclovir 200 mg PO 5 times per day for 5 days
- Acyclovir 400 mg PO tid for 5 days
- Acyclovir 800 mg PO bid for 5 days

Daily Suppressive Therapy

Another approach for patients with frequent and severe recurrences is the use of daily acyclovir therapy. Studies have shown that individuals with frequent recurrences of HSV (defined as six or more outbreaks per year), may have a 75% reduction in the number of recurrences on daily suppressive therapy. Chronic suppression appears to be safe for a 3-year period, but the U.S. Public Health Service recommends a 1-year course, followed by reassessment of the need for daily therapy. Acyclovir-resistant HSV has been isolated from patients on suppressive therapy, but this has not been clearly associated with treatment failures. One limitation of daily suppressive therapy is its lack of long-term benefit; the frequency of outbreaks often returns to baseline once acyclovir has been discontinued.

Either of the following are recommended regimens for daily suppressive therapy:

- Acyclovir 400 mg PO bid for 1 year
- Acyclovir 200 mg PO 3–5 times per day for 1 year

Because the safety of acyclovir in pregnancy has not been established, daily suppressive acyclovir *should not* be used for recurrent genital HSV in pregnant women, nor should recurrent episodes be treated individually unless life-threatening.

Genital HSV and AIDS

Severe, progressive HSV infections are commonly seen in patients with AIDS. Progressive genital and perianal ulcers with proctocolitis may be due to either HSV-1 or HSV-2. HSV proctitis is often quite debilitating, with anorectal pain, bloody stools, and fever. Because recurrences are the rule, these patients are often placed on chronic acyclovir suppression. This has led to the emergence of acyclovir-resistant HSV mutants. Recurrent episodes are often suppressed with daily acyclovir, especially if severe or associated with HSV proctitis. The dosage of acyclovir in this setting is controversial, with some experts recommending 400 mg 3–5 times per day. HSV isolates that are resistant to acyclovir may respond to foscarnet, which acts by a different mechanism than acyclovir or ganciclovir.

SYPHILIS (CAUSATIVE AGENT: *TREPONEMA PALLIDUM*)

PRIMARY SYPHILIS

Clinical Presentation of Primary Syphilis

Genital Lesion The incubation period ranges from 3–90 days (mean 21 days). The syphilitic chancre is typically a single, painless ulcer with raised and indurated borders. The base of the ulcer is clean, usually without purulence. Up to one-third of syphilitic ulcers, however, may be mildly painful. Development of the ulcer is usually slow. In the absence of treatment, chancres persist for up to 6 weeks.

Inguinal Adenopathy   Adenopathy is present in the majority of cases of primary syphilis (about 80%). The onset of adenopathy usually occurs at the same time as the genital lesion. Characteristically, the adenopathy is painless (like the chancre), and the nodes are firm. In 70% of cases, the adenopathy is bilateral.

Constitutional Symptoms   In primary syphilis, constitutional symptoms usually are absent.

Diagnosis of Primary Syphilis

The definitive methods for diagnosing early syphilis are dark-field examination and direct fluorescent antibody tests on active lesions or tissue biopsies. Serologic tests for syphilis, although commonly used, are not diagnostic. A *presumptive* diagnosis of active syphilis can be made using one of various serologic tests, which are classified as follows:

- Nontreponemal
  - Venereal Disease Research Laboratory (VDRL)
  - Rapid Plasma Reagin (RPR)
- Treponemal
  - Fluorescent Treponemal Antibody Absorbed test (FTA-ABS)
  - Microhemagglutination Assay for antibody to *T. pallidum* (MHA-TP)
  - *Treponema pallidum* Immobilization (TPI) test

Both a treponemal and nontreponemal test are generally necessary to presumptively diagnose primary syphilis. As a rule, the treponemal tests stay positive for life following the initial infection, whether or not appropriate therapy has been administered. Because treponemal tests do not correlate with disease activity, they are usually reported as either positive or negative. In contrast, nontreponemal tests *do* correlate with the activity of disease, reaching high titers with primary infection or recent reinfection, and falling over time following appropriate therapy. Nontreponemal tests are reported as quantitative titers. The adequacy of therapy can be determined using serial RPR (or VDRL) tests; ideally the same test in the same laboratory should be followed sequentially.

In primary syphilis, the VDRL is positive in about 70% of cases (treated or untreated), and the RPR is positive in about 80% of cases. Thus, it is important to realize that a substantial number of patients with a typical syphilitic chancre may have a negative nontreponemal test. In contrast, the VDRL and RPR are positive in nearly 100% of individuals with secondary syphilis, treated or untreated. The treponemal tests also may be falsely negative in primary syphilis. The percent positive for the FTA-ABS is 85%, for the MHA-TP, 65%, and for the TPI, 50%.

Treatment of Primary Syphilis

Primary, secondary, and early latent syphilis (defined as syphilis of less than 1 year's duration) are treated with benzathine penicillin G 2.4 million units IM (one dose). For the penicillin-allergic patient, the alternative is doxycycline 100 mg PO bid for 2 weeks.

SECONDARY AND TERTIARY SYPHILIS

As noted above, primary syphilis may produce genital ulceration with regional adenopathy. In the absence of specific therapy, however, further clinical manifestations may develop. Secondary syphilis may develop up to 2 years after initial infection. The common clinical manifestations of secondary syphilis are summarized in Table 12.2.

All patients with syphilis, regardless of stage, should be tested for HIV per CDC recommendations. Patients with syphilis with clinical signs suggesting either meningitis or uveitis should be fully worked up for neurosyphilis or luetic uveitis, including lumbar puncture and slit-lamp examination. During primary or secondary syphilis, invasion of the CSF by *T. pallidum* is common; abnormalities in the spinal fluid can often be demonstrated. However, only a small percentage of patients develop neurosyphilis *if treated appropriately*. The CDC does not recommend routine lumbar punctures in patients with primary or secondary syphilis unless there are signs or symptoms of neurologic involvement.

The natural history of untreated secondary syphilis is that the illness resolves spontaneously after 3–12 weeks, although viable organisms persist. In the absence of specific treatment, patients enter a stage of "latency." Patients are classified as having "early latent" disease if they are asymptomatic and have acquired infection within the preceding year. Those with no symptoms and infection of greater than 1 year's duration are said to have "late latent" syphilis. In the asymptomatic patient with a positive serology, it may sometimes be difficult to distinguish early from late latent disease. Tertiary syphilis

Table 12.2.   Clinical Manifestations of Secondary Syphilis

Manifestation	Percentage of Cases
Skin	90
Mouth and throat	35
Genital lesions	20
Constitutional symptoms	70
CNS	
Asymptomatic	8–40
Symptomatic	1–2

Modified from G.L. Mandell, J.E. Bennett, R. Dolin, eds. Principles and Practice of Infectious Diseases, 4th ed. New York: Churchill Livingstone, 1989:2117–2133.

may produce cardiac or neurologic disease, as well as a variety of less common manifestations.

The sensitivity of the specific diagnostic tests for syphilis are summarized in Table 12.3.

The recommended therapy for the respective stages of syphilis are summarized in Table 12.4.

Syphilis in the HIV-infected individual can be highly aggressive. Patients can progress from primary to tertiary syphilis over several years, as opposed to several decades in the individual without HIV. Several important caveats regarding syphilis in the HIV-infected patient include:

- Progression to tertiary syphilis may occur rapidly (several years).
- Neurosyphilis should always be considered if neurologic disease is present.
- When findings suggest syphilis at any stage but serologic tests are negative, pursue diagnosis with biopsy, dark-field examination, or direct fluorescent Ab staining.

- Treatment
  - Use penicillin
  - No changes in therapy for early syphilis
  - Consider CSF examination in all patients with lues and HIV.
  - Follow-up with VDRL or RPR at 1, 2, 3, 6, 9, 12 months. If titers fail to decrease fourfold after 6 months, retreat and perform LP.

CHANCROID (CAUSATIVE AGENT: *HAEMOPHILUS DUCREYI*, A GRAM-NEGATIVE COCCOBACILLUS)

Although chancroid has remained an uncommon STD in the U.S., its worldwide incidence may exceed that of syphilis. From 1971 to 1980, the number of cases of chancroid in the U.S. was fewer than 900 annually. In the 1980s, the incidence of chancroid increased markedly, with 3,418 cases reported in 1986. Chancroid is a known cofactor for HIV transmission and is endemic in many areas in the United States. From 1981 to 1987, nine major outbreaks of chancroid were reported in the U.S., primarily in Florida, New York City, California, Boston, and Dallas. Chancroid was seen mainly in Hispanic and black heterosexual men who patronized prostitutes. In Florida, chancroid was seen in highly sexually active men without clear prostitute exposure. In Boston, the outbreak may have been related to individuals who had been originally infected in endemic foreign countries, such as Haiti and the Dominican Republic.

CLINICAL PRESENTATION OF CHANCROID

Genital Ulcers

The incubation period for *H. ducreyi* is 1–21 days, with an average of 7 days. Chancroid ulcers are painful, deep, shaggy

Table 12.3. Diagnostic Tests for Syphilis

Test	Primary	Secondary	Late
Nontreponemal			
VDRL	70[a]	99[a]	1[b]
RPR	80	99	0
Treponemal			
FTA-ABS	85	100	98
TPHA or MHA-TP	65	100	95
TPI	50	97	95

[a] Treated or untreated
[b] Treated
Modified from G.L. Mandell, J.E. Bennett, R. Dolin, eds. Principles and Practice of Infectious Diseases, 4th ed. New York: Churchill Livingstone, 1989:2117–2133.

Table 12.4. Treatment for Syphilis

Stage	Recommended	Alternative
Primary Secondary Early latent (<1 year)	Benzathine PCN G 2.4 MU IM × 1	Doxycyline 100 mg PO bid × 2 weeks[a]
Late latent (>1 year) Gummas Cardiovascular	Benzathine PCN G 2.4 MU IM q week × 3	Doxycycline 100 mg PO bid × 4 weeks[a]
Neurosyphilis	Aqueous PCN G 12–24 MU IV qd × 14 days	Procaine PCN 2–4 MU IM qd + Probenecid 500 mg qid (both for 10–14 days)

[a] Avoid tetracyclines during pregnancy
Reprinted with permission from Centers for Disease Control and Prevention. U.S. Public Health Service Recommendations. MMWR 1993;42(RR-14):1–102.

and friable. The borders of the ulcer are undermined. In men, ulcers are more commonly single, whereas in women, the ulcers are multiple.

Inguinal Adenopathy

Regional adenopathy occurs simultaneously with the ulcer and is seen in 50–65% of cases. The nodes are quite tender and tend to be unilateral. In addition, they tend to be fluctuant and can easily fistulize. The combination of a painful ulcer with suppurative inguinal adenopathy is almost diagnostic of chancroid.

Constitutional Symptoms

Constitutional symptoms are uncommon.

DIAGNOSIS OF CHANCROID

Isolation of *Haemophilus ducreyi* from an active genital ulcer is the only definitive means of confirming a case of chancroid. Special media and culture techniques are required to culture this fastidious organism. The Gram stain of an ulcer specimen may be misleading because of the presence of polymicrobial flora colonizing genital ulcers, and culture confirmation remains the gold standard. The sensitivity of culture isolation of *H. ducreyi* from active genital ulcers is variable, ranging from 50–80% depending on the culture medium employed. It is important to note that *H. ducreyi* is almost never isolated from aspiration of inguinal buboes. Alternatives to culture confirmation have been described, but are investigational.

A probable diagnosis of chancroid can be made if all of the following criteria are met:

- One or more painful genital lesion(s)
- No evidence of syphilis (negative darkfield examination or negative RPR more than 7 days after onset of ulcer)
- No evidence of HSV (clinically or by HSV testing)

TREATMENT OF CHANCROID

Treat chancroid with azithromycin 1 g orally (single dose) or ceftriaxone 250 mg IM × 1, or erythromycin 500 mg PO qid for 7 days. For individuals coinfected with HIV and chancroid, some experts recommend the erythromycin regimen (close follow-up is necessary).

LYMPHOGRANULOMA VENEREUM (CAUSATIVE AGENT: *CHLAMYDIA TRACHOMATIS*, SEROVARS LI, L2, OR L3)

CLINICAL PRESENTATION OF LYMPHOGRANULOMA VENEREUM

Genital Lesions

The incubation period for lymphogranuloma venereum (LGV) is variable, ranging from 3 to 21 days. The LGV genital lesion

is not striking and may be missed by the patient or the physician. The lesion is usually single and painless; it may be a papule, a vesicle, or an ulcer. It resolves within several days.

Inguinal Adenopathy

The key to the diagnosis of LGV is the nature of the regional adenopathy, not the genital lesion. The inguinal nodes in LGV develop 2–6 weeks after the primary lesion, but in rare cases the genital lesion may still be present. The nodes are matted, fluctuant, and large. Typically they are unilateral (two-thirds of cases) and painful. Fistulae have been described, especially after diagnostic needle aspiration.

Constitutional Symptoms

These symptoms are often prominent, with complaints of fever, headache, myalgias, and malaise.

DIAGNOSIS OF LYMPHOGRANULOMA VENEREUM

Serologic titers for LGV may be useful in select cases. The complement fixation (CF) test is positive in most cases of active LGV at titers of 1:64 or higher. Such titers become positive between 1 and 3 weeks postinfection. Occasionally, high CF titers have been found in individuals with other chlamydial infections and in asymptomatic patients. Titers less than 1:64 are suggestive but not diagnostic of LGV. It is difficult to demonstrate a classical fourfold rise in specific antibody titer in LGV because of the late presentation of many patients.

TREATMENT OF LYMPHOGRANULOMA VENEREUM

Treat LGV with doxycycline 100 mg PO bid for 21 days. Alternatives include erythromycin 500 mg PO qid for 21 days or sulfisoxazole (or equivalent sulfonamide) 500 mg PO qid for 21 days. Treatment is the same in HIV-infected individuals.

GRANULOMA INGUINALE (CAUSATIVE AGENT: *CALYMMATOBACTERIUM GRANULOMATIS*, A GRAM-NEGATIVE BACILLUS)

Granuloma inguinale, also referred to as Donovanosis, is rare in the United States. In many developing countries, however, it is one of the most prevalent sexually transmitted diseases, and it is common in India, the Caribbean, and Africa. In 1984, an outbreak of 20 cases was identified in Texas. The epidemiology and pathogenesis of Donovanosis in the United States (and endemic countries as well) are poorly characterized. The precise role of sexual transmission is unclear, but repeated anal intercourse appears to be a risk factor for rectal and penile lesions in homosexual couples. Available data suggest that the infection is only mildly contagious.

CLINICAL PRESENTATION OF GRANULOMA INGUINALE

Genital Ulcers

The incubation period varies from 8 to 80 days. The lesions initially appear as subcutaneous nodules (either single or multiple), which later erode. The ulcerations that form above the nodules are painless, clean, and granulomatous. There is often a ''beefy-red'' appearance to the granulation tissue, along with occasional contact bleeding. The lesions are most common on the glans or prepuce of the male and the labial area in the female. The ulcers progressively enlarge in a chronic, destructive fashion. The ulcerations of Donovanosis may be misidentified as carcinoma of the penis, chancroid, condyloma lata of secondary syphilis (when perianal lesions are present), and other causes of genital ulceration.

Inguinal Adenopathy

Infection with *Calymmatobacterium granulomatis* does not produce true regional lymphadenopathy. Instead, the granulomatous process in the genitals may extend into the inguinal region, causing further fibrosis and granulation tissue (termed ''pseudobuboes''). Present in only 10% of patients with Donovanosis, these pseudobuboes are variably painful.

Constitutional Symptoms

These are usually absent.

DIAGNOSIS OF GRANULOMA INGUINALE

The diagnosis of granuloma inguinale can be confirmed by finding the characteristic ''Donovan bodies'' in a crush preparation. Fresh granulation tissue from a genital ulcer is spread over a clean microscope slide, air-dried, and stained with Wright's or Giemsa's stain. ''Donovan bodies'' are multiple, darkly-staining intracytoplasmic bacteria *(Calymmatobacterium granulomatis)* found within the vacuoles of large mononuclear cells. Donovan bodies can also be identified in formal biopsy specimens using standard light microscopy.

TREATMENT OF GRANULOMA INGUINALE

Granuloma inguinale responds well to the following first-line oral antibiotics (used singly):

- Tetracycline 500 mg PO qid
- Ampicillin 500 mg PO qid
- Trimethoprim-sulfamethoxazole DS PO bid

Antibiotics are continued until the lesions are completely healed, usually 21 days or more. In pregnancy, erythromycin 500 mg PO qid is recommended. The treatment for HIV-infected individuals with granuloma inguinale is the same.

URETHRITIS

Urethritis in the sexually active male is characterized by discharge of purulent material from the urethra and by dysuria. Urethritis in the male is traditionally divided into two types: gonococcal and nongonococcal. It is now recommended that testing be performed to determine the specific diagnosis of urethritis, because:

- Both of these infections are reportable to state health departments
- Treatment compliance may be better with a specific diagnosis
- Partner notification may be improved

The CDC recommends that if the diagnostic means are not available, patients should be treated for both infections (gonococcal and chlamydial), although establishing a specific diagnosis is preferred.

NONGONOCOCCAL URETHRITIS

ETIOLOGY

Chlamydia trachomatis is the most common cause of nongonococcal urethritis (NGU), accounting for approximately 50% of the cases. A variety of other pathogens can account for about 15% of cases:

- *Ureaplasma urealyticum*
- *Trichomonas vaginalis*
- Herpes simplex virus

Nearly 35% or more of cases have no etiologic diagnosis.

CLINICAL PRESENTATION OF NONGONOCOCCAL URETHRITIS

NGU is characterized by a mucoid or watery discharge from the urethra and may be asymptomatic in up to 25% of men. The incubation period is about 1–3 weeks.

DIAGNOSIS OF NONGONOCOCCAL URETHRITIS

In the presence or absence of a urethral discharge, NGU may be diagnosed by $\geq$ 5 polymorphonuclear leukocytes per immersion field on a smear of a urethral swab. More recently, the leukocyte esterase test (LET) has been used by clinicians to screen urine from asymptomatic males, looking for urethritis. Although this test is convenient, a positive LET must be confirmed with a Gram stain smear of a urethral swab specimen.

TREATMENT OF NONGONOCOCCAL URETHRITIS

The recommended regimen for NGU is doxycycline 100 mg PO bid for 7 days. Alternative regimens include:

- Erythromycin base 500 mg PO qid for 7 days
- Erythromycin ethylsuccinate 800 mg PO qid for 7 days

Patients who cannot tolerate high doses of erythromycin can try erythromycin base 250 mg PO qid for 14 days or erythromycin ethylsuccinate 400 mg PO qid for 14 days.

COMPLICATIONS OF NONGONOCOCCAL URETHRITIS

Complications of NGU include epididymitis and Reiter's syndrome. Partner notification is important because the female sex partner is at high risk for chlamydial infection and its complications.

MUCOPURULENT CERVICITIS

ETIOLOGY OF MUCOPURULENT CERVICITIS

The major infectious causes of mucopurulent cervicitis (MPC) include *Chlamydia trachomatis*, *Neisseria gonorrhoeae*, and Herpes simplex virus. In many cases, no organism will be isolated. The CDC recommends that patients with MPC have cervical specimens tested for *C. trachomatis* and cultured for *N. gonorrhoeae*.

CLINICAL PRESENTATION OF MUCOPURULENT CERVICITIS

MPC in the sexually active female is the counterpart to urethritis in men. It is characterized by a yellow endocervical exudate, which can be seen in the endocervical canal or in a swab of cervical secretions. In many females, the infection can be minimally symptomatic or completely asymptomatic; others may have abnormal vaginal bleeding following intercourse.

DIAGNOSIS OF MUCOPURULENT CERVICITIS

The diagnosis of MPC is supported by the visualization of yellow or green endocervical mucopus on a white swab (positive swab test). In one recent study, the presence of ten or more polymorphonuclear leukocytes per high-powered field of a Gram-stained specimen of endocervical mucopus correlated with the presence of recognized infectious causes of MPC. It is important to note that most women with *C. trachomatis or N. gonorrhoeae* do not have active MPC.

TREATMENT OF MUCOPURULENT CERVICITIS

Treatment of MPC should be based as much as possible on the results of specific testing for *C. trachomatis* or *N. gonorrhoeae*. If the patient is not likely to return for a follow-up visit, treatment for both should be initiated. If the likelihood of infection with either organism is very high in the particular population, both organisms should be treated as well. The CDC recommends:

- If there is a high prevalence of both *Chlamydia trachomatis* and *N. gonorrhoeae*, treat for both agents (as in many STD clinics).
- If the incidence of *N. gonorrhoeae* is low in the population and the likelihood of *Chlamydia* is high, treat for *Chlamydia* only.
- If both infections are uncommon and compliance for a return visit is good, await test results.

COMPLICATIONS OF MUCOPURULENT CERVICITIS

Serious complications may occur, such as pelvic inflammatory disease, tubal infertility, ectopic pregnancy, and chronic pelvic pain.

CHLAMYDIA TRACHOMATIS INFECTIONS

As discussed previously, *Chlamydia trachomatis* may produce a variety of clinical syndromes, including urethritis, cervicitis, and proctocolitis in the homosexual male. In addition, *C. trachomatis* may be a contributing pathogen in some women with pelvic inflammatory disease. Recent data suggest that there is a high prevalence of *C. trachomatis* in young adults in the United States. Because many chlamydial infections are asymptomatic, the CDC recommends aggressive treatment of both patients with *C. trachomatis* infections and their partners, even if the partners are asymptomatic. The CDC also recommends screening asymptomatic women who are at high risk for chlamydial infection, such as those with multiple sex partners. Some females with apparently uncomplicated cervical infections are likely to have subclinical upper-reproductive-tract infection and are thus at high risk for pelvic inflammatory disease (PID), ectopic pregnancy, and infertility. Treatment of such cervical infections likely reduces these sequelae, although this has not been formally established in clinical trials.

Treatment regimens for uncomplicated chlamydial infections include one of the following:

- Doxycycline 100 mg PO bid for 7 days
- Azithromycin 1 g orally in a single dose

Azithromycin, a new recommendation by the CDC, has the advantage of a single-dose administration that is particularly effective in noncompliant patients. However, doxycycline has a longer history of safety, efficacy, and use and is much less expensive. Azithromycin should not be used in persons younger than 15 because the safety and efficacy of this agent have not yet been established in this group.

Alternative regimens include:

- Ofloxacin 300 mg PO bid for 7 days
- Erythromycin base 500 mg PO qid for 7 days
- Erythromycin ethylsuccinate 800 mg PO qid for 7 days
- Sulfisoxazole 500 mg PO qid for 10 days (relatively poor efficacy)

Ofloxacin, also a new recommendation, is the only quinolone with proven efficacy against chlamydial infection. Ofloxacin is expensive and has no dosing advantages over doxycycline, however, and should not be given to persons younger than 18 or during pregnancy.

Sex partners of those with chlamydial infections should be referred for evaluation and treatment. Partners of symptomatic patients with *C. trachomatis* infection should be treated if the last sexual contact with the index patient is less than 30 days from the onset of the index patient's symptoms. If the index patient is without symptoms, the sex partner, whose last sexual contact with the index patient was within 60 days of diagnosis, should be evaluated and treated. In any case, the *most recent* sex partner should be treated even if the last sexual intercourse took place before these foregoing time intervals.

To manage chlamydial infections in pregnancy, erythromycin base 500 mg PO qid for 7 days is recommended. Doxycycline, ofloxacin, and sulfisoxazole are contraindicated for women during pregnancy and for women who are nursing. The safety of azithromycin in pregnancy is unknown.

GONOCOCCAL INFECTIONS

Despite measures for infection control, more than one million new cases of *Neisseria gonorrhoeae* infection occur in the U.S. annually. In males, gonococcal infections cause serious-enough symptoms for the patient to seek medical care. In females, many infections are asymptomatic, and thus these individuals are at risk for complications, such as PID leading to infertility and ectopic pregnancy. Because of this, the CDC recommends screening high-risk women for gonorrhea, even if they are asymptomatic.

A number of factors influence the therapy of patients with suspected or confirmed gonococcal infections. Over the last 10 years, resistant strains of *N. gonorrhoeae* have become increasingly common. These include penicillinase-producing *N. gonorrhoeae*, tetracycline-resistant *N. gonorrhoeae*, and strains with chromosomally-mediated resistance to multiple antimicrobials. In addition, patients with gonococcal infections are frequently also infected with *C. trachomatis*, making empiric therapy for this infection mandatory in most individuals. The new therapeutic recommendations for uncomplicated urethral, endocervical, or rectal gonorrhea include:

- Ceftriaxone 125 mg IM × 1
- Cefixime (Suprax) 400 mg PO × 1

- Ciprofloxacin 500 mg PO × 1
- Ofloxacin 400 mg PO × 1

Each regimen above should be given with an agent active against C. trachomatis, *such as doxycycline 100 mg PO bid for 7 days*. In the past, the recommended dosage of ceftriaxone was 250 mg IM × 1; the updated recommendation of 125 mg is based on clinical data that show good efficacy with this regimen.

Alternative regimens for uncomplicated gonococcal infections include:

- Spectinomycin 2 g IM × 1
- Injectable cephalosporins (ceftizoxime, cefotaxime, cefotetan, or cefoxitin)
- Cefuroxime (Ceftin), 1 g PO × 1
- Cefpodoxime (Vantin) 200 mg PO × 1
- Quinolones (enoxacin, lomefloxacin, norfloxacin)

Each regimen above should be given with an agent active against C. trachomatis, *such as doxycycline 100 mg PO bid for 7 days*.

All sex partners of symptomatic individuals with gonococcal infection should be evaluated and treated for both *N. gonorrhoeae* and *C. trachomatis* if their last sexual contact with the index patient was within 30 days of the onset of the patient's symptoms. If the index patient has no symptoms, sex partners whose last sexual contact with the index patient was less than 60 days from the diagnosis should be evaluated and treated. In any case, the *most recent* sex partner should be treated, even if the last sexual intercourse took place before these time periods.

DISSEMINATED GONOCOCCAL INFECTION

Disseminated gonococcal infection (DGI) is a unique clinical syndrome. Clinical manifestations include:

- Common manifestations
  Fever
  Leukocytosis
  Skin lesions
  Tenosynovitis
  Polyarthralgias
  Oligoarthritis
  Hepatitis
  Myopericarditis
- Unusual manifestations
  Endocarditis
  Meningitis
  Perihepatitis
- Rare manifestations
  Pneumonia
  ARDS
  Osteomyelitis

In the past, DGI was invariably produced by penicillin-susceptible strains of *N. gonorrhoeae*. In recent years, however, well-documented cases of DGI due to penicillinase-producing strains have been described. The differential diagnosis of patients with suspected DGI includes:

- Infections, such as meningococcemia, endocarditis, septic arthritis, infectious tenosynovitis
- Other bacteremias
- Seronegative arthritides, such as Reiter's syndrome, ankylosing spondylitis, psoriatic arthritis, dermal vasculitis
- Collagen vascular diseases, such as systemic lupus erythematosus

The diagnosis of disseminated gonococcal infection should be suspected in patients with the classic hemorrhagic pustules *and* symptoms of tenosynovitis or oligoarthritis. Skin lesions may be relatively asymptomatic and should be carefully sought. (Usually fewer than ten lesions are evident.) Patients with suspected DGI should have cultures for *N.*

gonorrhoeae obtained of skin lesions, joint fluid, blood, and mucosal surfaces, such as the urethra, cervix, rectum, and pharynx. The diagnostic sensitivities of these respective cultures are summarized in Table 12.5.

VAGINAL INFECTIONS

Vaginal discharge, a common complaint, accounts for up to 10% of all office visits to physicians in private practice. Unfortunately, vaginal signs and symptoms are nonspecific in the diagnosis of vaginitis, and other more serious conditions—such as cervical neoplasia, mucopurulent cervicitis, and pelvic inflammatory disease—must be excluded. The most common causes of vaginitis include bacterial vaginosis (i.e., nonspecific vaginitis), *Trichomonas vaginalis* vaginitis, and yeast vulvovaginitis, due to *Candida albicans* and other yeasts.

The symptoms of vaginitis are rarely specific enough to suggest a precise etiologic diagnosis. Nevertheless, the common clinical manifestations of the respective etiologies of vaginitis are summarized in Table 12.6.

The diagnostic evaluation of the patient with suspected vaginitis should include microscopic examination of vaginal secretions, testing of secretions for pH, and analysis for a fishy odor after the addition of 10% potassium hydroxide to vaginal secretions ("whiff test"). The results of these tests, summarized in Table 12.7, may distinguish the respective etiologies of vaginitis.

BACTERIAL VAGINOSIS

Bacterial vaginosis is produced by *Gardnerella vaginalis,* mycoplasmas, and occasionally anaerobic bacteria. The clinical criteria for the diagnosis of bacterial vaginosis include:

- Gray homogeneous discharge adherent to vaginal epithelium and cervix

Table 12.5. Diagnosis of Disseminated Gonococcal Infection (DGI)

Percent of Patients with Positive Test

Site	Culture	Gram Stain	Immunofluorescence
Skin lesions	10	10	60
Joint fluid	20–30	10–30	25
Blood	10–30	—	—
Mucosal	80–90	—	—
Pharynx			
Urethra			
Cervix			
Rectum			

Table 12.6. Clinical Manifestations of Vaginal Infections

	Normal Vagina	*Yeast Vaginitis*	*Trichomoniasis*	*Bacterial Vaginosis*
Etiology	—	*C. albicans*, other yeasts	*T. vaginalis*	*G. vaginalis,* mycoplasmas, anaerobes
Symptoms	—	Itching, irritation, discharge	Malodorous discharge often profuse	Malodorous discharge
Discharge				
Color	Clear or white	White	Yellow	White or gray
Consistency	Nonhomogeneous, floccular	Clumped, adherent plaques	Thin, homogeneous, frothy	Homogeneous, coats vaginal mucosa
Inflammation of Vulva/Introitus	—	Vaginal erythema, vulvar dermatitis	Vaginal erythema, strawberry cervix	None

Modified from Paavonen J. Sexually transmitted diseases. Lower genital tract infections in women. Inf Dis Clin N Am 1987;1:179.

Table 12.7. Diagnosis of Vaginal Infections

	Normal Vagina	*Yeast Vaginitis*	*Trichomoniasis*	*Bacterial Vaginosis*
pH	<4.5	<4.5	≥4.5	≥4.5
Ammonia odor with 10% KOH	None	None	Usually present	Present
Microscopy	Epithelial cells, lactobacilli	Leukocytes, epithelial cells. Yeast, mycelia, pseudomycelia in up to 80%	Leukocytes, motile trichomonads in 80–90%	Clue cells, few leukocytes, profuse mixed flora

Modified from Paavonen J. Sexually transmitted diseases. Lower genital tract infections in women. Inf Dis Clin N Am 1987;1:179.

- Fishy odor
- pH ≥ 4.5
- Clue cells
- Positive whiff test (vaginal fluid + KOH = fishy odor)

Treatment regimen for bacterial vaginosis include:

- Recommended treatment: metronidazole 500 mg PO bid for 7 days
- Alternative treatment: metronidazole 2 g PO × 1
- Other treatment (effective in clinical trials, but limited experience):
  - Clindamycin 2% cream 5 g intravaginally at bedtime for 7 days
  - Metronidazole 0.75% gel 5 g intravaginally bid for 5 days
  - Clindamycin 300 mg PO bid for 7 days

No treatment is required for sex partners. The following are recommended during pregnancy (metronidazole is contraindicated during the first trimester):

- First trimester
  - Clindamycin vaginal cream
- Second & third trimesters
  - Metronidazole gel
  - Clindamycin cream
  - Oral metronidazole

TRICHOMONIASIS

Treatment regimen for trichomoniasis include:

- Recommended: metronidazole 2 g PO × 1
- Alternative: metronidazole 500 mg PO bid for 7 days

Sex partners should be treated (same regimen as above). The following are recommended during pregnancy (metronidazole is contraindicated during the first trimester):

- First trimester: The CDC states that metronidazole is contraindicated but makes no recommendations for alternative therapies. Some experts have used intravaginal clotrimazole tablets (100 mg daily) for 2 weeks.
- Second and third trimester: metronidazole 2 g PO × 1

Metronidazole gel has not been studied for trichomoniasis.

VULVOVAGINAL CANDIDIASIS

Treatment regimen for vulvovaginal candidiasis include:

- Recommended
  - Butaconazole 2% cream 5 g intravaginally for 3 days
  - Clotrimazole 1% cream 5 g intravaginally for 7–14 days
  - Clotrimazole 100 mg vaginal tablet for 7 days
  - Clotrimazole 100 mg vaginal tablet, two tablets for 3 days
  - Clotrimazole 500 mg vaginal tablet, one tablet in a single application
  - Miconazole 2% cream 5 g intravaginally for 7 days
  - Miconazole 200 mg vaginal suppository for 3 days
  - Miconazole 100 mg vaginal suppository for 7 days
  - Tioconazole 6.5% ointment 5 g intravaginally in a single application
  - Terconazole 0.4% cream 5 g intravaginally for 7 days
  - Terconazole 0.8% cream 5 g intravaginally for 3 days
  - Terconazole 80 mg suppository for 3 days
  - Alternative: Fluconazole 150 mg PO × 1

No treatment is required for sex partners (unless balanitis is present). Treatment during pregnancy is the same as for nonpregnant females.

REVIEW EXERCISES

1. A 19-year-old male presents with a low-grade fever, tender inguinal adenopathy, and the lesions shown in Figure 12.1. He has never had an STD before and he has a new female partner.

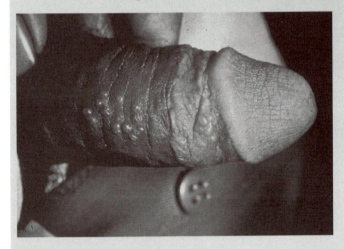

    How should this patient be managed?

    a. Zovirax cream to lesions tid until resolved
    b. No therapy, because trials have failed to demonstrate efficacy in this setting
    c. Acyclovir 200 mg PO 5×/day
    d. Acyclovir 5 mg/kg IV q 8 hours
    e. None of the above

2. A 26-year-old male presents with a several-week-old penile lesion with new inguinal adenopathy. On examination, there is a single nontender ulcer shown in Figure 12.2. There are bilateral palpable inguinal nodes, also nontender. RPR is negative.

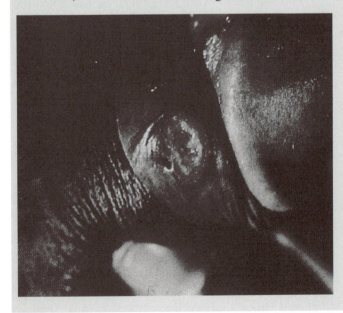

    The most likely diagnosis is:

    a. Gonorrhea
    b. Chancroid
    c. Primary syphilis
    d. Variant herpes simplex
    e. Granuloma inguinale

3. A 44-year-old male presents with several weeks of a painful penile ulcer. He is HIV negative but has frequent prostitute exposure. He has tender inguinal lymph nodes on the right that appeared at the same time as the genital ulcer. He has seen several physicians, apparently without a diagnosis. On examination, the node is fluctuant and has a fistula with pus. The ulcer is shown in Figure 12.3.

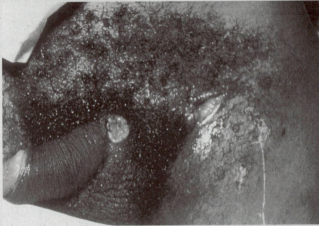

    Which of the following would be effective treatment?

    a. Azithromycin 1 g PO, once
    b. Ceftriaxone 250 mg IM, once
    c. Erythromycin 500 mg PO qid for 7 days
    d. All of the above
    e. None of the above

4. A 60-year-old female is referred to you for a positive VDRL. She is asymptomatic except for mild memory loss. She recalls having syphilis as a teenager, but was never treated. CSF examination shows 0 WBCs, normal protein, and normal glucose; CSF VDRL is nonreactive.
    How should she be managed next?

    a. Erythromycin 250 mg PO qid for 2 weeks
    b. Hospitalize and start aqueous crystalline penicillin G at 12 million units IV qd for 14 days
    c. Benzathine penicillin G 2.4 million units IM × 1
    d. Benzathine penicillin G 2.4 million units IM q week × 3

5. Which of the following statements about secondary syphilis is FALSE?

   a. Rash is the most common clinical manifestation.
   b. Erythromycin is the treatment of choice in the penicillin-allergic patient.
   c. Up to 20% of patients will have a genital lesion evident.

6. A 19-year-old sexually active male (HIV negative) presents with dysuria and a urethral discharge. He has a new partner. The Gram stain of the discharge is shown in Figure 12.4.

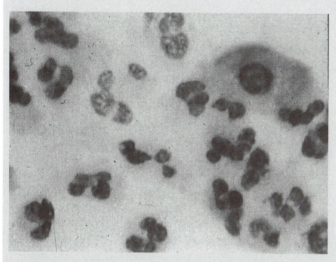

Which of the following statements is FALSE?

   a. He should be specifically tested for *C. trachomatis*.
   b. He should be specifically tested for *N. gonorrhoeae*.
   c. If the patient is unreliable for follow-up, he should be treated with antibiotics empirically.
   d. This condition could be caused by herpes simplex virus.
   e. Asymptomatic infection is rare.

7. A 19-year-old white male presents with a painful urethral discharge. He denies any history of prior sexually transmitted diseases. The Gram stain of the discharge is shown in Figure 12.5.

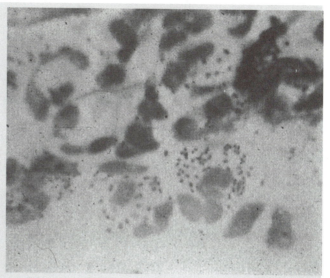

The next step is:

   a. No treatment until cultures of the discharge are finalized
   b. Doxycycline 100 mg PO bid for 7 days
   c. Ceftriaxone 125 mg IM × 1 alone
   d. Ceftriaxone 250 mg IM × 1 alone
   e. None of the above

8. A 35-year-old white female presents with a several-day history of malodorous vaginal discharge. On pelvic examination, there is a gray homogeneous discharge. Examination of the discharge reveals a pH of 6. The Gram's stain is shown in Figure 12.6.

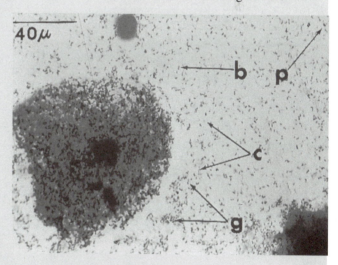

The most likely diagnosis is:

   a. Trichomoniasis
   b. *Chlamydia trachomatis* infection
   c. Bacterial vaginosis
   d. Yeast vulvovaginosis
   e. Other

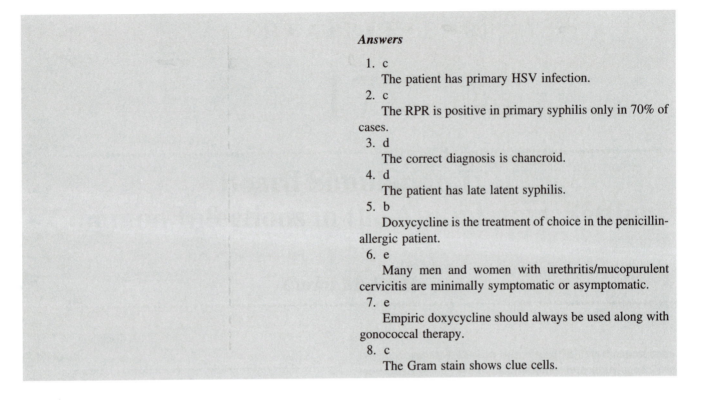

Answers

1. c

    The patient has primary HSV infection.
2. c

    The RPR is positive in primary syphilis only in 70% of cases.
3. d

    The correct diagnosis is chancroid.
4. d

    The patient has late latent syphilis.
5. b

    Doxycycline is the treatment of choice in the penicillin-allergic patient.
6. e

    Many men and women with urethritis/mucopurulent cervicitis are minimally symptomatic or asymptomatic.
7. e

    Empiric doxycycline should always be used along with gonococcal therapy.
8. c

    The Gram stain shows clue cells.

SUGGESTED READINGS

1. Centers for Disease Control and Prevention. 1993 Sexually transmitted diseases treatment guidelines. MMWR 1993; 42(RR-14):1–102.
2. IDCP Guidelines: Sexually transmitted diseases, Part I. Infectious diseases in clinical practice. 1995;4(6): 407–418.
3. IDCP Guidelines: Sexually transmitted diseases, Part II. Infectious diseases in clinical practice. 1996;5(1):6–11.
4. IDCP Guidelines: Sexually transmitted diseases, Part III. Infectious diseases in clinical practice. 1996;5(2):85–93.
5. Drugs for sexually transmitted diseases. The Medical Letter December 22, 1995;37(964):117–122.
6. Mandell GL, Bennett JE, Dolin R, eds. Principles and practice of infectious diseases, 4th ed. New York: Churchill Livingstone, 1989:1055–1103.

HIV Infection and AIDS

Susan J. Rehm

The acquired immunodeficiency syndrome (AIDS) was recognized as a distinct clinical entity in 1981, when unusual clusters of cases of Kaposi's sarcoma and *Pneumocystis carinii* pneumonia were observed in California and New York. The causative agent, human immunodeficiency virus (HIV), was described in 1983, and serologic tests for HIV antibodies were available in 1985.

Since 1981, more than 600,000 individuals have died of AIDS in the United States. AIDS was the leading cause of death of 25 to 44-year olds in the United States in 1995 (15.6/100,000), but the mortality rate dropped 26% in 1996 (11.6/100,000). (This is primarily attributed to the availability of combination therapies for patients with HIV and AIDS.) At present, approximately one million Americans are infected with HIV.

ETIOLOGY OF HIV INFECTION

Like other retroviruses, the HIV genome contains three major genes coding:

* Viral structural proteins (gag)
* Reverse transcriptase (pol)
* Envelope glycoproteins (env)

Analysis of HIV isolates from individual patients has shown that the genome differs substantially from one person to another, particularly in the portion that encodes the viral envelope. Thus, different strains of HIV have biologically important differences in their envelope antigens. Strains in individual patients appear to mutate with time; in addition, patients may be infected with several HIV strains. These factors complicate attempts to develop effective vaccines.

EPIDEMIOLOGY OF HIV INFECTION

The proportion of AIDS cases in the major exposure groups remained stable for the first 5 years of the epidemic, but new trends have been recognized. Homosexual and bisexual males originally accounted for nearly three-quarters of AIDS cases; now these risk groups compromise just over 50% of the total. IV drug users, the heterosexual contacts of infected people, and neonatal patients now make up an increasing share of the total AIDS cases in the United States. The prevalence of HIV infection is highly variable in various communities and regions in the U.S., ranging from 0.1 to 7.8%.

The HIV epidemic is particularly significant with regard to the health of women (who comprise almost 20% of adult patients with AIDS) and children. More than 90,000 American women have been diagnosed with AIDS, and many thousands of women may be infected with HIV yet unaware of their infection. The growth in AIDS cases is more rapid in women than in any other epidemiologic group. The risk for continued perinatal spread of infection is obvious: More than three-quarters of women with AIDS are age 13–39.

Several healthcare workers have been infected in workplace accidents. The number of patients with AIDS due to transmission of HIV infection through blood or blood-product transfusion, however, is declining.

LIFE CYCLE OF HIV

HIV preferentially infects CD4 + cells, primarily T-helper/inducer lymphocytes, but it may also infect other cells that carry the CD4 receptor, such as monocytes and macrophages. Infected monocytes are felt to act as important cellular reservoirs for HIV-1, allowing viral infection to spread to the brain and other organs. HIV attaches to the CD4 receptor via its gp120 envelope protein. The viral DNA is incorporated into the host cell DNA and is reproduced, along with normal cellular components, every time the cell divides. Using host cell components, HIV produces a DNA copy of its RNA genome through its unique enzyme, reverse transcriptase. Production of HIV virions usually proceeds at a low level for long periods after establishment of infection, but there is a progressive loss of CD4 + lymphocytes with time because of the cytopathic effect of viral reproduction. It is postulated that at some point in the infection, an event (possibly an intercurrent infection) may trigger rapid HIV production and subsequent development of severe immunodeficiency.

Mathematic models have been used to further characterize the life cycle of HIV and to guide antiviral chemotherapy. The average generation time for HIV (defined as the time from release of a virion to infection of another cell with release of a new generation of viral particles) is 2.6 days. This includes the life span of a productively infected cell (2.2 days) plus the life span of a virion in the excellular phase (6 hours). The estimated average total HIV production is 10.3×10^9 virions daily. HIV-1, which contains 10^4 base pairs, mutates at a rate of 3.4×10^{-5} per base pair per replication cycle; thus, every mutation at every position in the genome may occur numerous times each day. This calculation has important implications with regard to antiretroviral therapy because it means that combinations of potent agents must be used to prevent the development of resistance. Another challenge of therapy is that approximately 1% of HIV resides in other "compartments," such as tissue macrophages and latently infected cells that are not readily accessible to currently available drugs.

IMMUNOPATHOGENESIS OF HIV INFECTION

The protean clinical manifestations of HIV infection are related to its devastating effect on the immune system, primarily owing to a selective infection of the CD4 + lymphocytes (Table 13.1). These lymphocytes are responsible for the generation of most specific human immune responses, so there are functional defects in virtually all limbs of the system. The severity of the defects depends on the host, the stage of infection, and unknown variables.

TRANSMISSION OF HIV INFECTION

HIV has been isolated from a number of body fluids, including blood, semen, vaginal secretions, breast milk, saliva, urine, cerebrospinal fluid, and tears. In addition, tissues from lymph nodes and from the brain and other organs with large numbers of infected lymphocytes and macrophages are considered potentially infectious. The concentration of virus, or number of infective particles, varies widely in body fluids and tissues and is largely related to the number of lymphocytes in the body fluid. Blood and semen are the fluids that usually contain the highest concentrations of HIV.

Transmission of virus potentially occurs with parenteral or mucosal contact with body fluids that contain high concen-

Table 13.1.   Immune Dysfunction in HIV Infection

Lymphopenia
  Predominantly due to a selective defect in the CD4 lymphocyte subset
Decreased in vivo T-cell function
  Susceptibility to neoplasms and opportunistic infections
  Decreased delayed hypersensitivity
Altered in vitro T-cell function
  Decreased blast transformation
  Decreased alloreactivity
  Decreased specific and nonspecific cytotoxicity
  Decreased ability to provide help to B lymphocytes
Polyclonal B-cell activation
  Elevated levels of total serum immunoglobulins and circulating immune complexes
  Inability to mount a de novo serologic response to a new antigen
  Increased numbers of spontaneous immunoglobulin-secreting cells
  Refractoriness to the normal in vitro signals for B-cell activation

Adapted from Fauci, et al. Acquired Immunodeficiency Syndrome: Epidemiologic Clinical Immunologic and Therapeutic Considerations. Ann Intern Med 1984;100:92–106.

trations of virally infected cells. It is clear that sexual contact and inoculation with infected blood through IV drug use, perinatal exposure, or transfusion are the primary modes of spread of HIV. The risk of perinatal transmission of HIV infection is 25–30%; transmission may occur during gestation or during the birth process (the risk of transmission increases over 1.5-fold with rupture of membranes over 4 hours before delivery of the child). Postnatal transmission via breast milk has also been demonstrated.

Thus, bloodstream or mucous membrane contact with infected fluid can result in transmission of HIV. The concentration and strain of virus, duration and type of exposure, and unknown host factors probably determine whether infection takes place. There have been several reports of seroconversion after a single sexual encounter or significant needlestick exposure. On the other hand, some regular sexual partners of infected individuals have inexplicably remained seronegative. All blood products in the United States have been screened for HIV since the spring of 1985. Because of the rare false-negative testing of a donor who has not yet developed antibodies to HIV, there remains a small risk of seroconversion (estimated at 1 in 680,000 units) after transfusion of a screened unit of blood.

Numerous studies have demonstrated that HIV is not routinely spread to casual household contacts of an infected patient. A few cases of transmission in household settings have been reported, primarily in the context of cutaneous or percutaneous exposure during the course of care of an individual with advanced HIV infection. Surveys of healthcare personnel with intense exposure to AIDS patients have shown no increased incidence of HIV infection unless there was a percutaneous exposure to infected materials. When percutaneous exposure does occur, the average risk of HIV seroconversion is 0.3%

CLINICAL PRESENTATION OF HIV INFECTION

PRIMARY HIV INFECTION

Up to one-half of patients infected with HIV will develop an infectious mononucleosis-like syndrome now recognized as primary HIV infection or retrovirus syndrome. This is observed 3–6 weeks after exposure and resolves spontaneously. Transverse myelitis, lymphocytic pneumonitis, and other more severe manifestations have also been described in the setting of acute HIV infection. HIV seroconversion occurs approximately 8–12 weeks after exposure to the virus. Without antiretroviral therapy, seropositive individuals will eventually develop long-term sequelae of infection, with an incubation period ranging from 18 months (rapid progressors) to more than 10 years. Higher viral load measurements around the time of seroconversion have been associated with increased risk for rapid clinical progression. Patients with persistently elevated viral loads may be appropriate candidates for early initiation of antiretroviral therapy. Rapid disease progression has also been associated with the presence of syncytium-inducing HIV-1, low lyphocyte function, and certain HLA types in the infected individual.

The CD4 + lymphocyte counts in a small percentage of people with HIV infection remain in the normal range for more than 15 years after infection. These individuals, called "long-term survivors," have few clinical symptoms and signs associated with HIV infection. Genetic factors that influence immunity, as well as strain variations in viral virulence, apparently account for the benign clinical course of infection in these rare individuals. An association between heterozygosity for a 32-nucleotide deletion in the C-C chemokine receptor 5 gene and delayed disease progression has recently been described.

RECOGNITION OF HIV INFECTION

Most HIV-infected individuals look and feel well, so recognition of patients with early HIV infection is potentially a challenge for primary-care physicians. Experience in counseling patients at risk and the availability of rapid and accurate testing for HIV infection has eased the process. In the 16 years since AIDS was described, clinicians have become more aware of the subtle signs that may indicate underlying immunodeficiency. For example, women with recurrent vaginal candidiasis and those with carcinoma of the cervix should be screened for HIV infection. Also, young people who have more than one episode of shingles should be offered HIV testing, as should individuals with unusually severe or recur-

rent herpes simplex infections. Because a variety of dermatologic disorders, including severe seborrheic dermatitis, psoriasis, warts, molluscum contagiosum, and particular types of folliculitis, have been associated with HIV infection, testing should also be considered when these conditions are diagnosed. In particular, a constellation of findings (e.g., thrush in a patient with seborrheic dermatitis and venereal warts) may suggest the presence of subtle problems with the cellular immune system. Because treatment with AZT greatly reduces HIV transmission to the fetus, all pregnant women should be screened for HIV and treated if they are found to be infected.

DIAGNOSIS OF HIV

HIV TESTING

The overwhelming majority of infected individuals develop a detectable antibody to HIV within 6 months of exposure. The ELISA test currently used for screening carries a false-negative rate of less than 1% (usually individuals who are in an early stage of infection). ELISA test results should not be reported to the patient until they have been confirmed by Western blot or other confirmatory testing. False-positive rates vary, depending on the prevalence of infection in the population studied. The most common causes of a false-positive ELISA test are multiparity, multiple blood transfusions, infections, and autoimmune diseases.

The Western blot test, immunofluorescent antibody studies, p24 antigen determinations, qualitative polymerase chain reaction (PCR) studies, viral cultures, and other techniques are used to evaluate suspected false-positive and false-negative test results. The p24 antigen test and PCR techniques may be used to detect HIV infection before an antibody has formed or in infants, in whom a maternal antibody may make results difficult to interpret.

In the past year, new methods of determining the HIV viral load have become commercially available. Quantitative PCR and DNA-branched chain methodology determine the number of HIV RNA copies in the plasma of infected individuals. These new tests may be used to measure viral activity and predict disease progression. They also may help to guide antiretroviral therapy, as discussed in that section.

CLASSIFICATION FOR HIV INFECTION AND THE DEFINITION OF AIDS

The CDC classification system for AIDS was modified in 1993 to include the CD4 + lymphocyte count as well as various clinical conditions associated with HIV infection. The system designated three categories for CD4 + lymphocyte counts:

- Category 1: $\geq$ 500 cells/μL ($\geq$ 29%)
- Category 2: 200–499 cells/μL (14–28%)
- Category 3: < 200 cells/μL ($\leq$ 14%)

These categories are to be used in conjunction with one of three clinical categories to assess morbidity associated with the infection. The categories are hierarchical: once a higher (worse) category has been reached, the person remains in the higher category. The clinical categories are:

- Category A
  - Asymptomatic HIV infection
  - Persistant generalized lymphadenopathy
  - Acute (primary) HIV infection or history of acute HIV infection
- Category B
  - Bacillary angiomatosis
  - Candidiasis: oropharyngeal, vaginal (persistent, frequent)
  - Cervical dysplasia (moderate or severe)/carcinoma in situ
  - Constitutional symptoms (fever $> 38.5°$ C; diarrhea lasting > 1 mo.)
  - Hairy leukoplakia, oral
  - Herpes zoster (shingles), involving at least two distinct episodes or more than one dermatome
  - Idiopathic thrombocytopenic purpura
  - Listeriosis
  - Pelvic inflammatory disease, particularly if complicated by tubo-ovarian abscess
  - Peripheral neuropathy
- Category C: AIDS-defining conditions (see Table 13.1)

The CDC surveillance definition of AIDS is designed to identify individuals with the most severe manifestations of HIV infection. In January 1993, the definition was changed; now any HIV-infected individual whose CD4 + lymphocyte count is less than $200/\mu L$ is classified as having AIDS (subcategories A3, B3, and C3). The presence of one of the specified "indicator diseases" is also diagnostic of AIDS, regardless of the CD4 count (subcategories C1, C2, and C3) (Table 13.2). Invasive cervical cancer, recurrent bacterial pneumonia, and pulmonary tuberculosis were added to the list of indicator diseases in the early 1990s.

Used together, the CD4 + lymphocyte and clinical categories can help guide clinical decision-making. For example, individuals in subcategories A3, B3, and C3 (CD4 + lympho-

cyte count $< 200/\mu L$, various clinical stages) would all meet the CDC surveillance definition for AIDS; consequently, prophylaxis against *Pneumocystis carinii* pneumonia and other pathogens should be instituted.

TREATMENT OF HIV INFECTION
ANTIRETROVIRAL THERAPY

Extraordinary progress in HIV therapy has been achieved, particularly in the past year. It is remarkable to reflect that until late 1986, prophylaxis/treatment of opportunistic infections, antineoplastic chemotherapy, and measures aimed at symptom relief were the only modalities available for the treatment of HIV infection. Now there are three classes of drugs available for treatment of HIV infection:

- Nucleoside reverse transcriptase inhibitors
- Nonnucleoside reverse transcriptase inhibitors
- Protease inhibitors

The first specific antiretroviral agent, AZT (zidovudine, Retrovir), became available for general use in April 1987. AZT is the prototype drug for the nucleoside analogue reverse transcriptase inhibitors, which act as chain terminators for HIV reverse transcriptase when they are incorporated in the elongating strand of viral DNA (Table 13.3). As a single agent, AZT usually has been effective in transiently raising the CD4 lymphocyte count, but clinical and virologic resistance have became a problem in many cases. In pregnant women, monotherapy with AZT has reduced fetal infection with HIV from 26% to 8%.

Over the next few years, other nucleoside reverse transcriptase inhibitors (NRTIs)—ddI (Videx), ddC (Hivid), d4T (Zerit), and 3TC (Epivir)—became available for use in HIV-infected patients whose CD4 + lymphocyte count was less than 500 cells/mL. The major side effects of each of the nucleoside RTIs are listed on Table 13.3. Resistance has remained a problem with the newer reverse transcriptase inhibitors.

The availability of protease inhibitors—saquinavir (Invirase), ritonavir (Norvir), indinavir (Crixivan), and nelfinavir (Viracept)—has contributed to new successes in HIV therapy

---

Table 13.2. **AIDS Indicator Diseases**

Candidiasis, invasive	Isosporiasis of > 1 mo. duration
Cervical cancer, invasive	Kaposi's sarcoma
Coccidioidomycosis, extrapulmonary	Lymphoma: primary CNS, immunoblastic, or Burkitt's
Cryptococcosis, extrapulmonary	Mycobacterial disease, disseminated or extrapulmonary
Cryptosporidiosis of > 1 mo. duration	Mycobacterium tuberculosis infection
CMV disease outside lymphoreticular system	*Pneumocystis carinii* pneumonia
Encephalopathy, HIV-related	Pneumonia, recurrent (> 1 episode in a year)
Herpes simplex infection of > 1 mo. duration or visceral	Progressive multifocal leukoencephalopathy
Salmonella bacteremia, recurrent	Toxoplasmosis, cerebral
Histoplasmosis, extrapulmonary	Wasting syndrome due to HIV

Table 13.3. Nucleoside Reverse Transcriptase Inhibitors

Generic Name	Brand Name	Dose[a]	Common Side Effects
AZT (zidovudine, ZDV)	Retrovir	200 mg tid or 300 mg bid	Bone marrow suppression; neurologic, hepatic abns
ddI (didanosine)	Videx	≥ 60 kg: 200 mg bid < 60 kg: 125 mg bid	Pancreatitis; peripheral neuropathy
ddC (zalcitabine)	Hivid	0.75 mg tid	Pancreatitis; mucosal ulcers; peripheral neuropathy
d4T (stavudine)	Zerit	≥ 60 kg: 40 mg bid	Pancreatitis
3TC (lamivudine)	Epivir	≥ 50 kg: 150 mg bid < 50 kg: 2 mg/kg bid	Headache, nausea, nasal symptoms

[a] Dose adjustment may be required for patients with renal dysfunction; consult reference.

Table 13.4. Protease Inhibitors

Generic Name	Brand Name (Tablet Size)	Dose	Major Side Effects[a]
Saquinavir	Invirase (200 mg)	600 mg tid, with meals	Nausea, diarrhea, abdominal discomfort
Indinavir	Crixivan (400 mg)	800 mg tid, between meals	Nephrolithiasis, abdominal discomfort, incr. bilirubin
Ritonavir	Norvir (100 mg)	600 mg bid, with food	GI symptoms, paresthesias, numerous drug interactions
Nelfinavir	Viracept (250 mg)	750 mg tid, with food	Diarrhea, nausea

[a] Therapy with any of the protease inhibitors has been associated with diabetes mellitus.

(Table 13.4). Acting at the stage of viral release from the host cell, the protease inhibitors prevent the action of proteases essential to production of mature, infectious viral particles. Protease inhibitors are able to reduce production of infectious viruses from chronically infected host cells. In contrast, reverse transcriptase inhibitors act primarily on newly infected cells. When used in combination with reverse transcriptase inhibitors, protease inhibitors often stabilize or raise patients' CD4 counts and reduce the viral load. Prerelease studies have revealed that viral resistance may develop with any of the agents, and cross-resistance between the protease inhibitors has been demonstrated. Their oral bioavailability is only fair. Significant drug interactions between the protease inhibitors and other therapeutic agents may also influence their utility. In particular, rifamycins (i.e., rifampin and rifabutin) cause acceleration of the metabolism of the protease inhibitors through induction of hepatic P450 cytochrome oxidases. Protease inhibitors also retard the metabolism of rifamycins, resulting in elevated serum levels and enhanced potential for toxicity. Table 13.4 provides additional information on side effects and drug interactions.

Two nonnucleoside reverse transcriptase inhibitors—nevirapine (Viramune) and delavirdine (Rescriptor)—were released within the past year (Table 13.5). In contrast to the NRTIs, the nonnucleoside reverse transcriptase inhibitors are not incorporated into HIV's DNA; instead they act by binding noncompetitively with viral reverse tran-

scriptase. HIV rapidly develops resistance to NNRTIs when they are used alone; however, these isolates are not cross-resistant to the nucleoside reverse transcriptase inhibitors. Both nevirapine and delavirdine cause a rash in up to a third of the patients receiving therapy. The incidence of nevirapine-associated rash is diminished if the dose is gradually escalated. There are significant drug interactions with the protease inhibitors, precluding concomitant therapy without dose reductions of the protease inhibitor. The role of NNRTIs is evolving, but it is likely that they will be used as part of combination therapy for selected HIV-infected individuals.

Currently, combination therapy with three antiretroviral agents is recommended when therapy is initiated. Most clinicians are using two nucleoside reverse transcriptase inhibitors and a protease inhibitor, but the International AIDS Society-USA Panel suggests that combining two nucleoside RTIs with a nonnucleoside reverse transcriptase inhibitor is also acceptable. The choice of specific agents will depend on individual compliance, treatment history, drug tolerance, concomitant therapy, and patient preference. Currently, the most commonly used combination is AZT, 3TC, and indinavir. If treatment is changed because of clinical progression of disease, rising viral load, falling CD4 count, or adverse drug effects, it is desirable to change all drugs in the regimen. Genotypic and phenotypic analysis of the patient's isolate is necessary to guide therapy through specific information about drug resistance.

Table 13.5. Nonnucleoside Reverse Transcriptase Inhibitors

Generic Name	Brand Name (Tablet Size)	Dose	Major Side Effects
Nevirapine	Viramune (200 mg)	200 mg daily for 2 wks, then 200 mg bid	Rash, abnormal liver function tests, fever, nausea, headache
Delavirdine	Rescriptor (100 mg)	400 mg tid	Rash

Limited data are available for combination therapy with protease inhibitors.

Table 13.6. HIV Viral Load Markers in Clinical Practice

Plasma HIV RNA level suggesting that treatment be initiated
 > 5,000–10,000 copies/mL
Target HIV RNA level after initiation of treatment
 < 500 copies/mL
 1.5 to 2 log reduction from pretreatment levels
Change in HIV RNA level that suggests treatment failure
 > 2,000–5000 copies/mL
 Return to pretreatment level
Suggested frequency of HIV RNA measurement
 Baseline: Two measurements, 2–4 weeks apart
 Every 3–4 months or in conjunction with CD4 + cell counts
 Shorter intervals as critical decision points are approached
 Three or 4 weeks after initiation or change of therapy

Modified from Carpenter et al. Antiretroviral therapy for HIV infection in 1997: updated recommendations of the International AIDS Society—US Panel. JAMA 1997;277:1962–1969.

Newer RNA- and DNA-based quantitative PCR tests for "viral load" or "viral burden" have also been critical to advances in HIV therapy. There are slight variabilities among the assays (RT-PCR, bDNA, NASBA) that preclude setting an absolute plasma HIV RNA threshold for initiation or changes in treatment. Table 13.6 summarizes current indications for their use.

POSTEXPOSURE PROPHYLAXIS

The average risk of HIV seroconversion after percutaneous exposure to blood is 0.3%. When larger volumes of infected materials or fluids with high titers of HIV are involved, the risk is likely to be higher. Conclusive information demonstrating the efficacy of antiretroviral prophylaxis are not available, but in one study AZT postexposure prophylaxis was associated with a 79% reduction in the risk for HIV seroconversion. Prophylaxis with a combination of AZT and 3TC for 4 weeks after the high-risk exposure is recommended; however, the potential for multiply resistant strains of HIV in source patients complicates the picture. In high-risk exposures (those with large volumes, high viral titers, or a potentially resistant HIV strain), a protease inhibitor, such as indinavir, may be added to the regimen. Recommendations for antiretroviral therapy after high-risk sexual exposures are being developed.

PRIMARY CARE OF THE HIV-INFECTED PATIENT

With infection now diagnosed and treated earlier, health maintenance for individuals with HIV infection has assumed an increasingly important role. Increasingly, the chronic illness model is appropriate to their ongoing care. Education of patients with regard to prevention of HIV transmission, proper use of medications, and food/environmental precautions is essential to their care. Likewise, ongoing assessment and support of the patient's psychosocial needs are critical.

In addition to the usual recommendations for health maintenance in adults, patients with HIV infection—depending on their stage of illness—may require additional vaccinations, examinations, and preventive care. A thorough health history, including travel and exposures, should be sought from all newly diagnosed patients. Review of the history of sexually transmitted diseases is particularly important because of the risk of reactivation of central nervous system syphilis during the course of HIV infection. A 5 tuberculin unit purified protein derivative (TU PPD) test with controls should be administered; a PPD response of ≥ 5mm induration is considered positive in HIV infected patients. HIV-infected women should undergo Pap smears every 6 months because of the risk of rapidly progressive HPV-associated cervical neoplasia.

In general, the risk of serious complications of cellular immune deficiency is inversely proportional to the CD4 + T-lymphocyte count, so prophylaxis recommendations are linked to the CD4 + lymphocyte count. Table 13.7 summarizes current recommendations for prophylaxis. The role of oral ganciclovir for prevention of cytomegalovirus (CMV) infection remains controversial. Evidence indicates that the incidence of CMV disease is reduced in HIV-infected persons whose CD4 + lymphocyte count is less than 50 cells/mm^3 who receive oral ganciclovir prophylaxis. Concerns about the cost of CMV prophylaxis and the potential for the development of resistance in this patient population, however, have limited widespread use.

As immune deficiency progresses, major infectious complications may dominate the clinical picture; however, patients receiving antimicrobial prophylaxis against infections

Table 13.7.   Primary Prophylaxis Against Opportunistic Diseases

Pathogen	Indication	Drug of Choice	Alternatives
Pneumocystis carinii	CD4+ count < 200/μL or oral thrush or FUO > 2 weeks	TMP-SMZ, 1 SS or DS tab daily	Low-dose TMP-SMZ; dapsone; aerosol pentamidine
Mycobacterium tuberculosis[a]	PPD + ($\geq$ 5 mm) or contact with active case	INH, 300 mg daily plus pyridoxine 50 mg daily for 12 months; others	Rifampin
Toxoplasma gondii	CD4+ count < 100/μL, and IgG AB to Toxo	TMP-SMZ, 1 DS tab daily	Low-dose TMP-SMZ; dapsone/pyrimethamine/leucovorin
Varicella zoster virus (VZV)	Significant exposure in seronegative patient	VZIG, 5 vials IM, $\leq$ 96 h after exposure	Acyclovir, 800 mg PO 5 times/d $\times$ 3 wks
Streptococcus pneumoniae	All patients	Pneumococcal vaccine, 0.5 mL, IM $\times$ 1	None
Mycobacterium avium complex	CD4+ count < 50/μL	Clarithromycin, 500 mg bid or azithromycin, 1200 mg weekly	Rifabutin or azithromycin + rifabutin
Bacteria[b]	Neutropenia	G-CSF, 5–10 mcg/kg SC daily $\times$ 2–4 weeks	GM-CSF, 250 mcg/m^2 IV over 2 h
Candida spp.[b]	CD4+ count < 50/μL	Fluconazole, 100–200 mg q d	Ketoconazole
Cryptococcus neoformans[b]	CD4+ count < 50/μL	Fluconazole, 100–200 mg q d	Itraconazole
Histoplasma capsulatum[b]	CD4+ count < 50/μL, endemic area	Itraconazole, 200 mg q d	Fluconazole
Coccidioides immitis[b]	CD4+ count < 50/μL, endemic area	Fluconazole, 200 mg q d	Itraconazole
CMV[b]	CD4+ count < 50/μL and antibody positivity	Ganciclovir, 1 g PO tid	None
Hepatitis B[c]	All susceptible pts	Hepatitis B vaccine	None
Influenza[c]	All patients, annually	Whole or split-virus vax	Rimantadine; amantadine

[a] Consult USPHS/IDSA document for recommendations on prophylaxis of INH-resistant or multidrug-resistant *Mycobacterium tuberculosis*.
[b] Indicates recommendations for selected patients.
[c] Generally recommended.

may develop HIV-related disease of the central nervous system, intestinal tract, liver, kidney, or other major organs systems.

COMPLICATIONS OF ADVANCED HIV INFECTION

Patients with advanced HIV infection experience a variety of concomitant infections and other disorders. Some are due to opportunistic pathogens; others are related to infection with common organisms that cause severe disease in the face of underlying immune abnormalities. Infections may be diagnosed in an isolated organ system, but disseminated disease is often present. No matter the cause of infection, there is considerable overlap in symptoms.

RESPIRATORY TRACT DISEASE

Cough and dyspnea are common symptoms in persons with AIDS. Despite major advances in prophylaxis and treatment, *Pneumocystis carinii* continues to be the most frequent cause of pneumonia in this patient population. In the past, the organism has been classified as a protozoan; DNA analysis indicates it is closely related to the fungi. It is a ubiquitous pathogen with which most people have become infected by age 5.

Reactivation of infection occurs in the presence of profound suppression of T lymphocytes; in persons with AIDS, the risk of pneumonia increases significantly when the CD4 lymphocyte count dips below 200/mm^3. Clinically, *Pneumocystis carinii* pneumonia (PCP) usually presents insidiously, with progressive fever, nonproductive cough, weight loss, and dyspnea on exertion. The diagnosis is established by the demonstration of typical cysts on silver stain of induced sputum or material obtained through bronchoscopy. Chest films, DLCO measurements, and gallium scans may be useful adjuncts to diagnosis but do not provide definitive information.

Treatment with either trimethoprim/sulfamethoxazole or pentamidine for 14–21 days appears to be equally effective; there is no benefit to using the agents concomitantly. The rate of significant cutaneous or systemic reaction to trimethoprim/ sulfa is over 50% when high doses are used to treat persons with AIDS. Trimetrexate/leukovorin therapy may be used for patients who are unresponsive to, or intolerant of, standard regimens. Combination therapy with clindamycin and primaquine is another alternative. Patients with milder cases of PCP may be treated with oral trimethoprim/sulfa or the combination of dapsone and trimethoprim. Atovaquone therapy is usually reserved for individuals with mild to moderate cases of PCP who are intolerant to trimethoprim-sulfamethoxazole and dapsone. Absorption of atovaquone is enhanced by concomitant oral intake of fat; individuals with diarrhea may absorb inadequate amounts of the drug, resulting in failed therapy. The use of liquid atavaquone may reduce absorption problems.

Patients with moderate to severe PCP may benefit from the adjunctive administration of corticosteroids. Because recurrent pneumonia is common, patients who have had one episode of PCP should receive prophylaxis against recurrence with low-dose trimethoprim/sulfamethoxazole, aerosol pentamidine, or dapsone. Most HIV-infected patients receive ''primary prophylaxis'' (prophylaxis before the first clinical episode of PCP) when the CD4 lymphocyte count drops below 200/mm^3. Pneumonia confined to the upper lobes of the lung has been described with both primary and recurrent PCP in patients receiving aerosol pentamidine. This, along with the fact that trimethoprim-sulfamethoxazole prophylaxis affords some protection against cerebral toxoplasmosis, has led to preferential use of oral trimethoprim-sulfamethoxazole prophylaxis by many practitioners.

PCP is by no means the only type of pneumonia seen in HIV-infected persons. Bacterial pneumonia owing to *Hemophilus influenzae, Streptococcus pneumoniae, Staphylococcus aureus, Branhamella catarrhalis,* and other common pathogens is being recognized with increasing frequency. In contrast to PCP, the onset of bacterial pneumonia is usually more sudden and the cough is often productive; the chest x-ray may show a well-defined infiltrate. Examination of the sputum gram stain and culture, along with blood cultures, usually establishes the diagnosis. *Nocardia* pneumonia, which is less common than the other bacterial pneumonias, can also be diagnosed by these methods.

The incidence of pulmonary tuberculosis is rising in the face of the AIDS epidemic. It should not be forgotten as part of the differential diagnosis of pneumonia in an HIV-infected person. Even in a profoundly immunosuppressed patient, the tuberculin skin test is occasionally positive. (Five millimeters of induration constitutes a positive skin test in an HIV-infected person.) PPD-positive patients who are infected with HIV should receive prophylaxis with INH. Multiple drug-resistant tuberculosis is spreading rapidly among persons with AIDS in New York and Florida.

The role of *Mycobacterium avium-intracellulare (Mycobacterium avium* complex) and other nontuberculous mycobacteria in producing pulmonary symptomatology remains controversial, although a recent report documented the importance of *Mycobacterium kansasii* pneumonitis in persons with AIDS. Although CMV is often isolated from the bronchoalveolar lavage fluid of patients with PCP, it does not appear to cause clinical pneumonitis in the majority of patients. It is possible that a positive BAL culture for CMV has the same significance as positive urine or saliva cultures in immunosuppressed patients: it often represents reactivation of viral secretion without parenchymal invasion.

Fungal pneumonias owing to *Histoplasma capsulatum, Cryptococcus neoformans,* and *Coccidioides immitis* have been described in persons with HIV infection and AIDS. Pulmonary aspergillosis is quite uncommon, but has been observed in individuals who are neutropenic and/or receiving corticosteroid therapy. Lastly, several noninfectious disorders, such as visceral Kaposi's sarcoma and various lymphocytic pneumonitis syndromes, may be associated with respiratory tract symptoms.

Sinusitis has been recognized as another serious respiratory tract complication of HIV infection. It is usually associated with infection with common bacteria, but unusual fungal pathogens or suprainfection with resistant bacteria may complicate treatment. A sector computed tomography (CT) of the sinuses is a quick and relatively cost-effective way to evaluate this area. Parenteral antibiotic therapy and/or surgical drainage may be required in serious cases of sinusitis.

ORAL LESIONS

Thrush (oral candidiasis) is a well-recognized complication of HIV infection, but it is not diagnostic of AIDS. Therapy with clotrimazole or nystatin topical preparations (troches or mouthwash) is usually adequate; azole therapy should be reserved for patients with recalcitrant disease. Severe gingivitis and periodontitis, related to impaired local immunity in the gingivae, are common. Cases of acute necrotizing ulcerative gingivitis have been described. Some of these disorders can be avoided or ameliorated by careful attention to daily dental hygeine and regular dental prophylaxis. This should be in place well before severe immunosuppression intervenes.

Hairy leukoplakia is a characteristic heaped-up, white lesion on the lateral borders of the tongue. Epstein-Barr viral particles have been identified within these lesions. This disorder is of some clinical significance in that it indicates significant immune dysfunction. No treatment is necessary, but acyclovir has been shown to reduce the bulk of the lesion. Patients with AIDS sometimes experience severe aphthous ulcers; when antiseptic mouthwashes fail, topical steriod therapy may be of benefit. ''Noninfectious'' diseases of the mouth are less common. Macular or papular purple lesions in the oral cavity should raise the suspicion of Kaposi's sarcoma.

GASTROINTESTINAL DISEASE

Dysphagia is a frequent complaint among patients with AIDS. Although candidal esophagitis is the most frequent cause, the presence of thrush in a patient with esophageal symptoms is not predictive of candidal esophagitis. CMV and herpes simplex infections may also be observed, and ulcers due to AZT and "giant aphthous ulcers" of uncertain etiology may cause the same symptoms. If the patient does not respond to empiric antifungal therapy, endoscopy and biopsy are indicated.

Whether due to opportunistic infection, neoplasms, or the HIV infection itself, diarrhea is a ubiquitous problem in HIV-infected individuals. Infections with opportunistic pathogens, such as *Cryptosporidium, Microsporidium, Isospora belli,* cytomegalovirus, and nontuberculous mycobacteria, are frequent and document the diagnosis of AIDS. Other more common microorganisms such as *Salmonella, Shigella, Campylobacter, Giardia lamblia,* and *Entamoeba histolytica* may also cause diarrhea in HIV-infected patients, but their presence does not imply immunodeficiency. The same is true for diarrhea secondary to *Clostridium difficile* toxin. Noninfectious causes of diarrhea in this patient population include gastrointestinal lymphomas and Kaposi's sarcoma. Many patients with HIV infection, however, experience gastrointestinal symptoms in the absence of infections or malignancy. This appears to be due to HIV infection of the gastrointestinal (GI) tract itself, known as HIV enteropathy. There is a spectrum of clinical manifestations of HIV enteropathy. The GI tract infection is asymptomatic in some patients, whereas others experience varying degrees of diarrhea, malabsorption, weight loss, or abdominal pain. Malabsorption may be noted even in patients without gastrointestinal symptoms. Endoscopic findings are negligible in the absence of coexistent infection with another pathogen. Treatment is directed at symptom control after active infectious processes have been sought and ruled out.

Many patients with HIV infection have abnormal liver function tests, even in the absence of infection with hepatitis A, B, or C virus. The reasons for liver dysfunction have not been elucidated fully, and liver biopsy has not been particularly helpful. Biliary tract disease has been described, usually associated with disseminated CMV infection. Lastly, various medications have been associated with hepatobiliary dysfunction; for example, AZT therapy may be associated with reversible hepatic dysfunction; drugs used to treat mycobacterial infections can induce liver dysfunction; and pentamidine use may cause pancreatitis.

NEUROMUSCULAR MANIFESTATIONS

Persons with AIDS may experience headaches, seizures, cranial nerve dysfunction, hemiparesis, peripheral paresthesias,

dementia, and other symptoms. In evaluating patients with neurologic disorders, it is important to determine whether the lesion is peripheral or central.

If a central nervous system abnormality is suspected, the physician should determine whether an intracranial mass lesion is present, as further diagnostic and therapeutic considerations are dependent on the result of the initial CT or MRI scan of the brain. Peripheral blood VDRL, cryptococcal antigen, and toxoplasmosis titers may be helpful in evaluation. For patients who are not receiving trimethoprim-sulfamethoxazole for prophylaxis against *Pneumocystis carinii* infection, toxoplasmosis has been the most common cause of ring-enhancing cerebral mass lesions in HIV-infected persons. Empiric treatment for toxoplasmosis (either a sulfonamide antibiotic or clindamycin in conjunction with pyramethamine) is recommended when the clinical and radiographic findings are compatible and no other diagnosis has been confirmed. If the patient does not respond to therapy for toxoplasmosis, a brain biopsy should be performed. Lymphoma and progressive multifocal leukoencephalopathy (a rapidly progressive white matter disease caused by the JC virus and associated with nonenhancing lesions on CT scan) are other relatively common causes of cerebral mass lesions in HIV patients.

In the absence of mass lesions that cause a midline shift, lumbar puncture is indicated in the evaluation of HIV-infected patients with significant neurologic symptoms. The following evaluations should be performed: cerebrospinal fluid cell counts; protein and glucose determinations; routine, fungal, and mycobacterial cultures; and cryptococcal antigen and Venereal Disease Research Laboratories (VDRL) titers. Cryptococcal meningitis may produce a paucity of symptoms, and a high index of suspicion is warranted. Because treatment failures have been reported with primary fluconazole therapy, initial therapy with intravenous amphotericin B (with or without 5-FC) should be followed with long-term oral fluconazole suppression.

Syphilis is now recognized as an important cause of neurologic and systemic symptoms in HIV-infected persons, and it is clear that HIV infection profoundly influences the individual's response to treatment. Many patients who develop symptoms during the course of their HIV infection were treated for syphilis years earlier; the infection is reactivated in the nervous system because of inadequate CNS penetration of benzathine penicillin. Many authorities recommend cerebrospinal fluid (CSF) analysis for all HIV-infected individuals with a positive serum RPR or HA-TP. Those with a positive CSF VDRL titer should receive several days of intravenous or daily intramuscular penicillin therapy, as outlined in CDC guidelines.

HIV infects the central nervous system early in the course of disease. Up to 90% of persons with AIDS have evidence of HIV encephalopathy at autopsy, and rigorous testing reveals that 70% of AIDS patients develop mental deterioration consistent with AIDS dementia complex. (Severe HIV-associated dementia is observed in a minority of patients.) HIV encephalopathy is an ''indicator disease'' and is diagnostic of AIDS in an otherwise healthy HIV-infected patient. In its early stages, HIV encephalopathy may be confused with depression. Memory loss, changes in affect and judgement, and disruption of normal sleep patterns progress at variable rates. The diagnosis is established when dementia is present in an HIV-infected person and all other causes have been ruled out via brain imaging, lumbar puncture, and appropriate serologic tests.

Myelopathy and peripheral neuropathy are often associated with HIV infection, antiretroviral therapies or intercurrent infections. Treatment with nucleoside analogues, such as ddI and ddC, has been associated with painful peripheral neuropathy. CMV infection may cause myelopathy and assorted unusual neurologic manifestations. Myalgia is a common symptom and myositis a common finding in HIV-infected persons; whether this is due to HIV infection itself, or to therapy such as AZT, is not clear. Pyomyositis has been described in patients with AIDS, and careful examination is necessary to detect mass lesions within muscles. Magnetic resonance imaging (MRI), followed by aspiration and culture of the material in the mass lesion, will aid in the diagnosis of pyomyositis. *Staphylococcus aureus* has been the most common isolate.

OPHTHALMOLOGIC DISORDERS

The most common retinal manifestation of AIDS is CMV retinitis. Affected patients, most of whom have advanced immune dysfunction, may notice progressive ''floaters,'' visual field deficits, or cloudiness in the field of vision. Usually one eye is more involved than the other, but bilateral disease may be found in the absence of symptoms when the periphery is involved. Characteristic fluffy white lesions associated with hemorrhage are visualized along blood vessels of the retina. Early lesions must be distinguished from cotton-wool spots. Uveitis is usually mild compared to the degree of retinitis; severe retinal disease, however, may be associated with diffuse vitreal inflammation. Progression of the lesions results in retinal necrosis. CMV retinitis usually responds to therapy with ganciclovir or foscarnet, but lifelong suppressive antibiotic therapy is required to prevent recurrent disease. Blindness often develops despite aggressive treatment. When visual disturbances progress during therapy, a trial of combined treatment with both ganciclovir and foscarnet is warranted. The release of cidofovir (Vistide) for patients with major intolerance to other treatments or treatment-resistant disease provides another therapeutic option, but the nephrotoxicity of this agent is significant. (It sometimes causes irreversible renal failure.)

Toxoplasma retinitis and *Pneumocystis carinii* choroiditis are less common causes of visual symptoms in patients with AIDS. Pneumocystis choroiditis, a manifestation of disseminated infection, may develop in patients receiving aerosol pentamidine prophylaxis. Toxoplasma retinitis usually responds well to treatment with sulfonamides; experience with treatment of pneumocystis choroiditis is limited, but some patients have responded to infusions of intravenous pentamidine. Several forms of keratitis may also complicate the course of a patient with AIDS. Bacterial keratitis has been observed in individuals who wear contact lenses when the lenses are not cleansed properly. Corneal infection with herpes simplex or varicella zoster may lead to blindness. Microsporidia (protozoal) keratitis, for which there is no known effective antimicrobial therapy, has been described. Uveitis may be due to *Treponema pallidum* or other infections; it has also been described as a side effect of rifabutin therapy.

DERMATOLOGIC DISEASE

Most patients with HIV infection experience several types of skin lesions in the course of their illness. Many eruptions—such as cold sores, genital *Herpes simplex* infections, shingles, warts, condyloma acuminata, and molluscum contagiosum—represent reactivation of old infections due to immunosuppression. Others may be associated with cutaneous manifestations of systemic disease: cryptococcosis, bacillary angiomatosis, CMV, nontuberculous mycobacteria, and other etiologies have been identified. In addition, a number of common skin disorders (most notably seborrheic dermatitis, folliculitis, and psoriasis) may become severe as HIV infection progresses. Most of these skin disorders can be distinguished from Kaposi's sarcoma without difficulty, but clinical manifestations may overlap, making skin biopsy and cultures useful adjuncts to the usual battery of diagnostic tests. In the context of HIV infection, Kaposi's sarcoma (KS) is primarily a disease of individuals who acquired infection sexually; as safer sex practices were used more frequently in the gay population, the incidence of KS has fallen dramatically, leading to speculation that it is a manifestation of a sexually transmitted disease. This theory has been corroborated by the recent discovery of human herpes virus 8 (HHV-8) viral particles within Kaposi's sarcoma lesions.

DISSEMINATED PROCESSES

The clinical manifestations of advanced HIV infection have been modified because of the use of antimicrobial prophylaxis against common opportunistic pathogens. Patients with profound CD4 + lymphocyte depletion may present with undifferentiated wasting, characterized by weight loss, fevers, and night sweats. Although a number of conditions may be associated with this nonspecific syndrome, the most common causes are disseminated *Mycobacterium avium* (MAC) infection and non-Hodgkin's lymphoma.

SUGGESTED READINGS

NATURAL HISTORY

Donaldson YK, Bell JE, Ironside JW, et al. Redistribution of HIV outside the lymphoid system with onset of AIDS. Lancet 1994;343:382–385.

Mellors JW, Rinaldo CR Jr, Gupta P, et al. Prognosis in HIV-1 infection predicted by the quantity of virus in plasma. Science 1996;272:1167–1170.

O'Brien WA, Hartigan PM, Marin D, et al. Changes in plasma HIV-1 RNA and CD4 + lymphocyte counts and the risk of progression to AIDS. N Engl J Med 1996;334:426–431.

O'Brien TR, Blattner WA, Waters D, et al. Serum HIV-1 RNA levels and time to development of AIDS in the Multicenter Hemophilia Cohort Study. JAMA 1996;276:105–110.

Pantaleo G, Graziosi C, Demarest JF, et al. HIV infection is active and progressive in lymphoid tissue during the clinically latent stage of disease. Nature 1993;362:355–358.

Perelson AS, Neumann AU, Markowitz M, Leonard JM, Ho DD. HIV-1 dynamics in vivo: virion clearance rate, infected cell life-span, and viral generation time. Science 1996;271: 1582–1586.

EPIDEMIOLOGY

Centers for Disease Control and Prevention. U.S. HIV and AIDS cases reported through June 1997. HIV/AIDS Surveillance Report 1997;9:1–37.

Centers for Disease Control and Prevention. Update: Trends in AIDS incidence, deaths, and prevalence—United States, 1996. MMWR 1997;46:165–173.

Karon JM, Rosenberg PS, McQuillan G, et al. Prevalence of HIV infection in the United States, 1984 to 1992. JAMA 1996; 276:126–131.

IMMUNOPATHOGENESIS

Fauci AS, Pantaleo G, Stanley S, Weissman D. Immunopathogenic mechanisms of HIV infection. Ann Intern Med 1996; 124:654–663.

Greene WC. The molecular biology of human immunodeficiency virus type 1 infection. N Engl J Med 1991;324: 308–317.

TRANSMISSION

Centers for Disease Control and Prevention: Human immunodeficiency virus transmission in household settings—United States. MMWR 1994;43:347, 353–356. (Reprinted in JAMA 1994;271:1897–1899.)

Friedland GH, Klein RS. Transmission of the human immunodeficiency virus. N Engl J Med 1987; 317:1125–1135.

Lackritz EM, Satten GA, Aberle-Grasse J, et al. Estimated risk of transmission of the human immunodeficiency virus by screened blood in the United States. N Engl J Med 1995;333: 1721–1725.

Landesman SH, Kalish LA, Burns DN, et al. Obstetrical factors and the transmission of human immunodeficiency virus type 1 from mother to child. N Engl J Med 1996;334: 1617–1623.

PRIMARY HIV INFECTION

Cooper DA, Gold J, Maclean P, et al. Acute AIDS retrovirus infection: definition of a clinical illness associated with seroconversion. Lancet 1985;1:537–540.

de Roda Husman A-M, Koot M, Cornelissen M, et al. Association between CCR5 genotype and the clinical course of HIV-1 infection. Ann Intern Med 1997;127:882–890.

Mellors JW, Kingsley LA, Rinaldo DR, et al. Quantitation of HIV-1 RNA in plasma predicts outcome after seroconversion. Ann Intern Med 1995;122:573–579.

Schaker T, Collier AC, Hughes JH, Shea T, Corey L. Clinical and epidemiologic features of primary HIV infection. Ann Intern Med 1996;125:257–264.

HIV TESTING

Centers for Disease Control. Interpretation and use of the Western blot assay for serodiagnosis of human immunodeficiency virus type 1 infections. MMWR 1989;38(S-7):1–7.

Davey RT, Lane HC. Laboratory methods in the diagnosis and prognostic staging of infection with human immunodeficiency virus type 1. Rev Infect Dis 1990;12:912–930.

Owens DK, Holodniy M, Garber AM, et al. Polymerase chain reaction for the diagnosis of HIV infection in adults: a meta-analysis with recommendations for clinical practice and study design. Ann Intern Med 1996;124:803–815.

US Public Health Service recommendations for human immunodeficiency virus counseling and voluntary testing for pregnant women. MMWR Morb Mortal Wkly Rep 1995;44(RR-7):1–14.

CLASSIFICATION

Centers for Disease Control. 1993 revised classification system for HIV infection and expanded surveillance case definition for AIDS among adolescents and adults. MMWR 1993; 41(RR-17):1–20.

Centers for Disease Control. Revised classification system for human immunodeficiency virus (HIV) infection in children under 13 years of age. MMWR 1994;43:1–7.

ANTIRETROVIRAL THERAPY

Carpenter CCJ, Fischl MA, Hammer SM, et al. Antiretroviral therapy for HIV infection in 1997. Updated recommendations of the International AIDS Society-USA panel. JAMA 1997; 277:1962–1969.

Collier AC, Coombs RW, Schoenfeld DA, et al. Treatment of human immunodeficiency virus infection with saquinavir, zidovudine, and zalcitabine. N Engl J Med 1996;334: 1011–1017.

Connor EM, Sperling RS, Gelber R, et al. Reduction of maternal-infant transmission of human immunodeficiency virus type 1 with zidovudine treatment. N Engl J Med 1994;331: 1173–1180.

D'Aquila RT, Johnson VA, Welles SL, et al. Zidovudine resistance and HIV-1 disease progression during antiretroviral therapy. Ann Intern Med 1995;122:401–408.

Deeks SG, Smith M, Holodniy M, Kahn JO. HIV-1 protease inhibitors: a review for clinicians. JAMA 1997;277:145–153.

Fessel WJ. Human immunodeficiency virus (HIV) RNA in plasma as the preferred target for therapy in patients with HIV infection: a critique. Clin Infect Dis 1997;24:116–122.

Hammer SM, Katzenstein DA, Hughes MD, et al. A trial comparing nucleoside monotherapy with combination therapy in HIV-infected adults with CD4 cell counts from 200 to 500 per cubic millimeter. N Engl J Med 1996;335:1081–1090.

Kopp JB, Miller KD, Mican JAM, et al. Crystalluria and urinary tract abnormalities associated with indinavir. Ann Intern Med 1997;127:119–125.

McDonald CK, Kuritzkes DR. Human immunodeficiency virus type 1 protease inhibitors. Arch Intern Med 1997;157: 951–959.

McLeod GX, Hammer SM. Zidovudine: Five years later. Ann Intern Med 1992;117:487–501.

Murray M, Lumpkin MD. FDA Public Health Advisory: Reports of diabetes and hyperglycemia in patients receiving protease inhibitors for the treatment of human immunodeficiency virus (HIV). Bethesda, MD: Food and Drug Administration; 1997.

O'Brien WA, Hartigan PM, Daar ES, Si mberkoff MS, Hamilton JD. Changes in plasma HIV RNA levels and CD4 + lymphocyte counts predict both response to antiretroviral therapy and therapeutic failure. Ann Intern Med 1997;126: 939–945.

Saag M, Holodniy M, Kuritzkes DR, et al. Viral load markers in clinical practice. Nature Medicine 1996;2:625–629.

Spooner KM, Lane HC, Masur H. Guide to major clinical trials of antiretroviral therapy administered to patients infected with human immunodeficiency virus. Clin Infect Dis 1996; 23:15–27.

Wilfert C. Prevention of perinatal transmission of human immunodeficiency virus: a progress report 2 years after completion of AIDS Clinical Trials Group Trial 076. Clin Infect Dis 1996;23:438–441.

PROPHYLAXIS

Centers for Disease Control and Prevention. Case-control study of HIV seroconversion in health-care workers after percutaneous exposure to HIV-infected blood-France, United Kingdom, and United States, January 1988–August 1994. MMWR 1995;44:929–933.

Centers for Disease Control and Prevention. Provisional Public Health Service recommendations for chemoprophylaxis after occupational exposure to HIV. MMWR 1996;45: 468–472. (Reprinted in JAMA 1996;276:90–92.)

Forseter G, Joline C, Worsmer GP. Tolerability, safety, and acceptability of zidovudine prophylaxis in health care workers. Arch Intern Med 1994;154:2745–2749.

Gerberding JL. Management of occupational exposures to blood-borne viruses. N Engl J Med 1995;332:444–451.

Gerberding JL. Prophylaxis for occupational exposure to HIV. Ann Intern Med 1996;125:497–501.

Katz MH, Gerberding JL. Postexposure treatment of people exposed to the human immunodeficiency virus through sexual contact or injection-drug use. N Engl J Med 1997;336: 1097–1100.

PRIMARY CARE OF HIV INFECTED INDIVIDUALS

Bozzette SA, Finkelstein DM, Spector SA, et al. A randomized trial of three antipneumocystis agents in patients with advanced human immunodeficiency virus infection. N Engl J Med 1995;332:693–699.

Carr A, Tindall B, Brew BJ, et al. Low-dose trimethoprim-sulfamethoxazole prophylaxis for toxoplasmic encephalitis in patients with AIDS. Ann Intern Med 1992;117:106–111.

Girard PM, Landman R, Gaudebout C, et al. Dapsone-pyrimethamine compared with aerosolized pentamidine as primary prophylaxis against *Pneumocystis carinii* pneumonia and toxoplasmosis in HIV infection. N Engl J Med 1993;328: 1514–1520.

Havlir D, Dubé MP, Sattler FR, et al. Prophylaxis against disseminated *Mycobacterium avium* complex with weekly azithromycin, daily rifabutin, or both. N Engl J Med 1996; 335:392–398.

Havlir D, Torriani F, Dubé M. Uveitis associated with rifabutin prophylaxis. Ann Intern Med 1994;121:510–512.

Jacobson MA, Besch CL, Child C. Toxicity of clindamycin as prophylaxis for AIDS-associated toxoplasmic encephalitis. Lancet 1992;339:333–334.

Jacobson MA, Besch CL, Child C, et al. Primary prophylaxis with pyrimethamine for toxoplasmic encephalitis in patients with advanced human immunodeficiency virus disease: Results of a randomized trial. J Infect Dis 1994;169:384–394.

Jewett JF, Hecht FM. Preventive health care for adults with HIV infection. JAMA 1993;269:1144–1153.

Nightingale SD, Cameron W, Gordon FM, et al. Two controlled trials of rifabutin prophylaxis against *Mycobacterium avium* complex infection in AIDS. N Engl J Med 1993;329: 828–833.

Powderly WG, Finkelstein DM, Feinberg J, et al. A randomized trial comparing fluconazole with clotrimazole troches for the prevention of fungal infection in patients with advanced human immunodeficiency virus infection. N Engl J Med 1995; 332:700–705.

Public Health Service Task Force on Prophylaxis and Therapy for Mycobacterium avium Complex. Recommendations on prophylaxis and therapy for disseminated *Mycobacterium avium* complex disease in patients infected with the human immunodeficiency virus. N Engl J Med 1993;329:898–904.

USPHS/IDSA 1997 guidelines for the prevention of opportunistic infections in persons infected with human immunodeficiency virus. MMWR Morb Mortal Wkly Rep 1997;46(RR-1):1–48. (Reprinted in Ann Intern Med 1997;127:922–946.)

MANAGEMENT OF COMPLICATIONS OF ADVANCED HIV INFECTION

Drugs for AIDS and associated infections. The Medical Letter 1996;37:87–94.

Hoover DR, Saah AF, Bacellar H, et al. Clinical manifestations of AIDS in the era of Pneumocystis prophylaxis. N Engl J Med 1993;329:1922–1926.

Lane HC, Laughon BE, Falloon J, et al. Recent advances in the management of AIDS-related opportunistic infections. Ann Intern Med 1994;120:945–955.

Smith GH. Treatment of infections in the patient with acquired immunodeficiency syndrome. Arch Intern Med 1994;154: 949–973.

Wachter RM, Luce JM, Hopewell PC. Critical care of patients with AIDS. JAMA 1992;267:541–547.

PULMONARY COMPLICATIONS

Barnes PF, Bloch AB, Davidson PT, Snider DE Jr. Tuberculosis in patients with human immunodeficiency virus infection. N Engl J Med 1991;324:1644–1650.

Beck-Sagué C, Dooley SW, Hutton MD, et al. Hospital outbreak of multidrug-resistant *Mycobacterium tuberculosis* infections: factors in transmission to staff and HIV-infected patients. JAMA 1992;268:1280–1286.

Caumes E, Roudier C, Rogeaux O, Bricaire F, Gentilini M. Effect of corticosteroids on the incidence of adverse cutaneous reactions to trimethoprim-sulfamethoxazole during treatment of AIDS-associated *Pneumocystis carinii* pneumonia. Clin Infect Dis 1994;18:319–323.

Centers for Disease Control. Guidelines for preventing the transmission of tuberculosis in health-care settings, with special focus on HIV-related issues. MMWR 1990;39(RR-17): 1–27.

Centers for Disease Control. Management of persons exposed to multidrug-resistant tuberculosis. MMWR 1992;41(RR-11): 61–71.

Clindamycin and primaquine therapy for mild-to-moderate episodes of *Pneumocystis carinii* pneumonia in patients with AIDS: AIDS Clinical Trials Group 044. Clin Infect Dis 1994; 18:905–913.

Daley CL, Small PM, Schecter GF, et al. An outbreak of tuberculosis with accelerated progression among persons infected with the human immunodeficiency virus: an analysis using restriction-fragment-length polymorphisms. N Engl J Med 1992;326:231–235.

Dooley SW, Villarino ME, Lawrence M, et al. Nosocomial transmission of tuberculosis in a hospital unit for HIV-infected patients. JAMA 1992;267:2632–2635.

Dohn MN, Weinberg WG, Torres RA, et al. Oral atovaquone compared with intravenous pentamidine for *Pneumocystis carinii* pneumonia in patients with AIDS. Ann Intern Med 1994;121:174–180.

Edlin BR, Tokars JI, Grieco MH, et al. An outbreak of multidrug-resistant tuberculosis among hospitalized patients with the acquired immunodeficiency syndrome. N Engl J Med 1992; 326:1514–1521.

Johnson MP, Coberly JS, Clermont HC, et al. Tuberculin skin test reactivity among adults infected with human immunodeficiency virus. J Infect Dis 1992;166:194–198.

Kramer F, Modilevsky T, Waliany AR, Leedom JM, Barnes PF. Delayed diagnosis of tuberculosis in patients with human immunodeficiency virus infection. Am J Med 1990;89: 451–456.

Masur H, Lane HC, Kovacs JA, Allegra CJ, Edman JC. Pneumocystis pneumonia: from bench to clinic. Ann Intern Med 1989;111:813–826.

Masur H. Prevention and treatment of Pneumocystis pneumonia. N Engl J Med 1992;327:1853–1860.

Meduri GU, Stein DS. Pulmonary manifestations of acquired immunodeficiency syndrome. Clin Infect Dis 1992;14: 98–113.

Minamoto GY, Barlam TF, Vander Els, NJ. Invasive aspergillosis in patients with AIDS. Clin Infect Dis 1992;14:66–74.

Monno L, Angarano G, Carbonara S, et al. Emergence of drug-resistant *Mycobacterium tuberculosis* in HIV-infected patients. Lancet 1991;337:852.

Murray JF, Mills J. Pulmonary infectious complications of human immunodeficiency virus infection. Am Rev Infect Dis 1990;141:1356–1372, 1582–1598.

The National Institutes of Health-University of California Expert Panel for Corticosteroids as Adjuctive Therapy for Pneumocystis Pneumonia. Consensus statement on the use of corticosteroids as adjuctive therapy for Pneumocystis pneumonia in the acquired immunodeficiency syndrome. N Engl J Med 323:1500–1504.

Polsky B, Gold JWM, Whimbey E, et al. Bacterial pneumonia in patients with the acquired immunodeficiency syndrome. Ann Intern Med 1986;104:38–41.

Pursell KJ, Telzak EE, Armstrong D. *Aspergillus* species colonization and invasive disease in patients with AIDS. Clin Infect Dis 1992;14:141–148.

Sattler FR, Frame P, Davis R, et al. Trimetrexate with leucovorin versus trimethoprim-sulfamethoxazole for moderate to severe episodes of *Pneumocystis carinii* pneumonia in patients with AIDS: a prospective, controlled multicenter investigation of the AIDS Clinical Trials Group Protocol 029/031. J Infect Dis 1994;170:165–172.

Selwyn PA, Sckell BM, Alcabes P, Friedland GH, Klein RS, Schoenbaum EE. High risk of active tuberculosis in HIV-infected drug users with cutaneous anergy. JAMA 1992;268: 504–509.

Small PM, Schecter GF, Goodman PC, Sande MA, Chaisson RE, Hopewell PC. Treatment of tuberculosis in patients with advanced human immunodeficiency virus infection. N Engl J Med 1991;324:289–294.

White DA, Matthay RA. Noninfectious pulmonary complications of infection with the human immunodeficiency virus. Am Rev Respir Dis 1989;140:1763–1787.

ORAL COMPLICATIONS

Schulten EAJM, tenKate RW, van der Waal I. The impact of oral examination on the Centers for Disease Control classification of subjects with human immunodeficiency virus infection. Arch Intern Med 1990;150:1259–1261.

Shiboski CH, Hilton JF, Neuhaus JM, et al. Human immunodeficiency virus-related oral manifestions and gender: a longitudinal analysis. Arch Intern Med 1996;156:2249–2254.

Weinert M, Grimes RM, Lynch DP. Oral manifestations of HIV infection. Ann Intern Med 1996;125:485–496.

GASTROINTESTINAL DISEASE

Asmuth DM, DeGirolami PC, Federman M, et al. Clinical features of microsporidiosis in patients with AIDS. Clin Infect Dis 1994;18:819–825.

Blanshard C, Francis N, Gazzard BG. Investigation of chronic diarrhea in acquired immunodeficiency syndrome: a prospective study of 155 patients. Gut 1996;39:824–832.

Bissuel F, Cotte L, Rabodonirina M, Rougier P, Piens M-A, Trepo C. Paromomycin: an effective treatment for cryptosporidial diarrhea in patients with AIDS. Clin Infect Dis 1994:18: 447–449.

Bonacini M, Young T, Laine L. The causes of esophageal symptoms in human immunodeficiency virus infection: a prospective study of 110 patients. Arch Intern Med 1991;151: 1567–1572.

Cello JP. Acquired immunodeficiency syndrome cholangiopathy: spectrum of disease. Am J Med 1989;86:539–546.

Goodgame RW. Understanding intestinal spore-forming protozoa: *Cryptosporidia, Microsporidia, Isospora,* and *Cyclospora.* Ann Intern Med 1996;124:429–441.

Laine L, Bonacini M. Esophageal disease in human immunodeficiency virus infection. Arch Intern Med 1994;154: 1577–1582.

Sharpstone D, Gazzard B. Gastrointestinal manifestations of HIV infection. Lancet 1996;348:379–383.

Smith PD, Quinn TC, Strober W, Janoff EN, Masur H. Gastrointestinal infections in AIDS. Ann Intern Med 1992;116: 63–77.

Wilcox CM, Schwartz DA, Clark WS. Esophageal ulceration in human immunodeficiency virus infection: causes, response to therapy, and long-term outcome. Ann Intern Med 1995; 122:143–149.

NEUROLOGIC COMPLICATIONS

Arribas JR, Storch GA, Clifford DB, Tselis AC. Cytomegalovirus encephalitis. Ann Intern Med 1996;125:577–585.

Chaisson RE, Griffin DE. Progressive multifocal leukoencephalopathy in AIDS. JAMA 1990;264:79–82.

Chuck SL, Sande MA. Infections with *Cryptococcus neoformans* in the acquired immunodeficiency syndrome. N Engl J Med 1989;321:794–799.

Cohn JA, McMeeking A, Cohen W, Jacobs J, Holzman RS. Evaluation of the policy of empiric treatment of suspected *Toxoplasma* encephalitis in patients with the acquired immunodeficiency syndrome. Am J Med 1989;86:521–527.

Dannemann B, McCutchan A, Israelski D, et al. Treatment of toxoplasmic encephalitis in patients with AIDS: A randomized trial comparing pyrimethamine plus clindamycin to pyrimethamine plus sulfadiazine. Ann Intern Med 1992;116:33–43.

Gordon SM, Eaton ME, George R, et al. The response of symptomatic neurosyphilis to high-dose intravenous penicillin G in patients with human immunodeficiency virus infection. N Engl J Med 1994;331:1469–1473.

Kalayjian RC, Cohen ML, Bonomo RA, Flanigan TP. Cytomegalovirus ventriculoencephalitis in AIDS. Medicine 1993;72:67–77.

Lipton SA, Gendelman HE. Dementia associated with the acquired immunodeficiency syndrome. N Engl J Med 1995;332:934–940.

McCutchan JA. Cytomegalovirus infections of the nervous systems in patients with AIDS. Clin Infect Dis 1995;20:747–754.

Musher DM, Hamill RJ, Baughn RE. Effect of human immunodeficiency virus (HIV) infection on the course of syphilis and on the response to treatment. Ann Intern Med 1990;113:872–881.

Porter SB, Sande MA. Toxoplasmosis of the central nervous system in the acquired immunodeficiency syndrome. N Engl J Med 1992;327:1643–1648.

Saag MS, Powderly WG, Cloud GA, et al. Comparison of amphotericin B with fluconazole in the treatment of acute AIDS-associated cryptococcal meningitis. N Engl J Med 1992;326:83–89.

Simpson DM, Tagliati M. Neurologic manifestations of HIV infection. Ann Intern Med 1994;121:769–785.

van der Horst CM, Saag MS, Cloud GA, et al. Treatment of crytpococcal meningitis associated with the acquired immunodeficiency syndrome. N Engl J Med 1997;337:15–21.

OPHTHALMOLOGIC COMPLICATIONS

Jacobson MA. Treatment of cytomegalovirus retinitis in patients with the acquired immunodeficiency syndrome. N Engl J Med 1997;337:105–114.

Lalezari JP, Stagg RJ, Kuppermann BD, et al. Intravenous cidofovir for peripheral cytomegalovirus retinitis in patients with AIDS: a randomized, controlled trial. Ann Intern Med 1997;126:257–263.

Lowder CY, Meisler DM, McMahon JT, Longworth DL, Rutherford I. *Microsporidia* infection of the cornea in an HIV-positive man. Am J Ophthalmol 1990;109:242–244.

Masur H, Whitecup SM, Cartwright C, Pois M, Nussenblatt R. Advances in the management of AIDS-related cytomegalovirus retinitis. Ann Intern Med 1996;125:126–136.

Musch DC, Martin DF, Gordon F, et al. Treatment of cytomegalovirus retinitis with a sustained-release ganciclovir implant. N Engl J Med 1997;337:83–90.

Weinberg DV, Murphy R, Naughton K. Combined daily therapy with intravenous ganciclovir and foscarnet for patients with recurrent cytomegalovirus retinitis. Am J Ophthalmol 1994;117:776–782.

DERMATOLOGIC DISEASE

Chang Y, Cesarman E, Pessin MS, et al. Identification of herpesvirus-like DNA sequences in AIDS-associated Kaposi's sarcoma. Science 1994;266:1865–1869.

Foreman KE, Friborg J Jr, Kong WP, et al. Propagation of a human herpesvirus from AIDS-associated Kaposi's sarcoma. N Engl J Med 1997;336:163–171.

Zalla MJ, Su WPD, Fransway AF. Dermatologic manifestations of human immunodeficiency virus infection. Mayo Clin Proc 1992;67:1089–1108.

DISSEMINATED DISEASE

Cohen OJ, Stoeckle MY. Extrapulmonary *Pneumocystis carinii* infections in the acquired immunodeficiency syndrome. Arch Intern Med 1991;151:1205–1214.

Horsburgh CR Jr. *Mycobacterium avium* complex infection in the acquired immunodeficiency syndrome. N Engl J Med 1991;324:1332–1338.

Kemper CA, Meng TC, Nussbaum J, et al. Treatment of *Mycobacterium avium* complex bacteremia in AIDS with a four-drug oral regimen: rifampin, ethambutol, clofazimine, and ciprofloxacin. Ann Intern Med 1992;116:466–472.

Koehler JE, Tappero JW. Bacillary angiomatosis and bacillary peliosis in patients infected with human immunodeficiency virus. Clin Infect Dis 1993;17:612–624.

Markowitz N, Hansen NI, Hopewell PC, et al. Incidence of tuberculosis in the United States among HIV-infected persons. Ann Intern Med 1997;126:123–132.

Public Health Service Task Force on Prophylaxis and Therapy for *Mycobacterium avium* Complex. Recommendations on prophylaxis and therapy for disseminated *Mycobacterium avium* complex disease in patients infected with the human immunodeficiency virus. N Engl J Med 1993;329:898–904.

Pulido F, Pena J-M, Rubio R, et al. Relapse of tuberculosis after treatment in human immunodeficiency virus-infected patients. Arch Intern Med 1997;157:227–232.

Raviglione MC. Extrapulmonary pneumocystosis: The first 50 cases. Rev Infect Dis 1990;12:1127–1138.

Telzak, EE, Cote RJ, Gold JWM, Campbell SW, Armstrong D. Extrapulmonary *Pneumocystis carinii* infection. Rev Infect Dis 1990;12:380–386.

COMPLICATIONS OF HIV INFECTION IN WOMEN

Carpenter CC, Mayer KH, Fisher A, Desal MB, Durand L. Natural history of acquired immunodeficiency syndrome in women in Rhode Island. Am J Med 1989;86:771–775.

Centers for Disease Control and Prevention. Update: AIDS among women—United States, 1994. MMWR 1995;44: 81–84.

Centers for Disease Control. Risk for cervical disease in HIV-infected women—New York City. MMWR 1990;39: 846–849.

Gwinn M, Pappaioanou M, George JR, et al. Prevalence of HIV infection in childbearing women in the United States: surveillance using newborn blood samples. JAMA 1991;265: 1704–1708.

Rhodes JL, Wright C, Redfiled RR, Burke DS. Chronic vaginal candidiasis in women with human immunodeficiency virus infection. JAMA 1987;257:3105–3107.

RENAL DISEASE

Bourgoignie JJ. Renal complications of human immunodeficiency virus type 1. Kidney Internat 1990;37:1571–1584.

Cantor ES, Kimmel PL, Bosch JP. Effect of race on expression of acquired immunodeficiency syndrome-associated nephropathy. Arch Intern Med 1991;151:125–128.

Rao TKS, Friedman EA, Nicastri AD. The types of renal disease in the acquired immunodeficiency syndrome. N Engl J Med 1987;316:1062–1068.

MUSCULOSKELETAL AND RHEUMATOLOGIC MANIFESTATIONS

Berman A, Esponoza LR, Diaz JD, et al. Rheumatic manifestations of human immunodeficiency virus infection. Am J Med 1988;85:59–64.

Buskila D, Gladman D. Musculoskeletal manifestations of infection with human immunodeficiency virus. Rev Infect Dis 1990;12:223–235.

Calabrese LH. Vasculitis and infection with the human immunodeficiency virus. Rheum Dis Clin N Am 1991;17:131–147.

Kaye BR. Rheumatologic manifestations of infection with human immunodeficiency virus (HIV). Ann Intern Med 1989; 111:158–167.

NEOPLASMS AND HEMATOLOGIC DISEASE

Beral V, Peterman TZ, Berkelman RL, Jaffe HW. Kaposi's sarcoma among persons with AIDS: a sexually transmitted infection? Lancet 1990;335:123–128.

Beral V, Peterman T, Berkelman R, Jaffe H. AIDS-associated non-Hodgkin lymphoma. Lancet 1991;337:805–809.

Fine HA, Mayer RJ. Primary central nervous system lymphoma. Ann Intern Med 1993;119:1093–1104.

Groopman JE. Management of the hematologic complications of human immunodeficiency virus infection. Rev Infect Dis 1990;12:931–937.

Levine AM. Therapeutic approaches to neoplasms in AIDS. Rev Infect Dis 1990;12:938–943.

Moore RD, Kessler H, Richman DD, Flexner C, Chaisson RE. Non-Hodgkin's lymphoma in patients with advanced HIV infection treated with zidovudine. JAMA 1991;265: 2208–2211.

Pluda JM, Yarchoan R, Jaffe ES, et al. Development of non-Hodgkin's lymphoma in a cohort of patients with severe human immunodeficiency virus (HIV) infection on long-term antiretroviral therapy. Ann Intern Med 1990;113:276–282.

C·H·A·P·T·E·R

14

Infective Endocarditis

Thomas F. Keys

Following is the classic description of the characteristics of infective endocarditis:

- Remittent fever
- Old valvular heart lesion
- Embolic features
- Skin lesions
- Progressive cardiac changes

ETIOLOGY OF INFECTIVE ENDOCARDITIS

The pathogenesis of infective endocarditis begins with endothelial trauma, such as might occur from regurgitant blood flow or a high pressure gradient. Microorganisms that have adherence factors are preferentially attracted to these lesions. They proliferate within a fibrin meshwork, resulting in an endovascular vegetation. Adherence appears to be promoted by dextran-producing streptococci. For example, *Streptococcus mutans,* which produces large concentrations of dextran, is commonly associated with endocarditis, but it is rarely caused by nondextran-secreting group-A beta-hemolytic streptococci.

EPIDEMIOLOGY OF INFECTIVE ENDOCARDITIS

With the introduction of effective chemotherapy in the early 1940s and surgical intervention beginning in the late 1960s, the outcome of infective endocarditis is not nearly as bleak as in the preantibiotic era when mortality approached 100%. Nevertheless, mortality today remains around 20% (Table 14.1). In part, this is because more patients are living longer with prosthetic heart valves and because of continuing problems of intravenous drug abuse. Furthermore, the resulting

complexities of our technologically advanced health care system expose patients to nosocomial bloodstream infections that may cause endocarditis.

Death from infective endocarditis is related to the following:

- Congestive heart failure
- Embolic phenomenon
- Ruptured mycotic aneurysm
- Cardiac surgery
- Antibiotic failure
- Prosthetic valvular heart disease

It has been estimated that 8,000 cases of infective endocarditis occur annually in the United States. Although historically rheumatic valvulitis was considered the most common form of native heart disease predisposing to infective endocarditis, times have changed. Mitral valve prolapse, aortic sclerosis, and even bicuspid aortic valvular heart disease are now more frequently associated with the diagnosis (Table 14.2). Furthermore, prosthetic valve heart disease underlies about one-third of all cases of infective endocarditis. This complication occurs in 1–3% of all patients with implanted heart valves. Twenty years ago, prosthetic valve endocarditis (PVE) occurring within 2 months of surgery was often fatal; surgeons were reluctant to operate on patients who had active endocarditis on freshly implanted heart valves. Mortality was reported as high as 88%. Prosthetic valve endocarditis most often resulted from intraoperative contamination by nosocomial bacteria, especially *Staphylococcus epidermidis,* as well as inexperience with the newer surgical techniques. Despite advancing surgical expertise and standard antibiotic prophylaxis, early-onset PVE continues to be a problem. However, mortality has been lowered to 20–30%, largely because of aggressive surgical intervention combined with antibiotic therapy.

Table 14.1. Declining Incidence of Death from Infective Endocarditis

Series	Years	Cases	Deaths (%)
Cates and Christie	1945–1949	442	44
Lerner and Weinstein	1939–1959	100	37
Pelletier and Petersdorf	1963–1972	125	37
Keys et al.	1974–1983	90	21
Bayliss et al.	1981–1982	577	14
Sandre and Shafron	1985–1993	135	19

Table 14.2. Underlying Heart Disease in 60 Patients with Native Valve Endocarditis

Lesion	Cases	Incidence (%)
Mitral valve prolapse	14	23
Aortic sclerosis	12	20
Bicuspid aortic valve	6	10
Miscellaneous	6	10
Rheumatic	5	8
Unknown	17	28

Late-onset PVE (LO-PVE), that is, occurring at least 2 months after surgery, is a greater problem because more patients with prosthetic heart valves are surviving longer. Fortunately, however, LO-PVE is usually caused by the same organisms that cause native valve endocarditis; cure rates are nearly as good; and reoperation is usually not necessary.

CLINICAL PRESENTATION OF INFECTIVE ENDOCARDITIS

Clinical findings in patients presenting with PVE do not differ significantly from those with native valve endocarditis (Table 14.3). Fever, skin lesions, a newly appreciated heart murmur, and splenomegaly occur with equal frequency. However, weight loss may be a more common feature in patients with native valve endocarditis, presumably because they are likely to be sicker for a longer period of time before seeking medical attention.

DIAGNOSIS OF INFECTIVE ENDOCARDITIS

LABORATORY STUDIES

Certain laboratory studies are helpful in the diagnosis of infective endocarditis. Nonspecific findings such as an elevated erythrocyte sedimentation rate, a positive rheumatoid factor, proteinuria, and circulating immune complexes are suggestive of the diagnosis. However, the most important laboratory studies are repeated positive blood cultures. In a landmark study reported by Werner and colleagues in 1967, a clear majority of patients suspected of having bacterial endocarditis, provided they had not received antimicrobial agents recently, had positive blood cultures within a period of 24–48 hours. Therefore, one should not need to collect more than three sets of blood cultures over this period, unless the patient has been on recent antibiotic therapy (within 2 weeks).

ECHOCARDIOGRAPHY

Echocardiography, although not a precise diagnostic test for endocarditis, can detect a variety of associated cardiac lesions, such as vegetations, aortic root, and septal and prosthetic ring abscesses, which are very suggestive of the diagnosis (Table 14.4). However, this procedure is overused, especially to ''rule out'' a diagnosis when there is little to suggest the diagnosis at the bedside. The serum bactericidal titer (SBT), which measures the ability of the patient's serum-containing antibiotics to kill the blood isolate, has been a traditional method for measuring in vivo effectiveness of therapy. Unfortunately, the SBT has never been standardized and remains controversial. In our own experience, the SBT has not been a reliable predictor of outcome.

ENDOSCOPY AND COLONOSCOPY

Streptococci, especially viridans streptococci and Group D streptococci (*Enterococcus fecalis* and *Streptococcus bovis*),

Table 14.3. Clinical Findings in 90 Patients with Infective Endocarditis

Symptom	NVE (n = 60)%	PVE (n = 30)%
Fever	75	87
Weight loss	52	20
Skin lesions	51	47
New murmur	33	33
Splenomegaly	20	20

Table 14.4. Echocardiogram Detection of Vegetations in Patients with Infective Endocarditis

Study	Year	N	Sensitivity (%) TTE	(Sensitivity %) TEE
Daniel	1987	69	78	94
Mugge	1989	91	58	90
Shively	1991	16	44	94
Birmingham	1992	31	30	88

Table 14.5.   Native Valve Endocarditis Microbiology

Organism	% of Cases
Streptococcus viridans	30–40
Enterococcus species	5–10
Other streptococci	10–25
Staphylococcus aureus	10–27
Coagulase-negative staphylococci	1–3
Gram-negative bacilli	2–13
Fungi	2–4
Other	5
''Culture negative''	5–24

continue to account for the largest percentage of cases of infective endocarditis (Table 14.5). An interesting association of *Streptococcus bovis* endocarditis with certain forms of gastrointestinal disease, especially cancer and polyps, was reported by Murray and colleagues in 1978. Because of this concern, diagnostic procedures including endoscopy and colonoscopy should be considered in patients with endocarditis owing to *S. bovus,* especially if the patient has any symptoms referable to this area.

The HACEK group of fastidious gram-negative microorganisms occasionally cause endocarditis. HACEK is an all inclusive term for endocarditis due to (*Hemophilus, Actinobacillus, Cardiobacterium, Eikenella* and *Kingella species* of bacteria.) Clinically, these cases are characterized by a subacute-to-chronic course and are often associated with large vegetations that tend to embolize.

When endocarditis occurs within 60 days of cardiac valve implantation, *Staphylococcus epidermidis* and *Staphylococcus aureus* are the most frequent organisms. The problem usually appears related to intraoperative contamination by skin bacteria, but bacteremia from vascular catheters and wound infections in the immediate postoperative period may also be the source of infection. Infection as a result of gram-negative bacteria and yeasts, although rarer, may even be more worrisome because surgical intervention is almost always required to cure the infection.

DIAGNOSTIC CRITERIA FOR INFECTIVE ENDOCARDITIS

The diagnostic criteria as described by Sir William Osler in 1908—remittent fever plus an old valvular heart lesion, embolic features, skin lesions, and progressive cardiac changes—remain true today. Recently, however, transesophageal echocardiography has provided additional criteria that were not appreciated in the past. For example, Durack et al. reported that patients who had at least two of the following three criteria had probable infective endocarditis: a typical organism, persistent bacteremia, and a positive echocardiogram for vegetations, abscess, or valve dehiscence. The added echocardiogram criterion appears to improve the specificity

of the diagnosis previously lacking using the standard clinical criteria of Von Reyn. Transesophageal echocardiography clearly improves the sensitivity of detecting vegetations in patients with endocarditis versus transthoracic studies.

The Von Reyn criteria for the diagnosis of infective endocarditis are as follows:

- Positive valve culture or histology
- Persistent bacteremia with new regurgitant heart murmur, or valvular heart disease and vasculitis
- Negative or intermittent bacteremia and fever; new regurgitant heart murmur and vasculitis

The Duke criteria for the diagnosis of infective endocarditis are as follows:

- Positive valve culture or histology
- Two major criteria: typical organism, persistent bacteremia; positive echocardiogram for vegetations, abscess, or valve dehiscence
- Five or six minor criteria: predisposing lesions or intravenous drug abuse, temperature over 38°C, vasculitis, skin lesions, suggestive echocardiogram, microbiology
- One major and three minor criteria

TREATMENT OF INFECTIVE ENDOCARDITIS

PHARMACOLOGIC TREATMENT

In the preantibiotic era, infective endocarditis was a fatal disease. Now, penicillin, often in combination with gentamicin, remains the cornerstone of therapy for endocarditis due to streptococci. For the penicillin-allergic patient, vancomycin is substituted. Intravenous ceftriaxone has recently been reported to cure penicillin-sensitive streptococcal endocarditis. This agent need be given only once a day and has been used to complete a course of antibiotic therapy at home. When gentamicin is given in combination with penicillin, only 2 weeks of therapy is needed to produce a cure. However, for all cases of prosthetic valve endocarditis and those due to penicillin-''insensitive'' streptococci, a 4–6 week course of therapy is recommended. Table 14.6 summarizes the pharmaceutical treatment of native valve endocarditis.

Therapy for native valve endocarditis due to staphylo-

Table 14.6.   Therapy of Native Valve Endocarditis: PCN-Sensitive Streptococci (M ≤ 0.1 μg/mL)[a]

Antibiotic	Regimen	Duration
PCN-G	12–18 MU IV daily	4 weeks
Ceftriaxone	2 g IV/IM daily	4 weeks
PCN-G	12–18 MU IV daily	2 weeks
+ gentamicin	1 mg/kg IV/IM q 8 hr	
Vancomycin	1 g IV q 12 hr	4 weeks

[a] Doses assume normal renal function

cocci susceptible to methicillin is oxacillin or cefazolin for a 4–6-week course of therapy. If the isolate is methicillin-resistant, vancomycin is substituted. Gentamicin may be added for the first 3–5 days to reduce the burden of bacteremia. However, it does not improve the cure rates and, if continued longer, may cause significant aminoglycoside toxicity.

Antibiotic therapy for staphylococcal endocarditis on prosthetic heart valves must be more aggressive because of the greater likelihood of treatment failure or relapse (Tables 14.7 and 14.8). When the isolate is methicillin-susceptible, oxacillin plus rifampin is prescribed for 6 weeks, and gentamicin is prescribed for the first 2 weeks. When the isolate is methicillin-resistant, vancomycin is substituted for oxacillin, and rifampin and gentamicin are prescribed as noted above.

The current recommended treatment for the HACEK group of gram-negative bacteria is ceftriaxone alone or ampicillin plus gentamicin for 4 weeks of therapy. It should be noted that even cases of late-onset prosthetic valve endocarditis due to HACEK microorganisms have been cured with this type of medical therapy.

On the other hand, patients with yeast endocarditis do not do nearly as well. In 1975, Rubenstein reported that only 31% of patients who received medical combined with surgical therapy were cured. Nguyen and colleagues reported in 1996 that the cure rate was 50% whether or not surgery was combined with medical therapy. With the newer, more effective oral antifungal agents, it has become standard practice to in-

definitely continue patients on oral azole agents after they have received an initial course of IV amphotericin-B therapy. In our experience, fewer than 10% of patients with clinically-suspected endocarditis will have negative blood cultures. Such patients might deserve a trial of empiric therapy such as ampicillin with gentamicin for native valve endocarditis and vancomycin, ampicillin, and gentamicin for prosthetic valve endocarditis. In one study, nearly 50% of patients responded to this type of empiric therapy. However, if the patient is not responding, consider such rare organisms as *Chlamydia psittaci, Coxiella burnetii, Bartonella species, Brucella abortus, Yersinia enterocolitica,* and *Legionella pneumophila.*

Persistent fever during treatment of endocarditis need not be discouraging. In the majority of cases, the fever is benign and may reflect responsiveness to appropriate therapy, drug reactions, or superimposed nosocomial infections (Table 14.9). The most dreaded complication is myocardial abscess, which is an indication for surgical debridement.

SURGICAL TREATMENT

Death from infective endocarditis is less common than in the early antibiotic era, but current data still show mortality rates around 19–21%. Death usually is due to congestive heart failure, frequently complicated by valve dysfunction. Other causes in lesser frequency are major embolic complications,

Table 14.7. Early-Onset Prosthetic Valve Endocarditis Microbiology

Organism	% of Cases
Staphylococcus epidermidis	35
Staphylococcus aureus	17
Streptococcal species	8
Diphtheroids	10
Gram-negative bacilli	16
Fungi	11
Other	3

Table 14.9. Cause of Persistent Fever in 26 Patients with Endocarditis

Cause	Incidence (%)
Myocardial abscess	27
Drug treatment	19
Nosocomial infection	19
Persistent infection	12
Cardiac	12
Postcardiotomy syndrome	4
Splenic abscess	4
Unknown	15

Table 14.8. Therapy of Prosthetic Valve Staphylococcal Endocarditis[a]

Isolate	Antibiotic	Regimen	Duration
MSSA or MSSE	Oxacillin	2 g IV q 4 hr	≥6 weeks
	+ gentamicin	1 mg/kg IV/IM q 8 hr	First 2 weeks
	+ rifampin	300 mg PO q 8 hr	≥6 weeks
MRSA or MRSE	Vancomycin	1 g IV q 12 hr	≥6 weeks
	+ gentamicin	1 mg/kg IV/IM q 8 hr	First 2 weeks
	+ rifampin	300 mg PO q 8 hr	≥6 weeks

[a] Doses assume normal renal function

ruptured mycotic aneurysm, and failure of antibiotic treatment. Today, aggressive surgery is the most important advance in treatment. Surgery during the acute infection does not increase hospital mortality; in fact, restoration of a failing pump will improve the outcome. Valve failure causing moderate to severe congestive heart failure (NYH Class III or IV) is the most important indication for immediate surgery, as are abscesses of the aortic root, prosthetic ring, or ventricular septum. Less pressing indications for surgery are large vegetations (over 1 cm in diameter), predictably resistant organisms such as *Pseudomonas aeruginosa* or *Candida albicans,* and microbiologic relapse after medical therapy.

Even if surgery is not needed acutely, it may be required at a later date when the patient is cured medically but develops heart failure as a result of valve damage. In one study, 47% of patients required corrective valvular heart surgery, usually within 2 years of medical therapy.

COMPLICATIONS OF INFECTIVE ENDOCARDITIS

Major neurologic complications from endocarditis are fortunately rare, but they can present difficult and sometimes vexing management dilemmas. Leading causes are stroke, intracranial hemorrhage, brain abscess, and mycotic aneurysms. As a general rule, anticoagulation should be avoided because of the increased risk of intracranial bleeding. One may elect to continue anticoagulation in patients with mechanical heart valves, but dosing should be ''low therapeutic'' to minimize the hazards of bleeding. Fortunately, most cases of mycotic aneurysms do not require surgery but resolve after appropriate medical therapy.

PREVENTION OF INFECTIVE ENDOCARDITIS

The need for and the adequacy of antibiotic prophylaxis to prevent infective endocarditis continue to be debated. In 1986, Bayliss and colleagues pointed out that a dental portal of entry was recognized less than 20% of the time in their series of 582 cases of endocarditis. Two-thirds of the time, no portal of entry could be found. Myths concerning dental-induced endocarditis include:

- Most physicians and dentists comply with AHA guidelines on antibiotic prophylaxis.
- Most cases of oral origin are caused by dental procedures.
- The risk of endocarditis is almost always greater than the risk of antibiotic side effects.

The American Heart Association recently updated recommendations for prophylaxis (Table 14.10). Indications have been stratified into high, moderate, and negligible risk categories. Examples of those in the high-risk category include patients with prosthetic heart valves and previous infective endocarditis; moderate-risk patients include those with acquired valvular heart disease and mitral valve prolapse with regurgitation. The negligible-risk category includes patients with previous coronary artery bypass surgery, mitral valve prolapse without valvular regurgitation, and cardiac pacemakers:

For high-risk and moderate-risk patients undergoing dental, oral, respiratory tract, or esophageal procedures, amoxicillin (2.0 g orally) is recommended 1 hour before the procedure. For penicillin-allergic patients, clindamycin (600 mg orally), cephalexin (2.0 g orally), or azithromycin (500 mg orally) may be substituted. No postprocedure dose is needed.

For high risk patients undergoing genitourinary and other gastrointestinal procedures, ampicillin (2.0 g) IM or IV plus Gentamicin (1.5 mg per kg, but not to exceed 120 mg), should be given within 30 minutes of the procedure, and a single dose of amoxicillin (1.0 g orally) 6 hours later. For penicillin-allergic patients, vancomycin (l.0 g IV) is substituted for ampicillin. A second dose is not needed. For moderate-risk patients, amoxicillin (2.0 g orally) should be given 1 hour before the procedure, or ampicillin (2.0 g IM or IV) within 30 minutes of the procedure. Vancomycin (1.0 g IV) is suggested for penicillin-allergic patients.

For patients undergoing heart surgery with cardiac valve implantation, standard perioperative antibiotic prophylaxis is a first- or second-generation cephalosporin given with the infusion completed 30 minutes before the procedure and continued for no longer than 48 hours. If the operation is longer than 4 hours, another dose should be given at that time. When hospitals have a high prevalence of methicillin-resistant staphylococci, vancomycin should be substituted for the cephalosporin.

Table 14.10. Examples of AHA Recommendations for Prophylaxis During Procedures

Yes	*No*
Dental extractions	Dental restorations
Periodontal procedures	Adjustment of braces
Dental implants	Flexible bronchoscopy
Prophylactic cleaning	GI endoscopy
Tonsillectomy	C-section deliveries
Rigid bronchoscopy	Urethral catheterization[a]
Esophageal dilatation	Cardiac catheterization
Sclerotherapy	
Cystoscopy	
Urethral dilatation	

[a] When urine is sterile

REVIEW EXERCISES

CASE 1

A 40-year-old woman presents with a 2-month history of fever, night sweats, and weight loss. She has not visited her dentist recently and denies IVDA. Her temperature is 38.5°C, and a loud holosystolic murmur is noted at the cardiac apex.

QUESTIONS

1. The most helpful laboratory test to confirm the diagnosis is

   a. Echocardiography
   b. Rheumatoid factor
   c. CBC with ESR
   d. Blood culture

2. The most likely organism causing this infection is

   a. *Staphylococcus epidermisis*
   b. HACEK group
   c. *Streptococcus viridans*
   d. *Staphylococcus aureus*

CASE 2

A 65-year-old man who underwent AVR for RVHD returns 1 month after discharge with daily fevers and fatigue. His temperature is 38.0°C. A systolic ejection murmur is noted at the cardiac base with radiation to the neck. There are wet bibasilar crackles and bilateral pedal edema.

QUESTIONS

3. The best test to follow this patient through treatment is

   a. Serial blood cultures
   b. Echocardiography
   c. Serum bactericidal test
   d. Erythrocyte sedimentation rate

4. The most important indication for cardiac surgery is

   a. Congestive heart failure
   b. Aortic root abscess
   c. Major emboli
   d. Stroke

5. All of the procedures below are indications for prophylaxis in patients at risk, except which one?

   a. Tonsillectomy
   b. Rigid bronchoscopy
   c. Dental cleaning
   d. Routine cavity filling

Answers

1. d
2. c
3. b
4. b
5. d

SUGGESTED READINGS

Bayliss R, Clarke C, Oakley, et al. Incidence, mortality, and prevention of infective endocarditis. J Royal Coll Phys London 1986;20:15–20.

This paper reports an epidemiologic study of infective endocarditis in the United Kingdom that examined the incidence and mortality of the disease and identified possible methods to prevent it.

Dajani AS, Taubert KA, Wilson W, et al. Prevention of bacterial endocarditis: recommendations by the American Heart Association. JAMA 1997;277:1794–1801.

This article provides current recommendations for the appropriate use of antibiotic prophylaxis for patients at risk of endocarditis during invasive procedures and certain surgeries.

Durack DT, Lukes AS, Bright DK, et al. New criteria for diagnosis of infective endocarditis: utilization of specific echocardiographic findings. Amer J Med 1994;96:200–209.

This article proposes new criteria, including echocardiography findings, which improve the sensitivity without reducing the specificity of the diagnosis.

Murray HW, Roberts RB. *Streptococcus bovis* bacteremia and underlying gastrointestinal disease. Arch Intern Med 1978; 138:1097–1099.

In this study, which includes 26 cases of endocarditis, the majority of cases had underlying GI disease (including neoplasms) that were thought to be the source of the bacteremia.

Nguyen MH, Nguyen ML, Yu VH, et al. *Candida* prosthetic valve endocarditis: prospective study of six cases and review of the literature. Clinic Infect Dis 1996;22:262.

This article, which includes a review of the literature, reports that patients with uncomplicated endocarditis did as well with medical therapy alone as they did when therapy was combined with surgery.

Von Reyn CF, Levy BS, Arbeit RD, et al. Infective endocarditis: an analysis based on strict case definitions. Ann Int Med 1981;94:505–518.

A landmark study in which strict definitions, applied to 123 cases of infective endocarditis, were found useful for their management.

Werner AS, Cobbs CG, Kaye D, et al. Studies on the bacteremia of bacterial endocarditis. JAMA 1967;202:127–131.

A classic study that showed the frequency of positive blood cultures and the quantity of microorganisms during presentation of streptococcal and nonstreptococcal endocarditis.

Pneumonias

Steven K. Schmitt

Sir William Osler described pneumonia as the "captain of the men of death." Although the advent of the antimicrobial age has somewhat reduced this rank, pneumonia remains the sixth leading cause of death in the United States. In 1993, the age-adjusted death rate due to pneumonia was 13.5 per 100,000 persons, reflecting a 20.5% rise from 1979–1993. Estimates of the incidence of pneumonia range from 3–4 million cases per year, with about 20% requiring hospitalization. Because pneumonia crosses the boundaries of all internal medicine subspecialties, a discussion of difficult issues regarding diagnosis, antimicrobial selection, treatment setting, and prevention is appropriate.

ETIOLOGY OF PNEUMONIA

PATHOGENESIS

Five mechanisms have been identified in the pathogenesis of pneumonia in immunocompetent adults:

- Inhalation of infectious particles
- Aspiration of oropharyngeal or gastric contents
- Hematogenous deposition
- Invasion from infection in contiguous structures
- Direct inoculation

Inhalation of infectious particles is probably the most important pathogenetic mechanism in the community. It is thought to be particularly contributory in pneumonia due to *Legionella* species and *Mycobacterium tuberculosis.*

Aspiration of oropharyngeal or gastric contents is by far the most prevalent pathogenetic mechanism in cases of nosocomial pneumonia, with a variety of factors contributing to this risk. Swallowing and epiglottic closure may be impaired by neuromuscular diseases or stroke. States of altered con-

sciousness, such as in chemical sedation, delirium, coma, or seizures, can also depress swallowing, the gag reflex, and closure of the epiglottis. In addition, endotracheal and nasogastric tubes may interfere with these anatomic defenses. Finally, impaired lower esophageal sphincter function and nasogastric and gastrostomy tubes increase the risk of regurgitation of gastric contents. Fortunately, aspiration rarely leads to overt bacterial pneumonitis. It is probable that the nature of the resident flora, the size of the inoculum, and underlying diseases may determine which aspirations result in lung infection.

Direct inoculation rarely occurs as a result of surgery or bronchoscopy but may play a role in the development of pneumonia in patients supported with mechanical ventilation. Hematogenous deposition of bacteria in the lung is also uncommon but is responsible for some cases of pneumonia due to *Staphylococcus aureus, Pseudomonas aeruginosa,* and *Escherichia coli.* The direct extension of infection to the lung from contiguous areas such as the pleural or subdiaphragmatic spaces is rare.

Once bacteria reach the tracheobronchial tree, infectivity may be enhanced by defects in local pulmonary defenses. The cough reflex can be impaired by stroke, neuromuscular disease, sedatives, or poor nutrition. Mucociliary transport is depressed with the aging process, dehydration, morphine, atropine, prior infection with influenza virus, tobacco smoking, and chronic bronchitis. Anatomic derangements including emphysema, bronchiectasis, and obstructive mass lesions can also hinder clearance of organisms. Proteolytic enzymes such as neutrophil elastase are released by inflammatory cells recruited to infected areas of the pulmonary tree, altering the bronchial epithelium and ciliary clearance mechanisms, as well as stimulating excess mucus production.

Bacteria in the tracheobronchial tree may encounter a

blunted cellular and humoral immune response, increasing the risk of pneumonia. For example, granulocyte chemotaxis is reduced with aging, diabetes mellitus, malnutrition, hypothermia, hypophosphatemia, and corticosteroid administration. Absolute granulocytopenia may be caused by cytotoxic chemotherapy. Alveolar macrophages may be rendered dysfunctional by corticosteroids, cytokines, viral illnesses, and malnutrition. Diminished antibody production or function can be sequellae of hematologic malignancies such as multiple myeloma or chronic lymphocytic leukemia.

PATHOLOGIC AGENTS

Despite the emergence of several newer pathogens as causes of community-acquired pneumonia, *Streptococccus pneumoniae* remains the most commonly identified pathogen. A variety of other pathogens have been reported to cause pneumonia in the community, with their order of importance dependent on the location and population studied. These include long-recognized pathogens such as *Haemophilus influenzae, Mycoplasma pneumoniae,* and influenza A, along with newer pathogens such as *Legionella* sp. and *Chlamydia pneumoniae.* Other common causes in the immunocompetent patient include *Moraxella catarrhalis, Mycobacterium tuberculosis,* and aspiration pneumonia.

Following are the causative agents in the 50–70% of cases in which they are identified (Bartlett 1995):

Streptococccus pneumoniae	20–60%
Haemophilus influenzae	3–10%
Staphylococcus aureus	3–5%
Gram-negative bacilli	3–10%
Legionella sp.	2–8%
Mycoplasma pneumoniae	1–6%
Chlamydia pneumoniae	4–6%
Viruses	2–15%
Aspiration	6–10%
Others	3–5%

Whereas pneumonias arising in the nursing home can be caused by community-acquired pathogens, a higher percentage are caused by pathogens seen with relatively low frequency in the community. *Staphylococcus aureus* should be sought in the setting of aspiration or as a sequella of influenza in the nursing home. Gram-negative organisms are also more prominent.

Because of the different pathogenetic mechanisms leading to its development, nosocomial pneumonia is caused by a group of microorganisms quite different from those causing community-acquired pneumonia. Organisms known to colonize the respiratory tree of hospitalized patients, such as *Staphylococcus aureus* and enteric gram-negative organisms of the genuses *Pseudomonas, Enterobacter, Citrobacter, Serratia, Acinetobacter,* and *Stenotrophomonas,* are commonly isolated. Outbreaks of *Legionella* pneumonia and tuberculosis have also occurred in nursing homes and hospitals.

DIAGNOSIS OF PNEUMONIA

Because the clinical syndromes characterizing pneumonic infections caused by various agents frequently overlap with each other and with many noninfectious processes, the diagnosis of pneumonia can be challenging. However, the diligent clinician can narrow the differential diagnosis by considering the place of acquisition and patient characteristics along with diagnostic tests.

PLACE OF ACQUISITION

The differential diagnosis of pneumonia acquired in the community is quite different from that acquired in the nursing home or hospital.

A residence and travel history can help focus the differential diagnosis of pneumonia. Coccidioidomycosis should be considered in patients developing pneumonia upon return from the southwestern U.S. A patient developing pneumonia after a trip to southeast Asia may mave melioidosis or tuberculosis. An HIV-infected patient living in New York City with cough, fever, and nightsweats may have multidrug-resistant tuberculosis. Residents of the desert southwestern U.S. with pneumonia and exposure to rodent excreta should be evaluated for the hantavirus pulmonary syndrome.

CLINICAL PRESENTATION

''Typical'' bacterial pathogens such as *S. pneumoniae, H. influenzae,* and the enteric gram-negative organisms usually present acutely with high fever, chills, tachypnea, tachycardia, productive cough, and examination findings localized to a specific lung zone. In contrast, ''atypical'' pathogens such as *Mycoplasma, Chlamydia,* and viruses can present in a subacute fashion with low-grade fever, nonproductive cough, constitutional symptoms, and absent or diffuse findings on lung examination. Rapid progression of disease can be seen in severe pneumococcal or *Legionella* pneumonia. However, the overlap between the presentations of typical and atypical pathogens weakens the specificity of these categorizations considerably.

Certain extrapulmonary physical findings can provide clues to the diagnosis. Poor dentition and foul-smelling sputum may indicate the presence of a polymicrobial lung abscess. Bullous myringitis can accompany infection with *M. pneumoniae.* An absent gag reflex or altered sensorium raises the question of aspiration. Encephalitis can complicate pneumonia with *M. pneumoniae* or *L. pneumophila.* Cutaneous manifestations of infection can include erythema multiforme (*M. pneumoniae*), erythema nodosum (*C. pneumoniae and M. tuberculosis*), or ecthyma gangrenosum (*Pseudomonas aeruginosa*).

PATIENT CHARACTERISTICS

The *age* of the patient can play an important role in disease etiology and presentation. Older patients often have humoral and cellular immunodeficiency as a result of underlying diseases, immunosuppressive medications, and aging. They are more frequently institutionalized with anatomic problems that inhibit pulmonary clearance of pathogens. The presentation is often more subtle than in youger adults, with more advanced disease and sepsis despite minimal fever and sputum production. More prolonged antimicrobial therapy is often required.

The *occupation* and *hobbies* of the patient can provide important clinical clues. For example, exposure to construction sites or old buildings with accumulations of bat or bird droppings can predispose to pneumonias due to *Histoplasma capsulatum* or *Cryptococcus neoformans*. Hunters who skin their own rabbits may be exposed to *Francisella tularensis*. Farmers working with stored hay may be exposed to *Aspergillus* species, as may patients who smoke marijuana.

Underlying diseases are a critical part of the history of the patient with pneumonia. Risk factors for HIV infection should be sought. HIV increases the risk for pneumonias because of common bacterial pathogens, as well as opportunistic pathogens such as *Pneumocystis carinii*, cytomegalovirus, and *Mycobacterium avium-intracellulare*. Fungal pneumonias caused by *H. capsulatum, Coccidioides immitis,* and *C. neoformans* have been seen in HIV patients in appropriate epidemiologic settings and can have especially severe courses. Neutropenic patients are especially prone to fungal pneumonias, such as those caused by *Aspergillus* species. Patients treated with prolonged courses of immunosuppressive medications such as corticosteroids are at risk for pulmonary infections with various viral, fungal, and mycobacterial agents. Alcoholism predisposes individuals to aspiration pneumonia, with mixed gram-positive and gram-negative aerobic and anaerobic flora, as well as tuberculosis. *M. catarrhalis, H. influenzae,* and *S. pneumoniae* are more likely in those with chronic obstructive pulmonary disease. Diabetic patients are more prone to staphylococcal infections. Patients with functional or surgical asplenia are prone to infection with encapsulated organisms such as *S. pneumoniae* and *H. influenzae*.

RADIOGRAPHY

A cornerstone of diagnosis is the chest x-ray, which usually reveals an infiltrate at presentation. However, this finding may be absent in the dehydrated patient during the first 24–48 hours of rehydration. Also, the radiographic manifestations of chronic diseases such as congestive heart failure, chronic obstructive pulmonary disease (COPD), and malignancy may obscure the infiltrate of pneumonia.

Although radiographic patterns are usually nonspecific, they can suggest a microbiologic differential diagnosis. Lobar consolidation or a large pleural effusion suggests a bacterial pathogen. Cavitation suggests a bacterial (abscess), mycobacterial, fungal , or nocardial cause. Pneumonias caused by the pneumococcus may present as a lobar or bronchopneumonia. Gram-negative and staphylococcal pneumonias can cause consolidation and cavitation. The infiltrate that progresses rapidly from a single lobe to multiple lobes should raise suspicion of *Legionella pneumophila.*

Although aspiration more commonly affects the right lung because of tracheobronchial anatomy, both lungs can be affected simultaneously. The affected site may depend on position at the time of aspiration. Aspiration while recumbent will commonly lead to clinical and radiographic pneumonia in the posterior segments of the upper lobes and superior segments of the lower lobes. Upright aspiration usually affects the lung bases.

When diffuse interstitial infiltrates predominate in the absence of clinical evidence of fluid overload, pneumonias caused by viruses or *Pneumocystis carinii* should be considered in the differential diagnosis.

CULTURES

A Gram-stained sputum specimen also can provide critical information in choosing empiric therapy. Unfortunately, sputum is frequently difficult to obtain from elderly patients because of a weak cough, obtundation, and dehydration. Inhaled nebulized saline may help mobilize secretions. Nasotracheal suctioning can sample the lower respiratory tract directly but risks oropharyngeal contamination and is therefore of lesser value. A sputum specimen is thought to reflect lower respiratory secretions when more than 25 white blood cells and less than 10 epithelial cells are seen in a low-powered microscopic field. When such a specimen also shows a predominant organism, it lends a high positive predictive value for choice of appropriate antimicrobial therapy. Other stains, such as the acid-fast stain for mycobacteria, modified acid-fast stain for *Nocardia,* or the toluidine blue and Gomori methenamine silver stains for *Pneumocystis carinii* may prove useful when historically indicated. Direct fluorescent antibody staining of sputum, bronchoalveolar lavage fluid, or pleural fluid may help identify *Legionella* species.

The sputum culture remains a controversial tool but is still recommended to help tailor therapy. It may prove particularly helpful in identifying resistant nosocomial bacterial pathogens. Expectorated morning sputum specimens can also be sent for mycobacterial culture when the history suggests exposure.

When these procedures fail to yield a microbiologic diagnosis and when the patient fails to respond to empiric antibiotic therapy, more invasive diagnostic techniques may be indicated. The value of transtracheal aspiration depends on the operator's skill. This procedure can have dangerous complications. It has been largely supplanted by fiberoptic bronchoscopy in the diagnosis of pneumonia. Several techniques are employed by the bronchoscopist. Bronchoalveolar lavage with saline can obtain deep respiratory specimens for the gamut of stains and cultures mentioned above. Transbronchial biopsy of infiltrated lung parenchyma can reveal alveolar or interstitial pneumonitis, viral inclusion bodies, and invading fungal or mycobacterial organisms. The protected brush catheter is utilized to quantitatively distinguish between tracheobronchial colonizers and pneumonic pathogens. When recovered secretions contain 10^3 CFU/mL of a bacterial pathogen, lower respiratory infection should be suspected.

A newer method being employed in the diagnosis of nosocomial pneumonia in some centers is "mini" bronchoalveolar lavage performed by nonbronchoscopic passage of a telescoping catheter through the endotracheal tube. Several recent articles have suggested a high culture concordance between this method and the bronchoscopic protected-brush catheter technique.

A more substantial amount of lung tissue may be obtained for culture and histologic examination by thorascopic or open-lung biopsy. Because these procedures can carry substantial morbidity, their timing in the diagnostic algorithm is controversial. They are usually reserved for the deteriorating patient who defies diagnosis by less invasive techniques.

SEROLOGIC TESTING

Serologic testing for such pathogens as *Legionella* species, *Mycoplasma* species, and *Chlamydia pneumoniae* should include sera drawn in both the acute and convalescent phases for comparison. A fourfold rise in the IgG titer is suggestive of recent infection with these organisms.

A sensitive enzyme immunoassay has been developed for the detection of *Legionella pneumophila* antigen in urine. Because the antigen persists for prolonged periods of time after infection, it is difficult to differentiate between past and current infections when using this assay.

MOLECULAR TECHNIQUES

Powerful molecular techniques are now being applied to the early diagnosis of pneumonia. DNA probes have been used for the detection of *Legionella* species, *Mycoplasma pneumoniae,* and *Mycobacterium tuberculosis* in sputum. These probes have excellent sensitivity and specificity but can produce some false-positive results. The polymerase chain reaction (PCR) has been shown to be a sensitive tool for the early detection of *Mycobacterium tuberculosis* in sputum specimens. It is currently a research technique and is not available in most clinical laboratories.

TREATMENT OF PNEUMONIA

HOSPITALIZATION

Health-care budgetary constraints have given rise to a number of studies addressing the issue of hospitalization in community-acquired pneumonia. A recent study (Fine et al., 1997) validated a risk scale for mortality in community-acquired

pneumonia. Patients less than 50 years of age without significant coexisting diseases or vital sign abnormalities were assigned to risk group I. All others were grouped in classes II ($\leq$ 70 points), III (71–90 points), IV (91–130 points), and V (> 130 points) using a system assigning points for age, coexisting diseases, physical examination findings, and laboratory abnormalities:

- Age: Males: 1 point per year; females: 1 point per year minus 10.
- Coexisting illnesses: Neoplastic disease (30 points), chronic renal disease (10 points), congestive heart failure (10 points), chronic liver disease (20 points), cerebrovascular disease (10 points).
- Physical findings: Respiratory rate $\geq$ 30/min (20 points), systolic blood pressure < 90 mmHg (20 points), pulse $\geq$ 125 beats per minute (10 points), temperature $\geq$ 40°C or < 35°C (15 points), altered mental status (20 points).
- Diagnostic tests: PaO_2 < 60mmHg (10 points), hematocrit < 30% (10 points), blood urea nitrogen > 30 mg/dL (20 points), pleural effusion on chest radiograph (10 points), sodium <130mmol/L (20 points), glucose > 250 mg/dL (10 points), arterial pH < 7.35 (30 points).

Patients in the first three risk classes had less than 1% mortality, with steep rises to 9.3% in class IV and 27.0% in class V. Fewer than 6% of patients in the first three groups treated as inpatients required ICU admission, and fewer than 10% of patients in the first two groups treated as outpatients were subsequently hospitalized. Whereas these data can help in patient assessment, the decision to admit must ultimately be individualized to each patient encounter.

PHARMACOLOGIC TREATMENT

When the history, chest radiograph, and a Gram-stained sputum fail to suggest a specific cause for pneumonia, a trial of empiric antibiotics is warranted. Antibiotic therapy is best initiated after obtaining appropriate specimens for culture, when appropriate. The choice of antimicrobial is dictated by severity of illness, treatment setting, and comorbid diseases. Table 15.1 provides a reasonable framework for initial therapy of community-acquired pneumonia.

In the outpatient treatment of younger patients without comorbidity, an oral macrolide or tetracycline should provide adequate coverage. When outpatient therapy is deemed appropriate in older patients or those with comorbid disease, an oral second-generation cephalosporin or beta lactam/beta lactamase inhibitor combination provides excellent coverage. When *S. aureus* is not suspected, trimethoprim/sulfamethoxazole (TMP/SMX) provides an inexpensive but effective alternative. When atypical pathogens are suspected, a macrolide should be added to this regimen. If HIV infection is a suspected comorbidity, then strong consideration should be given to the inclusion of TMP/SMX in the treatment regimen.

Table 15.1.   Antibiotic Therapy for Community-Acquired Pneumonia in Immunocompetent Adults

Setting	Patient	Common Pathogens	Empiric Therapy
Outpatient	<60 years old No comorbid diseases	S. pneumoniae M. pneumoniae C. pneumoniae Viruses H. influenzae	A macrolide[a] or a tetracycline[b]
	> 60 years old or having comorbid disease	S. pneumoniae Viruses H. influenzae Gram-negative bacilli[c] S. aureus[c]	A second-generation cephalosporin or trimethoprim/sulfamethoxazole
Inpatient	Not severely ill	S. pneumoniae H. influenzae Polymicrobial Anarerobes S. aureus C. pneumoniae Viruses	A macrolide[a] and either a second- or third-generation cephalosporin or a beta-lactam/beta lactamase inhibitor
	Severely ill	S. pneumoniae[d] Legionella Gram-negative bacilli M. pneumoniae Viruses S. aureus	A macrolide and: an antipseudomonal cephalosporin or an antipseudomonal penicillin or ciprofloxacin or aztreonam or imipenem

[a] Erythromycin is the drug of choice; use clarithromycin or azithromycin for patients who smoke or are intolerant of erythromycin.
[b] Many isolates of S. pneumoniae are resistant to tetracyclines, and they should be used only if the patient cannot tolerate macrolides.
[c] In most cases, patients with infections due to these organisms should be hospitalized. Rifampin may be added in Legionella infection.
[d] Critically ill patients in areas with significant rates of high-level resistance to vancomycin and a suggestive sputum Gram's stain should receive vancomycin.
Modified from American Thoracic Society. Guidelines for the initial management of adults with community-acquired pneumonia: diagnosis assessment of severity, and initial antimicrobial therapy. Am Rev Resp Dis 1993;148:1418–1426.

When patients with community-acquired pneumonia require hospitalization, intravenous therapy with a second- or third-generation cephalosporin or a beta-lactam/beta-lactamase inhibitor combination is warranted. A macrolide should be included when atypical pathogens are a consideration. When the pneumonia is severe, empiric coverage should be broadened to include an agent possessing antipseudomonal activity and high-dose erythromycin.

Because gram-negative organisms predominate in pneumonia acquired in hospital settings, an agent possessing antipseudomonal activity (such as an antipseudomonal cephalosporin or penicillin, beta-lactam/beta lactamase inhibitor, imipenem, ciprofloxacin, or aztreonam) and an aminoglycoside are usually used. When nosocomial pneumonia is severe and the institution has a significant percentage of methicillin-resistant staphylococci, consideration should be given to the empiric addition of vancomycin until culture data excluding the presence of these pathogens can be obtained. If the hospitalized patient is also neutropenic and the response to antibacterials is suboptimal, some consideration should be given to the early addition of antifungal therapy.

Clindamycin is preferred over penicillin for the treatment of community-acquired aspiration pneumonia because of its superiority in the treatment of oral anaerobes such as *Bacteroi-*

des melaninogenicus. When large-volume aspiration is documented in the hospital, a beta-lactam/beta-lactamase inhibitor combination or the combination of clindamycin and an antipseudomonal agent should be employed.

When diagnostic techniques described above yield a specific causative agent for the pneumonia, special effort should be made to narrow the spectrum of activity used as early as possible. Overuse of broad-spectrum agents encourages the development of resistance and should be avoided whenever possible.

In many cases of community-acquired pneumomia, 10–14 days of therapy should cure the infection. However, certain organisms (*Legionella, S. aureus, Pseudomonas,* or *C. pneumoniae,* for example) may require longer courses. Similarly, patients with comorbidities that compromise local (COPD) or systemic (hematologic malignancy) immunity may take longer to clear their illness.

SPECIFIC PATHOGENS

Certain emerging pathogens have been the subject of considerable research in recent years. Given their importance, they are worthy of special attention.

STREPTOCOCCUS PNEUMONIAE

Although the pneumococcus is a familiar enemy, it has become even more formidable in recent years. The exact incidence of pneumococcal pneumonia is unknown, but it has been estimated at 1–2 per 1000 persons per year in the United States. It is more common in the elderly, with incidence estimates ranging from 14–46 per 1000 persons per year. Untreated mortality has been estimated at about 30%.

While pneumococci have traditionally been exquisitely sensitive to penicillin, strains of the organism possessing low- or high-level resistance to penicillin have established a foothold in several communities. A recent report from the Centers for Disease Control and Prevention found that a full 25% of pneumococcal isolates exhibited penicillin resistance (penicillin-nonsusceptible pneumococci, or PNSP), 7% with high-level resistance (penicillin-resistant *S. pneumoniae,* or PRSP). Some of these strains are multiply resistant, with resistance to multiple cephalosporins, erythromycin, and TMP/SMX. No strains resistant to vancomycin have been isolated. This has led to the recommendation by several authorities that empiric therapy for life-threatening disease suspected or proven to be due to pneumococci include vancomycin until susceptibility patterns are known. If sputum culture yields pneumococci that are inhibited by a minimum concentration of 0.12–2.0 mcg/mL of penicillin, then high-dose penicillin (150,000–200,000 U/kg/day in divided doses) or a cephalosporin are recommended therapy. If the penicillin MIC is more than 2.0 mcg/mL (PRSP), then vancomycin is the treatment of choice. Whenever possible, vancomycin should be changed to beta-lactam therapy, because of both improved efficacy and the continuing emergence of vancomycin resistance among gram-positive pathogens such as enterococci and staphylococci.

LEGIONELLA *SPECIES*

Although difficult to visualize on sputum Gram's stain and slow to grow even on specialized culture media, members of the *Legionella* genus frequently leave several epidemiologic clues helpful to the diagnosis of Legionnaire's disease. Most frequently occurring in the spring or summer months, Legionnaire's disease can occur sporadically or in epidemics in settings with recirculated air, such as hotels, airplanes, and hospitals. It can occur in adults of all ages but is more common in middle-aged and elderly persons. There is frequently a prodrome of malaise, myalgia, and headache, sometimes accompanied by gastrointestinal symptoms such as watery diarrhea, nausea, or abdominal pain. The pneumonia is often explosive, with nonproductive cough, high fever, shaking chills, tachycardia, and tachypnea. Focal findings on lung examination and chest x-ray (initially patchy areas of bronchopneumonia) can progress within hours to a multilobe process. Confusion and disorientation can be present.

Laboratory evaluation can also yield information useful in the diagnosis. There may be left-shifted leukocytosis on the complete blood count. Elevated liver function tests, azotemia, hypophosphatemia, hyponatremia, and hypoxemia may be seen, but none of these findings are pathognomonic for legionellosis. Urinalysis may reveal hematuria.

The sputum Gram's stain in *Legionella* pneumonia usually reveals many white blood cells but no predominant organism. Culture is best attempted with charcoal-yeast extract (CYE) agar, but sensitivities of 50–70% are common. Therefore, a variety of alternative tests have been developed to support the diagnosis. Serology is 70–96% sensitive and more than 95% specific, but results may not be available for several days. Sputum-direct fluorescent antibody testing is likewise highly specific, but quite technique-dependent, with sensitivities of 25–80% reported. DNA probing of sputum specimens is expensive, available only in a few laboratories, and relatively insensitive (50–65%). Urinary antigen testing is sensitive (75–90%), uniformly specific, and may turn positive as early as 72 hours into the illness. However, it only detects *Legionella pneumophila* type 1, which account for 80% of cases of legionellosis. The test fails to distinguish acute from remote infection because antigenuria may be present for up to a year after infection. It is clear that, given these vagaries, empiric therapy for legionellosis may still be warranted when the clinical setting is appropriate, despite extensive negative testing.

Standard therapy consists of a macrolide, typically erythromycin, intravenously at a high dose (1 g IV q6h). A lengthy course (at least 3 weeks) may be required for cure. Many authorities advocate the addition of rifampin, which also offers good intracellular penetration. For patients who are macrolide-intolerant, doxycycline offers an alternative. Recent reports have emphasized the efficacy of quinolones, especially ciprofloxacin, in legionellosis, although clinical experience is somewhat limited.

CHLAMYDIA PNEUMONIAE

Only recognized as a cause of respiratory infection in 1986, this obligate intracellular pathogen was originally designated as the TWAR agent from the laboratory numbers of the first two strains: TW-183 and AR-39. Predicted over 40 years ago by epidemiologic studies of psittacosis-like infections with no exposure to birds, *C. pneumoniae* is now classified as a pathogen distinct from *C. psittaci* with person-to-person respiratory transmission. Current seroepidemiology suggests that *C. pneumoniae* accounts for about 10% of all cases of community-acquired pneumonia, with a seroprevalance in the United States of about 50%. Data indicate that most adults are exposed during the teenage years, outside the home. Outbreaks have been reported to spread somewhat more slowly than influenza through closed populations such as military recruits and college students.

The clinical presentation of respiratory infections due to *C. pneumoniae* is frequently nonspecific. Cough (productive or nonproductive) and sore throat are common, occurring in more than 80% of patients. A clinical clue present in only 30% of cases is hoarseness, but this finding is present in less than 5% of patients with mycoplasmal or viral infections. Mild fever and leukocytosis are common. The presentation on lung examination and chest radiography is usually that of a localized infiltrate. The illness is usually indolent, although severe pneumonias can occur in elderly and immunocompromised adults.

Culture diagnosis is uncommon because the organism is difficult to cultivate. The diagnosis is made more commonly by serology, with IgM titers $\geq 1:16$, IgG titers $\geq 1:512$, or a fourfold titer rise considered diagnostic.

Both tetracyclines and macrolides have been shown to have excellent in vitro activity against *C. pneumoniae* and are considered the treatment agents of choice despite a relative paucity of clinical data. Alternatives to these agents may include quinolones such as ofloxacin, although ciprofloxacin appears to be less active.

MYCOPLASMA PNEUMONIAE

Like *C. pneumoniae*, *M. pneumoniae* accounts for 5–20% of community-acquired pneumonia, with slow spread through closed populations. It produces a syndrome of low-grade fever, nonproductive cough, and pharyngitis. Headache and otalgia are also frequently reported. The most common respiratory syndrome is bronchitis, with up to one quarter of these patients proceeding to pneumonia. Radiographic presentations range from single to multilobe, with patchy infiltrates. Uncommon but sometimes severe extrapulmonary manifestations can include hemolytic anemia, myocarditis, pericarditis, meningoencephalitis, monoarthritis or polyarthritis, and erythema multiforme.

Culture of *M. pneumoniae* requires broth medium and a 7–10-day span of time, so it usually is not performed. Diagnosis is serologic, with specific IgM positivity, IgG $\geq 1:256$, or a fourfold rise in IgG titer considered diagnostic. The cold agglutinin test is nonspecific but supports the diagnosis of mycoplasmal infection when a high titer ($\geq 1:128$) is present.

Therapy consists of administration of a macrolide or tetracycline agent for at least 14 days. Ciprofloxacin and ofloxacin have some activity but are second-line alternatives.

INFLUENZA AND OTHER VIRUSES

In some series of community-acquired pneumonia, no etiologic agent was established in 40–50% of cases. It is likely that a portion of these are due to viral agents, which are an underdiagnosed cause of pneumonia. Among immunocompetent adults, influenza viruses (especially influenza A) are the most common causes of viral pneumonia. Mainly occurring between October and March, influenza pneumonia is characterized by nonproductive cough, wheezing, myalgia, sore throat, and fever. Chest radiographs may show localized or diffuse patchy infiltrates. The diagnosis is established by serology or by swab collection of nasophayngeal cells for culture or direct immunofluorescent staining. This latter method, which can provide an answer in minutes to hours, is perhaps

most useful when treatment is being contemplated. Standard treatment of influenza A pneumonia has been amantidine, but it may be supplanted by the newer rimantidine because of its more favorable side-effect profile. If given soon after the onset of symptoms, these drugs can shorten the duration of symptoms and viral shedding by 1–2 days.

When the patient with suspected or documented influenza develops a secondary, more acute phase of illness with high fever and productive cough, bacterial superinfection must be considered. *S. aureus*, *S. pneumoniae*, and *H. influenzae* are the most common causes of pneumonia in this setting.

Adenoviruses have been demonstrated to cause pneumonia in military recruits. Along with adenoviruses, respiratory syncytial virus, influenza virus, and parainfluenza virus can cause viral pneumonia in immunocompromised patients. Direct immunofluorescent staining of nasopharyngeal cells provides the most rapid diagnostic method.

HANTAVIRUS PULMONARY SYNDROME

In May and June, 1993, a cluster of 24 patients living in the Four Corners area of New Mexico, Arizona, Colorado, and Utah developed acute respiratory failure following an influenza-like illness. Twelve of these patients died, sparking an epidemiologic investigation that led to the isolation of a new pathogen in the hantavirus family, the Muerto Canyon virus. Subsequent characterization of the illness caused by this agent suggests that it is transmitted to humans by exposure to the excreta of the deer mouse (*Peromyscus maniculatus*).

The prodromal phase of the disease, lasting 3–6 days, is marked by fever, myalgia, nausea, vomiting, and abdominal pain. Upper respiratory symptoms are uncommon. The cardiopulmonary phase is heralded by progressive cough and dyspnea, with tachypnea, tachycardia, fever, and severe hypotension. Laboratory evaluation reveals thrombocytopenia, abnormal coagulation parameters, and leukocytosis, sometimes with atypical lymphocytosis. Renal failure is rare but ventilatory failure is common, with 88% of patients requiring mechanical ventilation. The chest x ray progresses rapidly to diffuse interstitial edema. Lung pathology reveals evidence of vascular permeability without parenchymal necrosis.

Diagnosis is serologic, with demonstration of IgM or a fourfold rise in IgG antibodies. Treatment is largely supportive. Ribavirin, either in the intravenous or aerosolized form, has been proposed by some as a potential therapy, but controlled data to support the use of this toxic drug are lacking.

PREVENTION OF PNEUMONIA

Given increased resistance among pneumococci and the undiminished importance of influenza as a respiratory pathogen, emphasis on immunization against these agents should be intensified. Immunization can play a critical role in the prevention of pneumonia, particularly in immunocompromised and older adults. The influenza vaccine is formulated and administered annually. Given the risk of postinfluenza bacterial super-infection in elderly and immunocompromised individuals, this vaccine should be given to all patients in these groups except those allergic to eggs.

The pneumococcal vaccine, containing polysaccharide antigens of the 23 strains responsible for 88% of cases of bacteremic pneumococcal disease, has been shown to be 60–70% effective in immunocompetent patients. Side effects are rarely serious and consist of local pain and erythema, which occur in up to 50% of recipients. Patients who are immunosuppressed and those with severely debilitating cardiovascular, pulmonary, renal, hepatic, or diabetic disease may not have sustained titers of protective antibody and should be considered for revaccination after 6 years.

Selective digestive decontamination (SDD) employs a combination of antibacterial and antifungal agents in an at-tempt to reduce gastrointestinal and oropharyngeal colonization with microorganisms. The simultaneous administration of these agents as an oral paste and a nasogastric suspension has been shown to reduce the incidence of nosocomial pneumonia in some studies but without a convincing improvement in morbidity, mortality, or length of intensive care unit (ICU) stay.

Nosocomial aspiration is frequently preventable. Many hospitals now employ teams to evaluate swallowing function and aspiration risk. The modified barium swallow can help establish the types of liquid and solid foodstuffs likely to be aspirated. Elevation of the upper airway to above the level of the stomach and the use of jejunostomy (rather than gastrostomy) tubes for enteral feeding can help diminish aspiration risk in patients with incompetent lower esophageal sphincters. Finally, careful attention to pulmonary toilet can assist debilitated persons in clearing tracheobronchial secretions.

REVIEW EXERCISES

1. A 58-year-old woman presents with a 3-week history of nonproductive cough and hoarseness. She reports a temperature of 100.4°F. She is not short of breath and has no chills or sweats. She has a 20-pack per year smoking history but quit 20 years ago. She lives at home with her husband, who is asymptomatic. She has had several antibiotics in the past week, of which she comments, ''I felt a little better after the clarithromycin, but not much, so my doctor changed me to cefuroxime, and I felt worse.'' Physical examination reveals apparent health. She has a low-grade fever at 38.0°C, but her vital signs are otherwise normal. The rest of the physical examination is unremarkable. Laboratory evaluation is remarkable only for normal white blood cell (WBC) count with a mild left shift. Chest x-ray reveals a subtle right-sided infiltrate.

   The most appropriate next step in the care of this patient would be:

   a. Admission for high-dose IV erythromycin
   b. Oupatient therapy with oral doxycycline
   c. Admission for observation and treatment with IV cefuroxime
   d. Oupatient therapy with oral cephalexin
   e. Home intravenous antibiotic therapy with ticarcillin/clavulanic acid

2. A 23-year-old college student presents in late December with a 5-day history of nonproductive cough and shortness of breath. He notes that a number of fellow students have had respiratory illnesses over the past 2 months. He has recently tested HIV-negative.

   Physical examination shows he is in good physical condition. His temperature is 38.3°C, his heart rate is 120/minute, his respiratory rate is 22/minute, and his blood pressure is 90/60 mmHg. The examination otherwise is remarkable only for a few scattered rales at the lung bases.

   On laboratory evaluation, he is hypoxemic with a pO_2 of 76. The WBC count is 14,000/mm^3, with a marked left shift. His hemoglobin is 8.3 g/dL, and his peripheral smear shows red cell fragments. Chest x-ray reveals bilateral patchy lower lobe infiltrates. The sputum Gram's stain shows many WBCs but no organisms.

   The patient deteriorates soon after admission, requiring mechanical ventilation and pressors. Chest radiography reveals progression of the infiltrates to involve all five lung lobes. A Swan-Ganz catheter is placed, revealing a high systemic vascular resistance but a low cardiac output.

   The most appropriate empiric antimicrobial therapy for this patient is:

   a. Trimethoprim-sulfamethoxazole 5 mg/kg IV q6h
   b. Erythromycin 500 mg IV q6h and ciprofloxacin 400 mg IV q12h
   c. Ticarcillin/clavulanic acid 3.1 g IV q6h
   d. Erythromycin 1 g IV q6h and ceftazidime 1 g IV q8h
   e. Piperacillin 3 g IV q4h and gentamicin 120 mg IV q8h

Answers

1. b

The patient presents with a subacute, indolent illness and radiographic evidence of community-acquired pneumonia. There are no risk factors for mortality, and admission is probably not warranted. Cephalexin and ticarcillin/clavulanic acid have no activity against *Legionella*, *Mycoplasma*, or *Chlamydia*. The correct therapy is an oral tetacycline or macrolide. In this case, the symptom of hoarseness and partial response to clarithromycin create suspicion for pneumonia with *C. pneumoniae*. Tetracycline is preferred in this setting, given the higher rate of treatment failure seen with macrolides.

2. d

The patient is acutely and severely ill with a community-acquired process. By ATS guidelines, appropriate therapy consists of high-dose IV erythromycin and an antipseudomonal agent. As he is HIV negative and acutely ill, trimethoprim/sulfamethoxazole would not provide adequate coverage for either atypical or serious gram-negative pathogens. Likewise, neither ticarcillin/clavulanic acid or the combination of piperacillin and gentamicin would cover atypical pathogens. Erythromycin at 500 mg IV q6h is insufficient to treat severe *Legionella* pneumonia, which is in the differential diagnosis.

This patient presents with several clinical clues to the correct diagnosis. He presents with a nonproductive cough and low-grade fever, suggesting an ''atypical'' pathogen. His sputum Gram's stain shows no predominant organism, despite a fulminant process. He has evidence of hemolytic anemia and cardiac dysfunction. His *Mycoplasma* IgM titer was strongly positive, illustrating the potentially severe complications of this ordinarily indolent pathogen.

SUGGESTED READINGS

American Thoracic Society. Guidelines for the initial management of adults with community-acquired pneumonia: diagnosis, assessment of severity, and initial antimicrobial therapy. Am Rev Respir Dis 1993;148:1418–1426.

Bartlett JG, Mundy LM. Community-acquired pneumonia. N Engl J Med 1995;333:1618–1624.

Butler JC, Peters CJ. Hantaviruses and hantavirus pulmonary syndrome. Clin Infect Dis 1994;19:387–395.

Fine MJ, Auble TE, Yealy DM, Hanusa BH, Weissfeld LA, Singer DE, Coley CM, Marrie TJ, Kapoor WN. A prediction rule to identify low-risk patients with community-acquired pneumonia. N Engl J Med 1997;336:243–250.

Friedland IR, McCracken GH. Management of infections caused by antibiotic-resistant *Streptococcus pneumoniae*. N Engl J Med 1994;331:377–382.

Grayston JT, Campbell LA, Kuo CC, Mordhorst CH, Saikku P, Thom DH, Wang S. A new respiratory tract pathogen: *Chlamydia pneumoniae* strain TWAR. J Infect Dis 1990;161: 618–625.

Marrie TJ. Community-acquired pneumonia. Clin Infect Dis 1994;18:501–513.

Marrie TJ. *Mycoplasma pneumoniae* pneumonia requiring hospitalization, with emphasis on infection in the elderly. Arch Intern Med 1993;153:488–494.

Meeker DP, Longworth DL. Community-acquired pneumonia: an update. Cleve Clin J Med 1996;63:16–30.

Murray HW, Masur H, Senterfit LB, Roberts RB. The protean manifestations of *Mycoplasma pneumoniae* infection in adults. Am J Med 1975;58:229–242.

Nguyen MH, Stout JE, Yu VL. Legionellosis. Infec Dis Clinics N Amer 1991;5:561–584.

Rello J, Quintana E, Ausina V, et al. Incidence, etiology, and outcome of noscomial pneumonia in mechanically ventilated patients. Chest 1991;100:439–444.

Scheld WM, Mandell GL. Nosocomial pneumonia: pathogenesis and recent advances in diagnosis and therapy. Rev Infect Dis 1991;13:S743–S751.

16

New and Emerging Infectious Diseases

Steven M. Gordon

Despite predictions earlier this century that infectious diseases would soon be eliminated as a public health problem, infectious diseases remain the major cause of death worldwide and a significant cause of death and morbidity in the United States. The United States' public health system has been challenged by several newly identified pathogens (e.g., HIV, *E. coli* 0157: H7, and hepatitis C) as well as a resurgence of old diseases that had been presumed to be under control (e.g., tuberculosis and syphilis). In addition, control and prevention of infectious diseases are undermined by the emergence of multiple-drug-resistant strains of pneumococci, gonococci, enterococci, staphylococci, salmonella, and mycobacteria.

Emerging infections can be defined as those infectious diseases that have recently appeared in the population or have existed but are rapidly increasing in incidence or geographic range. Recent examples of emerging diseases in various parts of the world include outbreaks of plague in Surat, India, and the Ebola virus in the central African nation of Zaire.

This chapter provides an overview of some old and new emerging infectious diseases of significance to the internist:

- Cyclosporiasis
- Parvovirus B19
- *Escherichia coli* 0157:H7
- Babesiosis
- *Chlamydia pneumoniae*
- Bacillary angiomatosis and other *Bartonella-* (formerly *Rochalimaea*) associated diseases
- Hantavirus pulmonary syndrome (HPS)
- Primary HIV infection
- Ehrlichiosis

CYCLOSPORIASIS

In the summer of 1996, several food-borne outbreaks of *Cyclospora* diarrheal disease, involving more than 1,000 per-

sons, occurred in the United States and Canada. Previously, *Cyclospora cayetanensis,* the causative parasite, had been associated with only three recognized outbreaks of human infection in the United States. *Cyclospora* is not a "new" organism, but it is now recognized as an emerging pathogen.

ETIOLOGY OF *CYCLOSPORA*

Cyclospora is a protozoan parasite in the same suborder as four other human pathogens: *Cryptosporidium, Isospora, Toxoplasma,* and *Sarcocystis. Cyclospora* oocysts are 8–10 μm in diameter, almost twice the size of *Cryptosporidium,* and are often referred to as "*Cryptosporidium* Grande." Within each oocyst are two sporocysts, each containing two sporozoites. In the past, the parasite has been referred to as cyanobacterium-like, coccidia-like, and *cyclospora*-like.

Epidemiology of Cyclosporiasis

Although *Cyclospora* infections have been documented worldwide, the parasite is endemic to Nepal, Haiti, and Peru, and most of our epidemiologic knowledge comes from studies in these countries. Cyclosporiasis appears to be seasonal, with peak incidence during the rainy seasons that occur between April and June in Peru, and May and September in Nepal.

Risk Factors of Cyclosporiasis

Although all age groups can acquire the disease, the highest attack rates occur among children older than 18 months of age. There is no apparent immunity to infection, and reinfection can occur at all ages.

Pathogenesis of Cyclosporiasis

Cyclospora is an increasingly recognized cause of traveler's diarrhea, causing up to 11–20% of cases of diarrhea in studies of expatriates in Nepal. Documentation of infection acquired in the United States is increasing. The earliest recorded outbreak of diarrheal disease associated with *Cyclospora* in the United States occurred in 21 resident physicians in a Chicago hospital in 1990 and was epidemiologically linked to a contaminated water supply. In the summer of 1996, more than one thousand confirmed cases from the United States and Canada were reported to the Centers for Disease Control and Prevention.

TRANSMISSION OF CYCLOSPORIASIS

Cyclospora infection occurs most commonly through contaminated water. *Cyclospora*, like *Cryptosporidium,* is resistant to chlorination and is not readily detected by methods that are currently used to assure the safety of drinking water. Epidemiologic evidence also exists of transmission by contaminated food; trace-back studies from a multistate cyclosporiasis outbreak of 1996 indicate that raspberries imported from Guatemala were served at the events related to clusters of cyclosporiasis. *Cyclospora* oocysts are excreted unsporulated in the stool and require a period of time for maturation and infectivity; therefore, direct transmission from an infected patient to another person is unlikely. The infective dose necessary to cause disease in man is unknown.

CLINICAL PRESENTATION OF CYCLOSPORIASIS

Infection by *C. cayetanensis* can be asymptomatic, cause self-limited diarrhea, or cause chronic diarrhea. *Cyclospora* has an incubation period of 2–10 days (median of 7 days). The diarrhea is usually watery and nonbloody, clinically indistinguishable from other types of noninvasive secretory infectious diarrhea. The infection is often accompanied by abdominal cramps, and patients may report a rapid loss of weight. The clinical picture may sometimes be dominated by severe fatigue and at times fever, anorexia, and chills. These nonspecific symptoms often lead to delay in diagnosis while the practitioner pursues other possible etiologies of fatigue. There are no specific findings on physical examination.

DIAGNOSIS OF CYCLOSPORIASIS

The diagnosis of Cyclosporiasis is made by direct examination of stool samples. A combination of wet mount and modified acid-fast stain on stool should be ordered when *Cyclospora* is suspected. Under modified acid-fast stain, the organism has variable staining characteristics from dark red to transparent

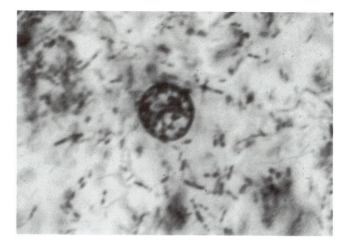

Figure 16.1. Cyclospora revealed through acid-fast stain of stool sample (see color plate).

(Fig. 16.1). It is important to realize that the diagnostic yield correlates with the experience of the laboratory personnel; the false-negative rate is high in laboratories in which technicians are not specifically trained to look for this pathogen.

TREATMENT AND PROPHYLAXIS OF CYCLOSPORIASIS

Trimethoprim-sulfamethoxazole is the only drug that has shown efficacy against *C. cayetanensis* so far. Two prospective trials have documented the efficacy of oral trimethoprim-sulfamethoxazole (160 mg of TMP and 800 mg of SMX twice daily for 7 days) in the treatment of Cyclosporiasis.

PARVOVIRUS B19

Parvovirus B19 was discovered by serendipity in 1975 by electron microscopy during the study of transfusion-associated hepatitis.

ETIOLOGY OF PARVOVIRUS B19

A single-stranded DNA virus, parvovirus B19 is the smallest DNA virus to infect mammalian cells (approximately 25 nm) compared with Herpes simplex virus (160 nm) and HIV (225 nm). The virus replicates only in human erythroid progenitor cells; in the laboratory it has been propagated in bone marrow, peripheral blood, fetal liver, and a few hematopoietic cell lines with erythroid characteristics. The virus is heat-stable and may be transmitted via blood products.

In contrast to most viruses, parvovirus B19 is trophic for one highly differentiated cell type, the human erythroprogenitor. The P antigen, a cellular receptor on the erythrocyte, has recently been identified as the B19 virus receptor. Persons without the P antigen on their erythrocytes are naturally resistant to B19 infection. Of note, endothelial cells may also be targets of viral infections that may mediate transplacental transmission and contribute to the facial rash of Fifth's disease. (See *Erythema infectiosum* below.)

CLINICAL PRESENTATION OF PARVOVIRUS B19

The only known pathogenic human parvovirus, parvovirus B19 causes a wide spectrum of human illnesses, including:

- *Erythema infectiosum* (Fifth's disease)
- Polyarthralgia syndrome (adulthood)
- Aplastic crisis
- Hydrops fetalis (gestational infection)

Erythema infectiosum (Fifth's Disease)

This illness has been recognized since the late 19th century. At that time, communicable rash illnesses were classified using a numbering system (1, measles; 2, scarlet fever; 3, rubella; 4, Duke's disease or epidemic *pseudoscarlatina;* 5, *erythema infectiosum;* and 6, roseola), hence the name "Fifth's disease." *Erythema infectiosum* (also called "slap-face disease" because of the red cheeks that occur when children are infected) is usually a mild childhood illness characterized by a facial rash and a lace-like rash on the trunk and extremities. Reappearance of the rash may occur following nonspecific stimuli, such as a change in temperature, sunlight, and emotional stress. Typically, the patient is otherwise well at the rash onset, but gives a history of mild systemic symptoms 1–4 days before the rash onset. Symptoms are usually self-limited, but may persist for several months.

Polyarthralgia syndrome (adulthood)

Arthritic symptoms, more common in adults, may occur as a sole manifestation of infection. The differential diagnosis of infectious arthritis appears in Table 16.1. Rubella and parvovirus B19 cause a similar clinical syndrome in young women; with a falling incidence of rubella and modification of rubella vaccines to eliminate arthritogenic strains, however, parvovirus arthropathy may now be more common. Adults seldom have the typical "slapped-cheek" appearance and only 50% have a rash. Within several days, a sudden onset of a symmetrical, self-limited polyarthritis occurs, most often affecting the hands. Like other viral arthritidies, the arthritis is thought to be immune mediated.

Aplastic Crisis

Aplastic crisis may occur in patients with hemolytic anemia or chronic anemia (red cell aplasia) from persistent infection in immunocompromised patients. The virus preferentially parasitizes the erythroid precursors in the bone marrow, with a transient suppression and production of red blood cells. This will usually have no measurable consequence in the hematocrit of a normal individual, as the erythroid precursor infection is self-limited and of short duration. In patients who have a chronic hemolytic disorder dependent on a high rate of production of erythrocytes, however (e.g., patients with thalassemia, sickle cell, or HIV), parvovirus B19 infection may result in an acute aplastic anemia.

Hydrops fetalis (gestational infection)

Parvovirus infection in pregnancy can lead to hydrops fetalis (gestational infection) and fetal loss or congenital infection. In the immunocompetent patient, the illness is usually self-limited; currently there is no recommendation for routine screening of pregnant women for B19 virus. An infection in pregnancy is not an indication for therapeutic termination of the pregnancy.

DIAGNOSIS OF PARVOVIRUS B19

A diagnosis of parvovirus infection may be made by isolation of parvovirus DNA from peripheral white blood cells using PCR technology or serologic testing for IgG or IgM (using radioimmunoassay and enzyme immunoassay based on the antibody-capture principle with solid-phase polystyrene beads). The presence of a giant pronormoblast in a bone marrow aspirate in a patient with anemia and a low reticulocyte count is also very suggestive of parvovirus B19 infection.

TREATMENT OF PARVOVIRUS B19

Immunoglobulin therapy has been used to treat the aplastic anemia associated with parvovirus B19 infection in the immunocompromised patient.

ESCHERICHIA COLI 0157:H7

Escherichia coli 0157:H7 is a pathogenic gram-negative bacterium first identified as a cause of illness in 1982 during an

Table 16.1. Differential Diagnosis of Infectious Arthritis

Pathogen	Characteristics	Diagnosis
S. aureus	Pyogenic; monoarticular	cx of synovial fluid
N. gonorrhoeae	Polyarticular	cx of extraarticular site
B. burgdorferi	Migratory small joints	Serology; PCR
Mycobacterial and Fungal	Chronic monoarticular	Culture or biopsy
T. Whippelli	Polyarticular; migratory	Small bowel bx; PCR
Hepatitis B	Polyarticular	Serology
Parvovirus B19	Migratory; Polyarticular	Serology

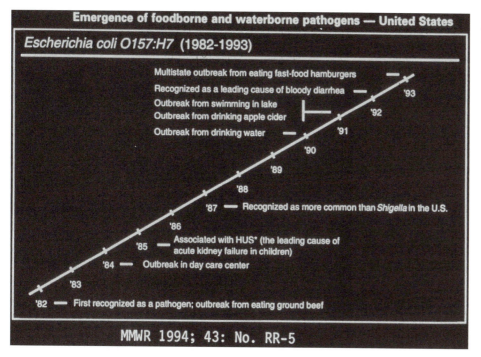

Figure 16.2. Time-line of emergence of *E. coli* 0157:H7 as a foodborne and waterborne pathogen in the United States.

outbreak of severe bloody diarrhea traced to contaminated hamburgers. Subsequently, in January 1993, a large outbreak (700 persons) of *E. coli* 0157:H7 infection was associated with undercooked hamburgers served in certain fast-food outlets in the Puget Sound area in Washington State. A time line of the emergence of *E. coli* 0157:H7 as a foodborne and waterborne pathogen in the United States is shown in Figure 16.2.

BACTERIOLOGY OF *ESCHERICHIA COLI* 0157:H7

The letters and numbers 0157:H7 identify certain antigens found on the surface of *E. coli* in the same way that the surface antigens can be explored at the serologically classified strains of salmonella. Three types of antigens are useful in the classification of *E. coli*. The first group of antigens, O antigens, are somatic antigens associated with lipopolysaccharide cell wall. The second group of antigens, the capsopolysaccharide or K antigens, are heat-stable. The third group of useful antigens, the H antigens, are flagellar antigens, which are heat-labile proteins. Accordingly, *E. coli* 0157:H7 has a 157 serotype O antigen in the seven-serum type H or flagellar antigen. This strain differs from other strains of *E. coli* by *not* fermenting sorbitol in under 24 hours and by *not* producing a beta-glucuronidase. Also, it does not grow well (if at all) at 44°–45°C and does not have any unusual heat resistance.

CLINICAL PRESENTATION OF *ESCHERICHIA COLI* 0157:H7

The differential diagnosis of infectious diarrhea is shown in Table 16.2. *E. coli* 0157:H7 causes abdominal pain and watery

Table 16.2. Differential Diagnosis of Infectious Diarrhea

Often Bloody	*Not Bloody*	*Either*
Shigella	Viral	*Salmonella*
EHEC	ETEC	*Campylobacter*
(*E. coli* 0157:H7)	EPEC	*Vibrio*
Amebiasis	*V. cholerae*	parahemolyticus
EIEC	*B. cereus*	*C. difficile*
	Giardia	
	Cryptosporidium	
	Cyclospora	

diarrhea followed within a few days by bloody diarrhea: hence the name hemorrhagic colitis. The bloody diarrhea corresponds to the dysentery phase of shigellosis, although as 0157:H7 does not invade enterocytes, it does not cause true dysentery. Sequelae include both the hemolytic uremic syndrome and thrombotic thrombocytopenic purpura (TTP). The organism is particularly pathogenic for children, and about 5% of children who get diarrhea from this organism develop HUS. In those who survive, renal damage and insufficiency may persist. *E. coli* 0157:H7 is a Vero toxigenic *E. coli* (VTEC). However, because the clinical sign of infection by this bacteria involves a hemorrhagic colitis, the organism is referred to as an enterohemorrhagic *E. coli* (EHEC). Vero toxins cause diarrhea and are similar to Shiga toxin produced by *Shigella* in classic dysentery. Of note, in an ongoing study of bloody diarrhea at the CDC, the number of infections attributed to *E. coli* 0157:H7 (8%) is higher than that of *Shigella*.

DIAGNOSIS OF *ESCHERICHIA COLI* 0157:H7

Isolation of this organism is possible only during the acute phase of the illness; the organism may not be detectable 5–7 days after the onset. Screening for the organism requires sorbitol MacConkey (SMAC) medium in which the *nonsorbitol-fermenting* O157:H7 organisms form white colonies. This screen is usually performed by the clinical microbiology laboratory only upon a doctor's request or upon receipt of a grossly bloody stool.

TREATMENT OF *ESCHERICHIA COLI* 0157:H7

Antibiotics have no favorable effect on the course of the bloody diarrhea or the sequela of the infection. In fact, there is some evidence that suggests poor outcomes for patients treated with antibiotics with O157:H7 HUS syndrome.

PREVENTION OF *ESCHERICHIA COLI* 0157:H7

Outbreak investigations have linked most cases with consumption of undercooked ground beef, although other food vehicles (including roast beef, raw milk, salami, water, and apple cider) have been implicated. Internal temperature of commercially cooked hamburger needs to meet federal guidelines of 140°F just before it is removed from the grill.

BABESIOSIS

The genus *Babesia* comprises dozens of species of tick-transmitted protozoa that infect a wide variety of wild and domestic animals. *Babesia* were actually the first organisms shown to be transmitted by an arthropod (Texas cattle fever).

ETIOLOGY OF BABESIOSIS

Babesia parasites are called *piroplasms* because of their pear-shaped intraerythrocytic stages. Until recently, only two species—*Babesia microti* (in the United States) and *B. divergens* (in Europe)—have been identified as human pathogens. Because humans are accidental hosts, it is a relatively rare protozoan infection. The distribution in animals is worldwide, although most *B. microti* infections have occurred in persons living in Nantucket and Martha's Vineyard, Massachusetts, and Long Island and Shelter Island, New York. *B. divergence*, sporadic worldwide, is a parasite of cattle.

A newly identified babesia-like organism (designated WA1 because it was first identified in Washington State) has caused infections in humans in the western United States. The clinical spectrum associated with this protozoan ranges from asymptomatic or influenza-like illness to fulminant, fatal disease (in splenectomized patients). Diagnosis is made by demonstration of significant antibody titers to WA1 using indirect

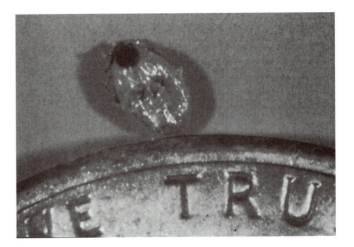

Figure 16.3. Hard-body tick that transmits spirochete of Lyme disease (see color plate).

immunofluorescent-antibody slides. An arthropod vector for the organism is suspected but has not yet been identified.

The ixodid or "hard body" ticks ingest babesia, which multiply and are subsequently transmitted to the vertebrate host by saliva. In the hosts, they invade red blood cells (RBCs) without an exoerythrocytic stage (unlike malaria), and multiply by budding. Of note, the Ixodes vector also transmits the spirochete of Lyme disease, accounting for reports of erythema chronicum migrans in patients with babesiosis (Fig. 16.3).

CLINICAL PRESENTATION OF BABESIOSIS

Clinically, most infections are asymptomatic; severe infections occur usually in older or asplenic patients. *B. microti* infections generally have a gradual onset of intermittent fevers, chills, diaphoresis, and fatigue after an incubation period of 1–3 weeks. Physical examination discloses fever, pallor, and hepatosplenomegaly. The level of parasitism rarely exceeds 10% of the RBCs. The illness usually has a low mortality but lasts from weeks to a month or more, with low-level parasitism lasting up to 4 months.

B. divergence is much more severe and usually follows a fatal course, with a rapid onset of fever, chills, nausea, vomiting, and severe hemolytic anemia, leading to jaundice, hemoglobinemia, and renal failure. Most reported incidents of *B. divergence* have occurred in the Old World and in patients who have had splenectomies.

DIAGNOSIS OF BABESIOSIS

The diagnosis should be considered in any patient with a fever and a history of tick exposure, especially if they are asplenic or have suggestive travel. In thin- and thick-smear Giemsa stains, babesiosis can be confused with malaria, as the predominant form resembles the malaria ring forms. However, the brownish pigment hemozoin seen in red blood cells parasitized by malaria is absent in babesiosis. Also absent are the schizont and gametocyte forms of malaria. The presence of tetrads of merozoites is a rare but specific feature of babesiosis.

TREATMENT OF BABESIOSIS

Oral quinine with clindamycin for 5–10 days is efficacious. There is a question whether pentamidine may also be efficacious. For *B. microti* infections, treatment may be required only in asplenic persons. There are only two reported cases of patients surviving *B. divergence* infections.

CHLAMYDIAE PNEUMONIAE, TWAR STRAIN

ETIOLOGY AND EPIDEMIOLOGY OF CHLAMYDIAE PNEUMONIAE, TWAR STRAIN

Chlamydiae pneumoniae has now been established as the third species of chlamydia on the basis of DNA, immunologic, and ultrastructural studies. Only one strain, TWAR, has been identified–first isolated in 1965 from the eye of a Taiwanese child, then in 1983 from a college student with pharyngitis.

Because isolation of *Chlamydiae pneumoniae* is difficult and may be hazardous, the development of a TWAR-specific monoclonal antibody microimmunofluorescent test has played a key role in defining the epidemiology of this disease. The test can differentiate between IgM and IgG serum fractions; the former is usually lost 2–6 months after infection, but IgG antibody persists. The seroprevalence rates are low in children and increase with age. Several studies have correlated TWAR with an acute respiratory disease, including pneumonia, bronchitis, pharyngitis, and sinusitis. During a 5-year period at the University of Washington Student Health Center, *Chlamydiae pneumoniae* infection was diagnosed in 22 students, representing almost 10% of all diagnosed pneumonias and 20% of radiographically proven pneumonias. Two studies of community-acquired pneumonia in Canada and Pittsburgh demonstrated TWAR antibodies in 6% of 660 patients, making TWAR the third or fourth most common recognized cause of pneumonia in these studies. Pathologic studies of uncomplicated TWAR pneumonia are limited because the illness is usually not fatal.

CLINICAL PRESENTATION OF CHLAMYDIAE PNEUMONIAE, TWAR STRAIN

TWAR can cause a variety of relatively mild respiratory infections that lack any distinctive clinical presentation. To date, pneumonia has been the illness most often associated with TWAR infection. Rales are almost invariably present, but

Table 16.3.   Community-Acquired Pneumonias

Atypical Bacterial	Typical Bacterial	Miscellaneous
L. pneumophilia	*S. pneumonia*	TB
L. micdadei	*H. influenza*	Influenza
C. pneumonia	Aspiration	Fungal
M. pneumonia	*Klebsiella*	*Coxiella burnetti*
		staphylococcal
		PCP
		Psittacosis
		Tularemia

signs of consolidation are less common. Hoarseness is found in about 10% of cases; if present, it is a useful clinical clue.

DIAGNOSIS OF CHLAMYDIAE PNEUMONIAE, TWAR STRAIN

Chest x-ray films usually reveal a modestly sized, single, pneumonic infiltrate. The microbiology laboratory is of little help in establishing the diagnosis at present. TWAR-specific antibody tests are the easiest way to confirm a diagnosis. Because the clinical syndrome of pneumonitis caused by TWAR is not distinctive, it is included in the differential diagnosis of the array of agents producing generally mild pneumonia among young adults (Table 16.3). The most common pathogen producing a similar illness is *Mycoplasma pneumoniae*.

TREATMENT OF CHLAMYDIAE PNEUMONIAE, TWAR STRAIN

No studies of antibiotic therapy for TWAR infections have been performed, but there is limited clinical experience suggesting that erythromycin may not be adequate. Based upon experience with other chlamydial infections, tetracycline at 2 g/day for 10–14 days is suggested, although doxycline and the newer macrolides (clarithromycin and azithromycin) are probably effective as well.

BACILLARY ANGIOMATOSIS AND OTHER BARTONELLA- (FORMERLY ROCHALIMAEA) ASSOCIATED DISEASES

Bacillary angiomatosis (BA) is a newly recognized infectious disease, primarily affecting immunocompromised patients, especially those infected with HIV. BA derives its name from the vascular proliferation seen on the histologic examination of affected tissues (including skin, bone, liver, spleen, and brain) and from the presence of bacillary organisms on silver stain or electron microscopy.

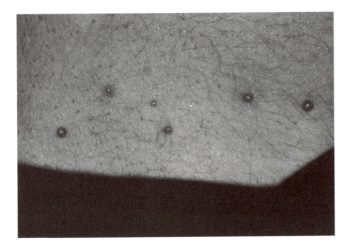

Figure 16.4. Nodular, tender, raspberry-like *Bartonella* lesions (see color plate).

ETIOLOGY OF BACILLARY ANGIOMATOSIS AND OTHER *BARTONELLA*-ASSOCIATED DISEASES

Recent molecular microbiologic investigations confirmed that at least two organisms, *Bartonella henselae* and *Bartonella quintana* (the louse-born agent of trench fever), can cause BA. *Bartonella* are rod-shaped, gram-negative bacteria that can cause febrile disease in humans.

Epidemiology of Bacillary Angiomatosis and Other Bartonella-*Associated Diseases*

The incidence of infection is unknown. It is probably a zoonosis associated with cat exposure (or fleas on the cats). The most commonly described cutaneous lesions are nodular "raspberry-like" tender papules or subcutaneous nodules that occasionally resemble Kaposi's sarcoma (Fig. 16.4).

The epidemiology and natural history of opportunistic infections caused by *Bartonella* continue to unfold. Recent reports of *B. quintana* bloodstream infections and infective endocarditis in HIV-negative, alcoholic, homeless men emphasize the need for heightened clinical awareness as well as increased surveillance for the detection and characterization of these fastidious pathogens.

Cat-Scratch Disease Connection: A Synthesis

Isolation of both *Afipia felis* and *Bartonella* species organisms has been reported from cases of cat-scratch disease. The development of an indirect fluorescent antibody test for *Bartonella henselae,* developed at the CDC, has advanced our understanding of the epidemiology of cat-scratch disease. In a recent study of 60 patients with cat-scratch disease in Connecticut, 94% of case patients had positive serology, versus 4% of age-matched, cat-owning, control patients. In addition, *B. henselae* has been isolated from the lymph nodes of patients with cat-scratch disease as well as from the blood and fleas from cats

that are suspected of transmitting cat-scratch disease. Thus, it would appear that cat-scratch disease and BA may be different manifestations of the same infection. The causative organism in most cases appears to be *Bartonella sp.* The serologic test is now commercially available.

CLINICAL PRESENTATION OF BACILLARY ANGIOMATOSIS AND OTHER *BARTONELLA*-ASSOCIATED DISEASES

Clinical manifestations associated with these organisms include BA, bacillary peliosis or hepatitis, relapsing fever with bacteremia, infective endocarditis, and cat-scratch disease.

DIAGNOSIS OF BACILLARY ANGIOMATOSIS AND OTHER *BARTONELLA*-ASSOCIATED DISEASES

The differential diagnosis of subcutaneous and cutaneous lesions in the HIV-infected patient is broad and includes a variety of disseminated opportunistic infections, as well as neoplastic and dermatologic conditions. The differential diagnosis of the cutaneous vascular lesions include pyoderma gangrenosum, Kaposi's sarcoma, verruga peruana (a late manifestation of infection with *Bartonella bacilliformis*), and BA (Table 16.4). The presence of bacillary organisms on the Warthin-Starry stain suggest the diagnosis of BA, but a definitive diagnosis depends upon the demonstration of the organisms in tissue or culture. The organism is a small curved gram-negative rod that grows best in 5% carbon dioxide with high humidity on solid tryptic soy agar containing rabbit blood. Isolator-lysis tubes and a prolonged incubation time (up to 6 weeks) are necessary for the isolation of *Bartonella* from blood.

TREATMENT OF BACILLARY ANGIOMATOSIS AND OTHER *BARTONELLA*-ASSOCIATED DISEASES

Excellent clinical response has been reported to erythromycin, rifampin, doxycycline, as well as quinolones and gentamicin. Beta-lactamase activity has been reported in some strains.

Table 16.4. Distinction Between Bacillary Angiomatosis (BA) and Kaposi's Sarcoma

Characteristics	*BA*	*KS*
Circumscription	Good	Poor
Capillary proliferation	lobular	Slit-like
Endothelial cell shape	Plump	Spindled
Neutrophils	Present	Absent
Infectious agent	*Bartonella*	?HHV-8
Warthin-Starry	Bacillary forms	Absent
Response to antiinfective	Yes	?

HANTAVIRUS PULMONARY SYNDROME (HPS)

Hantavirus infection in the United States has recently been recognized and may be characterized as an "old virus with a newly recognized clinical illness."

ETIOLOGY

Hantaviruses, members of the *bunyaviridae* family, are about 100 nm in diameter, with a lipid envelope (which makes them susceptible to alcohol and other lipid solvents).

Classically, hantavirus, in its most severe form, causes hemorrhagic fever with renal syndrome (HFRS) associated with hypotension and shock. (HFRS is endemic in Eurasia and Scandinavia.) A milder form of the disease, without shock and hypotension, is called *Nephropathia epidemica.*

In the recent outbreak of Hantavirus pulmonary syndrome, centered in the four-corner area of the United States (Arizona, Colorado, New Mexico, and Utah), at least 28 people have died. Additional cases have now been confirmed in California, Texas, Louisiana, and New York (Figure 16.5).

TRANSMISSION OF HANTAVIRUS PULMONARY SYNDROME (HPS)

Outbreaks of HFRS in Eurasia and Scandinavia have been associated with increased exposure to rodent populations in whom prolonged excretion of the virus in saliva, urine, and feces are suspected to be the reservoir. In the United States, the reservoir appears to be deer and mice; transmission presumably is via aerosolization of infected rodent droppings, although ingestion of contaminated food, or a direct bite or scratch, are also a possible means of transmission. To date, there has been no evidence of person-to-person transmission of HPS.

CLINICAL PRESENTATION OF HANTAVIRUS PULMONARY SYNDROME (HPS)

The biggest difference between the disease in the United States and previously described hanta infection has been the clinical manifestations. The U.S. cases have been more severe and associated with shock and pulmonary involvement. Most patients presented with adult respiratory distress syndrome following a flu-like prodromal illness.

DIAGNOSIS OF HANTAVIRUS PULMONARY SYNDROME (HPS)

The differential diagnosis of HPS is broad and includes all causes for acute respiratory distress syndrome. The geographic location and the history of rodent exposure should suggest a possibility of Hantavirus infection. A diagnosis of HPS may be made from one of the following:

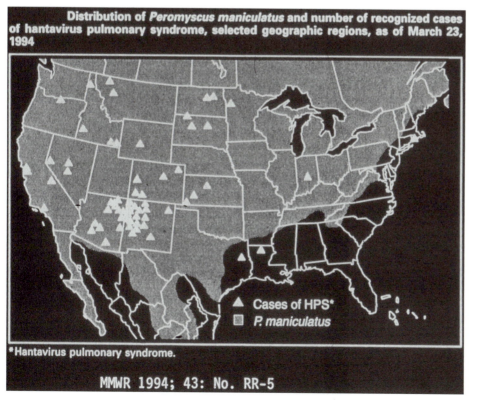

Figure 16.5. Distribution of Hantavirus pulmonary syndrome (HPS) cases in the United States.

- Serology—an elevated IgM titer or seroconversion
- A positive immunohistochemistry stain of formalin-fixed lung tissue
- PCR amplification of Hantavirus nucleotide sequences from frozen tissue

TREATMENT OF HANTAVIRUS PULMONARY SYNDROME (HPS)

Ribavirin has been used, but its efficacy is not proven.

PREVENTION OF HANTAVIRUS PULMONARY SYNDROME (HPS)

One should try to decrease exposure to the rodent population, including rodent-control measures (such as elevating tents and using zippers when camping).

PRIMARY HIV INFECTION

Primary HIV infection causes significant and progressive immunologic and virologic changes in the host.

ETIOLOGY OF PRIMARY HIV INFECTION

Recent studies of quantitative viral burden of patients with acute HIV infection (seroconversion) have led to a greater understanding of the natural history of HIV infection. High levels of infectious virus are detectable in the cerebrospinal fluid (CSF), peripheral-blood mononuclear cells, and plasma before the development of antibodies to HIV (Fig. 16.6). This brief period of p24 core antigenemia and viremia undergoes a rapid and spontaneous decline. A decline in viral burden coincides with an increase in the levels of antiviral antibodies, an increase in the CD4 count, and the resolution of symptoms, which suggests an "effective" initial immune response. However, this apparent clearance of virus and the restoration of CD4 cell count becomes less effective over time. These phenomena were initially believed to be accompanied by viral latency, with little or no viral replication until late in the course of infection. *It is now known that viral replication persists throughout all phases of HIV disease.*

CLINICAL PRESENTATION OF PRIMARY HIV INFECTION

More than half of the patients with primary HIV infection have an acute symptomatic illness. Common signs and symptoms are fever, adenopathy, pharyngitis, and a rash. As many as 70% of the patients with primary HIV experience dermatologic signs. In the skin, there is commonly an erythematous nonpruritic macular-papular eruption of the face, neck, or upper trunk. In the mucous membranes, aphthous-like ulcers with surrounding erythema may be observed. More than 80% of patients with symptomatic primary HIV infection complain of having symptoms of mononucleosis; therefore, primary HIV infection is in the differential diagnosis of "monospot-negative mononucleosis," which includes:

Ebstein-Barr virus
Cytomegalovirus
Toxoplasmosis

Figure 16.6. Generalized virologic and immunologic course of HIV disease.

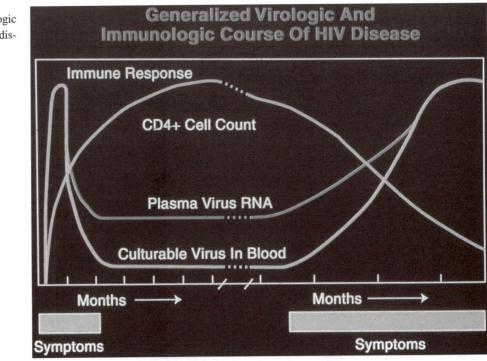

Primary HIV infection
Syphilis
Human herpes virus 6

DIAGNOSIS OF PRIMARY HIV INFECTION

A diagnosis of primary HIV infection during the period of acute infection that precedes the development of antibodies to HIV is made by detecting serum HIV p24 antigen. Viral cultures for HIV may also be positive from peripheral blood mononuclear cells.

TREATMENT OF PRIMARY HIV INFECTION

The utility of antiretroviral therapy is unclear at this time for primary HIV infection, especially in view of the recent reports of primary infection with zidovudine (AZT)-resistant HIV strains.

EHRLICHIOSIS

Ehrlichia are tick-borne rickettsial organisms that infect the leukocytes of susceptible mammalian hosts. *Ehrlichia canus* causes a canine illness characterized by fever, weight loss, bleeding, and pancytopenia.

ETIOLOGY OF EHRLICHIOSIS

In 1987, an Arkansas man with fevers, disorientation, pancytopenia, and a history of a tick bite was determined to be the first case of human ehrlichiosis in the western hemisphere.

Rickettsial-like organisms in inclusion bodies were observed among circulating leukocytes; in addition, he had positive serologic studies to *E. canus.* Subsequently, investigators determined that *E. chaffeensis,* closely related but not identical to *E. canus,* is the sole causative agent of human ehrlichiosis in the United States.

Since the initial case description, more than 350 cases of human ehrlichiosis have been reported in the United States; most cases are reported from the South Central and South Atlantic states, particularly Oklahoma, Missouri, and Georgia (Fig. 16.7).

Of note, a novel species of *Ehrlichia* that causes human disease has recently been described among 12 patients in the upper-Midwest region of the United States. This disease entity has been termed Human Granuloctyic Ehrlichiosis (HGE) because, unlike *E. chaffeensis,* the morulae of *E. phagocytophila* appear in the cytoplasm of neutrophils (granulotropic) but not in mononuclear white blood cells.

CLINICAL PRESENTATION OF EHRLICHIOSIS

The differential diagnosis of "summertime flu" is shown in Table 16.5. The most characteristic features of ehrlichiosis are high fevers and headaches; other common features include malaise, nausea, and vomiting. Approximately 90% of the patients will have a history of a tick bite or exposure within the preceding 3-week period; after an incubation period of 7 days, ehrlichiosis will present as a nonspecific febrile illness that resembles Rocky Mountain Spotted Fever (RMSF). Both are diseases of the outdoors with the highest incidence in the summertime months of May, June, and July.

Some epidemiologic and clinical differences exist between RMSF and ehrlichiosis. A rash develops in only approx-

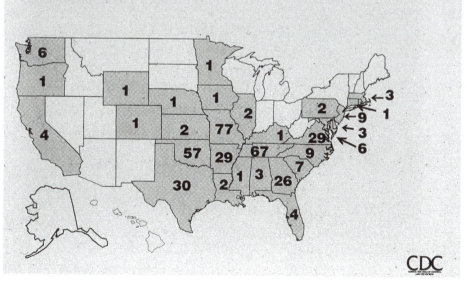

Reported Cases of HME, United States, 1986-1994 (Cases=386)

Figure 16.7. Reported cases of HME in the United States, 1986–1994.

imately 20% of cases of ehrlichiosis (vs. 80% of RMSF), and, when observed in ehrlichiosis, the rash usually *does not* involve the soles and the palms. Thrombocytopenia is common in both, but neutropenia with an absolute lymphopenia is more commonly observed in ehrlichiosis than in RMSF.

DIAGNOSIS OF EHRLICHIOSIS

A summertime flu-like illness following a tick bite should immediately raise the clinical suspicion of tick-borne illnesses that can result from infections with pathogens that include bacteria, rickettsia, viruses, and protozoa. The geographic setting and the occurrence of thrombocytopenia and lymphopenia in absence of a rash with negative serologies to RMSF, together with a clinical response to tetracycline, should suggest a clinical diagnosis of ehrlichiosis. A positive serology test confirms a diagnosis of ehrlichiosis.

The Centers For Disease Control and Prevention now use an IFA against *E. chaffeensis* for their assay. A single titer of 1:64 or four-fold rise or fall confirms a diagnosis. For HGE,

Table 16.5.   Differential Diagnosis of Infectious Etiologies for "Summertime Flu"

Viral	Bacterial	Rickettsial
Influenza	Mycoplasma	*Coxiella burnetti*
CMV	Syphilis	RMSF
Ebstein-Barr	TWAR	Erhlichiosis
HIV	Lyme disease	
HSV		

an antibody titer of > 1:80 for *E. phagocytophila* suggests infection.

TREATMENT OF EHRLICHIOSIS

Treatments of choice include tetracycline or chloramphenicol for 5–7 days. Most cases are self-limited, although one fatal case of seronegative ehrlichiosis (an Arkansas woman with AIDS) was recently reported.

REVIEW EXERCISES

1. All of the following are true about parvovirus B19 infections except:

   a. They may cause a polyarthralgia syndrome in adults
   b. They may cause *erythema infectiosum* (slap-cheek rash in children)
   c. Persons with the globoside receptor on the surface of the erythrocytes are resistant to B19 infections
   d. Diagnosis is made by serology (IgM/IgG) or PCR

2. The differential diagnosis of monospot-negative mononucleosis includes all of the following except:

   a. Cytomegalovirus
   b. Epstein-Barr virus
   c. Primary HIV infection
   d. Babesiosis
   e. Human Herpes Virus 6

3. All of the following are true about *E. coli* 0157:H7 infections except:

   a. Outbreaks have been associated with undercooked hamburger meat.
   b. Sequela of infection may include hemolytic uremic syndrome and thrombotic thrombocytopenic purpura.
   c. Isolation of the organism from stool cultures does not require any special medium.
   d. The diarrhea is usually bloody.

Answers

1. c
2. d
3. c

SUGGESTED READINGS

OVERVIEW

Addressing emerging infectious disease threats: a prevention strategy for the United States. MMWR 1994;43:1–18.

Satcher D. Emerging infections: getting ahead of the curve. Emerging Infectious Diseases 1995;1:1–6.

CYCLOSPORIASIS

Centers for Disease Control and Prevention (CDC). Update: outbreaks of cyclospora cayetanensis infection—United States and Canada MMWR 1996;45:611–612.

Soave R. Cyclospora: an overview. Clin Infect Dis 1996;23:429–437.

PARVOVIRUS B19

Anderson LJ. Human Parvoviruses. J Infect Dis 1990;161:603.

Brown KE, Anderson S, Young NS. Erythrocyte P antigen: cellular receptor for B19 parvovirus. Science 1993;262:114.

Brown KE, Hibbs JR, et al. Resistance to parvovirus B19 infection due to lack of virus receptor (erythrocyte P antigen) N Engl J Med 1994;330:1192–1196.

Kurtzman G, et al. Pure red-cell aplasia of 10-years duration due to persistent parvovirus B-19 infection. N Engl J Med 1989;321:519.

ESCHERICHIA COLI 0157:H7

Slutsker L, Ries AA, Greene KD, et al. *Escherichia coli* 0157:H7 diarrhea in the United States: clinical and epidemilogic features. Ann Intern Med 1997;126:505–513.

Tauxe RV. The epidemiology of infections caused by *E. coli* 0157:H7 and other enterohemorrhagic *E. coli,* and the associated HUS. Epidemiol Rev 1995;13:60–98.

BABESIOSIS

Benach JL. Clinical characteristics of human babesiosis. J Infect Dis 1981;144:481.

Meldrum SC, et al. Human babesiosis in New York State: an epidemiologic description of 136 cases. Clin Inf Dis 1992;15:1019–1023.

Persing DH, Herwaldt BG, et al. Infection with a Babesia-like organisms in Northern California. N Engl J Med 1995;332:298–303.

CHLAMYDIA PNEUMONIA, TWAR Strain

Grayston JT, et al. A new respiratory tract pathogen: *Chlamydia* pneumoniae strain TWAR. J Infect Dis 1990;161:618.

Pneumonia associated with the TWAR strain of *Chlamydia.* Ann Intern Med 1987;106:507.

BACILLARY ANGIOMATOSIS AND OTHER *BARTONELLA*-ASSOCIATED DISEASES

Drancourt M, Luc Mainardi J, et al. *Bartonella* (Rochalimaea) Quintana endocarditis in three homeless men. N Engl J Med 1995;332:419–423.

Regnery R, Tappero J. Unraveling mysteries associated with cat-scratch disease, Bacillary angiomatosis, and related syndromes. Emerg Infect Dis 1995;1:16–21.

Slater LN, Welch DF, Hensel D, et al. A newly recognized fastidious gram-negative pathogen as a cause of fever and bacteremia. New Engl J Med 1990;323:1587–1593.

Spach D, Kanter A, Dougherty M, et al. *Bartonella* (Rochalimaea) Quintana bacteremia in inner-city patients with chronic alcoholism. N Engl J Med 1995;332:424–428.

Zangwill KM, et al. Cat-scratch disease in Connecticut: epidemiology, risk factors, and evaluation of a new diagnostic test. N Engl J Med 1993;329:8–13.

HANTAVIRUS PULMONARY SYNDROME (HPS)

Duchin JS, et al. Hantavirus pulmonary syndrome: a clinical description of 17 patients with a newly recognized disease. N Engl J Med 1994;330:949–955.

Management of patients with suspected viral hemorrhagic fever. MMWR Supplement 1988;37(5-3).

Yanagihara R. Hantavirus infection in the United States: epizootiology and epidemiology. Rev Infect Dis 1990;12:449.

PRIMARY HIV INFECTION

Daar ES, et al. Transient high levels of viremia in patients with primary human immunodeficiency virus type 1 infection. New Engl J Med 1991;324:961–964.

Clark SJ, et al. High titers of cytopathic virus in plasma of patients with symptomatic primary HIV-1 infection. New Engl J Med 1991;324:954–958.

Piatak M, Saag M, et al. High levels of HIV-1 in plasma during all stages of infection determined by connective PCR. Science 1993;254:1011–1018.

EHRLICHIOSIS

Bakken JS, Dumler S, et al. Human granulocytic ehrlichiosis in the upper midwest United States: a new species emerging? JAMA 1994;272:212–218.

Fishbein DB, et al. Human ehrlichiosis: prospective active surveillance. J Infect Dis 1989;160:803.

Harkness JR, et al. Human ehrlichiosis in Oklahoma. J Infect Dis 1989;159:576.

McDade JE. Ehrlichiosis: a disease of animals and humans. J Infect Dis 1990;161:609.

Spach DH, et al. Tick-borne diseases in the United States. New Engl J Med 1993;329:936–947.

Board Simulation I:
Common Infections in the Ambulatory Setting

Carlos M. Isada

CASE 1

Patient Information

A previously healthy 28-year-old female presents with a sore throat, myalgia, low-grade fever, and headache. The patient has a new male sexual partner who reportedly is in good health. On examination, the patient appears fatigued but not acutely ill. The pharynx is injected and tonsils are enlarged. Generalized lymphadenopathy is present in the cervical, axillary, and inguinal areas. The liver is mildly enlarged, and a spleen tip is palpable. No rash is present. A CBC shows a 2900 WBC with 11% reactive lymphocytes and platelet count of 114,000. The SMA is significant for an SGOT of 120. A monospot test is negative.

QUESTION

1. Choose the one best statement:

   a. Patient requires immediate steroid therapy.
   b. Infectious mononucleosis is ruled out because of the negative monospot test.
   c. Primary CMV or toxoplasmosis can both mimic EBV infection, but testing is not appropriate since the patient is an otherwise healthy host.
   d. A plasma HIV RNA test is appropriate.
   e. None of the above is true.

Discussion and Answer Explanation

The Syndrome of Infectious Mononucleosis

Infectious mononucleosis is a common clinical syndrome characterized by the "classic triad" of fever, sore throat, and lymphadenopathy. Epstein Barr virus (EBV) is the most common cause of this syndrome, but other infectious agents can produce a nearly identical illness including cytomegalovirus and human immunodeficiency virus (HIV-1). The correct etiologic diagnosis is important since treatment and prognosis are variable.

Mononucleosis Secondary to Epstein Barr Virus Infection

Epstein Barr virus, a double-stranded DNA virus, can cause a broad spectrum of illness, including asymptomatic infection and infectious mononucleosis. Epstein Barr virus-induced mononucleosis is an acute clinical syndrome characterized by the "classic triad" described above, but other symptoms are often present such as fatigue, headache, and myalgia. Lymphadenopathy is noted on physical examination in nearly 95% of cases, although patients rarely complain of it themselves. Other physical signs include pharyngitis in more than 80% of cases, splenomegaly in 50%, and hepatomegaly in 10%. A rash is noted on presentation in 5–10% of cases. A peripheral blood smear characteristically shows a mononuclear lymphocytosis, often with greater than 10% reactive ("atypical") lymphocytes. Other common laboratory abnormalities include: leukopenia, often in the 2000-3000/mm^3 range, thrombocytopenia in 50% of cases, usually mild and clinically insignificant although occasionally more severe, and increased hepatocellular enzymes.

Several antibody tests are useful in confirming the diagnosis of acute EBV infection:

- **Heterophile antibody, or "monospot" test.** Heterophile antibodies are present in more than 90% of EBV cases at some point during the illness, and can appear at the onset of infection or may be delayed. The presence of heterophile antibodies was originally described in 1932, when it was noted that serum from patients with acute infectious mononucleosis caused agglutination of sheep erythrocytes (after absorption of the serum by guinea pig kidney). Heterophile antibodies are transiently present during acute EBV infection, but vary, ranging from asymptomatic infection to a mononucleosis-like illness with pharyngitis, adenopathy, lymphocytosis, and rash. The ''standard'' HIV-1 antibody test (by EIA or Western blot) is usually negative at presentation and may require weeks to months to become positive. Accurate diagnosis requires a plasma HIV-1 RNA test; if this is not available, the HIV-1 p24 antigen test is often positive but is probably less reliable. It is extremely important to obtain a sexual history on all patients with mononucleosis and to consider primary retroviral syndrome in at-risk individuals or persons with a new sexual partner. A missed diagnosis of HIV infection results in long- and short-term consequences. Recent studies support early intervention in the primary retroviral syndrome with antiretroviral therapy.

- **EBV-induced mononucleosis.** EBV should still be considered even if the heterophile is negative (EBV-specific serologies may be helpful).

Other causes of heterophile-negative mononucleosis include acute hepatitis (B or C), group A streptococcal pharyngitis, and rubella. These are usually more easily distinguished from EBV.

The answer to Question 1 is d.

CASE 2

Patient Information

A 28-year-old female presents with acute onset of urinary frequency and burning. The patient has not been sexually active for 6 months and has had only two urinary tract infections in the past. On examination the patient appears well and is afebrile. The patient has suprapubic tenderness but no CVA tenderness. Urine dipstick is positive for leukocyte esterase.

QUESTION

2. Which of the following statements is true?

   a. A urine culture should be sent prior to starting antibiotic therapy.
   b. Patient should be treated with Bactrim for 7 days.
   c. Patient should be placed on prophylactic antibiotics for prevention of recurrent UTIs.
   d. Ampicillin should be avoided as empiric therapy.
   e. If a urine culture is sent, there must be $> 10^5$ cfu/ml of a bacterial species for this to be considered a true UTI.

Discussion and Answer Explanation

Acute Cystitis in Women

Acute lower urinary tract infections (UTIs) are still one of the most prevalent reasons for a physician's office visit. The following discussion pertains to young women with uncomplicated bacterial cystitis, the most common presentation of UTI in ambulatory settings. The organisms responsible for bacterial cystitis in young females have remained predictable:

- *E. coli* in about 80% of cases
- *Staphylococcus saprophyticus,* a coagulase-negative staphylococcus species of increasing clinical significance, in over 10% of cases
- Others (2–3% each): *Proteus mirabilis, Klebsiella* species, enterococci

The first step in the pathogenesis of UTI involves colonization of the periurethral area and vagina with potentially uropathogenic bacteria originating from bowel flora. The ability of certain uropathogenic bacteria (particularly *E. coli* with type 1 pili) to adhere to uroepithelial cells is a complex situation and may sometimes be mediated by a specific receptor on uroepithelial cells. A variety of local host defense factors act to prevent infection, including: urinary Tamm-Horsfall protein, which interferes with bacterial attachment, local and systemic immunoglobulins, and mechanical flushing of the bladder with micturition. The short distance from the distal urethra to the bladder in women predisposes to infection. This ascending route of infection is by far the most common scenario, with a hematogenous route of infection occurring only rarely.

Clinically, women with cystitis present with the sudden onset of dysuria, urinary frequency and urgency, and suprapubic discomfort. The presence of flank pain, fevers, nausea, and vomiting is more characteristic of an upper UTI (such as pyelonephritis) than a lower UTI. However, studies using bacterial localization techniques suggest that distinguishing upper from lower UTIs on clinical grounds is not always accurate: a subset of patients (perhaps as high as 20%) with upper UTI will not manifest flank pain or fever and will present only with dysuria. Since localization techniques are not available in clinical practice, the presence of fever and costovertebral angle tenderness remains the most useful predictor of the level of the infection, although imperfect.

Not all females who present with symptoms of acute dysuria have bacterial cystitis. Other conditions should be considered in the differential diagnosis, including:

- **Acute urethritis, usually from *Chlamydia trachomatis*, herpes simplex virus, *Neisseria gonorrhoeae*.** A urinalysis is often positive for numerous WBCs, but RBCs are rare. The onset of symptoms may be more gradual than with acute cystitis, possibly with vaginal discharge or bleeding. Obtaining a sexual history is particularly important if urethritis is suspected.

- **Vaginitis, usually from Candida species but also trichomonas and "bacterial vaginosis."** Patients may complain more of "external dysuria" then the "internal dysuria" of cystitis and commonly also have vaginal itching, odor, or discharge.

A pelvic examination should be performed if either urethritis or vaginitis is suspected.

Most cases of uncomplicated cystitis require only a limited laboratory evaluation. A urine dipstick for leukocyte esterase (LE) testing is rapid and inexpensive and may be done in a busy clinic. Most commercial tests are reasonably sensitive (70-90%) for the detection of significant pyuria (10 WBCs/mm^3 urine), which is present in the vast majority of patients with symptomatic cystitis. However, it should be noted that pyuria is not specific for infection, and significant pyuria may be seen without infection. A urinalysis with microscopic analysis of spun urine sediment is the next step in laboratory diagnosis: this adds additional specificity to the dipstick LE test. A midstream urine sample may be examined either centrifuged or not centrifuged, with or without a Gram stain. Bacteria can be best identified on a centrifuged specimen that has been Gram stained. A woman with acute dysuria and a negative urine LE test should have a formal urinalysis done with microscopic examination, a urine culture, and a pelvic examination.

A urine culture is not necessary in most cases since the microbiology of cystitis in young women is still predictable and the degree of antibiotic resistance is still low. Urine culture should be reserved for the following situations:

- Atypical presentation (e.g., suspected urethritis)
- Recurrent UTIs
- Recent failed antimicrobial therapy
- Known anatomic or structural genitourinary abnormalities
- Underlying diabetes mellitus
- Immunocompromised status
- Pregnancy
- Elderly women
- Systemic symptoms
- Prolonged symptoms (more than 1 week)
- Diaphragm use

Otherwise, in uncomplicated cases an empiric course of antibiotics without a urine culture is acceptable.

Note that a bacterial UTI may be associated with low numbers of bacteria in the urine. Although most women with acute cystitis have large numbers of bacteria in the urine, a bacterial UTI is not defined by a urine culture with $> 10^5$ cfu of bacteria/ml. In some studies, up to 50% of women may have a symptomatic UTI with less than the cut-point of 10^5 bacteria/ml. This has been termed the "acute urethral syndrome." Studies have shown that as few as 100 cfu bacteria/ml as detected on a mid-void urine culture can cause a lower tract UTI in young females. Pyuria is still present on a urinalysis. In addition, an important cause of acute dysuria in young

women is *Staphylococcus saprophyticus,* one species of coagulase negative staphylococci. This organism may often be present in low numbers on urine culture and should not be automatically dismissed as a contaminant.

The optimal duration of therapy for uncomplicated cystitis in women is 3 days: there appears to be no advantage of a 7-day regimen in this setting. The 7-day regimen also results in a higher incidence of drug rash and vaginal candidiasis; however, a 7-day course is indicated in women with cystitis who have one of the above listed complicating factors. An alternative approach is "single dose therapy" (SDT), in which a single dose of oral antibiotics is administered: the rationale for SDT is lower cost, near 100% compliance, and less drug toxicity. SDT has been successful in some settings but in most trials appears inferior to the standard 3-day regimen. SDT is contraindicated in many situations, including suspected pyelonephritis and anatomic abnormalities; it should not be administered to men.

Most authorities still recommend trimethoprim-sulfamethoxazole as the agent of choice for empiric therapy of cystitis (i.e., without knowledge of the organism). Other preferred agents include trimethoprim alone, norfloxacin, and ciprofloxacin. Trimethoprim-sulfamethoxazole and trimethoprim alone are superior to the beta-lactam antibiotics, such as ampicillin. The incidence of antibiotic-resistant *E. coli* as a cause of community-acquired cystitis is increasing. The following drugs are not recommended for empiric therapy: amoxicillin, ampicillin, or sulfonamides (alone).

Lower UTIs: Special Situations

Recurrent Infections   Recurrent infections in women may be due to either relapses or reinfections. Relapses soon after therapy may be a result of: unsuspected upper tract infection (pyelonephritis), anatomic abnormality of the GU tract (obstruction, reflux, stricture, etc.), or presence of a renal calculus. However, more than 90% of recurrent infections are because of reinfections and not relapses. The yield of diagnostic tests such as ultrasonography, IVP, and cystoscopy in women with reinfections is very low. Risk factors for reinfection should be sought, such as the use of diaphragms and spermicides. Genetic factors may play a role. Several strategies for prevention of recurrent infections have been employed:

- Continuous antibiotic prophylaxis
- Postcoital prophylaxis
- Patient-initiated antibiotic prophylaxis

Recurrent UTIs may be frequent in postmenopausal women, probably due to several factors including incomplete voiding and low estrogen levels (which allow *E. coli* to become part of the vaginal flora). Intravaginal topical estradiol preparations have been effective in UTI prevention in postmenopausal females.

Asymptomatic Bacteriuria   Asymptomatic bacteriuria in adults without indwelling bladder catheters is a frequent problem in clinical practice and occurs in older women. This condition is best defined by a patient with $> 10^5$ cfu of bacteria/ml on two or more consecutive urine cultures, who has none of the typical symptoms of dysuria, urinary frequency, etc. The finding of asymptomatic bacteriuria in an adult is not an immediate indication for therapy except in two situations: (1) the pregnant female (owing to the high risk of acute pyelonephritis in the mother and prematurity in the infant), and (2) before GU tract manipulation or surgery (to decrease the incidence of bacteremia). Asymptomatic bacteriuria as defined here is quite common in both elderly men and women. However, only a few such patients ultimately develop symptomatic cystitis, and even fewer develop urosepsis or pyelonephritis. The literature regarding the management and significance of asymptomatic bacteriuria is extensive but conflicting. Most authorities feel that asymptomatic bacteriuria in the elderly is a benign condition that does *not* warrant routine antimicrobial therapy.

The answer to Question 2 is d.

CASE 3

Patient Information

A previously healthy 53-year-old male sustained a dog bite injury to his hand 12 hours ago. The dog was a domestic pet that was provoked. A deep bite on the dorsal surface of the nondominant hand, with a significant edema but no apparent cellulitis, is present on examination. The patient has moderately severe pain and diminished range of motion at the wrist.

QUESTION

3. Which of the following statements is true?

    a. *Pasteurella multocida* is a likely pathogen.
    b. Radiographs of the hand are indicated.
    c. Dicloxacillin and erythromycin should be avoided.
    d. Patient should be admitted for IV antibiotic therapy.
    e. All of the above are true.

Discussion and Answer Explanation

Animal Bites

It is estimated that more than two million animal bites occur in the United States each year. Approximately 50% of Americans will suffer a significant cat or dog bite in their lifetime. Although bite wounds comprise about 1% of emergency room visits, most of those bitten do not seek formal medical attention. Those who do are usually concerned with bites to the extremities, especially if the dominant hand is involved. Animal bites to the face are less common than bites to the extremity but may be potentially life-threatening, particularly in children.

If a patient seeks treatment within 8 hours after the bite, it is usually motivated by a concern for tetanus or rabies treatment, for an extensive crush injury, or for care of a cosmetically disfiguring bite (e.g., involving the face). The wound is usually not clinically infected but does contain a mixture of aerobes and anaerobes. A variable number of such wounds (1–30%) seen within 8 hours become infected, nevertheless. However, if a patient presents more than 8 hours after a bite, the likelihood of infection is significantly higher.

Typical symptoms of established infection include: moderate to severe local pain, edema, drainage, low-grade fever, adenopathy in the draining regional nodes, and cellulitis or lymphangitis. Evaluating the patient for underlying osteomyelitis is important, especially in bites to the extremities: this is a common complication, and patients complain of a markedly decreased range of motion or deep pain. A bite close to a joint may also lead to septic arthritis. Local abscess formation and tenosynovitis may occur. Patients at high risk for complications of animal bites include the following:

- Splenectomized persons
- Immunocompromised hosts
- Patients with chronic edemas of the legs or upper extremities (especially postmastectomy)
- Patients with a total joint arthroplasty

Dog Bites About 85% of dog bites are considered provoked attacks: the dog is usually known to the victim. Approximately 15% of dog bites become infected, in contrast with cat bites that are puncture wounds that frequently become infected. Infecting organisms in dog bites reflect the normal canine oral flora:

- Streptococci species (alpha, beta, and gamma hemolytic)
- Pasteurella species, especially *P. Multocida* (about 20-50% of cases)
- *Staphylococcus aureus* (20-40% of cases)
- Coagulase negative staphylococci
- Anaerobes (up to 40% of cases, in mixed culture): Bacteroides (*Prevotella*) species and *Fusobacterium nucleatum*

An important dog-bite pathogen is *Capnocytophaga canimorsus,* previously known as dysgonic fermenter 2 (DF-2). This is a fastidious organism that often requires special laboratory techniques for isolation. It has been associated with fulminant and rapidly fatal sepsis in patients who have been splenectomized or who have underlying liver disease.

The use of "prophylactic" antibiotics is an important management decision and refers to the administration of antibiotics (usually oral) for patients who present early with wounds that are clinically uninfected. Potential pathogens are present in more than 85% of wounds, and predicting which wounds will become infected may be difficult.

Gram stains taken from bite wounds have poor sensitivity but good specificity for the etiologic organism(s). Gram stains and cultures of a wound are not useful or cost effective before the onset of a clinically apparent infection and need not be obtained. However, Gram stains and culture may be useful in established infections to guide antimicrobial therapy, especially with severe crush injuries and bone or joint penetration. If the possibility of a bone puncture or fracture exists, obtaining a radiograph of an extremity is important.

Prophylactic antibiotics are usually *not* indicated following dog bites due to the low incidence of significant infections. Consider prophylactic antibiotics only in selected situations:

High risk hosts:

- Asplenic patients
- Immunocompromised patients
- Patients with liver disease
- Patients with chronic limb edemas

High risk bites:

- Distal extremity puncture wounds
- Moderate to severe crush injuries
- Wounds less than 8 hours old with edema, possible joint space infection, or possible osteomyelitis
- Wounds near a prosthetic joint
- Genital area wounds
- Injury to a cosmetically sensitive area such as the face
- Any significant hand wound

The organisms to be included are *S. Aureus, Pasteurella* sp., and anaerobes. Several oral antibiotics may be used for prophylaxis, including amoxicillin-clavulanate, amoxicillin alone, or doxycycline in the penicillin-allergic patient. Duration of prophylaxis is 5 days.

For infected dog bite wounds, therapy should be directed toward the same pathogens as prophylaxis, pending culture results. Studies suggest that the types of bacteria cultured from early presenting and late presenting wounds are essentially identical (and are the same as contaminated but not infected wounds). The decision to use oral or intravenous antibiotics is based on the severity of the injury and its location. The outpatient antibiotic treatment for mild to moderate established infection is amoxicillin and clavulanate (Augmentin) for 10–14 days. If the patient is allergic to penicillin, use doxycycline (contraindicated in children). The outpatient parenteral antibiotic treatment for moderate established infection is ceftriaxone as a single-dose regimen (popular in many emergency room protocols).

In some cases, hospitalization is necessary, especially with fever and sepsis, worsening cellulitis, immunocompromised hosts, significant crush injury or pus, joint space involvement, or extensive edema.

Cat Bites A cat bite is a tiny, deep, highly infectious puncture: estimates of infection range from 25–50%. Common pathogens include *Pasteurella multocida, Staphylococcus aureus,* and anaerobic streptococci. Unlike dog bites, cat bites require routine antibiotic prophylaxis. Patients should be examined carefully for involvement of a joint space or bone penetration, common with cat bites. Outpatient oral and parenteral regimens are the same as for dog bites.

Other factors important for management of bite wounds include:

- Irrigation
- Debridement
- Suturing
- Immobilization
- Elevation
- Immunizations:
  - Tetanus
  - Rabies prophylaxis: immune globulin and human diploid cell vaccine.

The answer to Question 3 is e.

C·H·A·P·T·E·R

18

Board Simulation II:
Infectious Diseases

J. Walton Tomford and David L. Longworth

CASE 1

Patient Information

A 60-year-old African-American male originally from Alabama is transferred from his home in southern Ohio to a Cleveland Hospital. The patient has been a foundry worker for many years though he has never had a tuberculin skin test. The patient has chronic obstructive pulmonary disease (COPD): he has received corticosteroids for the past 6 months. The patient was admitted 1 week ago, to a local hospital, with worsening respiratory failure and possible pneumonia requiring mechanical ventilation.

A week later the patient's condition has worsened on broad-spectrum antibiotics for gram-negative bacilli, which grew from the sputum. He is transferred for ''weaning.'' His chest radiograph is shown in Figure 18.1.

QUESTIONS

1.1. Endotracheal tube sputum should be sent for:

   a. Giemsa stain
   b. Wright stain
   c. Polymerase chain reaction (PCR)
   d. Ziehl-Neelsen stain
   e. Papanicolaou stain

1.2. If the above stain was positive for many beaded red staining organisms, what would be the correct treatment plan?

   a. Isoniazid (INH), B6, Rifampin, Pyrazinamide (PZA), and Ethambutol
   b. Ethionamide, Cycloserine, Streptomycin, Ethambutol

   c. INH, B6
   d. Wait for cultures
   e. Ciprofloxacin

Discussion

This case illustrates the importance of considering mycobacteria, especially *Mycobacterium tuberculosis,* in any case of pneumonia that fails to respond to antibacterial therapy. Corticosteroid therapy for COPD has been associated with a variety of infectious complications. The patient's silica exposure in a foundry should have prompted a baseline tuberculin skin test years ago and certainly prior to the initiation of steroids for COPD.

The presence of gram-negative rods in the sputum culture does not necessarily indicate a true gram-negative pneumonia: clinical judgement, knowledge of the sputum gram stain result, and additional laboratory data are necessary to distinguish colonization from infection from disease. Acid-fast bacilli are sometimes weakly gram positive, but gram stain is not a reliable way to exclude tuberculosis.

Once acid-fast bacilli are found on the sputum smear, one has to decide the likelihood of *Mycobacterium tuberculosis* versus other nontuberculous mycobacteria (also termed atypical mycobacteria or mycobacteria other than tuberculosis [MOTT]). In a clinically serious situation such as this, *M. tuberculosis* must be at the top of the list, although *M. kansasii, M. avium intracellulare,* and rapidly growing mycobacteria such as *M. chelonei* also can produce serious acute pulmonary disease.

The decision to treat this pulmonary process as tuberculosis is a wise one. Therapy should begin promptly with a very aggressive multidrug regimen. In regions of the United States where the incidence of multidrug-resistant (MDR) tuberculosis is less than 5%, three drug regimens of INH, RIF, and PZA are probably adequate, but it is probably safer to include

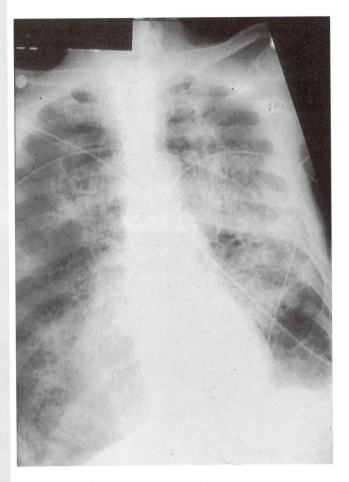

Figure 18.1. Chest radiograph of patient in Case 1.

ethambutol as well until sensitivities can be obtained. Vitamin B6 in a dose of 50 mg to 100 mg orally per day should be given with INH to prevent peripheral neuropathy.

Answers and Explanations

1.1. d.

A Giemsa stain is not usually requested for sputum. It is useful in detecting malarial parasites or Babesia. A Wright stain of the sputum would detect eosinophils suggestive of asthma or allergic bronchopulmonary aspergillosis. At present PCR cannot be performed on expectorated sputum in most commercial laboratories, though direct detection in sputum of *M. tuberculosis* by PCR is being developed. A Ziehl-Neelsen stain properly decolorized on a carefully collected and handled endotracheal sputum specimen would be strongly indicated in this patient receiving steroids. It would likely be positive and clinically suggestive of severe infection from *M. tuberculosis*. A Papanicolaou stain on sputum might be useful if one were looking for malignant cells. In addition, an alerted cytologist can sometimes recognize certain fungal organisms such as *Blastomyces dermatiditis* or *Histoplasma capsulatum,* two organisms that are epidemiologically possible causes of pneumonia in this case and could be especially virulent in the presence of steroids. Fungi are best seen with a potassium hydroxide prepared Calcofluor white fluorescence stain.

1.2. a.

The regimen in answer choice b includes two second-line drugs, ethionamide and cycloserine, which are toxic and often poorly tolerated. Therapy with isoniazid and B6 alone would be foolish in the presence of obvious active disease and would lead to the development of secondary resistance. To withhold therapy pending cultures in a patient with severe illness and positive sputum smears would be inappropriate. Monotherapy with ciprofloxacin may be appropriate in selected patients with certain types of gram-negative pneumonia but would be inappropriate in someone with suspected or proven tuberculosis. Ciprofloxacin is sometimes used in combination with other agents in the therapy of certain types of nontuberculous mycobacterial infection, such as *M. chelonae.*

CASE 2

Patient Information

A 50-year-old Indian physician presents with a right neck mass. The patient received Bacillus-Calmette–Guerin (BCG) immunization as a child. A tuberculin skin test was strongly positive 10 years ago upon immigration to the United States. A computerized tomographic (CT) scan of the neck is shown in Fig. 18.2. Two major surgical procedures and a prolonged

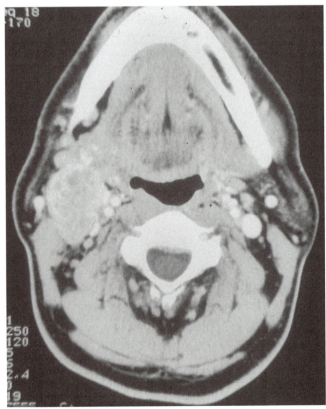

Figure 18.2. CT scan of neck of patient in Case 2.

course of expensive medications were required to produce a successful clinical and cosmetic result.

QUESTION

2.1. In retrospect, what should have been done a decade ago?

a. Offer INH/B6 for 6–9 months
b. Offer INH/PZA/Streptomycin for 1 year
c. Exclude active disease
d. Observation, especially since the patient has a history of being hepatitis B surface antigen positive
e. a and c

Discussion

This case illustrates the importance of understanding concepts of INH prophylaxis. Current American Thoracic Guidelines address issues regarding Bacillus-Calmette-Guerin (BCG) vaccination and skin test conversions. It is always important to exclude active disease since monotherapy with INH will quickly produce resistance in such situations. In fact, when in doubt, treat as if there is active disease. If this is a possibility, one needs to start at least two new drugs to which the patient's mycobacteria have not been previously exposed.

Remote BCG vaccination is neither a contraindication to nor a reason not to offer INH prophylaxis in appropriate clinical situations as outlined below.

Answer and Explanation

2.1. e.

The exclusion of active disease by history, a compulsive physical examination, and routine laboratory studies such as a CBC, chest radiograph, and urinalysis to exclude silent sterile pyuria are the first order of business. The presence of active disease would require multidrug therapy as outlined above. Once active disease is excluded, the need for prophylaxis is determined by weighing a number of considerations, including whether the skin test conversion is recent and within 2 years; the size of the skin test reaction; the risk of INH hepatitis; the risk of disease reactivation; and the presence or absence of certain underlying disorders which, if present, increase the risk of disease reactivation. In most circumstances INH plus B6 is the recommended prophylactic regimen. If the contact person has drug-resistant TB, then recommendations are different and include the use of combinations of rifampin, PZA, and ciprofloxacin, depending on the susceptibility profile of the organism in the contact source. In this case, answer choice b would be inappropriate, since drug-resistant disease is not a concern. Hepatitis from INH and rifampin is not predictable, so close education and compliance are of great importance.

CASE 3

Patient Information

A 35-year-old construction worker from southern Ohio is transferred to your hospital for meningitis. The patient was sick with fever and malaise for 3 weeks prior to admission and received an empiric course of therapy with trimethoprim-sulfamethoxazole for possible sinusitis. The patient is known to be HIV-negative. Spinal fluid, upon admission to the patient's local hospital, shows 85 WBC/ mm^3 with 95% polys, glucose of 45mg/dl, and a protein of 180 mg/dl. The patient's condition worsens despite therapy with vancomycin and ceftriaxone. Cryptococcal antigen in the CSF is negative on the initial and follow-up spinal taps. The patient's condition again worsens, and a CT scan shows hydrocephalus, meningeal enhancement, and a basal ganglia infarct. The patient is transferred to your hospital and dies shortly after arrival. A postmortem examination shows chronic meningitis with caseating granulomas.

QUESTION

3.1. Which of the following two diseases would be likely causes for this patient's demise?

a. *M. tuberculosis, C. neoformans*
b. *M. kansasii, Brucella* species
c. *M. tuberculosis, H. capsulatum*
d. *Mycobacterium avium intracellulare* (MAI), sarcoidosis

Discussion

This case illustrates the varied presentations of tuberculosis. This patient's presentation is not atypical for tuberculous meningitis, which can occur alone or as a manifestation of miliary disease. In suspected cases, even if smear-negative, empiric therapy should not be withheld pending culture and may be life saving if initiated in a timely fashion. The polymorphonuclear predominance in this patient's CSF is not uncommon in tuberculous meningitis and occurs in 20%–30% of cases in the early stages of the disease. This patient's CT findings are very characteristic of tuberculosis involving the meninges. Basilar meningitis can lead to obstructive hydrocephalus and inflammatory vasculitis, which results in infarcts. The pathologic finding of granulomas should always make one think of mycobacteria, especially TB. While caseation is often said to be almost pathognomonic for TB, it can be seen in histoplasmosis, blastomycosis, cryptococcosis, and coccidioidomycosis. Sarcoidosis is rarely associated with caseation necrosis in the meninges. However, in patients with chronic or basilar meningitis, the distinction between tuberculosis and sarcoidosis and can be extremely difficult. In addition, tuberculosis and the other fungal infections discussed above can occasionally coexist with or complicate sarcoidosis and its treatment.

Table 18.1.   Recommendations for Isoniazid Preventative Therapy

Category	Under 35 Years Old	Over 35 Years Old
+ risk factor	Treat all ages if PPD > 10 mm* or > 5 mm and recent contact with active case, +HIV or chest radiograph with scar compatible with old TB or untreated TB	
− risk factor + high incidence	Treat if PPD > 10 mm	No treatment
All other situations	Treat if PPD > 15 mm	No treatment

* Measurements refer to diameter of induration at 48–72 hours

Table 18.1 lists recommendations for isoniazid preventive therapy for tuberculosis.

Following are groups at high risk for tuberculosis reactivation:

- Persons from Asia, Africa, Latin America
- Medically under-served groups: African-Americans, Hispanics, Native Americans
- Residents of prisons, nursing homes, institutions
- Health care workers in high incidence jobs or institutions

Following are the risk factors for tuberculosis reactivation:

- HIV-positive
- Recent close contact with active pulmonary case
- Recent PPD conversion (within 2 years):
  - 10 mm* or greater when under age 35
  - 15 mm or greater when over age 35
- PPD 10 mm or greater when under age 4 regardless
- Old TB scar or history of pulmonary TB untreated
- Selected underlying disorders or medications:
  - Corticosteroid use
  - Diabetes mellitus
  - Gastrectomy
  - Disorders requiring chronic immunosuppression (e.g., transplant recipients)
  - Malignancy
  - Silicosis
  - Chronic renal failure
  - Injection drug use

Answer and Explanation

3.1. c.
The CSF cryptococcal antigen is very sensitive and is positive in up to 95% of patients with cryptococcal

meningitis. While *C. neoformans* can produce caseating granulomatous necrosis, the spinal fluid usually tests positive for antigen. Brucellosis would be an unlikely consideration in this setting, given the absence of any history of travel, animal exposure, or unusual food ingestion. Most of the mycobacteria besides *Mycobacterium tuberculosis* do not disseminate to the meninges even in the presence of HIV infection. While sarcoidosis is possible, it is rarely this fulminant. Histoplasmosis can present with meningitis as seen in this patient.

CASE 4

Patient Information

A 25-year-old fisherman from the Gulf Coast of Florida presents to your office with a 1-day history of erythema of the hand, fever to 39°C, and shaking chills. There is no lymphangitis. History is notable for chronic hepatitis C.

QUESTION

4.1.   Choose the least likely agent for the cellulitis.

   a. *Aeromonas hydrophila*
   b. *Vibrio vulnificus*
   c. *Streptococcus pyogenes*
   d. *Mycobacterium marinum*
   e. *Erysipelothrix rhusiopathiae*

Discussion

This case involves the differential diagnosis of cellulitis acquired in a marine environment. While most organisms on the skin are gram-positive cocci, most organisms in water are gram-negative bacilli. *Aeromonas* and *Vibrio* cellulitis occur following skin trauma in individuals who are exposed to water contaminated with these organisms. Secondary bacteremia is common with both organisms, and *Vibrio* infections have a propensity for individuals with underlying liver disease. *Erysipelothrix* cellulitis occurs in meat handlers and fisherman following minor skin trauma. The localized cutaneous form tends to be subacute and classically has a serpiginous purple-red appearance. Fever may be absent. Diffuse cellulitis is less common and may evolve from erysipeloid. In cases presenting with diffuse cellulitis, fever is common. *Mycobacterium marinum* produces a chronic cellulitis, often with nodular lymphangitis, and is usually seen in fishermen or owners of aquaria. Fever is uncommon. Salient facts regarding waterborne cellulitis are summarized in Table 18.2.

Answer and Explanation

4.1. d.
Although this organism can produce cellulitis in fishermen, it produces a chronic cellulitis. The patient described has an acute rather than a chronic cellulitis. All of the other

Table 18.2. Features of Cellulitis Acquired in a Marine Environment

Organism	Epidemiology	Clinical	Therapy
Aeromonas hydrophila	Fresh or brackish H$_2$O; leeches	Acute cellulitis after trauma	TMP-SMX
V. vulnificus	Salt H$_2$O; liver disease	Acute cellulitis; septicemia in immunocompromised	TCN or Cefotaxime
Erysipelothrix rhusiopathiae	Fishermen, fish or meat handlers handlers	Erysipeloid Diffuse cellulitis	PCN G
M. marinum	Swimming pools, Aquaria, marine exposure, fish spines	Subacute, chronic; papules, ulcers; tenosynovitis, nodular lymphangitis	Rif + Etham

organisms would be common causes of acute cellulitis in this setting.

CASE 5

Patient Information

A 23-year-old female undergoes cytomegalovirus donor positive/recipient negative (CMV D + /R-) allogeneic bone marrow transplantation for acute myelogenous leukemia (AML). The patient presented 1 year ago with fever, petechiae, and gingival bleeding and was found to have AML. Induction therapy with high-dose cytosine arabinoside and daunorubicin achieved remission. Treatment course was complicated by *E. coli* bacteremia during patient neutropenia. No source was found. Six months later the patient had a relapse and underwent reinduction with the same regimen. This time treatment course during neutropenia was complicated by transient candidemia for which 1 gram of amphotericin B was given. Remission was achieved and a Hickman catheter was placed in preparation for allogeneic bone marrow transplantation.

The patient is admitted and receives a preparative regimen of busulfan, Cytoxan, and etoposide on days 7 through 10, which produce considerable vomiting. Prophylaxis with oral ciprofloxacin is begun on day 0 at the time of allogeneic transplantation. She is treated with granulocyte colony stimulating factor, cyclosporine, and prednisone. She becomes absolutely neutropenic on day +2.

On day +3 she develops fever to 39.4°C. On examination she appears chronically but not acutely ill and is vomiting. There is mild oral mucositis. The remainder of the physical examination is normal. The WBC is 100 and the alkaline phosphatase is elevated at 235 IU/ml. A chest radiograph raises the question of a vague right middle lobe infiltrate.

QUESTIONS

5.1. Which is the least likely diagnosis?

    a. Cytomegalovirus (CMV) pneumonia
    b. Aspiration pneumonia
    c. Hickman-related bacteremia
    d. Fever from mucositis
    e. Gram-negative bacteremia with early adult respiratory distress syndrome

Therapy with vancomycin, piperacillin, and tobramycin is begun. Blood cultures grow streptococci viridans in one set of peripheral cultures. Blood cultures obtained via the Hickman are negative. The chest radiograph does not evolve. She promptly defervesces but is slow to engraft. On day 15 she spikes to 40°C. She has diarrhea, and the physical examination is normal. The white blood count is 250 with 5% polymorphonuclear leukocytes. The alkaline phosphatase is 600 IU/ml, AST 42 IU/ml, ALT 55 IU/ml, and bilirubin 1.5 mg%. A computerized tomographic scan of the abdomen discloses ill-defined areas of mottling in the liver.

5.2. Which is the most likely diagnosis?
    a. Graft versus host disease
    b. Veno-occlusive disease
    c. Hepatic candidiasis
    d. Liver abscess from prior bacteremia
    e. *C. difficile* colitis

Blood cultures grow *Candida albicans* and amphotericin B is given. The patient engrafts at day 20 and is discharged to complete 100 days of outpatient ganciclovir and 2.5 grams of amphotericin B. Trimethoprim-sulfamethoxazole is begun. Patient is maintained on cyclosporin A and prednisone 30 mg per day, and does well until day +120 when a fever to 38.5°C. and a dry cough develop. A chest radiograph discloses a large left upper lobe cavity. The patient has forgotten to take prescribed Bactrim for the past month and has returned to work as a supervisor on construction sites. The patient also recalled that an uncle with whom she had lived as a child had died of tuberculosis.

5.3. Which is the least likely diagnosis?

    a. Nocardia pneumonia
    b. Pneumocystis pneumonia
    c. CMV pneumonia
    d. Pulmonary tuberculosis
    e. Cryptococcal pneumonia

Bronchoscopy is performed. For each potential finding shown in Figures 18.3 through 18.6, choose the best therapy.

    a. Trimethoprim-sulfamethoxazole
    b. Amphotericin B + flucytosine
    c. Isoniazid + Rifampin + Pyrazinamide + Ethambutol
    d. Amphotericin B at 1 mg/kg/d
    e. Erythromycin

5.4. Pathogen in Figure. 18.3:_____
5.5. Pathogen in Figure. 18.4:_____
5.6. Pathogen in Figure. 18.5:_____
5.7. Pathogen in Figure. 18.6:_____

Discussion

This case deals with the differential diagnosis of fever in the bone marrow transplant recipient. The differential diagnosis of fever in such patients is invariably broad, but several impor-

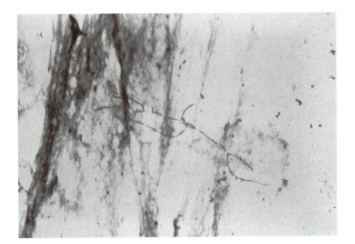

Figure 18.5. Finding for Case 5. (See color plate)

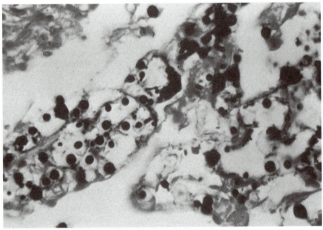

Figure 18.6. Finding for Case 5. (See color plate)

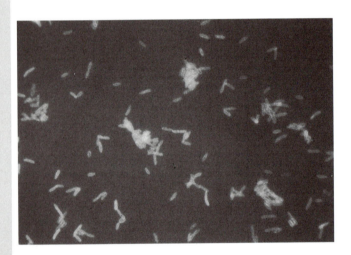

Figure 18.3. Finding for Case 5. (See color plate)

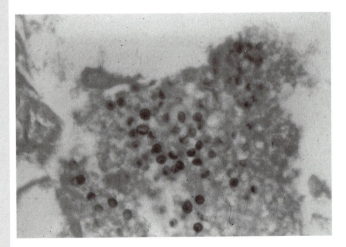

Figure 18.4. Finding for Case 5. (See color plate)

tant considerations are helpful in approaching a microbial differential diagnosis:

- Time of onset relative to transplantation
- Presence or absence of neutropenia
- CMV donor-recipient status
- Prior infections or exposures
- Autologous versus allogeneic transplant
- Immunosuppressive regimen
- Presence of GVHD
- Prophylactic regimens

The temporal onset of infectious complications following allogeneic bone marrow transplantation are summarized in Table 18.3.

In general, the first month following transplantation is the period associated with neutropenia and thus with invasive bacterial infections, such as bacteremias, line-related infections, *C. difficile* colitis (given the use of empiric antimicrobi-

Table 18.3.   Timing of Complications in Patients Undergoing Allogeneic Bone Marrow Transplantation

Risk Factor	Neutropenia	Acute GVHD	Chronic GVHD
		Immunosuppression	Chronic immunosuppression
Bacterial Infections	Bacteremias Lines C. difficile Pneumonia Mucositis		Encapsulated organisms, pneumonia, sinusitis
Fungal	Candida and Aspergillus		
Viral	HSV	CMV and Adeno	VZV
Pneumonia	Bacterial	CMV Interstitial	TB, Nocardia Encapsulated bacteria
0	1	4	12

Month

als), and bacterial pneumonias. Oral herpes simplex virus infections and fungal infections such as candidiasis or aspergillosis may also be encountered. The use of growth factors has shortened the duration of neutropenia and thus the incidence of these infectious complications.

In months 1–4, CMV becomes a diagnostic consideration in patients with unexplained fever, cytopenia, or pneumonia, especially in those with concomitant graft versus host disease. Cytomegalovirus donor positive/recipient negative patients are at highest risk of CMV disease. CMV disease is rare in autologous bone marrow transplant recipients, who do not require long-term immunosuppression. Beyond month 4, allogeneic recipients are at risk of infectious complications associated with chronic immunosuppression, such as *Pneumocystis carinii* pneumonia, herpes zoster, cryptococcosis and reactivation tuberculosis.

Answers and Explanations

5.1. a.

Cytomegalovirus is the least likely diagnosis given that the patient is only at day +3.

5.2. c.

Hepatic candidiasis is the best answer. Clues to this diagnosis in the history include the prior candidemia, the abnormalities on CT scan of the abdomen, and the elevated alkaline phosphatase out of proportion to the transaminases, which is characteristic of hepatic candidiasis. Graft-versus-host disease often produces diarrhea when it involves the gut, but occurs after engraftment and rarely produces fever. Veno-occlusive disease may occur early but is usually associated with jaundice. Antibiotic-associated colitis is a reasonable concern but does not account for the liver function abnormalities. Bacteremic seeding of the liver occurs but is very rare and thus this is not the best answer.

5.3. c.

Cytomegalovirus is the correct answer because CMV

pneumonia, although not unexpected at day +120, does not cavitate. All of the other choices can produce cavitary pneumonia in the immunocompromised patient and might occur at this point following allogeneic bone marrow transplant.

5.4 to 5.7

Transbronchial biopsy might conceivably show one of several pathogens depicted in Figures 18.3 to 18.6, which could produce a cavity. Figure 18.3 shows *Legionella* species for which erythromycin would be appropriate therapy. While not a common pathogen in allogeneic bone marrow transplant recipients, the construction site exposure and cavitary infiltrate necessitate its inclusion in the differential diagnosis. Figure 18.4 shows *Pneumocystis carinii*, which rarely may cavitate, though generally with small rather than large cavities. The patient stopped taking prescribed trimethoprim-sulfamethoxazole, making this a concern. Trimethoprim-sulfamethoxazole would be the best therapy of the choices offered for *Pneumocystis carinii* pneumonia. Figure 18.5 shows weakly acid-fast branching filamentous bacilli typical of *Nocardia asteroides*, for which trimethoprim-sulfamethoxazole is the best choice. Figure 18.6 shows *Cryptococcus neoformans*, for which amphotericin B and flucytosine would be appropriate.

CASE 6

Patient Information

A 23-year-old male undergoes CMV D + /R + bilateral lung transplantation for cystic fibrosis. He receives postoperative cyclosporin A and prednisone. There is a history of exposure, during childhood, to a brother with active pulmonary tuberculosis. A pretransplant tuberculin skin test was negative.

On day 5 postoperatively, fever develops to 39.0°C. On physical examination the patient appears ill. The incision is clean. There are a few rales along the right parasternal border.

The white blood count is 18,000/mm^3 with 90% granulocytes. A chest radiograph discloses a subtle right basilar infiltrate.

QUESTIONS

6.1. Which of the following is the least likely consideration?

   a. CMV pneumonia
   b. Anastomotic leak from the right mainstem bronchus
   c. Mediastinitis
   d. *Pseudomonas cepacia* pneumonia
   e. Acute rejection
   f. *Hemophilus parainfluenza* pneumonia from the donor.

The patient is bronchoscoped and found to have *H. parainfluenzae* pneumonia and responds to a course of parenteral antibiotics. Ganciclovir is given for 4 weeks postoperatively. The patient is compliant with trimethoprim-sulfamethoxazole prophylaxis maintenance. At 5 months posttransplant the patient presents with fever and a left upper infiltrate.

6.2. On a statistical basis, what is the most likely diagnosis?

   a. *Pneumocystis carinii* pneumonia
   b. CMV pneumonia
   c. Tuberculosis
   d. Bacterial pneumonia
   e. Cryptococcal pneumonia

Discussion

This case deals with the differential diagnosis of fever in patients undergoing solid organ transplantation. In approaching such patients, several important considerations directly affect the differential diagnosis:

- Type of organ transplanted
- Timing of fever relative to transplantation
- CMV donor-recipient status
- Prior and current epidemiologic exposures

In general, infectious complications occurring within the first month are most often attributable to postoperative bacterial infections involving the allograft (or surrounding structures), wound infections, or nosocomial bacterial infections (e.g., intravascular lines, urinary tract infections from Foley catheters, etc.). Cytomegalovirus disease most often presents from months 1–4 posttransplant and is especially problematic in CMV D + /R- transplant recipients. Infectious complications beyond month 4 are often attributable to pathogens associated with impaired cellular immunity, which occur in the setting of chronic immunosuppression. An exception to this occurs in lung transplant recipients: bacterial pneumonia is the most common infectious complication, regardless of posttransplant time. The common infectious complications and their temporal onset following transplantation are summarized by organ transplant in Figures 18.7, 18.8, and 18.9.

Answers and Explanations

6.1. a.

Although at risk for CMV pneumonia, day +5 would be very early in the course. Most patients with CMV pneumonia would present at 1–4 months posttransplant. Mediastinitis, anastomotic leak at the bronchial anastomosis, and acute rejection would all be major concerns. In addition, cystic fibrosis patients may seed their new lungs with organisms that continue to colonize their native trachea and sinuses, such as *Pseudomonas cepacia, Pseudomonas aeruginosa* and *Staphylococcus aureus*. Finally, some studies have shown that colonizing organisms in the donor bronchus may produce postoperative pneumonia in the transplanted lung, as occurred in this patient.

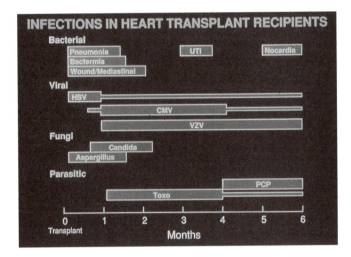

Figure 18.7. Infections in heart transplant recipients.

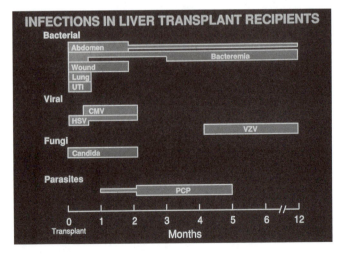
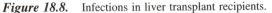

Figure 18.8. Infections in liver transplant recipients.

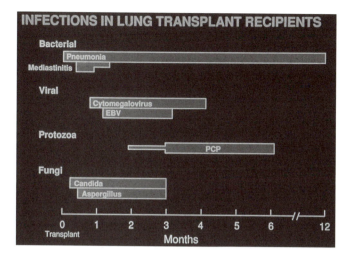

Figure 18.9. Infections in lung transplant recipients.

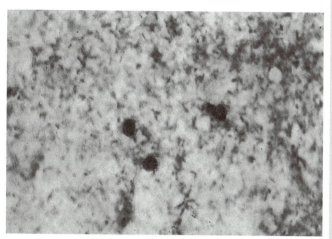

Figure 18.10. Pathogen in Case 7. (See color plate)

6.2. d.

As noted above, bacterial pneumonia is the correct answer and is the leading cause of infection in lung transplant recipients in all time periods posttransplant. All of the other answers, however, would be appropriate concerns at 5 months, in view of the cellular immunodeficiency from chronic immunosuppression.

CASE 7

Patient Information

A 42-year-old HIV-positive businessman consults you for periumbilical crampy abdominal pain and nonbloody, watery diarrhea. He has recently returned from a 2-week trip to Moscow and St. Petersburg. His CD4 count is 560/mm^3, and his history is otherwise unremarkable.

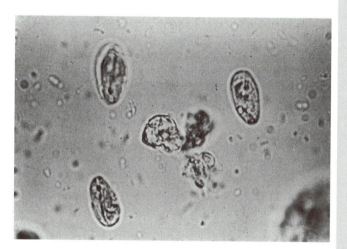

Figure 18.11. Pathogen in Case 7. (See color plate)

QUESTIONS

7.1. All of the following would be likely causes of diarrhea except:

  a. Enteropathogenic *E. coli*
  b. Giardiasis
  c. Cryptosporidiosis
  d. Microsporidiosis
  e. Amebiasis

Stool examinations for ova and parasites demonstrate several organisms. Select the appropriate therapy for each pathogen shown in Figures 18.10, 18.11, and 18.12:
  a. No therapy.
  b. Paromomycin 500 mg orally 2 times a day for 1 week
  c. Metronidazole 250 mg orally 3 times a day for 7 days

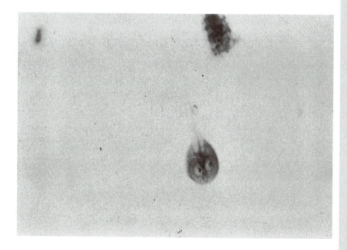

Figure 18.12. Pathogen in Case 7. (See color plate)

d. Metronidazole 750 mg orally 3 times a day for 5–10 days *plus* Diloxanide Furoate 500 mg orally 3 times a day for 10 days

7.2. For the pathogen in Figure. 18.10: _____
7.3. For the pathogen in Figure. 18.11: _____
7.4. For the pathogen in Figure. 18.12: _____

Discussion

This case involves the differential diagnosis of diarrhea in an HIV-positive traveler. The most important consideration in the differential diagnosis is the patient's CD4 count, which is normal. Opportunistic pathogens such as *Mycobacterium avium intracellulare* complex (MAIC), microsporidiosis and cytomegalovirus would not be considerations in an individual with a normal CD4 count. These infections are usually seen in patients with advanced immunodeficiency and CD4 counts below 100 cells/mm³. In this patient, all of the common causes of nonbloody traveler's diarrhea would be appropriate concerns, including enterotoxigenic *E. coli,* giardiasis, cryptosporidiosis (a self-limited disease in immunocompetent individuals) and amebiasis (though in most homosexual males, entamoebas detected in stool usually represent the nonpathogenic zymodeme *Entamoeba dispar).*

Answer and Explanations

7.1. d.
As described above, this would not be a concern in an HIV + individual with a normal CD4 count.

7.2.
Figure 18.10 demonstrates acid fast organisms of *Cryptosporidium.* Although paromomycin has been beneficial in some HIV-infected patients with advanced immunodeficiency and chronic cryptosporidiosis, its usefulness in the therapy of acute cryptosporidiosis in immunocompetent individuals and HIV-infected individuals with normal CD4 counts has not been proven. Quinacrine and metronidazole are not effective in cryptosporidiosis.

7.3. and 7.4.

Figures 18.11 and 18.12 show a cyst and trophozoite of *Giardia lamblia.* Metronidazole 250 mg orally 3 times a day for 1 week would be appropriate. High-dose metronidazole and diloxanide furoate are the recommended treatment for intestinal amebiasis. A trophozoite and cyst form of *E. histolytica* are depicted in Figures 18.13 and 18.14, respectively.

Salient facts concerning cryptosporidiosis, giardiasis, microsporidiosis, and amebiasis are summarized in Tables 18.4 through 18.11.

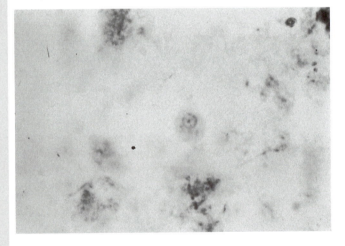

Figure 18.13.   *E. histolyticia* trophozoite. (See color plate)

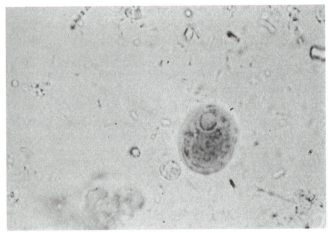

Figure 18.14.   *E. histolytica* cyst. (See color plate)

Table 18.4.   Cryptosporidiosis

	Immunocompetent	*Immunocompromised*
High Risk	Travelers, day care workers, veterinarians, gay males, health care workers, household contacts	AIDS, congenital immunodeficiency, immunosuppression
Incubation Period	1–12 days (Mean = 7)	Same
Clinical	Self-limited gastroenteritis	Intractable secretory diarrhea, weight loss, malabsorption, bronchial and biliary
Duration	2–26 days (Mean = 12)	Prolonged

Table 18.5. Cryptosporidiosis: Diagnosis

- Conventional stool exam unreliable
- Special techniques
  - Sugar-coverslip flotation
  - Kinyoun or Giemsa stains
  - Phase contrast microscopy
- Small bowel biopsy

Table 18.6. Cryptosporidiosis: Therapy

Immunocompetent	Immunocompromised
Supportive	Reverse immunosuppression
	Hydrate, sometimes TPN
	Antimotility agents
	Paromomycin

Table 18.7. Giardiasis: Transmission

- Known reservoirs include man, dogs, beavers
- Transmission via person-to-person spread or via food or water
- Groups at high risk:
  - Travelers to areas with poor sanitation
  - Campers who drink from streams
  - Male homosexuals
  - Children in day care centers
  - Institutionalized patients
  - Communities with inadequate or faulty water purification systems
  - Hypogammaglobulinemia or achlorhydria

Table 18.8. Giardiasis: Clinical Manifestations

Illness	Manifestations
Asymptomatic	Passes organisms
Acute illness	Incubation period 1–3 weeks
	Watery nonbloody diarrhea
	Anorexia, nausea, distension, flatulence
	Sulfur burps, crampy pain
	Duration more than 1 week
Chronic illness	Evolves from acute illness or insidiously alternating diarrhea and constipation
	Distension, belching, flatulence common
	Malabsorption and weight loss on occasion

Table 18.9. Giardiasis: Diagnosis

Test	Sensitivity	Comment
Stool O & P × 3	40%–80%	
UGI sampling	80%–100%	
• String test		
• Aspirate		
• Small bowel biopsy		
Serology	>95%	Not widely available
• ELISA (serum & stool)		
• IFA (serum)		
UGI series	Poor	Nonspecific

CASE 8

Patient Information

You are a general internist in a small community in Oklahoma. A family, long-time patients in your practice, presents to your office again with febrile illnesses. They have recently returned from another extended exotic vacation. Six weeks ago they traveled to the Amazon basin in central Brazil, where they worked for 3 weeks in a rural missionary hospital. Three weeks ago they returned to the United States and spent 1 week vacationing at their private home on Nantucket. While there, they cared for a neighbor's infant daughter who had an unexplained febrile illness. Two weeks ago they returned to their ranch in Oklahoma where they spent several days working with their dogs herding cattle. Several family members recall removing ticks from the dogs.

Patient 1 is a healthy 52-year-old male business executive. The patient developed falciparum malaria last year following a trip to Nigeria. Ten days ago the patient complained of the gradual onset of fever, shaking chills, headache, lethargy and cough. These symptoms have waxed and waned but persist. Physical examination is notable for a temperature of 39.0°C, heart rate of 78, mild diaphoresis, hepatosplenomegaly, and a faint cluster of pink macules on the abdomen. The WBC is 3000 cells/mm³.

Patient 2 is a 48-year-old female school teacher, previously healthy except for a bout of babesiosis acquired on Martha's Vineyard. Two days ago the patient noted gradual onset of fever to 38.7°C, arthralgias, anorexia, chills, fatigue and headache. Physical examination is notable for a temperature of 38.7°C, a heart rate of 104, tender nonswollen joints of the hands, cervical lymphadenopathy, and a faint reticular rash on the trunk and limbs. The WBC is 3500 cells/mm³.

Patient 3 is an 18-year-old male college freshman who was healthy previously, except for a bout of ehrlichiosis last year. The patient presents with a 3-day history of fever to 38.5°C, headache, diarrhea, myalgia, and arthralgia. Temperature is 38.4°C, and physical examination is normal.

Patient 4 is a 16-year-old male junior in high school who

Table 18.10.   Giardiasis: Therapy

Agent	Regimen	Efficacy	Comment
Quinacrine	100 mg tid × 5d	~90%	Side effects: toxic psychosis, liver necrosis, dermatitis Contraindicated in psoriasis Limited availability
Metronidazole	250 mg tid × 5d	80%–100%	Antabuse effect
Furazolidone	100 mg qid × 7–10d	90%–95%	Elixir available Brown urine, rash, antabuse effect, GI, hemolysis in G6PD deficiency
Tinidazole Lactose–free diet	1.5–2 g × 1	90%	Not available in the United States

Table 18.11.   Clinical Features of Microsporidiosis in HIV-Infected Patients

Enterocytozoon
   CD4 Counts <100
   Chronic diarrhea, anorexia, weight loss most common
   Cholecystitis, cholangitis, sinusitis, bronchitis rare
Encephalitozoon
   CD4 counts <100
   Keratoconjunctivitis, bronchiolitis, pneumonitis
   Sinusitis, nephritis, cystitis, ureteritis
S. intestinalis
   Enteritis, cholecystitis
Diagnosis
   Microscopic visualization in tissues or body fluids using
      Gram, Weber, and Giemsa stains
   Reliable serodiagnostic tests lacking
Therapy
   Albendazole may be effective for *S. intestinalis*,
      Encephalitozoon, and Enterocytozoon gastrointestinal
      illness
   Fumagillin or propamidine for ocular Encephalitozoon

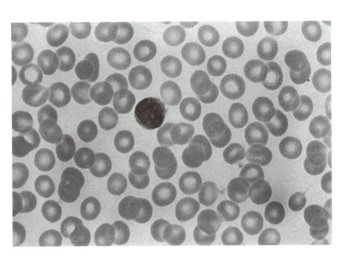

Figure 18.15.   Smear for patient 1. (See color plate)

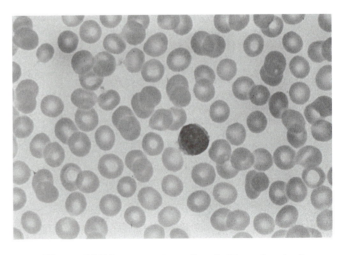

Figure 18.16.   Smear for patient 2. (See color plate)

is previously healthy as well, except for a football injury last year which led to a splenectomy. Five days ago the patient complained of fever, chills, myalgia, and headache. Physical examination is notable for a temperature of 38.7°C and a healed left upper quadrant scar.

Patient 4 is a 14-year-old male foreign exchange student from Scotland spending the year with the family. The patient presents with a 4-day history of fever to 38.8°C, headache, myalgia, and arthralgia. Temperature is 38.6°C and examination is normal. The patient's WBC is 3900 cell/mm³ (65P, 30L, 5M), platelet count is 105,000/mm³, and AST and ALT are 115 U/L and 135 U/L, respectively.

Because of the extensive travel history, you obtain peripheral thick and thin smears on the family, which are shown in Figures 18.15 through 18.19.

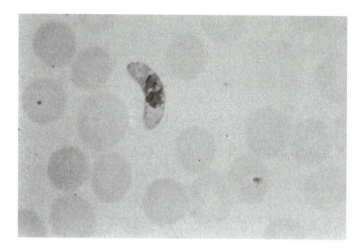

Figure 18.17. Smear for patient 3. (See color plate)

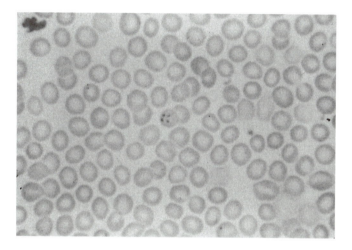

Figure 18.18. Smear for patient 4. (See color plate)

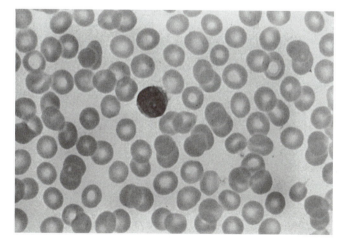

Figure 18.19. Smear for patient 5. (See color plate)

QUESTIONS

Based upon the history, findings, laboratory studies, and blood smear results, choose the best therapy for each of the patients.

a. Chloroquine phosphate 1 g followed by 500 mg in 6 hours, then 500 mg/day for 2 days
b. Clindamycin 600 mg orally 3 times a day and quinine sulfate 650 mg orally 3 times a day for 7–10 days
c. Ciprofloxacin 500 mg orally 2 times a day
d. Tetracycline 500 mg orally 4 times a day
e. Quinine sulfate 650 3 times a day for 3–7 days and pyrimethamine-sulfadoxine 3 tabs at once on last day of quinine
f. No therapy

8.1. Patient 1: _____
8.2. Patient 2: _____
8.3. Patient 3: _____
8.4. Patient 4: _____
8.5. Patient 5: _____

Discussion and Answer Explanations

The patients present with acute febrile illnesses in the setting of extensive travel to the Amazon basin, Nantucket, and subsequently home to Oklahoma, where several of them recall tick bites. The patients also recall exposure to an infant with an unexplained febrile illness. This places them at risk for a number of acute infectious diseases.

8.1.
　　Patient 1: illness could be mistaken for a viral illness, especially given the leukopenia. Malaria and ehrlichiosis are major concerns; blood smear (Fig. 18.15) is normal, however, and the presence of hepatosplenomegaly and rose spots should suggest the diagnosis of typhoid fever, which is endemic in the tropics. Of the offered choices, the correct treatment for Patient 1 is ciprofloxacin, answer c. In the past, chloramphenicol has been the treatment of choice, but resistance to this drug, as well as to ampicillin and trimethoprim-sulfamethoxazole, has emerged in some parts of the world. Third-generation cephalosporins such as ceftriaxone and quinolones such as ciprofloxacin have excellent activity against *S. typhi*.

8.2.
　　Patient 2: peripheral blood smear (Fig. 18.16) is normal, arguing against a diagnosis of malaria. Rash, cervical lymphadenopathy, and tender joints should suggest a diagnosis of parvo B19, likely acquired from the infant on Nantucket. No therapy is available for this illness, and answer choice f is correct.

8.3.
　　Patient 3: illness could easily be confused with acute gastroenteritis, a viral illness, or typhoid fever. His peripheral smear, however, shows the typical banana gametocyte of *P. falciparum* (Fig. 18.17). His illness is a medical emergency. It is imperative to consider the diagnosis of malaria in all

patients with an acute febrile illness returning from a malaria-endemic part of the world, even if they have taken prophylaxis. Malaria may be accompanied by diarrhea, which should not dissuade one from considering the diagnosis. Chloroquine resistance occurs throughout South America. The correct treatment for the patient is therefore a combination of quinine sulfate and pyrimethamine-sulfadoxine, answer e.

8.4.

Patient 4: peripheral smear demonstrates the tetrad of *Babesia microti* (Fig. 18.18), which was likely acquired during his sojourn on Nantucket. Clinically severe babesiosis occurs more commonly in splenectomized individuals. Appropriate therapy consists of clindamycin plus quinine sulfate, answer choice b. In severe cases, exchange transfusion may be necessary.

8.5.

Patient 5 has a febrile flu-like illness, a normal peripheral smear (Fig. 18.19), leukopenia, thrombocytopenia, and mild hepatitis. These findings are nonspecific and raise numerous possibilities. In someone residing in Oklahoma with a history of tick exposure, however, this should suggest the diagnosis of ehrlichiosis or Rocky Mountain spotted fever, for which doxycycline, tetracycline, or chloramphenicol would be appropriate therapy. Answer choice d is correct.

Key points concerning typhoid fever, parvo B19, malaria, babesiosis, ehrlichiosis, and Rocky Mountain spotted fever are summarized in Tables 18.12 through 18.22

CASE 9

Patient Information

A 42-year-old male insulin-dependent diabetic archaeologist presents to your office with a 6-week history of intermittent fever, dry cough, a 10-pound weight loss, and nights sweats. In the past 6 months the patient has worked on various digs at Indian burial sites in New Mexico, Wisconsin, and southern Ohio. In addition, the patient traveled to rural Thailand 4 months ago for a 2-week holiday.

Table 18.12. Babesiosis

Epidemiology
  Etiology in North America is usually *B. microti*
  Transmission occurs via ixodid ticks and, rarely,
    transfusion
  Most cases contracted on Nantucket, Martha's Vineyard,
    Long Island, Shelter Island
Clinical manifestations
  Incubation period 1–4 weeks
  Many do not recall a tick bite
  Spectrum of illness ranges from asymptomatic to
    prolonged severe illness
  Splenectomy predisposes to more severe illness with
    higher levels of parasitemia
Diagnosis
  Thick and thin smears stained with Giemsa
  Serology
Therapy
  Clindamycin 1.2 g IV BID or 600 mg PO TID × 7 days
    plus Quinine sulfate 650 mg PO TID × 7 days
  Consider exchange transfusion in critically ill patient

Table 18.14. Features Suggesting *P. Falciparum*

Banana gametocytes
High grade parasitemia
Double applique forms
Multiply parasitized red blood cells
Absence of trophozoites or schizonts in periphery

Table 18.13. Biologic and Clinical Characteristics of Human Malaria

	Falciparum	Vivax	Ovale	Malariae
Prevalence	Common	Common	Uncommon	Uncommon
Incubation	7–27 days	10–40 days	12–26 days	18–76 days
RBC Cycle	48 hours	48 hours	48 hours	72 hours
Hepatic relapse	No	Yes	Yes	No
Persistence	<3 years	<3 years	<3 years	Many years
Parasitemia	Up to 60%	<1%	<1%	<1%
Morbidity	Hemolysis	Hemolysis		Nephrosis
	ATN	Splenic rupture		
	Pulmonary edema			
	CNS			
Mortality	Common without therapy	Uncommon	Rare	Rare
Chloroquine Resistance	Widespread	Rare	No	No

Table 18.15. Therapy of Malaria: All Forms Except Chloroquine-Resistant *P. Falciparum*

Route	Drug	Adult Dose	Pediatric Dose
Oral	Chloroquine phosphate	600 mg base (1g), then 300 mg base (.5 g) at 6, 24, and 48 hours	10 mg base/kg (max. 600 mg), then 5 mg base/kg at 6, 24, and 48 hours
Parenteral	Quinidine gluconate	10 mg/kg loading dose (max. 600 mg) in NS over 1 hour, followed by continuous infusion 0.02 mg/kg/min. × 3d maximum	Same as adult
	or Quinine dihydrochloride	20 mg salt/kg loading dose in 10 ml/kg D5W over 4 hours, then 10 mg salt/kg over 2–4 hours Q8H (max. 1800 mg/d) until oral Rx	Same as adult

Table 18.16. Therapy of Malaria: Chloroquine-Resistant *P. Falciparum*

Route	Drug	Adult Dose	Pediatric Dose
Oral	Quinine SO$_4$	650 mg po tid × 3–7 days	25 mg/kg/day in 3 doses × 3 days
	+		
	Pyrimethamine-sulfadoxine	3 tabs × 1, last day of Quinine SO$_4$	<1 yr.: ¼ tab 1–3 yrs: ½ tab 4–8 yrs: 1 tab 9–14 yrs: 2 tab
	or + Tetracycline	250 mg qid × 7 day[1]	20 mg/kg/day Q6 × 7d
	or + Clindamycin	900 mg tid × 3d	20–40 mg/kg/d Q8 × 3 days
Oral Alternatives	Mefloquine	1250 mg × 1	25 mg/kg once
	Halofantrine	500 mg Q6H × 3 doses	8 mg/kg Q6H × 3 doses
Parenteral	Quinidine gluconate	As before	As before
	Quinidine dihydrochloride	As before	As before

[1] Avoid in children <8 yrs old

Table 18.17. Prevention of Malaria Relapses: *P. vivax* **and** *P. ovale*

	Adult Dose	Pediatric Dose
Primaquine Phosphate	15 mg base (26.3 mg)/day × 14 days or 45 mg base (79 mg)/wk × 8 wk	0.3 mg base/kg/day × 14 days

Table 18.18. Malaria Chemoprophylaxis: Chloroquine-Sensitive Areas

Drug	Adult Dose	Pediatric Dose
Chloroquine Phosphate	300 mg base (500 mg salt) PO Q wk, beginning 1 week before and continuing 4 weeks after last exposure	5 mg/kg base (8.3 mg/kg salt) Q week, up to adult dose

Table 18.19.   Malaria Chemoprophylaxis: Chloroquine-Resistant Areas

Drug	Adult Dose	Pediatric Dose
Mefloquine	250 mg PO Q wk	15–19 kg: 1/4 tab Q wk 20–30 kg: 1/2 tab Q wk 31–45 kg: 3/4 tab Q wk >45 kg: 1 tab Q wk
Doxycycline	100 mg daily	>8 yrs old: 2 mg/kg/d QD up to adult dose
Chloroquine phosphate plus Fansidar	As before 3 tabs for presumptive diagnosis	As before Adjust as before
or Proquanil	200 mg QD during exposure and for 4 weeks thereafter	<2 yr: 50 mg QD 2–6 yr: 100 mg QD 7–10 yr: 150 mg QD >10 yr: 200 mg QD

Table 18.20.   Human Ehrlichiosis Versus Rocky Mountain Spotted Fever

	Ehrlichiosis	Rocky Mountain Spotted Fever
Vector	D. variabilis A. americanum	D. variabilis
Organism	E. chaffeensis	R. rickettsii
Seasonality	Late spring, summer	Same
Geography	Oklahoma, Arkansas, Missouri, Georgia, Carolinas	Same plus South Atlantic
Peak Age	Children	Adults
Symptoms	Fever, headache, myalgias	Same
Rash	<35%	>90%
Leukopenia	Common	Rare
Thrombopenia	Common	Occasional
Hepatitis	Common	Common
Therapy	Tetracycline, Doxycycline, Chloroquinine	Same

Table 18.21.   Typhoid Fever

Incubation period 5–21 days
Onset may be insidious
Fever, constitutional symptoms typical; diarrhea in only 20%–40%, neuropsychiatric symptoms in 10%
Signs include: relative bradycardia (50%), rose spots (30%), hepatosplenomegaly (50%)
Anemia and leukopenia common
Blood cultures positive in 50%–70%
Blood, bone marrow or stool cultures positive in over 90%
Serologic tests unreliable
Resistance to chloramphenicol, ampicillin, and trimethoprim-sulfamethoxazole increasingly common
Third generation cephalosporin or quinolone are drugs of choice

Table 18.22.   Clinical Syndromes of Parvo B19

Host	Disease
Children, adults	Erythema infectiosum
Adults, children	Arthritis
Chronic hemolysis	Aplastic crisis
Immunocompromised hosts	Chronic anemia
Fetuses	Hydrops fetalis, fetal death
Various hosts	Isolated reports of cardiac, neurologic, vasculitic disease

Temperature is 38.0°C and physical examination is normal. A chest radiograph discloses a left upper lobe cavitary lesion with surrounding infiltrate. A bronchoscopy is performed. For each potential finding shown in Figures 18.20, 18.21, and 18.22, choose which answer is incorrect about the associated disease.

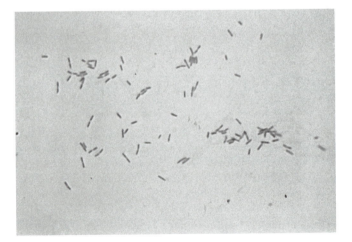

Figure 18.20.   Pathogen in Case 9. (See color plate)

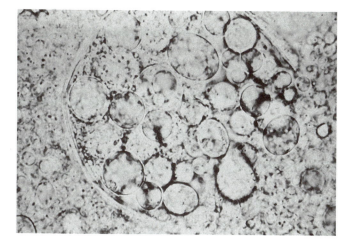

Figure 18.21.   Pathogen in Case 9. (See color plate)

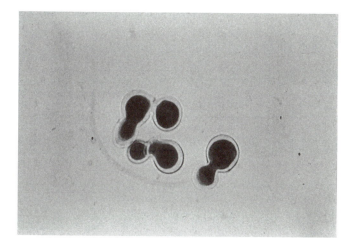

Figure 18.22.   Pathogen in Case 9. (See color plate)

QUESTIONS

9.1. Choose the incorrect statement for Figure 18.20.

  a. This disease is produced by *Pseudomonas pseudomallei.*
  b. Amoxicillin-clavulanate 1 g 3 times a day would be an appropriate antibiotic in this setting.
  c. This disease can produce acute, subacute and chronic illness and may mimic pulmonary tuberculosis.
  d. Trimethoprim-sulfamethoxazole 2 DS tabs 2 times a day would be appropriate therapy.
  e. Prolonged therapy for several months is indicated.

9.2. Choose the incorrect statement for Figure 18.21.
  a. Diabetics and those with compromised immunity are at higher risk of developing this form of the disease.
  b. Surgical removal of cavitary disease is indicated for persistent, severe or recurrent hemoptysis; rupture

into the pleura; or enlargement of the cavity despite therapy.
  c. The skin test will likely be positive and is helpful in confirming the diagnosis.
  d. Therapy is indicated.
  e. Triazole may be efficacious, and therapy should be continued at least 6 months beyond resolution of disease activity.

9.3. Choose the incorrect statement for Figure 18.22.
  a. A careful examination for subcutaneous nodules and skin lesions should be performed, since these are commonly seen.
  b. Genitourinary disease is common in males, and urine culture may yield the organism after prostatic massage.
  c. A complement fixation test may help confirm the diagnosis.
  d. Ketoconazole or itraconazole is appropriate for patients with mild to moderate pulmonary disease.
  e. Amphotericin B is indicated for those with life-threatening disease or central nervous system disease, and for those who are immunocompromised.

Discussion and Answer Explanations

This question examines the differential diagnosis of a subacute respiratory illness together with a cavitary infiltrate in a diabetic archaeologist with an extensive travel history.

9.1.
    Figure 18.20 shows gram-negative bacilli. The travel history to Thailand should suggest the diagnosis of melioidosis, produced by the gram-negative bacillus *Pseudomonas pseudomallei.* Melioidosis may produce a variety of syndromes, including subacute pulmonary disease mimicking tuberculosis, acute pneumonitis, septicemia, chronic localized suppurative infection involving a variety of organs (including the lung), and acute localized suppurative infection. In patients with localized disease who are not toxic, amoxicillin-clavulanate, trimethoprim-sulfamethoxazole, chloramphenicol or tetracycline have been shown to be effective. For septicemic patients, trimethoprim-sulfamethoxazole plus ceftazidime is recommended. Melioidosis is not endemic in the United States. This disease would have been acquired in Thailand, where fewer than 20% of strains are susceptible to trimethoprim-sulfamethoxazole. The incorrect statement is d, trimethoprim-sulfamethoxazole.

9.2.
    Figure 18.21 shows a spherule of *Coccidioides immitis.* This illness is consistent with acute pulmonary coccidioidomycosis evolving into chronic cavitary disease. Diabetics and immunocompromised hosts are at increased risk of developing chronic pulmonary disease. Diagnosis is based upon visualization of spherules in sputum, bronchoscopy specimens, or other tissue or fluid samples, as well as culture isolation. Serum IgM precipitins are present in 75% of individuals 1–3 weeks into the acute illness. Complement-fixing IgG antibodies are

present in 50%–90% of patients with symptomatic primary coccidioidomycosis by 3 months. Elevated complement fixation titers are characteristic of disseminated disease. Skin tests with coccidioidal antigens are positive in most individuals by 1 month, but do not in themselves confirm the diagnosis in the absence of serologic or microbiologic evidence of infection (thus answer choice c is incorrect). Therapy is indicated for those with severe primary infection, high complement fixation antibody titers, symptoms persisting beyond 6 weeks, pregnancy, progressive pulmonary disease, or significant underlying diseases (diabetes, immunosuppressed, asthma, etc).

Amphotericin B is indicated in patients with extrapulmonary disease, and the triazoles can be employed in those with non-meningeal disease. Prolonged therapy is indicated for at least 6 months beyond resolution of clinically apparent disease.

9.3.

Figure 18.22 shows the broad-based yeast form of *Blastomyces dermatitidis*. All of the statements above, except answer choice c, are true statements about North American blastomycosis. Complement fixation tests are neither sensitive nor specific for serologic diagnosis.

Hematology and Medical Oncology

Oncologic Emergencies

David J. Adelstein

Malignancies produce many special problems resulting from both local and metastatic involvement. This discussion will focus on several common structural problems associated with malignancy. The metabolic, hematologic, endocrinologic, and paraneoplastic complications of malignancy will not be addressed.

SUPERIOR VENA CAVA SYNDROME

The superior vena cava is a thin-walled, low-pressure, vascular structure rigidly confined in the mediastinum and surrounded by lymph nodes. It is readily occluded or thrombosed by any distortion of the normal architecture. Fortunately, an extensive collateral network exists, allowing for decompression and venous return. Patients with superior vena cava obstruction usually present with:

- Complaints of neck and facial swelling
- Dyspnea
- Cough

Physical examination is notable for:

- Distended jugular veins
- Prominent superficial venous collaterals
- Edema of the face, shoulders, and arms

The diagnosis is usually made at bedside. A chest radiograph may reveal mediastinal widening or a right hilar mass. Further delineation of the anatomic abnormality can be obtained with computerized tomography (CT) or contrast venography. Differential diagnosis includes:

- Congestive heart failure
- Pericardial tamponade/constriction
- Pulmonary hypertension

Although the clinical presentation of superior vena cava syndrome is often dramatic, death from superior vena cava obstruction alone is not well described. Overall, the prognosis of patients with this syndrome depends entirely on the prognosis of their underlying disease.

Symptomatic measures, such as diuretics and elevation of the head of the bed, are usually sufficient and will allow time for an accurate etiologic diagnosis.

The etiology of superior vena cava syndrome includes:

- Malignancy
  - Lung cancer
  - Small cell carcinoma
  - Lymphoma
- Thrombosis
- Fibrosis
- Substernal goiter
- Syphilitic aneurysm

Most patients with superior vena cava obstruction have malignancy. Lung cancer, particularly small-cell carcinoma, is the cause in most of these cases. Malignant lymphoma is also commonly responsible. Many patients are now developing superior vena cava syndrome as a result of the more frequent use of central venous catheters and from pacemaker wires.

An accurate etiologic diagnosis is crucial, and tissue confirmation will be required to verify the presence of malignancy. Despite fears to the contrary, invasive diagnostic procedures carry little additional risk in these patients. Although it was recommended in the past, radiotherapy before the histologic confirmation of malignancy is inappropriate and confusing. Several cancers commonly implicated are potentially curable with appropriate treatment, thus justifying an aggressive diagnostic and therapeutic approach.

Clinical improvement occurs in most patients, although this improvement may largely result from the development of adequate collateral circulation. Anticoagulation has not been used extensively, despite the presence of thrombosis in many patients. The treatment plan should, in general, be based on the tumor histology and disease extent, not just on the presence of superior vena cava obstruction. Radiation therapy is most appropriate in those patients with non-small-cell lung cancer or other neoplasms unresponsive to chemotherapy. Patients with small-cell lung cancer or lymphoma, however, can be treated primarily with chemotherapy, with the expectation of a rapid response.

Although clinical improvement can be expected in 70–95% of patients, radiologic evidence of recannulation and patency of the superior vena cava at autopsy are much less frequent. It is the development of adequate collateral circulation that allows for this symptomatic resolution, despite continued superior vena caval obstruction.

SPINAL CORD COMPRESSION

Spinal cord compression resulting from malignancy usually occurs in patients with incurable disease, and is responsible for serious morbidity but not mortality. Indeed, treatment success is usually measured by whether a patient remains ambulatory and continent. The diagnosis of spinal cord compression must be anticipated: once neurologic dysfunction develops, it is rarely reversible.

Most often, spinal cord compression arises from a metastasis that involves the vertebral body and extends to produce an anterior epidural cord compression. Hematologic neoplasms, however, such as lymphoma and myeloma, may produce epidural cord compression by direct extension from a paravertebral mass without bone involvement. The thoracic spine represents the most common site of cord compression, and the lesions are often multiple. The most common tumors responsible include:

- Lung cancer
- Breast cancer
- Prostate cancer
- Myeloma
- Lymphoma

The gastrointestinal tumors metastasize to bone less frequently, and are therefore relatively less likely to cause this syndrome.

The symptomatic hallmark of spinal cord compression is back pain. Although a common symptom, its presence in association with known spinal metastases mandates further evaluation. The presence of a symptomatic radiculopathy or myelopathy in a patient with malignancy is also a clear indication for further evaluation. Although epidural cord compression is the most common cause of myelopathic symptomatology in a patient with malignancy, the following etiologies must also be considered:

- Intradural or intramedullary tumor
- Carcinomatous meningitis

- Radiation myelopathy
- Paraneoplastic syndrome

Diagnostic options include:

- Neurologic examination
- Plain films
- Bone scan
- Complete myelogram
- CT
- Magnetic resonance imaging

The neurologic examination is often normal in these patients. If abnormal, however, it may be very useful in localizing the level of cord disease. Either a magnetic resonance imaging (MRI) scan or complete myelography is required for diagnosis (Fig. 19.1). While most patients with spinal metastases and a radiculopathy or myelopathy will have evidence of epidural lesions, cord compression will also be found in a significant number of patients with spinal metastases and back pain alone.

Once myelopathic signs have developed, the treatment of spinal cord compression is imperfect. Nonambulatory patients rarely recover the ability to ambulate. When diagnosed early, however, preservation of neurologic function is the rule. Radiation therapy has proven as effective as surgery in most cases, and corticosteroids appear to have a short-term benefit. Surgical decompression should be reserved for the following situations:

- Diagnosis is unclear
- Tumor involved is radioresistant
- Progression occurs during radiotherapy
- Recurrence develops after completion of radiotherapy
- Spinal instability

In general, the key to a successful outcome in this neurologic emergency is early diagnosis, although a patient's overall prognosis is more dependent on the natural history of the malignancy. While spinal cord compression from metastatic bronchogenic carcinoma has a very poor prognosis and a very limited survival, patients with lymphoma, myeloma, breast

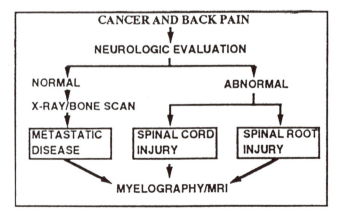

Figure 19.1. Cancer and back pain neurologic evaluation.

cancer, or hormone-sensitive prostate cancer are more readily treatable and may survive for protracted periods. The preservation of neurologic function is of obvious importance in this group of patients.

BONE METASTASES

Bone metastases may develop in up to 50% of patients with malignancy, and between 5–10% of patients with bone metastases will develop pathologic long bone fractures. The most frequent primary tumors metastasizing to bone are:

- Breast cancer
- Prostate cancer
- Lung cancer
- Multiple myeloma (almost invariably involves bone)
- Kidney cancer
- Malignancies of gastrointestinal origin

Marrow-containing bone, such as the vertebral bodies, pelvis, ribs, and femurs, are the most common sites of bone involvement.

Pain is the most common manifestation of bone metastases and is found in up to 75% of patients. Asymptomatic bone disease may be found during staging procedures, or at another unsuspected site during an evaluation for bone pain.

Radionuclide bone scans are very sensitive in the detection of bone metastases but are relatively nonspecific. Patients with purely lytic bone disease, however, as in multiple myeloma, may have normal bone scans. Plain radiographs, while considerably less sensitive, are quite specific. Radiographic abnormalities have been described as purely lytic (myeloma, kidney, thyroid), predominantly blastic (prostate), or mixed lytic and blastic (breast, lung). Computed tomography and MRI scans may be useful for specific indications, particularly in better defining disease of the spine and pelvis.

Biopsy confirmation of a bone metastasis may be required if the abnormality represents the first sign of tumor recurrence or in the presence of a single or otherwise unusual bone abnormality. Multiple bone lesions, in the setting of widely disseminated disease, do not require histologic verification.

The treatment of bone metastases is considered palliative. Treatment goals include relief of pain and preservation of function.

Surgery is usually required for adequate repair of a pathologic fracture and is often recommended for those patients with radiographic evidence of an impending fracture. The indications for prophylactic surgical intervention, particularly involving a weight-bearing bone (such as the femur), include a lytic bone lesion with a diameter of greater than 2–3 centimeters or with more than 50% cortical destruction.

Radiation therapy will relieve pain in up to 90% of patients and may prevent progression of bone destruction or even allow for healing. Its value is limited, however, in patients with widespread bone involvement.

Hormonal therapy in patients with breast and prostate cancer, and chemotherapy in patients with hematologic neoplasms and other chemotherapy-sensitive diseases, are often very effective in achieving temporary control.

In widespread disease with multiple sites of painful bone involvement, hemibody radiation or systemic administration of radioisotopes have been utilized.

MALIGNANT EFFUSIONS

PLEURAL EFFUSIONS

Malignant pleural effusions may develop in one of two ways:

- Direct deposition of tumor metastases on the pleural surface, with a resultant exudation of pleural fluid
- Tumor involvement of mediastinal lymph nodes producing lymphatic obstruction and pleural fluid accumulation

The second mechanism has been described in some patients with lymphoma and lung cancer.

The most common diagnoses in patients with malignant pleural effusions include:

- Breast cancer
- Lung cancer
- Lymphoma
- Ovarian cancer
- Adenocarcinoma of unknown primary site

Although the effusion may be asymptomatic in up to 25% of patients, the clinical presentation includes:

- Dyspnea
- Cough
- Chest pain

Patients may have a preexisting malignancy or may present with a malignant effusion as the first manifestation of disease. Accurate diagnostic confirmation and differentiation from a benign pleural effusion are of obvious prognostic and therapeutic importance.

A thoracentesis with pleural fluid cytology is often the easiest diagnostic maneuver. Biochemical analysis of the pleural fluid may be suggestive, but is nonspecific. A closed pleural biopsy may add to the diagnostic yield. Thoracoscopy has recently emerged as an excellent diagnostic tool for pleural effusions. If neoplastic, appropriate treatment is often possible at the time of thoracoscopy as well. It is important to recognize the diagnostic difficulty posed by patients with mesothelioma. Cytology and needle biopsy are often nondiagnostic or confusing in such patients, and thoracoscopy, or even thoracotomy, are usually needed.

Treatment strategies include:

- Thoracentesis
- Pleural sclerosis
- Pleurectomy
- Pleuroperitoneal shunt

- Radiation therapy
- Systemic chemotherapy/hormones

Patients with malignant pleural effusions are usually incurable, and their management strategy should be a palliative one. Only in those patients with lymphoma does the potential for disease-free, long term survival exist. Thoracentesis alone is of only temporary benefit unless effective systemic treatment is available, such as in lymphoma or breast cancer. Patients with non-small-cell lung cancer will usually require chest tube drainage and pleural sclerosis if permanent control of the effusion is to be expected. The intrapleural instillation of agents such as doxycycline, talc, quinacrine, bleomycin and various other chemotherapeutic agents, has been associated with a successful outcome in 70–85% of patients. Those patients with continued fluid reaccumulation despite pleural sclerosis may require pleurectomy or the use of a pleuroperitoneal shunt. Radiation therapy is unfortunately of limited value, except when administered to the mediastinum in patients with extensive mediastinal lymphoma.

MALIGNANT PERICARDIAL EFFUSIONS

Cardiac involvement by malignancy is often an asymptomatic autopsy finding, and has been reported in 10–15% of patients with malignancy. It is clinically important only if it results in cardiac dysfunction, the most common manifestation being pericardial tamponade. This complication is not usually the first manifestation of malignancy and has been reported most frequently in patients with:

- Lung cancer
- Breast cancer
- Leukemia/lymphoma
- Melanoma
- Sarcoma

The etiology may reflect either direct extension from mediastinal tumor (as in lymphoma and lung cancer) or hematogenous dissemination. Despite the dramatic presentation of patients with pericardial tamponade, several of the responsible malignancies are potentially curable, even when involving the heart. As such, an aggressive approach to diagnosis and management is imperative. It is also important that malignant pericarditis be distinguished from both the acute and chronic pericarditis occurring after radiation therapy and from the cardiomyopathy that can result from anthracycline use.

The presence of clinical signs or symptoms suggestive of pericarditis or pericardial tamponade mandates urgent evaluation. Diagnostic options include:

- Echocardiogram
- Pericardiocentesis
- Pericardial biopsy

Echocardiogram is usually diagnostic and can be followed rapidly by a diagnostic/therapeutic pericardiocentesis. Cytologic examination may be positive in 80% of patients with neoplastic involvement. In those patients with lymphoma, however, especially after radiation therapy, pericardial biopsy may be needed for diagnosis.

Treatment strategies include:

- Closed drainage/intrapericardial sclerosis
- Pleuro-pericardial window/subxiphoid pericardiotomy
- Pericardiectomy
- Radiation therapy
- Systemic chemotherapy

Multiple treatment options have been described. Closed pericardial drainage and intrapericardial sclerosis with doxycycline, talc, or any of several chemotherapeutic agents has proven remarkably effective and often represents the procedure of first choice. If unsuccessful, or if the diagnosis is uncertain, a surgical approach using either a pleuro-pericardial window or a subxiphoid pericardiotomy has been recommended. Patients with radiosensitive tumors can often be effectively treated with mediastinal radiation therapy. Systemic chemotherapy is appropriate in those patients with sensitive diseases.

MALIGNANT ASCITES

The development of ascites in any patient requires a vigorous evaluation for etiology. Ascites is considered malignant if it arises from the metastatic deposition of tumor on peritoneal surfaces with the resultant exudation of fluid. However, ascites may develop in a patient with malignancy from a number of other causes, including:

- Hepatic failure due to tumor replacement
- Chemotherapy toxicity
- Myocardial or pericardial disease
- Vena-caval/hepatic-venous obstruction
- Infection

The therapeutic approach taken will obviously depend on the etiology of the ascites.

In patients with ovarian or gastrointestinal cancer, malignant ascites may be either the presenting manifestation of the disease or an end-stage complication. In other tumors, such as breast cancer or lymphoma, malignant ascites usually reflects progression of an established malignancy.

Diagnostic evaluation includes paracentesis with cultures and cytologic analysis. Abdominal CT scan or ultrasound is often needed to define the presence of any hepatic abnormality. Rarely, an open peritoneal biopsy may be required.

Therapeutic options in patients with cytologically positive malignant ascites have been limited and relatively unsuccessful:

- Medical management
- Paracentesis
- Intracavitary radiocolloids
- Intraperitoneal chemotherapy

- Systemic chemotherapy
- Peritoneovenous shunts

Unlike patients with malignant pleural or pericardial effusions, palliation is difficult. Medical management, including diuresis and salt restriction, has provided only marginal benefit. Repeated paracentesis is an unsatisfactory solution; it is inconvenient for patients and results in significant protein loss and also the risk of infection. Intracavitary administration of radioactive colloids has been attempted in the past with mixed results. Intracavitary sclerosing agents, such as those used for pleural effusions, make little theoretical sense and are generally not beneficial.

There has been some interest in the use of intraperitoneal chemotherapy, particularly in neoplasms such as ovarian cancer. Drug penetration, however, is very limited, and in the presence of bulky, intraperitoneal tumor, this intervention has not been terribly successful. In patients with breast cancer, ovarian cancer, or lymphoma, systemic chemotherapy may be very effective and is indicated.

For those patients with refractory ascites unresponsive to other measures, peritoneovenous shunting has been moderately effective. Generally such patients have limited life expectancy and achieve significant palliative benefit from this procedure. While shunt occlusion is frequent, the development of carcinomatosis, or of a coagulopathy has not been common.

REVIEW EXERCISES

Case presentation:

A 55-year-old female smoker is seen in the Emergency Room complaining of several days of increasing facial fullness, orthopnea, and swelling in her neck and hands. Physical examination is notable for obvious facial swelling with conjunctival edema, jugular venous distention, and symmetric swelling of both upper extremities. There is fullness in both supraclavicular fossae, but no clear lymph node enlargement and the lungs are clear. The patient is tachycardic, but there is no gallop, murmur, or rub. There is no hepatomegaly, ascites, or pedal edema. Chest radiograph reveals a right hilar mass.

1. The patient is admitted to the hospital at midnight and you order:
   a. An emergency upper extremity venogram
   b. An emergency CT scan of the chest
   c. An emergency echocardiogram
   d. Diuretics and elevation of the head of the bed until the morning

2. The next morning, the patient feels better, although she remains quite edematous and cannot lie flat. You order the following test to determine the etiology of the patient's superior vena cava syndrome:
   a. CT scan of the chest
   b. Thyroid scan
   c. Serologic test for syphilis
   d. Upper extremity venogram
   e. All of the above

3. You are called by the radiologist that afternoon with the results of the chest CT scan. This study reveals a large right hilar and mediastinal mass, with evidence of compression of the superior vena cava. Your response is to:
   a. Expeditiously proceed to bronchoscopy or mediastinoscopy to establish the tissue diagnosis
   b. Recognize the risk of invasive diagnostic procedures in patients with superior vena cava syndrome and order sputum cytologies.
   c. Identify this as an incurable malignancy and refer the patient for urgent radiation therapy
   d. Identify this as an incurable malignancy and refer the patient for hospice care

4. The patient proves to have squamous cell carcinoma of the lung and receives a course of mediastinal radiation therapy. The patient does quite well, noting rapid improvement in both the symptoms and signs of her superior vena cava obstruction. A staging work-up subsequently demonstrates evidence of asymptomatic bone metastases in rib, femur, and multiple vertebral bodies. Because the patient is feeling well, she declines any discussion of chemotherapy and is followed in your office. Four months later the patient calls you with the complaint of a two week history of increasing midback pain. The patient is fully ambulatory, but the pain is causing difficulty sleeping. The patient specifically denies any weakness in the lower extremities, radicular pain, or incontinence. You would do the following:
   a. Suggest a course of Tylenol with codeine
   b. Order an elective bone scan
   c. Refer the patient for radiation therapy to the spine
   d. Order an MRI of the entire spine

5. Your patient has heard about MRI scans and does not want one. Angry that you suggested it, the patient cancels her appointment, and begins to take her husband's analgesics. Three days later you call the patient and are told by her husband that she has fallen several times and is now having difficulty walking. You insist that the patient come to the hospital and obtain an emergent MRI scan, which she then does. The MRI reveals extensive midthoracic vertebral body replacement by tumor, with evidence of spinal cord compression. Unfortunately, by the time the patient gets to the hospital, she is unable to walk and has had a single episode of urinary incontinence. You begin high dose corticosteroids, hospitalize the patient and recommend:
   a. Immediate neurosurgical intervention
   b. Intravenous morphine and hospice referral
   c. Immediate radiation therapy

6. The patient is treated with radiation therapy and, somewhat to your surprise, makes a significant recovery. The patient regains almost full leg strength and can ambulate with minimal assistance. Physical therapy has been started, but during treatment new discomfort is noted in the patient's right hip. You order plain films that reveal a large lytic lesion of the right hip with cortical involvement, but no fracture. In consideration of the patient's deteriorating medical condition, limited ambulatory ability and life expectancy, you recommend:
   a. Pain medication with continued physical therapy and partial weight bearing
   b. Pain medication, physical therapy with partial weight bearing, and radiation therapy to the affected hip
   c. Surgical stabilization of the right hip with pain medication and subsequent physical therapy

7. Your patient elects to not have surgery, but undergoes the radiation and physical therapy with some success. The patient has limited ambulation, but is managing at home with a walker. Over the next six weeks the patient gradually improves but then returns to see you in the office concerned about increasing exertional dyspnea. On exam the patient is afebrile, has a resting tachycardia, but has no facial swelling and no jugular venous distention. There is no pleural or pericardial rub, although diminished breath sounds are noted at the right base. Hepatomegaly, ascites, or pedal edema are not identified. Hemoglobin is 11.2 g/dl, and a chest radiograph reveals a new, large, right-pleural effusion. The most likely diagnosis is:
   a. Malignant pleural effusion
   b. Radiation-induced pleuritis
   c. Congestive heart failure
   d. Radiation-induced pericardial constriction
   e. Pulmonary embolus with infarction

8. In the office you perform a one-liter thoracentesis for slightly bloody fluid, which on analysis proves exudative. Cultures are negative, and cytologies are not diagnostic. The patient feels immediately better after the thoracentesis, but is back in the office three days later with increasing dyspnea and recurrence of this effusion. Your next step is to:
   a. Repeat the thoracentesis with cytology
   b. Repeat the thoracentesis with cytology and perform a closed pleural biopsy
   c. Refer the patient for thoracoscopy
   d. Refer the patient for chest tube drainage and pleural sclerosis

Answers

1. d
The clinical diagnosis of superior vena cava syndrome seems clear.

2. a

3. a

4. d

5. c

6. b or c
The best treatment option is unclear, although either radiation therapy (b) or surgery (c) seems reasonable.

7. a
8. d
In a patient this sick, the best answer is probably chest tube drainage and pleural sclerosis.

SUGGESTED READING

Adelstein, DJ. Managing three common oncologic emergencies. Cleve Clin J Med 1991;58:457–458.

Adelstein, DJ, Hines JD, Carter SG, Sacco D. Thromboembolic events in patients with malignant superior vena cava syndrome and the role of anticoagulation. Cancer 1988;62: 2258–2262.

Aelony Y, King R, Boutin C. Thoracoscopic talc poudrage pleurodesis for chronic recurrent pleural effusions. Ann Intern Med 1991;115:778–782.

Ahmann, FR. A reassessment of the clinical implications of the superior vena cava syndrome. J Clin Oncol 1984;2: 961–969.

Alcan KE, Zabetakis PM, Marino ND, et al. Management of acute cardiac tamponade by subxiphoid pericardiotomy. JAMA 1982;247:1143–1148.

Byrne TN. Spinal cord compression from epidural metastases. N Engl J Med 1992;327:614–619.

Gilbert RW, Kim JH, Posner JB. Epidural spinal cord compression from metastatic tumor: diagnosis and treatment. Ann Neurol 1978;3:40–51.

Glover DJ, Glick JH. Managing oncologic emergencies involving structural dysfunction. CA-A Cancer J Clin 1985;35: 238–251.

Gough IR, Balderson GA. Malignant Ascites. A comparison of peritoneovenous shunting and nonoperative management. Cancer 1993;71:2377–2382.

Hausheer FH, Yarbro JW. Diagnosis and treatment of malignant pleural effusion. Semin Oncol 1985;12:54–75.

Helms SR, Carlson MD. Cardiovascular emergencies. Semin Oncol 1989;16:463–470.

Lacy JH, Wieman TJ, Shively EH. Management of malignant ascites. Surg Gynecol Obstet 1984;159:397–412.

Maranzano, Latini P, Checcaglini F et al. Radiation therapy in metastatic spinal cord compression. Cancer 1991;67: 1311–1317.

Markman M. Common complications and emergencies associated with cancer and its therapy. Cleve Clin J Med 1994; 61:105–114.

Markman, M. Intraperitoneal chemotherapy. Semin Oncol 1991;18:248–254.

Nielsen OS, Munro AJ, Tannock IF. Bone metastases: pathophysiology and management policy. J Clin Oncol 1991;9: 509–524.

Okamoto H, Shinkai T, Yamakido M, Saijo N. Cardiac tamponade caused by primary lung cancer and the management of pericardial effusion. Cancer 1993;71:93–98.

Posner MR, Cohen GI, Skarin AT. Pericardial disease in patients with cancer: The differentiation of malignant from idiopathic and radiation-induced pericarditis. Am J Med 1981;71: 407–413.

Press OW, Livingston R. Management of malignant pericardial effusion and tamponade. JAMA 1987;257:1088–1092.

Rodichok LD, Harper GR, Ruckdeschel JC, et al. Early diagnosis of spinal epidural metastases. Am J Med 1981;70: 1181–1188.

Ruckeschel JC, Moores D. Lee JY, et al. Intrapleural therapy for malignant pleural effusions: A randomized comparison of bleomycin and tetracycline. Chest 1991;100:1528–1535.

Sahn MA. Malignant pleural effusions. Clin Chest Med 1985; 6:113–125.

Schraufnagel DE, Hill R, Leech JA, Para JAP. Superior vena caval obstruction–is it a medical emergency? Am J Med 1981; 70:1169–1174.

Spiess JL, Adelstein DJ, Hines JD. Multiple myeloma presenting with spinal cord compression. Oncol 1988;45:88–92.

Tong D, Gillick L, Hendrickson FR. The palliation of symptomatic osseous metastases. Final results of the study by the Radiation Therapy Oncology Group. Cancer 1982;50: 893–899.

Weissman DE. Glucocorticoid treatment for brain metastases and epidural spinal cord compression: a review. J Clin Oncol 1988;6:543–551.

Willson JKV, Masaryk TJ. Neurologic emergencies in the cancer patient. Semin Oncol 1989;16:490–503.

Gynecologic, Prostate, and Testicular Cancers

Maurie Markman

GYNECOLOGIC CANCERS

CANCER OF THE CERVIX

It is interesting that once, carcinoma of the cervix was the most common cause of cancer death in women. The mortality rate from this malignancy has decreased more than 50% over the past 30 years, largely due to the widespread use of the Papanicolaou (Pap) smear in routine gynecologic medicine, internal medicine, and family practice.

Several etiologic factors are associated with carcinoma of the cervix, including:

• Early initial sexual activity
• Multiple sexual partners
• Prior venereal infections

Recent experimental and epidemiologic data have provided strong evidence that infection with the human papilloma virus, particularly subtypes 16 and 18, is important in the pathogenesis of this malignancy. Recently, it has been shown that individuals with AIDS have a high risk for the development of carcinoma of the cervix.

The development of cervix cancer proceeds along a well-defined pathway, from dysplasia to carcinoma *in situ* (cytologic features of neoplasia, but without an invasion through the basement membrane), to invasive carcinoma. The Pap smear is 90–95% accurate in detecting early intraepithelial neoplastic changes. False negative smears can be observed in the presence of inflammation, necrosis, or hemorrhage, so that *all areas observed to be abnormal on visual inspection must be biopsied, regardless of the Pap smear findings.*

Standard treatment of carcinoma *in situ* of the cervix is surgery (total abdominal hysterectomy). Young women wanting to have children may be treated with cervical conization and extremely careful follow-up. More locally advanced cases of carcinoma of the cervix are treated with surgery, radiation

therapy, or a combination of the two modalities. Chemotherapy is used mainly in patients with far advanced and metastatic disease. Although responses are observed, they are generally of short duration (< 4–6 months).

The importance of finding cancerous changes as soon as possible in the natural history of this disease is highlighted by the fact that the long-term survival for individuals who are diagnosed as having carcinoma *in situ* is more than 98–99%. The survival rate for invasive carcinoma is much less. For patients with advanced cervix cancer, the chances for long-term disease-free survival are limited.

ENDOMETRIAL CANCER

Uterine cancer is the most common gynecologic cancer, causing approximately 9% of all malignancies in women. The incidence of the disease is about three times higher than cervix cancer. Suggested risk factors include:

• Age
• Late menopause
• Obesity
• Diabetes
• Hypertension

Unopposed exogenous estrogen use has been shown to increase the incidence of endometrial cancer. In contrast, the risk of the disease appears to be *decreased* by the administration of progesterone. Thus, the use of *combination estrogen and progesterone* may decrease the risk of endometrial cancer in women receiving this regimen.

The Pap smear identifies approximately 15–20% of women with endometrial carcinoma. In most patients, the diagnosis is made by more extensive evaluation of evacuated tissue following a fractional dilatation and curettage, or direct biopsy. The most common symptom of endometrial cancer is abnormal bleeding in postmenopausal woman.

Fortunately, endometrial cancer is generally diagnosed at an early stage, a point at which surgery with or without radiation therapy is curative. As with carcinoma of the cervix, chemotherapy plays only a limited role in the management of this disease.

OVARIAN CANCER

While ovarian cancer is less common than either cancer of the cervix or uterus, it causes more deaths each year in the United States than both of the other gynecologic malignancies combined. Because currently no effective screening test for detecting *early stage* disease exists, fewer than 10–20% of patients are diagnosed with localized disease. Recently, intensive research efforts have been undertaken at a number of centers to find a reliable screening test for ovarian cancer. These have focused on vaginal ultrasound and circulating tumor antigens (e.g., CA-125). While screening may be employed with patients who have an increased risk for the development of ovarian cancer (i.e., strong family history), such a strategy should not be considered standard clinical practice in most clinical settings.

While many etiologic factors have been proposed for the development of ovarian cancer (including disordered endocrine function), none have been strongly associated with the disease. Recently, it has been noted that approximately 2% of all women with ovarian cancer will have a *strong* family history of the malignancy, suggesting the importance of genetic factors. In the rare circumstance where a woman has two first-degree relatives with ovarian cancer, she will have as much as a 50% chance of developing the malignancy during her lifetime. Unfortunately, the ultimate risk to women with one first-degree relative with ovarian cancer is currently unknown.

Ovarian cancer tends to remain largely confined to the peritoneal cavity for most of its natural history. However, the disease can be quite widespread throughout the abdomen at the time of diagnosis.

A recently completed randomized controlled trial has revealed that the combination of cisplatin plus Taxol results in a superior objective response rate, progression-free survival, and overall survival compared to the previous standard treatment regimen of cisplatin and cyclophosphamide. Thus, the majority of ovarian cancer researchers currently consider a platinum agent (cisplatin or carboplatin) plus taxol to be the ''standard therapy'' for women with advanced ovarian cancer. In patients with persistent or recurrent disease following initial chemotherapy, salvage chemotherapy regimens can be employed, but the impact of such treatment on ultimate survival is uncertain.

In the unusual situation where ovarian cancer is found to be confined to one ovary (Stage 1), surgery without adjuvant chemotherapy can be a reasonable treatment option. Long-term survival in Stage 1 ovarian cancer is more than 80–90%.

For patients with more advanced disease, 80–90% will experience objective evidence of a response to chemotherapy, and 50% will be found to have no clinical evidence of disease at the completion of therapy. Unfortunately, the disease ultimately recurs in most of these patients. Long-term disease-free survival for patients with advanced ovarian cancer is only 15–30%.

PROSTATE CANCER

Prostate cancer is the leading cause of cancer in American males. Approximately 1 in 11 males will have this malignancy during their lifetime. Prostate cancer is the third leading cause of cancer mortality in men.

The digital rectal exam is extremely important in screening for prostate cancer as 70% of tumors are located peripherally and can potentially be felt on physical examination. Prostate cancer can present as a single nodule, or may be multifocal in origin.

Local presenting signs of prostate cancer include:

- Palpable nodule (50% or more of the cases)
- Dysuria
- Cystitis or prostatitis
- Frequency of urination
- Urinary retention
- Decreased urinary stream

Signs of advanced prostate cancer include:

- Pain (particularly bone pain)
- Uremia (due to ureteral obstruction and subsequent renal failure)
- Weight loss

Distant metastatic disease in prostate cancer involves the bone in more than 90% of cases. An uncommon, but difficult, complication of advanced prostate cancer is systemic bleeding due to the development of disseminated intravascular coagulation.

Subclinical prostate cancer is even more common than clinical disease with 15–45% of autopsies in males without any known history of cancer during their life demonstrating the malignancy. This observation raises the important question of the clinical relevance of finding asymptomatic prostate cancer on screening tests in older males. Overall, prostate cancer is a slowly growing malignancy. Thus, simply finding microscopic cancer in an elderly individual should not necessarily be an indication to treat.

One of the more controversial areas in oncology is the issue of the role of screening for the presence of prostate cancer. Considering screening for this disease is reasonable as prostate cancer is a common malignancy, the prostate is accessible on examination, and a serum diagnostic test is available (prostate-specific antigen, PSA).

As previously noted, the digital rectal examination is the most sensitive and cost-effective method of diagnosing prostate cancer and should be part of a regular physical examination in adult males.

The American Cancer Society recommends the following for prostate cancer screening:

- Men over the age of 40 should have a digital rectal exam as part of their regular physical checkup.
- A digital rectal exam and a PSA test should be obtained once a year for men 50 years of age and older.
- Men in high-risk groups, such as African Americans or those with a strong family history of prostate cancer, may start having these tests at a younger age.

It should be noted that an enlarged prostate gland from benign prostatic hypertrophy (BPH) can raise PSA levels two-to-three times higher than normal. In addition, infected or inflamed prostate glands can cause a two-to-three times increase in the PSA level.

Any suspicious area (e.g., hard nodule) felt on digital rectal examination requires biopsy. Techniques for biopsy include transurethral resection of the prostate (TURP) and fine-needle aspiration.

Treatment of local prostate cancer includes several options:

- Surgery (radical prostatectomy)
- External-beam radiation therapy
- Interstitial implantation of radioactive seeds

The patient must participate in the discussion and decision as to the optimal treatment strategy for the management of local disease.

The major treatment of advanced prostate cancer is hormonal manipulation, including chemical androgen blockade or orchiectomy. Approximately 40–80% of patients with advanced prostate cancer will respond to hormonal therapy with rapid decreases in bone pain being common. Responses to hormone therapy generally last 9–18 months.

TESTICULAR CANCER

Testicular cancers are the most common solid tumors in males aged 15–35. Approximately 5,500 new cases occur in the United States each year. This is a highly curable group of malignancies, with a >99% survival rate for local/regional disease and 80 + % survival rate in advanced stage disease. Several factors have contributed to the overall success of therapy in testicular cancer, including:

- Accurate surgical staging

- Availability of highly sensitive tumor markers for the malignancy (beta-HCG, alpha-fetoprotein)
- Highly effective chemotherapy (cisplatin-based)

The majority of testicular neoplasms (more than 95%) are of germinal origin. Testicular cancers are divided into two general types: seminoma (classic, anaplastic, and spermatocytic subtypes), and nonseminomas (teratoma, embryonal cell carcinoma, endodermal sinus tumor, choriocarcinoma).

Pure seminoma is the most common testicular neoplasm, accounting for 40% of the total cancers of this organ. Nonseminomas may have several cellular elements present (i.e., mixed tumor type). Teratomas can be mature, immature, or contain elements of carcinoma or sarcoma.

Treatment of testicular tumors is directed at the element with the worst prognosis. For example, a patient with a Stage 1 seminoma (low risk of relapse, excellent prognosis) who is found to have a small portion of endodermal sinus tumor (high risk of relapse) would receive intensive chemotherapy.

The most common presentation of a germ-cell tumor is the finding of an asymptomatic (painless) firm testicular nodule or mass. The abnormal testis should be compared to the contralateral testis to determine differences in size, shape and consistency.

Testicular pain is uncommon and is more likely the result of acute epididymitis. However, after treatment for a presumed infection, the testicle should be examined to be certain it has returned to normal size. Ultrasound can be helpful in the diagnosis of suspected testicular cancer. A hypoechogenic mass within the testicle is highly suspicious for cancer.

When a testicular cancer is suspected, both the testis and spermatic cord should be removed through the inguinal canal (radical orchiectomy). It is important to remember that a transscrotal biopsy should not be performed due to the risk of scrotal contamination by tumor, which can complicate further management options. Following surgical removal of the testicular mass, patients with pure seminomas may be treated with local radiation only (seminomas are exquisitely sensitive to radiation) and should receive cisplatin-based chemotherapy if there is evidence of metastatic disease.

Patients with nonseminomas that appear to be confined to the testis may be observed (and treated with chemotherapy with any evidence of tumor marker elevation) or can receive several courses of cisplatin-based adjuvant chemotherapy.

Any patient with a nonseminoma germ cell tumor with evidence of tumor marker elevation or persistent masses following surgery will received cisplatin-based (cisplatin, etoposide plus bleomycin) chemotherapy.

REVIEW EXERCISES

Gynecologic Cancers

1. A 68–year-old woman is seen in your office for the first time. Which statement concerning the risk of development of cervix cancer in this patient and the role of screening in this population is correct:
   a. The risk of developing cervix cancer is low and screening is not necessary.
   b. The risk of developing cervix cancer is high and the patient should be screened yearly at least until age 80.
   c. The risk of developing cervix cancer is related to the patient's prior screening history.
   d. The risk of developing cervix cancer is high, but screening is of no value in the elderly.
   e. None of the above

2. Which of the following statements concerning cancer of the cervix is incorrect:
   a. Having a large number of sexual partners protects against the development of cervix cancer.
   b. Carcinoma-in-situ is essentially 100% curable.
   c. Cervix cancer has been associated with AIDS.
   d. Treatment of metastatic cervix cancer is designed principally to palliate symptoms rather than result in long-term disease-free control.
   e. None of the above

3. A 54–year-old patient is started on estrogens because of significant postmenopausal symptoms. Due to the association between estrogens and endometrial cancer, this patient should:
   a. Undergo a hysterectomy
   b. Undergo an endometrial biopsy at least every 3–4 months while on estrogen therapy
   c. Never be given progesterone
   d. Undergo a hysterectomy and bilateral oophorectomy
   e. None of the above

4. A 42–year-old patient asks about screening for ovarian cancer. She has no symptoms suggestive of the disease and has a normal physical examination. You should:
   a. Ask about her family history of ovarian and breast cancers.
   b. Strongly recommend yearly screening until at least age 70.
   c. Recommend a CA-125 blood test and vaginal ultrasound to be performed within the next 3–5 days.
   d. Inform the patient screening has been proven to be of no value in this disease.
   e. None of the above

5. A 53–year-old patient is found to have advanced ovarian cancer. She asks for your recommendation regarding treatment. Which one of the following would be inappropriate statements concerning possible treatment options:
   a. Cisplatin or carboplatin plus taxol is the standard chemotherapy treatment strategy in this clinical setting.
   b. Assuming the patient can tolerate intensive therapy, very high dose chemotherapy with bone marrow transplantation has been proven to result in the best overall outcome in this disease.
   c. Surgical tumor removal prior to starting chemotherapy is attempted in most patients with advanced ovarian cancer.
   d. Approximately 80% of patients with advanced ovarian cancer achieve at least temporary improvement of symptoms following chemotherapy.
   e. None of the above

6. A 19–year-old patient has an advanced germ-cell tumor of the ovary, which has spread to the omentum. All gross disease is removed at the time of surgery. Which one of the following statements concerning this tumor is correct:
   a. With cisplatin-based chemotherapy this individuals' chances of survival are between 10–20%.
   b. The administration of chemotherapy will almost certainly result in sterility.
   c. Compared to epithelial ovarian cancers, germ cell tumors of the ovary have a superior survival.
   d. Dysgerminomas have the worst prognosis among the germ cell tumors of the ovary.
   e. None of the above

Prostate Cancer

7. An 87–year-old male presents to you with a 9-month history of urinary frequency. The patient has no other major medical problems and specifically denies bone pain. Physical examination is remarkable only for a nontender prostatic mass. The serum PSA is 69 ng/ml. The remainder of the laboratory evaluation is unremarkable except for a modest increase in alkaline phosphatase (two times normal). A transurethral resection is able to completely relieve the patient's symptoms. Unfortunately, pathology review reveals the patient to have a Gleason's grade 3/10 prostate cancer. A CT scan of the pelvis is unremarkable. A bone scan reveals several "hot spots" in the lumbar spine and iliac bone. At this point in time how would you manage this patient.

a. Bilateral orchiectomy
b. Radiotherapy to the pelvis
c. Interstitial implants
d. "Total chemical androgen blockage"
e. Observation with treatment when symptoms develop

8. A 55-year-old asymptomatic African-American male undergoes a routine physical examination, his first in more than 10 years. On prostate exam you discover a diffusely enlarged gland, but one area does feel "firmer" than other areas of the gland. The PSA is 10.8 ng/ml. At this point you would:
a. Repeat the exam and PSA in 2 months
b. Recommend a transrectal prostate biopsy.
c. Obtain a pelvic CT scan
d. Obtain a bone scan
e. Initiate hormonal therapy

9. A 62-year-old male presents to his physician with diffuse back pain (requiring narcotic analgesia), and a 1-month history of urinary hesitancy. Diagnostic evaluation and biopsy confirms the presence of prostate cancer. A bone scan reveals diffuse bony involvement with the malignancy. The PSA is 75 ng/ml. At this point you would recommend:
a. Comfort measures only (including narcotic analgesia)
b. Radiation therapy to areas of bony involvement
c. Hormonal therapy (orchiectomy or androgen blockade)

d. Cytotoxic chemotherapy
e. Continuous intravenous infusion of morphine

Testicular Cancer

10. A 22-year-old male is found to have a right testicular mass. A right-sided radical orchiectomy is performed which reveals a pure seminoma. Treatment should include:
a. Combination cisplatin-based chemotherapy
b. Observation only
c. Radiation therapy
d. High-dose chemotherapy with bone marrow transplantation
e. A left radical orchiectomy

11. A 27-year-old male is found to have a localized nonseminomatous germ cell tumor at surgery. The patient elects to be observed (no chemotherapy administered). Three months later the beta-HCG increases to three times normal. At this time you would:
a. Initiate cisplatin-based combination chemotherapy
b. Continue to observe the patient until the B-HCG is > 5 times normal
c. Suggest an exploratory laparotomy
d. Initiate chemotherapy only if the alpha-fetoprotein is also elevated
e. Recommend a high dose chemotherapy regimen

Answers

1. c
Women who have undergone appropriate Pap smear testing throughout their life do *not* require continued testing beyond the age of 70. However, if testing has not been performed regularly, there remains a significant risk of cervix cancer even beyond age 70. Such individuals should continue to undergo Pap smear testing for cervix cancer.

2. a
One of the major risk factors for developing cervix cancer is a large number of sexual partners. This fact provides strong supportive evidence for the sexual transmission of an infectious agent which has an important role in the development of this malignancy.

3. e
A specific recommendation for the follow-up of women receiving estrogen replacement as a result of postmenopausal symptoms is not possible based on currently available data. However, there is no convincing evidence that surgery or routine endometrial biopsy is required in women receiving treatment with this agent.

4. a
There is currently no evidence that screening for ovarian cancer reduces mortality from this malignancy. However, for women with a *strong* family history of ovarian and breast cancer, it certainly can be argued that screening at least has the potential for detecting the disease at an earlier point in time where therapy may be more effective.

5. b
The standard treatment for advanced ovarian cancer is surgical debulking, followed by a cisplatin or carboplatin, plus paclitaxel chemotherapy regimen. There is *no* evidence that "high-dose therapy" does anything except increase the toxicity of treatment.

6. c
The overall prognosis of germ cell tumors of the ovary is excellent, certainly compared to epithelial ovarian cancer.

7. e
In this clinical setting, treatment is palliative in nature. The patient's symptoms have been relieved with the surgery. Thus, there remains little reason to initiate treatment at the present time. With evidence of disease progression, treat-

ment can certainly be started. The specific treatment will depend on the nature of the symptoms (e.g., radiation therapy for localized painful bony lesions).

8. b

This individual has an abnormal prostate gland on physical examination, with an elevated PSA test. A biopsy is indicated.

9. c

This patient is quite symptomatic with diffuse body involvement with cancer. Hormonal therapy has a > 50% chance of improving symptoms and should be initiated.

10. c

Seminomas are extremely sensitive to radiation. In this clinical setting the remaining testicle can be shielded from the radiation. Symptoms from treatment are very limited and the prognosis is excellent.

11. a

The elevated B-HCG is essentially diagnostic of recurrent disease in this clinical setting. Standard cisplatin-based chemotherapy should be initiated. The anticipated outcome is excellent.

SUGGESTED READING

GYNECOLOGIC CANCERS

Cannistra SA: Cancer of the ovary. N Engl J Med 1993;329:1550.

Cannistra SA, Niloff JM: Cancer of the uterine cervix. N Engl J Med 1996;334:1030.

Koss LG: The Papanicolaou test for cervical cancer detection: a triumph and a tragedy. JAMA 1989;261:737.

Markman M, Hoskins W, eds: Ovarian Cancer. New York: Raven Press, 1992.

PROSTATE CANCER

Albertsen PC, et al: Long-term survival among men with conservatively treated prostate cancer. JAMA 1995;274:626.

Catalona WJ, et al: Measurement of prostate-specific antigen in serum as a screening test for prostate cancer. N Engl J Med 1991;324:1146.

Gittes RF: Carcinoma of the prostate. N Engl J Med 1991;324:236.

Johansson J-E, et al: High 10-year survival rate in patients with early, untreated prostatic cancer. JAMA 1992;267:2191.

Krahn MD, et al: Screening for prostate cancer; a decision analytic view. JAMA 1994;272:773.

Kramer BA, et al: Prostate cancer screening: What we know and what we need to know. Ann Intern Med 1993;119:914.

Litwin MS, et al: Quality–of-life outcomes in men treated for prostate cancer. JAMA 1995;273:129.

TESTICULAR CANCER

Einhorn LH: Treatment of testicular cancer: a new and improved model. J Clin Oncol 1990; 8:1777.

Lange PH, et al: Serum alpha fetoprotein and human chorionic gonadotropin in the diagnosis and management of nonseminomatous germ cell testicular cancer. N Engl J Med 1976;295:1237.

Williams, SD, et al: Treatment of disseminated germ cell tumors with cisplatin, bleomycin and either vinblastine or etoposide. N Engl J Med 1987;317:1435.

21

Leukemia

Brad Pohlman

A rare malignancy, leukemia accounts for only 2% of new cancer cases and 4% of cancer deaths. The American Cancer Society estimates that approximately 28,300 new cases of leukemia will be diagnosed within the United States in 1997:

- 9,200 cases of acute myelogenous leukemia (AML)
- 7,400 cases of chronic lymphocytic leukemia (CLL)
- 4,300 cases of chronic myelogenous leukemia (CML)
- 3,000 cases of acute lymphoblastic leukemia (ALL)
- 4,400 other leukemias

Most leukemia (except ALL) occurs in adults.

ACUTE LEUKEMIA

ETIOLOGY OF ACUTE LEUKEMIA

Acute myelogenous leukemia accounts for 90% of acute leukemia in adults. The risk of AML increases with age and 50% of patients are older than 60. In contrast, the maximal incidence of ALL occurs in early childhood, although a second, more gradual rise in frequency also occurs later in life.

Several factors have been associated with the development of acute leukemia:

- Both chronic benzene exposure and extreme radiation exposure are known to cause acute leukemia.
- Human T-cell lymphotropic virus type I (HTLV-1) has been implicated in the development of one form of adult T-cell leukemia. This virus is endemic to parts of Japan, the Caribbean, and Africa, but is also present in the United States. It is spread from mother to fetus, through sexual contact, and by blood products. Less than 1% of those infected with the virus develop leukemia, generally many years after exposure. In the United States, blood is routinely screened for antibodies to HTLV-1.
- For some individuals, a genetic predisposition may

exist. For example, the identical twin of a patient with childhood leukemia has a 20% chance of also developing leukemia. Rarely, multiple members of a family have developed an identical form of leukemia.

- Patients with Down's syndrome (trisomy 21), autosomal recessive disorders associated with chromosomal instability (e.g. Bloom's syndrome and Fanconi's anemia), and other congenital disorders (e.g. Bruton's X-linked agammaglobulinemia, hereditary ataxia-telangiectasia, severe combined immune deficiency, and Wiscott-Aldrich syndrome) are predisposed to acute leukemia.
- Li-Fraumeni cancer family syndrome is an autosomal-dominant trait, which in some families is due to mutations of the P53 gene on chromosome 17p and is associated with the development of leukemia and also multiple other solid tumors.
- AML may evolve from myelodysplastic syndromes and myeloproliferative disorders.
- Patients who receive chemotherapy for treatment of certain malignancies (e.g. Hodgkin's disease, lymphoma, myeloma, and ovarian and breast carcinoma) may develop AML several years later. Alkylating agents, (e.g. chlorambucil, melphalan, and nitrogen mustard), and epipodophyllotoxins, (e.g. etoposide), have been implicated in the pathogenesis of these secondary malignancies.

Although the cytogenetic and molecular abnormalities for many leukemias have been explained, the details of leukemogenesis remain poorly understood (Table 21.1).

PATHOPHYSIOLOGY OF ACUTE LEUKEMIA

Acute leukemia results from the proliferation of hematopoietic cells that have lost their capacity to differentiate. The malig-

Table 21.1. Cytogenetic and Molecular Abnormalities in Leukemia

Cytogenetics	Genes	Consequence	Leukemia
t(8;21)	ETO and AML1	fusion gene	AML
inv(16)	CBFβ and MYH11	fusion gene	AMML w/ eos
t(15;17)	PML and RARα	fusion gene	APL
t(9;22)	BCR and ABL	fusion gene	Ph′ ALL
t(8;14)	IGH and cMYC	overexpression	L3 ALL

AML = acute myelogenous leukemia
AMML w/ eos = acute myelomonocytic leukemia with eosinophils
APL = acute promyelocytic leukemia
Ph′ ALL = Philadelphia chromosome positive acute lymphoblastic leukemia
ALL = acute lymphoblastic leukemia

nant clone expands at the expense of normal hematopoiesis, and the manifestations of the disease result from the proliferation of leukemic cells and the ensuing pancytopenia.

CLINICAL PRESENTATION OF ACUTE LEUKEMIA

Clinical manifestations of acute leukemia result from: decreased marrow function and invasion of organs by leukemic blasts.

Signs and symptoms may be owing to:

- Anemia (e.g. fatigue, pallor, headache, angina, and CHF)
- Thrombocytopenia (e.g. petechiae, ecchymosis, mucosal bleeding, and frank hemorrhage)
- Neutropenia

Up to one-third of patients have significant or life-threatening infections at diagnosis. Infiltration of organs with enlargement of lymph nodes, liver, and spleen is more common in ALL (50%) than in AML.

Leukemic meningitis occurs in less than 5% of patients at diagnosis but is a frequent site of relapse, particularly in ALL. Acute monocytic and myelomonocytic leukemia are the most likely to have extramedullary involvement, for example gum infiltration. Acute promyelocytic leukemia is often associated with a coagulopathy.

DIAGNOSIS OF ACUTE LEUKEMIA

Acute leukemia is defined by the presence of more than 30% blasts in the bone marrow. The peripheral blood smear usually has obvious blasts; however, the lack of blasts does not exclude the diagnosis. The distinction between AML and ALL is important because of differences in clinical behavior, prognosis, and treatment. Historically, leukemias have been classi-

fied by the French/American/British (FAB) system, which is based on morphology and cytochemistry (Table 21.2).

More recently, surface antigen expression (by flow cytometry) has been used to determine phenotype (Table 21.3). In addition, cytogenetics and molecular studies (as noted above) have been used to distinguish different subtypes of leukemia.

TREATMENT AND COMPLICATIONS OF ACUTE LEUKEMIA

At diagnosis, some situations require urgent management. Patients with fever and neutropenia need a thorough evaluation (including blood cultures), in an attempt to identify a source of infection, and should be started on broad-spectrum antibiotics in earnest. Bleeding associated with thrombocytopenia requires platelet transfusions. Bleeding associated with disseminated intravascular coagulation (DIC) requires fresh frozen plasma (to replace coagulation factors) and cryoprecipitate (to replace fibrinogen), and may be improved with low-dose heparin. Leukostasis associated with a blast count greater than 100–200,000 may respond quickly to leukopheresis and/or hydroxyurea.

Once the patient has been stabilized, specific anti-leukemic therapy should begin: usually within 24–48 hours of diagnosis. The treatment of ALL consists of:

- Induction chemotherapy
- Post-remission (consolidation and maintenance) chemotherapy
- Central nervous system (CNS) prophylaxis

Hematopoietic growth factors administered immediately after myelosuppressive induction chemotherapy for ALL have been shown to decrease the period of neutropenia, the number of infections, and mortality, especially in elderly patients.

The treatment of AML consists of:

- Induction chemotherapy
- Post-remission (consolidation) chemotherapy.

Table 21.2. FAB Classification of Acute Leukemia

FAB	Subtype	Morphology	Cytochemistry
L1		Small lymphoblasts	TdT +, PAS +
L2		Large lymphoblasts	TdT +, PAS +
L3	Burkitt's	Basophilic lymphoblasts	TdT −, PAS −
M0		Undifferentiated	
M1		Immature myeloblasts	MP + −
M2		Mature myeloblasts, Auer rods	MP + +
M3	APL	Hypergranular promyelocytes multiple Auer rods	MP + + +
M4	AMML	≥20% monocytes	MP + +, NSE + +
M5	AMoL	Monoblasts	MP − +, NSE + + +
M6	AEL	Erythroblasts	
M7	AMKL	Dysplastic megakaryocytes myelofibrosis	

FAB = French/American/British
MP = myeloperoxidase
APL = acute promyelocytic leukemia
AMML = acute myelomonocytic leukemia
NSE = Non-specific esterase
AMoL = acute monocytic leukemia
AEL = acute erythroblastic leukemia
AMKL = acute megakaryocytic leukemia

Table 21.3. Pathologic Criteria to Distinguish ALL and AML

Characteristic	ALL	AML
Morphology		
Cytoplasmic granules	−	+
Auer rods	−	+
Cytochemistry		
Myeloperoxidase	−	+
TdT	+	−
Surface antigens		
CD 3	T cell	
CD 19	B cell	
CD 13		+
CD 33		+

More intensive consolidation regimens have been shown to improve overall survival, especially among younger patients. In AML, CNS prophylaxis or maintenance chemotherapy does not improve overall survival. In randomized studies, the use of hematopoietic growth factors following chemotherapy for AML has reduced the period of severe neutropenia; however, the effect on severe infections, antibiotic usage, duration of hospitalization, remission rates, and overall survival has been inconsistent. Importantly, these growth factors have not appeared to increase the risk of leukemia recurrence. Nevertheless, their routine use is not considered standard therapy at this time.

Acute promyelocytic leukemia (APL) is unique because daily oral all-*trans*-retinoic acid (ATRA) leads to remissions in approximately 90% of patients. While this treatment may avoid marrow ablation and the complications of cytotoxic therapy (i.e., neutropenia, thrombocytopenia, and DIC), remissions are short and subsequent postremission chemotherapy is necessary. Among patients with APL, a randomized study has demonstrated that inclusion of ATRA for induction or maintenance improves survival.

Specialized supportive care for patients receiving intensive chemotherapy is essential:

- Neutropenic fever should be treated with broad-spectrum antibiotics until recovery of neutrophils.
- In 50% of patients, bacterial infections (most commonly *Staphylococci* species and gram negative bacilli) are documented.
- The risk of fungal infections increases with the duration of neutropenia, and therefore, persistent fever should be treated empirically with Amphotericin B. These patients are also at risk for *Pneumocystis carinii* pneumonia, cytomegalovirus, and Herpes simplex infections.
- The risks of serious spontaneous bleeding increases rapidly as the platelet count falls below 10,000. Platelet transfusions for platelet counts less than 10,000–20,000 are therefore warranted. These compromised patients are at risk for transfusion-associated graft-versus-host disease due to the transfer of lymphocytes in blood products; these patients, especially bone marrow transplant (BMT) candidates, should receive irradiated blood products. Patients may acquire cytomegalovirus (CMV) through blood transfusions, and therefore

previously unexposed patients, especially BMT candidates, should receive CMV-seronegative or leukocyte-reduced blood products.

- Refractory thrombocytopenia due to alloimmunization may occur in approximately 20% of patients with acute leukemia; the incidence may be decreased by transfusing only leukocyte-reduced blood products.

PROGNOSIS OF ACUTE LEUKEMIA

Among adults with ALL, 50–85% will achieve a complete remission; however, only 20–35% remain disease free at 5 years. A worse prognosis is associated with:

- WBC greater than 30,000–50,000
- Increasing age over age 10–30
- CNS involvement
- Lymphadenopathy
- Hepatosplenomegaly
- Time to remission greater than 4 weeks
- Cytogenetics t(9;22) or t(4;11)

Fifty to eighty percent of patients with AML achieve a complete remission, but only 15–50% are cured. Elderly patients and those with secondary leukemia or a preceding myelodysplastic syndrome or myeloproliferative syndrome have a poor prognosis. Cytogenetic analysis provides an important predictor of outcome in AML:

- Patients with t(8;21) or inversion 16 have a good prognosis
- Patients with t(15;17)—characteristic of acute promyelocytic leukemia—or a normal karyotype have an intermediate prognosis
- Patients with any other cytogenetic abnormalities have a poor prognosis.

These three prognostic groups are increasingly used to determine management.

Less than 50% of patients with relapsed acute leukemia achieve a second remission. Few, if any, of these patients are cured with conventional chemotherapy. In contrast, BMT may cure 10–40% of patients who fail to achieve an initial remission or who relapse after initial complete remission. Patients in first complete remission—but at high risk for relapse—who receive a BMT have a 40–60% five year disease-free survival.

MYELODYSPLASTIC SYNDROME

ETIOLOGY OF MYELODYSPLASTIC SYNDROME

The myelodysplastic syndrome (MDS) is a group of heterogeneous clonal neoplasms of pluripotent stem cells characterized by dysfunctional and/or deficient hematopoietic cell production with a variable tendency to evolve to acute leukemia. The MDS usually occurs in elderly patients, although 10–20% of

patients are younger than 50 years old. As with AML, prior chemotherapy is a predisposing factor.

CLINICAL PRESENTATION AND DIAGNOSIS OF MYELODYSPLASTIC SYNDROME

Patients with MDS may be:

- Asymptomatic
- Symptomatic
  - Anemia
  - Thrombocytopenia
  - Neutropenia

The MDS diagnosis is based on the characteristic blood and bone marrow findings. Morphologic abnormalities seen in the peripheral blood include:

- Macrocytic and poikilocytic red cells
- Agranular, hypogranular, hypersegmented and hyposegmented neutrophils
- Giant, hypogranulated platelets

Even though these patients have anemia, bicytopenia, or pancytopenia, the bone marrow is typically hypercellular and by definition has less than 30% blasts. Cytogenetic abnormalities (often involving chromosomes 5, 7, or 8) are identified in 40–70% of patients and may help to confirm the diagnosis.

TREATMENT OF MYELODYSPLASTIC SYNDROME

Since most of these patients are elderly, treatment is mainly supportive, such as transfusions and antibiotics. For patients with neutropenia and recurrent infections, use of hematopoietic growth factors may be helpful, at least temporarily. This therapy does not appear to accelerate the progression to overt leukemia.

Treatment with conventional AML-type chemotherapy is often associated with a poor outcome because it is especially toxic in elderly patients, infections are common, and remissions, if achieved, are short. For some young patients, aggressive treatment may be appropriate despite these limitations. Bone-marrow transplantation for young patients offers the only curative treatment. Some studies have suggested that patients receiving transplants early in the disease have a better outcome.

PROGNOSIS OF MYELODYSPLASTIC SYNDROME

The FAB classification, which is based in part on the percentage of blasts in the peripheral blood and bone marrow, has prognostic significance (Table 21.4). Approximately one half of patients progress to acute myeloid leukemia; however, many patients die from infection or bleeding.

Table 21.4. FAB Classification of Myelodysplastic Syndromes

Type	Blasts in BM %	Blasts in Blood %	Progression to AML %	Death from Hemorrhage or Infection (%)	Median Survival (mo)
RA	< 5	≤ 1	11–20	27–57	17–65
RARS	< 5	≤ 1	4–20	10–43	14–76
CMML	≤ 20	< 5	13–40	13–20	5–22
RAEB	5–20	< 5	28–56	37–88	10–14
RAEB-T	21–30 or	≥ 5	47–60	36–83	3–11

RA = refractory anemia
RARS = refractory anemia with ringed sideroblasts
CMML = chronic myelomonocytic leukemia
RAEB = refractory anemia with excess blasts
RAEB-T = refractory anemia with excess blasts in transformation

CHRONIC LYMPHOCYTIC LEUKEMIA

ETIOLOGY OF CHRONIC LYMPHOCYTIC LEUKEMIA

Chronic lymphocytic leukemia is a B-cell malignancy characterized by the abnormal proliferation of mature lymphocytes. Patients are usually more than sixty years old at diagnosis. No specific etiologies have been identified, but familial clustering is more common than with other leukemias.

CLINICAL PRESENTATION OF CHRONIC LYMPHOCYTIC LEUKEMIA

Typical clinical presentation of CLL includes:

- Asymptomatic (a minority of patients)
- Symptomatic
  - Fatigue
  - Lethargy
  - Loss of appetite
  - Weight loss
  - Decreased exercise tolerance

Lymphadenopathy is present in 67% and splenomegaly in 40% of patients. The absolute lymphocyte count (by definition greater than 5,000) is usually 40,000–150,000. Despite even a very high WBC, leukostasis is uncommon. A small minority of patients have normochromic normocytic anemia and/or thrombocytopenia at diagnosis. The peripheral smear shows mature-appearing lymphocytes and characteristic smudge cells.

DIAGNOSIS OF CHRONIC LYMPHOCYTIC LEUKEMIA

The presentation, absolute lymphocytosis, and peripheral smear are usually adequate to make the diagnosis. Flow cytometric analysis of the peripheral blood is useful in confirming the diagnosis. These B-cells co-express pan B-cell antigens, (e.g., CD 19, CD 20, and CD 23) and CD 5, a pan T-cell antigen. For patients with mild lymphocytosis, evidence of monoclonality (e.g., kappa/lambda light-chain restriction or immunoglobulin gene rearrangement) may distinguish a benign process from a malignant process. Bone marrow aspirate and biopsy are generally not required to make the diagnosis of CLL.

TREATMENT OF CHRONIC LYMPHOCYTIC LEUKEMIA

Treatment of early-stage disease has not been shown to prolong survival; therefore, patients with early-stage disease should only be treated to control symptoms. In contrast, patients with advanced-stage disease may benefit from early treatment. Other indications to initiate treatment include:

- Progressive organ and/or nodal enlargement
- Anemia
- Thrombocytopenia
- Neutropenia with infection
- Lymphocyte doubling time of less than 6–12 months

Autoimmune hemolytic anemia and immune thrombocytopenia (without other indications for treatment) usually respond to steroids alone.

Although aggressive chemotherapy regimens may result in higher remission rates than single-agent chemotherapy, they have not been shown to improve survival. Fludarabine, a nucleoside analog, produces approximately a 50% response in patients refractory to alkylating agents and an approximately 80% response in previously untreated patients. Unfortunately, these excellent response rates have not yet been shown to improve survival.

COMPLICATIONS OF CHRONIC LYMPHOCYTIC LEUKEMIA

Potential complications of CLL include:

- Infections due to neutropenia, hypogamma globulinemia, and T-cell deficiency or dysfunction

Table 21.5.   Staging Systems for Chronic Lymphocytic Leukemia

Clinical Features	Rai	Modified Rai	Binet	Survival (yrs)
Lymphocytosis only	0	Low risk		> 10
Enlargement of < 3 areas*			A	> 10
Enlarged lymph nodes	I			8
Enlarged liver and/or spleen	II			6
Enlarged lymph nodes + spleen + liver		Intermediate risk		7
Enlargement of ≥ 3 areas*			B	5
Hgb < 11	III			2.5
Plts < 100K	IV			2.5
Hgb < 11 and Plts < 100K		High risk		1.5
Hgb < 10 and/or Plts < 100K			C	2.5

* The three areas include cervical, axillary, and inguinal lymph nodes, spleen, and liver.

- Autoimmune hemolytic anemia
- Immune thrombocytopenic purpura
- Richter's phenomenon (the development of diffuse large cell lymphoma)

PROGNOSIS OF CHRONIC LYMPHOCYTIC LEUKEMIA

The prognosis of patients with CLL is predicted by the Rai, modified Rai, and Binet staging systems (Table 21.5).

Patients with early-stage disease have a median survival of greater than 8–10 years, while those with advanced-stage disease—that is anemia and/or thrombocytopenia not due to immune mechanisms—have a median survival of 1.5–2.5 years. Other prognostic features include:

- Diffuse pattern of bone marrow infiltration
- Abnormal karyotype
- Advanced age
- Male sex
- Lymphocyte doubling time of less than one year

CHRONIC MYELOGENOUS LEUKEMIA

ETIOLOGY AND PATHOPHYSIOLOGY OF CHRONIC MYELOGENOUS LEUKEMIA

CML is a clonal myeloproliferative disorder of a primitive hematopoietic stem cell that has a peak incidence in the fifth decade of life. Exposure to radiation increases the risk; survivors of the atomic-bomb explosions in Japan had an increased incidence of CML that peaked 5–10 years after exposure.

The hallmark of CML is the Philadelphia chromosome, which is present in 90–95% of patients. This chromosomal abnormality is the result of a reciprocal translocation, t(9; 22)(q34;1), in which the *ABL* oncogene from chromosome 9 is juxtaposed with the *BCR* gene on chromosome 22. This translocation results in the transcription of a chimeric *bcr/abl*

mRNA, which is translated into a fusion protein, p210, with enhanced tyrosine kinase activity. These molecular events occur in a pluripotent stem cell such that erythrocytes, monocytes, macrophages, less commonly B-lymphocytes, and rarely T-lymphocytes, are involved in the malignant transformation. On the other hand, bone marrow stroma cells, such as fibroblasts, are not involved. These molecular events lead to expansion of the malignant clone, the clinical manifestations of chronic phase CML, the progressive accumulation of secondary genetic alterations, and eventually, the development of the accelerated phase and terminal blast crisis.

Five to ten percent of patients with the characteristic manifestations of CML lack the Philadelphia chromosome. In these patients, techniques such as Southern analysis, Northern analysis or the polymerase chain reaction (PCR), Western blot or other assays may detect *BCR* gene rearrangement, *bcr/abl* mRNA, and/or p210, respectively. Patients in whom these molecular alterations are present (even though the Philadelphia chromosome *per se* may be lacking) have a course and prognosis identical to patients with Philadelphia–chromosome-positive CML and should be treated the same.

CLINICAL PRESENTATION OF CHRONIC MYELOGENOUS LEUKEMIA

The typical clinical presentation of patients with CML in chronic phase includes:

- Asymptomatic (incidental diagnosis)
- Symptomatic
  - Anemia
  - Splenomegaly
  - Increased metabolic rate

Less commonly, leukostasis may lead to dyspnea or neurologic changes, thrombocytopenia or platelet dysfunction may lead to bleeding, and thrombocytosis may lead to thrombosis. Infections are infrequent since neutrophil function is relatively normal. Splenomegaly is usually present, but hepatomegaly and lymphadenopathy are uncommon. The white count ranges from 10,000–1,000,000 and consists predominantly of myeloid cells with a characteristic left shift extending to blasts. Basophilia are present and sometimes eosinophilia. Mild anemia may be present but platelets are often elevated. The bone marrow is characteristically hypercellular with a myeloid/erythroid ratio of 15:1–20:1 (normal 2:1-3:1). The leukocyte alkaline phosphatase (LAP) score is usually very low.

The progression to accelerated phase is characterized by:

- B symptoms (i.e., fever, night sweats, and weight loss)
- Progressive leukocytosis
- Basophilia
- Splenomegaly uncontrolled by previously adequate therapy

The bone marrow may show dysplastic changes, increased blasts, increased basophils, myelofibrosis, and additional chromosomal abnormalities (e.g., duplication of the Philadelphia chromosome, trisomy 8, and isochromosome 17).

DIAGNOSIS OF CHRONIC MYELOGENOUS LEUKEMIA

CML can usually be differentiated from a leukemoid reaction. Characteristics of a leukemoid reaction include:

- The clinical history suggests an etiology
- Neutrophils contain toxic granulation and Döhle bodies
- Basophilia is absent
- The LAP score is normal or increased
- The Philadelphia chromosome and/or its molecular equivalents are lacking

The diagnosis of CML must be confirmed by the identification of the characteristic cytogenetic and/or molecular abnormalities described above.

TREATMENT OF CHRONIC MYELOGENOUS LEUKEMIA

Chronic-phase CML is treated with hydroxyurea or interferon α. While hydroxyurea may effectively alleviate symptoms, control leukocytosis, and diminish spleen size, it does not alter the natural history of the disease. In contrast, interferon, which is increasingly used for initial treatment and equally effective in producing hematologic remissions, may also induce cytogenetic remissions. Some studies have suggested that it is more effective than hydroxyurea and may prolong survival. The only proven curative treatment for CML is allogeneic BMT; unfortunately, most patients are not candidates for this therapy because of their age or lack of an acceptable marrow donor.

Patients who relapse following allogeneic BMT may be salvaged with reinfusion of donor lymphocytes. This ''adoptive immunotherapy'' is proof of the previously hypothesized graft versus leukemia effect.

PROGNOSIS OF CHRONIC MYELOGENOUS LEUKEMIA

Among newly diagnosed patients in chronic phase who do not receive a BMT, the median survival is approximately 5 years. The median survival after evolution to the accelerated phase is 6-18 months. Subsequent transformation to blast crisis—essentially acute leukemia (myeloid in 75% and lymphoid in 25%)—is frequently a terminal event.

Patients in chronic phase, accelerated phase, or blast crisis who receive marrow from a matched sibling donor have a 5-year disease-free survival of approximately 50%, 30%, and 15%, respectively. A recent analysis of data from the National Marrow Donor Program shows that patients in chronic phase, accelerated phase, or blast crisis who receive marrow from an unrelated donor have a 3-year disease-free survival of 40%, 19%, and 1%, respectively. The best candidates for unrelated donor BMT (i.e., younger than 35, HLA-matched donor, first chronic phase, and BMT less than 1 year from diagnosis), have a 3-year disease-free survival of 61%.

HAIRY-CELL LEUKEMIA

Hairy cell leukemia is an uncommon, chronic, B-cell malignancy with unique features. Four to six hundred cases are diagnosed in the United States each year, with a median age of 50 and a 4:1 male predominance. Symptoms due to pancytopenia and/or splenomegaly are often present. The leukocyte differential and peripheral smear demonstrate a relative or absolute lymphocytosis with characteristic hairy cells. The bone-marrow biopsy is usually hypercellular with a diffuse infiltrate of hairy cells and increased reticulin, collagen, and fibrosis. Although immunoglobulin levels are normal, antibody-dependent cellular cytotoxicity and cellular immunity are impaired. These immune defects, in association with neutropenia and a characteristic monocytopenia, often lead to unusual infections (e.g. mycobacterial and fungal infections).

Splenectomy improves pancytopenia in two-thirds of patients. Although this procedure temporarily removes the site of platelet and white cell sequestration, it does not prevent continued malignant lymphocyte proliferation, marrow infiltration, or eventual relapse. Patients treated with interferon obtain a partial remission but relapse within one to two years following the discontinuation of therapy. More recently, nucleoside analogs have demonstrated promising results. A single cycle of 2-chlorodeoxyadenosine (2-CDA) induces prolonged complete and partial remissions in 80% and 20% of patients, respectively.

REVIEW EXERCISES

CASE 1

A 35–year-old female clerical worker from Cleveland presents to the Emergency Room with 24 hours of fever and chills. In addition, she complains of increasing fatigue, dyspnea on exertion, and spontaneous bruising.

Her past medical history is significant for choriocarcinoma, which was diagnosed at age 33. She was treated with cyclophosphamide, actinomycin, methotrexate, vincristine, cisplatin, and etoposide (VP-16). She obtained a complete remission and has had no evidence of recurrence. She has received no blood transfusions. She has no family history of cancer and she has four siblings that are in excellent health.

Physical examination: ill-appearing woman; T 39.5°C, BP 80/40, P 140, RR 22; petechiae on soft palate; no lymphadenopathy; clear lungs; tachycardia, I/VI SEM; no abdominal mass or hepatosplenomegaly; scattered petechiae, especially on lower extremities.

Labs: Hemoglobin 8.7, Platelets 14K, WBC 3,000 with 2% neutrophils, 45% lymphocytes, and 53% blasts; PT INR 1.1, PTT 23, fibrinogen 345.

Peripheral blood smear: normochromic, normocytic anemia; thrombocytopenia; rare neutrophils, many blasts.

1. Which pathologic characteristic is least likely to characterize this woman's blasts?
   a. Cytoplasmic granules and Auer rods
   b. Myeloperoxidase-containing granules
   c. CD 33 immunophenotype
   d. t(8;14)

2. Which one of the following interventions is not indicated for the woman?
   a. Fluid resuscitation
   b. Blood cultures followed by broad spectrum IV antibiotics
   c. Transfusion of red blood cells and platelets
   d. Transfusion of fresh frozen plasma and cryoprecipitate

3. What is the long-term prognosis of this woman if she receives standard chemotherapy?
   a. Good
   b. Poor

CASE 2

A 25–year-old male city hall employee is referred to you for evaluation of anemia. He was told he was anemic two years earlier. He complains of dyspnea on exertion for several months. Recently, he has noted frequent nasal congestion and occasional epistaxis. He denies fevers, night sweats,

weight loss, or bruising. His past medical history is remarkable for severe acne since age 22. He denies any hospitalizations or history of transfusions.

Physical examination: Well developed male in no acute distress; T36.8 P60 126/74 RR 16; skin of face, shoulders, upper trunk, and proximal arms are covered with severe pustular acne; no palpable lymphadenopathy or splenomegaly; otherwise normal.

Labs: Hemoglobin 8.3, platelets 32K, WBC 1,100 with 28% neutrophils, 53% lymphocytes, 13% monocytes, and 1% eosinophils.

Peripheral smear: Pancytopenia, macrocytic erythrocytes, bilobed neutrophils, and hypogranular platelets.

Bone marrow aspirate and biopsy: Hypercellular with 21% blasts

4. This man will inevitably die from acute myelogenous leukemia?
   a. True
   b. False

CASE 3

A 29–year-old woman presents to your office for a PAP smear. She is asymptomatic and has a normal physical examination except for a moderately enlarged spleen.

Lab results: Hemoglobin 11.9, platelets 671K, WBC 227,000 with 55% neutrophils, 7% metamyelocytes, 19% myelocytes, 2% promyelocytes, 2% blasts, 1% eosinophils, 7% basophils, and 3% lymphocytes.

You confidently make the diagnosis of CML but are surprised when the bone marrow chromosome analysis shows only 46XX.

5. The patient's next clinic visit should include which one of the following:
   a. Tell the patient she does not have CML
   b. Discontinue hydroxyurea
   c. Cancel plans for a bone marrow transplantation
   d. Order *BCR/ABL* gene studies to confirm the suspected diagnosis

CASE 4

A 51–year-old man is referred to your office with new, asymptomatic cervical adenopathy. Physical examination is remarkable only for several < 1 cm cervical lymph nodes.

Lab results: Hemoglobin 14.5, platelets 235K, and WBC 35,000 with 10% neutrophils, 87% lymphocytes, 2% monocytes, and 1% eosinophils.

Peripheral blood smear: Increased number of mature-appearing lymphocytes

6. Which one of the following is most characteristic of this patient's leukemia cells?

	Cell surface antigen	Immunoglobulin gene rearrangement
a.	CD 5+, CD 19+	present
b.	CD 5−, CD 19+	absent
c.	CD 5+, CD 19−	present

7. What is the most appropriate management of the patient at this time?
   a. Observation
   b. Prednisone
   c. Chlorambucil
   d. Fludarabine

Answers

1. d

This woman most likely has secondary AML as a result of prior chemotherapy, in particular, etoposide (VP-16). The blasts in AML are characterized morphologically by cytoplasmic granules and Auer rods, cytochemically by myeloperoxidase-staining, and flow cytometrically by CD 33 positivity. The t(8;14) is characteristic of ALL (L3) and Burkitt's lymphoma—not AML.

2. d

This patient has life-threatening sepsis and needs fluid resuscitation, a quick evaluation including blood cultures, and administration of empiric, broad-spectrum IV antibiotics. She is anemic and thrombocytopenic with spontaneous bruising and is at risk for life-threatening hemorrhage, and therefore, she needs transfusion with red blood cells and platelets. Her coagulation tests are normal; based on the information provided, she does not need fresh frozen plasma or cryoprecipitate.

3. Poor

Patients with secondary AML have a poor prognosis, and in fact, are incurable with conventional chemotherapy.

4. True

This patient has refractory anemia with excess blasts in transformation (RAEB-T), which is a subtype of myelodysplastic syndrome. Various studies have shown that up to 83% of these patients will die a median of 3–11 months after diagnosis from complications of pancytopenia, such as infection and/or hemorrhage. Only 47–60% of these patients will progress to AML (by definition > 30% blasts in the bone marrow).

5. d

This patient's signs, symptoms, CBC, and bone marrow are characteristic of CML. Five to ten percent of patients presumed to have CML have a normal karyotype and no Philadelphia chromosome. Among these patients with "Philadelphia–chromosome-negative CML," approximately one half will have the molecular abnormalities characteristic of the Philadelphia chromosome, such as BCR gene rearrangement, bcr/abl message, or p210. Patients with these molecular equivalents of the Philadelphia chromosome should be treated the same as patients with Philadelphia–chromosome-positive CML, such as hydroxyurea, interferon, or BMT.

6. a

This patient has a history, physical examination, CBC, and peripheral smear characteristic of CLL. The leukemic B cells in these patients usually express CD 19 (a B-cell antigen) and CD 5 (a T-cell antigen) and are monoclonal (i.e., an immunoglobulin gene rearrangement is present). Normal B cells are CD 19 + but CD 5 − and are polyclonal (i.e., immunoglobulin gene rearrangement is absent). Normal T cells are CD 5 + but CD 19 − and are polyclonal (i.e., immunoglobulin gene rearrangement is absent).

7. a

According to the Rai, modified Rai, or Binet staging systems, this patient is stage I, intermediate risk, or stage A, respectively. Treatment of early stage disease has not been shown to improve survival; therefore, this patient should be observed.

SUGGESTED READING

Bloomfield CD, Herzig GP, Caligiuri MA, eds: Acute Leukemia. Semin Oncol 1997;24:1–151.

Cheson BD, Bennett JM, Grever M, et al: National Cancer Institute-sponsored working group guidelines for chronic lymphocytic leukemia: Revised guidelines for diagnosis and treatment. Blood 1996;87:4990–4997.

Copelan EA, McGuire EA: The biology and treatment of acute lymphoblastic leukemia in adults. Blood 1995;85:1151–1168.

Grinani F, Fagioloi M, Alcalay M, et al: Acute promyelocytic leukemia: From genetics to treatment. Blood 1994;83:10–25.

Kantarjian HM, Deisseroth A, Kurzrock R, et al: Chronic myelogenous leukemia: A concise update. Blood 1993;82: 691–703.

Kantarjian HM, O'Brien S, Anderlini P, Talpaz M: Treatment of chronic myelogenous leukemia: Current status and investigational options. Blood 1996;87:3069–3081.

Koeffler HP, ed: Myelodysplastic syndromes. Hematol Oncol Clin North Am 1992;6:485–728.

O'Brien S, del Giglio A, Keating M: Advances in the biology and treatment of B-cell chronic lymphocytic leukemia. Blood 1995;85:307–318.

Preti A, Kantarjian HM: Management of adult acute lymphocytic leukemia: present issues and key challenges. J Clin Oncol 1994;12:1312–1322.

Rozman C, Montserrat E: Chronic lymphocytic leukemia. New Engl J Med 1995;333:1052-1057.

Saven A, Piro L: Newer purine analogues for the treatment of hairy-cell leukemia. New Engl J Med 1994;330:691–697.

Warrell RP, deThé H, Wang Z, Degos L: Acute promyelocytic leukemia. New Engl J Med 1993;329:177–189.

22

Platelet and Clotting Disorders

Steven W. Andresen

DISSEMINATED INTRAVASCULAR COAGULATION

Disseminated intravascular coagulation (DIC) is a potentially lethal coagulopathy associated with a variety of medical and surgical disease states. Whatever the inciting event, when coagulation mechanisms are activated, intravascular fibrin is produced, small vessel thrombosis occurs, and ischemic organ damage results. A compensatory fibrinolysis develops, and with the exhaustion of coagulation factors and thrombocytopenia, a hemorrhagic diathesis may occur.

Conditions associated with the development of DIC include obstetrical problems such as abruptio placenta and retained dead fetus, and sepsis, malignancy, tissue injury typically produced by burns, and connective tissue diseases.

CLINICAL PRESENTATION OF DISSEMINATED INTRAVASCULAR COAGULATION

The clinical manifestations of DIC are most frequently thrombotic, although hemorrhagic events may predominate. Most patients with hemorrhage bleed from several different sites. In addition, from the ongoing microvascular thrombosis that occurs, ischemic injury to the lung, kidney, liver, and heart may ensue.

DIAGNOSIS OF DISSEMINATED INTRAVASCULAR COAGULATION

The prothrombin time (PT) and the activated partial thromboplastin time (APTT) are usually prolonged in patients with DIC. The fibrinogen is diminished, and if the patient is bleed-ing associated with DIC it is usually less than 100. Fibrin degradation products (FDP) are present. The most accurate fibrin degradation product is the D-dimer. The D-dimer is released only when thrombin is activated to produce fibrin from fibrinogen, and secondarily this fibrin is degraded by plasmin. Monoclonal antibodies to this fused region have been developed that do not cross-react with fibrinogen or other fibrin-degradation products. Antithrombin III is also consumed in the process of disseminated intravascular coagulation, and thus its levels are also diminished. The thrombin time is prolonged by the presence of fibrin degradation products. Platelets are consumed during intravascular coagulation, and thrombocytopenia, often severe, results. In addition, red cells that encounter strands of fibrin laid across the vessel lumen are sheared, and microangiopathic hemolysis results.

Following is a summary of the laboratory results seen in DIC:

CBC	Anemia, thrombopenia
Smear	Microangiopathic hemolysis
PT	↑
PTT	↑
Fibrinogen	↓
Thrombin time	↑
d-Dimer	↑
Antithrombin III	↓

Disseminated intravascular coagulation may exist in a chronic form, such that the increased consumption of clotting factors is compensated for by increased production. The usual screening laboratory tests may be normal, although the fibrinogen is often slightly depressed. Hemorrhage may occur when the coagulation mechanisms are stressed either by trauma or some other stress such as a surgical procedure. In this chronic form of DIC, thrombotic complications may predominate.

TREATMENT OF DISSEMINATED INTRAVASCULAR COAGULATION

The cornerstone of therapy for DIC is identification and amelioration of the precipitating cause. Should the inciting event be rapidly reversible, supportive therapy may suffice. If bleeding should occur while this goal is pursued, transfusion therapy with cryoprecipitate as a source of fibrinogen, fresh frozen plasma as a source of clotting factors, and platelets to correct the resulting thrombopenia may be effective. If the pathologic process that produced this coagulopathy is not readily reversible, or serious refractory bleeding occurs, anticoagulation with heparin may be considered. Heparin in this situation interrupts the consumption of coagulation factors and fibrinogen and may cease clinical bleeding. The goal of therapy is to allow the fibrinogen to increase to a level above 100–150 mg/dl. Central nervous system bleeding or severe thrombocytopenia contraindicates the use of heparin. Continued replacement with cryoprecipitate and fresh frozen plasma is indicated. Antithrombin III levels have been used to monitor the effectiveness of anticoagulant therapy in this situation. Antithrombin III is commercially available and has been used in the treatment of DIC.

In patients who have thrombotic events associated with chronic DIC, particularly in association with a malignancy, anticoagulation with warfarin is often unsuccessful in preventing further thrombotic events. In this situation, the use of subcutaneous heparin should be considered.

Deficiency of vitamin K-dependent factors may be associated with bleeding and, in the laboratory, result in a prolonged PT and PTT. The fibrinogen and other laboratory abnormalities associated with DIC are usually normal. Any form of liver disease may decrease the production of these factors. With vitamin K deficiency, a lack of carbamylation of vitamin K-dependent factors leads to the formation of nonfunctioning molecules. Vitamin K deficiency may develop in patients on prolonged antibiotic therapy, which may sterilize the gut and cause malnutrition and malabsorption. Oral anticoagulants interfere with the in vivo utilization of vitamin K and produce similar coagulation abnormalities. The distinction between decreased production of K-dependent factors by the liver and vitamin K deficiency may not be easy. Both have a prolonged PT and PTT. Both have decreased vitamin K-dependent factors, and both may improve with vitamin K administration.

THROMBOTIC THROMBOCYTOPENIC PURPURA

Thrombotic thrombocytopenic purpura (TTP) is a multisystem disorder produced by a microvascular thrombotic phenomenon. It is included in a broader category of disease states termed thrombotic microangiopathies, which besides TTP includes the hemolytic uremic syndrome.

PATHOPHYSIOLOGY OF THROMBOTIC THROMBOCYTOPENIC PURPURA

Pathophysiologically, platelet fibrin thrombi involve multiple organ systems. These thrombi produce ischemic necrosis and, the resultant clinical manifestation neurologic symptoms. The origin of the platelet agglutination that begins this process is unclear. Plasma from patients with TTP has demonstrated an increase in platelet-aggregating activity, which may be related to a platelet aggregating factor (PAF). In addition, unusually large von Willebrand multimers have also been described and in some patients are involved in the process. It is possible that the plasma in some patients with TTP lacks an inhibitor to either one of these molecules.

DIAGNOSIS OF THROMBOTIC THROMBOCYTOPENIC PURPURA

The characteristic clinical triad of TTP is microangiopathic hemolytic anemia, thrombocytopenia, and fluctuating neurologic symptoms. Renal disease and fever complete the classic pentad. Neurologic signs and symptoms are varied, ranging from mild headache to dense coma. Renal manifestations are also varied and may include minor changes in sediment to minor elevations in renal function tests. The degree of renal dysfunction is generally not as severe as that seen in the hemolytic uremic syndrome.

As the anemia is microangiopathic in nature, schistocytes are present in the peripheral blood, and the lactate dehydrogenase (LDH) level is elevated. In addition, the indirect bilirubin and reticulocyte counts are also increased. Thrombocytopenia is universally present and often severe. In the absence of a secondary problem, sepsis or respiratory failure, laboratory manifestations of disseminated intravascular coagulation are extremely unusual.

Disease entities that most commonly make the differential diagnosis of TTP problematic include the vasculitides and critically ill patients with sepsis. When the diagnosis of TTP cannot be excluded, treatment for this disorder should be instituted as it is a potentially reversible disorder.

TREATMENT OF THROMBOTIC THROMBOCYTOPENIC PURPURA

The treatment of choice in patients with TTP is plasma exchange, generally by the technique of plasmapheresis. This therapy should be undertaken despite the severity of symptoms and the overall status of the patient. It should be continued until a remission occurs or the patient expires. Replacement must be with fresh frozen plasma. If the equipment necessary for pheresis is unavailable, therapy with large volumes of fresh frozen plasma may be instituted until arrangements can be made for plasmapheresis. In some hands, the use of vincristine has led to increased response rates. Anecdotal reports of therapeutic benefit have been seen with high doses of gammaglobulin, corticosteroids, antiplatelet agents, splenectomy, and the infusion of cryosupernatant. The goal of therapy is normalization of the neurologic signs and symptoms, a decrease in LDH level which signifies improvement in hemolysis, and a platelet count increase to >100,000. If evidence of a therapeutic response is not seen in 3–5 days, the use of other measures, high doses of gammaglobulin or corticosteroids, should be considered. When other modalities are selected, they should be used in conjunction with the continued daily plasmapheresis. Aggressive supportive measures are often required, and a period in the intensive care unit setting is frequently needed. Platelet transfusions should be avoided because they may aggravate the underlying pathologic process.

PROGNOSIS OF THROMBOTIC THROMBOCYTOPENIC PURPURA

In the past, the mortality rate of TTP approached 90%. The response rate to modern therapy is now approximately 60%. As more and more patients survive, a distinct entity known as chronic relapsing TTP has been described. Hematologic abnormalities predominate in these relapsing situations. Patients who relapse are treated similarly, and often prophylactic measures of periodic pheresis or plasma infusion are necessary. Splenectomy may be helpful in this setting.

AUTOIMMUNE THROMBOCYTOPENIC PURPURA

Acute immune thrombocytopenic purpura (ITP) occurs most frequently in children but may occur in adults. This syndrome often follows a viral illness, and spontaneous remissions in children are commonly seen.

PATHOPHYSIOLOGY AND DIAGNOSIS OF ITP

Chronic ITP is generally a disease of adults. Females are affected more frequently than males, with peak incidences between the ages of 20 and 40. In most adults with chronic ITP, platelet-associated IgG antibodies may be found. These antibodies may be directed against specific membrane glycoproteins such as GPIIIa, IIb, or Ib. Because of these glycoprotein specificities, a superimposed qualitative platelet abnormality may be present. Platelet-associated IgG is not specific for chronic ITP, but may be found in other entities: solid tumors and lymphoproliferative disorders. Other disorders associated with immune thrombocytopenia need to be excluded: connective tissue diseases, lymphoproliferative disorders, and HIV infection. Immune thrombocytopenia is common in patients with HIV infection and results from an immune–complex-related phenomenon. Drugs that may be associated with immune thrombocytopenia—quinidine, cimetidine, and trimethoprim-sulfamethoxazole—should also be included in the differential diagnosis.

TREATMENT OF ITP

Corticosteroids are the initial treatment of choice in adults with chronic ITP. If the platelet count is less than 50,000 or bleeding is present, treatment should be started. A response to steroids is generally seen within 7–14 days. If a response is seen, treatment should be continued for 2–4 additional weeks, and then a slow taper of the steroid begun. In patients primarily refractory to corticosteroids, or in those patients whose maintenance dose of steroid is greater than 10 mg of prednisone equivalent daily, alternative treatment options should be considered. Approximately 50–60% of patients who respond well, but incompletely, to steroids will respond to splenectomy. Pneumococcal and *Hemophilus influenza* vaccines should be administered 2–3 weeks before splenectomy if possible. Splenic irradiation may be considered in patients who are not medically fit for an operation or who defer the procedure. In those patients not responding to splenectomy or who relapse subsequent to an initial response, other treatment options are available. The use of high doses of intravenous gammaglobulin have produced remissions in autoimmune thrombocytopenic purpura. The most satisfactory results are seen in children with acute ITP, but short-term responses may be seen in adults.

In the unusual patient with ATP who has a serious bleeding diathesis, the use of high-dose intravenous gammaglobulin may both provide therapy for the primary illness and increase increments to platelet transfusions. The exact mechanism of action of gammaglobulin in this situation is unknown, but its effectiveness most likely results from a blockade of Fc receptors on reticuloendothelial cells. A second possible mechanism of action would be the down regulation of antiplatelet antibody production. Rho (O) immune globulin also appears to have activity in ITP. Danazol, an attenuated androgen, has been associated with therapeutic responses in ITP. It may be particularly useful in elderly patients who are not good candidates for splenectomy. Protracted therapy of several months duration is often necessary before a therapeutic response is seen. It may also be helpful in patients who have relapsed following splenectomy. In patients refractory to the modalities described above, immunosuppressive agents, vincristine, azathioprine, and cyclophosphamide, have been effective. Their use in association with corticosteroids generally allows the dose of the latter to be significantly reduced. They have the disadvantage, however, of significantly greater toxicities including myelosuppression and neurotoxicity.

If the patient is not bleeding, platelet transfusions are not indicated. However, should serious bleeding problems result, platelet transfusions should not be withheld, and increments to these transfusions may be seen. As noted above, prior therapy with intravenous gammaglobulin may increase the therapeutic benefit of platelet transfusions.

In the setting of immune thrombocytopenia in a patient with HIV infection, the use of antiretroviral agents has often produced significant amelioration of the thrombocytopenia. As noted above, the underlying pathophysiology of immune thrombopenia in HIV infection may be related to immune complex deposition with antibody and viral antigen. If the amount of viral antigen can be reduced, the immune complex deposition may also be reduced and fewer platelets affected.

Many patients with ITP will have unsatisfactory responses to all of the therapeutic modalities above. However, they may get by relatively well with moderate thrombopenia in the range of 30,000–60,000, and if such is the case no specific therapy is required. However, periodically they may undergo surgical procedures or suffer trauma. During these periods, reinstitution of high-dose steroid therapy, high-dose intravenous gammaglobulin, and platelet transfusions generally will provide significant benefit when needed.

HEPARIN-INDUCED THROMBOCYTOPENIA

Heparin-induced thrombocytopenia (HIT) is an important form of immune thrombocytopenia. Because of heparin's widespread use as an anticoagulant, many patients are at risk for the development of this disease.

Approximately 5% of patients treated with bovine heparin and 1% of patients treated with porcine heparin will become thrombocytopenic. It is most commonly seen in patients receiving standard therapeutic doses of heparin, but has also been described in patients receiving low-dose prophylaxis and in patients receiving heparin flushes to keep indwelling access catheters patent.

In practice, HIT should be suspected when any patient receiving heparin becomes thrombocytopenic or sustains a significant decrease in total platelet count. It is estimated that approximately 20% of patients with HIT have arterial and venous thromboses including: myocardial infarction, peripheral arterial thromboses, and pulmonary emboli. High levels of circulating IL-6, endothelial damage, and activation of platelets have induced thromboembolism in the presence of heparin immune complexes. Sepsis, surgery, and atherosclerotic vascular disease are associated with the above noted phenomena and increase the risk of thrombosis in HIT. The development of HIT usually occurs within 8–10 days of initiation of heparin anticoagulation but may occur in as early as 5 days in patients with a previous exposure.

PATHOPHYSIOLOGY OF HIT

Patients with HIT have IgG-heparin complexes that bind to platelet FC receptors resulting in the clearance of platelets from the circulation. Platelet activation increases the density of FC receptors, and a high level of receptor expression seems to produce the most severe forms of thrombosis with HIT. Heparin-induced antibodies have also been demonstrated to increase platelet activation by binding to the platelet factor 4 (PF4) heparin sulfate complex and by inducing endothelial cell damage. This may heighten the potential for thrombosis.

DIAGNOSIS OF HIT

In the laboratory the patient's plasma is mixed with patient platelets, heparin is added, and aggregation studies are performed. Should aggregation occur, this is a positive test for a heparin-associated antibody. The test, however, is not 100% sensitive, particularly in the situation where the patient is thrombocytopenic enough that other target platelets are used.

TREATMENT OF HIT

Heparin should be discontinued as soon as the diagnosis is entertained as thrombotic events cannot be predicted in the individual patient and serious morbidity and death has been reported in up to 50% of patients with HIT who develop thrombosis. At present the heparinoids (e.g., Organon-10172) and the thrombin inhibitors (e.g., argatroban) have the most clinical utility for ongoing anticoagulation. When hirudin another thrombin inhibitor is more readily available this agent will be helpful also. Although the low molecular weight heparins have been used widely in the past, the high degree of cross reactivity with the heparin-associated antibody suggests that these agents should be avoided. In addition, utilization of a vena cava filter in the setting of lower extremity thrombotic events may be considered. Thrombolytic agents have also been used in some settings. Ancrod a defibrinating agent has been used in patients with HIT, however, the newer agents available are superior in their efficacy and easier to use with less potential toxicity.

QUALITATIVE PLATELET DISORDERS

The platelet forms the primary hemostatic plug by adhering to vascular endothelium and by the process of aggregation. Adherence to the endothelium or adhesion is accomplished by employing a protein intercellular bridge that attaches to receptors both on the platelet and the endothelium. Activation of the platelet produces ADP, which upon its release facilitates aggregation. Qualitative platelet disorders, which may be primary or secondary, result from abnormalities in one or more of the above noted processes.

PATHOPHYSIOLOGY OF QUALITATIVE PLATELET DISORDERS

Von Willebrand's protein acts as the intercellular bridge between the platelet and subendothelium. In its absence or in the presence of an abnormal protein, as in von Willebrand's disease, a failure of adhesion occurs. In Bernard-Soulier's syndrome, platelet glycoproteins I-A and I-B, which function as receptors for von Willebrand's protein, are absent, and accordingly, a deficiency in adhesion results. The abnormal protein that occurs in diseases associated with a monoclonal gammopathy such as multiple myeloma or Waldenstrom's macroglobulinemia may attach to platelet glycoprotein receptors and also interfere significantly with adhesion.

Sufficient platelet production of ADP and its subsequent release is necessary for normal aggregation. Storage pool disease results from a decrease in the number of platelet-dense granules, which are ADP storage granules. Aspirin irreversibly acetylates cyclo-oxygenase, which decreases the production of thromboxane A-2, also resulting in defective ADP release. Platelet glycoproteins IIB and IIIA are absent in Glanzmann's thromboasthenia. These receptors interact with ADP to produce aggregation, and accordingly as in the above noted disorders, abnormal aggregation and potential bleeding may occur.

Secondary disorders causing acquired platelet dysfunction include:

- Drugs
- Uremia
- Liver Disease
- Myeloproliferative and myelodysplastic disorder
- Paraproteinemias
- Autoimmune disorder
- Cardiopulmonary bypass

Drugs are the common cause of acquired platelet dysfunction. Common drugs that interfere with platelet membrane function include the tricyclics, Thorazine, cocaine, lidocaine, propranolol, cephalosporins, penicillins, and alcohol. Common drugs that interfere with platelet prostaglandin synthesis include aspirin, the nonsteroidal anti-inflammatory agents, furosemide, verapamil, hydralazine, methyl-prednisolone, and cyclosporine A. Drugs that inhibit platelet phosphodiesterase activity include caffeine, dipyridamole, aminophylline, and theophylline. Vincristine, vinblastine, and colchicine interfere with thrombosthenin, a platelet contractile protein.

Platelet dysfunction during cardiopulmonary bypass surgery is often severe and results from many factors. Patients who have ingested drugs known to interfere with platelet function compound the defects produced by cardiopulmonary bypass.

Patients with acute and chronic liver disease often have platelet dysfunction that may occur because of elevated levels of fibrin degradation products that compromise platelet function. Abnormalities in aggregation have also been noted.

Platelet dysfunction in uremia is common. This may result from altered prostaglandin metabolism, abnormalities in the interaction between von Willebrand's protein and platelet receptors, or perhaps elevated circulating levels of such compounds as hydroxyphenolic acid, which is known to decrease platelet factor 3 activity. Dialysis, desmopressin (DDAVP), estrogenic compounds, and cryoprecipitate are modes of therapy that have in some instances corrected the bleeding associated with uremia. Platelet transfusion, however, is necessary in instances of life-threatening hemorrhage.

As noted above, platelet dysfunction occurs commonly in disorders associated with a paraprotein. In addition, platelet function abnormalities are commonly seen in the myeloproliferative and myelodysplastic disorders. Combinations of platelet aggregation defects are observed.

DIAGNOSIS OF QUALITATIVE PLATELET DISORDERS

Bleeding time is the screening test used to assess for platelet function abnormalities. However, this test is not sensitive and does not correlate with the risk of bleeding, particularly in operative settings. An abnormal bleeding time is investigated by the use of platelet aggregometry using the aggregating agents ADP, epinephrine, collagen, ristocetin, and arachidonic acid. In many situations the specific abnormalities seen in this form of testing will reveal the specific platelet dysfunction. Unfortunately, despite the use of these sophisticated techniques, the specific mechanism of platelet dysfunction often remains undetermined.

TREATMENT OF QUALITATIVE PLATELET DISORDERS

Life-threatening hemorrhage secondary to platelet dysfunction should be treated with platelet transfusion. Other specific therapy, plasmapheresis in the paraprotein-related disorders and dialysis in uremia, must be considered. If a drug is being used that is associated with platelet dysfunction, its use should be discontinued.

HEMOPHILIA A

In the second century the Talmud described kindred whose males displayed recurrent severe hemorrhage. This may be the first description of the disease known today as hemophilia A. Hemophilia results from a deficiency or defect of Factor VIII. The predominant site of synthesis of Factor VIII remains unknown, although recent studies suggest that endothelial cells are a major source. Factor VIII is complexed to, and stabilized by, von Willebrand Factor (vWF) which transports it intravascularly and, through interaction with platelets and endothelium, is responsible for its availability in the coagulation process. Hemophilia A is an X-linked recessive disorder, making it a disease of males, all of whose sons will be normal and daughters will be obligatory carriers of the trait. There is a relatively high mutation rate for this disease, and as many as one-quarter to one-third of hemophiliacs may not have a family history of the disorder. Diagnosis of the carrier state may be made by analyzing familial restriction fragment length polymorphisms, ratios of plasma Factor VIII to von Willebrand factor, or the ratio of antigenic Factor VIII to procoagulant Factor VIII.

PATHOPHYSIOLOGY OF HEMOPHILIA A

The Factor VIII molecule is not absent in patients with hemophilia A, but the coagulant portion is either missing or dysfunctional, which produces the manifestation of the disease. When the Factor VIII:C level is less than 1%, the disease is considered to be severe, and spontaneous hemorrhage results. The disease is considered mild with Factor VIII:C levels greater than 5%, and spontaneous hemorrhages are unusual. However, when patients with mild disease become active, for example, by engaging in sports, hemarthroses or hematomas may result and prompt them to seek medical attention. Patients with levels of 1–5% have moderate disease. The severity of the disease remains uniform among kindred.

CLINICAL PRESENTATION OF HEMOPHILIA A

Hemarthroses and muscle hematomas are the most common manifestations of hemophilia A. They are the most difficult to deal with, and disabling sequelae may result. As platelet function is normal, bleeding from minor cuts or abrasions is unusual. The joints most frequently involved are the knees, elbows, ankles, and shoulders. Small intramuscular hematomas are common and may resolve spontaneously, although if they are large, they may cause compression of vital structures, i.e., compartment syndromes. Hematuria is frequent. Intracranial hemorrhage accounts for approximately 20–30% of deaths in hemophiliacs.

DIAGNOSIS OF HEMOPHILIA A

Patients with severe hemophilia A have a prolonged activated partial thromboplastin time (APTT). The prothrombin time (PT) and bleeding time are normal. The definitive diagnosis rests on the specific assay for Factor VIII.

TREATMENT OF HEMOPHILIA A

Therapy of hemorrhagic episodes revolves around replacement of Factor VIII. A suitable Factor VIII:C level for the control of mild hemorrhage is 30%. Advanced hemarthroses require replacement of levels of approximately 50%. For life-threatening hemorrhage, or in preparation for surgery, levels of 80–100% should be achieved. Although cryoprecipitate may still be used as a replacement source of Factor VIII, heat-treated or monoclonal– antibody-purified concentrates of Factor VIII are more commonly used at present. The cost is high; current prices are in the range of 8–20 cents per unit of Factor VIII. Desmopressin (DDAVP), when infused intravenously, causes release of endogenously synthesized Factor VIII from storage sites in endothelial cells. Patients with mild or moderate hemophilia A with nonlife-threatening hemorrhage may benefit from the use of this agent.

The major side effect of the use of these plasma products is the acquisition of A, B, or non-A/non-B hepatitis. Most hemophiliacs who have required therapy demonstrate some evidence of chronic liver disease. Approximately 80% of treated hemophiliacs have antibodies to HIV. About 5–10%

of such patients have developed AIDS, and the mortality from this approaches 1% in the total hemophiliac population. Nevertheless, bleeding remains the most significant source of morbidity and mortality, and treatment thus should remain aggressive.

Newer heat-treated or monoclonal antibody purified Factor VIII preparations have decreased the incidence of HIV infection. The use of human recombinant preparations should eliminate this problem.

Ten to 15% of severe hemophiliacs develop inhibitors to Factor VIII; this is discussed in detail in the later section on Acquired Inhibitors.

VON WILLEBRAND'S DISEASE

In 1924 Dr. Eric von Willebrand evaluated a family for what appeared to be a previously undescribed bleeding disorder. The observations he made at that time remain important features differentiating this new disorder from classic hemophilia. Bleeding was primarily mucocutaneous rather than the hemarthroses or muscle hematomas seen in hemophilia. Inheritance was autosomal dominant rather than X-linked recessive. Finally, patients of this kindred had prolonged bleeding times rather than the normal bleeding times seen in hemophilia. When he found that their platelet counts were normal, he hypothesized that a qualitative disorder of platelet function existed. Studies through the next several years demonstrated the following:

- Normal platelets did not correct the bleeding time
- Platelets from patients with von Willebrand's disease were effective when given as platelet transfusions
- Plasma from normal persons corrected the abnormal bleeding time seen in von Willebrand's disease

Thus, the abnormality in platelet function is apparently extrinsic to the platelet itself. While some patients have recurrent spontaneous hemorrhage, most patients with von Willebrand's disease (vWD) do not have frequent bleeding episodes except following trauma surgery. Estimates of the incidence of vWD range from 1:1000 to 1:100.

PATHOPHYSIOLOGY OF VON WILLEBRAND'S DISEASE

Endothelial cells and megakaryocytes synthesize von Willebrand's factor (vWF). This factor has two functions in hemostasis: (1) it is the intercellular bridge attaching platelets to vascular endothelium utilizing platelet gycloproteins Ib and IIb-IIIa and fibrillar collagen, and (2) vWF forms a stable complex with factor VIII, stabilizes the molecule, prolongs its intravascular half-life, and transports it intravascularly to sites of active hemostasis.

CLINICAL PRESENTATION OF VON WILLEBRAND'S DISEASE

Mucocutaneous bleeding is the most common symptom. Epistaxis, menorrhagia, gingival bleeding, and easy bruising are most frequent. Gingival bleeding after dental extraction occurs in about 50% of patients. Spontaneous hemarthroses are unusual and occur almost exclusively in patients with severe disease. Patients with the usual forms of the disease have hemarthroses only after major trauma. As opposed to hemophilia, the bleeding tendency tends to be variable in the same patient and in the same kindred.

DIAGNOSIS OF VON WILLEBRAND'S DISEASE

Von Willebrand's disease is most usually transmitted as an autosomal dominant trait, heterozygotes being moderately affected. Uncommonly, it may be transmitted as an autosomal-recessive trait. The laboratory evaluation of a person suspected of having von Willebrand's disease may be frustrating. Test results may vary in the same patient at different times; if they are normal but the index of suspicion is high, tests should be repeated on several occasions. There is a relationship between vWF levels and the ABO blood groups. Type O patients have the lowest levels, followed by types A, B, and AB. Stress and exercise transiently increase vWF levels, and the hormonal changes that accompany pregnancy may normalize vWF levels in even severely deficient patients. The bleeding time is usually prolonged. The partial thromboplastin time (PTT) is often prolonged yet may be normal in patients with mild disease. Depending on the subtype and severity of disease, decreased levels of factor VIII coagulant activity may be seen which in turn are responsible for the prolongation of PTT. Von Willebrand's factor antigen and von Willebrand's factor activity, as measured by the ristocetin cofactor assay, are sensitive and specific tests for the detection of von Willebrand's disease. Crossed immunoelectrophoresis determines the multimeric structure present and allows differentiation of the various types of von Willebrand's disease.

Type I vWD is the most common and accounts for approximately 80% of patients. It is inherited as an autosomal dominant trait. Bleeding is most often posttraumatic, and menorrhagia is also common. Levels of vWF and factor VIII are both reduced, and all sizes of vWF multimers are present.

Patients with type II-A von Willebrand's disease have normal or only slightly reduced levels of vWF and factor VIII but have low levels of high and intermediate molecular weight multimers in their plasma. Patients with type II-B disease have abnormalities of the protein which increase its affinity for platelet binding to glycoprotein Ib-IX which may result in mild thrombocytopenia. In type II-B disease there is a less marked loss of multimers. Type II forms of von Willebrand's disease are also inherited in an autosomal dominant manner.

Patients with type III vWD have severe bleeding and a marked reduction in vWF and factor VIII levels. These pa-tients frequently have hemarthroses secondary to their very low factor VIII levels. This form is inherited in an autosomal recessive manner.

A small group of patients has been described who have mutations in the factor VIII binding domain of vWF. These patients have normal multimeric distributions, normal levels of vWF, normal ristocetin cofactor activities, and very low factor VIII levels. Accordingly, the only abnormality relates to the decrease in factor VIII, and it is possible that some male patients who have previously been diagnosed as mild hemophiliacs may actually have this form of von Willebrand's disease. It is inherited as an autosomal recessive trait; the true frequency of this subtype is unknown.

Acquired vWD occurs with the development of inhibitors to vWF and has been described in association with various malignancies: nonHodgkin's lymphomas, Waldenstrom's macroglobulinemia, and multiple myeloma. These inhibitors have been associated with intestinal angiodysplasia and have developed in patients with type III vWD who have received multiple transfusions. Acquired vWD has also been described in myeloproliferative disorders.

TREATMENT OF VON WILLEBRAND'S DISEASE

Treatment options will depend on the extent of the bleeding problem and the severity and type of vWD. Desmopressin (DDAVP) raises vWF levels in plasma by promoting its release from endothelial cells. Not all patients will respond to the same extent, and the response diminishes over time as storage pools are depleted. Desmopressin DDAVP is most effective in patients with type I disease but has also been effective in those with type II-A disease. Ideally, an empiric trial of DDAVP to assess response should be performed prior to an anticipated operative procedure. Its use is not recommended in type II-B disease because an increase in this particular multimeric structure of vWF may produce excessive thrombopenia.

Patients with type III disease or other patients who have not responded appropriately to DDAVP must receive vWF employing plasma products. Older factor VIII preparations do not contain all multimeric forms of vWF and accordingly are insufficient for therapy. In addition, they have a high rate of viral disease transmission. Cryoprecipitate has been the mainstay of therapy but also may transmit viral disease. Newer factor VIII concentrates contain all multimeric forms of vWF and have a much lower incidence of viral disease transmission.

ACQUIRED COAGULATION INHIBITORS

Acquired inhibitors, also known as circulating anticoagulants, inhibit clotting factors or their reactions. They are generally immunoglobulins and occur most commonly in patients with hereditary bleeding disorders and arise as an immune response to foreign protein as a result of transfusion or factor replacement. Of those that arise de novo, factor VIII inhibitors are the most common and have been associated with autoimmune diseases: systemic lupus erythematosus, rheumatoid arthritis, and ulcerative colitis. They have also been seen in the lymphoproliferative disorders and multiple myeloma. Sulfonamides, phenytoin, and penicillin have also been associated with the development of VIII inhibitors. They may arise in the postpartum period and may develop de novo in the elderly.

DIAGNOSIS OF ACQUIRED COAGULATION INHIBITORS

In the laboratory, if a prolonged coagulation assay such as the partial thromboplastin time (PTT) is not corrected by a mixture of equal parts of patient and normal plasma, an inhibitor is assumed to be present. Specific factor assay is then performed to define the specificity of the inhibitor. In the case of factor VIII inhibitors, a specific titre is assayed and measured in Bethesda units: a low titre antibody is <5 units and a high titre antibody is >30. Inhibitors are also characterized as to whether or not they are inducible: will they increase anamnestically upon exposure to factor VIII? Factor VIII inhibitors that arise de novo are generally noninducible.

TREATMENT OF ACQUIRED COAGULATION INHIBITORS

The pattern of hemorrhage in patients with inhibitors generally is one of ecchymoses, intramuscular hematomas, and oozing from wounds or puncture sites. Therapy of the bleeding patient with a factor VIII inhibitor is difficult: it is determined by the titre of the inhibitor and the extent of hemorrhage. Minor local hemorrhage may be best approached with conservative local care. However, in serious or life-threatening hemorrhage, several treatment options are available:

- Use of high doses of factor VIII to "overwhelm" the inhibitor
- Plasmapheresis to decrease inhibitor titre in combination with high doses of factor VIII
- Use of porcine factor VIII
- Use of activated factor IX concentrates.

Immunosuppressive therapy with or without infusions of factor VIII have been used in an effort to induce tolerance and thus a decrease in inhibitor titre. Patients with nonhemophilia-related factor VIII inhibitors respond better to this type of therapy. Anecdotally, the use of high doses of gammaglobulin have been successful in those patients with factor VIII inhibitors that arise de novo.

Inhibitors to other coagulation factors including von Willebrand's factor, factor V, and factor IX have been described and are relatively rare.

LUPUS ANTICOAGULANT

Lupus anticoagulant was described in 1952 and determined to be an immunoglobulin with the ability to prolong phospholipid-dependent coagulation tests. Present in 5–15% of patients with systemic lupus erythematosus, this antiphospholipid is also seen in a variety of clinical conditions including malignancies and drug reactions, and in otherwise healthy individuals. It is seen in viral infections, particularly HIV. The partial thromboplastin time (PTT) is prolonged by the lupus anticoagulant, but this is a laboratory artifact in that the anticoagulant activity is directed against the phospholipid used in the test system. The inhibitor may uncommonly prolong the prothrombin time (PT), but one must be concerned that an associated hypoprothrombinemia may coexist. In addition, thrombocytopenia of an immune form may be associated with a lupus anticoagulant: the antiphospholipid antibody syndrome. Incubation of this inhibitor with normal plasma does not produce an increasing effect as is seen in inhibitors to specific clotting factors. A modified Russell Vipers Venom Time may be used as a confirmatory assay. There is a strong correlation between elevated anticardiolipid antibodies and the lupus anticoagulant, but the two are separate entities. Patients with the lupus anticoagulant do not have a hemorrhagic tendency unless another associated abnormality, hypoprothrombinemia or thrombocytopenia, is present. They do, however, as is the case with anticardiolipid antibodies, manifest a hypercoagulable state with recurrent thrombotic events of either arterial or venous origin and recurrent fetal loss.

An asymptomatic lupus coagulant does not need therapy, but patients with this disorder and a history of thrombosis require long-term anticoagulant therapy.

REVIEW EXERCISES

QUESTIONS

1. A 48-year-old female has had a stormy postoperative course after cholecystectomy. Today, bleeding and prolongation of her PT and PTT has occurred. Consult–R/0 DIC
Test results are as follows:

   PT 16 (control 12)
   INR 3.0
   PTT 56 (normal 28–32)
   Fibrinogen 326 (normal 200–450)
   Thrombin Time 10 (normal <15)
   Platelets 296,000

   The most likely diagnosis is:
   a. Intravascular coagulation
   b. Primary fibrinolysis
   c. Deficiency of K-dependent factors
   d. Heparin effect
   e. Antithrombin 3 deficiency

2. A recovering 22-year-old male patient with recent coryzal symptoms was lethargic and confused this morning and had a seizure in the emergency room. He is postictal, pale, icteric, and has petechiae. His laboratory results include HGB 6.0, platelets 6000, and LDH 3000. Coagulation studies are normal.

   The initial therapy should consist of:
   a. Heparinization
   b. Plasma infusion or exchange
   c. Platelet transfusion
   d. Splenectomy
   e. Plasmapheresis and replacement with salt-free albumin

3. A 21-year-old female presents to your emergency room with a dense hemiparesis. Platelet count is 3000. Her medical identification necklace says "I have ITP."

   Initial management should include which of the following?
   a. Platelet transfusion
   b. Intravenous corticosteroids
   c. High doses of gamma globulin
   d. Neurosurgical consultation
   e. All of the above

4. A 56-year-old male has an uneventful aortic valve replacement. Heparin anticoagulation is used. On the seventh postoperative day the patient develops a pale pulseless leg, and platelets are noted to be 5000.

   The most important step in initial management is which of the following?
   a. Obtain a vascular surgery consultation
   b. Increase the dose of heparin

c. Platelet transfusions
d. Discontinue the heparin
e. Decrease the dose of heparin

5. This 70-year-old female with a history of multiple myeloma develops a pathologic fracture of her femur. Preoperative PT, PTT, and platelet count are normal. A life-threatening hemorrhage occurs intraoperatively, and a bleeding time is markedly prolonged. PT and PTT remain normal.

   Which of the following diagnoses is most likely in this setting?
   a. Disseminated intravascular coagulation
   b. Vitamin K deficiency
   c. Lupus anticoagulant
   d. Platelet dysfunction secondary to dysproteinemia
   e. Acquired antithrombin 3 deficiency

6. The most appropriate initial therapy for the patient in the preceding question is:
   a. Plasmapheresis or exchange
   b. Fresh frozen plasma
   c. Platelet transfusion
   d. Heparin
   e. Aspirin

7. A 16-year-old male is injured playing high school football and experiences hemarthroses. His PT, PTT, and BT are normal. After returning to the field he experiences second hemarthroses. This time the PTT is prolonged. Of the following bleeding disorders, which may present with normal screening studies (PT, PTT, BT)?
   a. Mild von Willebrand's disease
   b. Mild hemophilia
   c. Platelet factor 3 deficiency
   d. Alpha 2-antiplasmin deficiency
   e. All of the above

8. A 22-year-old female has slammed her hand with a car door. A compartment syndrome develops, and in preparation for surgery a prolonged PTT is found. She has been evaluated for menorrhagia and easy bruising in the past without a specific diagnosis being made. Other family members have had similar problems.

   The most likely diagnosis is:
   a. Hemophilia
   b. Immune thrombocytopenic purpura
   c. Circulating anticoagulant
   d. von Willebrand's disease
   e. Deficiency of alpha 2 macroglobulin

9. An 82-year-old male is recovering from pneumonia. When an arterial line is removed, there is uncontrolled hemorrhage. PTT is markedly prolonged; PT and BT are normal. The most appropriate initial laboratory study is:

   a. Reptilase time
   b. Antiphospholipid antibody test
   c. Mixing study using a 1:1 mixture of normal and patient's plasma
   d. Bleeding time
   e. Dilute Russell viper venom time

Answers

1. c
2. b
3. e
4. d
5. d
6. a
7. e
8. d
9. c

C•H•A•P•T•E•R

23

Anemia

Robert J. Pelley

The red blood cell (RBC) mass is maintained in humans by a continuous production of differentiated erythrocytes generated by erythroid progenitors and stimulated by the hormone erythropoietin. Iron and nutrients, including vitamin B_{12} and folate, are necessary for RBC production. Energy sources are required to maintain the RBC membrane so that RBCs survive an average of 120 days.

Anemia is a reduction in the RBC mass, as measured by either the hematocrit or the hemoglobin concentration. Acquired anemia is not a disease per se, but a sign or symptom of an underlying disease. Since the severity of the anemia does not correlate with the seriousness of the underlying disorder, each patient with anemia deserves careful evaluation to learn the cause of the anemia.

CLINICAL PRESENTATION OF ANEMIA

Many clinical manifestations associated with anemia are determined by the cause of the underlying disease producing the anemia. However, if severe enough, all anemias will result in symptoms of tissue hypoxia: the consequence of a low oxygen-carrying capacity of the blood. Therefore, many of the signs and symptoms are common to all anemias. Headache, tinnitus, and exertional dyspnea are common nonspecific symptoms that may be mild if the anemia develops slowly. The presence of physical signs such as pallor and tachycardia can be severe but depend on the patient's previous cardiovascular status. Stress to the cardiovascular system may occur with mild anemia in patients with preexisting cardiovascular disease; however, even an ordinary individual begins to have cardiovascular stress at hemoglobin levels of <7 gm/dl due to the increased cardiac output required to compensate for the reduced oxygen-carrying capacity of the blood.

DIAGNOSIS OF ANEMIA

Normally the RBC mass is maintained by dynamic equilibrium: RBC production of 20 ml/day versus continual RBC destruction. Anemia results when this equilibrium cannot be maintained because of acute or chronic blood loss, failure to produce red blood cells, or a shortening of the RBC life span. When anemia is detected, it is analyzed by physical diagnostic and laboratory methods to classify and identify its underlying cause. The first step is always to exclude acute blood loss by history and physical examination, including stool guaiac for occult blood loss. Further analysis includes a complete blood count with red cell indices, including a calculation of the mean corpuscular volume (MCV), a review of the peripheral blood smear, and a corrected reticulocyte count. Results from these initial tests help determine whether more invasive or expensive testing is required: bone marrow aspiration and biopsy or immunoassays.

An important initial step in assessing an anemia involves examination of the peripheral blood smear (PBS), the most cost effective of hematologic tests. It is useful to correlate the PBS with RBC indices generated by an automated CBC. However, RBC indices should never substitute for examination of the PBS because the statistical averaging which occurs with an automated CBC loses valuable information about small populations of RBCs. Examination of the PBS will reveal more information about specific RBC morphology, dimorphic populations, inclusion bodies, and accompanying white blood cell (WBC) morphology—all of which is not available from an automated CBC.

The corrected reticulocyte count is a useful second test since it serves to divide anemias into two major categories: hyperproliferative anemias resulting from loss or destruction of RBCs with associated increased bone marrow activity, and hypoproliferative anemias resulting from decreased bone marrow production. When the underlying cause of anemia is not apparent, the reticulocyte count can be invaluable in blood smear interpretation and initial assessment as to the cause of the anemia.

Morphologically, hyperproliferative anemias are frequently macrocytic with high MCVs due to the large size of reticulocytes. However, some anemias caused by chronic hemolysis may result in normocytic morphology or MCVs that may be in the normal range because of averaging between macrocytic reticulocytes and smaller spherocytes. The PBS helps to identify hemolytic anemias rapidly. The presence of spherocytes or schistocytes and fragments may indicate such acquired disorders as immune hemolysis or disseminated intravascular coagulation (DIC). Inclusion bodies or sickle shapes may indicate hereditary disorders such as an enzymopathies or sickle cell disease. In hypoproliferative anemias the smear and MCV can be even more informative because RBC size can serve to organize the differential diagnosis. Furthermore, WBC morphology is more likely to be altered in hypoproliferative anemias in which multiple cell types within the bone marrow may be affected by the same disease process.

Table 23.1 outlines the differential diagnosis of anemia.

SPECIFIC ANEMIAS

HYPERPROLIFERATIVE ANEMIAS

Hyperproliferative anemias are simply divided between processes that remove blood cells (bleeding) and those that destroy blood cells (hemolysis). Discussed below are the two most common disorders resulting in RBC destruction: immune hemolysis and unstable hemoglobins.

Immune Hemolytic Disorders

Immune hemolytic processes can be crudely divided into autoimmune conditions in which the patient produces antibodies against RBC surface antigens, and drug-induced conditions in which the RBC is frequently an "innocent bystander" in an otherwise typical immune-mediated drug reaction.

All of these disorders are characterized by an indirect hyperbilirubinemia, reticulocytosis, marrow erythroid hyperplasia, hemoglobinemia, and perhaps hemoglobinuria. The peripheral blood smear may have spherocytes, and the haptoglobin protein level may be nearly undetectable as it is removed from circulation after binding free heme. The Coombs test will be "directly" positive if antibodies are detected on the patient's circulating RBCs, and it will be "indirectly" positive if antibodies capable of reacting to RBCs are only detected in the serum.

IgM-Induced Hemolysis   IgM antibodies produce "cold hemagglutinin" disease because they usually only bind or lyse RBCs at lower temperatures. The IgMs are frequently directed to the I antigen or related RBC antigens and result in complement fixation and lysis at temperatures usually below body

---

Table 23.1.   Differential Diagnosis of Anemia

A. Increased Reticulocyte Count
  1. Compensated acute blood loss occuring before depletion of iron stores
  2. Hemolytic anemias
     a. Immune and autoimmune
     b. Drug-induced
     c. Membrane defects
        1) Hereditary spherocytosis
        2) Hereditary elliptocytsosis
        3) Acquired PNH (paroxysmal nocturnal hemoglobinuria)
     d. Congenital enzymopathies
        1) PK deficiency
        2) G6PD Deficiency
     e. Hemoglobinopathies (sickle cell disorders)
     f. Mechanical hemolysis
        1) Heart valves
        2) DIC (Disseminated Intravascular Coagulation)
        3) TTP (Thrombotic Thrombocytopenic Purpura)
     g. Infections (malaria)
B. Decreased reticulocyte count
  1. Macrocytic anemias (MCV > 100)
     a. Pernicious anemia (vitamin B12 deficiency)
     b. Folate deficiency
     c. Alcoholism
     d. Malabsorption
     e. Liver disease
  2. Normochromic, normocytic (MCV > 80, MCV <100)
     a. Aplastic anemia
     b. Myelophthisic disorders
        1) Leukemias
        2) Lymphomas
        3) Myeloma
        4) Myelofibrosis
        5) Granulomatous diseases
        6) Lipid storage diseases
     c. Anemia of chronic disease (anemia of abnormal iron reutilization)
     d. Miscellaneous
        1) Anemia of chronic renal failure
        2) Anemia of endocrine diseases
        3) Anemia of hepatic failure
  3. Hypochromic microcytic (MCV < 80)
     a. Iron deficiency
     b. Sideroblastic anemia
     c. Lead intoxication
     d. Thalassemias
     e. Anemia of chronic disease (advanced)

temperature. The most common cause of cold agglutinins are cross-reactive IgMs resulting from infections (*Mycoplasma pneumoniae,* infectious mononucleosis, or Cytomegalovirus [CMV]). They are rarely clinically important. Lymphoproliferative diseases and connective tissue diseases can also produce cold agglutinins, some of which can generate difficult persistent hemolysis.

IgG-Induced Hemolysis

IgG antibodies also can produce hemolysis of RBCs; however, since they do so at body temperature, the hemolysis is clinically more serious. Also, since IgGs bind at warmer temperatures, they are referred to as ''warm antibodies.'' Although complement may be fixed by the IgGs, the antibody valency is inadequate to generate intravascular hemolysis. Generally, the RBCs are slowly converted into spherocytes and eventually removed extravascularly in the spleen.

Treatment of Immune Hemolytic Disorders

Warm antibody disease is much more likely to produce a clinically apparent anemia, which may be chronic and require treatment. Corticosteroids are the treatment of choice and are frequently used for treatment of the connective tissue disease or lymphoma that may be the cause of the warm antibody. Splenectomy is effective in more than half the patients who fail to respond to steroids. IgM hemolysis rarely requires therapy, but in exceptional instances when treatment is needed, plasmapheresis can effectively reduce the intravascular titer of the antibody. In either situation, transfusion of RBCs is seldom indicated and is always complicated by the difficulty of typing and crossing the patient's blood with compatible blood.

Drug-Induced Immune Hemolysis

Drugs can contribute to RBC hemolysis in four classical ways: hapten type, quinidine type, alpha-Methyldopa type (Aldomet), and nonspecific reactions. All are diagnosed with a careful history.

Hapten Type.   This occurs in patients receiving high doses of penicillins. The drug or its metabolites bind to the RBC and induce an immune response. The antibodies react to a RBC antigen/drug complex and therefore only bind to drug-coated RBCs.

Quinidine Type.   This IgM antibody reaction is directed most often to the drug quinidine when the drug binds to plasma proteins. The antibody then cross-reacts with RBC antigens, resulting in acute hemolysis.

alpha-Methyldopa Type (Aldomet).   This reaction is very similar to idiopathic ''warm antibody'' disease. By an unknown mechanism, one quarter of patients receiving Aldomet develop IgG autoantibodies directed against the Rh antigens, with 1% suffering some hemolysis. The drug itself is not involved in the antibody/RBC antigen reaction.

Nonspecific Reactions.   In unique instances, drugs such as cephalosporins can coat the RBC membrane, resulting in the nonspecific binding of plasma proteins, which may make the Coombs test positive. Hemolysis is uncommon.

Treatment of Drug-Induced Immune Hemolysis.   Removal of the inciting drug is the appropriate treatment and usually results in immediate improvement. Infrequently, corticosteroids are necessary.

The Unstable Erythron (Hereditary Disorders Causing Hemolysis)

The red blood cell is the most thoroughly studied entity in the human body because of its accessibility and quantity. The result has been a tremendous understanding at the genetic and biochemical level of hereditary disorders affecting hemoglobin (hemoglobinopathies), RBC enzymes (enzymopathies), and RBC structural proteins (hereditary spherocytosis). Nonetheless, the impact of this information on the therapy of these disorders has been disappointing.

Hemoglobinopathies: Sickle Cell Anemia

A point mutation of the β globin chain at residue 6 substitutes a valine for glutamic acid altering the net charge and local conformation of the hemoglobin molecule (Hb S). The alteration in charge results in an instability of hemoglobin S when in the deoxygenated state, resulting in insoluble aggregates. These aggregates will precipitate into polymers of long rod-like fibers if the concentration of Hb S is sufficiently high. Propagation of these polymers distorts the normally pliant red blood cell membrane into bizarre forms that resemble sickles. These sickle-shaped RBCs are the hallmarks of a series of unstable hemoglobins that produce a constellation of clinical problems including hemolytic anemia, small vessel infarction, painful crises, and a predisposition to infections.

Hb S mutations follow recessive inheritance patterns with the carrier state (sickle trait) being silent. However, patients heterozygous for Hb S who have an additional mutant hemoglobin such as Hb C, D or O, will manifest a clinically evident sickle syndrome. Diagnosis of Hb S or other Hb mutants is made by electrophoresis of purified Hb. Additionally, reducing agents that deprive cells of O_2 promote Hb polymerization and ''sickling,'' even in the cells of patients who are Hb AS heterozygotes, thus serving as a screening test (sickle prep).

Treatment of Sickle Cell Anemia.   Therapy of sickle cell anemia and crisis has been unaffected by our understanding of the disease. The cornerstones of treatment remain hydration and analgesia, early treatment of infections, and judicious transfusions.

Enzymopathies

Hereditary defects in more than six enzymes involved in glycolysis and ATP production have been identified that can induce hemolytic states. The most common is glucose-6-phosphate dehydrogenase (G6PD), which has more than 150 mutant forms. The mutations serve to decrease the half life of the G6PD protein, which is essential for maintaining the reduced state of the RBC cytoplasm. With time, lost activity allows for oxidation and precipitation of aging hemoglobin with subsequent development of inclusion bodies and hemolysis. Deficiency of G6PD is sex-linked and usually manifests in a male with episodic hemolysis following oxidative stresses associated with infections or drug ingestion. Since it is the ''aged'' RBCs that hemolyze, analysis for G6PD levels soon after the hemolytic episode may be misleading and should be delayed to allow the reaccumulation of older cells.

HYPOPROLIFERATIVE ANEMIAS

These disorders include diseases that interfere with RBC production or maturation and lead to a very low reticulocyte count. Historically, these anemias have been classified by RBC morphology and size. This classification frequently groups physiologically unrelated processes together, but this classification survives because it is an efficient means for clinically diagnosing these anemias.

MACROCYTIC ANEMIAS

The two most important disorders in which the MCV is elevated are vitamin B_{12} deficiency and folate deficiency. Macrocytosis may also be seen in myelodysplasia, alcoholism, and liver disease, as well as in individuals receiving chemotherapy or phenytoin. The peripheral blood smear is again valuable in identifying megaloblastic processes (B_{12} and folate deficiency) from processes that produce macrocytosis alone. Not only are hypersegmented neutrophils commonly present, but the RBCs are pleomorphic with fragments and other signs of dyserythropoiesis.

Vitamin B_{12} and Folate Deficiency

Both vitamin B_{12} and folate are involved in DNA synthesis. A deficiency in either leads to dyssynchrony in nuclear and cytoplasmic maturation, producing RBC macrocytosis and neutrophil hypersegmentation which are the hallmarks of these disorders. In addition, vitamin B_{12} plays an important role in myelin production, and B_{12} deficiency leads to serious neurologic disorders. Since B_{12} and folate metabolism are closely connected, administration of folate will bypass and correct the hematologic abnormalities of vitamin B_{12} deficiency without correcting the neurologic abnormalities. It is therefore essential to correctly diagnose B_{12} deficiency.

Vitamin B_{12} Deficiency
Vitamin B_{12} is found in animal products and is synthesized by intestinal bacteria. Upon ingestion, B_{12} is bound up by an intrinsic factor secreted by gastric parietal cells, and the B_{12}-intrinsic factor complex passes into the distal ileum where it is actively absorbed. Vitamin B_{12} is then transported by transcobalamins into the liver for storage and into the erythron. Absolute dietary deficiency is almost impossible, and most deficiencies are the result of malabsorp-tion. Parietal cell dysfunction occurs either through the autoimmune process of pernicious anemia or by surgical removal of the stomach. Ileal disease such as Crohn's disease or radiation enteritis, pancreatic insufficiency, blind loop syndromes, and ileal resections will also result in failure to absorb the B_{12}/intrinsic factor complex. The Schilling's test allows one to discriminate between a gastric disorder and an ileal disorder.

The clinical manifestations of B_{12} deficiency include symptoms attributable to anemia but also include disproportionate fatigue and subtle neurologic symptoms. Some B_{12}-deficient individuals manifest only mild anemia or macrocytosis, perhaps due to folate ingestion. Some of these patients may develop neuropsychiatric symptoms, neuropathies, or difficulties with unconscious proprioception. Vitamin B_{12} deficiency can lead to ''megaloblastic madness'' in which individuals may even be demented or disoriented.

Therapy for vitamin B_{12} deficiency is simply parenteral administration by monthly intramuscular injections of 100 ug of B_{12}, usually after initial repletion of body stores with an injection of 1 mg. This dose is sufficient to reverse the megaloblastosis within days. An improvement in erythropoiesis results in a lowering of serum iron as it is rapidly used and a lowering level of serum LDH, which is elevated due to ineffective erythropoiesis and intramedullary hemolysis.

Folate Deficiency
Many individuals are at risk for relative or absolute folic acid deficiency. Individuals who have diets poor in fresh vegetables, who have jejunal malabsorption, or who take antagonistic drugs may develop low folic acid levels. Pregnant women are especially susceptible. Folic acid, like B_{12}, is also necessary for DNA synthesis and is important in one carbon transfer, but unlike vitamin B_{12}, it is poorly stored by the body and needs to be continuously replenished. Unlike liver stores of vitamin B_{12}, which may be sufficient for 3 to 6 years, folate stores are minimal and florid deficiency can develop in 3 months or less.

The anemia of folate deficiency resembles the megaloblastosis of B_{12} deficiency. Diagnosis may be difficult because a small meal, blood transfusion, or intravenous multivitamins may be sufficient to elevate serum levels, making any subsequent testing ambiguous. Since RBC folate levels are the last compartment to be replenished and normalized, measuring RBC folate can be diagnostic in situations where treatment was initiated before diagnosis. Unfortunately, such testing is not universally available.

The most important aspect of folate deficiency is that folate is not involved in myelin production and cannot correct the neurologic deficit of B_{12} deficiency. Therefore, it is critical to not mistake vitamin B_{12} deficiency for folate deficiency.

NORMOCHROMIC NORMOCYTIC HYPOPROLIFERATIVE ANEMIAS

Anemia of Chronic Disease

The anemia of chronic disease can generate RBCs that are microcytic, but more frequently are normocytic. It is defined as an anemia associated with an underlying disorder when no other cause for the anemia can be identified. Not surprisingly, it is the most common category for anemias within institutions or hospitals. This disorder is characterized by low serum iron, low TIBC (transferrin), and a low percent saturation of iron, thus resembling iron deficiency. However, there is often a normal or high ferritin, which in the presence of a low TIBC is diagnostic of anemia of chronic disease. It has been labeled by some as ''the anemia of abnormal iron reutilization.'' Consistent with this, the bone marrow appears normocellular or slightly hypocellular with poor hemoglobinization but with significant iron within the marrow spaces. Patients with this anemia often have underlying neoplasms, inflammatory disorders, connective tissue diseases (lupus or rheumatoid arthritis), or infectious processes such as osteomyelitis or tuberculosis. There is increasing evidence that cytokines and inhibitory growth factors released during such disease processes may directly inhibit erythropoiesis or make RBC progenitors relatively resistant to normal or mildly elevated erythropoietin (EPO) levels. Efforts at treating these anemias with exogenous recombinant EPO have unfortunately met with only modest success. The only effective therapy for this anemia remains treatment of the underlying disorder.

Other forms of normochromic normocytic anemias tend to be uncommon and usually are associated with clinically obvious conditions such as hypothyroidism and renal failure, or are manifestations of pancytopenia. The anemia of renal failure deserves special mention as it represents the isolated deficiency of erythropoietin. Injections of recombinant EPO correct this anemia as long as iron is given to support erythropoiesis.

HYPOCHROMIC MICROCYTIC HYPOPROLIFERATIVE ANEMIAS

The microcytic anemias can all be characterized as anemias in which hemoglobin production is somehow deficient. This may be the result of hereditary inability to produce globin protein chains (thalassemia), to produce heme (sideroblastic anemias), or to supply the iron necessary for heme production (iron deficiency). Of these, iron deficiency is the most common form of impaired heme synthesis worldwide.

Iron-Deficiency Anemia

Worldwide, dietary insufficiency and parasite infestations are leading causes for iron-deficiency anemia. However, in the United States, the diagnosis of iron deficiency in an adult requires a careful and diligent search for a pathologic source of blood loss. Iron-deficiency anemia should be entertained in any anemic patient with microcytosis. However, iron deficiency can also accompany other anemias, and if presented with a macrocytic anemia, a dimorphic condition might exist with normocytic indices. The red cell distribution width (RDW) is a recently devised index that measures the variation

in RBC size. As the RDW increases, the variation in RBC size increases, making it likely that severe anisocytosis or a dimorphic population of RBCs are present. Examination of the peripheral smear is then essential. In iron deficiency, the RDW is high, reflecting the hypochromia, microcytosis, poikilocytes, and fragments that are often present.

People at risk of iron deficiency include infants with low dietary intake, pregnant women, adolescents, and the elderly. Symptoms of iron deficiency are common to other anemias: weakness, lassitude, palpitations, and dyspnea on exertion. However, iron deficiency also produces some unique symptoms in rapidly proliferating tissue: glossitis, stomatitis, gastric atrophy with abdominal pain, menorrhagia, and fingernail changes are all associated. Pica, or a craving to eat abnormal substances such as starch, ice, or dirt, occurs for unexplained reasons.

The serum ferritin is generally the best test for screening for iron deficiency. If the ferritin is below 30 ng/ml in a male or 10 ng/ml in a female, iron deficiency is present. Since ferritin is also an acute phase reactant, it may be falsely elevated. Even so, a value of less than 50 ug/ml in the face of inflammation is a strong indicator of iron deficiency. Iron deficiency can be further quantified by measuring the total iron-binding-capacity (TIBC) and total iron level, with calculated percent transferrin saturation. Finally, the absence of iron within the bone marrow or liver is the gold standard for confirming iron deficiency.

Treatment of Iron-Deficiency Anemia Therapy is straightforward. Iron salts such as ferrous sulfate, gluconate, or lactate can replete stores in 2–4 months. However, the initial step in treating iron-deficiency anemia is to identify the underlying disease and the source of blood loss.

Thalassemias

The thalassemias are hereditary diseases characterized by inadequate or unbalanced production of globin protein chains. Alpha thalassemia represents a deficiency in alpha chain production, and beta thalassemia a reduction in beta chains. The pathologic mechanisms responsible for decreased protein production generally are the result of hereditary mutations that totally delete the genes, or result in minimal or no globin RNA production. Afflicted individuals have a life-long microcytic, hypochromic anemia dependent on the severity of the deficiency. Four copies of the alpha globin gene and two copies of the beta globin gene generate vast variations in the production of, and the clinical spectrum of disease. For instance, the total lack of alpha globin results in death in utero in the second trimester. Lack of only one alpha gene, on the other hand, can be clinically silent and difficult to diagnose. In between are patients with 50% or less beta or alpha globin production who have mild anemias that resemble iron-deficiency anemia morphologically, but who obviously do not respond to iron therapy. Over the past century, clinicians have classified patients as having either thalassemia major, intermedia, or minor. These terms have no pathologic basis and only describe the severity of the patient's anemia.

In severe thalassemia, clinical symptoms present in early childhood and are the result of dyserythropoiesis and bone marrow hypertrophy rather than anemia. Patients develop bony deformities from marrow hyperplasia and organomegaly from extramedullary hematopoiesis. Strangely, the clinical manifestations of thalassemia relate more to the degree of imbalance between alpha and beta globin production: that leads to precipitation of abnormal hemoglobins in the developing RBC and lysis within the marrow. Patients with severe disease rarely survive to the age of 30. Fewer manifestations of hyperplastic bones and bone marrow, and more manifestations of the classic symptoms and problems of chronic anemia are common with less severe thalassemias.

The peripheral smear in thalassemia is usually remarkable for hypochromic microcytic cells. Patients with severe disease have manifestations of precipitating hemoglobin in their RBCs, including inclusion bodies and cell fragments resulting from dyserythropoiesis. Patients with only anemia or only thalassemia trait conditions will have increased numbers of RBCs (>5 million/ul) and target cells, but not fragmented cells from severe intracellular hemoglobin precipitation.

Treatment of Thalassemia Treatment of thalassemia in severely affected children involves transfusion of RBCs to reduce their own endogenous bone marrow activity and thus avoid bony hypertrophy and extramedullary hematopoiesis. In adults with anemia, transfusion is again beneficial but can lead to severe iron overload with consequent heart failure. Finally, the patient with thalassemia minor or trait seldom requires transfusion. However, accurate diagnosis is required to avoid unnecessary investigations for incorrectly diagnosed iron-deficiency anemia.

REVIEW EXERCISES

QUESTIONS

1. A 31-year-old woman presents with complaints of fatigue, dyspnea on exertion, and tinnitus: symptoms started 1 month ago. The patient had previously been in "perfect health," and has had three normal pregnancies.

   Physical examination is remarkable for pallor. Hemoglobin concentration is 7.5 gms/dL; WBC is 6,200, and platelet count is 550,000 /uL. Following the patient's last pregnancy 2 years ago, hemoglobin was normal.

   Which of the following tests is the most appropriate first test in the *initial* evaluation of this patient's anemia?
   a. Serum folate and vitamin B_{12} level
   b. Review of the peripheral blood smear (PBS)
   c. Serum ferritin determination
   d. Haptoglobin level
   e. Coombs' direct and indirect tests

2. A 58-year-old woman with a history of heart disease has taken quinidine for 1 year. The patient presents at an urgent care center with acute onset fever, cough, and diarrhea. You diagnose bronchitis and start oral amoxicillin. Two days later the patient is worse, with a productive cough, shortness of breath, and bilateral infiltrates on chest radiograph. You admit the patient to the hospital with a diagnosis of atypical pneumonia. The patient is anemic with a hemoglobin of 9 gms/dL. A peripheral smear shows polychromasia and RBC clumping without spherocytes. Coombs' direct test is positive for complement. Haptoglobin is low, and unconjugated bilirubin is 2.2.

   The most likely cause for this patient's hemolysis is
   a. Quinidine drug-induced hemolysis
   b. Penicillin drug-induced hemolysis
   c. Cold agglutinin associated with atypical pneumonia
   d. None of the above

3. A 24-year-old Lebanese exchange student presents to you in the college infirmary with a 3-day history of URI symptoms, cough, purulent sputum, and a low-grade fever. His chest exam is clear, and he is given available Bactrim "samples" for a clinical bronchitis.

   The following day he returns with shortness of breath, severe abdominal pain, a high spiking fever, and dark urine. A CBC reveals a Hgb of 7 g/dL and a WBC of 12,500. The peripheral blood smear has fragmented RBCs and distinct "bite cells" present. The chest radiograph is normal. The patient is admitted to the hospital.

   Which of the following statements is true?
   a. The Coombs' test direct will be positive.
   b. The haptoglobin will be undetectable.
   c. A sickle prep screen would be positive.
   d. All of the above

4. A 48-year-old white male presents with fatigue, weakness, diffuse nonlocalizing abdominal complaints, loss of libido, "funny sensations" in his arms and legs, and depression. The patient has attempted to medicate himself with high doses of B-complex vitamins as well as vitamin E and beta carotene. The patient denies any recent alcohol consumption, has had no diarrhea or steatorrhea, and has never had surgery. Physical examination is remarkable for a chronically ill-appearing middle-aged male. The only objective abnormalities include decreased sensation in the legs and decreased proprioception.

   The initial work-up includes a CBC with a Hgb of 13 g/dL, MCV of 120, and WBC of 4500. The platelet count is 220,000. The PBS confirms macrocytosis and rare hypersegmented polys. A reticulocyte count is 0.5%. You measure serum B_{12} and folate levels due to the macrocytosis. Folate level is greater than 14 (the normal is > 2.0), and B_{12} is 20 (the normal is >100).

   Which of the following statements is false?
   a. Administration of folate can correct the anemia of B_{12} deficiency.
   b. With severe vitamin B_{12} deficiency, pancytopenia can result.
   c. Folate administration cannot correct the myelin production defects and neurologic deficits.
   d. An oral vitamin B_{12} preparation (Geritol) would have been likely to prevent the above patient's neurologic deficits.

5. Match the following patients with these laboratory results (a–d):

	Serum Iron (60–160)	Trans-ferrin (TIBC) (250–460)	Trans-ferrin Satu-ration (25–45%)	Serum Ferritin (20–300)
Normal Values				
a	220	260	85%	2560
b	200	390	51%	840
c	40	210	19%	400
d	20	500	4%	12

5. A 65-year-old woman on NSAIDs for osteoarthritis with irregular, guaiac positive stools.

6. A 48-year-old man with polyarthritis, recent onset diabetes, hyperpigmentation, and cirrhosis.

7. A 59-year-old woman with long-standing rheumatoid arthritis and anemia.

8. A 35-year-old postal carrier with a history of alcohol abuse and acute bacterial pneumonia.

9. For a patient with a chronic autoimmune hemolytic anemia (warm IgG antibody) associated with a connective tissue disease, all of the following are appropriate therapy except:
   a. Daily oral Prednisone
   b. Plasmapheresis
   c. Treatment of the underlying autoimmune disorder
   d. Splenectomy

10. Which of the following is the most important factor in inducing HbS precipitation:
    a. pH
    b. O_2 partial pressure
    c. HbS concentration
    d. Osmolality

11. The least likely factor to produce Vitamin B_{12} deficiency is
    a. Pregnancy
    b. Crohn's disease
    c. Total gastrectomy for peptic ulcer disease
    d. Strict vegetarian diet

12. Which laboratory test is most likely to be elevated in iron-deficiency anemia?
    a. Homocysteine
    b. Transferrin saturation
    c. Platelet count
    d. Ferritin
    e. All of the above

13. Chronic transfusion for the treatment of thalassemia major is associated with which of the following?
    a. Cirrhosis
    b. Cardiomyopathy
    c. Hemosiderosis
    d. All of the above

Answers

1. b

Review of the peripheral blood smear is the single most valuable first step in evaluating acute anemia. Morphology of the RBCs, presence of polychromasia (reticulocytes), and platelet morphology can help to immediately focus the differential diagnosis and evaluation. The differential diagnosis for this patient's acute or subacute anemia is broad; it includes both gastrointestinal blood loss and diverse causes of hemolysis. The iron studies, folate and B_{12} levels, haptoglobin, and Coombs' test are premature and should be ordered according to results of the PBS review and reticulocyte count.

2. a

Quinidine is most likely responsible for the significant hemolysis, evidenced by the polychromasia on smear and the positive Coombs' test. Quinidine generates an "innocent bystander" situation by binding to serum proteins and inducing IgM antibodies, which then bind to RBCs and fix complement, resulting in intravascular hemolysis. Spherocytes rarely are generated by the binding of IgM and the fixing of complement and are instead more common with IgG antibodies. Penicillins provoke such a response but not at the low doses of amoxicillin used in this situation. The cold agglutinin associated with the atypical pneumonia can produce clumping of RBCs on the smear and also on the positive direct Coombs' test. However, these agglutinins do not produce significant hemolysis and are not a concern.

3. b

This patient has clinical G6PD deficiency with acute hemolysis as exhibited by the acute drop in hemoglobin, dark urine, and fragmentation on the peripheral blood smear. People of Mediterranean descent are more prone to rapid severe hemolysis, in contrast to people of African descent. The "bite cells" on the smear are pathognomonic for this condition, which was triggered by the oxidative stress of the sulfa drugs. The precipitating hemoglobin results in RBC stromal damage and acute hemolysis. The haptoglobin level will be low, if at all detectable, because of binding to free hemoglobin and removal by the liver.

The Coombs' tests, both direct and indirect, are negative since antibodies are not involved in this physical form of hemolysis. Although many antibiotics might produce immune hemolysis, the time course of an acute onset within 24 hours goes against any immune process. The sickle prep will be negative since the precipitation of hemoglobin results in inclusion bodies, but not polymerization with deformity of the RBC architecture. Sickle cells will not be seen unless this patient also has a hemoglobinopathy.

If the G6PD enzyme levels were measured, they would be near normal in the remaining young cells that survived and were not hemolyzed. As these cells age, the enzyme "decays" and enzyme levels drop, making these cells vulnerable to stress hemolysis. However, following acute hemolysis, the surviving cells usually have normal levels of enzyme.

4. d

This patient most likely has pernicious anemia, an autoimmune disease directed against the intrinsic factor-producing parietal cells of the gastric antrum. Almost all vitamin B_{12} deficiency is the result of malabsorption either because of a lack of intrinsic factor (pernicious anemia) or defective small bowel. Dietary deficiency is almost impossible and occurs almost exclusively with vegans, strict vegetarians who consume no animal products. Oral vitamin B_{12} administration cannot overcome the deficit in malabsorption. The Schillings test, which measures the absorption of oral vitamin B_{12} in the presence of exogenous intrinsic factor, can distinguish the cause of the malabsorption.

Folate administration circumvents the B_{12} defect in the production of thymidine and DNA synthesis. Therefore, anemia may be ameliorated and only macrocytosis may exist. However, folate does not correct the defect in myelin production so that flagrant neurologic deficits may exist without hematologic abnormalities.

5. d

Serum ferritin and iron levels are frequently used to diagnose iron-deficiency states. However, ferritin is an acute phase reactant and may be elevated to a degree seen in iron-overload states in response to inflammation and liver disease.

A low serum iron level in the presence of an elevated transferrin level and low ferritin level is diagnostic of some element of iron deficiency. The ferritin may be falsely elevated in the case of acute inflammation, but rarely is >50 ug/L in the face of iron deficiency. On the other hand, the iron level may be low, but if the transferrin level is not elevated and the ferritin is elevated or in the high normal range, the condition of anemia of chronic disease is most likely present. Rheumatoid arthritis is the best described disease producing this situation, but this anemia is associated with many others. Although the ferritin may be astronomically high in the iron-overload condition of hereditary hemochromatosis, the transferrin saturation is a much more sensitive and accurate test. Finally, the ferritin may be especially misleading in patients with ongoing or acute inflammation such as a patient with an acute infection.

6. a
7. c
8. b
9. b
10. c
11. a
12. c
13. d

SUGGESTED READING

Beutler E. The common anemias. JAMA 1988:259(16); 2433–2437.

Finch CA, Heubers H. Perspectives in iron metabolism. N Engl J Med 1982:306(25);1520–1528.

Freedman ML: Iron deficiency in the elderly. Hospital Practice 1996: March 30;115–137.

Henry DH, Thatcher, N: Patient selection and predicting response to recombinant human erythropoietin in anemic cancer patients. Seminars in Hematology 1996:33(1), Suppl 1:2–6.

Jongen-Lavrencic A, Peeters HRM, Vreugdenhil G, AJG Swaak: Interaction of inflammatory cytokines and erythropoietin in iron metabolism and erythropoiesis in anaemia of chronic disease. Clinical Rheumatology 1995:14:519–525.

Lindenbaum J, et al. Neuropsychiatric disorders caused by cobalamin deficiency in the absence of anemia or macrocytosis. N Engl J Med 1988:318(26);1720–1728.

Means Jr., RT, Krantz SB. Progress in Understanding the Pathogenesis of the Anemia of Chronic Disease. Blood 1992: 80(7);1639–1646.

Serjeant GR. Sickle cell disease. Oxford Medical Publishing Co., 1985.

Wallerstein RO. Laboratory evaluation of anemia. The Western Journal of Medicine. 1987:146;443–451.

Weatherall DJ, Clegg JB. The thalassemia syndromes, 3rd ed. Blackwell Scientific Publications, Oxford, 1981.

Welch HG, Meechan KR, Goodnough LT. Prudent strategies for elective red blood cell transfusion. Ann Intern Med 1992: 116;393–402.

Williams WJ, Beutler E, Erslev AJ, Lichtman MA, eds. Hematology, 4th ed. New York: McGraw-Hill Book Co., 1990.

C • H • A • P • T • E • R

24

Breast Cancer

Beth A. Overmoyer

Breast cancer, the most common malignancy among women in North America, accounts for 30% of all cancers. In 1997, an estimated 181,000 women will be diagnosed with breast cancer; an estimated 44,000 will die of the disease, making breast cancer the second most common cause of cancer-related deaths among women (17%), surpassed only by lung cancer. The incidence of breast cancer has been steadily rising by 3–4% per year since 1982, but the mortality rate has recently begun to decline:

- Increasing incidence, 1973–1991: 24% rise
  - Annual rise of 2% vs. baseline (1% since 1940)
  - Primarily among women > age 50 (29% vs. 9%)
  - With advent of mammography, 1982–1987: 4%/year increase
- Increasing 5-year survival rate
  - Overall survival 1973 = 72% vs. 1986 = 81%
  - Patients diagnosed 1983–1990
  - < age 45 = 76%
  - age 65–74 = 83%

Routine mammography screening and breast examinations may account for most of the increased incidence. Early detection, an increase in the diagnosis of non-invasive breast cancer, and adjuvant therapy have favorably affected the mortality rate.

ETIOLOGY OF BREAST CANCER

The exact etiology of breast cancer remains unknown. Although extensive research of genetic changes associated with breast cancer suggests a progression from benign breast disease to invasive carcinoma, the exact sequence of events has not been determined. It is suspected that the genetic changes

associated with the development of breast cancer are directly influenced by the duration of ovarian function.

The importance of hormones in breast cancer centers on two questions:

- Is estrogen important? The endocrine environment influences susceptibility to carcinogens, especially at times of unopposed estrogen. Risk factors include:
  - Reproductive timing
  - Obesity
  - Therapy with anti-estrogens

Is progesterone important? Peak mitotic activity occurs during a progesterone-dominant time.

EPIDEMIOLOGY OF BREAST CANCER

Epidemiologic studies suggest a link between diet and breast cancer development. This link has not been supported by controlled trials, and reducing fat intake has not been shown to significantly reduce breast cancer risk (Table 24.1).

A direct dose-relationship of alcohol use and the risk of developing breast cancer is apparent. The effects appear primarily to influence the development of breast cancer among women younger than 30.

Exposure to ionizing radiation from nuclear war or medical procedures is associated with increased breast cancer risk. The highest risk occurs when radiation exposure occurs before age 40. Associated treatments include thymic irradiation, "mantle" radiation for Hodgkin's disease, breast irradiation for mastitis, and multiple fluoroscopic procedures. Radiation-induced breast cancer has a long latent period.

Table 24.1. Cohort Studies of Fat Intake and Breast Cancer Risk

Nutrient (Daily)	CBSS	NLCS	NYSC	NHS	Pooled
Total fat	1.21	0.90	1.04	0.93	1.02
Saturated fat	1.07	1.08	0.90	0.99	1.03
Monosaturated fat	1.14	0.77	1.03	0.89	0.99
Polyunsaturated	1.38	0.94	1.09	0.93	1.03
Animal fat	1.01	1.00	0.91	1.03	1.00
Vegetable fat	1.08	0.98	1.04	0.93	1.01
Cholesterol	0.97	1.03	1.02	1.12	1.04

RISK FACTORS FOR BREAST CANCER

Risk factors of breast cancer include:

- Age
- Family history: 5%–10% with a genetic linkage (BRCA-1, BRCA-2)
- Hormonal factors
  - Early menarche (before age 12)
  - Late menopause (after age 55) [Relative risk (RR) = 2.0]
  - First-term birth after age 30 (RR = 2.0)
  - Nulliparity (RR = 1.4)
  - Exogenous estrogen (RR = 1.5)
- Diet
  - Alcohol (RR = 1.4)
  - Fat content—not related
- Therapeutic radiation exposure
- Proliferative breast disease (RR = 1.5)
  - With Atypia (RR = 4.0)

In the United States, a woman's lifetime risk of developing breast cancer is estimated to be 12.6%, or 1 in 8. Breast cancer continues to be a disease most commonly seen in older women. The incidence increases as a woman matures: median age at onset is 55 years. Although additional factors increase the risk of developing breast cancer, 50% of those diagnosed will have no identifiable risk factor except age and female gender. The greatest risk is conferred by a previous history of breast cancer. The risk of developing a second primary breast cancer is approximately 1% per year, or approximately 20% lifetime risk.

A family history of breast cancer is associated with an increased risk of developing the disease, though this risk is rarely greater than 30%. Women who have first-degree relatives, a mother or sister, with breast cancer may have an increased risk equaling 1.5 to 3.0 times that of women without affected first-degree relatives. The highest risk is conferred when a premenopausal family member has bilateral breast cancer.

Only 5–10% of all affected families will have a genetic linkage to breast cancer. These include germ-line mutations of tumor-suppressor genes, such as BRCA-1, and BRCA-2. These genes are transmitted autosomal dominantly and require a "second hit" or second mutation to progress to invasive carcinoma. The development of cancer associated with the inheritance of a cancer-related gene (i.e., BRCA-1 and BRCA-2) can occur in this manner:

1. Germ-line mutation: The person inherits a mutated tumor suppressor gene.
2. Somatic mutation: A mutation develops in the normal copy of the gene.
3. This "second hit" can be detected by changes in the genetic markers inherited with the cancer gene.

This is known as loss of heterozygosity.

BRCA-1, localized on chromosome 17q21, accounts for approximately 45% of all inherited breast cancers and >80% of inherited ovarian cancers. Mutations of BRCA-1 convey a 50% risk of developing breast cancer by age 45, and an 87% risk by age 80. Males who carry the abnormal BRCA-1 gene may have an associated increased risk of developing prostate cancer. There are more than 80 distinct mutations in the BRCA-1 genome. A specific mutation (185delAG) is present among 1% of the Ashkenazi Jewish population and in 20% of Ashkenazi Jewish women who are diagnosed with breast cancer before age 40. Women with mutated BRCA-1 genes have a 65% chance of developing a second primary breast cancer. Thirty-five percent of inherited breast cancers are associated with BRCA-2, localized to chromosome 13q12-q13. The BRCA-2 gene conveys an 85% lifetime risk of developing breast cancer but only a 10–20% risk of developing ovarian cancer, and may be associated with male breast cancer.

To summarize:

- BRCA-1
  - Isolated in 1994 on chromosome 17q1.1
  - Associated with 80% breast/ovarian families
  - Lifetime risk: breast–85%, ovarian–60%
  - Present in 5–10% of patients with breast cancer before age 40
- Ashkenazi Jews
  - 1% of population
  - 20% of the patients with breast cancer are < age 40
- BRCA-2
  - Isolated in 1995 on chromosome 13q
  - Lifetime risk: breast–88%, ovarian–25%, male breast cancer–6%
  - Accounts for 30–40% of inherited breast cancer

Other familial syndromes associated with an increased risk of developing breast cancer include:

- Li-Fraumeni Syndrome
- Cowden's Disease
- Ataxia telangiectasia

Genetic predisposition may be present in the following situations:

- Young women diagnosed with breast cancer (before age 40)
- Young women with bilateral breast cancer
- Women with many relatives diagnosed with breast and/ or ovarian cancer, such as:
  - Sister pairs with 2 breast, 2 ovarian, or 1 breast/1 ovarian cancer
  - Families with >3 cases of breast cancer diagnosed before age 50
- Families with >2 breast and >2 ovarian cancers diagnosed at any age

Although the sequence of the BRCA-1 and BRCA-2 genes are known, widespread genetic testing remains investigational. Deoxyribonucleic acid testing for cancer genes may be done in patients with a prior probability of BRCA-1 mutation >10%. These individuals may have:

- Family with >2 breast cancers and >1 ovarian cancer at any age
- Family with >3 breast cancers before age 50
- Sister pairs with two cancers diagnosed before age 50: 2 breast, 2 ovarian, or 1 breast and 1 ovarian

Hormonal factors also play a role in increasing a woman's risk for developing breast cancer. An early age of menarche (before age 12), late age of menopause (after age 55), nulliparity and a late first term pregnancy (after age 30), are associated with an increased risk of breast cancer. The mechanism is presumed to be linked with the duration of active ovulation. Exogenous estrogen use during the postmenopausal period is associated with a slight increased risk from 1.5 to 2.0. The length of estrogen use appears to be a factor (>10–20 years of use). A history of oral contraceptive use has not been demonstrated to be a definite risk factor. Hormone replacement therapy remains investigational in the breast cancer population (Table 24.2).

Benign breast lesions classified as "nonproliferative" (e.g., fibrocystic changes) do not increase the risk of breast cancer. "Proliferative" changes are associated with an increased risk (RR = 1.5), and atypical hyperplasia is presumed

Table 24.2. Hormone Replacement Therapy and Breast Cancer Risk

Hormone	Relative Risk (%)
None	1.0
Conjugated Estrogen	1.32
Estrogen	1.37
Estrogen + Progesterone	1.5
Progesterone	2.4

Table 24.3. Benign Breast Pathology and Risk of Developing Invasive Cancer

Increased Risk	No Increased Risk
DCIS	Fibroadenoma
LCIS	Cysts
Atypical hyperplasia	Adenosis
Papillary hyperplasia	Apocrine changes
	Epithelial hyperplasia

DCIS–Ductal carcinoma in situ.
LCIS–Lobular carcinoma in situ.

to be a marker for the development of breast cancer (Table 24.3).

PATHOPHYSIOLOGY OF BREAST CANCER

Breast cancers are classified as ductal or lobular, corresponding to the ducts and lobules of normal breast tissue, and then are divided into noninvasive or invasive. Noninvasive cancers (ductal or lobular) do not metastasize; rather, they remain confined within the basement membrane and are termed carcinoma in situ. Lobular carcinoma in situ (LCIS) may be a marker for increased breast cancer risk, rather than a premalignant lesion. More than 80% of women with LCIS do not develop breast cancer, but their risk for developing this disease is equal in both breasts. The risk of developing breast cancer persists indefinitely, and the cancer is primarily invasive ductal when it does occur.

Ductal carcinoma in situ progresses to invasive carcinoma primarily in the ipsilateral breast. Again, the primary invasive disease is usually ductal. Increased use of screening mammograms has contributed to the increased incidence of DCIS, which often presents as a cluster of microcalcifications, as a result of early detection. Unlike LCIS, DCIS is considered a pre-cancerous lesion. The comedo subtype appears to have greater malignant potential.

Eighty percent of all invasive breast cancers are ductal, and approximately 10% are lobular. Specific subtypes of invasive cancer have a more favorable prognosis, including:

- Medullary
- Mucinous (colloid)
- Tubular
- Papillary carcinoma

Inflammatory breast cancer is most often a clinical diagnosis, exhibiting characteristics of skin edema, erythema, and induration. Cancer involving the dermal lymphatics results in the clinical features of an inflammatory carcinoma. This subtype of breast cancer carries a poor prognosis.

DIAGNOSIS OF BREAST CANCER

PHYSICAL EXAMINATION, HISTORY, IMAGING, AND LABORATORY STUDIES

A complete evaluation is necessary to determine the stage of breast cancer. Pathologic examination of the tumor and ipsilateral axillary lymph nodes is mandatory for the evaluation of invasive breast cancer. The initial evaluation should also include a complete physical examination, CBC, liver function tests, and chest radiograph. Although a bone scan is positive in <5% of newly diagnosed breast cancer patients, a baseline bone scan may be necessary for comparison in case of future problems. The efficacy of liver scans (computed tomography or nuclear imaging) is low in early stage disease (Stage I or II), though the yield of detecting an abnormality increases with Stage III or in the presence of abnormal liver function tests.

The purpose of follow-up after the treatment of early-stage disease is mainly to detect a second primary breast cancer or an in-breast recurrence. Annual mammograms and physical examinations every 3–6 months for 2–3 years are recommended. Usually metastatic disease is associated with symptoms; therefore, extensive testing in an asymptomatic patient is not indicated. Annual chest x-ray, liver function tests, and CBC may be beneficial, in addition to annual mammography, history and physical examination. Unfortunately, there are no established serum markers to detect a recurrence of breast cancer.

SCREENING FOR BREAST CANCER

Characteristics of breast cancer appropriate for screening include:

- High prevalence and incidence
- Long preclinical stage of disease
- Effective treatment of early-stage disease

Screening mammograms and breast examinations are complementary means of diagnosis; they are not mutually exclusive. Breast cysts should be managed as follows:

- Fluid can be discarded unless
  - Grossly bloody (cytology evaluation)
  - Postmenopausal patients not on hormone replacement therapy
- Excisional biopsy after cyst aspiration when
  - Gross blood is aspirated
  - Reaccumulation of cyst in same location within 4–6 weeks
  - Residual mass is palpated after aspiration

A palpable breast mass should be surgically evaluated regardless of the mammographic findings:

- Fine-needle aspiration biopsy:
  - False positive rate is low (0.17%)
  - Any mass with atypical changes should be excised

- False negative rate is 0.4%–35%:
  - Inadequate sampling (6%–32%)
  - Tumor size <1 cm
  - Large amount of fibrosis, necrosis, edema

A fine-needle aspiration (FNA) or core biopsy can be performed in the office, although false-negative results can occur. An excisional biopsy is the standard method of diagnosing a breast mass. A suspicious finding on mammogram should be evaluated regardless of the physical examination. Nonpalpable lesions are evaluated by a needle-localized excisional biopsy or a stereotactic core-needle biopsy. Patients with suspicious findings in one breast should always have the contralateral breast evaluated by physical examination and mammogram.

The American College of Radiology Mammography Accreditation Program enforces the standardization of mammographic interpretation. Mammography screening statistics include:

- Most effective screening test for early breast cancer
- Sensitivity: 80%
- Specificity: 95%
- 10–20% of breast cancers are not detected by mammography

Recommendations for mammographic screening include:

- Annual mammograms for women > age 50
  - Reduce mortality from breast cancer by 30%
  - Baseline mammogram at age 40
  - No upper age limit for screening
- Mammograms for women age 40-49
  - Reduce mortality by 22–49% in some studies
  - >40% of years of life lost to breast cancer are from women < age 50
  - Screening recommendations are controversial

The endpoint of every screening trial is to determine whether the screening technique impacts significantly upon mortality. Yearly screening mammograms and breast examinations performed by a trained health professional have been shown to reduce the mortality from breast cancer by approximately 25% among women age 50 and older. However, the impact on mortality in younger women is still not known. For this reason, screening recommendations for women age 40 to 49 should be directed by the patent's risk of developing breast cancer and the physician's comfort in surveillance. The American Cancer Society suggests annual screening mammograms and breast examinations for this age group. A baseline mammogram should be obtained between the ages of 35–40. Annual mammograms should also be performed after age 50. There is no upper age limit to mammographic screening.

STAGING OF BREAST CANCER (T, N, M)

As shown in Table 24.4, the staging of breast cancer depends on:

Table 24.4. Staging of Breast Cancer (American Joint Committee on Cancer)

Primary Tumor (T)

T1 Tumor 2 cm
T2 Tumor >2 cm and ≤5 cm
T3 Tumor >5 cm
T4 Any tumor size with direct extension to chest wall or skin (includes inflammatory carcinoma)

Nodal Involvement (N)

N_0 No lymph node metastasis
N_1 Metastasis to moveable ipsilateral axillary lymph nodes
N_2 Metastasis to ipsilateral axillary lymph nodes that are fixed to each other or to other structures
N_3 Metastasis to internal mammary lymph nodes

Metastasis (M)

M_0 No distant metastatic involvement
M_1 Distant metastatic disease (includes metastasis to ipsilateral supraclavicular lymph nodes)

Early-Stage Breast Cancer

Stage I	T_1	N_0	M_0
Stage IIA	T_1	N_1	M_0
	T_2	$N_{0,1}$	M_0
Stage IIB	T_3	N_0	M_0

Locally Advanced Breast Cancer

Stage IIIA	$T_{1,2}$	N_2	M_0
	T_3	N_1	M_0
Stage IIIB	T_4	Any N	M_0
	Any T	N_3	M_0

Metastatic Breast Cancer

Stage IV	Any T	Any N	M_1

- The size of the tumor (T)
- Presence of axillary lymph node involvement (N)
- Detection of metastatic disease (M)

Only 10% of patients will initially present with metastatic disease:

- Bone (50–70%)
- Liver (50–60%)
- Lung (60–70%)
- CNS (10–20%)

Of the remaining 90%, 40% will have axillary lymph node involvement. The clinical detection of ipsilateral axillary lymph node involvement is extremely inaccurate:

- Clinically negative axilla (30% pathologically positive)
- Clinically positive axilla (25% pathologically negative)

These high-false-negative and high-false-positive rates make axillary lymph node dissection necessary in the staging

of breast cancer. A larger-size primary tumor also increases the probability of having pathologic axillary lymph node involvement.

TREATMENT OF BREAST CANCER

Breast cancer can be approached as if it were two diseases: the goal is to optimize local disease control and systemic disease control.

SURGICAL TREATMENT OF BREAST CANCER

The standard approach is local treatment with a *modified radical mastectomy:*

- Removal of the breast
- Ipsilateral axillary lymph node dissection
- Sparing of pectoralis muscle group

A comparable alternative for local control for Stage I and Stage II disease is *breast conservation:*

- The primary tumor is surgically removed (termed lumpectomy, quadrantectomy, or partial mastectomy)
- Level 1 and Level 2 axillary lymph nodes dissection
- Radiation therapy is given to the involved breast

There is no difference in disease-free survival or overall survival among Stage I or Stage II women who choose modified radical mastectomy or breast-conserving surgery with radiation therapy.

A *radical mastectomy* entails:

- Removal of the breast
- Removal of the pectoralis major and minor muscles
- Removal of the axillary lymph nodes

This technique is reserved for special circumstances. Noninvasive cancer is treated with the goal of preventing the development of invasive disease. Ductal carcinoma in situ is treated with a *simple mastectomy:*

- Removal of the breast
- No axillary lymph node dissection

Breast conservation is also offered as a treatment option for ductal carcinoma in situ. Lobular carcinoma in situ can be managed by either active observation including an annual mammogram, or with prevention strategy using bilateral simple mastectomy.

Reconstructive surgery is an option following a mastectomy. Options include a saline breast implant or a transverse rectus abdominis myocutaneous flap (TRAM).

RADIATION TREATMENT OF BREAST CANCER

Radiation is recommended in conjunction with breast-conserving surgery. Radiation to the chest wall and regional lymph nodes may also be necessary after mastectomy to prevent a local disease recurrence. Indications for postmastectomy radiation therapy are becoming broader; however, the currently accepted indications include:

- Large tumor (>5 cm)
- Lymph node involvement (>4 positive lymph nodes)
- Tumor extending close to surgical margin

Radiation is given after the completion of systemic chemotherapy.

CHEMOTHERAPY AND HORMONAL TREATMENT FOR BREAST CANCER

All patients with the diagnosis of invasive breast cancer should receive an evaluation by a medical oncologist to determine the risk of metastasis and the need for adjuvant systemic therapy to *reduce* the rate of systemic metastasis.

This recommendation is based upon the concept that occult micrometastatic disease is present at the time of diagnosis of invasive breast cancer. The greatest risk for metastasis is usually within the first five years after diagnosis, although the risk of developing metastatic disease never reaches zero. Patients with small tumors (<1.0 cm), negative axillary lymph nodes, and positive estrogen receptors have a low risk of metastasis, usually <10%.

Small, screening-detected, invasive breast cancer is characterized as:

- Tumor size (<1 cm)
- Estrogen-receptor-positive
- Risk for metastasis (<10%)
- May not benefit from adjuvant therapy

Patients with large tumors (>5 cm), many involved axillary lymph nodes (>10), and negative estrogen receptors, have a >90% chance of developing metastatic disease. Approximately 40% of patients with negative lymph nodes will develop metastatic disease. Therefore, among lymph-node-negative patients, adjuvant therapy options are dependent upon characteristics of hormonal responsiveness and tumor size (Tables 24.5 and 24.6).

The goal of adjuvant systemic therapy is to reduce circulating micrometastatic disease that may be present in early

Table 24.5.   Adjuvant Therapy: Lymph Node Negative

	Positive ER	*Negative ER*
Premenopausal	Chemotherapy Tamoxifen	Chemotherapy
Postmenopausal	Tamoxifen Chemotherapy	Chemotherapy

ER–Estrogen receptor

Table 24.6.   Adjuvant Therapy: Lymph Node Positive

	Positive ER	*Negative ER*
Premenopausal	Chemotherapy + Tamoxifen	Chemotherapy
Postmenopausal	Chemotherapy + Tamoxifen	Chemotherapy

ER–Estrogen receptor

stage breast cancer, and prolong survival. Treatment may be given as combination chemotherapy or hormonal therapy (tamoxifen). The application of this treatment depends on the individual tumor characteristics: estrogen receptor status, lymph node involvement, and tumor size.

Systemic therapy has been beneficial in patients with positive lymph node involvement. Patients usually receive approximately 4–6 months of chemotherapy, disregarding menopausal status. Patients with positive estrogen receptors usually receive 5 years of hormonal therapy with tamoxifen at the completion of chemotherapy. Investigational therapies using dose-intensity of chemotherapy are reserved for high risk patients: those with Stage III disease or with four or more lymph nodes involved.

Hormonal therapy with tamoxifen reduces the risk of recurrence among patients with positive estrogen receptors, menopausal status notwithstanding. The maximum duration of tamoxifen use for node-negative patients is 5 years. Additional benefits of tamoxifen exist: reducing the risk of developing a contralateral breast cancer by 40%, reducing osteoporosis among postmenopausal patients, and reducing cholesterol and LDL levels.

Chemotherapy reduces the risk of recurrence among patients with estrogen-receptor-negative tumors. Chemotherapy has also been found to benefit patients with larger tumors (>2 cm) and negative lymph nodes, despite the estrogen receptor status. Several options of combination chemotherapy are available:

- CMF–cyclophosphamide, methotrexate, 5-Fluorouracil
- CAF–cyclophosphamide, adriamycin, 5-Fluorouracil
- AC–cyclophosphamide, adriamycin
- Mitoxantrone/5-Fluorouracil
- Taxol
- Taxotere
- Vinorelbine (Navelbine)

PALLIATIVE TREATMENT OF METASTATIC DISEASE

Only 10% of patients will present with metastatic breast cancer at the time of diagnosis:

- 50%–75% destined to relapse within 2 years

- Late metastases occur more than 10 years from diagnosis
- Incurable with a median survival of 2–3 years

Most patients develop metastatic disease within the first 5 years after diagnosis, although late recurrences (>10 years) do happen. Once metastatic disease is diagnosed, it cannot be cured, only controlled with ongoing treatment. The treatment goals are relief of symptoms and prolongation of life.

Metastatic breast cancer treatment involves integration of surgery, radiation therapy, and systemic therapy with hormonal treatment and/or chemotherapy. The application of treatment depends on the location of recurrence, estrogen receptor status of the tumor, and characteristics of the patient (e.g., age and overall health). Breast cancer commonly recurs in bones, lungs, liver, and brain, although metastatic disease can be found anywhere (Table 24.7). Invasive lobular carcinoma often recurs along serosal surfaces: the peritoneal cavity and pelvic organs (ovaries).

Approximately 25% of patients with breast cancer will eventually develop metastatic involvement of the central nervous system: the brain, spinal cord, or cerebrospinal fluid. Radiation therapy can be given to patients with brain metastasis, spinal cord involvement, or bone metastasis. Intrathecal chemotherapy treats disease within the cerebrospinal fluid. Radiation therapy with or without surgery can be useful in controlling chest-wall or regional (axillary or supraclavicular) lymph node recurrences.

Patients with disseminated metastases usually benefit from systemic therapy. This can be in the form of either chemotherapy or hormonal therapy. Hormone therapy indications for metastatic breast cancer include:

- Hormone receptor positive (ER + or PR +)
- Indolent metastasis
- Long disease-free interval
- Sequential hormonal therapies often appropriate

Hormonal therapy for breast cancer includes:

- Tamoxifen
- Megestrol acetate (Megace)
- Arimidex
- Halotestin
- Ovarian ablation

Table 24.7. Sites of Initial Metastasis and Survival

Site	Clinical Detection	Autopsy Detection	Median Survival
Bone	29%	70%	14–34 months
Lungs	19%	66%	17–20 months
Liver	4%	61%	6–12 months
CNS	2%	65%	1–15 months

Overall, 30% of patients will respond to hormonal treatment; 50–60% of patients with estrogen-receptor-positive tumors will respond. The duration of response can be quite long, often lasting several years. Patients with disease progression following an initial response with one hormonal treatment often respond to another hormonal therapy. Ovarian ablation (chemical, surgical, or radiation) is also a treatment option for premenopausal patients with positive estrogen receptors, though it has no benefit for postmenopausal women.

Because at least 3 months of hormonal therapy is necessary to determine the efficacy of treatment, hormonal therapy is usually not given for rapidly progressing disease, or visceral involvement (e.g., liver). Approximately 70% of previously untreated patients will respond to chemotherapy for metastatic disease. Approximately 50% of patients with disease recurrences later than 1 year after adjuvant therapy will also respond to chemotherapy for metastatic disease. Chemotherapy indications for metastatic breast cancer include:

- Hormonal receptor negative
- Visceral metastasis
- Rapidly progressive disease
- Short disease-free interval
- Failure after sequential hormonal therapy

Chemotherapy for metastatic disease includes:

- Combination chemotherapy
  - Average response of untreated patients 40–75%
  - Extends median survival by 10%
- Doxorubicin (Adriamycin)
  - Most active single agent (43%)
  - Response rates 60–80% in combination
- Taxol/Taxotere (60% response rate among adriamycin failures)

Combination chemotherapy may be more effective than single-agent drugs. To date, Adriamycin is the most effective single agent in metastatic breast cancer. However, the taxanes, Taxol or Taxotere, appear to be effective among patients with disease progression following Adriamycin therapy. The *combination* of chemotherapy and hormonal therapy for metastatic breast cancer may play no treatment role: *sequential* treatment with hormonal agents and chemotherapy is optimal.

Two-to-three months of chemotherapy are necessary to determine disease response:

- 3-month duration to assess hormonal therapy response
- Assess chemotherapy response following 2–3 cycles
- Flare response of osseous metastasis

As noted, patients usually develop symptomatic relief well ahead of documented tumor response. Patients with bone metastasis often develop a ''flare,'' or exacerbation of symptoms, during the first few weeks of treatment. Hypercalcemia may complicate initial bone healing. Radiographic studies, such as the bone scan, may actually appear worse during the active healing stage. Patients who develop a flare are encouraged to remain on therapy and use narcotics to control pain.

High-dose chemotherapy followed by autologous bone marrow transplantation remains an investigational, but promising form of therapy for metastatic disease.

COMPLICATIONS

The toxicity of adjuvant therapy is low:

- Chemotherapy
  - No additional risk of acute leukemia
  - Amenorrhea
  - Weight gain
  - Second malignancies are rare
  - CHF 2% risk with Adriamycin
- Tamoxifen
  - Thromboembolic phenomena (1% risk)
  - Endometrial cancers (1% risk)

As noted, there is no increased risk of developing secondary leukemia following standard-dose adjuvant chemotherapy. The cardiac toxicity (congestive heart failure) associated with Adriamycin is approximately 2%. Other chemotherapeutic toxicities include leukopenia, alopecia, amenorrhea, nausea/vomiting, and weight gain.

Tamoxifen may increase the risk of developing endometrial cancer by 1%. There also may be an increased risk of thrombosis (1%), earlier onset of menopause, and vaginal discharge.

Lymphedema of the arm occurs in approximately 13% of the patients following breast-conserving surgery and radiation therapy. Secondary cancers, such as lung cancer or sarcoma of the breast, rarely occur following breast radiation.

PROGNOSIS OF BREAST CANCER

Established prognostic indicators include:

- Number of axillary lymph nodes involved
- Primary tumor size
- Histologic grade/nuclear grade
- Estrogen-receptor status
- Lymphatic/vascular invasion

The chance of developing metastatic disease increases with the number of axillary lymph nodes involved and with larger tumor size. Other factors that predict a poorer prognosis are negative estrogen receptors, high histologic grade (poor differentiation of the tumor), and lymphatic/or vascular invasion seen within the tumor.

PREVENTION

Currently, there is no specific prevention for breast cancer. Since tamoxifen has been shown to reduce the development of contralateral breast cancer by 40%, this drug is currently involved in clinical trials among women at high risk for the development of breast cancer:

- NSABP P-1: Tamoxifen vs. placebo (11,000 entered)
- ECOG: Tamoxifen vs. tamoxifen + 4-HPR
- NCI Milan: 4-HPR vs. placebo
- CCF: Perillyl alcohol vs. placebo

(NSABP: National Surgical Adjuvant Bowel and Breast Program; ECOG: Eastern Cooperative Oncology Groups; NCI: National Cancer Institute; CCF: Churchland Clinic Foundation)

Prophylactic simple mastectomies currently are the only acceptable means of cancer prevention. Prevention studies are often performed in conjunction with surveillance programs of high risk individuals. These include:

- Monthly self-breast examinations
- Annual mammograms
- Physical examination performed every 4–6 months

REVIEW EXERCISES

1. Which of the following are true statements concerning mammography:
   a. Annual screening mammograms are associated with reduced breast cancer mortality among women over 50 years of age.
   b. Radiation from mammograms is associated with causing cancer among women at high risk.
   c. Physical examinations can detect smaller cancers than mammograms.
   d. A small lesion seen on a mammogram should be watched until it reaches a palpable size for adequate biopsy.
   e. a and d

2. Which of the following is *not* considered a risk factor for the development of breast cancer:
   a. Ionizing radiation
   b. Inheritance of the BRCA-1 gene
   c. High dietary fat intake
   d. Estrogen replacement therapy
   e. Atypical hyperplasia present in a breast biopsy

3. The staging of breast cancer includes which of the following tests:
   a. Patient age
   b. Evaluation of the ipsilateral axillary lymph nodes
   c. Carcinoembryonic antigen level (CEA)
   d. Subtype of carcinoma:
      –Infiltrating ductal
      –Infiltrating lobular
   e. All of the above

4. A 36-year-old premenopausal woman is diagnosed with infiltrating ductal carcinoma. Tumor size is 2.5 cm, 2 axillary lymph nodes are positive, and there is no evidence for metastatic disease (Stage II, T2,N1,M0). Estrogen receptors are negative. Which of the following statements is true:
   a. A modified radical mastectomy will increase the patient's chance for overall survival when compared with a lumpectomy, axillary dissection, and radiation therapy.
   b. Adjuvant systemic therapy has not been shown to be beneficial following surgical excision.
   c. Surgical oophorectomy should be performed at the time of breast surgery.
   d. Chemotherapy should be given for 6 months after surgery.
   e. The patient is at high risk for systemic recurrence and should receive a bone-marrow transplantation.

5. A 40-year-old premenopausal woman has a routine bone scan 8 years after the diagnosis of Stage II (T2,N0) estrogen-receptor-positive breast cancer. A metastatic evaluation only finds involvement of the bone. The features of her disease that may influence the choice of therapies include:
   a. Absence of visceral involvement with metastatic disease
   b. Number of lymph nodes involved at the time of initial diagnosis
   c. Positive estrogen receptor status
   d. a and c
   e. All of the above

Answers

1. a
   Mammography has not been demonstrated to cause breast cancer. Data show that screening mammograms are associated with a reduced breast cancer mortality among women 50 and older. This has not been seen among women between ages 40–49 years. Screening mammograms do not replace the need for annual breast examinations: as many as 15% of breast cancers can be palpated but not visualized on mammogram. Needle-localization of abnormal findings on mammogram enables a surgical biopsy of nonpalpable lesions.

2. c

Therapeutic radiation for the treatment of other malignancies, e.g., Hodgkin's Lymphoma, has been associated with the development of breast cancer more than 10 years following treatment. The recent sequencing of two genes, BRCA-1 and BRCA-2, have permitted the identification of women with an 87% chance of developing breast cancer by age 70. Estrogen replacement therapy given for more than 15 years can increase the risk of developing breast cancer by 1.5–2.0. This small risk, however, does not necessarily outweigh its benefit to women at risk for developing heart disease or osteoporosis. Benign fibrocystic changes of the breast do not increase the risk of developing breast cancer, although atypical hyperplasia present within breast tissue is a marker for an increased risk of developing breast cancer.

3. b

The staging of breast cancer involves tumor size (T), ipsilateral lymph node involvement (N), and distant metastasis (M). Serum tumor markers (CEA, CA 15-3) are investigational in breast cancer. The type of invasive disease (lobular vs. ductal) does not influence stage nor prognosis, although lobular carcinoma metastasizes to unusual locations such as serosal surfaces.

4. d

The National Cancer Institute Consensus Conference of 1990 determined that in early stage breast cancer (Stage I and II), modified radical mastectomy or lumpectomy, axillary dissection, and radiation therapy are equal in their effect on overall survival. Adjuvant systemic therapy (i.e., chemotherapy or hormonal therapy) has been found effective in reducing the risk of systemic recurrence among node-negative and node-positive patients. Chemotherapy for 4–6 months is recommended for node-positive patients. Oophorectomy and bone marrow transplantation remain investigational in the adjuvant setting.

5. d

There is no standard treatment for metastatic breast cancer since this stage of disease is incurable. There is no advantage to concurrent use of chemotherapy and hormonal therapy, therefore sequential use of chemotherapy and hormonal therapy is preferable. Hormonal therapy with tamoxifen can be used in estrogen-receptor-positive disease that does not involve the viscera nor is rapidly progressing. Approximately 3 months of treatment is required to determine response.

SUGGESTED READINGS

Bartlett J: Breast cancer susceptibility genes: Current challenges and future promises. Ann Intern Med 1996:124:1088–1089.

Burke W, et al: Recommendations for follow-up care of individuals with an inherited predisposition to cancer. JAMA 1997:277:997–1003.

Carlson R, et al: NCCN Breast cancer practice guidelines. Oncology Supplement 10 1996:(11):47–75.

Donegan W: Tumor-related prognostic factors in breast cancer pathobiological considerations in DCIS. CA J Clin 1997: 47: 28–51.

Fisher B, et al: Re-analysis and results after 12 years of follow-up in a randomized clinical trial comparing total mastectomy with lumpectomy with or without radiation in the treatment of breast cancer. New Engl J Med 1995:333:1456–1461.

Fowble B: Postmastectomy radiation: Then and now. Oncology 1977:11: 213–240.

Goldhirsch A, et al: Meeting highlights: International consensus panel on the treatment of primary breast cancer. Journal of the National Cancer Institute 1995:87:1141–1445.

Harris JR, et al: Malignant tumors of the breast. In: DeVita VT, Hellman S, and Rosenberg SA, eds. Cancer: Principles and practice of oncology 5th Edition, 1197;1557.

Hudis C, Norton L: Adjuvant drug therapy for operable breast cancer. Seminars in Oncology 1996:23:475–493.

Smith G, Henderson I: New treatments for breast cancer. Sem Oncol 1996:23:506–528.

Hodgkin's , Non-Hodgkin's Lymphoma, and HIV-Associated Malignancies

Kevin R. Fox

HODGKIN'S DISEASE

Hodgkin's disease is a malignant neoplasm of lymphoid tissue. Although uncommon (Hodgkin's disease occurs in approximately 7,500–8,000 individuals each year in the United States), the approach to treatment serves as a model for a curative strategy in the treatment of adult malignancy.

ETIOLOGY, EPIDEMIOLOGY, AND PATHOGENESIS OF HODGKIN'S DISEASE

The diagnosis of Hodgkin's disease relies on the presence of the Reed-Sternberg cell within a lymphoid milieu of variable appearance. The diagnosis cannot be made without such cells in a background of accompanying lymphoid tissue. The cause of Hodgkin's disease is unknown, and the exact cellular origin of the Reed-Sternberg cell is unknown, although an infectious cause is suspected. When modern molecular techniques are used to study the Reed-Sternberg cell, the majority of cells will contain Epstein-Barr Virus (EBV) genomic material, and the EBV genome will be monoclonal. An undeniable relationship between EBV and Hodgkin's disease has never been conclusively proven.

A "bimodal" age peak occurs in the incidence of Hodgkin's disease: the first peak in young adulthood, the second peak in adults after age 45, and the peak incidence in the third decade of life. Although the disease befalls nearly all demographic and socioeconomic groups, it is more common in urban dwellers and in higher socioeconomic strata, and is more likely to occur in identical twins, siblings, and close relatives of affected patients.

CLINICAL PRESENTATION OF HODGKIN'S DISEASE

Patients may present in a variety of ways: a painless nodal mass in the neck (most common), or a painless nodal mass in the axilla or groin (less common).

Since two-thirds of these patients may present with intrathoracic disease, the diagnosis may be heralded by persistent cough or dyspnea, leading to a chest radiograph showing mediastinal, or less often, hilar, adenopathy, or rarely discrete pulmonary nodules.

The patient may manifest "B" symptoms, systemic symptoms including:

- Fever (>38° C) affecting nearly one-third of patients
- Drenching night sweats (requiring a change in bedclothes)
- Loss of more than 10% of body weight in the 6 months preceding the diagnosis

Patients may manifest only one of these "B" symptoms, however.

Pruritus, while uncommon and not prognostically a "B" symptom, is important in that the differential diagnosis of pruritus should always include Hodgkin's disease, particularly in young adults. While Hodgkin's disease patients may have subtle defects in cellular immunity at the time of diagnosis, clinical manifestations of such defects are rare before the diagnosis is made.

DIAGNOSIS OF HODGKIN'S DISEASE

Diagnosis and workup options of Hodgkin's disease include:
    Excisionial biopsy

- History of "B" symptoms
- Physical examination
- Laboratory studies (including erythrocyte sedimentation rate)
- CAT scans of chest, abdomen, and pelvis
- Bone-marrow biopsy
- Bipedal lymphangiogram (controversial)
- Staging laparotomy (controversial)

The initial diagnosis should be made by surgical excision or incisional biopsy of affected tissue. The entire lymph node mass in question should be surgically excised when possible. Reed-Sternberg cells are rarely abundant in Hodgkin's disease, and the pathologist must be provided with a reasonable quantity of lymphoid tissue to find such cells. For this reason, fine-needle aspiration or core biopsy of suspicious masses may not be adequate and cannot be routinely recommended when Hodgkin's disease is in the differential diagnosis. When patients are found to have incidental or symptomatic mediastinal or hilar masses on chest radiograph, a careful examination of the neck and axillae is required; any enlarged peripheral nodes should be biopsied first in an attempt to spare the patient an unnecessary surgical procedure.

The treatment of Hodgkin's disease is somewhat stage-dependent, and thus the staging evaluation must be exhaustive. After thorough physical examination, routine laboratory studies should be performed, including:

- CBC
- Liver-function tests
- Erythrocyte sedimentation rate
- Electrolytes and tests of kidney function

Computerized axial tomography scans of the chest and abdomen, and bone-marrow biopsies should be performed.

The traditional staging evaluation, although under question in many centers, requires that if the clinical presentation is above the diaphragm, which is usually the case, and if the abdominal CAT scan is normal, then a bipedal lymphangiogram should be done. If this study is nondiagnostic, a staging laparotomy should follow. The staging laparotomy requires sampling of retroperitoneal, pelvic, and celiac nodes, removal and careful inspection of the spleen, and liver biopsies. Ongoing research trials are questioning the need for staging laparotomy, a practice abandoned at many centers.

The patient's condition is evaluated as stage I through IV, and A or B, according to the Ann Arbor Staging classification:

- Stage I: Single lymph node area involved
- Stage II: Two or more sites of nodal involvement on same side of diaphragm
- Stage III: Involvement of nodal sites on both sides of diaphragm
- Stage IV: Involvement of any extranodal site (e.g., liver, lung, bone)
- Subheadings:
  - A: Absence of ''B'' symptoms
  - B: Presence of ''B'' symptoms
  - E: Involvement of a single extranodal site

Approximately 25–35% of patients with disease confined to sites above the diaphragm after thorough radiologic staging will have occult disease found at staging laparotomy.

TREATMENT OF HODGKIN'S DISEASE

Treatment Goals

The goal of treatment in Hodgkin's disease is cure. With conventional radiotherapeutic technique, approximately 80% of early-stage patients (stage I or II) will be cured. Early results of clinical trials suggest that combined-modality therapy in patients who are early-stage, but who did not undergo laparotomy, may be equally effective. Patients with more advanced stage disease may be cured up to 60% of the time by first-line chemotherapy alone, but this figure drops considerably for patients over age 50.

Standard Treatment Regimens

Although the treatment of early-stage Hodgkin's disease is undergoing a general reevaluation in ongoing clinical trials questioning the role of radiation therapy alone, traditional therapeutic approaches use radiation therapy alone in early stage patients (stage IA, IB, or IIA). For decades this has been the mainstay of treatment of such patients. Treatments are given to total doses of 3500 to 4500 cGy using supervoltage sources, and given to large fields encompassing many nodal groups. The ''mantle'' field includes:

- Axilla nodes
- Supraclavicular nodes
- Infraclavicular nodes
- Cervical nodes
- Mediastinal nodes
- Hilar nodes

The ''paraaortic'' field includes:

- Paraaortic nodes
- Splenic hilum (or the whole spleen if it has not been surgically removed)

These two fields of radiation are usually given sequentially in early stage patients.

In contrast, patients with stage IIIB or IV disease should be treated with chemotherapy:

- MOPP: Mechlorethamine (nitrogen mustard), Oncovin (vincristine), procarbazine, prednisone
- ABVD: Adriamycin, bleomycin, vinblastine, dacarbazine (DTIC)
- MOPP/ABVD: Alternating monthly treatments with the above
- MOPP/ABV ''hybrid'': Alternating weekly treatments with above, excluding DTIC

The standard chemotherapy for the treatment of Hodgkin's disease of this stage is some combination of the conventional ''MOPP'' regimen with the ''ABVD'' regimen in an alternating manner. Some centers believe that the ''ABVD'' regimen alone is therapeutically equivalent to ''MOPP/ABVD'' combinations, and thus have abandoned the use of ''MOPP'' altogether.

Depending upon institutional habits, severity of illness, and bulk of nodal disease, patients with stage IIB or IIIA disease may be treated with:

- Radiation therapy alone
  - Laparotomy-staged IA, IB, IIA, some IIB, and IIIA

- Non–laparotomy-staged IA, if nonbulky disease (particularly female)
- Chemotherapy alone
  - Any staged IIIB or IV, some IIB or IIIA
- Both
  - Bulky mediastinal masses, bulky stage III, possibly any early stage

The use of both chemotherapy and radiation therapy together, so-called "combined modality" therapy, is gaining wider acceptance for the treatment of early-stage disease. This approach affords the possibility of smaller fields and doses of radiation therapy, thus reducing the possibility of late complications of treatment.

Special Treatment Situations

Patients with large mediastinal masses that encompass more than one-third of the transverse chest diameter, although technically stage I or II in most cases, are not suitable candidates for radiation therapy alone and should be treated with some combination of chemotherapy followed by radiation.

Patients who relapse after radiation therapy alone may, in turn, receive conventional chemotherapy with curative intent. Patients who relapse after combination chemotherapy will usually be treated with "second-line" or "salvage" chemotherapy, using drugs different from initial treatment. Patients who respond to such "salvage" chemotherapy may be referred for "high-dose" chemotherapy, followed by stem-cell or bone-marrow rescue (or transplantation). A limited series of patients suggests that as many as 50% of patients responding to "salvage" chemotherapy may enter long-term remission with this technique.

COMPLICATIONS OF HODGKIN'S DISEASE

Late complications of Hodgkin's disease include:

- Sterility
- Hypothyroidism
- Acute myelogenous leukemia/myelodysplasia
- Solid tumors
- Coronary artery disease

Both chemotherapy and radiation therapy may cause sterility or may cause some risk of acute leukemia. Acute myelogenous leukemia or myelodysplasia may occur in up to 10% of patients, particularly those who received MOPP chemotherapy, and may not manifest itself until a decade after treatment. The exact contribution of radiation therapy to leukemia risk is uncertain. Sterility is virtually assured in men receiving MOPP chemotherapy but is considerably less likely in men receiving ABVD alone. Sterility in women, closely tied to age, is likely to occur in women receiving MOPP after age 30.

Hypothyroidism, either clinical or chemical, may occur in more than 30% of patients who received mantle-radiation

therapy, and patients should undergo regular measurements of serum TSH after completion of such therapy.

The occurrence of second tumors is increased in patients who receive radiation therapy: cancers of lung, stomach, breast, skin, bone, and sarcomas. A latency period of more than ten years may occur before the appearance of such tumors, and the incidence may continue to rise beyond this point. Breast cancer risk may be markedly increased in women treated during childhood, adolescence, or before age thirty.

NON-HODGKIN'S LYMPHOMA

The non-Hodgkin's lymphomas (NHL) are a diverse group of lymphoid neoplasms that may arise anywhere—in nodal or nonnodal tissue. Different types of NHL often exhibit few similarities and thus are not easily categorized. Most adult NHL in the United States are of B-cell origin, but lymphomas of T-cell origin and macrophage/monocyte origin and undifferentiated lymphomas are well-described.

ETIOLOGY, EPIDEMIOLOGY, AND PATHOGENESIS OF NON-HODGKIN'S LYMPHOMA

Certain types of lymphoma have known origins: the association of EBV and African Burkitt lymphoma and the association of the virus HTLV-1 with the T-cell leukemia/lymphoma syndrome seen in Japan and the Caribbean. Most lymphomas in the United States, however, are of unknown cause. The association between H. pylori infection and low-grade lymphomas of the stomach has been well-described. An increased risk of NHL has been reported in patients exposed to a variety of environmental agents, including:

- Phenoxyacetic acid herbicides
- Permanent hair dyes
- Organophosphates
- Ionizing radiation from nuclear mishaps

A variety of immunodeficiency states are associated with increased risk of the development of NHL, including:

- Congenital immunodeficiency states (e.g., ataxia-telangiectasia)
- Severe combined immunodeficiency disease
- Rheumatologic diseases
  - Sjögren's syndrome
  - Systemic lupus erythematosus
  - Rheumatoid arthritis
  - Sprue
  - Hashimoto's disease
- Immunodeficiency state associated with HIV infection
- Iatrogenic immunodeficiency states (particularly post-organ-transplant immunosuppression)

Chromosomal translocations of a predictable type have been recognized in certain NHLs: translocations between chromosome 8 and either chromosomes 14, 2, or, 22 in Burkitt lymphoma, and translocations between chromosomes 14 and 18 in follicular (low-grade) lymphomas. Overall, these translocations involve the apposition of immunoglobulin light-chain or heavy-chain genes and a variety of regulatory genes, such as MYC, BCL1, and BCL2. The etiologic agent in effecting these translocations remains unknown.

Unlike relatively uncommon Hodgkin's disease, NHLs account for more than 45,000 cases in the United States each year, and the incidence is increasing steadily. This increase has been observed particularly in adults > 60 years of age, although the incidence is rising in all age groups. The increased risk of NHL in HIV-infected patients accounts for most of the perceived increases in NHL.

Non-Hodgkin's lymphomas have no bimodal age peak, and can occur anytime after age one year. Their peak incidence may be in the fifth and sixth decades of life; the overall average age at diagnosis is 42.

CLINICAL PRESENTATION AND DIAGNOSIS OF NON-HODGKIN'S LYMPHOMA

The diversity of these lymphomas, with respect to mode of presentation and type, do not permit easily recognized patterns of presentation. Although NHLs may present themselves as painless adenopathy (as in the case of Hodgkin's disease), NHLs may arise virtually anywhere in the body. Presentation in extranodal sites, such as the brain, orbit, skin, sinus, and any visceral structure, helps to differentiate NHLs from Hodgkin's disease. Furthermore, NHLs may present themselves in nodal sites not often seen in Hodgkin's disease: Waldeyer's ring, mesenteric nodes, and lymphoid patches in the gastrointestinal tract. (Waldeyer's ring involvement may herald simultaneous involvement of the GI tract in 20% of cases.) As in Hodgkin's disease, "B" symptoms of fever, night sweats, or weight loss may be present, but are the exception rather than the rule.

The histologic diversity of NHL requires that precise pathologic subclassification be performed by the pathologist. For this reason, incisional or excisional tissue biopsy of abnormal nodal sites or affected organs is always preferable to fine-needle aspiration. Large-bore core needle biopsy is occasionally helpful, but the optimum diagnosis is usually established by the surgical removal of the greatest quantity of tissue within the confines of good clinical sense. Radical surgical procedures to remove whole viscera are rarely indicated and should be avoided unless absolutely essential for patient well-being.

The increasing reliance on molecular markers, immuno-histochemical staining, and cytogenetics by pathologists requires that the pathologist be notified when a biopsy of suspected lymphomatous tissue is undertaken. When the diagnosis is established, staging procedures are then addressed. Besides a history directed toward possible etiologic factors, "B" symptoms, and general organ-specific complaints, a thorough physical examination (including inspection of Waldeyer's ring, all nodal sites, skin, and the testes), is required.

Routine laboratory studies are required: complete blood count, liver chemistries, lactate dehydrogenase (LDH), renal function, and calcium. Computerized axial tomography scans of the abdomen and the pelvis (or alternatively, a chest radiograph) and CAT scans should be obtained, as well as bilateral bone marrow biopsies. Staging laparotomy is never required in the evaluation. Additional studies (bone scans, MRI scans, and lumbar puncture) should be reserved for special situations and should be discussed with the oncologist.

Staging of Non-Hodgkin's Lymphomas

Treatment of NHL is much less driven by stage than by histologic type. Nonetheless, the Ann Arbor Staging classification is usually ascribed to non-Hodgkin's lymphomas (see Hodgkin's disease above), although this system lacks clinical relevance under many circumstances. Recently, a new international staging system has been devised specifically for patients with aggressive lymphomas:

- International Staging System: Adverse prognostic features
  - Age >60
  - Ann Arbor Stage >II
  - Performance status >2
  - Elevated LDH
  - Extranodal involvement >1 site
- Applies to aggressive lymphoma
- Outcome worsens with higher number of adverse prognostic factors

In this system, patients are evaluated according to:

- Ann Arbor stage
- Age
- Performance status
- Serum LDH
- Number of involved extranodal sites

Patients are considered to be at greater risk for treatment failure with the following characteristics:

- Age >60
- Performance status greater than two
- Elevated serum LDH
- Stage greater than II
- More than one extranodal disease site

As expected, failure to achieve remission and survival decreases with increasing numbers of these risk factors. Patients who fall into poor-prognosis subgroups may be considered for experimental therapeutic protocols.

PATHOLOGICAL CLASSIFICATION OF NON-HODGKIN'S LYMPHOMA

The Working Formulation for lymphoma classification, developed in 1982, remains the mainstay of pathologic classification. However, it fails to encompass many unusual types of lymphoma and does not account for the molecular and immunochemical diagnostic aids used by modern pathologists. A new classification, the REAL classification, attempts to reorganize lymphoma classification according to these diagnostic methods, although clinicians continue to rely heavily on the Working Formulation in making clinical decisions.

It is neither necessary nor helpful to memorize these classification systems. A simplified version of the Working Formulation provides a framework for treatment considerations:

- Low-grade non-Hodgkin's lymphoma
  - Small lymphocytic (5%)
  - Follicular, small cleaved cell (25%)
  - Follicular, mixed small cleaved and large cell (15%)
- Intermediate-grade non-Hodgkin's lymphoma
  - Follicular, large cell (5%)
  - Diffuse, small-cleaved cell (10%)
  - Diffuse, mixed small-cleaved and large cell (10%)
  - Diffuse, large cell (cleaved or noncleaved) (30%)
- High-grade non-Hodgkin's lymphoma
  - Diffuse, large cell, immunoblastic type (<5%)
  - Lymphoblastic (<5%)
  - Small, noncleaved cell (Burkitt or non-Burkitt) (<5%)

For our purposes, one should consider lymphomas as low, intermediate, or high grade, as most treatment paradigms are chosen based on this distinction.

TREATMENT OF NON-HODGKIN'S LYMPHOMA

Low-Grade Lymphomas

Treatment options for low-grade lymphoma include:

- Early-stage treatment
  - Radiation therapy
- Advanced-stage treatment
  - Observation until symptoms appear
  - Oral alkylating agents
  - Combination chemotherapy
  - Fludarabine
  - Bone-marrow transplant

Under most circumstances, low-grade lymphomas will not be curable by any means. Instead, treatment should be directed at symptom relief. Although many, if not most, low-grade NHL patients will present with advanced stage (III or IV) disease, treatment is not mandatory for asymptomatic patients. Patients with low-grade lymphoma treated by observation alone (reserving treatment for symptomatic indications), will usually respond well to therapy and will have a median survival of 7–8 years. Chemotherapy may cause rapid disease remission when it is given to asymptomatic patients, but it is not curative and thus will not prolong survival when compared with patients first treated by observation alone. A possible

exception to this approach is the rare patient with low-grade lymphoma presenting with Stage I or II disease. These patients may experience prolonged disease-free survival when treated with radiation therapy alone. Such patients account for only 10% of all low-grade lymphoma patients.

When treatment is required for low-grade lymphoma, a variety of treatment options is available. Oral alkylating agents, such as chlorambucil or cytoxan, will induce remissions in the majority of patients, while combination chemotherapy programs, such as CVP (e.g., cytoxan, vincristine, and prednisone), may be reserved for patients who require more aggressive therapy. Newer agents, such as fludarabine, may have equivalent activity to oral alkylating agents and may be used as first-line or second-line therapy. Treatments of this type will produce remissions in the majority of patients, although the duration of these remissions will generally be less than 2 years. Younger patients with low-grade lymphoma, whose survival overall will necessarily be compromised despite the generally indolent behavior of their disease, may be considered for programs using high-dose chemotherapy with autologous or allogeneic stem-cell or bone-marrow transplantation. The long-term results of this approach are uncertain, however.

Intermediate-Grade Lymphomas

These lymphomas should be treated with curative intent. Treatment options for intermediate-grade lymphomas include:

- Early stage: Chemotherapy [cyclophosphamide (Cytoxan), hydroxydaunomycin (Adriamycin), Oncovin (vincristine), and prednisone (CHOP)], plus radiation
- Advanced stage: Chemotherapy (CHOP)

Although some patients with Stage I and II lymphomas are curable with radiation therapy alone, present care standards mandate that patients with early-stage lymphomas of this type receive 3–6 months of aggressive combination chemotherapy. The addition of radiation therapy to sites of disease involvement (rather than the large fields employed in the treatment of Hodgkin's disease) may improve the survival of early-stage patients.

Patients with more-advanced-stage disease (e.g., stage II with bulky disease greater than 10 cm and all stage III and IV) should receive combination chemotherapy for a period of approximately 6 months. Although the optimum chemotherapy regimen has not been defined, the "standard" regimen remains CHOP. More complex and more aggressive regimens have been devised for the treatment of intermediate grade NHL, however, none have clearly proven superior to CHOP.

The results of treatment in intermediate-grade NHL are stage-dependent. Patients with early-stage disease may be cured > 75% of the time, while cure rates for more advanced-stage patients will range from 30–50%.

High-Grade Lymphomas

Treatment paradigms for high grade lymphomas are modeled after treatment programs for pediatric patients:

- More aggressive treatments
- More frequent treatments
- Longer durations of therapy
- Larger numbers of drugs than employed in the CHOP regimen (CHOP therapy is inadequate in high-grade NHL.)

The patterns of presentation of high-grade NHL are variable and usually related to the development of symptoms in the anatomic regions occupied by these aggressive, rapidly growing masses. The lymphoblastic lymphoma, one subtype of high-grade NHL, is a T-cell neoplasm that usually presents with a mediastinal mass. Consequently, it must be considered in the differential diagnosis of such masses, along with Hodgkin's disease and diffuse large-cell NHL of the intermediate grade type.

All high-grade NHL have a propensity to relapse in the central nervous system (CNS); therefore, prophylactic treatment of the CNS with intrathecal chemotherapy, or less favorably, with radiation therapy, is a mandatory part of high-grade NHL management. Patients with poor prognostic features, such as bone-marrow involvement or an elevated serum LDH, will often be subjected to high-dose chemotherapy and autologous or allogeneic-stem-cell or bone marrow transplantation.

Like intermediate grade lymphomas, high-grade NHL should be treated with intent to cure. Although the overall cure rate for this disease subtype may approach only 50%, patients with limited-stage disease may be cured up to 90% of the time with appropriate therapy.

PROGNOSIS FOR NON-HODGKINS LYMPHOMA

Relapsed Disease

Disease relapses after treatment, expected in low-grade NHL, are generally treated with alternative chemotherapies in the considerable therapeutic armamentarium for these patients. Relapses after CHOP chemotherapy in intermediate-grade disease, however, have a very poor prognosis. This group of patients will often receive "salvage" chemotherapy with alternative agents; if they respond, they may be subjected to high-dose chemotherapy with autologous-stem-cell transplantation. Long-term remission rates of up to 50% have been reported for such patients, although 20–30% long-term remission may be a more realistic figure.

Transformed Disease

Any low-grade lymphoma is capable of transformation to a higher histologic grade. Such transformation, said to occur in 15–30% of low-grade NHL, is unrelated to prior therapy for low-grade disease. Patients typically will transform to an intermediate-grade NHL and will require treatment with CHOP chemotherapy or an equivalent regimen. Most of these patients will respond to appropriate treatment, but their curabil-

ity remains in question because of presumed persistence of low-grade elements.

Gastric Mucosally-Associated Lymphoid Tissue lymphoma

A particular subtype of low-grade B-cell lymphoma, known as mucosally-associated lymphoid tissue (MALT), may occur in the stomach and is frequently associated with H. pylori infection. Some patients with gastric MALT lymphoma and associated H. pylori infection have been treated with antibiotic therapy alone, leading in most cases to regression of lymphoma. This approach is best reserved for small lymphomas of this type and is not applicable to other histologies of gastric lymphoma.

HIV-ASSOCIATED MALIGNANCIES

Although many types of malignancies have been observed in AIDS patients, a true "causal" relationship between the malignancy in question and the HIV infection, the immunosuppressed state, or the sexual practices associated with HIV infection, has been defined for only three malignancies:

- Kaposi's sarcoma
- Non-Hodgkin's lymphoma
- Cervical carcinoma

KAPOSI'S SARCOMA

The development of this rare malignancy in homosexual men in the early 1980s helped spawn the clinical investigation that eventually led to the discovery of the pathogen responsible for the HIV syndrome. The frequency of Kaposi's sarcoma (KS) as the initial manifestation of AIDS has declined markedly since the mid-1980s and is now reported to be the index clinical manifestation in only 13% of patients. As of 1992, just 9% of HIV patients were known to develop this disease.

ETIOLOGY, EPIDEMIOLOGY, AND PATHOGENESIS OF KAPOSI'S SARCOMA

Kaposi's Sarcoma, in association with HIV infection, is essentially a disease of homosexual men, with more than 95% of the cases occurring in this risk group. The epidemiology of this neoplasm suggests a sexually transmitted "cofactor" as cause: it is seen predominantly in men practicing anal intercourse, it is more common in women who have had intercourse with bisexual men, and it is seen occasionally in men at risk for HIV (but without documentable HIV infection). The overall incidence of KS is declining among homosexual men, a fact perhaps attributable to "safe sex" practices.

The pathogenesis of KS in HIV patients is uncertain. The true cell of origin has not been fully defined, although indirect evidence suggests that it is of mesenchymal origin. In fact, KS may or may not be truly "clonal" as one would expect in human malignancy. Neither HIV infection alone nor the immunosuppressed state can adequately explain the origin and proliferation of KS, and recent evidence implicates a novel human herpes virus as cause, HHV8.

CLINICAL PRESENTATION OF KAPOSI'S SARCOMA

Human immunodificiency virus-associated KS is usually multicentric and may present in a variety of ways. The typical presentation is that of a small, red-to-purplish nodule on the skin, particularly in sun-exposed areas. Tumors may become patchy or plaque-like and may proliferate rapidly over the skin. The propensity for KS to involve the head and neck may cause such eruptions on the face, nose, oropharynx, or cervical nodes.

Lymphatic involvement may frequently lead to facial disfigurement from lymphedema, and the same phenomenon may cause significant morbidity in the legs and groin. In addition to nodal involvement, the gastrointestinal (GI) tract and lungs are the most common visceral sites of KS involvement. Gastrointestinal lesions, which may occur in up to half of KS patients, are less ominous than pulmonary lesions. Involvement of the GI mucosa may cause bleeding or, less often, obstruction; involvement of the biliary tract may cause obstruction and cholangitis. Pulmonary involvement may present with dyspnea with or without fever, and radiographic manifestations, which may include reticulonodular infiltrates, pleural effusions, or hilar nodes, is of dismal prognostic significance.

Diagnosis of Kaposi's Sarcoma

The diagnosis of KS is usually confirmed by punch biopsy of cutaneous lesions or instrument biopsies of GI or oral lesions. Lymph node excision may replace instrument biopsies, and the biopsy of pulmonary lesions should be avoided, because of hemorrhagic potential, if other sites are available for investigation. Many times, if bronchoscopy is necessary, the diagnosis is confirmed on clinical grounds alone owing to the characteristic appearance of the mucosal lesions.

Staging evaluation should include a thorough physical examination with attention to the oral cavity, anorectal region, nodal sites, and skin. A chest radiograph should be obtained, but no other radiographic studies are routinely necessary in the absence of clinical indications. Kaposi's Sarcoma does not lend itself to conventional staging evaluation. A method of staging proposed by the National Institute of Allergy and Infectious Diseases AIDS Clinical Trials Group follows:

- Good risk
  - Tumor
  - Confined to skin, nodes, or minimal oral disease
  - Immunity
  - CD4 count >200
  - Systemic symptoms

- No oral infections, including thrush
- No "B" symptoms
- Karnofsky PS >70
- Poor risk
  - Tumor
  - Any edema or ulceration
  - Extensive oral disease
  - GI or other visceral involvement
  - Immunity
  - CD4 count <200
  - Systemic symptoms
  - Oral infections present, "B" symptoms present
  - Karnofsky PS <70, any other AIDS manifestations

A poor prognosis is portended by:

- Lower CD4 counts
- Systemic "B" symptoms
- Prior opportunistic infections

Clinicians should keep in mind the fact that rapid proliferation of KS is often a harbinger of opportunistic infection and that such infections (not KS per se) remain the leading cause of AIDS mortality.

Treatment of Kaposi's Sarcoma

Treatment options for Kaposi's sarcoma include:

- Minimal disease
  - Observation appropriate
- Cosmetic problems, local symptoms
  - Radiation therapy
  - Cryotherapy
  - Intralesional vinblastine
- Extensive skin disease, nonthreatening visceral disease
  - Interferon
  - Extensive visceral disease
  - Single-agent chemotherapy
  - Combination chemotherapy
  - Liposome-encapsulated Adriamycin

Under some circumstances, KS lesions will remain indolent for many months and will not require any therapy. Since KS will account for only 10% of AIDS related deaths, therapy should be reserved for those who suffer significant cosmetic compromise, significant local symptoms, or who have widely disseminated, disease-causing, systemic symptoms. As responses to therapy are directly related to the CD4 count, optimization of the patients' antiretroviral therapy is mandatory before considering therapy, and excessively immunosuppressive therapies should be avoided.

When local therapy is considered for cosmetically significant lesions or for palliation of local symptoms, treatment with radiation therapy, intralesional vinblastine, or topical cryotherapy with liquid nitrogen can be considered. The local toxicity of radiation therapy to the oral and rectal mucosa is enhanced in these patients, a fact that should be taken into account before selecting this treatment.

Systemic treatment is reserved for those with widespread cutaneous disease for whom local therapies are impractical, or for those with symptomatic visceral disease. Interferon-alpha is particularly useful in patients with high CD4 counts and no opportunistic infections, and may produce response rates of 80% in this patient group. Cytotoxic chemotherapy, using single agents (such as vinblastine, vincristine, adriamycin, bleomycin or etoposide), may produce responses in 30–75% of patients and can be well tolerated. Combinations of adriamycin, bleomycin, and vinblastine have produced responses in the 90% range and should be considered in patients with life-threatening disease. The most recent chemotherapeutic advance in KS chemotherapy is liposome-encapsulated doxorubicin, in which response rates upwards of 70% have been described in a less toxic setting. In general, these patients should all receive prophylactic therapy against pneumocystis carinii.

Human immunodeficiency virus-associated KS is not a curable malignancy, and clinical trials do not generally suggest an improvement in survival. The palliative nature of these treatments should be kept in mind when making treatment selections.

NON-HODGKIN'S LYMPHOMA

The majority of lymphomas in the AIDS population are of B-cell origin, and are of the intermediate-grade to high-grade type. Low-grade lymphomas, which are rarely seen, by themselves do not constitute an AIDS-defining illness.

Etiology, Epidemiology, and Pathogenesis of Non-Hodgkin's Lymphoma

The occurrence of an intermediate-grade or high-grade NHL in an HIV-infected patient is an AIDS-defining illness in the absence of opportunistic infection or KS. Non-Hodgkin's lymphomas are the second most common malignancy in the AIDS population, and up to 10% of individuals with AIDS will ultimately develop NHL. The majority of these patients are homosexual and bisexual men, but unlike KS, HIV-associated NHL is known to occur in all AIDS risk groups, including IV drug users and hemophiliacs. In fact, the risk of developing NHL may be highest in HIV-infected hemophiliacs.

HIV infection per se is not the cause of NHL, but the consequences of the immunosuppressed state are responsible in a variety of possible ways. HIV-associated NHLs are not exactly like those seen in other immunosuppressed groups because:

* Not all HIV-associated NHLs are associated with EBV
* Burkitt lymphomas, while relatively common in HIV, are not seen in other groups
* HIV-associated NHLs have an unusual tendency to present in extranodal sites

It is hypothesized that the development of NHL will be affected by some combination of:

* EBV-induced or other microbially-induced B-cell polyclonal expansion
* Oncogene rearrangements
* HIV-induced cytokine stimulation of B-cell proliferation
* Suppression of T-cell surveillance

Clinical Presentation and Diagnosis of Non-Hodgkin's Lymphoma

Just as there exists no classic presenting pattern in non-HIV NHL, the same holds true in HIV-associated NHL, with the picture even more confounded by the unique ability of the latter NHL to present in extranodal sites. Approximately two-thirds of NHL patients will have an extranodal site at presentation, including the following common sites (virtually no site is spared):

* Bone marrow
* CNS
* GI tract
* Liver
* Anorectal mucosa
* Oropharynx

The CNS is the primary site of involvement in up to 20% of patients, including either brain parenchyma proper or the leptomeninges.

The predominant histologic subtypes of lymphoma in the HIV population are the Burkitt (small noncleaved cell) lymphomas, and large-cell lymphomas, either conventional or immunoblastic subtype. The various distribution of these subtypes varies among reports, but one can assume that 20–40% of these lymphomas will be of the Burkitt type, while the remainder will be of the large-cell variety. Virtually all of the primary CNS lymphomas are of the large-cell or large-cell-immunoblastic subtype.

The diagnostic workup of these patients should follow patterns established for non-HIV NHL. However, the frequency of "B" symptoms in these patients (80%) will often be confused with symptoms produced by other AIDS manifestations. Tissue biopsy is mandatory for diagnosis. As most of these lymphomas have a diffuse pattern of growth, fine-needle aspirates may be of greater value, although their use is discouraged in other patients with NHL. The staging evaluation should likewise follow that for other NHL patients, with the addition of particular attention to the CNS. Imaging studies of the brain for space-occupying lesions should be obtained routinely; if negative, lumbar puncture for the presence of leptomeningeal disease should be performed. Blood CD4 counts, which will have some prognostic significance in these patients, should also be obtained.

Patients with isolated CNS lesions present a particularly vexing problem in management, as most isolated CNS lesions in HIV patients are caused by toxoplasmosis, not NHL. Patients with this finding as their only disease manifestation may be treated expectantly with antimicrobial therapy, with biopsy of the lesion encouraged within two weeks if clinical improvement does not occur.

Treatment of Non-Hodgkin's Lymphoma

As HIV-associated NHL patients have an underlying incurable condition, treatment of NHL should be tempered by:

- Thoughtful evaluation of comorbid conditions
- Opportunistic infections
- Life expectancy

Untreated patients will usually die within 6 months of either lymphoma or other complications of AIDS.

In general, conventional chemotherapeutic approaches have been disappointing because of drastically reduced response rates (20–30%) and exacerbation of opportunistic infections by the immunosuppressive effects of chemotherapy. Overall, dose-intense approaches to treatment in these patients should be avoided. In fact, randomized trials have proven no advantage of conventional chemotherapeutic approaches over "low-dose" approaches specifically designed for these patients. Such a restrictive approach to treatment may not be appropriate, however, for patients with CD4 counts >200, and who have no other manifestations of AIDS.

Several general remarks may be made. The use of hematopoetic growth factors (G-CSF or GM-CSF) should be considered routine in these patients, as should infection prophylaxis. For patients presenting with no evidence of CNS involvement (60–80% of patients), prophylactic therapy of the CNS with intrathecal chemotherapy should be applied, particularly in patients with marrow involvement. Chemotherapy in standard doses should be used in patients with no other comorbid conditions, CD4 counts >200, and good performance status. Patients otherwise should receive a low-dose approach to therapy, with the expectation that responses will be limited and their duration short. Finally, severely ill patients with significant comorbid conditions and CD4 counts <100 may be candidates for supportive care without chemotherapy.

The same approach should be considered for patients with primary CNS lymphoma. These patients tend to be more compromised at diagnosis with lower CD4 counts (<100), and have more advanced underlying HIV disease. Their prognosis is generally poorer, and treatment should be restricted to steroids or radiation therapy designed to bring about short-term relief of CNS symptoms. The rare patient with CNS lymphoma and good performance status, with CD4 count >200, may be considered for a program of both radiation and chemotherapy.

Few patients with HIV-associated NHL will be cured. Patients with primary CNS lymphoma will have a median survival of less than 6 months, while patients with systemic lymphoma will have a median survival of less than a year. However, as response rates as high as 75% have been reported for good-risk patients, the palliative benefit of systemic chemotherapy remains a viable treatment option for many patients.

CERVICAL CARCINOMA

Cervix cancer in HIV-infected women was declared an AIDS-defining illness in 1993. It is assumed that the etiology and pathogenesis of cervix cancer in these patients relates to the transmission of oncogenic strains of human papillomavirus (HPV) through sexual practices, compounded by the immunosuppressive effects of the HIV-infected state.

EPIDEMIOLOGY OF CERVIX CARCINOMA

The female cervix is uniquely susceptible to infection with various strains of HPV:

- HIV-infected women may have not only higher rates of infection with HPV, but may be more susceptible to infection with the oncogenic subtypes of HPV.
- A significant percentage of young women with abnormal pap smears, preinvasive cervix cancer, and invasive cervix cancer may be HIV-seropositive in the absence of AIDS manifestations (up to 20%).
- Women known to be HIV-seropositive will have a high incidence of abnormal pap smears (up to 60%), cervical dysplasia (up to 40%), and most disturbingly, evidence of cervical intraepithelial neoplasia (CIN), despite a normal pap smear.

It is estimated that the risk of developing CIN may be as high as 50% in HIV patients. These noninvasive lesions tend to be more extensive and of higher grade than in non-HIV populations and seem to occur more often in women with lower CD4 counts.

Diagnosis and Treatment of Cervix Carcinoma

The prevalence of abnormal Pap smears in these patients has led to recommendations for screening at 6-month intervals for women infected with HIV. The failure of Pap smears to detect all cases of CIN has led some investigators to suggest routine screening colposcopy rather than Pap smears only.

Therapy of preinvasive disease using standard techniques of cryotherapy, conization, and laser therapy have been disappointing, as recurrence rates are high, and may exceed 50% for patients with CD4 counts under 50. Rates of transformation to invasive carcinoma are, in turn, higher than in non-HIV patients. A variety of new treatment strategies, including topical fluorouracil and interferons, are under investigation.

Patients with invasive cervical cancer and HIV infection have a higher recurrence rate and death rate than their non-HIV counterparts. As expected, patients with lower CD4 counts have a distinctly poorer outcome. Treatment strategies using either surgery, radiotherapy, or chemotherapy, based on stage of invasive cancer (which should mirror strategies employed in non-HIV patients), are beyond the scope of this chapter.

REVIEW EXERCISES

QUESTIONS

1. Which one of the following diagnostic procedures is most reliable in rendering the diagnosis of Hodgkin's Disease?

    a. Fine-needle aspiration of lymph node tissue
    b. Core-needle biopsy of lymph node tissue
    c. Excisional biopsy of lymph node tissue
    d. Bone-marrow biopsy

2. Which of the following is *not* a significant prognostic factor in patients with intermediate-grade non-Hodgkin's lymphoma?

    a. Age
    b. Serum LDH level
    c. Sex
    d. Ann Arbor stage

3. A thirty-year-old homosexual man presents with a 6 mm purplish lesion on the right cheek. Punch biopsy confirms Kaposi's sarcoma. The patient is seropositive for HIV, has a CD4 count of 498/ul, and has no other lesions on physical examination or chest radiograph. Which of the following does *not* constitute an acceptable therapeutic option for this patient:

    a. Intralesional vinblastine
    b. Cryotherapy with topical nitrogen mustard
    c. Observation without treatment
    d. Liposome-encapsulated doxorubicin

Answers

1. c

2. c

3. d

SUGGESTED READING

HODGKIN'S DISEASE

Canellos G, et al: Chemotherapy of advanced Hodgkin's disease with MOPP, ABVD, or MOPP alternating with ABVD. New Engl J Med 1992;327:1478.

DeVita V, Hubbard S: Hodgkin's disease. New Engl J Med 1993:328:560.

Mauch P: Controversies in the management of early stage Hodgkin's disease. Blood 1994;83:318.

Urba W, Longo D: Hodgkin's disease. New Engl J Med 1993; 328:678.

Van Leeuwen F, et al: Second cancer risk following Hodgkin's disease: A 20-year follow-up study. J Clin Oncol 1993; 11:2342.

NON-HODGKIN'S LYMPHOMA

Aisenberg A. Coherent view of Non-Hodgkin's lymphoma. J Clin Oncol 1995;13:2656.

Fisher R, et al: Comparison of a standard regimen (CHOP) with three intensive chemotherapy regimens for advanced Non-Hodgkin's lymphoma. New Engl J Med 1993;328:1002.

Harris N, et al: A revised European-American classification of lymphoid neoplasms: a proposal from the International Lymphoma Study Group. Blood 1994;84:1361.

The International Non-Hodgkin's Lymphoma Prognostic Factors Project. A predictive model for aggressive Non-Hodgkin's lymphoma. New Engl J Med 1993;329:987.

Nimer, S. et al: Bone marrow transplantation versus chemotherapy in Non-Hodgkin's lymphoma. New Engl J Med 1995; 333:728.

HIV-ASSOCIATED MALIGNANCIES

Bogner J, et al: Liposomal doxorubicin in the treatment of advanced AIDS-related Kaposi's sarcoma. J AIDS 1994;7: 463.

Kaplan, L. Human immunodeficiency virus associated neoplasia: changing spectrum? J Clin Oncol 1995;13:2684.

Maiman M, et al: HIV infection and invasive cervical carcinoma. Cancer 1993;71:402.

Mitsuyasu, R: Clinical aspects of AIDS-related Kaposi's sarcoma. Curr Opin Oncol 1993;5:835.

Pluda J, et al: Parameters affecting the development of non-Hodgkin's lymphoma in patients with severe human immunodeficiency virus infection receiving antiretroviral therapy. J Clin Oncol 1993;11:1099.

Reynolds P, et al: The spectrum of acquired immunodeficiency syndrome (AIDS)-associated malignancies in San Francisco 1980–1987. Am J Epidemiol 1993;37:19.

Board Simulation I: Hematology and Medical Oncology

Brian J. Bolwell

REVIEW OF PLASMA CELL DISORDERS

Plasma cell disorders are a group of neoplastic or potentially neoplastic diseases of plasma cells. The clinical manifestations of plasma cell disorders result from the uncontrolled and progressive proliferation of the cells, the effect of their replacement of normal bone marrow, and the manifestations of the overproduction of certain proteins.

Plasma cell disorders are characterized by the secretion of monoclonal proteins (M protein, or paraprotein). An M protein can be present when the total protein concentration and quantitative immunoglobulin values are within normal limits. The presence of an M protein suggests monoclonal gammopathy of undetermined significance (MGUS), multiple myeloma, primary amyloidosis, Waldenström's macroglobulinemia, or other lymphoproliferative diseases.

MONOCLONAL GAMMOPATHY OF UNDETERMINED SIGNIFICANCE

Monoclonal gammopathy of undetermined significance (MGUS) is a diagnosis of exclusion. It is characterized by:

- Serum and paraprotein concentration less than 3 gm/dl
- Fewer than 5% plasma cells in the bone marrow
- Absence of lytic bone lesions and renal insufficiency
- No other evidence of multiple myeloma
- Stability over time

A review from the Mayo Clinic described 851 patients presenting with a serum M protein (see Kyle and Lust, 1989). Two-thirds of these patients had MGUS as a clinical diagnosis:

MGUS	66%
Multiple myeloma (MM)	12%
Amyloidosis (AL)	9%
Non-Hodgkin's Lymphoma (NHL)	6%

Immunoglobulin G was the most common paraprotein, followed by IgM and IgA. Monoclonal gammopathy of undetermined significance is common, with 1% of the United States population more than age 50 having an abnormal paraprotein and 3% more than age 70.

The Mayo Clinic also has analyzed the long-term outcome of 241 MGUS patients (see Kyle, 1993). Median age at presentation was 64. Median M protein was 1.7 gm/dl. The outcome of the patients was as follows:

No change	24%
Progressed to MM, AL	22%
Died of unrelated cause	51%

Median time to progression was eight years: the longer patients lived, the more likely the risk of progression. Seventeen percent of the population had progressed at 10 years; thirty-three percent of the population had progressed at 20 years.

MGUS has no specific therapy; patients should have their protein values monitored every 3-12 months.

MULTIPLE MYELOMA

Multiple myeloma is characterized by neoplastic proliferation of a single clone of plasma cells. These abnormal cells grow in bone marrow and frequently directly invade adjacent skeletal tissue, resulting in bone destruction. The median age at presentation is 61. Multiple myeloma represents 1% of all malignancies. Eighteen to thirty-six percent of patients have cytogenetic abnormalities of the bone marrow. Interleukin 6 (IL-6) is a major myeloma cell growth factor in vivo and in vitro.

The clinical manifestations of myeloma can be divided into the following four broad categories:

1. Plasma cell growth in bone marrow:

    a. Hematologic changes

b. Bone destruction

c. Neurologic abnormalities

2. Immune deficiency

3. M protein itself

a. Hyperviscosity

b. Amyloid

c. Clotting disorder

4. Renal failure

Skeletal Disease and Plasma Cell Growth in Bone Marrow

The most common presenting symptom of multiple myeloma is bone pain. This most commonly involves the spine. The pain is often "rheumatic." The characteristic bone changes are lytic lesions (rounded, punched out areas of bones), most commonly in vertebral bodies, the skull, ribs, pelvis, humerus, and femur. Occasionally diffuse osteoporosis is seen on radiographs. Bone scans may or may not accurately reflect the destruction seen on plain x-ray films. It is likely that the mechanism of formation of lytic bone lesions is related to the release and interaction of a variety of cytokines. In early myeloma, osteoblastic recruitment and activation has been observed which may be related to a release of IL-1 and/or tumor necrosis factor (TNF) from myeloma cells. Osteoblasts in turn release large amounts of Interleukin 6, which is a myeloma cell growth factor that further stimulates the production of myeloma cells. Interleukin 6 also stimulates osteoclast formation. All these factors act in concert to promote excessive bone resorption, ultimately leading to osteolytic lesions.

A solitary plasmacytoma is found in 2% of patients. Solitary plasmacytomas usually present in vertebral bodies. Conventional treatment consists of radiation therapy. However, most patients ultimately progress to multiple myeloma. Disease-free survival at 10 years is only 15–25%.

Most of the neurologic abnormalities of multiple myeloma are a result of direct extension of the tumor from skeletal disease. Ten percent have spinal cord compression and many have nerve root compression. Peripheral neuropathy is not common and is usually caused by amyloidosis or hyperviscosity.

Hematologically, most patients ultimately develop anemia. This is generally secondary to poor red cell production. Rouleaux is often present, resulting from the increased amount of globulin in the plasma. Total leukocyte count is often normal, but mild neutropenia occurs in up to 50% of patients. Thrombocytopenia often develops at some point during the disease, either from the myeloma itself or from repeated courses of chemotherapy. When plasma cells predominate among the circulating white blood cells, the condition is known as plasma cell leukemia. This typically represents a terminal stage of the disease and is associated with a very short survival. Primary plasma cell leukemia, unlike multiple myeloma, is associated with lymphadenopathy, splenomeg-

aly, and fewer lytic bone lesions. Sixty percent of patients with plasma cell leukemia present as a primary manifestation of the disease, and 40% present as a transformation of multiple myeloma.

Immunologic Abnormalities

Myeloma patients often suffer repeated bouts of infection. The spectrum of infections is similar to those seen in patients with reduced levels of normal immunoglobulins. Encapsulated organisms, such as *Streptococcus pneumoniae* and *Hemophilus influenzae,* are frequent pathogens. After disease progression and therapy, *Staphylococcus aureus* is a common pathogen. More recent reports suggest that gram-negative organisms now account for up to 50% of septic events later in multiple myeloma.

Besides decreased levels of immunoglobulin, abnormalities of B-cells and T-cells exist, along with a loss of surface-immunoglobulin-positive B-cells. CD4 T-cell levels also are often reduced.

Effect of Abnormal Paraprotein

The hyperviscosity syndrome results from the presence of serum proteins with a high intrinsic viscosity. This is most commonly seen in Waldenström's macroglobulinemia, but it may occur in multiple myeloma with IgG or IgA paraprotein. The high viscosity interferes with efficient circulation to the brain, eyes, kidneys, and extremities. Headaches are common. Dizziness, vertigo, and symptoms as severe as stupor and coma can result secondary to intracerebral vascular occlusions. Seizures may develop. Peripheral neuropathy may result secondary to occlusive changes in small vessels. Occasionally, cardiac failure occurs. High levels of M protein can interfere with coagulation factors and lead to abnormal platelet aggregation and abnormal platelet function. Bruising and purpura are common. Bleeding from the mucous membranes of the mouth, nose, and intestinal tract may also be seen.

Renal Failure

Ninety percent of patients with multiple myeloma have proteinuria. Abnormal light chains (Bence-Jones protein) are present in 80% of patients. Fifty percent of patients have an elevated creatinine level at diagnosis. Proximal tubules are increasingly damaged by the large protein load. Additionally, large obstructing casts form along tubules. The combination of hyaline casts surrounded by epithelial cells or multinucleated giant cells, with interstitial fibrosis, constitutes the picture of "myeloma kidney." Besides Bence-Jones proteinuria, other factors are important causes of renal dysfunction: hypercalcemia and hypercalciuria secondary to bone destruction and immobilization, and hyperuricemia resulting from increased cellular turnover exists. Nephrotoxic drugs such as nonsteroidal anti-inflammatory drugs may precipitate renal failure. Finally, dehydration may exacerbate renal dysfunction.

Diagnosis of Multiple Myeloma

The criteria for a diagnosis of multiple myeloma are shown below:

I. A. Marrow >10% of plasma cells
    B. Plasmacytoma
II. A. Serum M Protein
    B. Urine M Protein
    C. Osteolytic bone lesions
IA or B + IIA, B, or C = Multiple Myeloma

Treatment and Prognosis of Multiple Myeloma

Radiation therapy is the treatment of choice for painful bone lesions. Radiation therapy is also indicated for lesions that impair the function of vital structures. For the overall treatment of multiple myeloma, chemotherapy is the treatment of choice. Most chemotherapeutic protocols employ alkylating agents. It is currently controversial whether multiple alkylating agents are superior to the standard Melphalan/Prednisone regimen. There is a 60% response rate with most chemotherapeutic schedules. Newer schedules using continuous infusion of Vincristine, Adriamycin, and Dexamethasone (VAD) may lead to improved response rates. Generally, chemotherapy is continued for about 12 months, and then stopped when paraprotein levels are stable. Newer therapy with both autologous and allogeneic bone marrow transplantation are promising in younger patients. The best results are seen in those treated earlier in the course of their disease.

Multiple myeloma is not curable with standard therapy, and the prognosis of multiple myeloma is generally poor. Survival is 6 months without therapy. The median survival with therapy is 2–3 years. Beta 2 microglobulin levels of less than 4 mg/ml correlate with a good prognosis. Beta 2 microglobulin levels greater than 6 mg/ml portend a poor prognosis. Prognosis is best with IgM disease and is worst with IgD myeloma. An elevated lactate dehydrogenase (LDH) level is associated with a poor prognosis.

WALDENSTRÖM'S MACROGLOBULINEMIA

Macroglobulinemia is a term used to describe a variety of clinical conditions associated with an abnormal M protein of IgM type. The primary disorder is Waldenström's macroglobulinemia, in which a clonal proliferation of abnormal lymphocytes with or without plasma cells leads to production of IgM paraprotein. Occasionally, an abnormal IgM paraprotein can be associated with non-Hodgkin's lymphoma. Low levels of IgM may be seen in MGUS.

The median age at presentation for Waldenström's macroglobulinemia is 65 years old. Symptoms are often related to hyperviscosity and include headaches, weakness, and bleeding. Forty percent present with hepatomegaly or splenomegaly. Thirty percent have lymphadenopathy. Seventeen percent have neurologic dysfunction. Renal disorders are not common in Waldenström's macroglobulinemia.

Patients are often anemic at presentation. Usually, white blood cell counts are normal, although occasionally a leukemic phase of macroglobulinemia is seen. Thrombocytopenia is found in approximately 50% of patients. The bone marrow biopsy shows increased numbers of lympho-plasmacytoid cells. These cells more closely resemble lymphocytes than plasma or myeloma cells. Less frequently, patients have a marrow more characteristic of myeloma.

No treatment is usually necessary in the early stage of the disease. When symptoms develop, treatment consists of chemotherapy similar to that used in multiple myeloma. Plasmapheresis is recommended for symptoms associated with hyperviscosity. Newer drugs, such as Fludarabine and Pentostatin, have been shown to have high response rates in small clinical trials. The median survival of Waldenström's macroglobulinemia is only 4–5 years. Death is secondary to the progression of the neoplastic process, infections, or cardiac failure.

QUESTIONS

1. Which of the following is true of monoclonal gammopathy of undetermined significance (MGUS)?

   a. Marrow plasma cells > 20%
   b. Lytic bone lesions
   c. Majority progress to multiple myeloma
   d. Reciprocal decreased normal serum immunoglobulin levels
   e. Serum paraprotein less than 3 g/dl

2. What condition is characterized by the following levels?

NA	130
K+	4.0
CL	105
HCO3	24

   a. Multiple myeloma
   b. Acute myelogenous leukemia
   c. Large cell lymphoma
   d. Breast cancer

3. Which of the following is true of multiple myeloma?

   a. While most people develop renal failure during their disease, only 10% present with renal failure at diagnosis.
   b. In contrast to non-Hodgkin's lymphomas, an elevated LDH is not an adverse prognostic sign.
   c. Most patients presenting with a solitary plasmacytoma are cured with radiation therapy.
   d. Newer chemotherapeutic regimens such as VAD (Vincristine, Adriamycin, Dexamethasone) cure approximately 30% of patients.

e. The most common presenting symptom of multiple myeloma is bone pain.

Patient Information for Questions 4–7

A 28-year-old internal medicine resident on vacation walks into the ER complaining of dyspnea, low-grade fever, and fatigue. The symptoms have been progressive more than 4 weeks.

Physical examination reveals no lymphadenopathy. Lungs reveal scattered rhonchi.

Hemoglobin is 11.0, white blood cell count is 14,000 with 85% neutrophils, and platelet count is 420,000. Lactate dehydrogenase level is 390. Beta HCG and aFP are normal. A chest radiograph reveals a large mediastinal mass.

4. What is the most likely diagnosis?

   a. Germ cell tumor
   b. Lymphoma
   c. Thymoma
   d. Lung cancer
   e. Sarcoidosis

5. What is your next step?

   a. Needle biopsy of mediastinum
   b. Follow the patient closely and repeat chest radiograph in 2 weeks
   c. Bronchoscopy
   d. Mediastinoscopy
   e. Thoracotomy

6. If the patient's mediastinal mass showed compression of the trachea, the correct procedure would be:

   a. Bronchoscopy first
   b. Proceed with mediastinoscopy
   c. Thoracotomy
   d. Deliver prebiopsy radiation therapy
   e. Immediate combination chemotherapy

7. The patient relapses after attaining a complete remission. The appropriate management is:
   a. Repeat a course of original chemotherapy protocol
   b. Combination chemotherapy with different drugs
   c. High dose chemotherapy with autologous progenitor cell rescue (transplant) after a second remission is obtained

8. A 42-year-old woman with follicular small cleaved cell lymphoma has had waxing and waning cervical and axillary lymphadenopathy since the condition was diagnosed 3 years ago. The patient presents with fever and a 1-week history of a rapidly enlarging right anterior cervical mass. The patient has a 4 × 6 cm mass on the right anterior cervical change and bilateral 1 × 2 cm axillary and inguinal enlarged lymph nodes. Except for a hemoglobin level of 10 and modestly elevated LDH, the results of laboratory studies are normal.

Which of the following would you recommend next?

   a. Combination chemotherapy
   b. CT scan of the abdomen
   c. Irradiation of the cervical mass
   d. Biopsy of the cervical mass
   e. CT scan of the neck

9. The following are toxicities of cisplatin except:

   a. Renal failure
   b. Decreased hearing
   c. Pulmonary fibrosis
   d. Myelosuppression
   e. Peripheral neuropathy

10. You have one last patient in clinic: a 30-year-old male with Stage IV Hodgkin's disease who is receiving MOPP chemotherapy (nitrogen mustard, vincristine, procarbazine, and prednisone). The patient's wife, who has never smiled in your presence, called this morning and demanded the patient be seen because he was "falling apart." You walk into the room and are greeted with a dazed look from the patient and a look of pure hatred from the spouse. You greet them as warmly as possible and ask what is the matter. The patient replies, "I don't know." The spouse says, "You have screwed him all up. Three months ago he was a vital 30-year-old man, on track to be a full partner in his law firm. Now he is mentally out of it, he has no hair, he complains of numbness of his hands and feet, he is always nauseated and has lost weight. He can't even have a glass of wine because it causes heavy sweating and headache. You did this to him. I want to know why, and what you propose to do about it."

    Reluctantly, you admit that the drugs you choose to treat his Hodgkin's disease probably did cause these symptoms. In fact, one drug can explain all of them. Which drug is it?

    a. Nitrogen mustard
    b. Vincristine
    c. Procarbazine
    d. Prednisone
    e. No one drug listed can cause all of the toxicities mentioned

11. All of the following are true of fludarabine except:

    a. It is the most active drug in chronic lymphocytic leukemia (CLL).
    b. It is extremely active in low grade lymphomas.
    c. The acute dose limiting toxic effect of fludarabine is myelosuppression.
    d. It causes B cell immunodeficiency.
    e. It can cause an irreversible neurotoxicity characterized by cortical blindness and coma.

12. You are caring for a 57-year-old woman with acute myelogenous leukemia. The patient has recently received

consolidation therapy consisting of high dose Ara-C (2gm/m2 every 12 hours for 12 doses) and Mitoxantrone. The patient's husband asks her to walk across the room, and unfortunately she clearly has an ataxic gait. The patient has no other significant problems and is fully alert.

Which of the following is true about this clinical situation?

a. The toxicity is likely a complication of antibiotic therapy.
b. You used the correct dose of Ara-C, and the ataxia is a well-described toxicity.
c. The patient's symptoms are probably metabolic in nature secondary to the well-described nephrotoxicity of Ara-C.
d. The patient's neurologic toxicity is probably a result of central nervous system involvement of leukemia.

13. A 50-year-old woman with gastric cancer has been in complete remission for 2 months following combination chemotherapy with 5FU, Adriamycin, and Mitomycin C (FAM). She now has early signs of renal failure. The HGB is 8.5, platelet count 25,000, and WBC 9,000 with a normal differential. Fibrinogen, PT, and PTT are normal. Peripheral blood smear shows RBC fragments. The most likely diagnosis is:

a. Disseminated intravascular coagulation
b. Bone marrow hypoplasia secondary to chemotherapy
c. Marrow involvement with cancer
d. Hemolytic uremic syndrome
e. Hepatic metastases with hypersplenism

14. Interleukin 2-based therapy has been shown to result in durable complete remissions in:

a. Breast cancer
b. Renal cell carcinoma
c. Testicular cancer
d. Colon cancer
e. Nonsmall cell lung cancer

15. The dose-limiting toxicity of Cyclophosphamide is:

a. Renal
b. Pulmonary
c. Hematologic
d. Cardiac
e. Neurologic

16. A woman with metastatic breast cancer presents with fever and shortness of breath. Four weeks ago the patient was discharged from another hospital after undergoing autologous bone marrow transplantation. The preparative regimen was high dose Cyclophosphamide, Cisplatin, and BCNU. Before the transplant, the patient had known metastatic disease of the lung and liver. The patient has had an increasing nonproductive cough and substernal discomfort. Physical examination and vital signs are normal. Hemoglobin is 11.8 and white count 5800 with 50%

neutrophils and 45% lymphocytes. Platelet count is 98,000. Hepatic enzymes and serum creatinine are normal. A chest radiograph is unremarkable. Pulse oximeter was 90% on room air. The patient's DLCO is 40% predicted.

The appropriate next step is:

a. Begin broad spectrum antibiotics.
b. Reassure the patient that she probably has a viral syndrome.
c. Begin prednisone.
d. Obtain a CT scan of the liver to document progression of hepatic metastases.
e. Obtain an echocardiogram to rule out pericarditis.

17. A 50-year-old woman with metastatic breast cancer presents to the emergency room with new onset hematemesis. The patient has had breast cancer for 18 months. The patient was progressing on hormonal therapy and was switched to Cyclophosphamide, Methotrexate, and 5FU 3 weeks ago. She has metastatic disease to her bone and lungs with a malignant right pleural effusion and is taking aspirin for bone pain. On physical examination temperature is 38.5°C, pulse is 120, and BP is 80/50 with orthostatic changes. The patient has a petechial rash. Right lung examination reveals dullness throughout half the examined field. Cardiac examination reveals normal first and second heart sounds with a I/VI systolic ejection murmur. Abdominal examination is unremarkable.

Hemoglobin is 7.5, white blood cell count 0.2, and platelet count 8000. Serum creatinine is 5.2 with a BUN of 65. Alkaline phosphatase is minimally elevated; AST is normal. The most likely diagnosis is:

a. Hemolytic uremic syndrome
b. Hepatorenal syndrome with hepatic dysfunction secondary to hepatic metastases
c. Bone marrow infiltration by metastatic breast cancer
d. Methotrexate toxicity
e. Cyclophosphamide toxicity

18. The combination of 5-FU and levamisole has been conclusively shown to reduce tumor recurrence in which stage of colon cancer?

a. Dukes A
b. Dukes B
c. Dukes C
d. Dukes D
e. None of the above; nothing has been shown to reduce tumor recurrences in colon cancer

19. A 65-year-old man with Dukes C colon cancer is being treated with adjuvant 5-FU and levamisole. The patient is normally an upbeat and optimistic person, but today comes into your office in a wheelchair. The patient's speech is slurred. His son tells you that the patient is not doing well. The son reports that the patient has experi-

enced frequent diarrhea with nausea, sensitivity to sunlight, hair loss, and recent problems with gait and slurred speech. The patient appears somewhat somnolent. A CBC shows a mild anemia, leukopenia, and cytopenia. SMA-16 reveals that SGOT is elevated twice the upper limit of normal.

You confidently tell the patient's son that everything will get better in the next 2 weeks, and the patient's next course of chemotherapy simply needs to be delayed.

Which of the following is true:

a. Your arrogance is getting the better of you; this patient is ill and not all of his symptoms can be explained by drug toxicity.
b. While 5-FU can certainly cause diarrhea, the remainder of the patient's symptoms (liver toxicity, myelotoxicity, cerebellar toxicity, and alopecia) are not caused by 5-FU.
c. While 5-FU can cause diarrhea and myelosuppression, the remaining toxicities are not from 5-FU.
d. 5-FU can cause all of the above toxicities except cerebellar dysfunction.
e. You are right, as all of the above mentioned toxicities can be caused by 5-FU and likely will improve if chemotherapy is delayed and the doses later reduced.

20. Which of the following is NOT true of alpha interferon?

a. While flu-like symptoms are the most common initial side effect, hepatic toxicity is the most common chronic toxicity.
b. Approximately 30% of patients with Kaposi's sarcoma have an objective response to alpha interferon.
c. Most patients have side effects to alpha interferon.
d. Interferon induces cytogenetic remissions in chronic myelogenous leukemia (CML) as evidenced by a decrease in the percentage of Philadelphia chromosome-positive cells in the bone marrow.
e. Nausea and anorexia are common initial toxicities.

21. You are STAT paged to the emergency room to see a patient. The patient is a 25-year-old man with CML who underwent allogeneic bone marrow transplant 3 months ago from a matched sibling donor. He has known graft vs. host disease of the skin and liver. The patient's current medications include Bactrim, fluconazole, acyclovir, cyclosporine, prednisone, and amoxicillin. The patient's father, who is with him in the room, gives you a medical history as the patient is obtunded. The father says, "My son lives in Los Angeles. He underwent his transplant at UCLA. He is visiting us. Today we were at a baseball game when he stated that he did not feel well and became progressively confused. I called his physician in Los Angeles and he said that I should bring him here and ask for you."

You state that more information is needed, and obtain some blood tests and radiographs. Fortunately, the patient does not have a neutropenic fever and has a nor-

mal chest radiograph. Hemoglobin is 8.1, white count 2400 with 90% neutrophils, platelet count 17,000. Peripheral blood smear is shown. Additionally, creatinine is 2.3, BUN 40, AST 2× elevated, bilirubin is 3, and LDH is 5× elevated. You should tell the father that:

a. Despite the fact that the patient has no physical symptoms and is afebrile, he likely has a central nervous system infection due to his profound myelosuppression, and this is likely the cause for his change in mental status.
b. The patient has hepatic failure, which explains his confusion.
c. The patient is experiencing a side effect of Prednisone.
d. The patient is experiencing a side effect of Cyclosporine.
e. The patient is experiencing a side effect of Acyclovir.

22. Taxol is known to cause all the following except:

a. A significant incidence of anaphylactic reactions
b. Neurotoxicity
c. Pulmonary toxicity
d. Hematologic toxicity
e. Nausea and vomiting

23. In addition to cardiac toxicity, all of the following are common toxicities of Adriamycin except:

a. Sterility
b. Radiation recall
c. Extravasation leading to local tissue necrosis
d. Mucositis
e. Neutropenia

24. A 45-year-old woman presents with a clinical history of bruising and a platelet count of 5000, with a normal hemoglobin and white count. Peripheral smear is unremarkable except for a paucity of platelets. The most likely diagnosis is:

a. Immune thrombocytopenia purpura
b. Glanzmann's thrombasthenia
c. Congenital thrombocytopenia
d. Acute leukemia
e. Posttransfusion purpura

25. The most frequent cause of death in polycythemia vera is:

a. Evolution to acute leukemia
b. Vascular thrombosis
c. Bleeding
d. Marrow fibrosis leading to leukopenia leading to infections
e. Cardiac failure

26. You are seeing a 29-year-old woman for pancytopenia. The patient presented to another hospital 4 weeks ago with jaundice. The patient's AST and ALT were over 2000, and bilirubin peaked at 12. All hepatic serologies

were negative. As her hepatic enzymes improved, the patient abruptly became pancytopenic. The patient was transferred to your institution, and at the time of consultation, hemoglobin was 6, white blood cell count 0.2 with 90% lymphocytes, and platelet count 25,000. The patient had received 5 units of packed red blood cells at the local hospital.

Physical examination was remarkable for only scattered ecchymoses and petechiae. A bone marrow aspirate was dry; a bone marrow biopsy showed a profoundly hypocellular marrow (cellularity less than 5%) with the majority of cells being plasma cells and lymphocytes.

The correct diagnosis is:

  a. Multiple myeloma
  b. Aplastic anemia
  c. Acute myelogenous leukemia
  d. Acute lymphoblastic leukemia
  e. Myelofibrosis

27. The most common cause of aplastic anemia is:

  a. Benzene
  b. Hepatitis
  c. Chloramphenicol
  d. Radiation
  e. Idiopathic or unknown

28. The therapy of choice for the patient in Question 26 is:

  a. Allogeneic bone marrow transplantation from a human leukocyte antigen (HLA)-matched sibling donor
  b. Antihymocyte globulin (ATG)
  c. Prednisone
  d. Androgens
  e. G-CSF

29. Completed prospective randomized trials published in medical journals have shown a statistically significant survival advantage for ABMT (autologous bone marrow/ stem cell transplantation) compared with ''standard'' doses of chemotherapy for which diseases?

  a. Relapsed intermediate grade NHL
  b. Metastatic breast cancer
  c. Multiple myeloma
  d. All of the above
  e. None of the above

30. A physician has asked you to evaluate his mother. The patient, unfortunately, has developed a diffuse large cell lymphoma. The physician elected to receive opinions concerning her treatment from physicians at five different cancer centers. All five opinions stated that the patient should receive CHOP chemotherapy. The patient has received five cycles of CHOP, but now presents with prolonged and severe leukopenia. Significant hematologic toxicity developed from chemotherapy after the third cycle and the patient was placed on G-CSF (Filgrastim).

The physician managing the treatment told her to continue her G-CSF daily, which the patient has done so for 40 consecutive days. The patient's last dose of chemotherapy was 4 weeks ago, but her white count is still only 1400 and the next course of chemotherapy has not been received as a result. The most likely cause of this clinical situation is:

  a. The patient is old and has expected hematologic toxicity from chemotherapy.
  b. The patient was treated with chemotherapy while taking G-CSF.
  c. The patient probably has marrow involvement of lymphoma.
  d. The patient is developing acute leukemia secondary to chemotherapy.

Discussion and Answer Explanations

1. e

Twenty percent or more plasma cells in the marrow, lytic bone lesions and reciprocal decreases in normal immunoglobulin levels are all characteristic of multiple myeloma. The majority of patients with MGUS do not evolve into multiple myeloma. Serum protein levels are less than 3 g/dl in MGUS.

2. a

The presence of a circulating paraprotein (''M'') is often associated with a decreased anion gap. At serum pH, these proteins act as cations binding chloride and reducing the sodium-chloride difference.

3. e

The most common presenting symptom of multiple myeloma is, in fact, bone pain, most commonly in the spine.
4–7; 4.b, 5.d, 6.d, 7.c

The chest radiograph shows a large mediastinal mass. In a patient of this age, lymphoma is far and away the most likely diagnosis. Hodgkin's disease, diffuse large cell lymphoma, and lymphoblastic lymphoma would be the most probable types of lymphomas.

A needle biopsy rarely gives a definitive diagnosis of a lymphoma, largely because the underlying cellular architecture is important for an accurate pathologic diagnosis. Thus, an appropriate open or excisional biopsy should be performed. If the chest CT scan revealed tracheal compression, pre-biopsy irradiation therapy should be administered to relieve the compression. The danger of proceeding with a biopsy in the face of external tracheal compression is the risk of tracheal collapse at extubation.

In the case presented, a diagnosis of large cell lymphoma was found. Large cell lymphoma is curable with primary therapy in approximately 40% of patients. However, a relapse would be incurable with conventional therapy. The only curative modality would be high-dose chemotherapy with autologous progenitor cell rescue.

8. d

This patient has stable adenopathy with the exception of an asymmetric enlarging nodal area. It is likely that this represents a transformation to a more aggressive histology. Biopsy confirmation is essential for additional management. The most likely result of the biopsy is a diffuse large cell lymphoma.

9. c

The following questions are related to the toxicities of chemotherapy. The American Board of Internal Medicine does not expect internal medicine graduates to know details of chemotherapy protocols: graduates are expected to know the toxicities of drugs with which they will be associated.

It is well known the Cisplatin can cause myelosuppression, including severe thrombocytopenia and renal failure. One of the main dose-limiting toxicities, however, is neurologic, which can include peripheral neuropathies or decreased hearing.

10. c

Procarbazine is an oral drug used in the treatment of Hodgkin's disease and is part of several chemotherapeutic regimens for non-Hodgkin's lymphoma. Hematologic toxicity is common, as well as nausea and vomiting. Procarbazine can cause direct and indirect neurologic effects. The drug itself is known to induce altered levels of consciousness including depression, psychosis, and peripheral neuropathy, usually reversible with discontinuation of the drug. Additionally, procarbazine inhibits the cytochrome P450 system. Drugs metabolized by hepatic microsomal enzymes have prolonged half-lives in patients who are receiving procarbazine; the sedative effects of barbiturates and narcotics are therefore potentiated. Some patients report headaches, sweating, and facial flushing when they consume alcohol while taking procarbazine. Procarbazine is also associated with hypersensitivity pneumonitis and is highly teratogenic. Corticosteroids have a number of known side effects, including gastrointestinal irritation, muscle weakness, fluid retention, glucose intolerance, and altered mental status. They do not cause myelosuppression. The main toxicity of vincristine is neurologic, which is dose-related, and is usually a peripheral neuropathy associated with sensory loss, pain, and weakness. Additionally, autonomic neuropathy can occur and may result in paralytic ileus. Vincristine can also cause local tissue irritation if extravasation occurs. Vincristine is not myelosuppressive. Nitrogen mustard is also a local vesicant. The main toxicities of nitrogen mustard are gastrointestinal (nausea and vomiting), hematologic, and reproductive (sterility).

11. d

Myelosuppression is common with fludarabine, and nausea, vomiting, and hepatocellular toxicity are also acute toxicities. The most serious side effect, however, is an irreversible neurotoxicity characterized by blindness, encephalopathy, and coma. Pathologic findings include a diffuse narcotizing leukoencephalopathy, especially in the occipital lobes. Fludarabine does cause T-cell immunodeficiency, but infections with *Pneumocystis carinii* are rare. It is extremely active in CLL and is also active in other low grade lymphoid malignancies.

12. b

Myelosuppression is the most common acute toxicity of Ara-C. However, high dose Ara-C can cause unique side effects including diarrhea, conjunctivitis, and possibly pneumonitis. Cerebellar toxicity is well described as a complication of high dose Ara-C. If patients begin to develop ataxia, the Ara-C should be discontinued. The neurologic toxicity is usually reversible. Ara-C is not known to cause nephrotoxicity. The doses used in the case are well described "high doses" for the treatment of acute leukemia.

13. d

Mitomycin C is known to be associated with hemolytic uremic syndrome (HUS), which may present weeks or months after administration of Mitomycin C. The clinical picture is consistent with HUS. This is not DIC because the PT, PTT and fibrinogen are normal. Bone marrow hypoplasia is not likely given the fact that the white blood cell count is normal. Bone marrow involvement with metastases would likely result in tear drop cells, not fragments. Hypersplenism rarely results from hepatic metastases and does not cause RBC fragments or renal failure.

14. b

Interleukin-2 in conjunction with LAK cells has been shown to lead to complete responses in 6%–13% of renal cell carcinoma. It is unclear whether the LAK cells contribute to this response. Interleukin-2 has no demonstrable activity in the other malignancies mentioned. There are many toxicities associated with IL-2. Patients receiving high dose IL-2 may get a capillary leak syndrome with severe peripheral edema, adult respiratory distress syndrome (ARDS), and hypotension. Severe rashes are common.

15. d

Cyclophosphamide has no known neurologic or renal toxicity. The latter point is often missed on board exams. Pulmonary toxicity is possible but rare. Hematologic toxicity is common. However, the dose-limiting toxicity, especially in the bone marrow transplant setting, is cardiac, with cardiomyopathy and cardionecrosis occurring with doses above 200 mg/kg.

16. c

The patient does not have any evidence of metastatic disease at present. Symptoms include substernal discomfort and cough. The patient has a severe reduction in her DLCO. All of this is consistent with lung toxicity secondary to BCNU containing high-dose chemotherapy regimens. This lung toxicity is commonly seen in women with breast cancer treated with high-dose BCNU. Untreated, pulmonary deterioration may be fatal. Prompt initiation of corticosteroids usually restores normal pulmonary function. The initiation of radiation therapy may precipitate this pulmonary toxicity.

17. d

Methotrexate has many toxicities: it is the most commonly seen chemotherapy drug mentioned on board exams. While aspirin is known to elevate methotrexate drug levels, the key to this question is the fact that the patient has a pleural effusion. Methotrexate will equilibrate into third space fluids within hours after intravenous therapy. However, clearance of methotrexate from third space fluids is slow, and retention of methotrexate in third space fluids results in a prolonged terminal plasma half life. This may result in serious methotrexate toxicity, which in this case includes serious hematologic and renal toxicity. The patient is critically ill and needs prompt initiation of intravenous antibiotics, fluids, red blood cells, and other intensive supportive care measures. Calcium leucovorin should be initiated and methotrexate levels followed.

18. c

Two studies have confirmed that the combination of 5-FU and levamisole reduce tumor recurrences and overall death rate for patients with Dukes C (those with involvement of regional lymph nodes) colon carcinoma. Levamisole is FDA-approved for this indication. The therapy of metastatic disease remains far from optimal, as 5-FU results in approximately 20% response rates and little, if any, improvement in overall survival. The addition of leucovorin to 5-FU has been shown to improve response rates in metastatic colon cancer, although studies are mixed as to whether or not overall survival is improved.

19. e

The most common toxicity of 5-FU is gastrointestinal and myelosuppression. The GI toxicity is more common when continuous infusions of 5-FU are given, producing stomatitis, nausea, vomiting, and diarrhea. Myelosuppression is more common when bolus 5-FU is given. Hyperpigmentation of the skin is frequently observed. Alopecia and conjunctivitis may occur as well. Cerebellar toxicity is a well known complication of 5-FU, with symptoms including somnolence, ataxia, slurred speech, and nystagmus.

20. a

Alpha interferon has a variety of toxicities. Most patients, in fact, experience a temporary flu-like illness within the first 2 to 3 weeks of initiation of therapy. However, chronic fatigue is the most common chronic toxicity. Many other organs may be effected by alpha interferon, but all toxicities resolve with discontinuation of therapy.

21. d

The peripheral smear and peripheral blood counts are consistent with thrombotic thrmobovytopenic purpura (TTP). Cyclosporine commonly causes renal toxicity and occasionally also causes TTP as manifested by thrombocytopenia, anemia, elevated LDH, altered mental status, and red blood cell fragments on the peripheral blood smear. Neurologic toxicity is an extremely uncommon side effect of acyclovir and is not associated with red blood cell fragments.

22. c

Taxol use in the treatment of breast and ovarian cancers is increasing. It is known to cause the above mentioned toxicities, except pulmonary toxicity.

23. a

While many chemotherapeutic drugs are known to cause sterility, it is unusual for Adriamycin to do so. Radiation recall is a phenomenon where a local injury may occur after the initiation of radiation therapy in a patient who has been previously exposed to Adriamycin. This is most commonly seen in radiation therapy above the diaphragm resulting in severe mucositis. Adriamycin extravasation is a serious problem that can lead to severe local necrosis and damage underlying nerves, tendons, and muscles. The use of a free-flowing intravenous line and avoidance of veins in the antecubital fossa is essential. If extravasation occurs, the drug should be stopped and an attempt made to aspirate blood from the IV line. Application of ice and steroid cream have been reported to reduce the severity of the reaction.

24. a

The only abnormality given is a low platelet count. In the absence of a congenital history, immune thrombocytopenic purpura is the most likely diagnosis. Glanzmann's thrombasthenia is a rare platelet disorder involving an abnormality of platelet membrane IIb/IIIa, which causes defective fibrinogen binding to the platelet surface. However, the platelet count is normal in this disorder. The patient has a normal hemoglobin and white count and an unremarkable peripheral smear which rules out acute leukemia. No clinical history of transfusions rules out posttransfusion purpura, a rare clinical syndrome in which acute thrombocytopenia develops 7–14 days after receiving a red blood cell transfusion.

25. b

All patients with polycythemia vera have abnormal platelet function. As a result, the most common manifestations of this myeloproliferative disorder are clotting and bleeding. Thrombosis is the cause of death in approximately 40% of patients with P. vera. Besides deep venous thrombosis of the lower extremities, pulmonary emboli, and cerebrovascular or coronary occlusions, developing thromboses at unusual anatomic sites is common for patients, including splenic, hepatic, and mesenteric vessels. In one series, 10% of patients presenting with Budd-Chiari syndrome had coexisting polycythemia vera: any patient developing Budd-Chiari syndrome should have polycythemia vera excluded. Bleeding is also common in this disease, but does not cause mortality as often as thrombotic events. Evolution to leukemia is a well-known complication, although the frequency of leukemic evolution is increased if patients have been treated with chlorambucil or P32. If patients are treated with phlebotomy alone, the incidence of progression to acute leukemia is approximately 2%. Myelofibrosis with resultant pancytopenia occurs in approximately 10% to 15% of patients and usually develops beyond 10 years after the initial diagnosis. Polycythemia vera does not have direct cardiac toxicity, although coronary artery disease may be exacerbated by the thrombotic tendency.

A diagnosis of polycythemia vera is made on the following clinical and laboratory criteria:

- An elevated red blood cell mass with a normal arterial oxygen saturation
- Splenomegaly
- Thrombocytosis
- Bone marrow hypercellularity
- Low serum erythropoietin levels
- Abnormal marrow proliferative capacity as shown by formation of erythroid colonies in the absence of exogenous erythropoietin

Therapy should attempt to maintain the hematocritic in the range of 42%–45%. Treatment generally consists of phlebotomy with or without hydroxyurea.

26. b

The patient has an aplastic anemia. Hepatitis is the most common infection preceding aplastic anemia, with 4%–6% of aplastic anemia patients having an antecedent infection. Serologic testing is usually negative.

27. e

The vast majority of patients presenting with aplastic anemia have no known etiologic factor. Benzene is known to cause acute leukemia and myelodysplasia, but it also may be associated with aplastic anemia. The actual incidence of aplastic anemia associated with chloramphenicol is exceptionally low. Chloramphenicol does cause dose-related bone marrow depression that is reversible. The actual incidence of chloramphenicol-associated aplastic anemia is 1 in 100,000 courses.

28. a

The therapy of choice is allogeneic bone marrow transplantation, which cures approximately 70% of patients with an HLA-matched sibling donor. Antihymocyte globulin is an immunologic therapy that leads to improvement in peripheral blood counts in approximately 50% of patients, although relapses are frequent, and the efficacy of ATG in patients with severe aplastic anemia is poor. Steroids have not been shown to be beneficial in this illness. Hematopoietic growth factors may temporarily improve neutrophil counts, although improvement is transient.

This case represents an actual patient treated several years ago. The problem encountered was HLA typing of the patient. The fact that the patient the white blood cell count was so low, coupled with the fact that the patient had received red cell transfusions, made for problematic tissue typing. Ultimately, we extracted DNA from hair follicles to perform HLA typing. The patient received an allogeneic bone marrow transplant and is alive and well 6 years later.

29. d

The first three references list three recently published trials that have demonstrated superiority of ABMT over conventional doses of chemotherapy for patients with relapsed non-Hodgkin's lymphoma, metastatic breast cancer, and multiple myeloma. Autologous bone marrow/stem cell transplantation is generally accepted as the treatment of choice for patients with relapsed intermediate and high-grade non-Hodgkin's lymphoma. There remains controversy as to whether ABMT should be the treatment of choice for selected populations of patients with metastatic breast cancer and multiple myeloma. The data cited are positive and provocative. However, two large, multi-institutional, intergroup, prospective randomized trials are being conducted in the United States to further examine the efficacy of ABMT for breast cancer and multiple myeloma, and the results of these two trials will further define the role of ABMT for these two diseases.

30. b

Filgrastim (G-CSF) stimulates granulocyte cells. It also stimulates the production and release of immature progenitor cells. Clinically, G-CSF has been very useful in autologous and allogeneic bone marrow transplantation to stimulate stem cells and to enhance neutrophil recovery. It also has been shown to reduce the incidence and severity of febrile neutropenia in selected patients receiving conventional doses of chemotherapy. However, given its ability to stimulate the granulocyte series at all levels of maturation, receiving G-CSF concomitantly with chemotherapy often causes profound and long-lasting neutropenia. As a result, patients receiving chemotherapy should not receive any hematopoietic growth factors for at least 48 hours.

SUGGESTED READINGS

Philip T, Guglielmi C, Hegenbeeck A: Autologous bone marrow transplantation as compared with salvage chemotherapy in relapses of chemotherapy-sensitive non-Hodgkin's lymphoma. N Engl J Med 1995;1540–1544.

Attal Mi, Harousseau J, Stoppa A, et al: A prospective randomized trial of autologous bone marrow transplantation and chemotherapy in multiple myeloma. N Engl J Med 1996; 91–97.

Bezwoda WR, Seymour L, Dansey RD: High-dose chemotherapy with hematopoietic rescue as primary treatment for metastatic breast cancer: A randomized trial. J Clin Oncology 1995;13(10):2483–2489.

Dunbar CE, Nienhuis AW. Multiple myeloma. New approaches to therapy. JAMA 1993; 269(18):2412–2416.

Gregory WM, Richards MA, Malpas JS: Combination chemotherapy versus melphalan and prednisolone in the treatment of multiple myeloma: an overview of published trials. J Clin Oncol 1992;10(2):334–342.

Greipp P: advances in the diagnosis and management of myeloma. Sem Hematol 1992;29(Suppl 2):24–44.

Kyle RA: Benign monoclonal gammopathy-after 20 to 35 years of follow-up. Mayo Clin Proc 1993;68:26–36.

Kyle RA, Lust JA: Monoclonal gammopathies of undetermined significance. Sem Hematol 1989;26(3):176–200.

Loeffler J, Leopold K, Recht A, et al: Emergency prebiopsy radiation for mediastinal masses: impact on subsequent pathologic diagnosis and outcome. J Clin Oncol 1986;4(5):716–721.

Board Simulation II: Cellular Morphology

Andrew J. Fishleder

This chapter reviews abnormal red blood cell and white blood cell morphology encountered in common hematologic disorders.

The opening case history questions allow you to test your knowledge of the correlation of cellular morphology and clinical findings. The morphology of red and white blood cells is then discussed in the following sections. Clinical conditions and their therapy are discussed in other chapters.

QUESTIONS

1. A 20-year-old male presents with weakness and fatigue. Complete blood count reveals a hemoglobin of 9.0 g/dl. The peripheral smear shown in Figure 27.1 (see also color plates) is most consistent with:

   a. Thalassemia minor
   b. Immune hemolytic anemia
   c. Cold agglutinin disease
   d. Postsplenectomy
   e. Unstable hemoglobin with oxidative hemolysis

2. A 35-year-old female presents to the emergency room with confusion. Laboratory data results: hemoglobin 7.0 g/dl, platelets $20.0 \times 10^3/\mu l$, and normal PT/PTT. The peripheral blood smear is shown in Figure 27.5 (see also color plates). The most likely diagnosis is:

   a. Immune thrombocytopenic purpura (ITP)
   b. Diffuse intravascular coagulation (DIC)
   c. Thrombotic thrombocytopenic purpura (TTP)
   d. Aortic valve disease
   e. Acute promyelocytic leukemia (M3)

3. A 25-year-old male presents with a hemoglobin of 10.0 g/dl at routine physical examination. The peripheral smear shown in Figure 27.7 (see also color plates) is most consistent with:

   a. Hemoglobin C trait
   b. Sickle cell trait
   c. Renal failure
   d. Iron deficiency
   e. Myelofibrosis

4. A 55-year-old male presents with a skin rash, pancytopenia, and mild splenomegaly. The peripheral smear shown in Figure 27.12 is most consistent with:

   a. Aplastic anemia
   b. Drug reaction
   c. Sézary syndrome
   d. Myelodysplasia
   e. Hairy cell leukemia

5. A 40-year-old female presents with fatigue, mild splenomegaly, lymphadenopathy, and a white blood cell count of $20.0 \times 10^3/\mu l$. The peripheral smear shown in Figure 27.17 is most consistent with:

   a. Acute lymphoblastic leukemia (ALL)
   b. Chronic lymphocytic leukemia (CLL)
   c. Infectious mononucleosis
   d. Adult T cell leukemia/lymphoma (ATL)
   e. Plasma cell leukemia

6. A 45-year-old male presents with mild splenomegaly and a white blood cell count of $30.0 \times 10^3/l$. The peripheral smear shown in Figure 27.19 is most consistent with:

   a. Bacterial infection
   b. Chronic lymphocytic leukemia (CLL)
   c. Chronic myelogenous leukemia (CML)
   d. Essential thrombocythemia
   e. Acute myelogenous leukemia (AML)

7. The patient is a 60-year-old male with a hemoglobin of 9.0 g/dl, an MCV of 110fl, and pancytopenia. A bone marrow for evaluation is performed. The cell demonstrated by Prussian Blue (iron) stain (Fig. 27.22) can be seen in all of the following except:

   a. Myelodysplasia
   b. Alcohol
   c. Megaloblastic anemia
   d. Hemochromatosis
   e. Postchemotherapy

Answers

1. b
2. c
3. a
4. e
5. a
6. c
7. d

RED BLOOD CELL MORPHOLOGY

The blood smear shown in Figure 27.1 (see also color plates) is remarkable for the presence of small, round red blood cells with dense hemoglobinization and no central pallor. These cells are called spherocytes. The larger, blue-gray red blood cells noted in the blood smear are reticulocytes, indicating a bone marrow response to this individual's anemia. Spherocytes are most commonly seen in cases of immune hemolysis and hereditary spherocytosis but can be seen in the following conditions:

- Immune Hemolysis
- Hereditary spherocytosis
- Postsplenectomy
- Posttransfusion
- Severe burns
- Oxidative hemolysis
- Fragmentation hemolysis

Remembering that immune hemolysis is associated with spherocytes but not with red blood cell fragments is important.

The blood smear in Figure 27.2 (see also color plates)

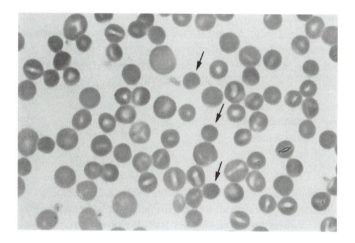

Figure 27.1.   (See color plate.)

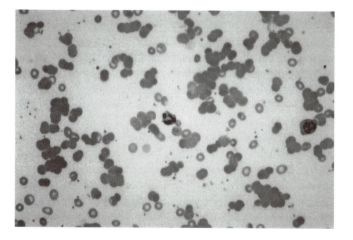

Figure 27.2.   (See color plate.)

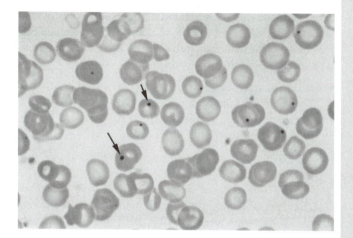

Figure 27.3.   (See color plate.)

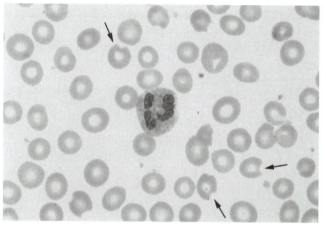

Figure 27.4.   (See color plate.)

shows variably sized clumps of red blood cells indicating the presence of a cold agglutinin in this patient. Spherocytes may be seen in cold agglutinin disease when an immune hemolytic component is present. Cold agglutinins can alter peripheral blood indices, causing a spurious decrease in red blood cell count and an increase in MCV, MCH, and MCHC. Red blood cell morphology and indices revert to normal following warming of the blood sample.

The blood smear in Figure 27.3 (see also color plates) displays dense, purple inclusions within red blood cells called Howell-Jolly bodies. These DNA inclusions are seen postsplenectomy and in conditions that compromise splenic function.

The smear in Figure 27.4 (see also color plates) demonstrates "bite cells" characteristic of oxidative hemolysis. Secondary to removal of denatured hemoglobin by the reticuloendothelial system, these red blood cells typically have one or more concave indentations in the red blood cell membrane. "Bite cells" can be seen in patients with oxidative hemolysis caused by unstable hemoglobins, red blood cell enzyme defects such as G6PD deficiency, or drugs with oxidative capacity such as sulfonamides.

The blood smear in Figure 27.5 (see also color plates) depicts many red blood cell fragments and only rare platelets. Red blood cell fragments can be seen in a variety of hematologic disorders, including the following:

- Diffuse intravascular coagulation (DIC)
- Thrombotic thrombocytopenic purpura (TTP)
- Hemolytic uremic syndrome (HUS)
- Heart valve disease
- Vasculitis
- Megaloblastic anemia
- Severe burns

The concomitant presence of thrombocytopenia and red blood cell fragments suggests TTP, DIC, or HUS, although megaloblastic anemia and autoimmune vasculitis cannot be excluded. Traumatic hemolysis secondary to heart valve disease, on the other hand, shows red blood cell fragments without thrombocytopenia. In contrast, immune thrombocytopenic purpura (ITP) is associated with decreased platelets but no evidence of red blood cell fragments.

As demonstrated in Figure 27.6 (see also color plates),

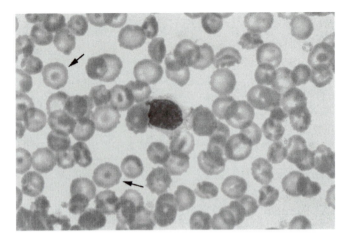

Figure 27.7. (See color plate.)

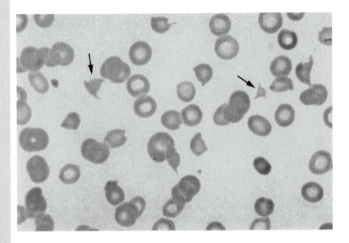

Figure 27.5. (See color plate.)

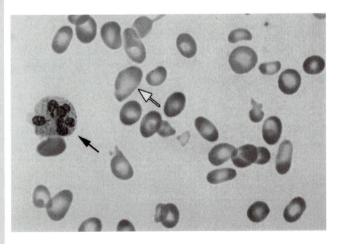

Figure 27.6. (See color plate.)

patients with megaloblastic anemia may also have decreased platelets and red blood cell fragments, although hypersegmented polymorphonuclear neutrophil leukocytes (arrow) and oval macrocytes (open arrow) are also typically seen.

The blood smear in Figure 27.7 (see also color plates) demonstrates abnormal red blood cells called target cells. These cells have a central core of dense hemoglobinization surrounded by a zone of otherwise normal red blood cell pallor. Target cells are a nonspecific finding and are seen in a variety of disorders, including the following:

- Liver disease
- Postsplenectomy
- Thalassemia
- Iron deficiency
- Hemoglobinopathies

Hemoglobin C disease, hemoglobin C trait, hemoglobin SC disease, and sickle cell anemia are all associated with target cells. Patients with sickle cell trait, however, have normal blood smear morphology. In addition, although iron deficiency may be associated with target cells, red blood cells in that disorder are typically pale and small. Target cells do not result from renal failure.

The smear in Figure 27.8 (see also color plates) demonstrates target cells and misshapen red blood cells consistent with sickle cells. Sickle cells are variable in shape, but diagnostic forms are typically elliptical with pointed ends. Sickle cells may be seen in sickle cell anemia, sickle beta thalassemia, and hemoglobin SC disease but are not seen in sickle cell trait.

The blood smear in Figure 27.9 (see also color plates) shows teardrop red blood cells most commonly associated with conditions causing bone marrow fibrosis: myeloproliferative disorders, myelodysplasia, and metastatic carcinoma. Teardrop red blood cells are also commonly seen in patients receiving cyclosporin therapy.

The smear in Figure 27.10 (see also color plates) demonstrates many pale red blood cells indicative of poor hemoglo-

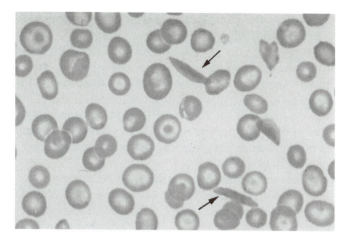

Figure 27.8.   (See color plate.)

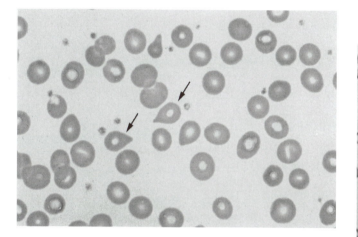

Figure 27.9.   (See color plate.)

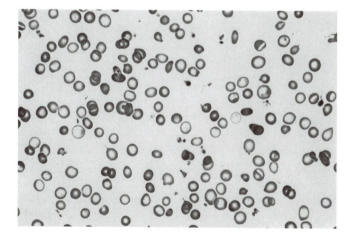

Figure 27.10.   (See color plate.)

binization. The associated variation in red blood cell size (as measured by an increased RDW) and shape is consistent with iron deficiency anemia.

Red blood cell hypochromasia and microcytosis are also seen in thalassemia minor, although the RDW is typically normal, indicative of a more uniform red blood cell size distribution, as shown in Figure 27.11 (see also color plates).

WHITE BLOOD CELL MORPHOLOGY

The lymphoid cell noted in Figure 27.12 is consistent with that seen in hairy cell leukemia. Classic "hairy cells" have a ragged cytoplasmic border, light blue-gray cytoplasm, and immature nuclear chromatin. Tartrate-resistant acid phosphatase activity can be shown cytochemically, and flow cytometry displays a characteristic immunophenotype of CD22+, CD11C+, and CD25+. Clinically, these patients typically present with pancytopenia and splenomegaly.

Pancytopenia with a significant hypocellular bone mar-

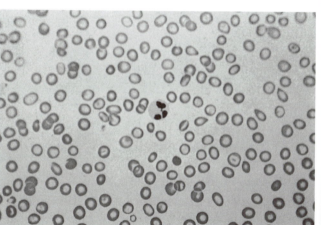

Figure 27.11.   (See color plate.)

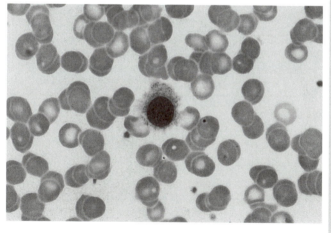

Figure 27.12.

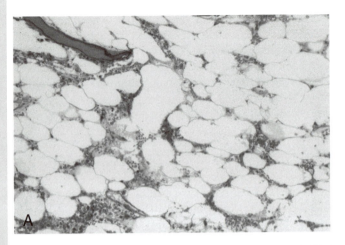

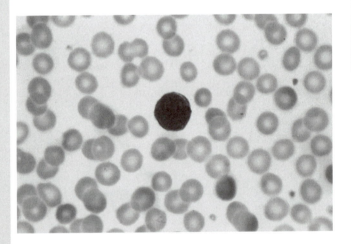

Figure 27.13.

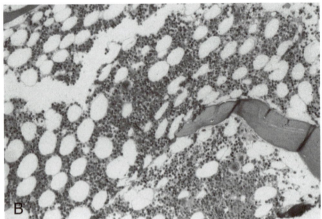

Figure 27.14.

positive for CD2, CD3, and CD4 but are negative for the pan T-cell marker CD7.

Figure 27.15 demonstrates a high white blood cell count with increased numbers of small mature lymphocytes (open arrow) consistent with chronic lymphocytic leukemia (CLL). "Smudged cells" (arrow) may be prominent in the blood smear, and there may be associated immune hemolysis or immune thrombocytopenia noted. Flow cytometry characteristically reveals an immunophenotype of CD19 +, CD23 +, and CD5 + in B-cell CLL.

The reactive lymphocytes seen in infectious mononucleosis and other viral infections (Fig. 27.16) typically have a low nuclear/cytoplasmic ratio with a moderate amount of cytoplasm. The cell nuclei are mature with smudged chromatin, although occasional immature nucleolated cells may be seen. Characteristically, reactive lymphocytes demonstrate scalloped cytoplasmic borders and often have dark blue cytoplasm. These reactive cells are seen in viral infections such as EBV and CMV, as well as in drug reactions. Serologic confirmation for diagnosis is necessary.

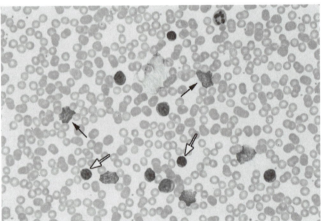

Figure 27.15.

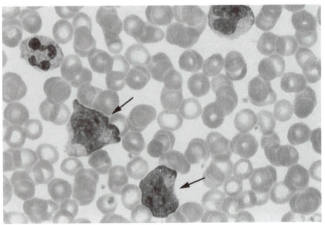

Figure 27.16.

row is typical of aplastic anemia (Fig. 27.13, a). In contrast, the cellularity of normal bone marrow typically ranges from 30%– 70% depending on the patient's age (Fig. 27.13, b).

Sézary cells (Fig. 27.14) are abnormal T-cells that typically demonstrate a high nuclear/cytoplasmic ratio with fine nuclear convolutions. Immunophenotypically, these cells are

Patients with myelodysplasia commonly have pancytopenia that may be accompanied by dysplastic granulocytes. These abnormal white blood cells may have nuclear hyposegmentation (Figure 27.20, a) or cytoplasmic hypogranularity (Figure 27.20, b).

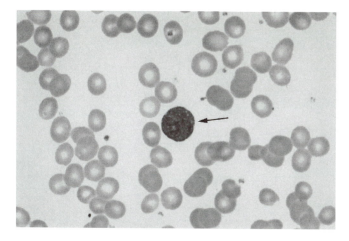

Figure 27.17.

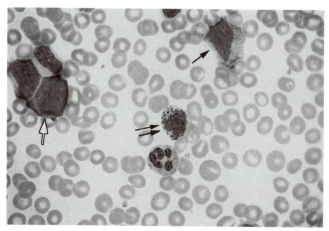

Figure 27.19.

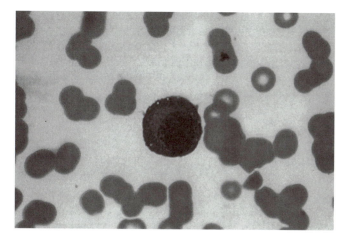

Figure 27.18.

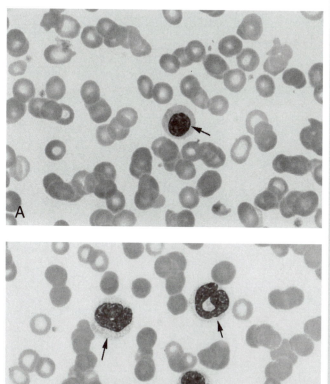

Figure 27.20.

Lymphoblasts seen in acute lymphocytic leukemia (ALL) Fab L_1 have a high nuclear/cytoplasmic ratio, and fine nuclear chromatin. The L_1 blasts, as demonstrated in Figure 27.17, are most commonly seen in childhood ALL.

In plasma cell leukemia, circulating plasma cells (Figure 27.18) are typically immature and comprise more than 20% of the circulating white blood cells (or an absolute count >2000/l). Circulating plasma cells have a low nuclear/cytoplasmic ratio, eccentric nucleus, and a pale, perinuclear golgi zone. Mature plasma cells may normally be found circulating in association with reactive processes.

The peripheral blood smear shown in Figure 27.19 is most consistent with chronic myelogenous leukemia (CML). Patients with CML typically have an elevated white blood cell count with a prominent granulocytic left shift including circulating metamyelocytes, myelocytes (arrow), promyelocytes, and scattered blasts (open arrow). Basophilia (double arrow) and sometimes eosinophilia are typically seen and help to distinguish CML from left shifted reactive processes such as bacterial infections.

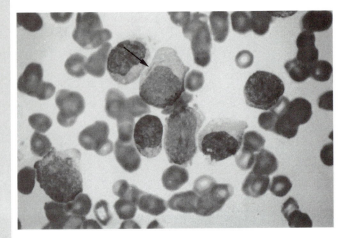

Figure 27.21.

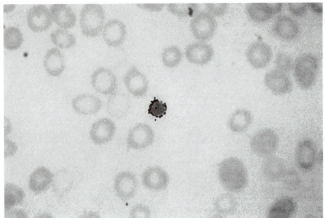

Figure 27.22.

The peripheral blood smear shown in Figure 27.21 is from a patient with acute myelogenous leukemia. Patients typically display circulating blasts with low nuclear/cytoplasmic ratios along with variable cytoplasmic granulation. The presence of Auer rods (arrow) is diagnostic of myelogenous origin.

The Prussian blue stain for bone marrow iron preparation demonstrates a classic ringed sideroblast in Figure 27.22. The blue granules surrounding the red nucleus represent iron accumulated within red blood cell mitochondria. Ringed sideroblasts are characteristically seen in myelodysplasia, although they may also be seen in other conditions: megaloblastic anemia and postchemotherapy.

S·E·C·T·I·O·N

IV

Rheumatology

28

Acute Monoarticular Arthritis

Brian F. Mandell

Acute monoarticular arthritis represents a medical urgency because of the possibility of joint infection, which can result in total loss of joint function. Additionally, septic arthritis may be the initial manifestation of systemic bacterial infection. An appropriate diagnosis of specific crystal-induced arthritis will help dictate long-term management decisions.

ETIOLOGY OF ACUTE MONOARTICULAR ARTHRITIS

In an unpublished series of 64 hospitalized and emergency room patients with acute monoarticular or oligoarticular arthritis, 17% had documented bacterial infection (Fig. 28.1)(1). The majority of patients had uric acid or calcium pyrophosphate crystal-induced arthritis. It is impossible to distinguish between crystal-induced and septic arthritis on clinical grounds alone. Hence, the possibility of bacterial infectious arthritis dictates the diagnostic approach to the patient with acute monoarticular or oligoarticular arthritis.

DIAGNOSIS OF ACUTE MONOARTICULAR ARTHRITIS

HISTORY

A thorough history should be obtained, with a focus on several specific issues. Quite frequently, patients will describe a history of trauma prior to their presentation with acute joint swelling and pain. Careful discussion regarding the mechanism and severity of injury, as well as the timing in relationship to the presentation with acute arthritis, is mandatory. Often, it can be determined that the history of trauma bears no relationship to the acute arthritis. Joint trauma rarely elicits a striking inflammatory articular response. General history

surrounding the onset of the arthritis should be explored. The presence of a migratory arthralgia prodrome is suggestive of infection, including rheumatic fever or disseminated gonorrhea. Prolonged systemic features prior to the onset of arthritis also suggests the presence of a chronic infection such as bacterial endocarditis or viral hepatitis. Patients should be questioned about prior episodes of arthritis in the same or different joints. Patients with *Borrelia* infection (Lyme disease), crystal disease, psoriasis, enteropathic arthritis, spondylitis, and other syndromes may have a history of prior episodes of acute arthritis. Careful questioning should be focused on exposure to intravenous drugs (or to sexual contact with partners with such exposure), exposure to prescribed medications, or potential exposure to viral hepatitis or HIV infection. Patients should be questioned regarding time spent during the spring, summer, or early fall months in an area endemic for Lyme disease.

PHYSICAL EXAMINATION

Careful physical examination should be undertaken. An entire musculoskeletal screening evaluation should be performed. Although the patient may complain of single joint pain, physical examination may reveal multiple inflamed joints or coexistent tenosynovitis or enthesitis. Mucosal surfaces should be carefully examined for the presence of ulcers or inflammation. The conjunctivitis of Reiter's syndrome (urethritis, arthritis, and conjunctivitis) is typically mild and asymptomatic. Extremities should be examined for purpura. Psoriatic lesions should be sought in typical but often unrecognized areas (gluteal crease, scalp, behind ears, and umbilicus).

Careful physical examination should be focused on distinguishing between bursitis and other soft-tissue, periarticular pain syndromes and true inflammatory arthritis (Fig. 28.2). Septic bursitis in these areas can be associated with a large degree of surrounding erythema and edema and can superficially mimic true joint involvement.

Certain syndromes have a predilection to involve the tendon sheath as well as the joint structures. Tenosynovitis should prompt consideration for the specific diagnosis of infection with *Neisseria* or *Haemophilus influenzae,* crystal disease, mycobacterial infection (particularly atypical infection such as *Mycobacterium marinum*), and specific fungal infections, such as sporotrichosis. Sausaging of digits suggests the diagnosis of psoriasis.

Constitutional markers of infection are not sensitive or specific enough to make the diagnosis of septic arthritis or distinguish this from crystal-induced arthritis. A study of 43 patients with documented bacterial arthritis predominantly due to *Staphylococcus aureus* revealed (2):

- Rigors present in 21%
- Temperature greater than 38°C in 41%
- Leukocytosis in 42%
- A sedimentation rate less than 30 mm/hr in 24%

A study of documented crystal-induced arthritis found (3):

- Temperature greater than 38°C in 29% of patients with documented gout (one patient with a maximal temperature of 39.4°C)
- Temperature greater than 38°C in 38% of patients with documented pseudogout
- Temperature greater than 38°C in 50% of patients with multiple joint involvement

Thus, fever and leukocytosis are neither sensitive nor specific findings in septic arthritis.

IMAGING AND LABORATORY STUDIES

Initial laboratory and radiographic studies should be kept to a minimum in evaluating the patient with acute monoarticular arthritis. The laboratory study of choice is synovial fluid analysis, as discussed below. The distinction between crystal- and bacterial-induced arthritis cannot be made using blood studies. Radiographs are of initial value *if* significant trauma or osteomyelitis is suspected; radiographs should play no role in the initial distinction of acute crystal-induced versus bacterial-induced arthritis.

Measurement of serum uric acid values is also of no diagnostic value in determining the etiology of acute arthritis. *The*

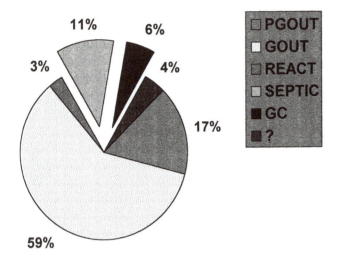

Figure 28.1. Etiology of acute arthritis. Graduate Hospital, Philadelphia: 64 hospitalized patients (1).

Figure 28.2. Acute soft-tissue problems.

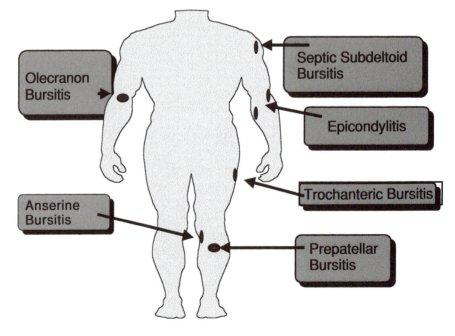

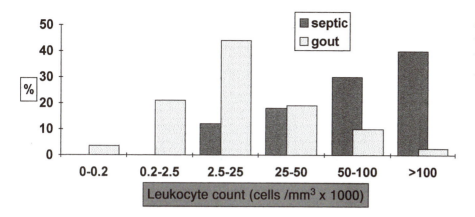

Figure 28.3. Diagnosis of septic arthritis synovial fluid leukocytosis. (Reprinted with permission from Krey PR, Bailen DA. Am J Med 1979;67:436–442.)

diagnostic test of choice in patients with acute monoarticular arthritis is synovial fluid analysis with cell count, polarized microscopy, and culture. Invariably, patients with infectious or crystal-induced arthritis will have synovial fluid leukocytosis with a striking neutrophil predominance (Fig. 28.3). However, the absolute cell count or neutrophil differential count will not distinguish between septic and gouty arthritis.

The initial accurate diagnosis of monoarticular arthritis rests entirely on the arthrocentesis and a few synovial-fluid studies. (A single drop of synovial fluid—as little as what is contained in the hub of the needle in what may initially be assumed to be a "dry tap"—may be sufficient to allow the diagnosis.) Use the following procedure:

1. Place a single drop of synovial fluid on a glass slide and cover with a cover slip.
2. Undertake a wet-preparation microscopic analysis using the 40x objective.
3. Estimate cell count with one cell per high-power field equaling 500 cells/mm³.
4. Undertake polarized microscopy on the same wet preparation.
5. Remove the cover slide, gently heat-fix the fluid, then perform a Gram's stain.

The Gram's stain will permit a differential cell count of polymorphonuclear neutrophils (PMNs) versus mononuclear cells and the actual Gram's stain itself. If the fluid is inflammatory with greater than 7500 cells/mm³ or more than 80% neutrophils and no crystals are seen, the fluid should be sent for culture and the patient treated for potential septic arthritis, unless there is an obvious alternative diagnosis. Common conditions such as uncomplicated osteoarthritis do not generally cause inflammatory fluids to this degree. If the fluid is not inflammatory by these markers and no crystals are observed, cultures should still be undertaken if the patient is febrile or there are other concerns for the possibility of infection, including potential periarticular osteomyelitis. If the fluid is bloody, evaluation for possible intraarticular injury or synovial tumor should be considered. Thrombocytopenia, unlike coagulation-factor deficiencies, usually is not associated with spontaneous

joint hemorrhage. Synovial fluid should be examined promptly, if at all possible, for the presence of crystals.

If prompt analysis is not possible, the fluid should be maintained in a sterile tube, in the absence of anticoagulants, pending polarized microscopic evaluation. Alternatively, the fluid can be placed on a glass slide and the cover slip sealed in place using nail polish, and the fluid can be examined the next day. It should be noted that crystals (especially calcium pyrophosphate) may be missed on examination as a result of observer inexperience, a limited number of crystals in the fluid, or other undetermined reasons. Hence, if no crystals are initially seen, repeated joint aspirations are mandatory, with repeated polarized microscopy. Special alizarin stain may aid in confirming the presence of calcium-containing crystals.

SPECIFIC ACUTE MONOARTICULAR ARTHRITIS CONDITIONS

GOUTY ARTHRITIS

Acute urate crystal arthritis is the most common cause of monoarticular arthritis in most reported series (see Fig. 28.1).

Etiology of Gouty Arthritis

Reviewing the natural history of gouty arthritis in older literature reveals that 90% of the first attacks of gouty arthritis are monoarticular, and 60% occur in the first MTP joints (podagra). About 60% of patients may have a recurrence within one year; however, 7% may never have another recurrence. The finding of subcutaneous uric acid deposits or radiographic findings of joint damage are extremely rare at the outset of disease, despite the fact that the synovial tissues are undoubtedly already saturated with uric acid. It is crucial to recognize that attacks of acute gout can be elicited by abrupt changes in the serum uric acid levels, whether up or down. Attacks frequently occur with a normal serum uric acid value. Figure

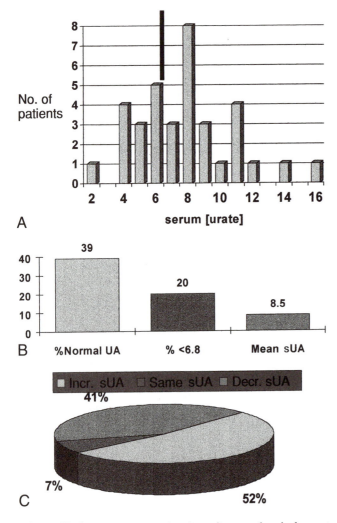

A

B

C

Figure 28.4.   **a,** Serum (urate) at time of acute polyarticular gout. **b,** Serum (urate) at time of acute articular gout in 59 male patients with documented gout. **c,** Serum urate at the time of an attack compared with intercritical period. (Reprinted with permission from [**a**] Hadler N et al. Am J Med 1974;56:715–716; [**b, c**] Schlesinger N et al. Arthritis and Rheumatism 1996;39S,8.)

erosive changes with reactive bone proliferation in these areas. The radiographs of patients with longstanding gouty arthritis may demonstrate the presence of erosions and reactive bone (the "overhanging edge") in the absence of significant joint space narrowing. This should be distinguished from the joint space narrowing seen in rheumatoid arthritis, which may occur prior to the onset of significant erosions. As the uric acid is leached out of the supersaturated synovium and cartilage and into the synovial fluid by such factors as a decrease in the serum uric acid value or microtrauma to the joint, it may crystallize into a phlogistic structure. The ability of the crystal to induce an inflammatory response can be modified by the coating of crystals with lipoproteins, immunoglobulins, or other proteins present within the synovial fluid. The crystals are phagocytized by synovial lining cells, neutrophils, or macrophages within the synovial fluid. Following phagocytosis of the crystals, these cells produce several cytokines that can elicit and amplify the inflammatory response. Defined inflammatory mediators include leukotriene B4, crystal-induced chemotactic factor, interleukin-8, interleukin-1, and possibly other granule contents. Release of many of these mediators has been shown to be suppressed by colchicine. Complement and Hageman factor, although activated by urate crystals, do not seem to be necessary for the development of the acute inflammatory response. Experimental injection of urate crystals under the skin or into the joints of humans is sufficient to elicit the acute inflammatory response (Fig. 28.5).

Syndromes of Gouty Arthritis   There are several distinct gout syndromes. Acute arthritis is usually monoarticular, but it may be oligoarticular or even polyarticular. The initial attacks are rarely polyarticular. Over time, untreated gout tends to increase in the frequency and severity of attacks. The attacks tend to last longer and involve additional joints. Initially, there is a predominance of lower-extremity joint involvement; however, over time, upper-extremity joints may become involved as well (Fig. 28.6). Sporadic case reports describe spine involvement. Flares may involve Heberden's nodes of osteoarthritis, causing inflammatory finger nodules in patients

28.4a summarizes baseline serum uric acid level data at the time of an acute polyarticular gouty attack. Figures 28.4b and 28.4c present data from additional studies (which focused on patients with monoarticular or oligoarticular attacks of gout), demonstrating again that patients may have a low, normal, or high serum uric acid value at the time of attack.

Pathogenesis of Gouty Arthritis   The pathogenesis of the acute gouty attack is reasonably well understood. The cartilage matrix and synovium are saturated with uric acid. This occurs over years of exposure to elevated levels of uric acid, above the saturation point in physiologic fluids. In some patients, this saturation will become extreme and result in subcutaneous deposits (tophi) or synovial deposits that set up a local inflammatory response that will invade adjacent bone, causing

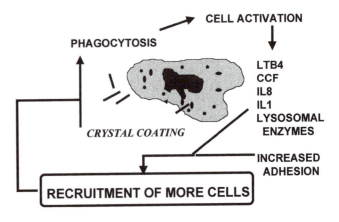

Figure 28.5.   Crystal-induced arthritis.

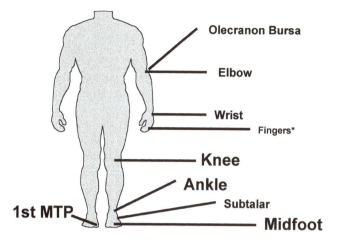

Figure 28.6. Gout: common sites of involvement.

with osteoarthritis. This has been well described to occur in postmenopausal, elderly women using thiazide diuretics.

Between attacks, in so-called intercritical periods, patients with gout may be totally asymptomatic. Nonetheless, if synovial fluid is obtained at these times, urate crystals may still be found floating in the slightly inflammatory synovial fluid, generally not within cells. Saturnine gout occurs in the setting of interstitial renal disease, historically in patients who have significant lead exposure resulting from ingestion of moonshine liquor.

As emphasized above, attacks of acute gouty arthritis can be precipitated by changes in serum uric acid values either up or down. Hence, documentation of hyperuricemia is not equivalent to the diagnosis of gouty arthritis in an individual patient. Many patients have laboratory evidence of hyperuricemia without ever having an attack of gouty arthritis. Additionally, hyperuricemia per se is not necessarily associated with any organ damage, including development of progressive renal disease. There is a statistical (population-based) association, however, with elevated levels of serum uric acid and development of urate nephrolithiasis and gouty arthritis.

Not all crystal-induced arthritis is due to uric acid. Calcium pyrophosphate crystals can cause attacks that totally mimic gout (pseudogout), but can also cause several other syndromes. Radiographic findings of calcium deposition within menisci and other intraarticular cartilage has been termed chondrocalcinosis and may be asymptomatic or associated with inflammatory arthritis. Attacks can be infrequent, or the syndrome of pseudorheumatoid disease may develop with a chronic symmetrical polyarthritis due to low-grade crystal-induced inflammation. Some metabolic diseases have been associated with atypical distribution and early onset of osteoarthritis owing to the presence of calcium pyrophosphate crystals; the best known of these is hemochromatosis, which causes low-grade inflammation in the wrists and second and third metacarpal-phalangeal (MCP) joints with a radiographic pattern consistent with osteoarthritis. Several systemic dis-

eases have been associated with the occurrence of calcium pyrophosphate deposition disease, including:

* Hyperparathyroidism
* Hypothyroidism
* Hypophosphatasia
* Hypomagnesemia
* Gout
* Amyloidosis
* Prior joint trauma
* Prior joint surgery
* Hemochromatosis

Both gout and pseudogout attacks are common in the postoperative setting.

Hemochromatosis should be significantly emphasized because the gene for hemochromatosis may be present in as high as 10% of the population. Manifestations include mildly inflammatory, osteoarthritis-like arthropathy with predominant MCP involvement, with or without chondrocalcinosis. Prominent MCP involvement is not typical of ''routine'' osteoarthritis. The arthropathy may precede the recognition of organ involvement due to iron overload. Unlike favorable liver and heart response to treatment, phlebotomy may not induce a remission in the hemochromatosis-related joint symptoms. Nonetheless, recognition of hemochromatosis due to the presence of the unique joint syndrome may preserve organ function by prompting early appropriate therapy. Skin pigmentation is due to deposition of melanin, not iron. Cardiomyopathy, hepatic cirrhosis, and endocrine disturbances including diabetes mellitus and hypogonadism are also manifestations of hemochromatosis.

Other crystal-induced arthropathies include oxalate-induced arthritis in patients on dialysis for treatment of chronic renal insufficiency and hydroxyapatite crystals. The last crystal has been associated with the entity of Milwaukee shoulder (a chronic disease with a tendency to affect elderly females) and is associated with chronic rotator cuff disease, shoulder effusions that may contain an enormous amount of synovial fluid containing few cells, and multiple aggregates of apatite crystals. The range of clinical manifestations include asymptomatic large effusions to severe pain and chronic disability due to shoulder dysfunction.

Treatment of Gouty Arthritis

Specific indications for treatment of hyperuricemia include prophylactic therapy to prevent the tumor lysis syndrome and treatment of recalcitrant gouty arthritis in patients in whom there is significant concern over the use of drugs for acute therapy. Patients who have documented soft tissue tophi or joint erosions due to uric-acid deposits should also be treated with hypouricemic agents. Some clinicians suggest that patients who have had more than two attacks of gouty arthritis should be treated with hypouricemic agents because it is implicit in the pathophysiology of the gouty attack that the joint structures are already saturated with uric acid. The concern over this therapy is the potential side effects of the hypouricemic therapy. Allopurinol, an inhibitor of xanthine oxidase (the key synthetic enzyme in the uric-acid pathway), is generally well-tolerated; however, the medication has been associated with life-threatening hypersensitivity reactions and the Stevens-Johnson syndrome. Uricosuric agents, such as probenecid, are well-tolerated but are harder to use effectively. For maximal efficacy, patients must ingest significant amounts of fluid and use the medication several times daily. Before initiating *any* therapy to lower the serum uric acid level, the clinician should be absolutely certain of the diagnosis of gout, which means synovial fluid analysis should have documented the presence of uric-acid crystals. Strong consideration should be given to simultaneous prophylactic anti-inflammatory therapy with medications such as colchicine or nonsteroidal anti-inflammatory drugs, because drug-induced hypouricemia may precipitate an attack of gout. Hypouricemic therapy should not be introduced in the setting of the acute attack, nor should hypouricemic therapy be discontinued while an attack is underway.

Exceedingly low levels of serum uric acid can be found in select clinical situations, including:

- The syndrome of inappropriate antidiuretic hormone secretion (SIADH)
- High-dose salicylate therapy
- Renal tubular diseases (such as Wilson's disease, Fanconi's syndrome)
- Starvation
- Alcohol withdrawal

Hypouricemia has also been described in a number of other cases:

- Xanthine oxidase deficiency syndromes
- Severe liver disease
- Overhydration
- In total parenteral nutrition
- Following the use of iodinated contrast agents

Agents that induce hyperuricemia include:

- Low-dose aspirin
- Diuretics
- Cyclosporine
- Organic acids
- Acute ethanol exposure
- Pyrazinamide
- Ethambutol

The majority of patients develop hyperuricemia because of renal underexcretion rather than overproduction. Disorders associated with hyperproduction of uric acid (> 1 g urate excreted daily) include hereditary enzymopathies such as HGPRTase deficiency and proliferative disorders such as psoriasis or Paget's disease of bone. Most commonly, the etiology for underexcretion of uric acid is not demonstrable. Polycystic kidney disease, Bartter's syndrome, Down's syndrome, starvation, and lead nephropathy have been associated with underexcretion of uric acid. The necessity of obtaining a 24-hour urine collection in all gouty patients to quantify uric acid excretion is controversial.

There are many treatment options for acute crystal arthritis. Probably any nonsteroidal anti-inflammatory drug (NSAID) in high doses is capable of treating the acute attack. Aspirin is generally avoided because it has striking effects on urate excretion. Concerns over the use of NSAIDs include renal and platelet dysfunction and gastric toxicity. Additionally, NSAIDs are general pyretics. Parenteral use of nonsteroidal drugs is no safer than oral use, and parenterally-available ketorolac is (in my opinion) a drug with a poor risk/benefit ratio since it is one of the most gastric toxic NSAIDs. Corticosteroid therapy, either oral or parenteral, is quite effective. There is no benefit in using adrenocorticotropic hormone (ACTH) injections, which are quite expensive, elicit variable cortisol secretion, and have more fluid retentive properties than prednisone. Concerns about corticosteroid use involve:

- Masking infection
- Exacerbation of diabetes
- Decreased wound healing in the postoperative setting (theoretical)
- Diagnostic confusion resulting from the leukocytosis induced by the corticosteroids

Intraarticular corticosteroids are effective; however, joint infection should be ruled out by synovial fluid culture prior to intraarticular administration in most cases. Colchicine is an effective prophylactic drug and can also be used as treatment of crystal-induced arthritis due to gout or pseudogout. The older oral administration regimen of one tablet (0.6 mg) every hour until relief or gastrotoxicity develops (usually diarrhea) is generally unacceptable to patients because the diarrhea ensues frequently at the same time, or slightly before, clinical relief is obtained. Intravenous colchicine is an effective therapy for many patients with acute attacks of crystal disease if used early in the attack, but *can be extremely toxic if inappropriate doses are used.* Colchicine should not be used in the acute therapy of patients with hepatic or renal disease without significant decrease in the dosage (if used at all). In patients who have had frequent attacks, there are multiple regimens that are potentially of value for prophylaxis. Colchicine (0.6–1.8 mg daily) can be used; diarrhea may limit the dosing. In patients with renal insufficiency, colchicine use can result in neuromuscular toxicity; this must be monitored for by history, examination, and occasional creatine phosphokinase (CPK) measurement, and the dosage decreased in this setting. Daily NSAIDs are not ideal as chronic prophylactic therapy due to their side-effect profile. Dietary manipulations, in general, are not likely to provide an enormous change in the serum uric acid value; the one exception to this is cautioning patients about intermittent binge ethanol use. The use of hypouricemic therapy was discussed above.

Gouty Arthritis in Transplant Patients

Special note should be made of the occurrence of severe gouty arthritis in transplant patients. Cyclosporine is seemingly the risk factor, as opposed to the transplant itself, because this therapy induces hyperuricemia. The course of gout in these patients is more rapidly progressive than in patients without cyclosporine. Tophi develop much earlier than expected, and frequently there is early of involvement of the joints of the upper extremity and axial skeleton. There are multiple potential toxicities in the treatment of transplant patients, including drug interactions between the NSAIDs and cyclosporine, and the interaction between allopurinol and azathioprine. These drug interactions must be closely monitored (4).

SEPTIC ARTHRITIS

Septic arthritis is an uncommon cause of arthritis; nonetheless, associated morbidity and potential mortality mandate its prompt exclusion as the cause of acute arthritis.

The summarized distribution of affected joints is shown in Figure 28.7. Fibrocartilage joints, such as the sternoclavicular, sacroiliac, and acromioclavicular joints, are involved with infections in specific settings. These joints are prone to infection following persistent bacteremias, particularly with gram-negative infections. Patients with a history of intravenous drug use, hemodialysis, or intravenous catheters (for total parenteral nutrition [TPN], apheresis, etc.) are at particular risk.

Etiology of Septic Arthritis

The most common organisms causing septic arthritis in most series are *Staphylococcus* or *Streptococcus* species. Disseminated gonococcemia is also a frequent cause of septic arthritis. The diagnosis of septic arthritis cannot be made with certainty without culture of the synovial fluid. The presence of fever, leukocytosis, rigors, or an elevated sedimentation rate are neither specific nor sensitive for the diagnosis of septic arthritis. Positive Gram's stains may be seen in only a slight majority

of cases of nongonococcal cases of septic arthritis; thus, a negative Gram's stain does not exclude the possibility of infection.

Disseminated gonococcal infection produces skin lesions and tenosynovitis more commonly than purulent arthritis. The arthritis often follows a syndrome of migratory myalgias and arthralgias. The synovial fluid Gram's stain is almost always negative in disseminated gonococcal arthritis, and usually is culture-negative as well. The explanation for the synovial fluid being culture-negative is complex and may relate in part to the difficulty in growing the organism, but may also relate to the pathophysiology by which arthritis can be induced by immune complexes containing gonococcal antigens, without live organism (Fig. 28.8).

Specific Conditions Related to Septic Arthritis

Lyme Disease   Lyme disease results from a tick-transmitted infection of a spirochete *Borrelia burgdorferi*. There is frequently a history of an initial characteristic rash, erythema chronicum migrans (ECM). ECM appears as single or multiple target-like lesions, with central clearing. Recent studies suggest that the overwhelming majority of patients with Lyme disease do have a rash at the onset of their illness. This rash may be associated with a flu-like syndrome and symptoms of aseptic meningitis. Fluctuating neurologic syndromes, including facial palsy, may develop shortly thereafter. Cardiac conduction disease, which can fluctuate but may be complete, also occurs. The joint involvement is a mono- or oligoarticular, remittent or intermittent, large-joint arthritis. It does *not* cause a symmetrical polyarthritis of small joints similar to rheumatoid arthritis. It is associated with inflammatory joint fluid. The diagnosis of Lyme disease must include:

* Opportunity for the patient to have been exposed to a suitable tick vector

Affected Joint Distribution

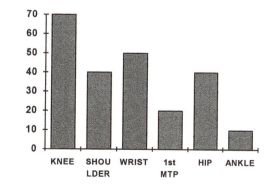

Figure 28.7. Septic arthritis in adults. (Reprinted with permission from Martens PB, Ho G. J Intensive Care Med 1995;10:246–252.)

Figure 28.8. Spectrum of disseminated GC infection.

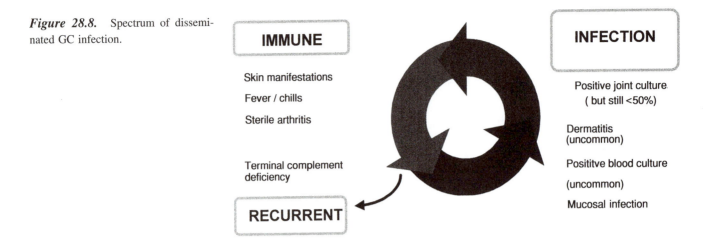

- Clinical pattern of symptoms consistent with described disease manifestations
- Positive ELISA assay supported by positive Western Blot

Seronegative Lyme disease is extremely uncommon, and the diagnosis of this should be entertained only with a great deal of trepidation. Fibromyalgia, although described in persons who have had lyme disease, is *not* a symptom complex suggestive of *active* infection.

Culture and Crystal Negative Acute Arthritis   In cases in which a cause for the monoarticular arthritis is not initially found to be due to crystals, and bacterial cultures are negative in the absence of prior antibiotic use, the differential diagnosis should include:

- Lyme disease (*if* potential exposure was possible—the absence of a concurrent rash does not exclude this diagnosis)
- Mycobacterial infection
- Fungal infection
- Reactive arthritis

Undiagnosed systemic diseases, such as psoriasis or inflammatory bowel disease, can also cause chronic monoarticular arthritis. Periarticular osteomyelitis should also be considered.

Reactive Arthritis   Reactive arthritis, in general, is a diagnosis of exclusion at the time of first presentation with monoarticular arthritis. The arthritis is presumably reactive to infection elsewhere in the body. The joint fluids are sterile, although some authors have suggested that specific bacterial antigens (including *Chlamydia*) may be present within the joint. Organisms associated with reactive arthritis include *Chlamydia, Salmonella, Clostridia difficile,* and *Yersinia.* Patients with reactive arthritis may have the other features of Reiter's syndrome, including mild conjunctivitis or uveitis, urethritis, which may be allergic or infectious, balanitis, psoriasiform

skin lesions, or oral ulcerations. The pattern of joint involvement is often large joints with a lower extremity predominance; joint fluid may be extremely inflammatory. Sausage digits, enthesitis, and sacroiliac involvement may also occur.

Viral Infections   Viral infections have also been associated with acute arthritis. Viral arthritis is often associated with a pseudorheumatoid pattern, although some forms of arthritis have been associated with mono- or oligoarticular arthritis (*Varicella*, cytomegalovirus [CMV], herpes simplex virus type 1 [HSV-1], human immunodeficiency virus [HIV]). Rubella-associated arthritis affects females more frequently than males, and occurs in 50–60% of patients following natural infection and perhaps 50% of patients following immunization. Approximately 1/3 of patients having joint symptoms retain these symptoms for approximately 1 year. *Parvovirus* (''fifth disease'' in children) has been associated with arthritis and arthralgias in adults, usually in a polyarticular pattern, in the absence of the typical skin eruption that is seen in children. Transient rheumatoid factor may occur in these patients. Parvovirus infection has also been associated with aplastic crises in patients with chronic hemolysis, or significant anemia. Hepatitis B and C have been associated with joint symptoms in the absence or presence of cryoglobulinemia, and can totally mimic acute rheumatoid arthritis. In one report there was an increased frequency of distal finger joint involvement with hepatitis B. The arthritis can be associated with the prodromal phase, or in the setting of chronic active hepatitis. It also can be associated with a polyarteritis nodosa syndrome. Hepatitis C-induced arthritis frequently occurs in association with cryoglobulinemia and high-titer rheumatoid factor; it may be present in patients who have only a minimal elevation in liver enzymes. HIV infection has been associated with an acute, extremely painful oligoarthritis associated with minimally or noninflammatory synovial fluid. There may be marked hyperesthesia of the joint capsule.

Diagnosis of Septic Arthritis

The diagnosis of gonococcal infection is frequently made by culturing alternative sites, predominantly the urogenital tract.

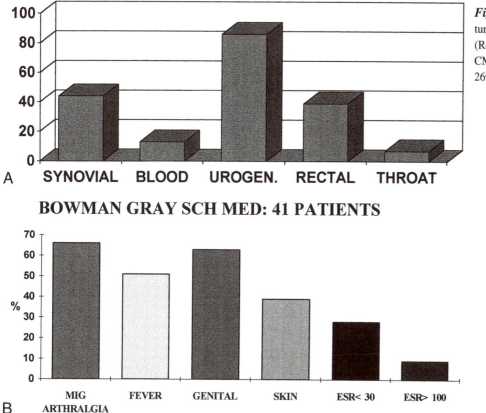

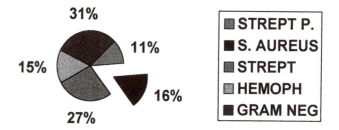

Figure 28.10. Polyarticular infections in patients without RA. Nongonococcal causative organisms. Six percent of all infected patients from a selected series had polyarticular diagnoses.

Figure 28.9. **a** and **b.** Positive culture results of patients with GC arthritis. (Reprinted with permission from Wise CM, et al. Arch Intern Med 1994;154: 2690–2695.)

It must be noted, however, that the absence of pelvic symptoms (or physical findings) in no way excludes the possibility of disseminated gonococcemia (Figs. 28.9a and 28.9b).

The appropriate evaluation of the patient with potential disseminated gonococcemia should include:

- Blood and joint-fluid cultures
- Cervical cultures (vaginal cultures in postmenopausal females)
- Rectal and pharyngeal cultures

The absence of rectal or pharyngeal symptoms does not obviate the need to obtain cultures from these areas. Patients with disseminated gonococcemia may have multiple joints involved. Other bacterial causes of nongonococcal polyarticular infections in patients without underlying rheumatoid arthritis (RA) are shown in Figure 28.10.

Treatment of Septic Arthritis

Treatment of suspected septic arthritis should not be delayed while waiting for culture results. If the diagnosis of infection is considered, the joints should be treated as a closed-space infection with parenteral systemic antibiotics and adequate local drainage. Percutaneous drainage of the joint is adequate if it can be performed efficiently. Hip joints are difficult to aspirate, and open drainage is usually utilized. Until a diagnosis is certain, percutaneous drainage of the affected joint(s)

should be performed daily, or as often as necessary to maintain an effusion-free joint. Successful antibiotic therapy is usually accompanied by a decrease in cell counts (the synovial WBC count generally decreases by 50% each day). The joint should be initially splinted for pain control and joint protection; however, as the inflammation resolves over subsequent days, passive and active physical therapy should be introduced as quickly as possible to preserve joint function. If disseminated gonococcemia is suspected, NSAIDs or other anti-inflammatory drugs should be withheld until the diagnosis is "solid," because a positive response to antibiotics may be necessary to support the diagnosis of gonorrhea when cultures are negative, and response to NSAID therapy may cause confusion.

There is no role for intraarticular antibiotics. At present, there are no data to suggest that any alternative drainage approach—such as lavage, arthroscopy, or arthrotomy—is superior to *adequate* percutaneous drainage in adults. Until a diagnosis is confirmed by culture, each aspirated joint fluid sample should be evaluated for the presence of crystals by polarized microscopy, because the crystals may have been missed on the initial evaluation. Recommended antibiotic regimens vary according to local bacteria-resistance profiles and patient demographics. One general initial antibiotic regimen for treating septic arthritis could be:

- Young healthy patients
  - Rx for gonococcus (GC)/*Staphylococcus/ Streptococcus*
- Patients with underlying joint disease, prolonged hospitalization, prior antibiotic use, urinary tract infections (UTIs), or prostate disease
  - Rx for methicillin-resistant *Staph* (MRSA) and gram-negative bacteria
- Patients with a history of intravenous drug abuse
  - Consider HIV issues
  - *Pseudomonas,* MRSA

After confirming Lyme disease and identifying the stage of the disease, treatment options include:

- ECM state—Rx on clinical grounds (21–28 days)
  - Doxycycline 100 bid
  - Amoxicillin 500 tid
  - Erythromycin 250–500 qid
- Stage 2 neurologic/cardiac disease (14–28 days)
  - Intravenous penicillin 20 million units qd
  - Intravenous ceftriaxone 1 g q12h
  - Doxycycline 100 bid

Thirty days of therapy in 38 patients with arthritis caused by Lyme disease produced the following results:

- Doxycycline 100 bid: 18/20 response
- Amoxicillin/probenecid 500 qid: 16/18 response

Note that although the majority of patients responded in less than 1 month to this regimen, response may take 3 months.

REVIEW EXERCISES

QUESTIONS

1. A 56-year-old white male presents to the emergency room with a 2-day history of increasing right wrist pain and associated swelling. He denies a history of prior episodes of arthritis or any antecedent trauma. His only medication is a diuretic for treatment of hypertension. He was recently hospitalized for a transurethral prostatic resection for benign prostatic hypertrophy. His older brother has been diagnosed with gout. The most useful diagnostic tests include:

   a. Radiograph of the wrist
   b. Serum uric acid level
   c. CBC with differential and ESR
   d. b and c
   e. None is particularly useful

2. A 56-year-old male is found to have a serum uric acid value of 9.4. Clear-cut indications for treatment with allopurinol include:

   a. A 24-hour urinary urate excretion > 1000 mg
   b. A creatinine value of 2.6
   c. A history of two episodes of documented gouty arthritis in the past 2 years
   d. A requirement for chronic HCTZ
   e. None of the above

3. All of the conditions below may be associated with hypouricemia except:

   a. Syndrome of inappropriate antidiuretic hormone (SIADH)
   b. High-dose salicylate therapy
   c. Wilson's disease
   d. Lactic acidosis
   e. Early alcohol withdrawal

4. Preoperative medical consultation was requested on a 56-year-old white, insulin-dependent, diabetic male with peripheral vascular disease and osteomyelitis/septic arthritis of the fourth toe. Pain, redness, and swelling was noted for 6 weeks and was only minimally responsive to medication with an oral antibiotic. Drainage of pus reportedly had increased over the previous week. ESR was 54 and WBC 10.5. Bone scan was positive in three phases, and radiographs showed periarticular PIP bone erosion with patchy sclerosis and demineralization of the phalanx. As the medical consultant, you recommend:

   a. Preoperative angiogram, an approach for glucose management, and consideration for spinal anesthesia
   b. Percutaneous (needle) bone cultures off antibiotics plus above preoperative evaluation
   c. Culture of sinus tract for sensitivities and 3 days preoperative intravenous (IV) antibiotics plus above preoperative evaluation
   d. Full reexamination of pus, including microscopy, before above preoperative evaluation

5. A 26-year-old African-American female presents with a chief complaint of foot pain. Examination reveals ankle-joint arthritis. She is afebrile and otherwise symptom free. She has a documented history of sickle cell anemia. Synovial fluid reveals a white count of 18,000 with 86% neutrophils. No crystals are seen. She is treated with broad-spectrum antibiotics, but 3 days later is only minimally improved. Synovial cultures after 72 hours are negative. The presumptive diagnosis is:

   a. Gout
   b. Salmonella arthritis
   c. Avascular necrosis (AVN)
   d. Gonococcal arthritis
   e. Reactive arthritis

Answers

1. e
   The major differential diagnosis is between acute crystal disease and infection. The only reliable way to distinguish these is by synovial fluid analysis and culture. Data are presented in the syllabus to support this.

2. e
   Asymptomatic hyperuricemia in general need not be treated. No firm evidence exists that treating hyperuricemia in this range prevents renal disease or other end-organ dysfunction in the absence of any symptoms, laboratory dysfunction, or related problems (e.g., nephrolithiasis).

3. d
   Organic acidosis produces mild hyperuricemia, not hypouricemia. Causes of hypouricemia include SIADH, renal tubular disorders, very-high-dose aspirin therapy, hydration, and administration of radiocontrast agents.

4. d
   As the medical consultant, it is worthwhile to review the primary data whenever possible. In this case, examination of the "pus" revealed that the infection was actually a draining uric acid tophus.

5. d
   Seventy-two hours is not always sufficient time to observe a dramatic response to antibiotics. Whereas salmonella or other routine bacterial infections would have been expected to have been recognized in bacterial culture, gonococcus often is not isolated from joint fluid. Gout is more common in sickle cell patients, but the diagnosis of gout should not be made in this setting in the absence of visualized crystals. AVN does NOT elicit an inflammatory synovial fluid response.

REFERENCES

1. Mandell BF. Unpublished.
2. Schlapbach P. Bacteria arthritis: are fevers, rigors, leuko-cytosis, and blood cultures of diagnostic value? Clin Rheumatol 1990;9:69–72.
3. Ho G, DeNuccio M. Gout and pseudogout in the hospitalized patient. Arch Int Med 1993;153:2787–2790.
4. George TM, Mandell BF. Gout in the transplant patient. J Clin Rheumatol 1996;1:328–334.

SUGGESTED READINGS

George TM, Mandell BF. Individualizing the treatment of gout. Cleve Clinic J Med 1996;63:150–155.

Pioro MH, Mandell BF. Septic arthritis. Rheum Dis Clin N.A. 1997;23:239–258.

The Differential Diagnosis of Polyarthritis

Gary S. Hoffman

RHEUMATOID ARTHRITIS

Rheumatoid arthritis (RA) is the most common form of chronic inflammatory polyarthropathy. Accordingly, it will be used as the reference point for comparison with other disorders in this overview.

All man's activities of daily living depend on normal ambulation and dexterity. Minor motor function abnormalities are immediately acknowledged and become a serious concern when lifestyles are compromised. Thus, it is not surprising that RA, the most obvious manifestation of rheumatoid disease, has been emphasized in the diagnosis, treatment, and basic research of this multisystem disorder. In fact, the 1987 Revised American College of Rheumatology Criteria for RA include among the seven useful criteria for diagnosis, five that specifically relate to joints:

1. Morning stiffness ≥1 hour
2. Arthritis of ≥3 joint *areas* (MCPs, PIPs, MTPs grouped as single areas)
3. Arthritis of hand joints
4. Symmetry (1–4 must be present for at least 6 weeks to rule out transient arthropathies, such as may be associated with viral illnesses)
5. Rheumatoid nodules
6. Serum rheumatoid factor
7. Radiographic changes

Four criteria generally indicate RA; more than four increases certainty.

Although most rheumatoid patients' complaints are musculoskeletal, some patients may present with:

- Lethargy
- Weight loss
- General malaise
- Fever
- Pleuropulmonary or cardiovascular symptoms
- ''Unsightly red palms''
- Painless periarticular nodule(s)
- Dry mucous membranes

These features constitute a few examples of the systemic nature of the aberrant rheumatoid immune diathesis.

Diagnosis of the patient with rheumatoid factor-positive, nodule-forming, erosive polyarthritic disease is not a problem. It is the slowly progressive or early-stage rheumatoid disease that is often difficult to diagnose and is most likely to be confused with other processes. Compounding the problem, early RA is often rheumatoid factor-negative and joint fluid may have noninflammatory qualities, although the synovium may be histologically abnormal.

DIFFERENTIAL DIAGNOSIS OF RHEUMATOID ARTHRITIS (1,2)

The differential diagnosis of symmetrical polyarthralgias and polyarthritis is often difficult. This chapter will attempt to distinguish the various illnesses that may present in this manner from other than obvious severe rheumatoid disease with established deformities. Table 29.1 represents a *partial* list of diseases that can be confused with RA. A minority of this group, shown in Table 29.2, has the potential to produce articular erosions and bony destruction. Most patients develop symptoms prior to showing swelling, inflammatory joint fluid, or erosions. As this is often the nature of these processes, a definitive diagnosis should be deferred until repeated examination elicits diagnostic findings.

The disorders discussed below fall into 3 groups (Table 29.1):

- Group 1. Arthritis with the potential to cause joint destruction.

Table 29.1. Polyarthralgias or Arthritis: Histologic and Roentgenographic Comparisons

Pannus with Potential for Articular Erosion	Pannus Without Articular Erosions	No Pannus or Erosions
RA	SLE, progressive systemic sclerosis, dermatomyosistis or polymyositis	Hypothyroidism

Septic
  Acute
    Insidious
      Fungal
      Tuberculous
	Vasculitis: polyarteritis nodosa, Henoch Schönlein purpura, Wegener granulomatosis, allergic angiitis, hepatitis B or C virus with vasculitis and/or cryoglobulinemia	Hyperparathyroidism
		Hemosiderosis/Hemochromatosis
		Osteoarthritis

Microcrystalline diseases Pseudo-RA	Essential cryoglobulinemia	Pancreatitis and periarticular fat necrosis
Ankylosing spondylitis	Hepatitis without vasculitis	Subacute bacterial endocarditis
Reiter's syndrome	Rubella, spontaneous and postvaccination	Rheumatic fever
Psoriatic arthritis	Other viruses	Polymyalgia rheumatica/giant cell arteritis
Arthritis of inflammatory bowel disease Postinfectious arthritis;† *Yersinia, Shigella, Salmonella* sp. Behçet's syndrome†	Lyme arthritis* Sarcoid arthritis* Leukemic arthritis Hypertrophic osteoarthropathy, 1° or 2°	Sickle cell disease
Mixed connective tissue disease and other ''overlap'' syndromes	Remote effects of solid tumors Amyloid, 1° or 2°	

* Erosions very rare, < 1% cases

† Erosions rare, < 5% cases

From Hoffman GS: Polyarthritis: The differential diagnosis of rheumatoid arthritis. Semin Arthritis Rheumatol 1979;8:115–141.

- Group 2. Arthritis with joint lining (synovial) proliferation, without destruction.
- Group 3. Arthritis with little or no synovial proliferation.

ARTHRITIS WITH THE POTENTIAL TO CAUSE JOINT DESTRUCTION

The following arthropathies have in common varying degrees of synovial proliferation. Articular erosion is common in RA and the spondyloarthropathies.

ACUTE ARTHRITIS

Acute Monarticular Process

An acute monarticular process should lead to consideration of microcrystalline (calcium pyrophosphate dihydrate or sodium urate) or septic arthritis. In each case, the synovial fluid will usually be inflammatory, and identification of crystals or infectious organisms is necessary for diagnosis. If neither crystals nor microorganisms are found on initial synovial analyses,

repeated aspiration and evaluation may prove diagnostic. Intra-articular steroids should *not* be used when the etiology of inflammatory monarticular arthritis is unclear and therefore potentially infectious. In a study of 293 rheumatoid patients, 1 patient in 6 presented with a monarticular arthritis (most often in a knee) lasting for at least one week before involvement of other joints became apparent. Similar observations have been made for other chronic inflammatory polyarthritides: ankylosing spondylitis, Reiter's syndrome, psoriatic arthritis (3).

Acute Polyarticular

Gout and septic arthritis may present as an acute polyarthritis. In one series, 102 cases of polyarticular gout were noted among 1830 gouty subjects (6% polyarticular) (4). In 12 of 34 crystal-proven cases, acute polyarthritis was the first manifestation of microcrystalline arthritis; eighty-three percent of involved joints were in the lower extremity, but in one-third of the cases the foot was spared. Asymmetric involvement tended to be the rule. In 40% (13 of 34) of those with documented crystal-induced synovitis, serum uric acid concentrations were less than 7.0 mg/dl, but 90% of these nor-

Table 29.2.   Erosive Polyarthritis: Differential Features

	Clinical Features	*Onset*	*Sex (M/F)*	*Laboratory*
RA	Bilateral, symmetric large and/or small joints. Less often monoarticular onset or asymmetric. Cervical and occasionally dorsal or lumbar spine. Nodules in 15%.	Variable Insidious-acute	1:3	RF in ~75%*
Septic	Nongonococcal, usually monoarticular, can be polyarticular; if polyarticular, asymmetric pauciarticular. Gonococcal often has polyarticular onset.	Acute, although TB, atypical TB, fungus usually insidious	No sexual preference in nongonococcal, gonococcal 1:8	Positive Gram stain or cultures
Gout	Usually monoarticular, can be polyarticular. Asymmetric symmetric if polyarticular. Weight-bearing joints most often.	Acute, occasionally chronic, tophaceous, polyarticular	19:1	Na urate crystals in fluid
Pseudogout	Similar to gout; infrequently can look like RA, as can gout (''pseudo-RA'')	Acute, infrequently subacute	1:1	CPPD crystals in fluid
Ankylosing spondylitis	Sacroiliitis, spondylitis, limb girdle joints, less often peripheral joints	Insidious-subacute	10:1	HLA-B27 present in ~90%
Reiter syndrome†	20%–80% spondylitis	Insidious-subacute	10:1	HLA-B27 present in ~80%
Psoriatic arthritis†	Peripheral arthritis-asymmetric tendency, affects 5% psoriatics and about 10%–20% of patients with IBD. About 2% of psoriatics and 5% IBD cases have axial skeleton disease.†	Insidious-subacute	1:1	HLA-B27 present in ~80% of those with spondylitis and sacroiliitis
Inflammatory bowel disease†		Insidious-subacute	1:1	

* RF (rheumatoid factor) usually negative in remaining erosive conditions.
† Associated with features of disease, i.e., skin, eyes, GU, GI tracts.
From Hoffman GS: Polyarthritis: The differential diagnosis of rheumatoid arthritis. Semin Arthritis Rheumatol 1979;8:115–141.

mouricemic patients were hyperuricemic before or after the polyarticular attack.

It should be apparent that gout can mimic other inflammatory polyarthritides, that definitive diagnosis depends on demonstration of sodium urate crystals from joints or tophi, and normal serum uric acid does not rule out gouty arthritis.

Calcium Pyrophosphate Dihydrate Microcrystalline Disease

Historically, calcium pyrophosphate dihydrate (CPPD) microcrystalline disease has most often been associated with acute monoarticular or pauciarticular arthritis. McCarty has stressed the varied presentations of CPPD deposition, including osteoarthritis, ''Charcot'' joints, and ''pseudo rheumatoid arthritis'' (5). About 5% of affected patients have subacute or

chronic polyarticular disease that may be associated with synovial proliferation and erosions in subchondral bone and, less often, at articular surfaces. Erosions may occur without radiographic evidence of chondrocalcinosis, in which case diagnosis depends on identification of crystals in synovial fluid, periarticular soft tissue, or cartilage. Along with clinical signs of inflammation (heat, synovial proliferation, inflammatory fluid), useful radiographic clues include:

• Subchondral cysts
• Sclerosis
• Osteophyte formation (osteoarthritis)

in the carpal bones and metacarpophalangeal (MCP) joints.

The MCP, wrist, and elbow joints are uncommon sites for osteoarthritic changes. Such changes suggest CPPD disease as a primary event leading to degenerative plus inflammatory events.

Septic Arthritis

Septic arthritis is usually not difficult to distinguish from rheumatoid disease. The onset of infection is usually acute and monarticular. Difficulty in diagnosis may arise in as many as 20% of nongonococcal septic cases in which pauciarticular disease and, less often, polyarticular disease occur. Such cases are usually asymmetric. Synovial fluid white blood cell (WBC) counts usually exceed 50,000/mm^3 and includes greater than 85% polymorphonuclear (PMN) cells. However, moderately inflamed synovial fluids with WBC counts of 5,000–10,000/mm^3; may also occur. Conversely, although rheumatoid disease is usually associated with synovial fluid WBC counts of 5,000–25,000/mm^3, WBC counts may occasionally exceed 100,000/mm^3.

Initial management of a case of possible septic arthritis may be confused by the knowledge that gram stains of synovial fluid are positive in only two-thirds of nongonococcal septic arthritis cases later proven to be septic by culture (6,7). Positive synovial fluid cultures occur in only 25%–50% of presumed gonococcal arthritis patients, perhaps in part because of reversion of the gonococcus to a protoplast or L form. Thus it is very important to try to identify and culture a primary source of infection (e.g., pharyngeal, respiratory, genitourinary, etc.) in all suspected cases.

SEPTIC ARTHRITIS IN RA

A superimposed infection should be suspected in the patient with known RA who develops progressively worsening problems in one or more joints. Most of the time, because such joint problems appear to be "out of phase" with the tempo of the patient's rheumatoid disease, they will eventually be proven to stem from rheumatoid arthritis and *not* infection. However, when the RA patient develops nongonococcal septic arthritis, mortality has been reported to vary from 23% to as high as 88%. In an extensive review, complete joint recovery occurred in only 43% of rheumatoid patients, compared with a 10% mortality and 73% complete recovery rate in the nongonococcal septic arthritis population as a whole (6). These data suggest that a rheumatoid joint "active" enough to be considered for corticosteroid injection should always be aspirated and synovial analyses conducted (including culture).

Survivorship studies have reported death from infection occurring 7–10 times more often in patients with rheumatoid disease than among age-matched controls. The high incidence of morbidity and mortality from infection has been related to (8,9,10):

- Delay in diagnosis
- Corticosteroid and other forms of immunosuppressive therapy
- Felty syndrome

- Impaired PMN cell chemotaxis
- Decreased bacteriolytic and bactericidal activity of rheumatoid serum and synovial fluid
- Impaired T lymphocyte function

VIRAL ARTHRITIS

Viral Infectious Arthritis

Rheumatoid arthritis and bacterial and fungal arthritis may produce erosive bony change, whereas viral infectious arthritis does not. Symptoms are generally of brief duration and require only symptomatic therapy. Naturally occurring rubella arthritis develops more often in adults than in children. Joint symptoms may occur before, after, or simultaneously with the onset of the rash. Although polyarthralgias usually last for several days, they can persist for months to more than a year. Frank arthritis would be unusual with such a long course. However, it is in this setting that confusion with RA may occur. When small effusions can be aspirated, the WBC count is usually noninflammatory or mildly inflammatory, consisting of a predominance of lymphocytes. This may also be the case in early RA, but in longstanding disease, an increased number of WBC with a predominance of PMN cells occurs. A generally milder process also occurs after vaccination with attenuated rubella virus. The onset of joint symptoms may occur from within days to more than 3 months after vaccination. The duration is usually not greater than 3 weeks, but in some cases may last several months and, more rarely, follows an intermittent recurrent course affecting the knees up to 6 years later (11–13).

Viral Hepatitis

Another form of viral polyarthritis that occasionally mimics RA occurs in about 10–15% of cases of viral hepatitis. Usually joint symptoms and myalgias appear before the onset of jaundice, although not always. Symmetric polyarticular disease often involves both small distal as well as larger proximal joints. Cervical and lumbar pain can be present. A valuable clue may be the appearance of maculopapular, urticarial, or petechial eruptions in the preicteric period. The likelihood of confusion with RA increases in anicteric persons with no rash. In these instances, abnormal liver function tests, especially transaminase elevations, should lead to the correct diagnosis. Examination of synovial fluid usually shows the WBC count to be noninflammatory or mildly inflammatory and consisting of a predominance of lymphocytes, similar to most viral arthritides. However, there are exceptions. The musculoskeletal symptoms of the hepatitis-arthritis syndrome rarely last more than several weeks. Currently, no long-term musculoskeletal morbidity has been known to occur. Hepatitis B and C virus infections have less often been associated with mixed cryoglobulinemia, systemic vasculitis, and chronic liver disease. These complications usually include myalgias, arthralgias and/or arthritis, positive rheumatoid factors, and hypocomplementemia.

LYME DISEASE

The peak incidence of Lyme disease is in summer and early fall. As many as 60–80% of patients have an expanding erythematous skin lesion on a proximal extremity or the trunk that precedes arthritis by 1 week to more than 6 months. The skin lesion is the best clinical marker of Lyme disease. Some patients recall having a tick (Ixodes species) bite at the site of the initial lesion. The typical rash begins as a red papule that expands into a large erythematous warm annular lesion (6–52 cm), often with central clearing. The eruption may last from several days to up to 4 weeks. Pain and itching are uncommon, but a burning sensation is frequently reported. Prominent systemic symptoms may follow appearance of the rash.

When arthritis follows skin disease, the pattern is no different from when it occurs de novo. Monarticular or asymmetric large joint oligoarticular disease is most common, particularly involving the knees. However, small joint arthritis and symmetric distributions can also occur. Recurrent attacks may last weeks to months. Intervening periods are usually associated with complete remission. Synovial analyses produce varying results, with WBC counts ranging from the noninflammatory range (500/mm^3) to what is often suspected as compatible with septic arthritis (98,000/mm^3). Polymorphonuclear cells predominate. Synovial biopsies, indistinguishable from those of RA, show synovial hypertrophy, vascular proliferation, and marked infiltration with monocytes and plasma cells. In spite of these findings, erosive disease has been extremely uncommon (14–16). The use of sensitive techniques, such as PCR, has led to detection of the causative organism, *Borrelia burgdorferi,* in synovium. Since the original descriptions by Steere et al in 1977, subsequent experience has also led to enhanced appreciation of cardiac and neurologic complications due to direct infection and the inflammatory response to Borrelia. Epidemiologic studies have revealed that the preferred host for Ixodes vectors are deer and mice; humans, in fact, are not necessary for the tick's life cycle.

It is easy to understand why many of these patients were initially misdiagnosed as having RA. Indeed, in the absence of a typical rash and geographic clustering, RA should be part of the differential diagnosis of such a clinical picture. The definitive diagnosis of Lyme disease is hindered by insensitive and not generally available bacteriologic isolation techniques. In a clinical setting in which the diagnosis is highly suspect, serology studies, although imperfect, may be confirmatory.

During the early stages of illness (e.g., isolated skin lesion), serologic studies are usually negative. Several weeks after disease onset, the IgM antibody response peaks (week 3–6) and then usually falls to normal by about 6 months. Immunoglobulin G antibody is often detectable after weeks 4–8, peaks 5–10 months later, and may remain elevated. Early

diagnosis is crucial to maximize treatment response. Later stages of disease may respond slowly or not at all. Specific therapeutic regimens that have recently been reviewed (16) will not be discussed in this analysis of differential diagnosis.

REACTIVE, POSTINFECTIOUS ARTHRITIS

Inflammatory joint disease may also occur after self-limiting enteric infections. Patients having the histocompatibility antigen HLA-B27 may be at higher risk than controls for developing postinfectious polyarthritis (17–20). The most frequently implicated organisms are:

- Shigella
- Salmonella
- Yersinia
- Campylobacter
- Chlamydia

Yersiniosis is common in Scandinavian countries but uncommon in the United States. The severity of the enteric phase of disease is quite variable and, if mild, may not be reported by the patient. Thus, a clue leading to stool cultures may be missed. Diagnosis would then likely be made by serologic identification of antibodies to suspected bacterial antigens. The nature of the inflammatory postinfectious polyarthritis may be nonspecific or less often include features of Reiter syndrome (such as, conjunctivitis, iritis, mucosal lesions, keratodermia blennorrhagica, circinate balanitis, urethritis, sacroiliitis, spondylitis, and aortic insufficiency). On the other hand, Reiter syndrome can occur in the absence of any features of gastrointestinal or genitourinary infection.

Men aged 20–40 years are most often affected, although young children and octogenarians are also known to have had Reiter syndrome. The polyarthritis tends to develop in an additive fashion and is usually asymmetrical. When symmetry occurs, the intensity is often different on the right and left sides. The lower extremities are more often involved than the upper, and sacroiliac involvement occurs variably in 20–80% of patients. Tendinitis, plantar fasciitis and periostitis (particularly in the os calcis) are seen more often with this process than with other inflammatory polyarthritides. Any of the myriad clinical features may recur episodically in up to 75% of cases. An increased likelihood of erosions, deformity and chronic permanent articular dysfunction occur with increasing numbers of recurrences and increased duration of each episode.

Early reports of Reiter syndrome insisted on the presence of the classical triad of urethritis, arthritis, and conjunctivitis or iritis. However, with the recognition of additional clinical features, most authorities accept this diagnosis when any two of the original triad are present, plus typical mucocutaneous lesions, including nonpitting onycholysis. The presence of the HLA-B27 antigen gives increased weight to the diagnosis in cases that would otherwise be considered "incomplete Reiter syndrome." This marker occurs in at least 75% of cases, compared to 4–8% of controls (21).

ANKYLOSING SPONDYLITIS

The HLA-B27 marker is at least as common (more than 90%) in ankylosing spondylitis (AS) as in Reiter syndrome. The lower prevalence of AS in blacks appears to relate to the absence of the B27 antigen and associated disease susceptibility factors in the pure African black population. The 4% of American blacks who are B27-positive purportedly obtained the gene for this antigen through past racial admixtures. Population studies of B27-positive individuals have suggested about a 20% risk of developing features of AS.

Patients presenting with symptoms eventually diagnosed as AS are predominantly young males. In about 75% of patients, low back pain is the presenting complaint, whereas 25% note peripheral arthritis first. Peripheral arthritis may be indistinguishable from RA, and in fact, both processes occasionally may coexist. With increased duration of disease, about 50% of ankylosing spondylitics develop peripheral arthritis: by definition, 100% develop sacroiliitis with or without spondylitis. The absence of mucocutaneous lesions, onycholysis, urethritis or preceding ''dysentery'' distinguishes AS from Reiter spondylitis.

PSORIATIC ARTHRITIS

About 5% of psoriasis patients have arthritis, and about half of these have axial skeleton involvement. In most cases, peripheral arthritis is asymmetrical. Onycholysis occurs, as in Reiter syndrome, but in psoriasis is distinguished by the presence of pitting. In a minority of patients, arthritis may be rheumatoid factor-positive, associated with nodules, and clinically indistinguishable from RA; both diseases may coexist in these patients. Except for this group, unequivocal diagnosis of psoriatic arthritis requires psoriatic skin or nail disease. Radiographs often show erosions with periosteal new bone formation, most typically seen in DIP joints and the calcaneus. In advanced cases, osteolysis can produce wide gaps between bones. While skin and peripheral joint changes may parallel each other, this is not so with axial skeleton disease, the course of which is independent of skin involvement. Some have asserted that the frequency of HLA-B27 is 45% in psoriatics with spondylitis, but when axial disease is absent, the frequency is not significantly greater than in controls (17–19).

INFLAMMATORY BOWEL DISEASE (IBD) ARTHROPATHY

Inflammatory bowel disease (IBD) (ulcerative colitis and Crohn's disease) shares the potential for developing peripheral inflammatory polyarthritis and sacroiliitis and also spondylitis with Reiter syndrome, ankylosing spondylitis, and psoriasis. As many as 20% of IBD patients develop arthritis, with one-fourth of these having spine involvement. Arthritis may precede overt bowel disease in 20% of cases. Peripheral involvement commonly is asymmetric and more common in large joints of the lower extremities. It may be migratory and intermittent, paralleling the severity of bowel disease. Destructive changes, such as those seen in RA or psoriatic arthritis, follow an independent course regardless of therapy and are more often associated with uveitis. Uncomplicated IBD, or IBD with only peripheral arthritis, does not have an increased incidence of HLA-B27. However, when both sacroiliitis and spondylitis occur, this marker may appear in 60%–89% of cases. When iritis complicates IBD it usually occurs in the B27 spondylitic group, suggesting that iritis and spine involvement share a common etiologic factor (20, 21).

In addition to the spondyloarthropathies already noted, Behcet syndrome and Whipple disease may affect peripheral joints, the axial skeleton and the eyes. Behcet syndrome is truly one of the ''great imitators.'' Since Behcet described the triad of iritis and painful oral and genital ulcers in 1937, it has become apparent that the majority of cases also include nonulcerative skin lesions and musculoskeletal symptoms. Among the 50–60% of the patients with musculoskeletal problems, three-fourths have an asymmetric inflammatory polyarthritis. Knees, ankles, and wrists are most often affected. Patients only occasionally develop sacroiliitis. Joint deformity and loss of motion is uncommon. Less often, central nervous system disease (about 20% of cases) and peripheral nervous system disease occurs, as well as thrombophlebitis, pulmonary infiltrates, hemoptysis and colitis. Since aphthous stomatitis, arthritis and inflammatory eye disease occur in both ulcerative colitis and Behcet colitis, distinguishing these two diseases may be difficult. Organic involvement of the central nervous system, genital ulcers, or the development of sterile pustular lesions at injection and venipuncture sites favor the diagnosis of Behcet syndrome.

The principal feature distinguishing B27-related processes from RA is the likely development of an enthesopathy of the axial skeleton that is inflammation of ligamentous attachments to bone. A postmortem study examination of many areas of different pathologic age suggested that inflammation was followed by formation of new bone in ligaments and disc margins. Synovitis of the vertebral apophyseal joints was common. While cervical arthritis is frequent in RA, subcervical axial arthritis is usually not a prominent clinical feature, although it is often noted at postmortem examination. If the dorsolumbar spine becomes an obvious problem in a known rheumatoid patient, consider intercurrent processes such as strain, osteoarthritis, disc herniation, vertebral collapse, malignancy and referred visceral pain.

CHRONIC NON-EROSIVE SYNOVITIS

The nonspondylitic, non-HLA-B27-related rheumatic diseases that are likely to be mistaken for RA include:

- Mixed connective tissue disease (MCTD)
- Systemic lupus erythematosus (SLE)
- Idiopathic inflammatory muscle disease (i.e., polymyositis (PM) or dermatomyositis (DM)

- Progressive systemic sclerosis (PSS)
- The vasculitides

When the classical features of these processes are lacking, the diseases may merely present as symmetric polyarthralgias or polyarthritis. The synovial process may be noninflammatory or inflammatory, with modest amounts of fluid produced (usually less than 15 cc in a large joint, such as a knee). Erosions of articular surfaces are rare. If polyarticular symmetric erosive disease occurs, it would be more appropriate to consider this an "overlap" syndrome of RA plus the other established rheumatic process. This is a clinically significant distinction because the therapeutic approach to the arthritis of RA would be more aggressive than that for the nonerosive mild synovitis seen in other noted conditions.

By the strictest criteria, MCTD should have features of SLE, PSS, and myositis. By definition, diagnosis of this syndrome also requires the presence of high titers of antibodies to an extractable nuclear antigen (ENA) obtained from calf thymus. This antigen (ENA) has since been found to be heterogeneous and composed of ribonucleoprotein (RNP), a ribonuclease-resistant protein (Sm), and still other as yet unidentified substituents. Patients with SLE may have high titers of antibodies to ENA, most specifically to the Sm protein. However, as many as 25–50% also have antibodies to RNP. High titers of antibodies to RNP are compatible with but not diagnostic of MCTD. The appropriate clinical features should also be present. The presence of anti-Sm antibodies would virtually rule out MCTD, and is felt by some to be diagnostic of SLE. Anti-Sm antibodies occur in 30–40% of SLE patients (22, 23).

Antinuclear antibodies (ANA), determined with fluorescein-tagged antisera (FANA), are noted for more than 95% of patients with both MCTD and SLE. When the FANA pattern is speckled and of high titer, a strong correlation exists with antibodies to the ENA antigens.

The reporting of clinical MCTD material has concentrated to a much greater extent on antibodies to ENA than on truly satisfying the clinical diagnosis of MCTD. Consequently, the largest series of these patients includes 37% lacking features of myositis and 67% lacking sclerodermatous skin changes. The most common clinical features include:

- Raynaud's phenomenon (81%)
- Polyarthralgias (90%)
- Polyarthritis (74%)
- Swollen hands (73%)

The following conditions are less frequent than reported in most lupus series:

- Renal disease (13%)
- CNS abnormalities (10%)
- Hypocomplementemia (20–25%)
- Positive lupus (LE cell) preparations (20%)

It is apparent that most of the features of MCTD also exist in SLE. Whether some of the MCTD population should

be considered distinct or a subset of SLE is probably not important. What is important is the observation that those patients who have high titers of anti-RNP antibodies have: a milder type of immune complex disease, a more predictable response to therapy, and a better prognosis compared with others with high titers of antinative DNA antibodies and hypocomplementemia. In these situations, different types of nucleic acids (RNP, DNA, etc.) form unique immune complexes with different pathogenetic potentials. That such processes are associated with different clinical pictures is also illustrated by comparing spontaneously occurring SLE with drug-induced disease. The latter has many features indistinguishable from spontaneous disease, but antibodies to native DNA, hypocomplementemia, and chronic renal or CNS disease would all be unusual in the drug-induced form. Of course, a medication history is very important in the patient with musculoskeletal symptoms and a positive FANA test. Merely stopping the offending drug is usually adequate therapy.

Criteria for SLE include:

1. Malar rash
2. Discoid rash
3. Photosensitivity (rash)
4. Oral (or nasopharyngeal) ulcers
5. Arthritis, nonerosive, peripheral joints
6. Serositis
7. Renal disease >500 mg proteinuria/24 hours or 3 + by dipstick or cellular casts
8. Neurologic disease, CNS: seizures, psychosis
9. Heme: hemolytic anemia, leukopenia <4K, lymphopenia <1.5K, platelets <100K
10. Immunologic disorder: +LE prep, anti-DNA or Sm or false positive test for syphilis
11. + ANA in absence of drugs known to produce + ANA

Diagnosis = $\geq$4

SARCOIDOSIS

The many faces of sarcoidosis have fascinated physicians of all interests. The incidence of rheumatic and other manifestations of sarcoid disease depend on the methods used to gather clinical material. In European studies, whites comprise the majority of most series; blacks predominate in American series gathered from large metropolitan centers. Men and women are affected with equal frequency.

The association of polyarthralgias or polyarthritis and bilateral hilar adenopathy strongly favors a diagnosis of sarcoid. In one series of 74 patients with bilateral hilar adenopathy, this association occurred in 15%. If erythema nodosum or uveitis occurred as well, the diagnosis of sarcoid was histologically confirmed in all patients. This constellation of findings did not occur in other patients with lymphoma, bronchogenic carcinoma, metastatic carcinoma to the lungs, or tuberculosis (24).

The most common musculoskeletal complaints of sarcoid disease are migratory polyarthralgias affecting large joints, particularly ankles and knees. Less often, the wrists, fingers, forefeet, elbows, shoulders, and heels are involved. Periarticular swelling and discomfort is more frequent than actual joint effusions. When effusions have been examined, there have been only several milliliters of fluid, which contained less than 1000 WBC/mm^3, chiefly the mononuclear type. Synovial biopsies have shown mild, focal-lining-cell proliferation and scattered round-cell infiltrates. The implied benignity of these observations is consistent with the self-limiting course of joint disease in more than 95% of cases. Chronic articular or skin disease is usually part of a chronic diffuse granulomatous process. Between 10–30% of all patients are positive for rheumatoid factor (Table 29.3) (25). This observation bears no relation to the severity of musculoskeletal disease. Confusion with RA should not occur since most patients have other features of sarcoidosis, particularly abnormal chest radiographs.

Table 29.3.   Rheumatoid Factor-Positive Results in Nonrheumatic Conditions

Conditions	*Latex Fixation Human F-11 Tests*	
	Number Sampled	*Positive (%)*
Age <29 years	2828	2
Age 30–59 years	2536	4
Age >60 years	413	24
SBE	58	48
Syphilis	215	13
Hepatitis	12	24
Leishmaniasis	10	100
Mononucleosis	70	4 (22°C)
	50	72 (4°C)
Monocryoprecipitates	20	100
Sarcoidosis	231	17
Tuberculosis	377	11
Leprosy	101	24
Bronchitis	105	62
Asthma	23	17
Idiopathic pulmonary fibrosis	66	32
Purpura hyperglobulinemia	5	100
Multiple myeloma	88	18
Liver cirrhosis	115	36
Macroglobulinemia		
Secondary	48	35
Primary	76	30
Leukemia and lymphoma	54	19
Cancer	151	22
Purpura cryoglobulinemia	13	90
Renal homograft	81	74
Myocardial infarction	55	12

Reprinted with permission from Annals of the New York Academy of Science. 1969;168:30.

MALIGNANCY AND ARTHRITIS

Numerous malignant processes, including solid tumors, leukemias and myelomas, have been associated with musculoskeletal problems. A symmetric polyarthritis of large and small joints has been reported to occur with (26–29):

- Bronchogenic adenocarcinoma
- Esophageal carcinoma
- Fibrous mesothelioma of the pleura
- Carcinomas of the:
  - prostate
  - kidney
  - thyroid
  - colon
  - rectum
  - larynx
  - breast
  - ovary
  - pancreas

The diagnosis and treatment of rheumatic complaints often precedes recognition of the associated malignancy. Although these patients have had joint swelling, rheumatoid factors were usually negative and articular erosions were not noted. In one case of metastatic lymphosarcoma to bone and skin, periarticular tumor deposits were responsible for erosions occurring along the shafts of long bones but not at the joint margins. Bennett et al (26) reported a case of ovarian adenocarcinoma presenting as rheumatoid-factor-positive, symmetric, inflammatory polyarthritis. No erosions were seen radiographically. Four days after tumor resection, complete remission occurred. A similar case, with pulmonary epidermoid carcinoma, was associated with high titers of rheumatoid factor and subcutaneous nodules, histologically compatible with the rheumatoid type of arthritis. The patient experienced remission of arthritis and disappearance of nodules and rheumatoid factor following resection of the tumor. Harrison and Scherbel (27) reported marked improvement of rheumatoid symptoms in cases of prostatic carcinoma treated with estrogens. Mackenzie and Scherbel (29) made the same observation in 8 of 11 cases of various solid tumors that were effectively treated. In many cases, it is uncertain whether improvement in rheumatic symptoms was directly related to chemotherapy, diminution of tumor, or both.

Hypertrophic Osteoarthropathy (HOA)

Patients in whom the relationship between tumor and rheumatic symptoms is more firmly established have hypertrophic osteoarthropathy (HOA). The presence of subperiosteal new bone formation along the shafts of long bones (especially tibia, fibulas, radii, ulnae and phalanges) and digital clubbing distinguishes the musculoskeletal symptoms of HOA from the previously discussed group of diseases. Complaints of pain relate to the long bones as well as the joints. Knees, ankles, wrists and fingers are most often involved. Relief from pain may follow use of nonsteroidal antiinflammatory agents. Mistaking this process for RA is usual, especially when no known tumor is present and clubbing is not present (or had been present since childhood). Pain along the shafts of tubular bones, the absence of articular erosions and rheumatoid factor, and the presence of noninflammatory synovial fluid also helps to distinguish HOA from RA (1).

Most clinicians are familiar with HOA being associated with primary pulmonary malignancies and metastatic disease to the lung. The incidence has been variably reported as 2–50% of pulmonary carcinomas: the 50% incidence relating to pleural mesotheliomas. Nonmalignant pulmonary disease (bronchiectasis, abscess, cysts, tuberculosis) as well as extrapulmonary inflammatory processes (liver abscesses, biliary and portal cirrhosis, inflammatory bowel disease, hydatid cysts) and chronic hypoxemic states have also been associated with HOA. Hypertrophic osteoarthropathy has also been associated with pregnancy: in one patient, HOA symptoms followed by prompt remission occurred in each of four pregnancies (30).

Most patients with secondary HOA improve if treatment is effective for the underlying process. A temporary or incomplete response suggests inadequate therapy. Thus, not only might HOA be the first sign of malignancy, it may also be the first sign of recurrence.

Multiple Myeloma

Multiple myeloma, a malignant plasma cell disorder, is known to cause osteopenia, vertebral collapse, and diffuse bone pain. Infrequently, it is associated with polyarthritis resembling RA, and may be so treated initially. Arthritis may precede other signs of myeloma or occur following that diagnosis. Synovial fluid analyses usually show noninflammatory or mildly inflammatory fluid, with mononuclear cells predominating. Occasionally fluid, especially if centrifuged, may contain tissue fragments with amyloid that can be identified by Congo red staining and characteristic green birefringence, as seen with polarized light microscopy. Synovial biopsies, as well as biopsies of periarticular tissues, have shown amyloid deposits that account for articular complaints. Such deposits may also occur with primary amyloidosis. Although involved joints may be quite swollen from amyloid infiltration, erythema and increased heat would be unusual and should lead to consideration of other processes. Joint radiographs may show the typical punched-out lytic lesions of myeloma along the shafts of long bones, but articular erosions, as seen in RA, usually do not occur. Observations confusing the approach to the patient with myeloma and polyarthritis are: some patients with RA can occasionally have M components without demonstrable myeloma or amyloidosis, and others may have well-established classic RA, later to be followed by myeloma.

Lymphocytic or Myelocytic Leukemias

Acute and, less often, chronic lymphocytic or myelocytic leukemias may be associated with arthritis that can be either monoarticular or polyarticular, static or migratory, symmetric or asymmetric. Children are affected up to 5 times more often than adults. Arthritis may precede overt leukemia or complicate the course of a known leukemic patient. Involved joints may be symptomatic but lacking objective findings, or may be warm, erythematous, and swollen. Synovial fluid analyses have shown noninflammatory or mildly inflammatory WBC counts, with either lymphocytes or polymorphonuclear cells predominating. Exceptional cases with WBC counts of 90,000/mm^3, and 99% polymorphonuclear cells in the absence of infection and microcrystalline disease, have also been reported. Synovial biopsies may occasionally show infiltrating leukemic cells. When metaphyseal periosteal elevation has been noted, leukemic infiltrates have also been found in that region. Periosteal involvement may result in complaints of pain along the length of an extremity rather than in the joints. When leukemic infiltrates affect the axial skeleton, back and chest wall pain can be severe (1, 31–33).

Radiographs are abnormal in 50–75% of cases. Periarticular demineralization does not help distinguish leukemic arthritis from nonmalignant inflammatory polyarthritis. However, osteolytic defects, cortical disruptions, and periosteal elevation are more compatible with the diagnosis of a malignant process. In immunologically handicapped leukemics, periosteal abnormalities may also indicate a superimposed osteomyelitis. Fever is not a helpful differential point in this setting. When uncertainty exists, a biopsy and cultures may be necessary to identify the true nature of this process.

The presence of a transverse radiolucent line beneath the metaphysis (''metaphyseal band'') of long bones is rare in diseases other than leukemia in children older than age 2. These radiolucent bands are not thought to be due to leukemic infiltration per se. Thomas et al noted metaphyseal banding in 88% of leukemic children and in 7% of leukemic adults. However, Calabro suggested that such changes may be seen in various conditions of disturbed osteogenesis, such as juvenile polyarthritis. Thus, although ''banding'' highly suggests leukemia, it is not pathognomonic (31).

METABOLIC ARTHROPATHIES

The following disorders are not usually associated with substantial synovial pannus formation or bony erosions, but polyarthralgias and myalgias are often a major feature of the symptom complex.

Hypothyroidism

Metabolic abnormalities, such as hypothyroidism, are usually recognized because of a constellation of generalized symptoms as well as occasional complaints relating to increased glandular size. Any one of a variety of rheumatic syndromes may be the principal manifestation of myxedema. Deposits of mucinous hyaluronic acid in the skeleton, muscle, and other soft tissues are probably responsible for:

- Stiffness
- Arthralgias
- Features of carpal tunnel syndrome
- Muscle cramps
- Nonspecific myalgias
- Weakness

Articular complaints most often occur in the knees, wrists, hands and feet. There are no characteristic radiograph changes, although diffuse osteopenia, chondrocalcinosis, and effusions may be noted. Swelling and large volumes of synovial fluid may occur. Fluid analyses have noninflammatory characteristics.

Exceptions to this rule have been seen in cases with associated chondrocalcinosis and pseudogout. Dorwart and Schumacher reported nine patients with severe hypothyroidism. Seven had radiographically coexistent CPPD deposition disease. In six of seven patients, synovial analyses showed typical CPPD crystals. These results suggest that the metabolic consequences of hypothyroidism predispose to the deposition of CPPD in cartilage. Subsequent alterations in cartilage may account for the occasional observation of premature degenerative changes that have been seen in weight-bearing joints. With the exception of secondary degenerative changes, the musculoskeletal manifestations of hypothyroidism are completely reversible with thyroid replacement.

Primary Hyperparathyroidism

The most common complaints among persons with primary hyperparathyroidism are weakness and fatigability. Myalgias occur in a minority of cases. Muscle enzymes are reportedly normal. Up to 10% of patients may have nonspecific arthralgias, and in some cases synovitis may occur secondary to superimposed CPPD crystal deposition and pseudogout. RA-like presentation has also been described with hyperparathyroidism. Longstanding untreated primary or secondary hyperparathyroidism may lead to severe diffuse bone resorption independent of pannus formation or CPPD deposition. Soft tissue and visceral calcifications may be present. Removal of the abnormal parathyroid gland(s) usually results in improvement of muscular and articular problems.

Hemochromatosis

Hemochromatosis most often presents as diabetes, liver disease, and increased skin pigmentation. The majority of patients have idiopathic or primary disease. Secondary iron overload has been associated with: alcoholic liver disease, refractory anemias requiring multiple transfusions, and chronic excessive oral iron ingestion. The association of arthropathy and hemochromatosis was established by Schumacher in 1964 (34). Since then, several large series of patients have been studied in which arthropathy, unrelated to other disorders, occurred in 20–56% of cases.

Although most patients manifest other features of iron overload before developing arthropathy, joint disease can be the presenting complaint. The peak incidence is between ages 50–60. The sites most often involved are the hands, particularly the second and third MCP joints, and in decreasing order of frequency: knees, ankles, wrists, hips, elbows, shoulders, symphysis pubis, and intervertebral discs are also affected.

The course of arthropathy is insidiously progressive, but it may be punctuated by acute inflammatory episodes of pseudogout. The mechanism by which ferritin and hemosiderin deposit in synovial lining cells, connective tissue, and cartilage to produce degradative changes is unknown. Inflammatory synovial pannus is not a feature of this process, as it is in RA. It has been suggested that an iron overload may inhibit the enzymatic activity of cartilage pyrophosphatases, thus leading to deposition of CPPD, chondrocalcinosis, acute and chronic arthritis, and finally, degenerative changes. Joint effusions, in the absence of superimposed microcrystalline arthritis, are noninflammatory. Chondrocalcinosis occurs in 30–60% of patients with hemochromatosis arthropathy.

Associated radiographic changes may include osteopenia and narrowed joint spaces with deformity of articular surfaces; rarely subchondral periarticular erosions are seen, as in RA. Bony sclerosis and osteophyte formation, however, characteristic of osteoarthritis, also occur. The occurrences of these changes in the MCP, carpal, and radioulnar joints would be atypical locations for osteoarthritis and should suggest CPPD-associated disorders: hemochromatosis, hyperparathyroidism, hypophosphatasia, Wilson's disease, ochronosis, diabetes, and hyperuricemia, with or without clinical gout. When these sites are symmetrically involved and chondrocalcinosis is not apparent, confusion with RA would not be surprising.

If hemochromatosis is considered in the differential diagnosis of atypical polyarthritis, determination of serum iron and iron binding capacity are inexpensive and reliable screening tests. In hemochromatosis, plasma iron binding protein is usually more than 75% saturated. Arthropathy may be a clue to the early diagnosis of iron-overload states. This is of more than academic interest, as phlebotomy therapy may protect or salvage other tissues at risk. Unfortunately, such therapy, in several reported cases, has had limited success in palliating joint symptoms. Synovial iron deposits poorly exchange with circulating iron pools compared to iron in liver and bone marrow. Whether or not prolonged phlebotomy therapy will be found ultimately to affect the course of arthropathy, will require long-term studies with larger numbers of patients, a very difficult objective considering the relative rarity of hemochromatosis joint disease.

ARTHRITIS AND PANCREATIC DISEASES

Diseases that present with periarticular and also articular symptoms (sarcoidosis, amyloidosis, leukemia, and hypertrophic osteoarthropathy) are a challenging aspect of differential diagnosis. These diseases highlight the importance of examining the periarticular soft tissues and bony structures.

On rare occasion pancreatic disease of any cause may produce periarticular abnormalities. In this instance, neither synovial pannus nor erosions occur (Table 29.1). Subcutaneous periarticular fat undergoes necrosis because of increased levels of circulating pancreatic lipase. Fat necrosis occurring elsewhere may produce multiple sites of visceral and bone-marrow injury, as well as tender erythema nodosum-like skin nodules suggestive of systemic vasculitis. Like those of erythema nodosum, these lesions frequently occur over the anterior tibias but are also common about all aspects of the thighs and buttocks. They appear less often on the trunk and upper extremities. Pancreatic abnormalities may be occult (carcinoma, pancreatic pseudocysts, pancreatic duct calculi) or bear obvious relationships to alcohol excess and abdominal trauma.

Periarticular and articular features of pancreatic disease may be symmetric (mimicking RA) or asymmetric. Warmth, tenderness, and swelling are common. Ankles, elbows, knees, and small joints of the hands, wrists, and feet are involved in a descending order of frequency. Joint effusions are probably secondary to periarticular tissue destruction. Although ''pus'' has been aspirated from such joints, in the few cases in which WBC counts were done there tended to be small volumes of fluid with noninflammatory characteristics. Gibson et al (35), suggested that this material is derived form adjacent necrotic debris, and they reported fat globules in the synovial fluid. Tannenbaum et al (36), however, reported a case with synovial fluid volumes up to 110 cc and WBC counts up to 17,000/mm^3 with a predominance of PMN leukocytes and the presence of fat globules.

Medullary fat necrosis may produce lytic lesions and periosteal changes in the long bones and digits. Linear and/or patchy areas of calcification may develop in sites of prior and ongoing lipolysis or bone infarction. Aseptic necrosis of articular bone may follow fat necrosis and subsequent extrinsic vascular compression or fatty embolization of medullary arterioles. The combination of history, physical findings, synovial analysis, and elevated serum amylase and lipase enable one to readily distinguish this process from RA and other inflammatory arthropathies. In general, symptomatic improvement rapidly occurs when amelioration of the pancreatic process is possible.

BACTERIAL ENDOCARDITIS

Patients with bacterial endocarditis are often initially suspected of having ''collagen vascular'' disorders. Arthralgias, arthritis, and myalgias occur in at least one-third of cases and may be the most common extravalvular manifestation of disease. In fact, 27% (52 of 192) of patients reported by Churchill et al (37) had musculoskeletal complaints as one of the first symptoms of endocarditis; 44% later developed similar symptoms that still preceded awareness of underlying valvular heart disease. Articular manifestations were usually mono- or oligoarticular, occurring most often in proximal large joints, such as shoulders, hips, and knees. Low back

pain occurred in 23%. Joints occasionally were swollen and became warm and tender. In the small number of cases in which synovial analyses have been done, fluid has varied from being noninflammatory to moderately inflammatory, with WBCs being predominantly mononuclear or polymorphonuclear.

Myalgias were either generalized, regional (especially lower limb girdle) or focal (such as in a single calf or thigh). Muscle biopsies have shown inflammatory infiltrates. In the great majority of cases, there has been no proof of septic emboli being responsible for these manifestations. Radiographs of peripheral joints were normal in two large series. However, Churchill et al (37) reported 5 of 192 cases (2.6%) in which low back pain was associated with radiographic features of disc space infection. These patients, as well as those with other musculoskeletal symptoms, experienced prompt relief following effective antibiotic therapy.

Extravalvular manifestations of endocarditis correlate with the presence of circulating immune complexes and hypocomplementemia. Although septic emboli are occasionally seen in skin and other lesions, immune complex formation and deposition is at least as important in the pathogenesis of noncardiac events. Patients having rheumatoid factors (33%) and antinuclear antibodies (25%) show progressive diminution of titers with resolution of illness. Fever and nonspecific rheumatic symptoms and serologies may precede other manifestations of endocarditis by months. Recognition of this association takes on great practical significance, leading to appropriate blood cultures, repeated careful cardiac examinations, and early treatment of a potentially fatal disease.

POLYMYALGIA RHEUMATICA AND GIANT CELL ARTERITIS

Polymyalgia rheumatica (PMR) is a disease only of the elderly (more than 50 years old). Pain, stiffness, and less often tenderness in proximal muscles are characteristic. Although patients often complain of weakness, objective weakness is usually minimal. The symmetric nature of this process often tempts the clinician to consider RA in the differential diagnosis. However, a careful history will usually localize symptoms to muscle groups more than to joints per se. Articular examination may show small effusions that are usually noninflammatory. Synovial biopsies have shown nonspecific changes. How often these changes are due to concurrent osteoarthritis is unclear. True inflammatory synovitis with synovial proliferation should lead to another diagnosis. Muscle enzymes and electromyography are normal. Rheumatoid factor occurs no more often than in age-matched controls (Table 29.3). A normal erythrocyte sedimentation rate (ESR) would place the diagnosis of PMR in doubt, since most (about 80%) patients have a Westergren ESR greater than 40 mm/hr.

Giant-Cell Arteritis (GCA)

The clinical features of PMR may precede or coexist with symptoms of giant cell arteritis (GCA). This observation has led several investigators to biopsy temporal arteries in patients having only myalgic symptoms. In 15–50% of cases, temporal arteritis was apparent. The yield for this procedure can be increased if the opposite temporal artery is biopsied when the initial result is negative. Giant cell arteritis is therefore multifocal and associated with ''skip lesions,'' as is true of other arteritides. The potential for any muscular artery to be involved is reflected by the diversity of symptoms and findings in patients with PMR/GCA. Many such patients undergo extensive evaluations for fever of unknown origin, occult malignancy, anemia of chronic disease, hepatic dysfunction, extremity claudication, and even functional illness before an elevated ESR leads to suspicion of PMR or GCA. In some unfortunate cases, diagnosis may not become apparent until after a major vaso-occlusive event has occurred.

This syndrome is exquisitely sensitive to corticosteroid therapy, which usually produces dramatic relief of symptoms within 24–36 hours. Because predicting which patients will respond to low doses (e.g., 10 mg prednisone daily) is impossible, starting with a high dose is advantageous (greater than or equal to 40 mg). A high dose would be effective for all, leaving few in jeopardy of permanent sequelae.

OSTEOARTHRITIS (OA)

Osteoarthritis most frequently develops in the absence of prior joint disease. Chronic trauma may play a role in some cases, but certainly not all. Aging is an important factor and is reflected in the observation that more than 85% of persons older than 75 have radiologic evidence of degenerative joint disease (DJD). Obesity may contribute to the increased occurrence of DJD in weight-bearing peripheral and axial joints. Hereditary factors may be the major determinants responsible for changes in PIP and DIP joints (Bouchard and Heberden nodes) of the hands. Such digital changes affect women ten times more

often than men. Primary osteoarthritic changes in the MCP joints and wrists would be very unusual and should suggest prior or coexistent inflammatory synovitis, including CPPD-related conditions. Radiographic manifestations of DJD include loss of joint space (cartilage), sclerosis, and formation of osteophytes (reactive new bone) and subchondral cysts. Synovial fluid analysis will show noninflammatory changes. There are no specific laboratory abnormalities. The presence of rheumatoid factor does not exceed that for age-matched controls (Table 29.3).

The clinical picture is usually that of an elderly patient with chronically evolving monoarticular or pauciarticular complaints. Joints most often involved are DIP, PIP, the first carpometacarpal joints of the hands, the first metatarsophalangeals of the feet, weight-bearing joints, and the cervical and lumbar spine. Systemic symptoms, if present, would not be related to primary osteoarthritis. Because osteoarthritis is so common, it is not unusual to encounter elderly patients with inflammatory joint diseases and coexistent, unrelated OA.

Treatment: Inflammatory vs. Mechanical Processes

In rheumatoid and other inflammatory joint diseases, it becomes extremely important to determine whether a patient's pain is related to:

- Inflammation, swelling, distention of a joint capsule
- Abnormal mechanical relationships
- Both factors occurring simultaneously

If inflammatory mechanisms are of primary concern, then antiinflammatory therapy should be the primary therapeutic approach. If the joint space is obliterated, the skin temperature overlying the joint is not increased, and synovial fluid, if present, is noninflammatory, then effective approaches to therapy will be analgesic and mechanical.

REVIEW EXERCISES

1. A 28-year-old female secretary presents with a history of daily joint pain for 6 months. Involved sites include the wrists, MCP joints, ankles and knees. Morning stiffness is present for at least one hour. ROS is significant only for cold sensitivity, without note of color change in the hands and feet. Physical examination does not reveal any features of synovial proliferation, warmth, swelling, or restricted motion. CBC, creatinine, hepatic enzyme studies, ESR, U/A, ANA, rheumatoid factor and chest radiograph are normal. The differential diagnosis should include:

    a. Osteoarthritis (OA)
    b. Psychogenic rheumatism
    c. Fibromyalgia
    d. Rheumatoid arthritis (RA)
    e. Microcrystalline arthropathies

2. The antinuclear antibody (ANA) test:

    a. Is specific for SLE
    b. Titers should be used to follow SLE disease activity and titrate therapy
    c. Is essential for the diagnosis of SLE
    d. Is not as sensitive as antibodies to double-stranded DNA or hypocomplementemia in patients with lupus
    e. All of the above
    f. None of the above

3. You are called to provide a consultation for a 68-year-old, male, cardiac-surgery patient. The day after a CABG procedure, the patient develops acute monarthritis of the right knee for the first time. It is tense, red and exquisitely painful. The patient will not allow you to move it. Temperature is 100°F; other vital signs are normal. Other medical problems include hypertension, insulin-dependent diabetes and chronic renal insufficiency (serum creatinine = 2.3 mg/dl). Serum uric acid is 8.3 mg/dl. The most appropriate options for diagnosis and treatment are:

    a. Obtain a radiograph. If it is normal, treat presumed gout with an NSAID such as Indocin, or use IV or oral colchicine.
    b. Because the knee is too tender to aspirate and the patient is too uncomfortable to move, treat presumed gout and get other studies if he does not respond in 2 to 3 days.
    c. Aspirate the joint and analyze gram stain and fluid for crystals, using polarizing lenses. If crystals are present, treat with NSAIDs.
    d. Aspirate the joint and if gram stain is negative and gout crystals are present, treat with intraarticular steroids.
    e. Take no chances and treat with both NSAIDs and antibiotics, being certain to cover for S. aureus.

Answers

1. d

The patient's age and distribution of joints are not compatible with OA. The joints involved are typical of chronic inflammatory joint disease. The chronicity and persistence of symptoms is not characteristic of microcrystalline disease. The specific reference to bilateral MCP joints, wrists and ankles is most typical of RA. The patient does not yet have adequate features to make a diagnosis of RA but can evolve into RA given time. It is less likely that she may evolve into SLE, scleroderma or myositis. Rheumatoid factor may only be present in 70% of bona fide RA patients, and its presence is not required for diagnosis.

2. f

The ANA is non-specific and can be present as a result of numerous inflammatory conditions, drug therapies, and aging. It is not a reliable guide to disease activity or treatment. Although approximately 90% of patients with SLE are ANA positive, ANA-negative lupus does occur. Antibodies to double-stranded DNA and hypocomplementemia are not sensitive tests for SLE. Antibodies to native DNA are more specific for SLE than are positive ANA reactions.

3. d

All acute monoarthritis problems of uncertain cause require aspiration and synovial analysis to rule in or out infection or microcrystalline arthritis. Nonsteroidal anti-inflammatory drugs are contraindicated in the setting of renal insufficiency. In the setting of microcrystalline monoarthritis and renal insufficiency the safest therapy is intra-articular steroid injection or a tapering course of prednisone (or equivalent) for 7–10 days.

REFERENCES

1. Hoffman GS: Polyarthritis: The differential diagnosis of rheumatoid arthritis. Semin Arthritis Rheumatol 1979;8: 115–141.
2. Cash JM, Hoffman GS: Rheumatoid arthritis. In: Lichtenstein LM, Fauci AS, eds. Current Therapy in Allergy, Immunology and Rheumatology. 5th ed. St Louis: Mosby, 1996:186–193.
3. Short CL, Bauer W, Reynold WE: Rheumatoid arthritis. Cambridge, MA: Harvard University Press, 1957.
4. Hadler NM, Franck WA, Bress NM, et al: Acute polyarticular gout. Am J Med 1974;56:715.
5. McCarty DJ: Diagnostic mimicry in arthritisCPatterns of joint involvement associated with calcium pyrophosphate dihydrate crystal deposits. Bull Rheum Dis 1975;25:804.
6. Goldenberg DL, Cohen AS: Acute infectious arthritis. A review of patients with non-gonococcal joint infections. Am J Med 1976;60:369.
7. Mitchell WS, Brooks PM, Stevenson RD, et al: Septic arthritis in patients with rheumatoid disease: A still under diagnosed complication. J Rheumatol 1976;3:124.
8. Baum J: Infection in rheumatoid arthritis. Arthritis Rheum 1971;14:135.
9. Mowat AG, Baum J: Chemotaxis of polymorphonuclear leukocytes from patients with rheumatoid arthritis. J Clin Invest 1971;50:2541.
10. Udden J, Kraus AS, Kelly HG: Survivorship and death in rheumatoid arthritis. Arthritis Rheum 1970;13:125.
11. Lerman SJ, Nankervis GA, Heggie AD, et al: Immunologic response, virus excretion, and joint reaction with rubella vaccine. Ann Intern Med 1971;74:67.
12. Spruance SL, Metcalf R, Smith CG, et al: Chronic arthropathy associated with rubella vaccination. Arthritis Rheum 1977;20:741.
13. Spruance SL, Smith CB: Joint complications associated with derivative of HPV-77 rubella virus vaccine. Am J Dis Child 1971;122:105.
14. Steere AC, Malawista E, Hardin JA, et al: Erythema chronicum migrans and Lyme arthritis. The enlarging clinical spectrum. Ann Intern Med 1977;86:685.
15. Steere AC, Malawista SE, Syndman DR, et al: Lyme arthritis. An epidemic of oligoarticular arthritis in children and adults in three Connecticut communities. Arthritis Rheum 1977;20:7.
16. Rahn DW: Lyme disease. In: Klippel JH, Dieppe PA, eds. Rheumatology. London: Mosby, 1994.
17. Calabro JJ, Garg SL, Khoury MI, et al: Reiter's syndrome. Am Fam Physician 1974;9:80.
18. Good AE: Reiter's disease: A review with special attention to cardiovascular and neurologic sequelae. Semin Arthritis Rheumatol 1974;3:253.
19. Good AE, Hyla JF, Rapp R: Ankylosing spondylitis with rheumatoid arthritis and subcutaneous nodules. Arthritis Rheum 1977;20:1434.
20. Brewerton DA, James DCO: The histocompatibility antigen HLA-B27 and disease. Semin Arthritis Rheum 1975; 4:191.
21. Morris RI, Metzger AL, Bluestone R, et al: HLA W 27—A useful discriminator in arthropathies of inflammatory bowel disease. N Engl J Med 1974;290:1117.
22. Tan EM: Immunospecificities of antinuclear antibodies. Arthritis Rheum 1977;20(Suppl..):187.
23. Reichlin M: Problems in differentiating SLE and mixed connective-tissue disease. N Engl J Med 1976;295:1194.
24. Winterbauer RH, Belic N, Moores KD: A clinical interpretation of bilateral hilar adenopathy. Ann Intern Med 1973;78:65.
25. Bartfeld H: Distribution of rheumatoid factor activity in nonrheumatoid states. Ann NY Acad Sci 1969;168:30.
26. Bennett RM, Ginsberg MH, Thomsen S: Carcinomatous polyarthritis. The presenting symptoms of an ovarian tumor and association with platelet activating factor. Arthritis Rheum 1976;19:953.
27. Harrison JW, Scherbel AL: Rheumatic musculoskeletal symptoms associated with carcinoma of the prostate gland. Postgrad Med J 1960;28:274.
28. Lansbury J: Collagen disease complicating malignancy. Ann Rheum Dis 1953;12:301.
29. Mackenzie AH, Scherbel AL: Connective tissue syndromes associated with carcinoma. Geriatrics 1963;18: 745.
30. Borden EC, Holling HE: Hypertrophic osteoarthropathy and pregnancy. Ann Intern Med 1969;71:577.
31. Calabro JJ: Cancer and arthritis. Arthritis Rheum 1967; 10:533.
32. Silverstein MN, Kelly P: Leukemia with osteoarticular symptoms and signs. Ann Intern Med 1963;59:637.
33. Spilberg I, Meyer GJ: The arthritis of leukemia. Arthritis Rheum 1972;15:630.
34. Schumacher HR: Hemochromatosis and arthritis. Arthritis Rheum 1964;7:41.
35. Gibson TJ, Schumacher HR, Pascual E, et al: Arthropathy, skin and bone lesions in pancreatic disease. J Rheumatol 1975;2:7.
36. Tannenbaum H, Anderson LG, Schur PH: Association of polyarthritis, subcutaneous nodules and pancreatic disease. J Rheumatol 1975;2:14.
37. Churchill MA, Geraci JE, Hunder GG: Musculoskeletal manifestations of bacterial endocarditis. Ann Intern Med 1977;87:754.

C·H·A·P·T·E·R

30

Systemic Autoimmune Diseases

Barri J. Fessler

The function of the immune system is to protect an individual from potentially harmful organisms. The immune system does not attack an individual's own tissues but rather targets and destroys substances perceived as foreign. This selective unresponsiveness to self is known as immunologic tolerance. When there is a breakdown in tolerance to self, an autoimmune reaction ensues.

Autoimmunity may be induced or develop spontaneously. Examples of induced autoimmune syndromes include hemolytic anemia associated with a mycoplasma infection, or drug-induced lupus following treatment with procainamide, both of which resolve once the exposure to the inciting agent has stopped. Spontaneous autoimmune syndromes are those in which the inciting agent or trigger has yet to be identified.

Autoimmune syndromes may be classified as organ-specific disease or systemic/multiorgan system disease. Examples of some organ-specific diseases include Hashimoto's thyroiditis, bullous pemphigoid, and myasthenia gravis.

Autoantibodies are usually directed against a single-organ system. Systemic autoimmune diseases, discussed in detail below, are characterized by inflammation and tissue damage in many areas and production of a wide array of autoantibodies. Factors that may contribute to the pathogenesis of autoimmune disease include:

- Genetic predisposition
- Hormonal factors
- Environmental triggers
- Infectious agents
- Drugs or toxins
- Diet

Autoantibody production, the hallmark of autoimmune disease, is caused by antigen-driven immune stimulation and/ or polyclonal B cell proliferation. Autoantibodies may be markers of a certain syndrome or merely the reflection of nonspecific immune stimulation. Autoantibodies may cause damage through direct cellular cytotoxicity or result in immune complex formation within the circulation, leading to activation of complement and inflammation. Immune complexes may also form *in situ* or circulate and deposit within tissue, leading to localized inflammation and destruction. However, not all autoantibodies are pathogenic.

In evaluating a patient with a suspected systemic autoimmune disease:

- A detailed history is *the* most important tool for establishing the diagnosis.
- Careful physical exam is necessary.
- Laboratory data is adjunctive–*not* the primary determinant of the diagnosis.

SYSTEMIC LUPUS ERYTHEMATOSUS

Systemic lupus erythematosus (SLE) is an autoimmune syndrome with a varied clinical presentation, ranging from very mild cutaneous disease and arthralgias to severe, life-threatening, multiorgan system involvement. Many autoantibodies are produced. The prevalence of SLE in the United States is estimated to be 50/100,000 caucasians, with the prevalence increasing to more than 200/100,000 in the african american population. Systemic lupus erythematosus is nine times more prevalent in women than men. It is typically a disease of the young, with the mean age at diagnosis of 30: more than 80% of the cases occur in women during their childbearing years.

PATHOGENESIS OF SYSTEMIC LUPUS ERYTHEMATOSUS

The pathogenesis of SLE has not yet been defined. Many factors are believed to influence the development of SLE, including genetic predisposition, as supported by:

- The increased incidence of the major histocompatibility complex, HLA DR2 and HLA DR3
- A 30% concordance rate for development of SLE in monozygotic twins
- A higher frequency of complement deficiency/complement C4 null alleles in patients with SLE
- 10% of relatives of SLE patients develop SLE

Several other factors are involved in the expression of the disease. Most patients with SLE are women, a fact that suggests hormones likely play an important role. In addition, environmental factors, such as ultraviolet light and infectious agents may play a role in triggering the disease onset. Drugs such as procainamide, hydralazine, and isoniazid have been implicated in triggering a drug-induced lupus syndrome in a small subset of patients receiving these medications.

CLINICAL PRESENTATION OF SYSTEMIC LUPUS ERYTHEMATOSUS

A diagnosis of SLE is based on characteristic clinical and laboratory abnormalities. The American College of Rheumatology has published criteria for the diagnosis of SLE, useful as a framework for understanding the protean manifestations of SLE and for standardizing patients for research protocols:

- Malar rash
- Discoid rash
- Photosensitivity
- Oral ulcers
- Arthritis
- Serositis (pleuritis or pericarditis)
- Renal disorder (proteinuria >500 mg/d or cellular casts)
- Neurologic disorder (seizures or psychosis)
- Hematologic disorder (hemolytic anemia or leukopenia [<4000/mm^3] or lymphopenia [<1500/ mm^3] or thrombocytopenia [<100,000/ mm^3])
- Immunologic disorder (Positive LE cell preparation, anti-DNA antibodies, anti-Smith antibodies, or false-positive serologic test for syphilis)
- Antinuclear antibody

A person has SLE if any four or more criteria are present, serially or simultaneously.

The most common manifestations of SLE affect the mucocutaneous and musculoskeletal systems. The cutaneous manifestations of SLE may be divided into 3 general categories: acute cutaneous lupus erythematosus (LE) (malar rash), subacute cutaneous LE (papulosquamous and annular-polycyclic variants) and chronic LE (discoid lesions). The classic malar rash is observed in 50% of patients and is described as an erythematous rash extending across the bridge of the nose, sparing the nasolabial folds. Other nonspecific mucocutaneous features that may be observed in more than half of SLE patients during the course of their illness include:

- Photosensitivity
- Alopecia
- Oral or nasal ulcers
- Urticaria
- Panniculitis
- Livedo reticularis

Muscle and joint complaints are frequently the presenting symptom of lupus. Arthralgias and arthritis are usually polyarticular, affecting both large and small joints. The arthropathy is typically nonerosive, as the inflammation usually affects the periarticular structures. A small percentage of patients may develop a deforming arthropathy called Jaccoud's arthropathy, which clinically mimics the deformities seen in rheumatoid arthritis, yet the characteristic bony erosions of rheumatoid arthritis are absent. Avascular necrosis may affect 5–10% of SLE patients. Fibromyalgia is being increasingly recognized in SLE patients.

Renal and neuropsychiatric manifestations result in the greatest morbidity and mortality associated with active lupus. The majority of patients with SLE have some degree of renal disease caused by localization of immune complexes within the kidney. The most sensitive screen for renal disease is the microscopic analysis of urine, which may reveal cellular casts before a rise in serum creatinine has developed. Glomerulonephritis is the most frequent renal manifestation of SLE, however interstitial nephritis and renal vein thrombosis may also occur. A renal biopsy, while not necessary in all clinical situations, is useful in establishing the diagnosis and useful in determining the severity of renal involvement. The types of glomerulonephritis associated with SLE include mesangial, focal proliferative, diffuse proliferative, membranous and advanced sclerosing glomerulonephritis.

Neuropsychiatric lupus encompasses a wide variety of abnormalities including:

- Seizure
- Neuropathies (peripheral, central and autonomic)
- Aseptic meningitis
- Transverse myelitis
- Stroke
- Psychosis
- Organic brain syndrome
- Neurocognitive dysfunction

Neurologic manifestations in SLE patients may also result from disease in other organs (e.g., metabolic or hypertensive encephalopathy associated with renal failure) and/or complications of therapy (e.g., drug-induced or infectious meningitis). Cerebrospinal fluid analysis, while not diagnostic of CNS lupus, is useful to rule out an underlying infection that can mimic CNS lupus. Magnetic resonance imaging of the brain is sensitive, especially in the setting of focal neurologic symptoms, but nonspecific.

Inflammation within the respiratory tract may result in: pleurisy and/or pleural effusions, acute pneumonitis, chronic interstitial lung disease, pulmonary hypertension, or pulmonary hemorrhage. Pleurisy is observed in more than 50% of SLE patients. Acute lupus pneumonitis and pulmonary hemorrhage syndromes are uncommon syndromes associated with high mortality rates if not identified and treated rapidly. The shrinking-lung syndrome, a condition of diaphragmatic dysfunction with resultant restrictive lung disease, is unique to SLE. The patient experiences shortness of breath, and the chest radiograph typically reveals an elevated hemidiaphragm without evidence of parenchymal lung disease.

Cardiac manifestations of SLE may involve the pericardium, myocardium, endocardium, or coronary vasculature. Pericarditis and pericardial effusions are common, although they rarely progress to cardiac tamponade. Libman-Sacks endocarditis and valvular heart disease are often asymptomatic, however, they may progress and result in hemodynamically significant lesions requiring surgery. Antibiotic prophylaxis for endocarditis should be considered in all SLE patients undergoing surgery as valvular disease may be occult. Compared with controls, SLE patients have a ninefold increase in the incidence of myocardial infarction. Contributing factors include accelerated atherosclerosis, antiphospholipid vasculopathy, arteritis, and in situ thromboses.

Cardiopulmonary manifestations can be summarized as:

- Serosal disease
  - Pleurisy/pericarditis +/ − effusions
- Parenchymal disease
  - Pneumonitis, acute or chronic
  - Alveolar hemorrhage
- Muscle disease
  - Shrinking lung syndrome
  - Myocarditis/myocardial dysfunction
- Valvular disease
  - Libman-Sacks endocarditis
  - Antiphospholipid associated valvulopathy
- Vascular disease
  - Pulmonary hypertension
  - Coronary arteritis (rare)

Constitutional symptoms such as malaise, fatigue, weight loss and low grade fevers are also frequent symptoms of SLE. In a patient with established SLE, new onset of fevers (especially if the patient is on immunosuppressive agents) should prompt a search for infection. Similarly, acute monarthritis in an SLE patient should not be assumed to be caused by the underlying inflammatory condition until other conditions such as infection, crystal disease, or avascular necrosis have been ruled out.

LABORATORY STUDIES

Cytopenias are common in patients with SLE. Although anemia of chronic disease is the most common finding, Coombs-positive hemolytic anemia may be observed in 15% of patients. Pure red-cell aplasia and aplastic anemia are rare associations. Leukopenia (between 2500 and 4000/mm^3) regularly occurs with active SLE, but the white blood cell count seldom falls below 1500/mm^3. Mild immune-mediated thrombocytopenia (100–150,000/ml) may affect one quarter of patients.

Severe thrombocytopenia (below 20,000 μl) occurs in fewer than 5% of patients. The presence of anti-platelet antibodies does not predict the occurrence of thrombocytopenia nor its severity. Rarely, patients with SLE may develop thrombotic thrombocytopenic purpura.

Autoantibody profiles are adjunctive tests, useful for confirming the clinical suspicion of SLE. Whereas a positive antinuclear antibody (ANA) is seen in more than 95% of patients with SLE, it is not a specific test, and occurs in a wide variety of other syndromes. A diagnosis of SLE can be made in the absence of a positive ANA if characteristic clinical features are present. Conversely, the presence of a positive ANA in the absence of appropriate clinical features is not sufficient to make the diagnosis of SLE.

The differential diagnosis of a positive antinuclear antibody includes:

- Rheumatic Diseases
  - Systemic lupus erythematosus
  - Rheumatoid arthritis
  - Sjögren's syndrome
  - Scleroderma
  - Polymyositis
- Drug-Induced Syndrome
  - Procainamide
  - Hydralazine
  - Isoniazid
  - Chlorpromazine
  - Methyldopa
  - Dilantin
  - Quinidine
  - Many more
- Hepatic Diseases
  - Chronic active hepatitis
  - Primary biliary cirrhosis
  - Alcoholic liver disease
- Pulmonary Diseases
  - Idiopathic pulmonary fibrosis
  - Primary pulmonary hypertension
- Endocrine Disorders
  - Type I diabetes mellitus
  - Grave's disease
- Neurologic Diseases
  - Multiple sclerosis
  - Myasthenia gravis
- Malignancy
  - Lymphoma
  - Leukemia
  - Melanoma
- Hematologic disorders
  - Idiopathic thrombocytopenic purpura
  - Autoimmune hemolytic anemia
- Chronic Infections
- Normal individuals
  - Women > men

- Increased frequency with age
- Relatives of patients with autoimmune diseases

The anti-double-stranded DNA antibody test, which correlates most closely with renal disease, is the most specific test (> 90% specificity) for SLE and is seen in approximately 70% of patients. In some patients, a rise in antibody titers to double-stranded DNA can herald a disease flare and titers may fluctuate with disease activity. Antibodies to single-stranded DNA are extremely nonspecific and should not be ordered. Anti-Smith antibodies, also a specific test, are observed in 30% of patients with SLE. Other autoantibodies (anti-Ro, anti-La, anti-RNP) are seen in association with various clinical manifestations but are not specific. Antiphospholipid antibodies, which may be seen in up to 50% of SLE patients, are associated with an increased incidence of recurrent arterial and venous thromboses, spontaneous miscarriages, and thrombocytopenia. Activation of the complement pathway as manifested by decreased levels of C3 and C4 often accompanies major flares of lupus. As complement proteins are also acute phase reactants, measurements may sometimes be normal, despite complement activation, thus complement split products may be a more accurate reflection of disease activity.

Serologies in SLE appear in Table 30.1.

TREATMENT OF SLE

Mild manifestations of arthralgias/arthritis, myalgias, and fatigue respond to treatment with nonsteroidal antiinflammatory drugs, low dose corticosteroids or antimalarial medications,

such as hydroxychloroquine. Hydroxychloroquine is useful for treatment of these symptoms and also the cutaneous manifestations of SLE. Hydroxychloroquine has also been found to have steroid-sparing properties and cholesterol-lowering properties, in addition to its anti-inflammatory properties, making it an important medication for the treatment of mild-to-moderate SLE. Side effects of hydroxychloroquine include gastrointestinal manifestations and a rare retinopathy. Dehydroepiandrosterone (DHEA), currently under investigation for treatment of mild symptoms of SLE, appears to be a promising new agent. Serositis often responds to nonsteroidal antiinflammatory medications or intermediate doses of prednisone. The arthritis associated with SLE may respond to treatment with corticosteroids, hydroxy-chloroquine or methotrexate.

Moderate-to-severe disease manifestations (e.g., proliferative glomerulonephritis, acute central nervous system disease, acute lupus pneumonitis, and severe cytopenias) requires treatment with high dose or pulse corticosteroids, cyclophosphamide, or azathioprine. Cyclophosphamide has been examined most closely for the treatment of active proliferative nephritis, in which it has been shown to be superior to corticosteroids alone. Side effects of cyclophosphamide include:

- Nausea
- Bone marrow suppression
- Hemorrhagic cystitis
- Potential for development of malignancies
- Premature ovarian failure

The 5-year survival rates in SLE patients has markedly improved over the past 4 decades, increasing from 50 to 90%. This is because of earlier recognition of the disease and more aggressive treatment. The leading causes of death in SLE patients are infectious complications, active lupus, and coronary artery disease.

DRUG-INDUCED LUPUS

Symptoms suggestive of SLE may develop in a subpopulation of people exposed to certain medications. Although reportedly more than 100 medications are implicated, the most common medications include:

- Procainamide
- Chlorpromazine
- Hydralazine
- Isoniazid
- Methyldopa
- Quinidine
- Penicillamine

Drug-induced lupus resembles systemic lupus, except that renal and central nervous system involvement are rare. Constitutional symptoms, arthralgias, serositis, and rashes are commonly observed. Serologic evaluation reveals ANA antibodies (99%) and antibodies to histones (95%). Antibodies to histones are not specific for drug-induced lupus, as they may also be observed in SLE (70%) and rheumatoid arthritis (RA).

Table 30.1. Autoantibodies in Systemic Lupus Erythematosus

Antibody	Frequency	Clinical Association
Anti-dsDNA	70%	Nephritis
Anti-Smith	30%	Nephritis/CNS disease
Anti-Ro (SS-A)	20–60%	Subacute cutaneous lupus
		Sjögren's syndrome
		Congenital heart block
		Thrombocytopenia
Anti-La (SS-B)	15–40%	Same as anti-Ro
Anti-Cardiolipin	30–50%	Arterial and venous thrombosis
		Recurrent fetal loss
		Thrombocytopenia
Anti-H2A,H2B		Drug-induced LE
Anti-RNP	10–30%	Mixed connective tissue disease
		Overlap syndromes
Anti-ribosomal P	15%	Psychosis
		Depression
Anti-ssDNA	90%	Non-specific

Antibodies to double-stranded DNA, hypocomplementemia and a false-positive VDRL test are rarely observed (<1%) in the drug-induced syndrome. Treatment consists of discontinuing the offending agent and symptomatic therapy with nonsteroidal antiinflammatory drugs or corticosteroids.

ANTIPHOSPHOLIPID ANTIBODY SYNDROME

The antiphospholipid antibody syndrome is characterized by arterial and/or venous thrombosis, recurrent fetal loss and thrombocytopenia in association with sustained titers of antiphospholipid antibodies (the lupus anticoagulant or anticardiolipin antibodies). This syndrome may occur as a primary entity or a secondary form associated with another autoimmune disease, most often SLE. Antiphospholipid antibodies may be drug-induced (e.g. phenothiazines or procainamide), may develop following certain infections. These antiphospholipid antibodies are generally not associated with an increased risk of thrombosis. Antiphospholipid antibodies may be seen in association with malignancies, neurologic diseases and other autoimmune diseases. Antiphospholipid antibodies may also be seen in normal healthy people, and the frequency increases with age. The presence of antiphospholipid antibodies in the absence of an associated clinical event does not constitute a disease state.

Antiphospholipid antibodies are composed of a heterogeneous array of antibodies that differ by isotype, phospholipid specificity, binding requirements for a protein cofactor, and pathogenicity. Antiphospholipid antibodies may bind to phospholipids, protein cofactors such as Beta-2 glycoprotein-1, or complexes of both. To evaluate for the presence of antiphospholipid antibodies, specific tests must be obtained. Prolongation of phospholipid-dependent coagulation tests (e.g. activated partial thromboplastin time (aPPT), kaolin clot time, dilute Russell's viper venom test, or tissue thromboplastin inhibition test) that do not correct with fresh plasma suggests the presence of the lupus anticoagulant. No single screening test is sensitive enough to be used alone. Anticardiolipin antibodies are assayed by isotype-specific ELISA techniques.

Clinical manifestations associated with the antiphospholipid antibody syndrome are diverse. Thrombosis may occur in venous or arterial vessels of any size. The most common site for deep venous thrombosis is in the lower extremities, however, axillary, ocular, and hepatic vein occlusions have been reported. The most common site for arterial occlusions is in the brain, with the majority of patients presenting with strokes or transient ischemic attacks. Recurrent spontaneous pregnancy loss is also associated with antiphospholipid antibody syndrome; it may occur at any time during pregnancy, but it is more common in the second and third trimester. Other less common clinical features associated with antiphospholipid antibodies include:

- Livedo reticularis
- Seizures
- Transverse myelitis
- Chorea
- Valvular heart disease
- Pulmonary hypertension
- Glomerulopathy
- Adrenal insufficiency
- Thrombocytopenia and hemolytic anemia

The catastrophic antiphospholipid syndrome, a rare syndrome, is characterized by acute multiorgan system deterioration caused by widespread thrombosis of small and large vessels.

Treatment of the thrombotic manifestations (arterial occlusions or deep venous thromboses) is with systemic anticoagulation. The use of corticosteroids, immunosuppressive agents or low dose aspirin does not prevent recurrence of thrombosis. Mild thrombocytopenia has been shown to improve with aspirin. In women who experience recurrent fetal loss, a regimen consisting of subcutaneous heparin and aspirin should be used. Asymptomatic antiphospholipid antibodies are *not* treated. The catastrophic antiphospholipid antibody syndrome is treated with anti-coagulation and immunosuppression.

SCLERODERMA (SYSTEMIC SCLEROSIS)

Scleroderma is an autoimmune syndrome characterized by cutaneous and visceral fibrosis, production of autoantibodies and a vasculopathy. Scleroderma is divided into 2 major categories:

- Diffuse scleroderma
- Limited scleroderma (CREST syndrome)

In addition, features of scleroderma may be found in association with other connective tissue diseases (overlap syndrome) or rarely occur with an abundance of visceral involvement and a paucity of cutaneous manifestations (scleroderma sine scleroderma). A rare disease, estimated to occur at a frequency of 2–10 per million population per year, scleroderma affects women three times more than men. The usual onset of scleroderma occurs in the fourth to fifth decade.

Scleroderma is classified as follows:

- Diffuse scleroderma
- Limited scleroderma (CREST syndrome)
- Scleroderma sine scleroderma
- Overlap syndromes
- Undifferentiated connective tissue disease
- Localized scleroderma (morphea, linear or eosinophilic fasciitis)

PATHOGENESIS OF SCLERODERMA

While the pathogenesis of scleroderma has not been defined, it is believed that a person with a genetic predisposition encounters an environmental stimulus, which results in immune activation and vascular injury. Viruses have been postulated to be the trigger. The immune activation induces cytokine release, vascular injury, endothelial and fibroblast proliferation and accelerated collagen (Type I and III) synthesis, ultimately resulting in end-organ damage.

CLINICAL PRESENTATION OF SCLERODERMA

Limited scleroderma (previously known as the CREST syndrome) is characterized by cutaneous fibrosis affecting the hands, feet, and face, without truncal involvement. The other manifestations that comprise the syndrome include:

- **C**alcinosis
- **R**aynaud's phenomenon
- **E**sophageal dysfunction
- **S**clerodactyly
- **T**elangiectasias

Raynaud's phenomenon is typically present for many years prior to onset of skin thickening. Telangiectasias are most prominent on the face and extremities. Subcutaneous calcium deposits are found in more than 50% of patients with limited scleroderma and may be located at the fingers, olecranon or prepatellar bursae. There is a significant incidence of pulmonary hypertension, with or without interstitial lung disease, in limited scleroderma. The anticentromere antibody is present in up to 70 % of patients with limited scleroderma. Cumulative survival at 10 years is approximately 70%.

Diffuse scleroderma is characterized by extensive acral, facial, and truncal cutaneous fibrosis. In addition, fibrosis significantly affects visceral organs, including the lungs, heart, kidneys and the gastrointestinal tract. Raynaud's phenomenon is usually noted within 1 year of onset of skin thickening. The combination of cutaneous fibrosis and severe Raynaud's phenomenon may lead to digital ulcers, cutaneous pitting, and bony resorption.

Gastrointestinal involvement is the third most common feature of both limited and diffuse scleroderma, following skin changes and Raynaud's phenomenon. Manifestations include:

- Esophageal dysmotility
- Decreased lower esophageal sphincter pressure
- Malabsorption
- Bacterial overgrowth
- Pseudo-obstruction
- Wide-mouth colonic diverticula

Pulmonary manifestations are now the major cause of death in scleroderma patients. The two major forms of lung involvement are fibrosing alveolitis/pulmonary fibrosis and pulmonary hypertension. Pulmonary fibrosis occurs in more than three quarters of patients with diffuse disease. High-resolution CT scanning helps define acute inflammatory alveolitis, which is believed to be treatment-responsive, as opposed to chronic fibrosing alveolitis, which is irreversible. Pulmonary hypertension occurs in 50%. Cardiac involvement may consist of conduction abnormalities, pericardial effusions, and a cardiomyopathy.

The sudden onset of hypertension, rapidly progressive renal insufficiency, microangiopathic hemolytic anemia and thrombocytopenia constitutes the syndrome called scleroderma renal crisis. In 10% of patients with scleroderma renal crisis, blood pressure may be normal. Scleroderma renal crisis typically occurs in the setting of rapidly progressive cutaneous fibrosis associated with diffuse scleroderma. Hyperreninemia is characteristic. The morbidity and mortality associated with this condition has significantly declined with increased recognition and the availability of angiotensin converting enzyme inhibitors which are used for treatment.

Musculoskeletal manifestations of scleroderma include arthralgias, myalgias, and an arthritis that may be erosive. Palpable tendon friction rubs may also be present. Calcinosis is less common in diffuse scleroderma compared with limited scleroderma. The characteristic autoantibody associated with diffuse scleroderma is anti-topoisomerase-1 or anti-SCL70, which is observed in 30–40% of patients. Other laboratory features may include:

- Antinuclear antibodies (90%)
- Hypergammaglobulinemia
- Cryoglobulins
- Rheumatoid factors

Survival of patients with diffuse scleroderma at 10 years is approximately 50%.

TREATMENT OF SCLERODERMA

There is no uniformly effective treatment for scleroderma. Treatment of Raynaud's phenomenon consists of calcium channel blockers, local protective measures, and topical nitrates. Some have advocated the use of aspirin, dipyridamole or pentoxifylline for more severe involvement. D-penicillamine or methotrexate may be helpful treatment for the cutaneous fibrosis. Cyclophosphamide is used to treat inflammatory alveolitis. Omeprazole is beneficial in the treatment of severe esophageal reflux disease. Prokinetic agents, such as cisapride and octreotide, are used for intestinal dysmotility, along with cyclic antibiotics, if bacterial overgrowth is present. Angiotensin converting enzyme inhibitors are used to treat scleroderma renal crisis.

EXPOSURE-ASSOCIATED SCLEROSING DISEASES

Sclerosing illnesses similar to scleroderma have been observed in patients exposed to agents such as bleomycin, vinyl chloride, and toluene. The toxic-oil syndrome, an epidemic consisting of pulmonary infiltrates, sclerodermatous skin changes, polyneuropathy, and myalgias that occurred in 1981 in Spain, followed ingestion of contaminated rapeseed oil. More recently, the Eosinophilia-myalgia syndrome, an epidemic that resulted in sclerodermatous skin thickening, myalgias, eosinophilia, neuro-cognitive dysfunction, arthralgias and a severe neuromyopathy, was associated with ingestion of contaminated L-tryptophan. In addition, a controversy exists regarding the induction of autoimmune diseases, such as scleroderma, following exposure to silicone breast implants.

SJÖGREN'S SYNDROME

Sjögren's syndrome, a systemic autoimmune disease characterized by infiltration of exocrine glands with lymphocytes, causes progressive symptoms of keratoconjunctivitis and xerostomia. Extraglandular manifestations of Sjögren's syndrome may affect the joints, kidneys, muscle, nerve, pancreas, lungs, and vasculature. It is an autoimmune disease with a 44-fold increased risk of transformation into lymphoma.

Primary Sjögren's syndrome is defined as the presence of keratoconjunctivitis sicca and an abnormal minor salivary gland biopsy demonstrating lymphoid aggregates, in the absence of another rheumatic disease. Secondary Sjögren's syndrome occurs in the setting of an underlying autoimmune disease, with rheumatoid arthritis being the most commonly associated illness. Sjögren's syndrome may also occur in the presence of:

- Rheumatoid arthritis
- SLE
- Scleroderma
- Myositis
- Primary biliary cirrhosis
- Thyroiditis
- Chronic active hepatitis

EPIDEMIOLOGY AND PATHOGENESIS OF SJÖGREN'S SYNDROME

Sjögren's syndrome occurs nine times more often in women, with the mean age at diagnosis of 50 years. The pathogenesis is unknown. There is an increased frequency of HLA B8, DR3 phenotype observed in 80% of patients with the primary syndrome, suggesting a genetic predisposition. Viruses such as Epstein Barr, herpes virus 6, and human intracisternal A type retrovirus have been suggested to play a role in the initiation and perpetuation of Sjögren's syndrome, although this has not been proven. The predominance of the disease in women suggests a role for hormones in the pathogenesis.

CLINICAL MANIFESTATIONS OF SJÖGREN'S SYNDROME

The clinical presentation of Sjögren's syndrome is a reflection of the abnormal infiltration of lymphocytes within exocrine glands. In primary Sjögren's, the presenting signs are generally acute-subacute onset of oral and ocular dryness, often accompanied by parotitis. Complaints of dental caries, difficulty swallowing, a gritty/sandy sensation in the eyes and scleral injection are common. The onset of secondary Sjögren's is often insidious. Infiltration of other exocrine organs

may result in dryness in the upper respiratory tract, decreased vaginal secretions, pancreatitis, and hypochlorhydria.

Extraglandular involvement in Sjögren's syndrome includes:

- Arthralgias (70%)
- Raynaud's Phenomenon (35%)
- Pulmonary manifestations (15%)
- Renal involvement (15%)
- Vasculitis (<10%)

Articular manifestations consisting of arthralgias, a nonerosive arthropathy or fibromyalgia may be observed. More than one third of patients will have Raynaud's phenomenon. Glomerulonephritis has been rarely reported. Renal manifestations consist of tubular abnormalities:

- Nephrogenic diabetes insipidus
- Renal tubular acidosis (Type II > Type I)
- Hyposthenuria
- Fanconi's syndrome

A small-to-medium vessel vasculitis is seen in fewer than 10% of patients with Sjögren's syndrome. The vasculitis may present as a purpuric rash, skin ulcerations, urticaria or mononeuritis multiplex. In addition, peripheral sensory or sensorimotor neuropathy, cranial neuropathy, and central nervous system disease has been observed. Pulmonary manifestations include xerotrachea, interstitial lung disease, and pseudolymphoma.

DIAGNOSIS OF SJÖGREN'S SYNDROME

The diagnosis of Sjögren's syndrome is based on the presence of sicca symptoms supported by objective evidence of salivary or lacrimal gland involvement. Sicca symptoms are not specific and may be medication-induced or age-related. Similarly, the finding of bilateral parotid swelling is nonspecific and the differential diagnosis includes:

- Infections
- Malignancy
- Hyperlipoproteinemia
- Sarcoidosis
- Cirrhosis

An abnormal Schirmer's test (wetting of filter paper placed under the lower eyelid) documents the presence of decreased tear production. Rose-Bengal staining of the eye will show devitalized corneal epithelium, and slit-lamp exam may reveal punctate or filamentary keratitis. Decreased salivary flow rates may be documented by sialometry, which measures salivary flow following stimulation. Minor salivary gland biopsy, the cornerstone for the diagnosis of Sjögren's syndrome, demonstrates focal lymphocytic infiltrates (predominantly CD4+ T cells) and destruction within the gland.

Laboratory testing may reveal anemia of chronic disease and, rarely, leukopenia. An elevated sedimentation rate and hypergammaglobulinemia are common, occurring in more than 80% of patients. Autoantibodies that may be observed in Sjögren's syndrome include:

- Antinuclear antibodies (90%)
- Rheumatoid factor (60%)
- Anti-Ro (SSA)
- Anti-LA (SSB)
- Cryoglobulins
- Antigastric parietal cell
- Antithyroglobulin
- Antisalivary duct

The histopathology observed in Sjögren's syndrome ranges from a benign lymphoepithelial lesion to pseudolymphoma to frank lymphoma. Conversion to lymphoma (predominantly B cell) occurs in 5% of patients with Sjögren's syndrome. The relative risk for the development of Non-Hodgkin's lymphoma is 44 times the expected rate. Waldenstrom's macroglobulinemia also appears to be more frequent in Sjögren's syndrome.

TREATMENT OF SJÖGREN'S SYNDROME

The treatment of Sjögren's syndrome is largely aimed at symptomatic relief:

- Lubrication of dry eyes with artifical tears
- Frequent ingestion of fluid and stimulation of salivary flow with sugar-free lozenges

Attention to dental hygiene is critical given the increased frequency of dental caries. Pilocarpine may help to increase salivary secretion. Treatment of sicca symptoms with hydroxychloroquine has met with variable success. Prednisone and cytotoxic agents are reserved for the treatment of extraglandular manifestations, such as vasculitis and severe pulmonary or renal involvement.

DIFFUSE INFILTRATIVE LYMPHOCYTOSIS SYNDROME ASSOCIATED WITH HIV

A syndrome resembling Sjögren's syndrome has been observed in some HIV-positive patients who present with xerostomia and parotid gland enlargement: Diffuse Infiltrative Lymphocytosis Syndrome (DILS) Associated with HIV. However, features that distinguish this syndrome from Sjögren's syndrome are the absence of autoantibodies, increased prevalence of HLA-DR5, infiltration of the CD8 + T cells within the salivary glands (in contrast to CD4 + cells seen in Sjögren's syndrome), and increased prevalence of lymphadenopathy.

INFLAMMATORY MYOPATHIES

The term inflammatory myopathy refers to a group of immune-mediated systemic muscle diseases that are idiopathic in nature and joined together by the common symptom of muscle weakness and the histologic finding of inflammatory cellular infiltrates in muscle:

- Polymyositis
- Dermatomyositis
- Childhood myositis
- Myositis associated with malignancy
- Myositis associated with another connective-tissue disease
- Inclusion body myositis

Polymyositis (PM) is the prototypic systemic inflammatory myopathy. Dermatomyositis (DM) is distinguished from polymyositis by its characteristic cutaneous findings. Both conditions may occur in children as well as adults and sometimes are associated with an underlying malignancy. Inclusion body myositis (IBM) is another form of idiopathic inflammatory myopathy, generally more refractory to treatment.

EPIDEMIOLOGY AND PATHOGENESIS OF INFLAMMATORY MYOPATHIES

As a group, inflammatory myopathies are rare, occurring with an annual incidence of 5–10 per million population. The mean age at diagnosis is 35. Inflammatory myopathies, excluding inclusion body myositis, are more common in women (approximately 2:1). Two peaks of incidence exist, one in childhood and another in the fifth decade. The cause of these syndromes is unknown. Incidence of the HLA-B8 DR3 phenotype is increased. It has been suggested that picornavirus and coxsackievirus trigger the onset of myositis in some patients, but this has not been firmly established.

CLINICAL PRESENTATION OF INFLAMMATORY MYOPATHIES

The most common manifestation of polymyositis is the gradual onset of painless proximal symmetrical muscle weakness. Oftentimes the onset of the weakness is preceded by a flu-like prodrome. The weakness generally starts in the hip and shoulder girdle and may also affect the neck flexors as the weakness progresses. Dysphagia due to involvement of the oropharyngeal striated muscles may be seen in more than 50% of patients. A summary of clinical presentation of inflammatory myopathies includes:

- Painless proximal muscle weakness for more than 3–6 months (55%)
- Acute/subacute proximal pain and weakness for 2–8 weeks (30%)
- Insidious proximal and distal weakness for years (10%)
- Proximal myalgia (5%)
- Dermatomyositis rash (< 1%)

Other features associated with polymyositis include:

- Arthralgias/inflammatory arthritis
- Pulmonary involvement (50%)
  - Respiratory muscle weakness
  - Interstitial lung disease
  - Aspiration pneumonia from pharyngeal muscle dysmotility
- Cardiac involvement (40%)
- Raynaud's phenomenon

Cutaneous lesions associated with dermatomyositis include:

- Heliotrope rash, (a violaceous discoloration occurring around the eyes)
- Gottron's papules, (erythematous papular, sometimes-scaly lesions occurring over the knuckles (sparing the phalanges), knees and elbows)
- V-sign rash (affects the V of the neck)
- Shawl sign rash (affects the upper back, shoulders and upper arms)
- Mechanic's hands (dry and cracking skin over the lateral and palmar aspects of the fingers)

Subcutaneous calcification is especially common in children with dermatomyositis. Raynaud's phenomenon is seen in 35–40% of patients. An inflammatory arthritis, interstitial lung disease, and cardiac involvement may also be observed. Patients with dermatomyositis, and to a lesser extent, polymyositis, have a higher incidence of malignancy than the general population (relative risk 3.4 and 1.7 respectively). Ten percent of patients with dermatomyositis have a malignancy diagnosed within the first year of diagnosis of the myositis.

Inclusion-body myositis is a distinct myopathy characterized by the muscle biopsy finding of intracytoplasmic and intranuclear inclusions and basophilic-lined vacuoles. It is distinguished from the polymyositis and dermatomyositis by its insidious course, with early (often asymmetric) involvement of distal as well as proximal muscles, low grade elevations in creatine kinase (CK), and relative resistance to treatment. It typically affects men over the age of 50, in contrast to inflammatory myopathies which more commonly affect women. There is no known association with autoantibodies.

DIAGNOSIS OF INFLAMMATORY MYOPATHIES

The hallmark of inflammatory muscle disease is an elevated creatine kinase and aldolase, but these tests are not specific. Other diagnostic tools include:

- Electromyogram
- Muscle biopsy
- Autoantibodies: ANA, anti-RNP (associated with mixed connective tissue disease), and anti-PM-Scl (observed in patients with an overlap of myositis and scleroderma)

The differential diagnosis of an elevated CK includes:

- Drugs: clofibrate, diclofenac, lovastatin, colchicine, pentobarbital, diazepam, cimetidine, tamoxifen, hydroxychloroquine sulfate, penicillamine, amphetamines, alcohol, cocaine, AZT, emetine
- Endocrinopathy: hypothyroidism, hyperthyroidism, and hypoparathyroidism
- Muscular dystrophies/enzymopathies
- Rheumatic disorders: polymyositis, dermatomyositis, systemic lupus erythematosus, scleroderma, and sarcoidosis
- Infection: toxoplasmosis, trichinosis, and pyomyositis
- Electrolyte abnormalities: hypokalemia and hypocalcemia
- Trauma: seizures, intramuscular injections, and runners

Elevations in SGOT, SGPT, and LDH in inflammatory muscle disease may also be observed. Antinuclear antibodies are commonly observed in up to 90% of patients. Several myositis-specific antibodies have been discovered and help to define homogeneous subpopulations of patients with myositis for research purposes. The most common myositis-specific antibody is the anti-Jo-1 antibody, which is observed in 15% of patients and is directed against histidyl tRNA synthetase. There is a wide array of other anti-synthetase antibodies; in general, they are associated with a clinical syndrome consisting of myositis, interstitial lung disease, inflammatory arthritis and mechanic's hands. The syndrome associated with anti-SRP (signal recognition particle) antibodies, another myositis-specific antibody, has an increased incidence of acute onset severe muscle weakness, distal muscle involvement, cardiac involvement, and poor outcome. Antibodies to Mi-2 are seen in 5–10% of patients and are associated with cutaneous manifestations and a good prognosis.

Electromyographic (EMG) recordings in suspected myositis is useful to distinguish myopathies from neuropathies. The EMG typically demonstrates increased spontaneous activity with fibrillations and complex repetitive discharges, polyphasic motor potentials of short duration and low amplitude, and positive sharp waves. However, this EMG pattern occurs in a variety of acute myopathic processes, and is not diagnostic for inflammatory myopathies. In inclusion-body myositis, both myopathic and neuropathic abnormalities may be found.

Magnetic resonance imaging of the extremities may reveal inflammation within muscle groups. The most definitive diagnostic tool, however, is the muscle biopsy. A muscle biopsy is useful to confirm the diagnosis of inflammatory muscle disease and rule out other diseases that may mimic myositis. A negative biopsy does not rule out a diagnosis of myositis because there may be patchy involvement of the muscles, resulting in sampling error on biopsy. In polymyositis, the biopsy shows:

- Inflammatory infiltrates (predominantly CD8+ lymphocytes) within the muscle fascicles
- Muscle necrosis and atrophy
- Degenerating and regenerating fibers

In dermatomyositis, the inflammatory infiltrates (predominantly CD4 + lymphocytes) are predominantly perivascular or around the muscle fascicles.

TREATMENT OF INFLAMMATORY MYOPATHIES

The first-line treatment for polymyositis and dermatomyositis are corticosteroids. If corticosteroids alone are ineffective, or if the myositis flares during steroid tapering, a second-line agent (methotrexate or azathioprine) is used. Recent reports have shown that intravenous immune globulin is effective treatment for refractory dermatomyositis. Hydroxychloroquine may be effective in the treatment of the cutaneous manifestations of dermatomyositis.

REVIEW EXERCISES

1. A 26-year-old woman with a 5-year history of SLE characterized by a malar rash, arthritis, pleurisy, and a positive ANA of 1:160 homogeneous pattern, presents for routine evaluation. Physical examination was remarkable for a malar rash and mild small joint synovitis. Labs reveal normal CBC and a serum creatinine of 1.4 mg/dl. Sedimentation rate was 47 mm/hour. Urinalysis revealed new onset hematuria and proteinuria. The next step in the evaluation is:

   a. Intravenous pyelogram
   b. Urine gram stain and culture
   c. Microscopic exam of urine to look for cellular casts
   d. Repeat ANA titer
   e. Cystoscopy

2. A 51-year-old man with an 8-month history of rapidly progressive diffuse scleroderma presents with severe headaches and weakness. On examination the patient is noted to have a blood pressure of 180/100. Laboratory testing reveals a serum creatinine 2.7mg/

dl, hemoglobin 10 g/dl with red blood cell fragments on peripheral smear, and a platelet count of 80,000/mm^3. The treatment of choice in this clinical setting is:

   a. Transfusion of platelets
   b. Pulse corticosteroids
   c. Angiotensin converting enzyme inhibitor
   d. Minoxidil
   e. Cyclophosphamide

3. A 46-year-old man presents with fatigue and bilateral parotid gland enlargement. All of the following may be associated with bilateral parotid enlargement *except:*

   a. Sarcoidosis
   b. Hyperthyroidism
   c. Sjögren's syndrome
   d. HIV infection
   e. Hyperlipoproteinemia

Answers

1. c

The finding of hematuria and proteinuria in a patient with SLE should raise the question of glomerulonephritis. However, hematuria may result from many other causes, such as a urinary-tract infection, cystitis, or malignancy, therefore microscopic examination of the urine is essential. Demonstration of red blood cell casts and dysmorphic red blood cells on microscopic examination of the urine suggests active glomerular disease and warrants further evaluation. Urine sediment will reflect changes in renal status before a rise in serum creatinine is observed.

2. c

The finding of new onset hypertension and progressive renal insufficiency associated with a microangiopathic hemolytic anemia and thrombocytopenia in a patient with rapidly progressive scleroderma indicates scleroderma renal crisis (SRC). It is also important to remember that in 10% of scleroderma patients with renal crisis, blood pressure is normal. Before the widespread use of angiotensin converting enzyme (ACE) inhibitors, mortality associated with scleroderma renal crisis was greater than 90%. Early recognition of the syndrome and aggressive treatment with ACE inhibi-

tors has significantly increased survival. Cumulative survival rates for ACE inhibitor-treated patients with SRC is more than 75% at 1 year versus 15% in untreated patients.

Immunosuppression with corticosteroids or cyclophosphamide has no role in the treatment of SRC. Minoxidil has not been shown to be useful in the treatment of SRC. Transfusions are only indicated if bleeding complications arise.

3. b

The differential diagnosis of bilateral parotid gland enlargement includes Sjögren's syndrome, sarcoidosis, viral infections (such as mumps), CMV and EBV, cirrhosis, diabetes mellitus, and hyperlipoproteinemia (Type IV and V). Human immunodeficiency virus infection has been associated with a condition called ''Diffuse Infiltrative Lymphocytosis Syndrome,'' which clinically mimics Sjögren's syndrome but lacks the autoantibodies commonly seen in Sjögren's syndrome. Unilateral parotid gland enlargement should raise suspicion for malignancy, bacterial infection or stones. Chronic sialoadenitis may also result in unilateral enlargement of the parotid gland. Hyperthyroidism is not associated with parotid gland enlargement.

SUGGESTED READING

SYSTEMIC LUPUS ERYTHEMATOSUS

Boumpas DT, Austin HA, Fessler BJ: Systemic lupus erythematosus: Emerging concepts, Part I: Renal, neuropsychiatric, cardiovascular, pulmonary and hematologic disease. Ann Intern Med 1995;22:940.

Boumpas DT, Fessler BJ, Austin HA: Systemic lupus erythematosus: Emerging concepts, Part II: Dermatologic and joint disease; pregnancy and hormonal therapy; morbidity and mortality; pathogenesis. Ann Intern Med 1995;23:42.

Cervera R, Khamashta MA, Font J, et al: Systemic lupus erythematosus: Clinical and immunologic patterns of disease expression in a cohort of 1000 patients. Medicine 1993;72:113.

Esdaile JM: Prognosis in systemic lupus erythematosus. Springer Semin Immunopathol 1994;16:337.

Gourley MF, Austin HA, Scott D, et al: Methylprednisolone and cyclophosphamide, alone or in combination, in patients with lupus nephritis. Ann Intern Med 1996:125:549.

Hill J: Systemic lupus erythematosus. N Engl J Med 1994;330:1871.

Pistiner M, Wallace DJ, Nessim S, et al: Lupus Erythematosus in the 1980's: A survey of 570 patients. Semin Arthritis Rheumatol 1991;21:55.

Schur PH: Genetics of systemic lupus erythematosus. Lupus 1995;4:425.

Von Mühlen CA, Tan EM: Autoantibodies in the diagnosis of systemic rheumatic diseases. Semin Arthritis Rheumatol 1995;24:323.

Yung RL, Richards BC: Drug-induced lupus. Rheum Dis Clin North Am 1994;20:61.

ANTIPHOSPHOLIPID ANTIBODY SYNDROME

Khamashta MA, Cuadrado MJ, Fedza MD, et al: The management of thrombosis in the antiphospholipid antibody syndrome. N Engl J Med 1995;332:993.

Love PE, Santoro SA. Antiphospholipid antibodies: Anticardiolipin and the lupus anticoagulant in systemic lupus erythematosus (SLE) and in non-SLE disorders. Prevalence and clinical significance. Ann Intern Med 1990:112:682.

Rosove MH, Brewer PMC: Antiphospholipid thrombosis: Clinical course after the first thrombotic event in 70 patients. Ann Intern Med 1992;117:303.

Sammaritano LR, Gharavi AE, Lockshin MD: Antiphospholipid antibody syndrome: Immunologic and clinical aspects. Semin Arthritis Rheumatol 1990;20:81.

Vianna JL, Khamashta MA, Ordi-Ros J, et al: Comparison of the primary and secondary antiphospholipid antibody syndrome: A European multicenter study of 114 patients. Am J Med 1994;96:3.

SCLERODERMA

Arroliga AC, Podell DN, Matthay RA: Pulmonary manifestations of scleroderma. J Thorac Imag 1992;7:30.

Helfrich DJ, Banner B, Steen VD, Medsger TA: Normotensive renal failure in systemic sclerosis. Arthritis Rheum 1989;32:1128.

Jimenez SA, Sigal SH: A 15-year prospective study of treatment of rapidly progressive systemic sclerosis with D-penicillamine. J Rheumatol 1991;18:1496.

Kaufman LD, Krupp LB: Eosinophilia-myalgia syndrome, toxic oil syndrome and diffuse fasciitis with eosinophilia. Curr Opin Rheumatol 1995;7:560.

Legerton, CW, Smith EA, Silver RM: Systemic sclerosis (scleroderma): clinical management of its major complications. Rheum Dis Clin North Am 1995;21:203.

LeRoy EC, Black C, Fleischmajer R, et al: Scleroderma (systemic sclerosis): Classification, subsets and pathogenesis. J Rheumatol 1988;15:202.

Steen VD, Costantino JP, Shapiro AP, et al: Outcome of renal crisis in systemic sclerosis: relation to availability of angiotensin converting enzyme (ACE) inhibitors. Ann Intern Med 1990;113:352.

Steen VD, Medsger TA: Epidemiology and natural history of systemic sclerosis. Rheum Dis Clin North Am 1990;16:1.

Wigley FM: Management of severe Raynaud's phenomenon. J Clin Rheumatol 1996;2:103.

SJÖGREN'S SYNDROME

Alexander EL, Lijewski JE, et al: Evidence of an immunopathogenetic basis for central nervous system disease in primary Sjögren's syndrome. Arthritis Rheum 1986;29:1223.

Anaya JM, McGuff HS, Banks PM, Talal N: Clinicopathological factors relating malignant lymphoma with Sjögren's syndrome. Semin Arthritis Rheumatol 1996;25:337.

Fox RI, Howell FV, et al: Primary Sjögren's syndrome. Clinical and immunopathologic features. Semin Arthritis Rheum 1994;14:77.

Itescu S, Winchester R: Diffuse infiltrative lymphocytosis

syndrome: a disorder occurring in human immunodeficiency virus-1 infection that may present as a sicca syndrome. Rheum Dis Clin North Am 1992;18:683.

Talal D: Sjögren's syndrome: Historical overview and clinical spectrum of disease. Rheum Dis Clin North Am 1992;18:507.

MYOSITIS

Dalakas MC: Polymyositis, dermatomyositis and inclusion body myositis. N Engl J Med 1991:325:1487.

Dalakas MC, Illa I, Dambrosia JM, et al: A controlled trial of high-dose intravenous immune globulin infusions as treatment for dermatomyositis. N Engl J Med 1993;329:1993.

Love LA, Leff RL, Fraser DD, et al: A new approach to the classification of idiopathic inflammatory myopathy: myositis-specific autoantibodies define useful homogeneous patient groups. Medicine 1991;70:360.

Oddis CV: Inflammatory myopathies. Bailliere's Clin Rheumatol 1995;9: 497.

Plotz PH, Dalakas M, Leff RL, et al: Current concepts in the idiopathic inflammatory myopathies: polymyositis, dermatomyositis, and related disorders. Ann Intern Med 1989;111: 143.

Sayers ME, Chou SM, Calabrese LH: Inclusion body myositis: analysis of 32 cases. J Rheumatol 1992;19:1385.

Schulman P, Kerr LD, Speira H: A reexamination of the relationship between myositis and malignancy. J Rheumatol 1991;18:1689.

31

Systemic Vasculitis

Leonard H. Calabrese

The term *vasculitis* generally is used interchangeably with the term *necrotizing vasculitis,* both referring to a heterogeneous group of disorders sharing, to varying degrees, the pathologic features of vascular inflammation and vascular necrosis. While vasculitis may stem from a variety of pathogenetic mechanisms, the primary necrotizing vasculitides generally encompass those syndromes either suspected or proven to be immune mediated. This review will detail our current understanding of the pathogenesis, classification, and clinical spectrum of these disorders, as well as provide a practical diagnostic and therapeutic approach.

ETIOLOGY OF SYSTEMIC VASCULITIS

PATHOGENESIS OF SYSTEMIC VASCULITIS

Over the past decade, considerable progress has been made in the understanding of vascular inflammation. Prior to the mid-1980s, most pathogenetic theories centered on the role of immune complexes. With refinement of assay techniques and the appreciation of the low specificity immune complex detection, however, broader mechanisms of vascular inflammation were searched for and elucidated. While specific etiologies are rare, there is support for at least four operative mechanisms in vasculitic diseases:

- Immune complexes (ICs)
  - Hypersensitivity group
  - Polyarteritis Nodosa (PAN)—some
- Antibody-mediated—antineutrophil cytoplasmic antibodies (ANCA), others
  - Wegener's, MPAN, Churg-Strauss, others
- Cell-mediated—endothelial focus
  - GCA, Takayasu's, others

- Immunoproliferative
  - Angiocentric immunoproliferative
  - Some viral-associated

Immune Complexes (ICs)

Supporting evidence for circulating immune complexes (CICs) in certain vasculitic conditions includes:

- Animal models of immune complex disease
- Identification of IC in tissues
- Identification of IC in the sera of patients with necrotizing vasculitis
- Identification of discrete antigens responsible for certain IC disorders

In humans, identification of IC in both sera and tissues is supportive of their importance in certain diseases. In particular, the diseases within the hypersensitivity vasculitis group have the strongest supported IC pathogenesis. True hypersensitivity vasculitis frequently follows the exposure to a discrete antigen by 7 to 10 days and is often accompanied by evidence of complement activation and immunoglobulin and/or complement deposition in involved tissues. Strong evidence for humoral immunity also is shared by Henoch-Schöenlein purpura, mixed cryoglobulinemia, urticarial vasculitis, and a fraction of patients with PAN.

Antibody-Associated Disease

Perhaps the greatest breakthrough in the field of vasculitic research since the development of combination immunosuppressive therapy was the discovery of antineutrophil cytoplasmic antibodies (ANCA). In 1982, ANCA were first identified, using immunofluorescent techniques, in a small number of patients with crescentic glomerulonephritis (GN) and vasculitis. This achievement was followed by the observations of a Scandinavian group that ANCA were frequently present in patients with Wegener's granulomatosis and seemed to correlate with disease activity. Since then, numerous investigators have confirmed and extended these findings, as well as documented their presence in patients with crescentic GN of the pauci-immune variety.

ANCA are divided on the basis of their immunofluorescent pattern and antigenic specificity. The patterns are C-ANCA for *diffuse cytoplasmic* pattern and P-ANCA for *perinuclear* pattern. The antigen responsible for the C-ANCA pattern more than 95% of the time (and correlated with vasculitic disease) is a serine protease of 29KD in size known as proteinase 3 (PR3). The antigen associated with the P-ANCA (associated with vasculitic disease) is the enzyme myeloperoxidase (MPO). Both substrates are located in the alpha or azurophilic granules of granulocytes and the cytosolic granules of monocytes. P-ANCA reactivity, by immunofluorescence alone, is highly nonspecific and, in the majority of cases, is owing to antinuclear antibody activity and/or other autoantibodies (i.e., anticatalase, anticathepsin). The C-ANCA pattern is much more specific for antibodies to PR3.

ANCA are not associated with a single disease, but are rather found in a family of diseases sharing certain pathologic features. The features include a vasculitis with some granulocytic component (at least early in the course) and a renal pathologic picture described as "pauci-immune" glomerulonephritis, implying little in the way of immune complex deposition. The glomerulitis also displays little in the way of capillary proliferation, segmental necrosis, and frequent crescent formation. Diseases with this pathologic picture include:

- Wegener's granulomatosis
- Microscopic polyarteritis nodosa
- Churg-Strauss
- Idiopathic rapidly progressive glomerulonephritis

Sensitivity of ANCA in these diseases varies but may exceed 90% in patients with active multisystem Wegener's granulomatosis. In general, anti-PR3 are found in patients with disease that is active, untreated and multisystem (i.e., Wegener's with upper and lower respiratory involvement and renal involvement). Antibodies to MPO are more likely to be found in patients with isolated renal disease (i.e., idiopathic RPGN). The specificity of these assays depends upon their technical performance attributes (whether done by immunofluorescence only or solid phase assay). In labs performing both immunofluorescence and solid phase assays to PR3 and myeloperoxidase, the specificity exceeds 95% for one of these conditions.

ANCA are useful in the diagnosis of one of the above described vasculitic conditions. Given their moderately high sensitivity and high specificity, antibodies against PR3 or MPO can replace the need for tissue confirmation under certain circumstances. These circumstances include a very high pretest probability of the likelihood of the disease being present (based on clinical grounds) and the absence of underlying infection. Some studies have suggested that these tests may be useful in monitoring disease activity, but it appears unlikely they can supersede clinical findings.

Many other conditions have been reported to have ANCA positivity, including:

- Kawasaki's disease
- Certain infections (i.e., HIV)
- Inflammatory bowel disease
- Sclerosing cholangitis

These reports have identified ANCA by immunofluorescence but have not confirmed that they represent reactivity to either PR3 or myeloperoxidase.

At present, it is uncertain whether ANCA are directly pathogenic, but growing evidence suggests this to be the case. ANCA, under certain circumstances, are capable of binding to neutrophils, causing release of their toxic products. Myeloperoxidase and PR3 may also bind to endothelial cells and serve as "innocent bystanders" for ANCA-mediated injury There are also data suggesting that endothelial cells may express PR3.

Cell-Mediated/Endothelial Focal Disease

Neither giant-cell arteritis nor Takayasu's disease demonstrate substantial evidence for either CIC or specific antibodies; their pathology is more suggestive of a cell-mediated process. The ability of endothelial cells to become "activated" and serve as antigen-presenting cells and sources of cytokine production suggests their ability to interact with immune competent cells even in the absence of injury. Endothelial cells also express multiple-adhesion molecules, which have the ability to interact with complementary ligands on immunocytes leading to leukocyte binding and emigration. Evidence currently exists for endothelial activation and adhesion molecule expression in the giant-cell disorders, as well as other forms of vasculitis.

Immunoproliferative Disorders

Several vascular inflammatory disorders demonstrate strong evidence of being lymphoproliferative disorders, in particular the syndromes of benign lymphocytic angiitis and lymphomatoid granulomatosis/polymorphic reticulosis. These conditions are angiocentric and predominantly T cell in nature, with little propensity for vessel necrosis. Frequently, they are the forerunners of frank T cell lymphomas within the vascular wall (i.e., angiocentric lymphoma). Recent studies using gene rearrangement have demonstrated the clonal nature of many of these cases, even in the presence of morphologically benign disease.

Finally, it should be appreciated that most vasculitic syndromes represent admixtures of these proposed mechanisms. For example, endothelium initially injured by antibody or IC may then become activated, secrete cytokines and/or display adhesion molecules and become the focus for cell-mediated pathologic damage. Other conditions such as Kawasaki's demonstrate strong evidence of endothelial activation and cytokine release, but also are associated with ANCA. A clearer understanding of the pathologic mechanisms involved in discrete syndromes will facilitate more specific therapies, including biologic response modifiers.

CLASSIFICATION OF SYSTEMIC VASCULITIS

Numerous classifications have been put forth in an effort to better understand the vasculitides. Most of these schemes have been plagued by inherent inconsistencies and lack of clinical utility. The following classification represents an admixture of several classification schemes, taking into account some features of vessel size and clinical features.

- PAN—classic (medium vessel)
- Pauci-immune (small-medium vessel)
  - Microscopic polyangiitis
  - Wegener's granulomatosis
  - Churg-Strauss
- Hypersensitivity vasculitis group (small vessel)
  - True hypersensitivity vasculitis
  - Henoch-Schöenlein purpura
  - Cyroglobulinemia
  - Vasculitis with malignancy
  - Hypocomplementemic vasculitis
  - Vasculitis of systemic disease
- Giant-cell group (large vessel)
  - Giant-cell arteritis
  - Takayasu's arteritis
- Overlap disorders
- Miscellaneous conditions
  - Primary angiitis of the central nervous system (PACNS)
  - Behcet's disease
  - Others

Recently, several newer classifications schemes have been proposed by the American College of Rheumatology and an international cooperative group, but neither group has significantly advanced our understanding of the relationships among these disorders.

CLINICAL PRESENTATION AND DIAGNOSIS OF SYSTEMIC VASCULITIS

As a group, the vasculitides remain formidable challenges to physicians from both diagnostic and therapeutic perspectives. Diagnostically, the signs and symptoms of vasculitis are generally nonspecific since they represent vascular ischemia regardless of the cause. Certain vasculitic syndromes represent greater diagnostic challenges than others because of the nature

and distribution of their target organ involvement. For example, when the skin is involved, such as in the hypersensitivity vasculitis group, it is apparent that vasculitis is the underlying process, but a greater challenge is to determine the precise etiology and thus, prognosis and treatment. In the absence of topical signs of vasculitis, such as a characteristic rash or signs of peripheral ischemia, systemic vasculitis may mimic a wide variety of nonvasculitic diseases. Warning signs or symptoms of systemic vasculitis include:

- FUO with constitutional symptoms
- Unexplained multisystem organ disease
- Unexplained inflammatory arthritis
- Unexplained myositis
- Suspicious rash
- Mononeuritis multiplex
- Unexplained end organ ischemia
- Glomerulonephritis

These findings should alert the clinician to the possibility of systemic vasculitis when a careful workup for other causes is unrevealing. Certain of these signs or symptoms have greater degrees of sensitivity or specificity depending upon the clinical situation. For example, mononeuritis multiplex in the absence of diabetes or trauma is highly specific and should always be considered indicative of vasculitis until proved otherwise. Other signs, such as unexplained myositis or arthritis, are relatively nonspecific and may be mimicked by a wide variety of conditions. Regardless, the appreciation that these clinical signs and/or symptoms are consistent with the diagnosis makes them reasonable starting places for the evaluation.

SPECIFIC SYSTEMIC VASCULITIS CONDITIONS

Descriptions of the following systemic vasculitis conditions follow.

- Polyarteritis Nodosa (PAN)
- Pauci-immune
  - Microscopic polyangiitis
  - Wegener's granulomatosis
  - Churg-Strauss disease
- Hypersensitivity vasculitis group (HVG)
  - Hypersensitivity vasculitis
  - Henoch-Schöenlein purpura
  - Cryoglobulinemia
  - Other conditions within the hypersensitivity vasculitis group
- Giant-cell arteritis
  - Temporal arteritis
  - Takayasu's arteritis
- Polyangiitis overlap syndrome
- Lymphomatoid granulomatosis and benign lymphocytic angiitis

POLYARTERITIS NODOSA (PAN)

PAN was first described more than 100 years ago by Kussmaul and Maier. PAN, which affects both the small- and medium-size muscular arteries, is an uncommon disease. General characteristics include:

- More common in males (sex ratio of about 2 : 1)
- All age groups affected
- Most common between the ages of 40 and 60

Pathophysiology of PAN

PAN has been reported in association with hepatitis B and has thus been considered immune complex in origin. Only about 5%–10% of patients with PAN have evidence of hepatitis B, while the remaining patients represent an admixture of idiopathic disease and those associated with other findings. Other underlying diseases that have been associated with a PAN-like syndrome include:

- Hairy-cell leukemia
- Endocarditis
- Connective tissue disease
- Drug abuse
- Drug abuse
- HIV infection

In the presence of these other systemic diseases, a diagnosis of PAN cannot be made.

Clinical Presentation and Pathologic Features of PAN

The clinical and pathologic features of PAN include:

- Medium-size vessel disease
- Cardiac, GI, central and peripheral nervous systems common
- Hypertension common
- Abdominal pain common
- Fever and constitutional symptoms common
- Livedo reticularis common
- Eosinophilia, allergy and lung disease uncommon

Common presenting complaints by patients with PAN include:

- Neuro signs/symptoms, 15%
- Malaise/weakness, 13%
- Abdominal pain, 12%
- Leg pain, 12%
- Fever, 8%
- Arthralgia/arthritis, 4%
- Skin involvement, 4%

Diagnosis of PAN

Angiography and Biopsy The diagnosis of PAN, which can be problematic, must first start with a high suspicion of its presence. The presence of the cardinal signs and symptoms of vasculitis may be the first clue to its presence. The diagnosis

must be based on either characteristic angiographic findings or biopsy (tissue evidence of necrotizing vasculitis).

There is significant debate as to which is the first test to choose when trying to diagnose this condition, but several generalizations can be made:

- Biopsy muscle and/or nerve if symptomatic
- Consider abdominal angiography if no accessible symptomatic site and risks are reasonable
- Consider other symptomatic sites if above strategy fails (i.e., testical, rectum, renal, other)

In the absence of any target-organ involvement (i.e., renal, GI, neurologic), abdominal angiography is the diagnostic modality of choice. Approximately 70%–80% of patients with PAN will have abnormal angiograms, with three-fourths of these patients demonstrating classical multiple microaneurysms.

Biopsy considerations should include:

- Skin
  - Nonspecific
  - May be useful when combined with other clinical findings
- Muscle
  - Specific
  - Poor sensitivity
  - Yield increases with clinical/EMG abnormalities
- Nerve
  - Specific
  - Poor sensitivity
  - Rarely demonstrative of ''necrosis''
  - Sensitivity increases with clinical/EMG abnormalities
- Testicular
  - Specific
  - Poor sensitivity
  - Invasive
- Rectal
  - Little data on sensitivity
  - Technique dependent
- Renal
  - Poor sensitivity
  - Rare extraglomerular vasculitis, FSGN

In the presence of documented peripheral neurologic disease by either clinical examination or EMG, a sural nerve biopsy has extremely high yield. Blind biopsies of muscle, kidney, and testicle in the absence of clinical signs and symptoms are rarely productive. Skin biopsy alone is inadequate evidence of the presence of PAN. Percutaneous renal biopsies may be employed, but it must be recognized that they will rarely demonstrate extraglomerular vasculitis, but rather a segmental necrotizing glomerulonephritis demonstrating little in the way of immune complex deposition (i.e., pauci-immune).

Diagnositic strategies of PAN must weigh safety, efficacy, and availability.

Laboratory Studies There are no specific laboratory tests for PAN. The most sensitive laboratory findings are the elevation of the acute-phase reactants, including erythrocyte sedimentation rate. Elevated white blood cell count and anemia are also frequently present. Without these findings, an individual suspected of having PAN likely does not have it. The presence of circulating immune complexes and hypocomplementemia are helpful when present, but are absent in the majority of patients. ANCA (both PR3 and MPO) are generally absent. To summarize laboratory tests:

- Mostly useful for ruling out other diagnoses
- Acute-phase reactants and CBC have high negative predictive value
- Immune complexes, complement, and autoantibodies of limited utility
- ANCA rarely positive

Treatment of PAN

Therapy of systemic vasculitis includes:

- Disease-associated variables
- Patient-associated variables
- Diagnosis
- Disease activity
- Treatment toxicity
  - PCP
  - Osteoporosis
  - Cancer
  - Bladder complications
  - Diabetes

Treatment of systemic vasculitis occurs in three phases:

1. Acute phase — initial control of disease
2. Subacute phase — tapering of immunosuppression to limit treatment and disease-associated comorbidities
3. Consolidation phase — minimizing long-term toxicity and ultimate discontinuation of therapy

Therapy of systemic vasculitis also includes:

- Corticosteroids (1 mg/kg) in the acute phase with taper
- Cyclophosphamide (2 mg/kg) orally
- Cyclophosphamide (0.5 gr–1 gr/meter) intravenously
- Methotrexate (15 mg to start) titrating to toxicity

Cyclophosphamide toxicity may cause:

- Infections, especially with steroids
- Hemorrhagic cystitis
- Gonadal dysfunction
- Bladder cancer
- Lympho and myeloproliferative disease
- Miscellaneous nausea, vomiting, rash, hepatitis, hypersensitivity reactions

Prognosis of PAN

Prognosis determinants in PAN include:

- Poor prognostic markers FFS:
  - Age > 50
  - GI involvement
  - Renal involvement (proteinuria, azotermia)
  - Cardiomyopathy
  - Central nervous system (CNS) involvement
- Mortality in 337 patients:
  - 0–12%
  - 1–26%
  - 2–46%
- May serve as a guide for treatment

If PAN is untreated, the 5-year survival rate is 10%–15% (Table 31.1). With the use of corticosteroids, the 5-year survival rate can improve to 50%. In recent years, the use of combination therapy with cyclophosphamide and high-dose steroids has been reported to increase the 5-year survival rate to 80% or more.

PAN in the presence of hepatitis B appears to have a more serious prognosis; a recent study from France suggests that therapy with interferon alpha may provide a higher rate of recovery for this subset (Lhote and Guillevin).

PAUCI-IMMUNE

The pauci-immune vasculitides are characterized by:

- Shared renal lesion of pauci-immune, necrotizing glomerulonephritis
- Propensity for both renal and pulmonary involvement (pulmonary-renal syndrome)
- Varying frequency of ANCA positivity
- High rate of relapse (especially when there is renal involvement)

The diseases may be clinically distinct or alternatively difficult to distinguish.

Microscopic Polyangiitis

The European literature is replete with descriptions of microscopic PAN or polyangiitis:

- Necrotizing, nongranulomatosis vasculitis, involving small and, at times, medium vessels

Table 31.1. Outcome in Patients with PAN

Intervention	*5-Year Survival*
None	< 15%
Corticosteroids	55%–70%
Corticosteroids & cyclophosphamide	> 80%

- Renal involvement common (RPGN)
- Pulmonary involvement common (hemorrhage)
- Neuropathy infrequent
- ANCA positive in 50%–80%
- Angiographic abnormalities uncommon

This generally refers to a vasculitis that involves small vessels (i.e., capillaries, venules, arterioles), with little immune complex deposition. The disease has a predisposition to involve the lungs; pathologically, they display a capillaritis without granuloma formation. It is frequently associated with ANCA (anti-MPO), particularly with the characteristic renal lesion of this group. Differentiation from Wegener's granulomatosis may at times be difficult when the pathology is not classic; at other times, it may resemble classic PAN, since larger vessels may also be involved in microscopic PAN by definition (see Jennette C, et al., 1994, and Lhote and Guillevin, 1995, in bibliography).

In contrast to classic PAN, microscopic polyangiitis:

- Involves small vessels (at times, medium vessels)
- Is frequently ANCA positive
- Is negative for HBsAg
- Tends to frequently involve the lungs

Wegener's Granulomatosis

Wegener's granulomatosis is a disease with distinctive clinical pathologic complex of necrotizing granulomatous vasculitis of the upper and lower respiratory system and glomerulonephritis. This disorder is particularly important because left untreated it has a uniformly fatal outcome. However, with the use of combined treatment with corticosteroids and cyclophosphamide, long-term remissions can be achieved in the vast majority of patients.

Clinical Presentation of Wegener's Granulomatosis Patients generally present with upper and/or lower respiratory tract symptoms such as sinusitis, cough, or shortness of breath. Renal disease is present in the majority at the onset. Involvement of the eyes, ears, CNS, skin, and joints can also be observed. To summarize:

- Common presentations include:
  - Prominent constitutional symptoms
  - Upper respiratory tract abnormalities
- Pulmonary and renal disease may be asymptomatic or clinically severe
- Other target organs include:
  - Skin
  - PNS
  - Eye
  - Joints

Diagnosis of Wegener's Granulomatosis In the past, the diagnosis of Wegener's granulomatosis depended upon the appropriate clinical picture and a diagnostic biopsy. Sampling

error and the patchy nature of the underlying pathology have made interpretation of biopsy material problematic:

- Diagnosis depends on identification of characteristic pathology
- Pathologic findings include:
  - Granuloma formation
  - Necrotizing vasculitis
  - Tissue necrosis
- Identification of characteristic findings in accessible tissue is rare (Devany AJ. Surg Path 1990;14:555)

Nasal biopsy often shows only nonspecific inflammation or necrosis and rarely shows necrotizing vasculitis. The renal biopsy generally demonstrates a segmental necrotizing crescentic glomerulonephritis of the pauci-immune variety (indistinguishable from that in PAN, microscopic PAN, and idiopathic rapidly progressive glomerulonephritis). Percutaneous renal biopsy rarely shows vasculitis outside the glomerulus. Lung biopsy is more invasive, but gives a higher yield. The use of antibody detection to PR3 (i.e., C-ANCA) can replace the need for tissue confirmation in limited circumstances when the "pretest" probability of the disease is high (Table 31.2). Meticulous attention must be taken to rule out underlying infection including the use of bronchoscopy.

The diagnosis of Wegener's has been greatly enhanced by the development of ANCA testing (see "Antibody-Associated Disease" above):

- Diagnosis
  - C-ANCA (PR3): Wegener's high sensitivity and specificity (70%–80% and > 98%) P-ANCA
  - P-ANCA: Varying sensitivity in several vasculitic conditions and specificity is technique dependent
  - Not a screening test
- Prognosis
  - C-ANCA and, to some degree, P-ANCA correlate with disease activity but of insufficient predicative value to serve as sole basis of therapy

Treatment of Wegener's Granulomatosis The treatment of this condition has relied upon the combination of corticoste-

Table 31.2. High "Pretest" Probability of Wegener's Granulomatosis

C-ANCA	*P-ANCA*
> 95% PR3	ANA 85%
5% other	MPO 10%
Cytoplasmic/ETOH	Non-MPO 5%
Cytoplasmic/formalin	Cathepsin G
	Lactoferin
	Others
	ETOH (P)
	Formalin (C)

roids and cyclophosphamide, similar to that used in polyarteritis nodosa (see ''Polyarteritis Nodosa'' above). Recent studies from the National Institutes of Health have suggested that methotrexate therapy may not only be a reasonable salvage treatment for patients either refractory or unable to tolerate cyclophosphamide, but also as primary therapy for patients without immediate life-threatening lung or kidney disease (see Hoffman, et al., 1993).

Lastly, numerous reports have suggested that trimethoprim-sulfamethoxazole may have therapeutic potential in patients with Wegener's granulomatosis. Most enthusiasm is currently held for using this agent in patients with localized disease (i.e., upper respiratory disease) that is not immediately life-threatening.

Prognosis of Wegener's Granulomatosis   Survival data include:

- Untreated mean survival of 5 months
- Survival greatly improved with combination treatment (cyclophosphamide and prednisone) and recognition of clinically less severe forms
- Treatment-related morbidity develops in 50% of the cases

Churg-Strauss Disease (Allergic Angiitis)

This condition was first described in 1951 when a group of patients with necrotizing vasculitis, a history of adult onset asthma, and striking eosinophilia was reported. This condition is clinically more rare than PAN. As with PAN, it has a predilection for medium-size muscular arteries, but in contrast to PAN, the lungs are nearly always involved in allergic granulomatosis. Skin involvement is also present in approximately two-thirds of patients, which is far more frequent than with PAN. The GI, cardiac, and renal systems also are frequently involved. The most striking clinical feature of this disorder is its predisposition for the peripheral nervous system with typical vasculitis neurophy. In fact, any person with recent-onset asthma who develops a peripheral neuropathic syndrome should be evaluated for Churg-Strauss.

To summarize the characteristics of allergic angiitis and granulomatosis:

- 62%–67% with neurologic involvement (Sehgal, et al. Mayo Clin Proc, 1995, Gullevin, et al. Br J Rheum 1988)—in 38% the dominant problem
- Mononeuritis multiplex > asymmetric polyneuropathy, distal symmetric polyneuropathy, lumbar radiculopathy
- Varying degrees of CNS involvement including, seizures, coma, infarction, confusion and hydrocephalus
- Asthma precedes the vasculitic phase by many years
- Disseminated vasculitis, asthma, eosinophilia
- Often preceded by allergic rhinitis then asthma
- Pathology of a small- to medium-size vessel disease associated with fibrinoid necrosis, eosinophilic infiltration and granuloma

- Wide-spread target organ damage with a preponderance of peripheral neurologic changes
- Consider in any patient with asthma developing neurologic symptoms

The laboratory hallmark of this disorder is the striking degree of peripheral eosinophilia, generally in excess of 1500 cells/mm^3.

The prognosis of this disorder is less well documented than that of PAN; some observers have considered it similar, while others consider it to be better because of its lower incidence of renal disease. The initial treatment is generally with high-dose steroids, reserving cytotoxic drugs such as cyclophosphamide for those with renal disease or refractory cases.

HYPERSENSITIVITY VASCULITIS GROUP (HVG)

The concept that hypersensitivity mechanisms could result in vasculitis was first proposed by Zeek and colleagues in 1948. The distinguishing features of the original condition were its frequent precipitation by drug or serum, prominent involvement of the skin, and pathologically, the tendency to involve small vessels and display leukocytoclasis (nuclear fragmentation):

- Skin involvement
  - Palpable purpura
  - Maculopapular
  - Other
- Small-vessel inflammation
- Leukocytoclasis

Pathogenesis of HVG

The etiology of these disorders is diverse, but within the hypersensitivity vasculitis group, there is strong evidence for a shared mechanism for vascular inflammation, namely, that mediated by immune complexes. Immune complexes can often be detected in the serum and tissues of afflicted patients.

Diagnosis of HVG

Diagnostic considerations in HVG include:

- Drug-induced ''hypersensitivity'' vasculitis
- Infection-associated vasculitis
- Henoch-Schöenlein purpura
- Cryoglobulinemia
- Malignancy-associated vasculitis
- Connective tissue-associated vasculitis
- Cutaneous manifestations of systemic vasculitis (i.e., PAN, Wegener's)
- Miscellaneous systemic diseases

Despite these distinguishing features, many patients with these features (e.g., cutaneous vasculitis or small-vessel involvement with leukocytoclasis) have no history of exposure to drug or toxin. Additionally, a wide variety of disorders with underlying mechanisms other than hypersensitivity have also been noted to have the same clinical and pathologic picture. These conditions include vasculitis secondary to connective tissue disease, Henoch-Schönlein purpura, malignancies, mixed cryoglobulins of essential origin and even occasional patients with other forms of systemic necrotizing vasculitis.

At present, the term *hypersensitivity vasculitis group* refers to a heterogeneous group of disorders, all displaying the clinical and pathologic features previously referred to. The presence of these findings (i.e., vasculitic rash that upon biopsy displays small vessel vasculitis with leukocytoclasis) should serve as a clinical starting point for a differential diagnosis of the disorders referred to in the classification scheme under this heading. To summarize the differential diagnosis:

- Idiopathic "hypersensitivity" vasculitis
- HSP
- CTD-associated
- Malignancy-associated
- Urticarial hypersensitivity
- Systemic vasculitis
- Cutaneous PAN
- Livoid vasculitis
- EED
- Others

Treatment of HVG

Key points in determining treatment for HVG include:

- Who to treat?
- Corticosteroids
- Cytotoxics
- Other, i.e., colchicine, dapsone, antihistamines
- Plasma exchange

Specific HVG Conditions

Hypersensitivity Vasculitis True hypersensitivity vasculitis owing to exposure to exogenous antigen is the most common syndrome within the hypersensitivity vasculitis group. Incriminate antigens that have been identified are diverse, but include:

- Drugs
- Infections
- Chemicals
- Immunizations
- A variety of miscellaneous exposures, such as:
  - Insect bites
  - Foreign proteins

To summarize the clinical pathologic features of hypersensitivity:

- Skin predominant organ — LCV, palapable purpura
- Visceral involvement variable

- Usually traced to a precipitating foreign antigen, i.e., drug, infection, toxin
- Usually occurs 7–10 days after exposure
- Skin lesions at same stage
- Evidence of immune complexes
- Self-limiting, but can be recurrent or chronic
- Treatment is best aimed at removing offending antigen

The clinical course of patients with hypersensitivity vasculitis is variable, but it is usually self-limited. Varying degrees of constitutional symptoms, including fever, malaise, and weight loss, may be observed. Occasionally, when more significant target-organ involvement may be seen (i.e., renal, pulmonary, or CNS), the course may be more severe. At times, the disorder may become chronic or recurrent. The treatment of true hypersensitivity vasculitis should primarily focus on removal of the inciting antigen. If the antigen is a drug, it should be discontinued, and if there is an incriminate infection, it should be treated. Many cases require no treatment at all, while more advanced cases may require the use of a variety of modalities including antihistamines, Colchicine, corticosteroids, and for severe cases, cytotoxic drugs.

Henoch-Schönlein Purpura Henoch-Schönlein purpura is a syndrome characterized by the presence of palpable purpura and varying degrees of GI ischemia and glomerulonephritis. Other symptoms such as arthritis, fever, and constitutional symptoms are not uncommon. The disorder is most common in individuals under the age of 18. Pathophysiologically, this condition is mediated by IgA-containing immune complexes, which have been identified within the tissues, especially in the kidney of afflicted patients. The treatment of this condition depends upon the severity of the syndrome, with mild disease requiring essentially no therapy, while life-threatening visceral disease may require corticosteroids and possibly even cytotoxic drugs. The use of these agents has not been demonstrated in controlled trials to either prevent or improve the course of nephritis in HSP. A recent study has suggested that intravenous gammaglobulin may be effective in stabilizing (but not improving) renal function in HSP and IgA nephropathy (see Rostoker, et al., 1994 in bibliography).

Cryoglobulinemia Much progress has been made in our understanding of cryoglobulinemia in the past three years:

- Type I — Monoclonal
  - B-cell malignancies
- Type II — Mixed/monoclonal
  - Hepatitis
  - Other
- Type III — Mixed
  - Immune complex disease

Recently, an association of hepatitis cryoglobulinemia C virus infection with Type-II mixed cryoglobulinemia has been established. Earlier, most patients with Type-II (mixed cryoglobulins containing both a monoclonal component and a polyclonal component of immunoglobulin) were believed to be idiopathic. Rare reports of hepatitis B associated with cryoglobulinemia had been noted, but these represented only a minority of cases. Numerous studies have now confirmed that hepatitis C virus RNA is found in the serum and cryoprecipitate of the majority of patients with Type II cryoglobulinemia. Estimates range from 30%–98% depending upon the techniques employed. By using molecular techniques (i.e., PCR), the virus has been identified and found to be enriched up to 1000-fold in the cryoprecipitate. It is controversial as to whether hepatitis C antibody can be identified within the cryoprecipitate or not.

As shown in Table 31.3, signs and symptoms of patients with hepatitis C-associated cryoglobulinemia include:

*   Palpable purpura
*   Arthralgias
*   Weakness
*   Peripheral neuropathy
*   Glomerulonephritis (most frequently membranoproliferative)
*   Hepatic and spleen enlargement
*   Skin ulcers

Hepatitis C has been identified in Type-II cryoglobulinemia:

*   Serologic evidence of exposure to hepatitis C in 90% of previous "essential" cases
*   Evidence of active hepatitis C infection
*   Concentration of hepatitis CRNA and antibodies in cryoglobulinemia
*   Hepatitis C in blood vessels or kidneys
*   Antiviral therapy leads to clinical improvement

This association has raised a possibility of a more direct form of treatment with interferon alpha, which has been approved to treat chronic active hepatitis secondary to this infection. Preliminary reports have suggested that the majority of patients with cryoglobulinemia and hepatitis C may favorably respond to treatment course lasting for 3 months or more. Some patients have sustained long-term remissions (up to 40 months) after discontinuing interferon. A recent controlled trial has demonstrated clinical improvement in the majority of patients, but unfortunately all patients relapsed after discontinuation of interferon.

Traditional therapies for Type-II cryoglobulinemia have been directed at decreasing the formation or deposition of the cryoglobulins and have relied on the use of immunosuppressives and apheresis. There is a moderate risk of developing lymphoproliferative disease after a period of time with this condition, and thus alkyators should be avoided wherever possible. While the overall prognosis for patients with this disorder is good, it depends upon the degree of visceral involvement, in particular the kidneys. There are no controlled trials of any of these agents in the treatment of these diseases. Most authorities would agree that apheresis is useful in controlling many of the acute manifestations of cryoglobulinemia, but levels are quick to rebound after its discontinuation. Other therapies reported for this condition include anti-inflammatories, antihistamines and intravenous immunoglobulin. To summarize the therapy of cryoglobulinemia:

*   No controlled studies of steroids, cytotoxics and/or apheresis
*   Morbidity and mortality related to the extent of target organ involvement
*   High rate of lymphoproliferative transformation
*   Several small controlled studies of IFN alpha demonstrate:
    *   Short-term benefit with brief courses of therapy
    *   60% clinical and virologic response with prolonged therapy (> 12 months)

Other Conditions Within the Hypersensitivity Vasculitis Group A variety of other conditions may present with a vasculitic skin rash (palpable purpura), which upon biopsy shows a small vessel vasculitis with leukocytoclasis. Conditions that should be kept in mind include connective tissue diseases, such as rheumatoid arthritis, systemic lupus erythematosis, and Sjögren's syndrome. Occasionally patients may present with vasculitis who have an underlying malignancy. These are most commonly lympho- or myeloproliferative disorders. In the majority of cases, the vasculitis antedates the malignancy by many months, but occasionally the vasculitis may appear after the malignancy. Urticarial vasculitis is another unique syndrome within this group. Generally, these patients have low serum-complement levels—the hallmark of the disorder—but occasional patients may have normal levels. Clinical clues to this condition are the presence of chronic urticaria, with attacks that frequently last for greater than 24 hours at a time. Constitutional symptoms include arthralgia and low-grade fever, and occasionally also may display angioneurotic edema. Occasional patients also may have renal involvement with this condition.

GIANT-CELL GROUP

Specific Giant-Cell Arteritis Conditions

There are two disorders in this group: temporal arteritis and Takayasu's arteritis.

Table 31.3. Mixed Cryoglobulinemia: Clinical Profile

Manifestation	Percent
Palpable purpura	80–100
Arthralgias	50–90
Weakness/fatigue	70–100
Glomerulonephritis	20–75
Polyneuropathy	20–70
Liver involvement[a]	60–90
Cryoglobulins in chronic hepatitis	40–70

[a] Lymphoproliferative disease (B cell NHL)

Temporal Arteritis Temporal arteritis, which affects the elderly, increases in frequency with age. Seldom seen before the age of 50, the disease is uncommon in blacks, but has been reported. Classical symptoms:

• Age over 50
• Unilateral headache
• Transient visual disturbances (amaurosis fugax)
• Jaw claudication
• Polymyalgia rheumatica (PMR) in 50% of the cases

This picture is even more characteristic when it occurs in a patient with polymyalgia rheumatica (PMR). The relationship between these two conditions is complex with pure examples of each being well recognized but an overlap state of being is not common. In the absence of signs or symptoms of temporal arteritis, temporal artery biopsies are not indicated in PMR.

The pathology in this disease is a granulomatous inflammation of the arterial wall with destruction of the internal elastic lamina and giant cell formation. The diagnosis is dependent upon a temporal artery biopsy. If the clinical suspicion is high and vision is threatened, this condition should be treated as a medical emergency with high-dose corticosteroids. Negative biopsies do occur since the lesions tend to be patchy in their nature. The only helpful laboratory test is the erythrocyte sedimentation rate, which is usually markedly elevated, although rare cases have been reported with normal sedimentation rates.

The treatment of this condition remains high-dose prednisone. Classically, the disease is treated with 40–60 mg a day for 6 weeks and then tapered to the lowest dose that would maintain freedom from symptoms and a suppression of the sedimentation rate. Many patients require treatment for many months to years.

Takayasu's Arteritis Takayasu's arteritis can be considered a generalized form of giant-cell arteritis that occurs mostly in young Asian females, but it has also been described in young individuals of other races including African-Americans and Caucasians. However, other than this demographic peculiarity, there is little to distinguish this as a nosologic entity from generalized giant-cell arteritis, which sometimes occurs in the elderly with or without temporal arteritis. Characteristics of Takayasu's arteritis:

• Large-vessel granulomatous arteritis affecting primarily the aorta and its branches

• Clinical features generally reflect end organ ischemia resulting from stenosis of involved arteries
• Female predominant
• Incidence of 2.6 per million
• 60 patients (median age 25) (Kerr G, et al. Ann Int Med 1994;120:919)
    • Variable presentation from asymptomatic to catastrophic
    • Only 33% had constitutional symptoms
    • Stenosis 98%; aneurysms 27%
    • ESR not a reliable guide for disease activity
    • Surgical specimens showed active disease in 44% of clinically inactive patients
    • Surgery was palliative but often followed by restenosis
    • Glucocorticoids with or without cytotoxics failed control disease in 25%

The clinical presentation of Takayasu's is entirely dependent upon the location of major involvement. The most common presentation is claudication of the upper extremities, but involvement of the aorta and its branches is not uncommon. Involvement of the aorta may lead to aneurysm formation and subsequent coronary artery involvement, and GI ischemia may be seen. The pathology is identical to temporal arteritis. Laboratory studies are not particularly helpful, and while the erythrocyte sedimentation rate is usually elevated, it may be normal in the presence of active disease.

Treatment of Giant-Cell Arteritis

The treatment of both of these conditions is corticosteroids. Cytotoxic drugs, including methotrexate, can be useful in refractory cases. Surgical intervention is often required in Takayasu's aortitis and has been reported to be successful.

POLYANGIITIS OVERLAP SYNDROME

In addition to PAN and allergic granulomatosis, the polyangiitis or overlap syndrome has been included under the heading of systemic necrotizing vasculitis. This condition bears the features of each of these conditions and may even demonstrate clinical features of other vasculitic syndromes such as hypersensitivity vasculitis or giant-cell arteritis. It is unclear whether this represents a distinct nosologic entity or not, and the prognosis is unclear at the present time. Patients fitting this description should be approached diagnostically and therapeutically as PAN.

REVIEW EXERCISES

QUESTIONS

1. Symptoms and signs that may lead to a diagnosis of underlying systemic necrotizing vasculitis include:

    a. Mononeuritis multiplex
    b. Fever of unknown origin
    c. Unexplained end organ eschemia
    d. RBC casts in the urine
    e. All of the above

2. A 50-year-old man was admitted with a 3-month history of fever, weight loss, abdominal pain and hypertension. A detailed FUO (fever of unknown origin) workup had thus been unrevealing. Pertinent physical findings included:

    • Blood pressure 220/120
    • Livedo reticularis on his legs
    • Foot drop on the left
    • Absent pin prick in the lower legs

    Laboratory studies include:

    • ESR: 100 mm/hr
    • Creatinine: 2.2 mg%
    • Microscopic hematuria
    • SGOT two times normal

    PAN is suspected. After weighing the diagnostic yield as well as the risks, the logical next step would be:

    a. Skin biopsy
    b. Percutaneous renal biopsy to demonstrate vasculitis of extraglomerular vessels.
    c. Abdominal angiography
    d. Sural nerve biopsy

3. The differential diagnosis for the rash shown in Figure 31.1 includes:

    a. Drug-associated vasculitis
    b. Vasculitis with malignancy
    c. Henoch-Schöenlein purpura
    d. Subacute bacterial endocarditis
    e. Answers a and b
    f. All of the above

4. The following may be said about the ANCA test:

    a. C-ANCA representing antibodies to proteinase-3 (PR-3) are highly correlated with a diagnosis of Wegener's granulomatosis.
    b. P-ANCA by immunofluorescence is less sensitive and specific for a diagnosis of Wegener's granulomatosis.
    c. A rise in ANCA titers alone should clearly justify an escalation of immunosuppressive therapy.
    d. Answers a and b
    e. Answers a, b, and c

5. The following statement about cryoglobulinemia is correct:

    a. The most common clinical finding is a vasculitic rash.
    b. If the cryoglobulin is composed only of a monoclonal immunoglobulin, it is generally associated with an underlying malignancy.
    c. The most common associated condition is an underlying infection of hepatitis B.
    d. Answer a and b
    e. Answer a, b, and c

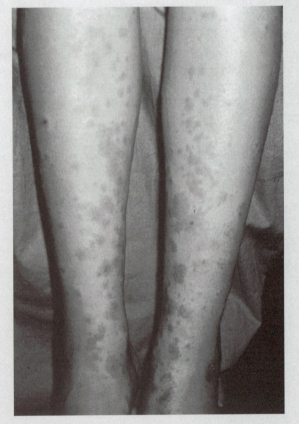

Figure 31.1. Rash (see color plate).

REVIEW EXERCISES

Answers

1. e.

The diagnosis of vasculitis begins with clinical suspicion. There are relatively few findings of high diagnostic specificity for systemic necrotizing vasculitis, but mounting suspicion should be appreciated in the presence of a number of presumptive signs or ''red flags'' for vasculitis. These include fever of unknown origin with constitutional symptoms, unexplained multisystem organ disease, unexplained inflammatory arthritis, unexplained myositis, a suspicious rash in particular palpable purpura, a variety of peripheral neuropathies especially mononeuritis multiplex, unexplained end organ ischemia, including cardiac, CNS and gastrointestinal, and lastly, glomerulonephritis. While none of these findings is specific for systemic vasculitis, the presence of any one or more should lead to increasing suspicion of the disease. (See the list of warning signs or symptoms of systemic vasculitis under ''Clinical Presentation and Diagnosis of Systemic Vasculitis'' above.)

2. d.

This patient has a diagnostic picture highly suspicious for systemic necrotizing vasculitis, in particular polyarteritis nodosa. Each diagnostic test outlined in the question should be considered in terms of sensitivity, specificity, and risk. A skin biopsy is sensitive but nonspecific, since vasculitis of the skin can be caused by so many different conditions. The percutaneous renal biopsy in this setting to demonstrate vasculitis of the extraglomerular vessels is insensitive, as vasculitis of the extraglomerular vessels is relatively rare by this technique. Abdominal angiography has an increasing sensitivity, but in the presence of severe hypertension and azotemia carries unacceptable risks. Lastly, sural nerve biopsy, while being somewhat morbid and invasive has an increasing diagnostic yield particularly in the presence of objective neurologic signs and symptoms.

3. f.

The rash shown in Figure 31.1 is palpable purpura. This rash is highly specific for small vessel cutaneous vasculitis but is unrevealing of an underlying nosologic diagnosis. Drug-associated vasculitis is an extremely common cause of small-vessel vasculitis. Vasculitis associated with malignancies is most frequently found in the setting of an underlying lymphoproliferative disease. A small-vessel vasculitis such as this would be characteristic. Henoch-Schöenlein purpura is characterized not only by such a rash, but also by the presence of abdominal pain and glomerulonephritis. This condition is seen most frequently in children, but can be seen in adults as well. Subacute bacterial endocarditis has a variety of extracardiac complications the majority of which are mediated by immune complexes. A small-vessel vasculitis would not be unusual in subacute bacterial endocarditis, though it is rare for this to be the dominant and

presenting finding of the disorder. Many other conditions can be seen with this type of rash, including a variety of connective tissue diseases such as rheumatoid arthritis and systemic lupus, other types of infections, cryoglobulinemia secondary to hepatitis C, and other disorders and a variety of miscellaneous systemic diseases.

4. d.

The ANCA test has been a great step forward in the diagnostic process for certain forms of systemic vasculitis. The test is generally performed by immunofluorescence and is increasingly performed by antigen-specific assays as well. An immunofluorescent pattern of C-ANCA is, in the majority of cases, associated with antibodies to the lysosomal enzyme proteinase-3 (PR-3). It is highly correlated with the diagnosis of Wegener's granulomatosis being more than 80% sensitive and more than 95% specific in the presence of active untreated and wide spread disease. P-ANCA by immunofluorescence, however, is not only less sensitive for the diagnosis of Wegener's being present in only a few percent of cases, but is relatively nonspecific. The P-ANCA pattern or perinuclear pattern can be mimicked by a variety of antibodies, including antinuclear antibodies. The antibodies of interest in the diagnosis of systemic vasculitis responsible for the P-ANCA pattern of immunofluorescence are those directed against myeloperoxidase, another lysosomal enzyme. A P-ANCA test result by immunofluorescence should always be confirmed by an antigen-specific assay. Lastly, while the major utility of ANCA are in the in the diagnosis and related conditions, there is some correlation with disease activity. ANCA titers are not in and of themselves justification for modification of therapy. Clinical evaluation of end organ damage is still the gold standard of determining modifications of therapy.

5. d.

Cryoglobulinemia and cryoglobulinemic vasculitis are owing to the presence of immunoglobulins and other proteins that precipitate from serum at temperatures less than 37° Centigrade. Cryoglobulins are characterized on the basis of their content including those that are monoclonal or containing a single immunoglobulin, those that are mixed containing a monoclonal component as well as polyclonal immunoglobulin and lastly those which are polyclonal. These are referred to as Type-I , Type-II, and Type-III:

Type-I cryoglobulins or monoclonal cryoglobulins are most often seen in the presence of lymphoproliferative diseases.

Type-II cryoglobulins or mixed were often considered to be of unknown or essential origin.

Type-III cryoglobulins represent circulating immune complexes.

The identification that the vast majority of cases of

mixed cryoglobulinemia are associated with underlying hepatitis C infection has been a major breakthrough in our understanding of this complex disease.

Patients with cryoglobulinemia of any underlying cause may have a variety of end organ manifestations. The presence of a small-vessel vasculitis most often manifesting as palpable purpura is the most frequent finding. Arthralgias and arthritis are also common. A significant number of patients also have glomerulonephritis, peripheral neuropathy and a variety of other complications.

SUGGESTED READINGS

Hoffman GS, Fauci AS. Emerging concepts in the management of vasculitic disease. Adv Int Med 1994;39:277.

Hoffman GS, Kerr GS. Recognition of systemic vasculitis in the acutely ill patient. In: Mandell BF, ed. Acute rheumatic and immunological disease. New York: Marcel Dekker, 1994: 279.

Savage COS, Adu LH. Primary systemic vasculitis. Lancet 1997;349:553–558.

Calabrese LH, Michel BA, Bloch DA, et al. The American College of Rheumatology 1990 criteria for the classification of hypersensistivity vasculitis. Arthritis Rheum 1990;33: 1108.

Callen JP, Ekenstam E. Cutaneous leukocytoclastic vasculitis: clinical experience in 44 patients. South Med J 1991;80:848.

White RHR. Henoch Schonlein purpura. In: Churg AC, Churg J, eds. Systemic vasculitis. New York: Ikagu-Shoin, 1991: 203–217.

POLYARTERITIS, MICROCOSPIC POLYARTERITIS, CHURG STRAUSS, OVERLAP

Calabrese LH, Guillivan, L, Hoffman, G. Therapy resistant systemic necrotizing vasculitis: PAN, Hypersensitivity Vasculitis Group and Wegener's granulomatosis. Rheumatic Dis Clin North 1995;21:41.

Guillivan L, et al. Treatment of polyarteritis nodosa related to hepatitis B virus with short-term steroid therapy with antiviral agents and plasma exchange. A prospective trial in 33 patients. J Rheum 1993;20:289–298.

Leavitt RY, Fauci AS. Polyangiitis overlap syndrome. Am J Med 1986;81:79.

Lhote F, Guillevin L. Polyarteritis nodosa, microscopic polyarteritis and Churg Strauss syndrome. Rheum Clin North Amer 1995;4:911.

Rosen S, Falk R, Jennette JC. Polyarteritis nodosa, microscopic form and renal vasculitis. In: Churg A, Churg J, eds. Systemic vasculitis. New York: Ikagu-Shoin, 1991.

HYPERSENSITIVITY VASCULITIS GROUP (HVG)

Agnello V, Romain P. Mixed cryoglobulinemia secondary to hepatitis C virus. Rheum Clin North Amer 1996;22:1–22.

Calabrese LH, Clough JD. Hypersensitivity vasculitis group (HVG): a case-oriented review of continuing clinical spectrum. Cleve Clin Q 1982;49:17.

WEGENER'S GRANULOMATOSIS, ANCA

DeRemee RA. Antineutrophil cytoplasmic autoantibody-associated disease: a pulmonologist's perspective. Am J Kidney Dis 1991;2:180–183.

Gross WL, Wilhelm HS, Csernok E. Antineutrophil cytoplasmic autoantibody-associated diseases: a rheumatologist's perspective. Am J Kidney Dis 1991;2:175–179.

Hoffman GS, et al. Wegener's granulomatosis: an analysis of 158 patients. Ann Intern Med 1992;116:488–498.

Jeannette JC. Antineutrophil cytoplasmic autoantibody-associated disease: A pathologist's perspective. Am J Kidney Dis 1991;2:164–170.

Jenette C, et al. Nomenclature of systemic vasculitis. Arthritis Rheum 1994;37:187–191.

Tervaert JW. The value of serial ANCA testing during follow up studies in patients with ANCA-associated vasculitides. A review. J Nephrol 1996;9:232–240.

GIANT CELL/TAKAYASU'S

Jacobs M, Allen N. Giant cell arteritis. In: Churg A, Churg J, eds. Systemic vasculitis. New York: Ikagu-Shoin, 1991: 143.

Kerr GS. Takayasu's arteritis. Rheum Clin North Amer 1995; 21:841–859.

32

Selected Musculoskeletal Syndromes

Brian F. Mandell

Musculoskeletal pain is one of the most frequently listed chief complaints of patients seeing family practice physicians and general internists. While some of these complaints relate to osteoarthritis or inflammatory joint disease, the majority are due to soft-tissue musculoskeletal syndromes. Many of these pain syndromes are self-limited or reversible with short-term therapy. Clinical recognition of specific syndromes limits the need for expensive diagnostic testing. In particular, recognizing specific syndromes may obviate the need for serologic laboratory evaluation or musculoskeletal imaging. Although the pathophysiology of many of these syndromes is poorly understood, accumulated clinical experience permits the clinical diagnosis of discrete syndromes and allows for empiric therapeutic interventions. Despite the common occurrence of these syndromes, controlled clinical outcome studies are rarely reported in the medical literature.

HIP SYNDROMES

Pain in the hip region in elderly patients is frequently attributed to hip osteoarthritis. However, in the elderly—as well as in young patients—a focused examination of the area may delineate one of several nonarticular pain syndromes. True hip joint discomfort classically is present in the inguinal crease or felt deep in this area. Occasionally, true hip pain is felt primarily in the deep gluteal area or radiating down the thigh as far as the knee. True hip joint pain can be elicited by passive range of motion of the hip joint, not usually reproduced by palpation. Examination should include:

• Passive internal rotation
• Passive external rotation
• Abduction
• Posterior extension

This last motion, undertaken with the patient lying on their abdomen, is frequently neglected. It is uncommon for hip (joint) disease to manifest only as lateral hip pain reproducible with pressure over the trochanteric area.

LATERAL HIP PAIN

The syndrome of lateral hip pain, reproduced with deep pressure to this area, has generally been termed *trochanteric* or *pseudotrochanteric bursitis*. There is a differential diagnosis of this lateral hip pain syndrome, but most commonly it is attributed to trochanteric bursitis.

Examination of the area is best undertaken with the patient lying on the contralateral side with the upper leg flexed toward the chest and adducted across the body with the medial aspect of the upper knee resting on the table. This pulls the soft tissue overlying the trochanteric area fairly taut, permitting examination. The superficial trochanteric bursa overlies the trochanteric prominence, and this area should be gently palpated. The deep trochanteric bursa area, which is proximal and slightly posterior and sits in a deep groove, can be easily palpated in this position. Reproduction of the patient's pain with firm pressure in these areas warrants a clinical diagnosis of "trochanteric bursitis."

This syndrome is exceedingly common and often does not respond to nonsteroidal anti-inflammatory therapy. It may respond dramatically to local infiltration with lidocaine and a deposit steroid. Injection should be made deep within this tissue, but not under the periosteum, which provokes extreme discomfort in the patient. (As with all steroid injections, the patient should be forewarned about the possibility of atrophy or skin discoloration.) Remember that the syndrome of trochanteric bursitis is often precipitated by other mechanical factors, including:

- Primary hip or knee disease
- Pes planus or other foot disorders
- Altered gait because of low back pain or new shoes

Mimics of this syndrome, with radiation of pain into the same anatomic area, include:

- High lumbar radiculopathy
- Hip abductor muscle strain
- Entrapment neuropathy
- Stress fractures of the femoral neck or pelvis

If the pain is owing to trochanteric bursitis, the local infiltration of several milliliters of lidocaine or marcaine will provide at least transient—and usually complete—relief of the discomfort. Patients will report that they are able to lie comfortably on this side, which they were not able to do before. Inclusion of corticosteroids in the injection provides lasting relief in approximately 70% of patients, perhaps for as long as several months. If a gait disturbance is present, the pain will likely return. For isolated trochanteric bursitis, pain relief may be indefinite following a single injection (or occasionally several injections). Failure of two (or at most, three) injections to relieve the pain should prompt an aggressive search for other etiologies of the pain.

The coexistence of trochanteric pain with degenerative disease of the spine or the hip must be noted, although the exact relationship between these conditions is not clear. If pain radiates down the leg from the trochanteric bursa and can be elicited by firm pressure along the fibrous tissue surrounding the muscle bundles (fascia lata), physical therapy directed at stretching this fibrous and muscle area should also be included.

The lasting value of physical therapy modalities—including ultrasound, TENs unit application, iontophoresis, or deep heat—remain unestablished.

GLUTEAL PAIN

Gluteal pain can be caused by either strain in the gluteal muscles or a bursitis involving the bursa overlying the ischial prominence or under the gluteal muscles.

Ischial bursitis is best diagnosed with the patient standing and forward-flexed at the hips; the area of tenderness can be easily palpated by pressure along the ischial prominence. Gluteal bursitis can be elicited by deep palpation along the gluteal muscles with the muscles pulled taut while the patient is in a lateral position.

Piriform syndrome is a controversial entity, presumably caused by spasm of the piriformis muscles. Patients complain of moderate, severe, or even disabling lateral buttock pain. Deep palpation of the piriformis muscle in the lateral upper quadrant of the buttock area, or more specifically by rectal wall examination, is considered to be diagnostic. Pain may radiate posteriorly to the upper portion of the thigh. Patients may walk with an antalgic gait. Pain may be elicited with forced internal rotation of the hip against resistance. Treatment, which also is controversial, may include physical therapy and/or local injection.

MERALGIA PARESTHETICA

Entrapment of the lateral femoral cutaneous nerve causes the syndrome of meralgia paresthetica. Entrapment usually occurs overlying the superior iliac spine under the inguinal ligament. The clinical syndrome is usually marked by an area of intense dysesthesia, often with numbness on careful pin-prick examination in a patch of skin in the anterior thigh. It can be associated with rapid weight gain, as can be seen in pregnancy, or with use of a tight, constraining belt. Treatment is generally supportive. No additional evaluation is necessary. It is not associated with systemic disease. It should be remembered, however, that zoster may be heralded by an area of dysesthesia without visible skin lesions.

KNEE PAIN

Similar to the situation in the hip, quite frequently all pain surrounding the knee is attributed to osteoarthritis of the knee, especially in the elderly. Pain in the knee area can be referred from the hip joint, the lumbar spine, and (rarely) from the foot in patients with significant pes planus with tightened calf muscles.

Examination of the knee should include evaluation for:

- Synovial thickening or fluid
- Reproduction of pain with pressure and movement of the patella
- Mechanical stability
- Popliteal fullness

An extremely common cause of regional knee pain, especially in patients with osteoarthritis of the medial compartment of the knee or with pes planus, is pain in the area of the pes anserine bursa. Patients with this syndrome frequently complain of pain localized to the medial aspect of the leg slightly below the joint line. Pain is frequently exacerbated by the act of arising from a low chair, walking up steps, and occasionally in bed at night as the two knee areas touch together. Patients may describe the need to sleep with a pillow between their legs at night to avoid the painful pressure of their knees touching together. Pain can be elicited by gentle palpation approximately 1 cm below the joint line on the medial aspect of the leg. It is most important to be certain that the pain that is elicited with palpation is the exact pain that the patient experiences; tenderness to palpation alone is not sufficient to make this diagnosis.

This syndrome frequently does not respond to nonsteroidal drug therapy, but again responds to local injection in a striking manner. The pain can be debilitating, but dramatically relieved by local infiltration of lidocaine. Inclusion of corticosteroid in the injection mixture is frequently done.

Prepatellar bursitis is a frequent cause of swelling in the

knee area. The area of swelling may appear as a fluctuant mass immediately anterior to the patella. This is frequently a result of trauma, and is an occupational hazard of patients who work in a kneeling position. Aspiration of fluid may relieve the discomfort; remember, however, that this bursa can be inflamed by infection (frequently *staphylococcus aureus*) or by gout disease. Infection frequently is associated with surrounding cellulitis and may mimic joint inflammation. The bursa does not communicate with the joint; care should be taken to distinguish this entity from actual arthritis. An attempt at true knee joint aspiration should not be undertaken unnecessarily, especially through an overlying cellulitis.

ELBOW AREA

The olecranon bursa separates the skin from the olecranon process. Frequently, following minor trauma (such as friction or resting of the elbow on a hard surface), the bursa may be distended with sterile, noninflammatory fluid. In this case, it may respond to drainage and injection of a local corticosteroid preparation. The bursa also may be involved with uric-crystal-induced inflammation or occasionally with infection, similar to the prepatella bursitis of the knee. Cell counts in septic bursitis are generally lower than in septic arthritis. Frequently there is a surrounding cellulitis with pitting edema of the soft tissue. *Staphylococcus aureus* is the most common infecting agent.

Specific pain syndromes in the area of the lateral or medial epicondyles of the elbow— ''tennis'' and ''golfer's'' elbow, respectively—are extremely common. Both of these pain syndromes are believed to be caused, in part, by frequent and vigorous use of the forearm muscles. Lateral epicondylitis may be reproduced by palpation to the specific area surrounding the lateral epicondyle but more specifically can be elicited by resisted, active extension of the middle finger. Pain will radiate specifically to the area of the lateral epicondyle and often to the forearm. Epicondylitis may respond to rest, use of a forearm band, and nonsteroidal anti-inflammatory therapy; frequently, infiltration of the area with a mixture of lidocaine and a low dose of deposit corticosteroid preparation may be of value. Surgical intervention is rarely required. Active physical therapy is often of therapeutic value. Care must be taken when injecting the medial epicondyle area to avoid to avoid the median nerve. Also remember that carpal tunnel syndrome can cause radiation of discomfort up the forearm toward the elbow region.

THE HAND

Carpal tunnel syndrome, compression of the median nerve as it travels through the carpal canal, is common. Its frequent associations include:

- Diabetes mellitus
- Pregnancy
- Hypothyroidism
- Repetitive palm trauma
- Synovitis of the wrist (most commonly from rheumatoid arthritis)

Association is also recognized with primary and dialysis-related (not secondary) amyloidosis. The development of carpal tunnel syndrome as an overuse syndrome is debatable.

Clinical recognition of the syndrome is by:

- Reproduction of dysesthesias in the appropriate distribution by pressure over the carpal canal (distal to the wrist crease at the base of the palm)
- Elicitation of the symptoms with percussion in the same area by finger or reflex hammer (Tinel's sign)
- Phalens maneuver

Early in the course of the syndrome, neurologic deficits are not present; however, two-point discrimination and sensory testing over the area of the thumb, index, and middle finger should be performed in detail and recorded accurately. The diagnosis can be confirmed, after it has been present for a significant period of time, by nerve conduction testing.

Initial treatment should be splinting the wrist in a slightly hyper-extended near-neutral position. Local injection of corticosteroid into the carpal canal may provide relief. Surgical treatment is usually curative if nerve damage has not occurred.

De Quervain's tenosynovitis, a common cause of pain on the radial aspect of the hand, is frequently described by the patient as thumb or wrist pain. This can occur as a sporadic pain syndrome but is frequently induced by repetitive or resisted motion of the thumb. The condition seems to occur with increased frequency in women caring for a newborn infant. Typical clinical presentation consists of pain overlying the radial styloid radiating into the thumb and occasionally up the forearm. There may be visible swelling and erythema over the tendon sheath of the extensor pollicis brevis. Pain can be elicited by resisted abduction of the thumb or by having the patient place the thumb inside a closed fist with movement of the fist by the examiner in an ulnar direction. Pain is elicited over the radial styloid. This syndrome should be distinguished from osteoarthritis of the MCP joint at the base of the thumb. Treatment of the tendonitis can initially be conservative with use of a resting thumb splint, and nonsteroidal anti-inflammatory therapy. Some authors have proposed primary infiltration of the tendon sheath with a corticosteroid-lidocaine mixture. Care should be taken with the injection to avoid the snuffbox area and the radial artery.

Trigger finger can occur owing to formation of non-inflammatory fibrous nodules in the flexor tendon sheath of the palmar tendons. Patients describe the finger(s) being stuck in a flexed position, with the need to be forcibly extended with a resultant sharp painful ''pop.'' Frequently, patients may awaken with the fingers ''stuck'' in a flexed position. Treatment can include passive splinting of the involved finger in an extended position, with or without local infiltration of corticosteroid into the flexor sheath nodule, resulting in shrinkage of the nodule and less triggering. Progressive fibrosis of the flexor tendons with contracture and nodularity of the palmar fascia results in Dupuytren's contractures. Most trigger fingers do not evolve into this syndrome. Nonsurgical treatment is usually effective, and surgical intervention is rarely required. Acute severe palmar fasciitis has been associated with carcinoma of ovary and lung.

SHOULDER AREA

Acute shoulder pain, in the absence of trauma, is most frequently because of rotator cuff disease (periarthritis) rather than true shoulder joint disease. Glenohumeral synovitis occurs frequently in the setting of rheumatoid arthritis and polymyalgia rheumatica (mild synovitis). Periarthritis can occur in young, active people, and in anyone following overuse of the musculature of the shoulder girdle. Pain is frequently described as worsened with specific motions, particularly with extension of the arm. Sharp pain with abduction or full arm motion is termed impingement, and is often caused by pressure of an inflamed tendon sheath on a bone or ligamentous structure in the area of the shoulder girdle. Attempts should be made at delineating the specific involved tendon with resistive stressing of the individual tendons of the rotator cuff. The most common form of rotator cuff tendonitis involves the supraspinatus tendon. This can be evaluated by having the patient elevate his or her arm, thumb pointed toward the ground, with the examiner applying downward pressure and the patient resisting this motion. Pain is often referred to the shoulder area, particularly to the deltoid and upper arm region.

Generally, pain with passive motion of the glenohumeral joint within the normal range of motion does not elicit pain in the absence of glenohumeral synovitis. Examination of the shoulder should also include palpation of the acromioclavicular and sternoclavicular joints. Cervical radiculitis can also refer to the shoulder area.

LUMBAR CANAL STENOSIS

Lumbar canal stenosis (spinal stenosis) occurs in the setting of degenerative joint and disc disease. It is characterized by the subacute or occasionally acute onset of bilateral leg and back discomfort. The leg discomfort frequently occurs in a pattern of pseudoclaudication of calves or thighs and can mimic vascular ischemia. Because this syndrome occurs in an elderly population, it frequently coexists with physical findings of peripheral vascular disease. Deep tendon reflexes may be preserved; specific nerve root symptoms are usually not elicited.

Diagnosis is generally made by MRI imaging of the lumbar canal. In the absence of cauda equina syndrome, marked neurologic deficits are not generally appreciated. The pain can be quite limiting to the patient's activity, and is frequently associated with lumbar pain.

Conservative treatment in many patients is successful with the focus on extension-oriented physical therapy. Surgical intervention is a reasonable option for patients who fail conservative therapy.

FIBROMYALGIA

Fibromyalgia is a generalized pain syndrome. It occurs in patients of all ages, and seemingly occurs at an increased frequency in patients with underlying systemic disease such as rheumatoid arthritis or SLE.

Neurologic complaints of dysesthesia are common; however, neurologic abnormalities on physical examination are generally absent. There are no inflammatory markers by laboratory testing or by physical examination. Synovitis is notably absent in primary fibromyalgia. Quite frequently there is an associated sleep disturbance with a complaint of not feeling refreshed in the morning. Patients frequently describe multiple awakenings during the night. Mild dryness of eyes or mouth is a frequent complaint. The presence of discrete myofascial tender points on examination is characteristic and required to make the diagnosis. Pressure should be applied to a degree that the fingernail of the examiner is noted to barely blanche with the pressure. Neutral points should also be evaluated. The number of involved tender points, and the intensity of tenderness may vary dramatically between different examinations. The tender points are frequently in areas of common myofascial pain syndromes previously described (trochanteric, gluteal, pes anserine), and the distinguishing characteristic of the fibromyalgia syndrome is the generalized nature of this pain sensitivity.

Recognition of this pain syndrome should dramatically limit the acquisition of laboratory testing. There is *no role for serologic testing* in a patient who has no features of specific autoimmune disease (e.g., SLE and rheumatoid arthritis). Care should be taken, however, when making this diagnosis, to exclude by detailed history and physical examination the presence of an underlying disorder, such as hypothyroidism or primary depression. Many patients with fibromyalgia have features of depression with somatization; however, not all patients are clinically depressed.

Treatment is directed at maintenance of normal activities, reversal of the abnormal sleep cycle with the use of soporific tricyclic antidepressants, if not contraindicated, and sparse, judicious use of medications such as Flexoril, acetaminophen and nonsteroidal anti-inflammatory drugs. Chronic use of nonsteroidal drugs should be discouraged. Narcotics, corticosteroids and other chronic pain medications should be avoided. Maintenance of aerobic exercise is felt to be of value in maintaining patient function. Distinction from chronic fatigue syndrome can be difficult, if not impossible.

REVIEW EXERCISES

QUESTIONS

1. A 56-year-old overweight female with radiographic osteoarthritis of the right knee presents with a chief complaint of increasing, limiting knee pain, most notable when arising from a chair or toilet, walking up stairs, and in bed at night. Examination reveals valgus deformity with walking; minimal cool-knee effusions; tenderness to palpation (which mimics the pain) at the medial aspect of the joint, approximately 2 inches distal to the joint line. You suggest:

   a. Full-dose NSAID trial (had been using OTCs)
   b. Quad-focused strengthening regime
   c. Intra-articular steroid injection
   d. Steroid injection of anserine bursa
   e. a and b

2. A 32-year-old previously healthy secretary complains of recent (3 months) onset of progressive pain in her right arm involving second and third fingers, forearm, and upper arm. It awakens her from sleep and worsens while driving. It is at times associated with painful tingling. Physical examination reveals normal neck motion, negative Spurling and Adson's tests, and normal shoulder exam. Pulses, DTRs, pin-prick, strength, and elbow are normal. A likely diagnostic test is:

   a. Nerve conduction of distal median nerve
   b. MRI of cervical spine
   c. Upper extremity angiogram
   d. Chemical sympathetic block

3. A 64-year-old former construction worker presents with increasing exertional bilateral calf pain and leg tingling. Leg symptoms have been present for 1 1/2 years but have worsened following his recent MI during cardiac rehabilitation. He could only walk 0.4 miles on the treadmill because of leg pain. He switched to an exercise cycle, on which he could ride for 3 miles. Physical examination demonstrated decreased left distal pulses and a left iliac bruit, with normal foot temperature, color, DTRs, pin-prick, and strength. The study with high yield for diagnosis is:

   a. Angiogram
   b. Abdominal ultrasound
   c. Spinal MRI
   d. EMG

4. A 28-year-old female presents 2 months postpartum complaining of 4 months of left-thigh burning pain. She was told of carpal tunnel syndrome during her pregnancy, and has been wearing wrist splints but is now concerned regarding the possibility of multiple sclerosis. Physical examination reveals bilateral wrist Tinel's with a positive Phalen's. Hip examination is normal with negative straight leg raise. DTRs are preserved. No motor weakness is detected. There is an area approximately the size of a hand with marked dysesthesias to light touch on the anterior lateral left thigh. In addition to clinical diagnosis, a positive test would be:

   a. EMG of sacral plexus
   b. Tinel's over the lateral inguinal ligament
   c. Pelvic CT scan
   d. CSF oligoclonal bands

5. A 42-year-old white female with a diagnosis of RA for 2½ years (fairly well controlled on Plaquenil, nabumetone, and 2.5 mg prednisone daily) 8 months following the birth of a healthy boy presents for a routine visit complaining of increasing ''pain all over.'' She describes an increase in AM stiffness of her back, neck and hands, trouble sleeping, and difficulties with painful flares following exposure to any drafts or physical exertion. ESR is 22, RF is present in high titre. Joint examination shows multiple tender, nonswollen joints; normal grip strength; bilateral trochanteric bursitis/gluteal tenderness/costochondritis, and anserine bursitis. Course of action:

   a. Increase prednisone for 10 days, then taper
   b. Add methotrexate
   c. Add a tricyclic/physical therapy
   d. b and c

Answers

1. d

Treat pes anserine bursitis. There are many causes of pain in patients with OA of the knee. Anserine bursitis is one of the more common nonarticular ones. It is particularly common in overweight patients with valgus deformity. Pain is reproduced by local pressure. It often does not respond to NSAIDs, but does respond to local injection. OA is not usually a cause of nocturnal pain in bed; however, patients with anserine bursitis get relief by relieving the pressure of their legs touching by sleeping with a pillow between their knees.

2. a

Carpal tunnel syndrome. Nerve conduction of the median nerve would likely provide the diagnosis. Local provocative testing with Tinel's, Phalen's or direct compression might also provide suggestive information. Prolonged keyboard typing may be a risk factor. Other tests are not warranted based on the history and examination, which do not suggest radiculopathy, thoracic outlet, or RSD/Raynaud's. Causes include:

- Wrist synovitis
- Hypothyroidism
- Diabetes mellitus
- Pregnancy
- Trauma
- Primary amyloidosis
- Acromegaly
- Polymyalgia rheumatica (perhaps)

3. c

MRI spine. Although MRI of the spine has limited specificity for diagnosing disc disease and back pain, it is excellent for diagnosing spinal stenosis (SS). This patient has PVD, but the positional aspects of claudication symptoms argue for the presence of neurogenic, not vascular claudication. SS frequently coexists with PVD, and neurological examination is often normal for age. OA of the spine is common. Physical therapy is often effective; surgery may be curative.

4. b

Meralgia paresthetica. Entrapment of the lateral femoral cutaneous nerve, often as it exits through the lateral inguinal ligament. It can be diagnosed clinically and usually requires no workup or treatment. It may accompany weight gain or constricting garments or seat belts. Often self-limiting, it may respond to local steroid injection. Another diagnostic thought here could be pre-zoster neuralgia.

5. c

Diagnosis fibromyalgia. The diagnosis is most likely secondary fibromyalgia, perhaps precipitated by the stress of a newborn child in the house. The symptoms will not respond to intensified therapy for the RA. Detailed examination will likely reveal additional myofascial trigger points. Education is another key element of the therapy.

SUGGESTED READINGS

Anderson BC. Treatment of Du Quervain's tenosynovitis with corticosteroids: a prospective study of the response to local injection. Arthritis Rheum 1991;34:793–798.

Goldenberg DL. Fibromyalgia and chronic fatigue syndrome: are they the same? J Musculoskel Med 1990;7:19–28.

Mandell BF. Avascular necrosis of the femoral head presenting as trochanteric bursitis. Ann Rheum Dis 1990;49:730–732.

Pace BJ. Piriform syndrome. Western J Med 1976;124:435–439.

Shbeeb MI. Evaluation of glucocorticosteroid injection for the treatment of trochanteric bursitis. J Rheum 1996;23:2104–2106.

Smith DL. Treatment of nonseptic olecranon bursitis: a controlled, blinded prospective trial. Arch Intern Med 1989;149:2527–2530.

Swezey RL. Pseudo-radiculopathy in subacute trochanteric bursitis of the subgluteus maximus bursa. Arch Phys Med Rehabil 1976;57:387–390.

Traycoff RB. "Pseudotrochanteric Bursitis": the differential diagnosis of lateral hip pain. J Rheum 1991;18:1810–1812.

C·H·A·P·T·E·R

33

....

Board Simulation: Rheumatic and Immunologic Disease

Raymond J. Scheetz

....

In the following questions, consider each possible answer and choose all that are correct. Many questions have more than one correct answer.

QUESTIONS

1. A 58-year-old diabetic man developed pain and swelling in his metacarpophalangeal joints and knees. The sedimentation rate is 27 mm/hr, the serum ferritin 862 mg%, and his rheumatoid factor negative. A synovial biopsy of his left knee stained for iron is shown in Figure 33.1. Appropriate actions by the physician would include:

   a. Family counseling
   b. Use of colchicine
   c. Use of methotrexate
   d. Institution of phlebotomies
   e. Use of a nonsteroidal anti-inflammatory drug (NSAID)
   f. Institution of radiation therapy

2. Which of the following statements is(are) true concerning hepatitis B infection?

   a. Acute polyarthritis usually follows the appearance of jaundice.
   b. Urticaria may accompany acute polyarthritis.
   c. Serum complement levels are usually elevated in patients with acute polyarthritis.
   d. Necrotizing vasculitis occurs in patients with persistent hepatitis B antigenemia.
   e. Glomerulonephritis may be associated with hepatitis B infection.

3. An 84-year-old woman is seen for severe right shoulder pain. She has a large effusion, and a radiograph shows erosive changes in the humeral head, which is displaced from the glenoid. Aspirated joint fluid stained with Alizarin red S shows the findings seen in Figure 33.2. Which of the following questions is(are) true in this case?

   a. These clumps of crystals contain apatite.
   b. Knees are never involved in this process.
   c. Both shoulders are affected in 50% of patients.
   d. Treatment may include NSAIDs, aspiration and/or injection, and surgery.
   e. Colchicine and allopurinol are effective treatments.

4. The laboratory reports that a patient in the hospital has a serum urate level of 1.6 mg%. This patient might have:

   a. Had a cholecystogram showing radiolucent stones
   b. Had an upper gastrointestinal Barium study showing a duodenal diverticulum
   c. Had a chest radiograph showing a right upper lobe mass
   d. Been taking colchicine
   e. Been taking glyceryl guaiacolate

5. A 42-year-old African-American woman presents with bilateral ankle and knee pain and swelling of 2 months' duration. She denies diarrhea and rectal bleeding. The synovial biopsy shown in Figure 33.3 is obtained from her right knee. In a patient with such a biopsy result you might expect which of the following?

   a. Normal delayed hypersensitivity skin tests
   b. An elevated level of angiotensin converting enzyme (ACE)
   c. A history of uveitis
   d. A primary Gohn complex and bilateral apical pleural thickening on chest radiograph

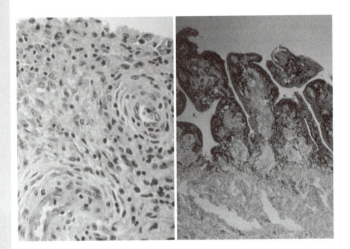

Figure 33.1. Synovial biopsy of knee stained for iron. (Reprinted with permission. Copyright Syntex [U.S.A.] Inc. All rights reserved.) (See color plate.)

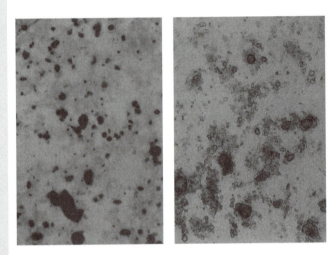

Figure 33.2. Aspirated shoulder joint fluid stained with Alizarin red S. (See color plate.)

e. Hyperpigmented maculopapular skin lesions
f. Sterile leukocyturia

6. The anemia of giant-cell arteritis responds to treatment with:

a. Prednisone
b. Vitamin B12
c. Oral iron
d. Parenteral iron
e. Salicylates

7. A 23-year-old woman complains of pain and swelling of the right elbow. A biopsy is eventually performed; the finding is shown in Figure 33.4. Based on these findings, you might expect:

a. Synovial fluid to contain an excessive number of red blood cells

b. A fairly good response to radiation therapy
c. A fairly good response to synovectomy
d. An excellent response to colchicine
e. A good response to isoniazid and rifampin
f. Cultures to reveal a definitive diagnosis

8. The differential diagnosis for sore throat, fever, and polyarthritis should include all of the following *except:*

a. Gonococcal arthritis
b. Rheumatoid arthritis
c. Dermatomyositis
d. Systemic lupus erythematosus
e. Psoriatic arthritis

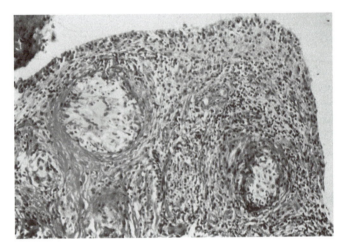

Figure 33.3. Synovial biopsy from knee. (Reprinted from the Clinical Slide Collection on the Rheumatic Diseases, Copyright 1991, 1995. Used by permission of the American College of Rheumatology.) (See color plate.)

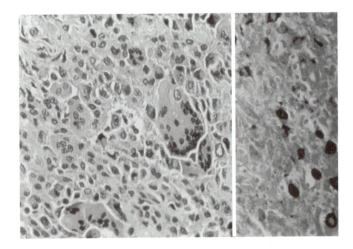

Figure 33.4. Elbow biopsy findings. (Reprinted with permission. Copyright Syntex [U.S.A.] Inc. All rights reserved.) (See color plate.)

9. Associated findings in patients with the disease seen in Figure 33.5 might include:

   a. Low serum phosphorus
   b. Elevated serum iron
   c. Hepatic cirrhosis
   d. Presence of HLA-B27
   e. Brown urine after alkalinization

10. Which one of the following tests is most likely to have abnormal results in a patient with carpal tunnel syndrome?

    a. Serum calcium
    b. Serum potassium
    c. Aspartate amino-transferase
    d. Latex for rheumatoid factor
    e. Alkaline phosphatase

11. A patient with the radiographic abnormality seen in Figure 33.6 might be found to have:

    a. A history of heavy alcohol consumption
    b. A high titer of native (double-stranded) anti-DNA
    c. An elevated marrow acid phosphatase
    d. An occupational exposure to vinyl chloride
    e. A history of salmonella osteomyelitis

12. Shoulder-hand syndrome may be associated with all of the following *except:*

    a. Myocardial infarction
    b. Cervical disc disease
    c. Laënnec's cirrhosis
    d. Cerebrovascular accident
    e. Anticonvulsant drugs

13. The findings shown in Figure 33.7 on physical examination should lead you to suspect:

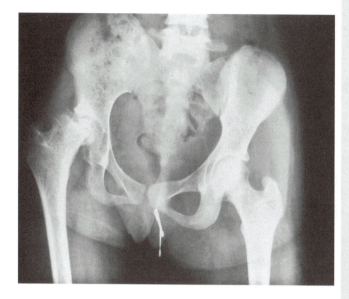

Figure 33.6.   Radiographic abnormality in Question 11.

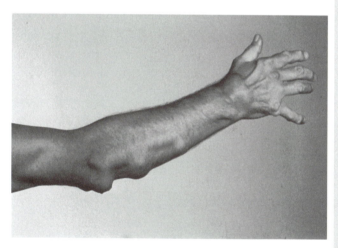

Figure 33.7.   Condition in Question 13.

    a. A high titer of rim-pattern antinuclear antibodies
    b. A good prognosis for joint integrity and function
    c. A high titer of sheep red cell agglutination
    d. A palindromic clinical course
    e. The possibility of pulmonary interstitial fibrosis

14. Management of Charcot's arthropathy of the knee in a tabetic would include all of the following *except:*

    a. Immobilization
    b. Total knee joint replacement
    c. Restriction of weight bearing
    d. Mechanical supports
    e. Arthrodesis

15. The radiographs shown in Figure 33.8 are characteristic of an arthritis that:

    a. May be polyarticular and symmetrical

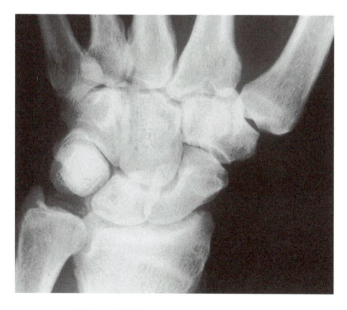

Figure 33.5.   Condition in Question 9.

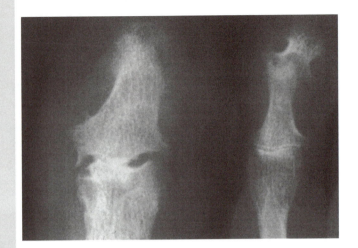

Figure 33.8.   Radiographs for Question 15.

other joint complaints. Appropriate evaluation might include:

a. Angiotensin converting enzyme (ACE) level
b. Chest radiograph
c. Muscle biopsy
d. Proctosigmoidoscopy
e. Synovial fluid aspiration and study

20. Treatment with penicillamine has been associated with:

b. Does not have an associated spondylitis
c. May be asymmetrical and pauciarticular
d. Does not cause primary involvement of distal interphalangeal joints
e. May have a severe mutilating form

16. Findings of sickle cell disease may include all of the following *except:*

a. Periostitis of the metacarpal, metatarsal, and proximal phalangeal bones
b. Oval phalangeal cysts parallel to the phalangeal axis
c. Osteonecrosis of the femoral head
d. Salmonella osteomyelitis
e. Severe diffuse polyarthralgias

17. With regard to the abnormality illustrated in Figure 33.9:

a. Cord compression is more common at C1–2 than at lower cervical areas.
b. The normal width of the preodontoid space is 3 mm or less.
c. Surgical intervention is always necessary.
d. It is not seen in rheumatoid factor negative patients.
e. It occurs in 20% of patients with rheumatoid arthritis with destructive arthropathy.

18. The individual in Figure 33.10 might be expected to have which of the following:

a. Aortic insufficiency
b. Auditory dysfunction
c. Glomerulonephritis
d. Tracheomalacia
e. Thrombocytopenia

19. An 18-year-old African American male presents with a swollen ankle as shown in Figure 33.11. He has no

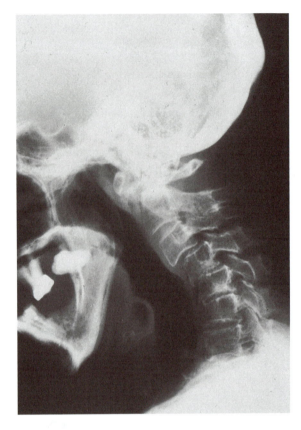

Figure 33.9.   Condition in Question 17.

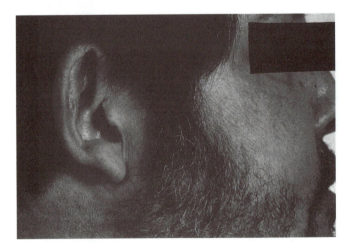

Figure 33.10.   Condition in Question 18. (See color plate.)

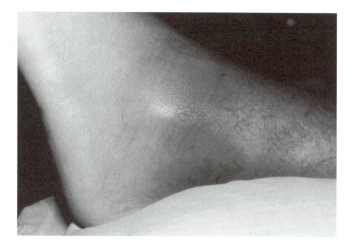

Figure 33.11. Condition in Question 19. (See color plate.)

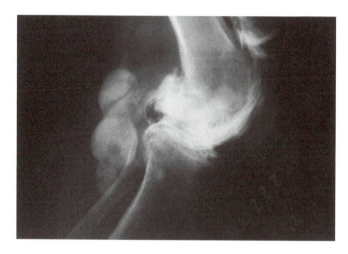

Figure 33.12. Arthrogram for Question 21.

a. Polymyositis
b. Pancytopenia
c. Myasthenia gravis
d. Deposition of mercury in the synovial lining cells

21. Proper treatment of the complication demonstrated by the arthrogram in Figure 33.12 would include:

 a. Anticoagulants
 b. Intra-articular corticosteroids
 c. Bed rest and elevation
 d. An intensive course of oral colchicine
 e. A short course of an immunosuppressive agent

22. In the complication of rheumatoid arthritis shown in Figure 33.13, pleural fluid findings would include:

 a. Low complement levels
 b. Very low glucose values
 c. Protein less than 3.0 gm%

d. Less than 5000 white blood cells /mm^3, mostly polymorphonuclear neutrophils
 e. A chylous appearance

23. Drug therapy in ankylosing spondylitis:

 a. Includes salicylates in most patients
 b. May have the best results with use of indomethacin
 c. May have the best results with use of naproxen
 d. Should generally be avoided, since it makes little or no difference in the outcome of the disease

24. The mucin string test shown in Figure 33.14 is compatible with a diagnosis of:

 a. Osteoarthritis
 b. Rheumatoid arthritis
 c. Pigmented villonodular synovitis

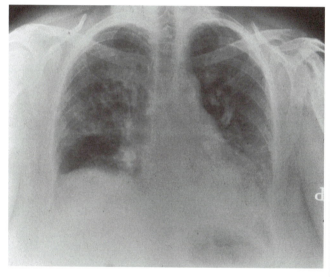

Figure 33.13. Condition in Question 22.

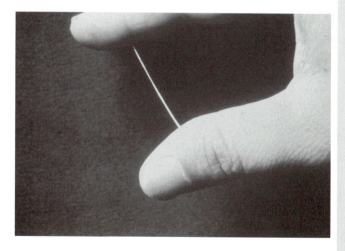

Figure 33.14. Mucin string test referred to in Question 24. (Used with the permission of Pharmacia & Upjohn Co.)

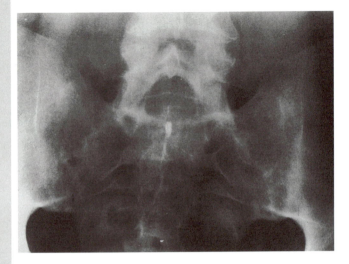

Figure 33.15. Radiograph for Question 25.

d. Rheumatic fever
e. Gout

25. The pelvic radiograph shown in Figure 33.15 is compatible with a diagnosis of:

   a. Reiter's syndrome
   b. Psoriatic arthritis
   c. Relapsing polychondritis
   d. Whipple's disease
   e. Ankylosing spondylitis

26. The abnormality demonstrated in the radiographs in Figure 33.16 may be found in a patient with:

   a. Keratoderma blennorrhagica
   b. Rheumatoid nodules
   c. Restricted chest expansion
   d. Upper and lower respiratory granulomas
   e. Thrombophlebitis and mucosal colitis

27. The histopathologic demonstration of aortitis seen in Figure 33.17 is found in patients with:

   a. HLA-B27
   b. Collapse of nasal and ear cartilage
   c. Circinate balanitis
   d. Nail pitting, discoloration, and onycholysis
   e. Oral and genital ulcerations, ocular inflammation, and arthritis

28. Crystals from the lesions shown in Figure 33.18:

   a. Would show strongly positive birefringence under compensated polarized microscopy (CPM)
   b. Would show strongly negative birefringence under CPM
   c. Would be yellow when parallel to the axis under CPM
   d. Would be blue when parallel to the axis under CPM

   e. Are never found intracellularly within synovial fluid

29. The eruption shown in Figure 33.19 is:

   a. Characteristic of Reiter's syndrome
   b. Typical of psoriasis
   c. Found only in Still's disease
   d. Often associated with joint pain and fever
   e. Usually associated with a fatal disease

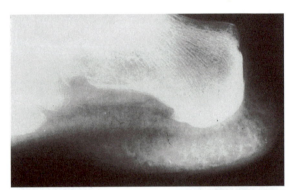

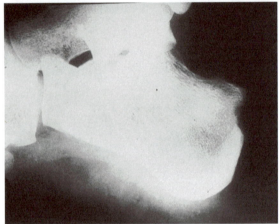

Figure 33.16. Radiographs for Question 26.

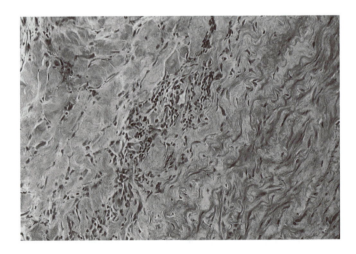

Figure 33.17. Condition in Question 27. (See color plate.)

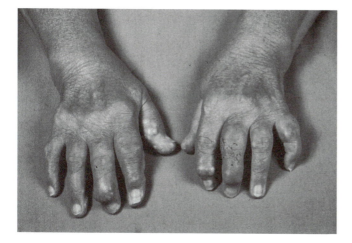

Figure 33.18. Condition in Question 28. (See color plate.)

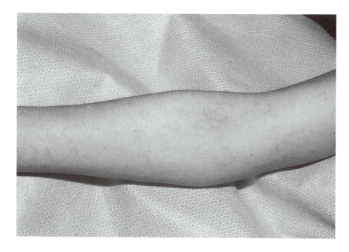

Figure 33.19. Condition in Question 29. (See color plate.)

30. Depending upon the situation, treatment of the illness shown in Figure 33.20 might include:

    a. Aspirin
    b. Colchicine
    c. Methotrexate
    d. Indomethacin
    e. Topical steroids

31. A 45-year-old carpenter reports malaise, weakness, weight loss, and generalized aching for 3 months. His temperature is 37.8°C, and blood pressure is 160/95 mm/hg. His knees are tender but not swollen. He has a right wrist drop, weakness of the right knee extensors, and absence of the right knee tendon reflex. Laboratory results are hematocrit, 35%; white blood cell count, 12,000/mm³; Westergren sedimentation rate, 54 mm/hr; aspartate amino-transferase, 45 mg%; creatine phosphokinase, normal; rheumatoid latex, negative; antinuclear antibody, negative; urine protein, 600 mg/

24 hrs; and urine red blood cells, 25/high-power field. The most likely diagnosis is:

    a. Rheumatoid arthritis
    b. Systemic lupus erythematosus
    c. Polymyositis
    d. Progressive systemic sclerosis
    e. Polyarteritis nodosa

32. A 25-year-old woman had pain on moving her left elbow for 1 day, then pain in her right third metacarpophalangeal joint followed by pain in her right knee. Examination discloses an uncomfortable young woman with a temperature of 37.2°C (99.0°F). Her right wrist is swollen and tender, and flexion and rotation of the left hip cause pain. Erythematous lesions with a central blister are noted on the dorsum of the left hand and on the left thigh. Aspirated fluid from her right wrist is cloudy and contains 37,000 leukocytes/mm³. Which of the following would be most likely to establish the diagnosis?

    a. A lupus erythematosus (LE) cell test
    b. A latex fixation test for rheumatoid factor
    c. Determination of the antistreptolysin-0 titer
    d. A culture of cervical secretions
    e. A smear and culture of synovial fluid

33. In a patient the joint fluid is found to have a poor

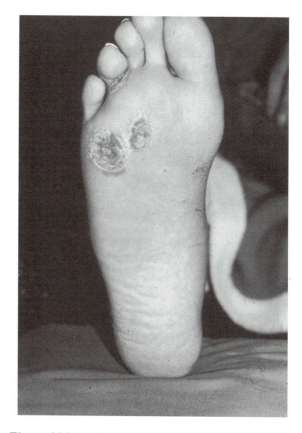

Figure 33.20. Condition in Question 30. (See color plate.)

mucin clot, 20,400 white blood cells (WBCs)/mm³, 90% neutrophils, 10% mononuclear cells, no crystals, decreased complement, and glucose of 45 mg%. The most likely diagnosis is:

a. Gout
b. Osteoarthritis
c. Rheumatoid arthritis
d. Pseudogout

34. In a patient, the joint fluid is found to have a poor mucin clot, 12,000 WBC/mm³, 72% neutrophils, 28% mononuclear cells, free and intracellular negative birefringent crystals, and normal complement. The most likely diagnosis is:

a. Gout
b. Osteoarthritis
c. Rheumatoid arthritis
d. Pseudogout

35. In a patient, the joint fluid is found to have a poor mucin clot, 85,000 WBC/mm³, 95% neutrophils, 5% mononuclear cells, no crystals, normal complement, and glucose of 15 mg%. The most likely diagnosis is:

a. Gout
b. Osteoarthritis
c. Rheumatoid arthritis
d. Pseudogout

36. In a patient, the joint fluid is found to have a normal mucin clot, 850 WBC/mm³, 25% neutrophils, 75% mononuclear cells, no crystals, and normal complement; cartilage fibrils are noted. The most likely diagnosis is:

a. Gout
b. Osteoarthritis
c. Rheumatoid arthritis
d. Pseudogout

37. In a patient, the joint fluid is found to have a fair mucin clot, 5000 WBC/mm³, 45% neutrophils, 55% mononuclear cells, free and intracellular weakly positive rhomboid birefringent crystals, and normal complement. The most likely diagnosis is:

a. Gout
b. Osteoarthritis
c. Rheumatoid arthritis
d. Pseudogout

38. A 20-year-old nurse complains of stiff, swollen fingers for 1 week. Examination discloses tenderness and slight swelling of the proximal interphalangeal joints of the second, third, and fourth digits bilaterally. The lab results are hematocrit, 39%; leukocyte count, 7000/mm³; Westergren sedimentation rate, 25 mm/hr; and rheumatoid latex, 1:40. The differential diagnosis should include:

a. Rheumatoid arthritis
b. Systemic lupus erythematosus
c. Acute viral hepatitis B
d. Postrubella vaccination reaction

39. A 28-year-old man has had rash, edema of his feet, and arthritis of knees and ankles for 6 weeks. He has had some recent upper abdominal pain, and his stools have been dark for 3–4 days. His rash is confined to the legs and consists of purpuric lesions varying from bright red to dark purple. Synovitis is present in both knees, and probably in both ankles, but is obscured by the edema. Platelets are normal in the peripheral blood smear. The most useful initial diagnostic test would be:

a. An LE cell preparation
b. A latex test for rheumatoid factor
c. A urinalysis
d. A synovial biopsy
e. A sedimentation rate

40. The basic pathologic lesion accounting for the skin and probably the gastrointestinal manifestations in Henoch-Schönlein purpura is:

a. Nerve fiber degeneration
b. A defect in platelet function
c. Degeneration of collagen fibers in the wall of blood vessels
d. A consumptive coagulopathy
e. A small vessel vasculitis

41. The most useful diagnostic test for determining the prognosis of Henoch-Schönlein purpura is:

a. A platelet count
b. A urinalysis
c. An electrocardiogram
d. A skin biopsy
e. A gastroscopy

42. Henoch-Schönlein purpura in children differs from its adult counterpart in that:

a. It is usually a mild or subclinical disorder in children.
b. Intussusception is common in children with the disorder but is rare or absent in adults.
c. The kidneys are rarely involved in adults.
d. The skin is rarely involved in children.
e. It is most common in adult males, but in children there is an equal sex distribution.

43. A young Arab from Jordan presents with severe headache and visual disturbances. He has bilateral papilledema, oral mucosal ulcers, and a single 4 cm scrotal ulcer. Bilateral uveitis is noted and is thought to have been present for several months. Oral and scrotal ulcers have been recurring over the past year.

Additional manifestations of this illness that might occur in the future include all of the following *except:*

a. Thrombophlebitis
b. Arthritis
c. Widespread amyloidosis
d. Skin lesions resembling erythema nodosum over the pretibial area
e. A syndrome resembling multiple sclerosis

44. For each of these circumstances, select the best treatment from the list following.

• 44A. The fifth day of an acute attack of gouty arthritis, not previously treated.
• 44B. A history of several attacks of acute gouty arthritis in a patient who has nephrolithiasis receiving no drugs.
• 44C. A patient with no signs or symptoms of renal or rheumatic disease, with serum urate of 8.2 mg% discovered on a routine screening test.
• 44D. A patient who has just recovered from his second attack of gouty arthritis whose serum urate was 10.4 mg% and urine urate excretion 486 mg/24 hrs, and who is receiving only colchicine.
• 44E. A patient who has just recovered from his second acute gouty attack in a month since starting therapy with allopurinol.
• 44F. A patient with a history of multiple acute gouty attacks who has a serum urate of 12.2 mg% and blood urea nitrogen of 48 mg%.

a. None
b. Probenecid 2 grams/day
c. Indomethacin 150 mg/day or more, as indicated
d. Allopurinol 300 mg/day
e. Colchicine 0.6 mg twice a day
f. Colchicine 0.6 mg every hour until diarrhea or vomiting occurs

45. The finding shown in Figure 33.21 can be present in:
a. Scleroderma
b. Systemic lupus erythematosus
c. Rheumatoid arthritis
d. Dermatomyositis
e. Polyarteritis nodosa

46. The condition of the patient shown in Figure 33.22:
a. Is frequently associated with headaches and visual changes
b. Is associated with rheumatoid factor
c. May be diagnosed by muscle biopsy
d. Responds dramatically to steroids
e. Need not be treated

Answers and Explanations

1. Figure 33.1 depicts positive synovial iron stain characteristic of hemochromatosis.

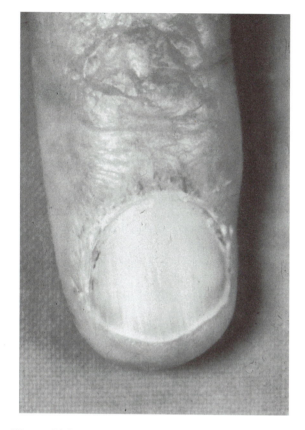

Figure 33.21. Condition in Question 45. (See color plate.)

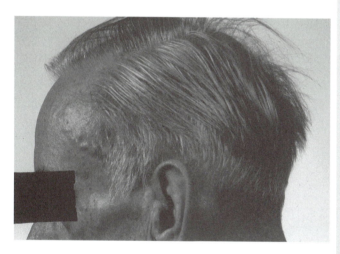

Figure 33.22. Condition in Question 46.

Correct answers:

a. Family counseling is appropriate because hemochromatosis is a hereditary disease.
d. Phlebotomy can be used to decrease the iron load.
e. Nonsteroidal anti-inflammatory drugs (NSAIDs) can improve joint symptoms.

Incorrect answers:

b. Colchicine is unlikely to improve joint symptoms.

c. Methotrexate could aggravate hepatic disease.

f. Radiation therapy has no role in treatment of hemochromatosis.

2. *Correct answers:*

b. Urticaria often accompanies acute polyarthritis prior to the onset of jaundice.

d. A significant percentage of patients with necrotizing vasculitis will have persistent hepatitis B antigenemia.

e. Immune complex glomerulonephritis may accompany hepatitis B infection.

Incorrect answers:

a. Polyarthritis precedes jaundice.

c. Complement levels will be depressed in this immune complex disease.

3. Figure 33.2 depicts "Milwaukee Shoulder" joint fluid findings.

Correct answers:

a. Crystals are primarily hydroxyapatite.

c. Often bilateral shoulder involvement is present.

d. All of these are appropriate treatments.

Incorrect answers:

b. Knees are often involved.

e. Colchicine and allopurinol do not have the same efficacy as in gout.

4. *Correct answers:*

a. Oral cholecystographic agents may have a uricosuric effect.

c. A lung tumor could secrete substances causing inappropriate antidiuretic hormone syndrome, leading to hypouricemia.

e. Mucolytic agents may also cause hypouricemia.

Incorrect answers:

b. Bowel contrast agents do not affect uric acid.

d. Colchicine does not affect urate levels.

5. The synovial biopsy in Figure 33.3 depicts noncaseating granulomas typical of sarcoidosis.

Correct answers:

b. Angiotensin converting enzyme is often elevated in sarcoidosis.

c. Uveitis occurs in sarcoidosis.

e. Hyperpigmented maculopapular skin lesions are typical of sarcoidosis.

Incorrect answers:

a. Delayed hypersensitivity skin tests are often abnormal with anergy in sarcoidosis.

d. Gohn complex and apical pleural thickening are characteristic of tuberculosis, not sarcoidosis.

f. Sterile leukocyturia is also characteristic of tuberculosis.

6. *Correct answer:*

a. Prednisone helps resolve the inflammation associated with giant-cell arteritis.

Incorrect answers:

b, c, d, e. None of these relieves anemia related to "inflammation."

7. Figure 33.4 depicts pigmented villonodular synovitis (PVS) with giant cells, red blood cells, and hemosiderin-laden macrophages.

Correct answers:

a. Synovial fluid in PVS is often hemorrhagic.

b,c. Radiation and/or synovectomy may be helpful for PVS.

Incorrect answers:

d, e. Neither colchicine nor antituberculous treatment is effective.

f. No infectious cause has been discovered.

8. *Correct answer:*

e. Psoriatic arthritis does not cause sore throat and would rarely cause fever.

Incorrect answers:

a. Disseminated gonococcal syndrome could cause polyarthritis, fever, and gonococcal pharyngitis.

b. Rheumatoid arthritis is often polyarticular and may cause fever and crico-arytenoid inflammation

c. Dermatomyositis may cause polyarthritis and fever and is often preceded by pharyngitis.

d. Systemic lupus erythematosus may cause polyarthritis, fever, and aphthous pharyngitis.

9. The patient in Figure 33.5 has chondrocalcinosis of pseudogout or calcium pyrophosphate crystal deposition disease.

Correct answers:

a. Hyperparathyroidism may be associated.

b. Hemochromatosis may be associated.

c. Cirrhosis may relate to hemochromatosis or Wilson's disease, which may be seen with chondrocalcinosis.

e. Alkaptonuria may also be associated with chondrocalcinosis.

Incorrect answer:

d. B27 is not seen with chondrocalcinosis.

10. *Correct answer:*

d. Rheumatoid arthritis is a common cause of carpal tunnel syndrome.

Incorrect answers:
a, b, c, e. No consistent abnormalities of calcium, potassium, or liver dysfunction are related to carpal tunnel syndrome.

11. The radiograph in Figure 33.6 shows avascular necrosis of bone.
    Correct answers:

    a. Alcoholism may cause elevated lipids, resulting in vascular obstruction.
    b. Lupus vasculitis may be causative.
    c. Gaucher's cells may block vessels.
    e. Salmonella osteomyelitis occurs in sickle cell disease, which may cause ischemic bone disease.

    Incorrect answer:
    d. Vinyl chloride is not related to avascular necrosis.

12. *Correct answer:*

    c. Cirrhosis is not associated with shoulder-hand syndrome.

    Incorrect answers:
    a, b, d, e. All of these have been associated with shoulder-hand syndrome by unknown mechanisms, but perhaps via neurovascular reflexes.

13. The patient in Figure 33.7 has rheumatoid nodules.
    Correct answers:

    c, e. A high titer of sheep red cell agglutination (rheumatoid factor) and other extra-articular disease (pulmonary fibrosis) would be associated with nodular rheumatoid arthritis.

    Incorrect answers:
    a. Rim-pattern antinuclear antibody is typical of anti-DNA seen in lupus
    b, d. Nodules do not portend a good functional prognosis or intermittent (palindromic) course.

14. *Correct answer:*

    b. Total joint replacement is not done ordinarily in a Charcot joint, since insensitivity to pain would lead to early prosthetic failure.

    Incorrect answers:
    a, c, d, e. All of these are acceptable treatments for a Charcot joint.

15. The radiographs in Figure 33.8 are typical of psoriatic arthritis.
    Correct answers:
    a, c, e. All of these forms may be seen in psoriatic arthritis.

    Incorrect answers:
    b, d. The characteristics described here are also typical of psoriatic arthritis.

16. *Correct answer:*

    b. Oval phalangeal cysts parallel to the phalangeal axis are typical of sarcoidosis, not sickle cell bone disease.

    Incorrect answers:
    a, c, d, e. All of these are typical of sickle cell bone and joint disease.

17. The abnormality pictured in Figure 33.9 is C1–2 subluxation in rheumatoid disease.
    Correct answers:

    b. True
    e. True

    Incorrect answers:
    a. Cord compression is more common at lower levels (e.g., at C3–4–5) because the available extra space is much less at these lower levels.
    c. Surgical intervention is necessary only if significant neurologic consequences or significant pain is present.
    d. Some seronegative rheumatoids and even psoriatic arthritics may have C1–2 subluxation.

18. The patient in Figure 33.10 has relapsing polychondritis (RPC) with saddle nose deformity.
    Correct answers:

    a. Valvular ring degeneration is common in RPC.
    b. Otic degeneration occurs in RPC.
    c. Glomerulonephritis has been reported in RPC.
    d. Tracheomalacia occurs frequently in RPC.

    Incorrect answer:
    e. Thrombocytopenia is not characteristic of RPC.

19. Figure 33.11 shows ankle synovitis.
    Correct answers:

    a. Sarcoidosis often involves ankles.
    b. Chest radiograph can be used to look for sarcoidosis.
    d. Inflammatory bowel disease may cause lower extremity synovitis.
    e. Synovial analysis can determine whether inflammatory or other type of synovial fluid.

    Incorrect answer:
    c. Myositis would be an unlikely cause of ankle swelling.

20. *Correct answers:*
    a, b, c. All of these can be seen in penicillamine therapy.

    Incorrect answer:

    d. This is not characteristic of penicillamine treatment.

21. The radiograph in Figure 33.12 shows a Baker's cyst.

Correct answers:

b. Steroid injection should help relieve the exudative process.

c. Bed rest and elevation help the fluid to resorb.

Incorrect answers:

a. This is not phlebitis, but pseudophlebitis.

d. Colchicine plays no role here as gout does not cause a Baker's cyst.

e. Immunosuppressives in short course will not help, even if caused by rheumatoid arthritis.

22. Figure 33.13 shows rheumatoid lung disease.
Correct answers:

a. Complement levels are low in rheumatoid pleural fluid.

b. Glucose values are often low in rheumatoid pleural fluid.

d. White blood cell (WBC) counts are low in rheumatoid pleural fluid.

Incorrect answers:

c. Protein values should be more than 3.0 gm% in rheumatoid fluids.

e. Rheumatoid pleural fluid is not milky.

23. *Correct answers:*

b. Indomethacin is often very effective in ankylosing spondylitis (AS).

c. Naproxen or other NSAIDs may be effective in some patients with AS.

Incorrect answers:

a. Salicylates do not work well in AS.

d. Anti-inflammatory drugs often provide relief of stiffness and pain, allowing better attempts at physical therapy.

24. The mucin string test in Figure 33.14 shows good synovial fluid (SF) viscosity.
Correct answers:

a, c, d. Osteoarthritis, pigmented villonodular synovitis, and rheumatic fever have viscous SF.

Incorrect answers:

b, e. Rheumatoid arthritis and gout have synovial fluid with decreased viscosity.

25. The pelvic radiograph in Figure 33.15 shows sacroiliitis.
Correct answers:

a, b, d, e. Reiter's syndrome, psoriatic arthritis, Whipple's disease, and ankylosing spondylitis may cause sacroiliitis.

Incorrect answer:

c. Relapsing polychondritis has not been associated with sacroiliitis.

26. A heel erosion is seen on the radiographs in Figure 33.16.
Correct answers:

a, b, c. Reiter's syndrome (keratoderma blennorrhagica), rheumatoid arthritis, and ankylosing spondylitis (restricted chest expansion) may cause calcaneal erosions.

Incorrect answers:

d, e. Wegener's granulomatosus (granulomas) and Behcet's syndrome (thrombophlebitis and colitis) do not cause calcaneal erosions.

27. The histomicrograph in Figure 33.17 shows aortitis.
Correct answers:

a, b, c, d, e. All conditions listed may cause aortitis (ankylosing spondylitis, relapsing polychondritis, Reiter's syndrome, psoriasis, and Behcet's syndrome).

28. Figure 33.18 depicts severe tophaceous gout.
Correct answers:

b,c. Uric acid crystals are strongly negative with respect to their birefringence and yellow when parallel to the axis of reference.

Incorrect answers:

a,d. These are characteristic of calcium pyrophosphate crystal deposition disease.

e. Uric acid crystals are often intracellular, especially with an acute attack.

29. The rash shown in Figure 33.19 is erythema marginatum characteristic of rheumatic fever.
Correct answer:

d. Rheumatic fever.

Incorrect answers:

a. This is not keratoderma blennorrhagica.

b. This is not psoriasis.

c. This is not the salmon-colored evanescent rash of juvenile rheumatoid arthritis.

e. Rheumatic fever is rarely initially fatal.

30. Figure 33.20 shows keratoderma blennorrhagica.
Correct answers:
a, c, d, e. All of these could be used.

Incorrect answer:

b. Colchicine does not help Reiter's syndrome.

31. Arthralgia, myalgia, fever, hypertension, wrist drop, peripheral neuropathy, anemia, leukocytosis, elevated sedimentation rate, proteinuria, and hematuria are very suggestive of polyarteritis nodosa.
Correct answer:

e. Polyarteritis nodosa.

Incorrect answers:
a. Proteinuria and hematuria would be unusual in rheumatoid arthritis.
b. Leukocytosis would be unusual in systemic lupus erythematosus.
c. Polyneuropathy and proteinuria would be unusual in polymyositis.
d. Fever and polyneuropathy would be unusual in progressive systemic sclerosis.

32. The case description is typical of gonococcal arthritis-dermatitis syndrome.
Correct answer:

d. Cervical cultures positive for gonococcus help to make the diagnosis.

Incorrect answers:
a. The skin lesions are atypical for systemic lupus erythematosus (SLE), and the synovial fluid white blood cell count is too high for SLE.
b. Rheumatoid arthritis joint pain is usually not so migratory, and rash would be atypical.
c. These skin lesions are not typical of rheumatic fever or poststreptococcal arthritis.
e. Gonococci are difficult to culture from synovial fluid.

33. *Correct answer:*

c. Rheumatoid arthritis (RA): Poor mucin clot, elevated white blood cell (WBC) count with increased neutrophils, low complement, and low glucose are typical of RA synovial fluid.

Incorrect answers:
a. No crystals seen.
b. WBC too high.
d. No crystals seen.

34. *Correct answer:*

a. Crystals described are typical of urate.

Incorrect answers:
b. WBC too high and crystals present.
c. Crystals present and complement normal.
d. Crystals not characteristic of calcium pyrophosphate.

35. *Correct answer:*

c. Poor mucin, high WBC, high neutrophils, no crystals, and low sugar are typical of rheumatoid arthritis.

Incorrect answers:
a. No crystals seen.
b. WBC too high, polys too high.
d. No crystals, glucose too low.

36. *Correct answer:*

b. Low WBC, low neutrophils, no crystals, normal

complement, and fibrils all suggestive of osteoarthritis.

Incorrect answers:
a. No crystals, WBC too low.
c. WBC and neutrophils too low, complement normal.
d. No crystals, WBC and neutrophils too low.

37. *Correct answer*

d. Crystals typical of calcium pyrophosphate crystal deposition disease.

Incorrect answers:
a. Wrong crystal description.
b. WBC and neutrophils too high, crystals present.
c. Crystals present.

38. The clinical description is that of acute synovitis.
Correct answers:
a, b, c, d. All of these illnesses could begin as acute synovitis in this fashion.

39. The case described is typical of Henoch-Schönlein purpura (HSP).
Correct answer:

c. It is helpful to know if renal involvement is present.

Incorrect answers:
a. The lupus erythematosus preparation is no longer used as a diagnostic test.
b. The purpuric rash is atypical for rheumatoid arthritis.
d. A synovial biopsy is not necessary for diagnosis and would probably be nonspecific.
e. Sedimentation rate is nonspecific.

40. In HSP, the basic lesion is leukocytoclastic vasculitis.
Correct answer:

e. Leukocytoclastic vasculitis is a small vessel vasculitis.

Incorrect answers:
a, b, c, d. None of these mechanisms is operative in HSP.

41. Renal involvement is the most serious complication in HSP.
Correct answer:

b. Hematuria is suggestive of renal involvement in HSP.

Incorrect answers:
a, c, d, e. None of these is helpful in determining prognosis in HSP.

42. HSP may behave differently in children.
Correct answer:

b. Intussusception characteristically occurs in children with HSP.

Incorrect answers:
a. HSP may be severe in children.
c. Renal involvement may be seen in adults.
d. The skin is frequently involved in children.
e. Male children are affected twice as often as female children.

43. The case described is typical of Behçet's syndrome (BS).
    Correct answer:

    e. A multiple sclerosis-like syndrome is not typical of BS.

    Incorrect answers:
    a, b, c, d. All of these may occur in BS.
    44A. *Correct answer:*
    c. NSAIDs are more effective than colchicine if treatment is delayed.
    44B. *Correct answer:*
    d. Allopurinol is indicated if gouty attacks are persistent and nephrolithiasis is already present (probenecid would further over expose the kidney to uric acid and potentially more stone formation).
    44C. *Correct answer:*
    a. No specific treatment indicated.
    44D. *Correct answer:*
    b. Probenecid is a reasonable choice to lower serum urate in nonoverexcreters.
    44E. *Correct answer:*

    e. Colchicine should be given as prophylaxis against acute attacks when initiating allopurinol therapy.
    44F. *Correct answer:*
    d. Allopurinol can be used with renal insufficiency, although lesser doses are needed with decreasing creatinine clearance.

45. Periungual capillary abnormalities are shown in Figure 33.21.
    Correct answers:
    a, b, d. Scleroderma, systemic lupus erythematosus, and dermatomyositis patients display these abnormalities.

    Incorrect answers:
    c, e. Rheumatoid arthritis and polyarteritis nodosa do not cause these changes.

46. Figure 33.22 shows a characteristic inflamed temporal artery as seen in giant-cell arteritis (GCA).
    Correct answers:

    a. Headaches and amaurosis are typical in GCA.
    d. Steroids create dramatic improvement in GCA.

    Incorrect answers:
    b. Rheumatoid factor is not ordinarily found in GCA.
    c. No abnormalities are seen in muscular arteries in GCA.
    e. GCA should be treated with steroids to avoid complications such as blindness.

SUGGESTED READINGS

Ben-Dov I, Berry E. Acute rheumatic fever in adults over the age of 45 years: an analysis of 23 patients together with a review of the literature. Semin Arthritis Rheum 1980;10:100.

Bluestone R. Rheumatological complications of some endocrinopathies. Clin Rheum Dis 1975;1:95.

Brogadir SP, Schimmer BM, Myers AR. Spectrum of the gonococcal arthritis-dermatitis syndrome. Semin Arthritis Rheum 1979;8:177.

Cream JJ, Gunpel JM, Peachey RDG. Schönlein-Henoch purpura in the adult. QJ Med 1970;39:461.

Dubois EL, Wallace DJ. Clinical and laboratory manifestations of SLE. In: Wallace DJ, Dubois EL, eds. Lupus erythematosus. Philadelphia: Lea & Febiger, 1987:317–449.

Edwards CQ, Griffen LM, Goldgar D, et al. Prevalence of hemochromatosis among 11,065 presumably healthy blood donors. N Engl J Med 1988;318:1355.

Espinoza LR, Spilberg I, Osterland CK. Joint manifestations of sickle cell disease. Medicine 1974;53:295.

Fam AG, Pritzker KPH, Stein JL, et al. Apatite-associated arthropathy: a clinical study of 14 cases and of 2 patients with calcific bursitis. J Rheum 1979;6:461.

Fauci AS, Haynes BF, Katz P. The spectrum of vasculitis: clinical, pathologic, immunologic, and therapeutic considerations. Ann Intern Med 1978;89:660.

Gilbert MS. Musculoskeletal manifestations of hemophilia. Mt Sinai J Med 1977;44:339.

Halverson PB, Carrera GF, McCarty DJ. Milwaukee shoulder syndrome. Fifteen additional cases and a description of contributing factors. Arch Intern Med 1990;150(3):677.

Hunder GG, Allen GL. Giant cell arteritis: a review. Bull Rheum Dis 1978–9;29:980.

Hurd ER. Extra-articular manifestations of rheumatoid arthritis. Semin Rheum Dis 1979;8:151.

Isenberg DA, Schoenfield Y. The rheumatologic complications of hematologic disorders. Semin Arthritis Rheum 1983;12:348.

MacKenzie AH. Differential diagnosis of rheumatoid arthritis. Am J Med 1985;85(Suppl4):2.

McCarty DJ. Calcium pyrophosphate dihydrate crystal deposition disease, 1975. Arthritis Rheum 1976;19:275.

McEwen C, DiTata D, Lingg C, et al. Ankylosing spondylitis and spondylitis accompanying ulcerative colitis, regional enteritis, psoriasis, and Reiter's disease: a comparative study. Arthritis Rheum 1971;14:291.

Michet CJ Jr., McKenna CH, Lutura HS, et al. Relapsing polychondritis. Ann Intern Med 1986;104:74.

Myers BW, Masi AT. Pigmented villonodular synovitis and tenosynovitis: a clinical epidemiologic study of 166 cases and literature review. Medicine 1980;59:223.

Smith PH, Beun RT, Sharp J. Natural history of rheumatoid cervical luxations. Ann Rheum Dis 1972;31:431.

Spilberg I, Siltzbach LE, McEwen C. The arthritis of sarcoidosis. Arthritis Rheum 1969;12:126.

Yu T. Diversity of clinical features in gouty arthritis. Semin Arthritis Rheum 1984;13:360.

Pulmonary and Critical Care Medicine

Deep Venous Thrombosis and Pulmonary Emboli

Jeffrey W. Olin

Deep venous thrombosis (DVT) and pulmonary embolism (PE) remain significant causes of morbidity and mortality in the hospitalized patient. Approximately 650,000 patients develop PE each year; in many cases (up to 70%), the diagnosis is not made antemortem (Fig. 34.1). Venous thromboembolic disease is the third most common cardiovascular disease (after ischemic coronary heart disease and stroke). In addition, it is one of the leading causes of sudden death in the United States and is a significant cause of in-hospital mortality. What is important: the mortality rate for PE is less than 8% when the condition is recognized and treated correctly, but approximately 30% when untreated.

Lindblad and colleagues have shown that the incidence of PE has not changed over the last 30 years (Table 34.1). In fact, in each of the last 3 decades, 21–26% of all autopsy patients had pathologic evidence of PE, and approximately 8–9% had fatal PE. One of the reasons for this extremely high incidence of PE is the failure of physicians to adequately prophylax patients with venous thromboembolism. Anderson, et al. evaluated the pattern of prophylaxis in 16 hospitals. Only 9–56% of *high-risk* patients were adequately prophylaxed. Prophylaxis occurred more commonly in teaching hospitals than nonteaching hospitals (44% versus 19%, p < 0.001).

Deep Venous Thrombosis

ETIOLOGY OF DEEP VENOUS THROMBOSIS

Most patients who develop DVT exhibit one or more of the following:

* Endothelial injury
* Venous stasis
* Hypercoagulability

The risk factors for DVT include:

* Increasing age
* Trauma
* Immobilization (including stroke)
* Obesity
* Malignancy
* Myocardial infarction
* Congestive heart failure
* Previous deep venous thrombosis
* Varicose veins
* Estrogen use
* Parturition

For any given risk factor, the risk of DVT increases as the age of the patient increases. For example, the risk of DVT in a patient with acute myocardial infarction may be 20% for individuals younger than 60, 40% for those older than 70, and 65% for patients age 80 or older.

CLINICAL PRESENTATION AND DIAGNOSIS OF DEEP VENOUS THROMBOSIS

The usual clinical signs used to diagnose DVT in the legs are notoriously inaccurate. For example, the most common physical finding in a patient with DVT is a completely normal examination. The presence of a swollen leg, dilated superficial veins, tenderness, a palpable cord, and a positive Homan's sign are suggestive, yet each of these may occur in other conditions. Therefore, a definitive study to confirm or rule out the presence of a DVT should be performed in every patient in whom this diagnosis is entertained.

Superficial thrombophlebitis can often be made on the basis of a good physical examination. Often an area of ery-

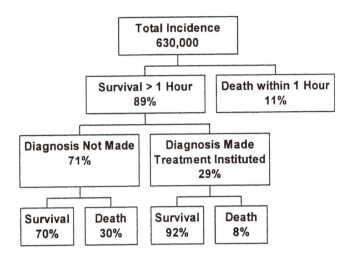

Figure 34.1. Incidence, survival, and death rates of PE. (Reprinted from Dale JE, Apert JS. Prog Cardiovasc Dis 1975;17: 259–270.)

Table 34.1. Incidence of Venous Thromboembolism by Necropsy (1987)	
Admissions to hospital	26,078
Number of deaths	1,293
Number with necropsy	994 (77%)
Venous thromboembolism	347 (35%)
Pulmonary embolism	260 (26%)
Fatal	93 (9.4%)
Contributory	90 (9.1%)
Incidental	77 (7.7%)

Adapted from Lindblad B, et al. BMJ 1991;302:709.

thema overlies a superficial vein, and a palpable venous cord is often present. These lesions, which are extremely tender, usually resolve in 1–3 weeks. Moist heat and analgesics, such as nonsteroidal anti-inflammatory agents, are the usual treatment for superficial thrombophlebitis. Anticoagulation for superficial thrombophlebitis is generally not recommended, unless the superficial thrombophlebitis is in the proximal thigh within 10 cm of where the greater saphenous vein enters the common femoral vein. Several reports have shown an association between the presence of superficial thrombophlebitis and DVT. Therefore, many investigators recommend that a duplex ultrasound be performed for patients with superficial thrombophlebitis, especially if the superficial phlebitis is located above the knee.

Approximately 15–25% of patients with untreated calf vein thrombosis have propagation of the thrombus to the more proximal segments. Most investigators believe that calf vein thrombosis does not lead to significant chronic venous insufficiency. Proximal venous thrombosis, if left untreated, leads to PE 50% of the time. Recurrent DVT or extension occurs

in less than 5% of individuals who have been adequately treated with anticoagulation therapy.

PE may also occur in patients with axillary or subclavian DVT. Therefore, patients with an axillary or subclavian DVT should receive anticoagulation therapy and/or thrombolytic therapy. Generally, these patients have either thoracic outlet syndrome or an indwelling central venous catheter (for total parenteral nutrition, cancer chemotherapy, long-term antibiotic therapy or dialysis therapy) as an etiology for the axillary subclavian DVT. The arm may become swollen, and dilated superficial veins or venules may be present over the upper arm and anterior chest wall. A duplex ultrasound or venogram will confirm this diagnosis.

Every patient suspected of having DVT needs a definitive study performed to confirm or rule it out. In the past, impedance plethysmography was almost exclusively used. Duplex ultrasound scanning has virtually replaced impedance plethysmography. Duplex scanning is quite accurate when performed by experienced physicians or technologists. The duplex ultrasound is positive for an acute DVT if a thrombus is visualized; the vein is noncompressible and/or the Doppler venous sounds lose their phasicity and do not respond normally to physiologic maneuvers (i.e., augmentation, Valsalva). With better ultrasound equipment and more experienced ultrasonographers, duplex ultrasound can now accurately detect calf vein thrombosis in most patients. However, the sensitivity and specificity of duplex ultrasound is not nearly as good when used for screening asymptomatic patients (i.e., those following total hip or knee replacement).

Venography, still the "gold standard" for diagnosing DVT, is rarely performed anymore because of the accuracy of duplex ultrasound. An intraluminal filling defect is diagnostic of an acute DVT on venography.

Several studies have measured D-dimer levels as a means of excluding the diagnosis of DVT or PE. D-dimer is a specific degradation product of cross-linked fibrin. Kits are now available to measure D-dimer at the bedside. Table 34.2 shows the sensitivity, specificity, and positive and negative predictive values of measuring D-dimer in patients with DVT and PE. These and other studies show that normal D-dimer levels have a high negative-predictive value for DVT or PE. However,

Table 34.2. D-dimer in DVT and PE			
	DVT[1]	*DVT*[2] *(Rehab Unit)*	*Pulmonary Embolism*[3]
Sensitivity	89%	79%	93%
Specificity	77%	78%	25%
PPV	56%	35%	30%
NPV	95%	96%	91%

[1] Wells PS, et al. Circulation 1995;91:2184–2187; [2] Harvey RL, et al. Circulation 1996;27:1516–1520; [3] Goldhaber SZ, et al. JAMA 1993;270: 2819–2822. DVT, deep venous thrombosis; PPV, positive predictive value; NPV, negative predictive value

the positive predictive values of high D-dimer levels are not very good.

TREATMENT OF DEEP VENOUS THROMBOSIS

The major complications of DVT include:

- PE
- Chronic venous insufficiency (postphlebitic syndrome)

Once a diagnosis of DVT is considered, intravenous heparin therapy should be started immediately (unless a contraindication to anticoagulation exists) until the diagnostic studies are complete. Patients with proximal venous thrombosis should be placed at bed rest for the first 24 hours. Raschke and associates recommend using a weight-based nomogram to initiate heparin therapy—a bolus of 80 units/kg, followed by a continuous infusion of 18 units/kg per hour with adjustment of the activated partial thromboplastin time between 50–80 seconds. Both heparin and low-molecular-weight heparin bind antithrombin, which binds to factor Xa, thus inactivating it. Unfractionated heparin also accelerates the rate at which antithrombin inactivates thrombin, thus preventing further clot propagation.

Several recent randomized, controlled trials have shown that patients with DVT can be safely and effectively treated at home subcutaneously with low-molecular-weight heparin (Enoxaparin 1mg/kg two times a day subcutaneously, or fraxiparine 8200–12,300 International Factor Xa Inhibitory Units per liter) (Table 34.3). In the study by Levine, et al., the mean number of hospital days was 0.9 in the LMWH group, compared with 6.7 in the standard heparin group. Many patients in both studies (in the LMWH group) were never admitted to the hospital. The incidence of DVT or PE recurrence was identical in those patients treated in the hospital with intravenous unfractionated heparin and those treated at home with subcutaneous low-molecular-weight heparin. Quality of life improved in both groups, while physical activity and social functioning were better in patients assigned to the low-molecular-weight heparin group. There was also no significant difference in bleeding rates between those randomized to unfractionated heparin or low-molecular-weight heparin.

Warfarin (Coumadin) is usually started on the first or second day of heparin therapy. Heparin and warfarin should be continued together for 4–5 days. Even if the International Normalized Ratio (INR) is in the therapeutic range, it is important to continue both drugs together because the half-life of Factor II is approximately 60–72 hours, and the patient will be unprotected if heparin is stopped too soon. A recent report by Harrison and associates demonstrated that a loading dose of 5 mg of warfarin produces less supratherepeutic INRs and depletes factor II levels to the same degree at 60–108 hours as when a loading dose of 10 mg of warfarin is used.

Individual laboratories use different thromboplastin reagents with various degrees of potency. This variability makes it difficult to monitor oral anticoagulant therapy in patients who have their prothrombin times drawn in different laboratories. The World Health Organization has attempted to standardize this technique by a calibration method called the International Sensitivity Index (ISI). This index is assigned to each batch of thromboplastin that each individual laboratory uses.

The INR (which most laboratories now calculate) has become the method of choice for following patients receiving warfarin anticoagulation:

$$INR = (PT\ patient/PT\ normal)^{ISI}$$

Generally, the goal for the treatment of venous thrombosis is an INR range between 2–3 with an INR target of 2.5 (Table 34.4).

While there is some controversy over how long to treat patients for an acute DVT, most clinicians recommend 3–6 months of warfarin therapy for the first DVT, 12 months of warfarin therapy for a second episode, and lifetime warfarin for the third episode of a DVT. Several recent studies have attempted to clarify the optimal duration of treatment for patients with DVT. Schulman and colleagues performed a multicenter, randomized trial comparing 6 weeks (N = 443) of oral anticoagulation with 6 months (N = 454) of therapy. The recurrence rate at 2 years was (odds ratio, 2.1, p < 0.001) (Fig. 34.2):

- 6-week group: 20.3%
- 6-month group: 10.8%

There was not a statistically significant difference in

Table 34.4.   Recommended Therapeutic Range for Warfarin

Situation	INR Range	INR Target
Treatment of DVT & PE	2–3	2.5
Prevention of recurrent DVT or PE	2.5–4	3

Table 34.3.   Low-Molecular-Weight Heparin vs. Unfractionated Heparin in DVT Treatment

Study	Recurrent VTE	Bleeding
Levine et al[1]		
LMWH (N = 247)	13 (5.3%)	5 (2%)
Standard heparin (N = 253)	17 (6.7%)	3 (1.2%)
Koopman et al[2]		
LMWH (N = 202)	14 (6.9%)	1 (0.5%)
Standard heparin (N = 198)	17 (8.6%)	4 (2%)

[1] N Engl J Med 1996;334:677–681.
[2] N Engl J Med 1996;334:682–687.

major hemorrhage between the two groups. There was no difference between the two groups if a temporary risk factor for thrombosis was present. However, if the risk factor was permanent, the recurrance rate was (odds ratio 2.3, p < 0.001):

- 6-week group: 24.8%
- 6-month group: 12.1%

Schulman, et al. recently conducted a study comparing 6 months (N = 111) of oral anticoagulation therapy with indefinite (N = 116) anticoagulation therapy in patients who had a second episode of venous thromboembolism. After 4 years of follow-up, the recurrence rate was (relative risk, 8.0, p < 0.001) (Fig. 34.3):

- 6-month group: 20.7%
- Indefinite group: 2.6%

There was a trend (not statistically significant) toward a higher hemorrhage rate in the indefinite group.

The major side effect of heparin and warfarin is bleeding. Other side effects of heparin include thrombocytopenia, which is immunologically mediated. Antibodies against heparin can cause peripheral destruction of the platelet. This occurs be-

tween 0.3–10% of all patients who are on heparin therapy, but it is clinically significant in only a minority of patients. A smaller percentage of patients will develop arterial and venous thrombosis on heparin while thrombocytopenic (the white clot syndrome). Patients who are on heparin for prolonged periods of time may develop osteoporosis. This complication appears to be less frequent with low-molecular-weight heparin.

Complications other than bleeding that may occur with warfarin include:

- Warfarin embryopathy syndrome
- Fetal hemorrhage
- Abortion
- Stillbirth

Consequently, patients should not receive warfarin during the first trimester of pregnancy. A more detailed discussion of the management of venous thromboembolic disease in pregnancy is beyond the scope of this chapter.

Warfarin-induced skin necrosis is an infrequent but devastating complication. When it occurs, the warfarin should be stopped, and vitamin K and/or fresh frozen plasma should be administered. Often a surgical consultation will be required to debride the necrotic tissue.

PROGNOSIS OF DEEP VENOUS THROMBOSIS

While standard anticoagulation is effective in preventing PE in patients with DVT, it probably is not very effective in preventing postphlebitic syndrome (chronic venous insufficiency). Venous thromboembolism may result in venous valvular scarring and incompetence or residual venous obstruction. The manifestations of the post-thrombotic syndrome include:

- Swelling
- Pain
- Pigmentation and induration of ankle and lower $\frac{1}{3}$ of leg
- Venous claudication
- Ulceration

In some series, edema occurs in 100% of patients and venous ulcerations in 80%. However, a more recently reported series shows a much lower incidence of induration and ulceration. Nicolaides and colleagues have shown a significant correlation between the ambulatory venous pressure and the presence of venous ulcers.

Several recent series have looked at the long-term outcome in patients with DVT. Beyth and colleagues evaluated 124 patients with DVT who were followed for 6–8 years. They reported that 15% of patients had recurrent venous thromboembolism and 6 patients had more than one recurrence. The cumulative incidence of DVT was:

- 3 months: 4%
- 12 months: 6%
- 60 months: 13%

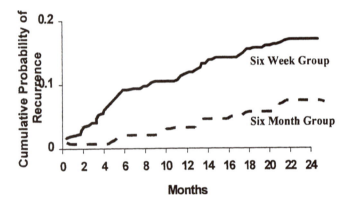

Figure 34.2.   Oral anticoagulation therapy for venous thromboembolism, 6 weeks versus 6 months. (Reprinted from Schulman S, et al. N Engl J Med 1995;332:1661–1665.)

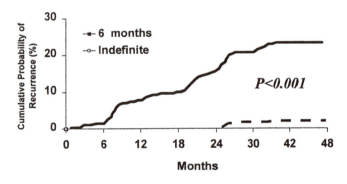

Figure 34.3.   Duration of anticoagulation after second episode of venous thromboembolism. (Reprinted from Schulman S, et al. N Engl J Med 1997;336:393–398.)

Over the course of follow-up, 52 (42%) patients died. Death was more frequent among patients older than 75 and those with cancer or stroke. The 5-year cumulative incidence of death in this subgroup of patients was 66%, compared with only 12% in patients who did not have cancer or stroke (p = 0.001).

More recently, Prandoni and colleagues evaluated the long-term clinical course of acute DVT. Three hundred fifty-five patients with the first episode of DVT were followed for 8 years. The recurrence rate was:

* 2 years: 17.5%
* 5 years: 24.6%
* 8 years: 30.3%

The incidence of post-thrombotic syndrome was:

* 2 years: 23%
* 5 years: 28%
* 8 years: 29.1%

The post-thrombotic syndrome was severe in 25 patients. The survival at 8 years was 70.2%.

Bergqvist and colleagues evaluated the cost of long-term complications of DVT. There were 242 post-thrombotic complications in a group of 257 patients who had DVT, compared with only 25 post-thrombotic complications in a control group of 241 patients. The overall cost of treating complications was substantially higher in the thrombosis group compared with the control group, and venous ulcerations made up a large portion of this cost.

ROLE OF THROMBOLYTIC THERAPY IN DVT

There are no randomized, prospective, controlled trials to definitively show that thrombolytic therapy prevents chronic venous insufficiency. However, most investigators believe that if a thrombus can be lysed quickly, venous valvular destruction and residual venous obstruction can be prevented.

Several retrospective studies have shown that patients receiving thrombolytic therapy experience fewer symptoms of chronic venous insufficiency than those receiving standard anticoagulation. Comerota has summarized the data in 13 studies comparing thrombolytic therapy with standard anticoagulation. Pooling of these data showed that in patients treated with anticoagulant therapy, 82% showed no improvement on repeat venography. However, of those patients treated with thrombolytic therapy, 47% had significant or complete thrombolysis and 21% had partial thrombolysis. In all likelihood, catheter-directed thrombolysis (similar to the technique used in the arterial circulation) will result in complete thrombolysis in a larger percentage of cases. A national registry has now been formed that will allow us to analyze the long-term outcome of patients treated with thrombolytic therapy.

It is our belief that young patients with iliofemoral DVT who do not have contraindications to thrombolytic therapy should receive catheter-directed thrombolytic therapy. In patients with phlegmasia cerulea dolens or venous gangrene, thrombolytic therapy is the therapeutic modality of choice.

DETERMINATION IF CANCER OR OTHER HYPERCOAGULABLE STATES ARE PRESENT

Patients who develop DVT or PE are at a greater risk for the future development of an underlying malignancy. Patients who develop a venous thromboembolic event with no underlying risk factors should have a careful search for an underlying neoplasm. Features of venous thrombosis that suggest an underlying neoplasm include:

* Phlegmasia cerulea dolens
* Migratory superficial thrombophlebitis
* Thrombophlebitis in unusual sites, such as the trunk and arms
* Highly inflammatory phlebitis
* Venous thrombosis that is resistant to anticoagulants

In the absence of an underlying neoplasm, a careful search should be undertaken for other hypercoagulable states. A hypercoagulability profile should include at least the following: antithrombin, protein C, protein S, circulating anticoagulant, homocysteine, anticardiolipin antibodies, and activated protein C (APC) resistance. APC resistance (factor V Leiden mutation) is the most common hypercoagulable state (other than malignancy) and is present in a large number of women who develop venous thromboembolism while taking oral contraceptive agents or other hormonal replacement therapy. The antiphospholipid antibody syndrome should be considered in patients with arterial and venous thrombosis and one or more of the following: thrombocytopenia, multiple miscarriages, unusual skin manifestations, or systemic lupus erythematosus. Patients who develop arterial or venous thrombosis while receiving heparin therapy should have a platelet count measured and a blood sample sent for serotonin release assay to look for the presence of heparin dependent platelet antibodies. The heparin should be discontinued when there is a clinical suspicion for heparin-induced thrombocytopenia. Indications to investigate for an underlying malignancy or hypercoagulable state include:

* Venous thromboembolism in the absence of usual risk factors
* Recurrent episodes of venous thromboembolism
* Patients experiencing both arterial and venous thrombosis
* Family history of venous thromboembolism
* Thromboembolism at a young age (< age 40–50)
* Thrombosis at unusual sites (e.g., trunk, arms, mesenteric veins, cerebral veins)
* Highly inflammatory thrombus
* Migratory thrombophlebitis
* Venous thrombosis resistant to anticoagulants
* Massive thromboembolism

- Multiple miscarriages
- Warfarin skin necrosis

Pulmonary Embolism

ETIOLOGY OF PULMONARY EMBOLISM

Ninety percent of patients who develop PE have a DVT in the lower extremities as a source. PE may also occur in patients with upper extremity venous thrombosis secondary to either thoracic outlet syndrome or indwelling central venous catheters.

Carson and colleagues prospectively studied the natural history of 399 patients with PE. Ninety-five patients (24%) died. The in-hospital mortality was 9.5%, and the 1-year mortality was approximately 24%. The most common causes of death were malignancy, infection, and cardiac or pulmonary disease (Table 34.5). Only 10.5% of the deaths were caused by PE.

CLINICAL PRESENTATION AND DIAGNOSIS OF PULMONARY EMBOLISM

The signs and symptoms of PE are quite nonspecific and may mimic those found in other diseases. Stein and colleagues have shown that there is no difference in the symptoms and signs in patients found to have PE by pulmonary arteriography compared with those patients who did not have PE (Tables 34.6 and 34.7). The classic triad of dyspnea, pleuritic chest pain and hemoptysis occurs infrequently. It is interesting to note that PE can present with syncope approximately 14% of the time.

A chest radiograph, ECG, and arterial blood gases are useful in ruling out other diseases, but these tests may show any number of nonspecific abnormalities or may be completely normal even in the presence of a PE. The arterial blood gases are especially misleading because it is possible to have a significant PE with a completely normal PO_2 and/or A-a oxygen gradient on room air. In an editorial titled "Diagnosis

Table 34.6. Symptoms of Acute PE

Symptom	PE (n = 117)	No PE (n = 248)
Dyspnea	85 (73%)	178 (72%)
Pleuritic pain	77 (66%)	146 (59%)
Cough	42 (37%)	89 (36%)
Leg swelling	33 (28%)	55 (22%)
Leg pain	30 (26%)	60 (24%)
Hemoptysis	15 (13%)	20 (8%)
Palpitations	12 (10%)	44 (18%)
Wheezing	10 (9%)	28 (11%)
Angina-like pain	5 (4%)	15 (6%)

Adapted from Stein PD, et al. Chest 1991;100:598–603.

Table 34.7. Signs of Acute PE

Sign	PE (n = 117)	No PE (n = 248)
Tachypnea (> 20/min)	82 (70%)	169 (68%)
Rales	60 (51%)	98 (40%)
Tachycardia (> 100/min)	35 (30%)	59 (24%)
S_3 or S_4	31 (27%)	44 (17%)
Increased P_2	27 (23%)	3 (13%)
Deep venous thrombosis	13 (11%)	27 (11%)
Diaphoresis	13 (11%)	20 (8%)
Temperature > 38.5°C	8 (7%)	29 (12%)
Wheezes	6 (5%)	21 (8%)
Homan's sign	5 (4%)	6 (2%)
Pleural Friction Rub	3 (3%)	6 (2%)

Adapted from Stein PD, et al. Chest 1991;100:598–603.

of Pulmonary Embolism (When Will We Ever Learn?)" (Chest 1995;107:3–4), Robin, et al. stated,

> In the present study in Chest, it is demonstrated conclusively that about 20% of patients with angiographically documented PE have a normal $P(A-a)O_2$ tension difference. Using a normal difference to exclude PE would lead to a large number of false negatives.

These studies underscore the fact that one cannot rely on the arterial blood gases to rule in or rule out PE. Blood gases should be obtained to determine the degree of hypoxemia present and to determine if supplemental oxygen is indicated.

An initial step in the diagnosis of PE is to obtain a six-view ventilation and perfusion lung scan: anterior, posterior, right lateral, left lateral, right posterior oblique, and left-posterior oblique. The lung scan is particularly helpful if there is completely normal perfusion, thus ruling out PE. Also, if there is a high probability scan, then 87% of the time the patient

Table 34.5. Causes of Death in 95 Patients with PE

Cause of Death	No. (%)	Relative Risk
Cancer	33 (35)	3.8
Infection	21 (22)	—
Cardiac	16 (17)	2.7
Pulmonary Embolism	10 (10.5)	—
Pulmonary	5 (%)	2.2
Stroke	5 (5)	—
Miscellaneous	5 (5)	—

Adapted from Carson JL, et al. N Engl J Med 1992;326:1240–1245.

Table 34.8. Probability of PE by Lung-Scan Findings	
Scan Category	*Probability of PE*
High	87%
Intermediate	30%
Low	14%

Adapted from PIOPED. JAMA 1990;263:2753.

Table 34.9.   Comparison of Spiral CT and Pulmonary Angiography in the Diagnosis of PE

• Sensitivity	39/43 (91%)
• Specificity	25/32 (78%)
• Positive Predictive Value	39/39 (100%)
• Negative Predictive Value	32/36 (89%)

Adapted from Remy-Jardin M, et al. Radiology 1996;200:699–706.

does have a PE (Table 34.8). However, in the Prospective Investigation of PE Diagnosis (PIOPED) study, only 42% of patients with a pulmonary embolus had a high-probability scan. It is important to remember that a low-probability or intermediate-probability scan does not rule out PE. In the PIOPED study, 14% of patients with low-probability scans in fact did have pulmonary emboli on pulmonary arteriography. The patient should be treated based on a high-probability lung scan as long as there are no contraindications to the use of anticoagulants.

The difficulty lies in patients with a low-probability, indeterminate, or nondiagnostic lung scan. If the lung scan is nondiagnostic, a duplex ultrasound of the leg veins can be obtained. If the duplex is negative, then serial duplex scans can be performed, and treatment can be withheld. However, if there is still a strong clinical suspicion, a pulmonary arteriogram could be performed. Pulmonary arteriography is still the gold standard in diagnosing pulmonary emboli. In the PIOPED study, the death rate associated with pulmonary arteriography in 1101 patients was 0.5%. The overall major complication rate was 1.3%, illustrating that pulmonary arteriography is a safe and effective means to diagnose pulmonary emboli in patients in whom the diagnosis is unclear.

Several newer imaging modalities have been used to diagnose pulmonary emboli in recent years. Transthoracic echocardiography may demonstrate one or more of the following:

• Right ventricular dilatation and/or hypokinesis
• Interventricular septal flattening and paradoxic motion
• Tricuspid valve regurgitation
• Pulmonary artery dilatation
• Decrease in inspiratory collapse of the inferior vena cava

Pruszczyk, et al. recently showed that transesophageal echocardiography (TEE) was a highly sensitive and specific test to diagnose pulmonary emboli. TEE showed unequivocal (20 patients) or suspected (3 patients) intraluminal thrombi in 88.5% of 26 patients with pulmonary emboli. The sensitivity of unequivocal pulmonary emboli was 80% and the specificity was 100% (no false positives). TEE is a very useful imaging modality in the critically ill patient in the intensive care unit who is too unstable to transport. TEE can be performed rapidly at the bedside with a high degree of accuracy.

Magnetic resonance imaging (MRI) has been used in some centers to diagnose PE. Erdman, et al. demonstrated:

• Sensitivity: 90%
• Specificity: 77%
• Positive predictive value: 86%
• Negative predictive value: 83%

MRI may take some time to perform, and does require breath holding (which may be difficult in unstable patients). Spiral computerized tomography (CT) scanning also appears to also be accurate in the diagnosis of PE. CT requires the administration of a bolus of contrast and some breath holding. The positive and negative predictive values were quite good when spiral CT scanning was compared with pulmonary arteriography (Table 34.9). Surprisingly, the sensitivity and specificity of spiral CT scanning was sensitive and specific in both the central and peripheral vascular zones of the lungs.

TREATMENT OF PULMONARY EMBOLISM

Figure 34.4 illustrates the pathophysiologic abnormalities that may be present in patients with acute PE. The acuity and severity of the cardiopulmonary hemodynamics will help to determine what therapy is most appropriate in an individual patient. Once the diagnosis of PE is considered, a bolus of heparin should be administered (as long as there are no contraindications to anticoagulation) and a heparin drip started. The patient should then undergo the necessary diagnostic test(s) to rule in or out PE.

Thrombolytic therapy has proved to be a useful therapeutic modality in patients with pulmonary emboli. Reasons to consider administering thrombolytic therapy in acute PE include:

• Acute hemodynamic instability
  • Reverse abnormal hemodynamics
  • Lower mortality
• Reverse acute and subacute right ventricular dysfunction
• Prevent (? reverse) chronic thromboembolic pulmonary hypertension

Thrombolytic therapy currently is recommended for patients with:

• PE-causing hemodynamic instability
• Massive pulmonary embolus
• PE-causing right ventricular dysfunction

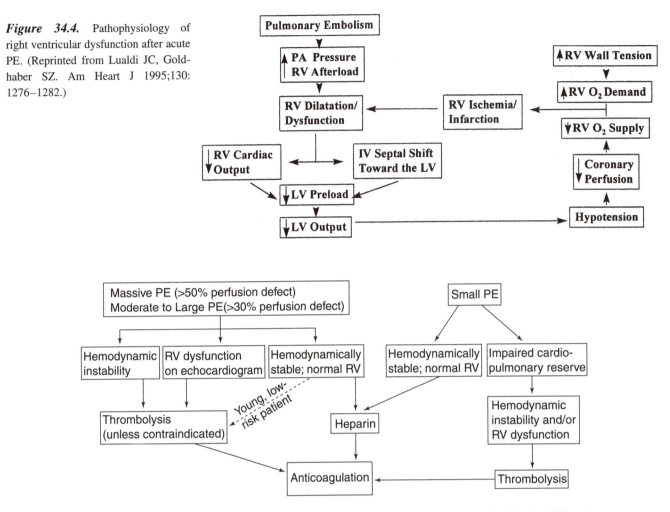

Figure 34.4. Pathophysiology of right ventricular dysfunction after acute PE. (Reprinted from Lualdi JC, Goldhaber SZ. Am Heart J 1995;130:1276–1282.)

Figure 34.5. Treatment of acute PE. (Adapted from Wolfe MW, et al. Curr Prob Cardiol Oct 1993; and Lualdi JC, Goldhaber SZ. Am Heart J 1995;130:1276–1282.)

• Pulmonary embolus of any size plus cardiac or pulmonary hemodynamic compromise

An algorithm for the treatment of patients with acute PE appears in Figure 34.5.

The streptokinase/urokinase PE trials have shown that thrombolytic therapy successfully decreased pulmonary artery pressures acutely and that there was improvement in the lung scan and arteriogram at 12 and 24 hours. However, there was no overall decrease in mortality in those patients who received thrombolytic agents compared with those who received heparin therapy. The recently published Management and Prognosis of Pulmonary Embolism Registry showed that the death rate in the thrombolysis group (n = 169) was 4.7% and in the heparin group (n = 550) was 11.1%, p = 0.016. Most of the deaths were related to PE.

Echocardiography may be useful in the diagnosis of pulmonary emboli and can help to determine to what degree the pulmonary embolus is causing an impairment in right ventricular function. A prospective, randomized trial comparing heparin therapy with intravenous t-PA (100 mg over 2 hours)

Table 34.10.   Alteplase vs. Heparin in Acute PE

	Echocardiographic Results	
	Improved	*Worsened*
rt-PA (n = 18)	89%[a]	6%
Heparin (n = 18)	44%[a]	28%

[a] P = 0.03

Adapted from Goldhaber SZ, et al. Lancet 1993;341:507–511.

demonstrated that t-PA was superior to heparin in reversing right ventricular dysfunction after an acute pulmonary embolus. Table 34.10 shows the likelihood of reversing right ventricular dysfunction in a subgroup of 36 patients who had RV hypokinesis prior to randomization.

Preliminary data suggest that pulmonary capillary blood volume and diffusing capacity, pulmonary artery pressures, and pulmonary vascular resistance are better at 2 weeks, 1 year, and 7 years after a PE in patients treated with thrombo-

Table 34.11.   Major Bleeding in Patients Treated with Thrombolytic Therapy after Pulmonary Angiography

Author	Heparin + Thrombolytic	No. (%) with Major Bleeding	Bleeding Complications
Verstraete (1988)	Yes	4/34 (11.7%)	≥ 2 units blood
PIOPED (1990)	Yes	1/9 (11.1%)	≥ 2 units blood
Dalla-Volta (1992)	Yes	4/20 (20%)	1 IC bleed, 2 pericardial, 1 retroperitoneal
Goldhaber (1988)	No	4/22 (18.2%)	≥ 10% drop in Hct
Goldhaber (1992)	No	5/44 (11.4%)	2 IC, 3 ≥ 2 units of blood

Modified from Stein PD, et al. Ann Intern Med 1994;121:313.

lytic therapy compared with heparin therapy. This may be important, since 25% of patients demonstrate unresolved PE on repeat lung scans, and at least some of these individuals may go on to develop chronic thromboembolic pulmonary hypertension. The subset of patients who do go on to develop chronic thromboembolic pulmonary hypertension may require a pulmonary thromboendarterectomy or else die of right-sided heart failure. The pulmonary thromboendarterectomy is performed via a median sternotomy and cardiopulmonary bypass, hypothermia, and cardioplegia. In Moser's series, this operation was successful in decreasing pulmonary artery pressures and in improving functional class.

Goldhaber, et al. performed a randomized, controlled trial comparing tissue plasminogen activator with urokinase in the treatment of acute PE. This initial study, which compared 100 mg of t-PA with 4400 u/kg/hr of urokinase, determined that t-PA was more effective in the short term (2 hours) compared with urokinase. The dosage between these two drugs was not really comparable. A more recent randomized trial by Goldhaber and colleagues compared 100 mg of t-PA with 3 million units of urokinase. One million units of urokinase was given initially as a bolus over 10 minutes and the remaining 2 million units were given over the next 2 hours. Both drugs were delivered via a peripheral vein. There was no difference in the amount of thrombolysis at 2 hours or in the improvement in the perfusion lung scan at 24 hours in patients randomized with urokinase or tissue plasminogen activator. Both drugs were equally effective, and the side effect profile was similar. Several studies have shown that bolus t-PA therapy (0.6 mg/kg, not to exceed 50 mg) was as good as the standard dose of 100 mg of t-PA infused over 2 hours. Major bleeding in patients treated with thrombolytic therapy for PE has been summarized by Stein and colleagues (Table 34.11).

Thrombolytic therapy should not be used in patients with active internal bleeding or a recent stroke (less than 2 months). It also should not be used in patients who have an intracranial process such as neoplasm or abscess. Relative contraindications include recent surgery or organ biopsy (10 days), uncontrolled hypertension, and pregnancy. The major complication associated with thrombolytic therapy is bleeding, and this can be minimized by careful patient selection and avoidance of

Table 34.12.   Prophylaxis for Deep Venous Thrombosis and PE

Operation or Condition	Prophylaxis
• General abdominal or thoracic surgery	Heparin 5000 U 2 hours before OR and Q 12 hours
• Medical patients (CHF, MI, stroke)	Heparin 5000 U Q 12 hours
• Eye surgery, neurosurgery, open prostatectomy	Pneumatic compression stockings
• Total hip or knee replacement	Low-molecular-weight heparin Adjusted-dose heparin Pneumatic CS Warfarin

Table 34.13.   Incidence of Thromboembolism by Patient Risk Categories

Thrombotic Event	Low Risk	Moderate Risk	High Risk
Calf vein thrombosis	~ 2%	10%–20%	40%–70%
Proximal VT	~ 0.4%	2%–4%	10%–20%
Fatal PE	< 0.02%	0.2%–0.5%	1%–5%

Modified from Hirsh J, Hoak J. Circulation 1996;93:2212–2245.

invasive procedures. Vessels that cannot be directly compressed should not be invaded.

For various reasons, some patients cannot receive anticoagulation therapy. In these individuals, an inferior vena cava filter should be placed. The indications for inferior vena cava interruption include:

• Prevention in patients with venous thromboembolism who have a poor cardiopulmonary reserve and who would not survive even a small PE
• Chronic recurrent PE

- Contraindication to anticoagulation in a patient with DVT or PE
- Major complication with anticoagulation
- Recurrence of PE or extension of DVT despite adequate anticoagulation
- Massive PE with severe cardiovascular instability

Prophylaxis

The most important aspect in the management of patients with venous thromboembolic disease is to assure that every patient receives adequate prophylaxis when indicated. Studies have shown this not to be the case. The principles outlined in the Fourth ACCP Consensus Conference on Antithrombotic Therapy (Chest 1995;108(Suppl):312S–334S) and in the American Heart Association /Scientific Statement (Circulation 1996;93:2212–2245) should be followed. General guidelines for prophylaxis appear in Table 34.12.

Hirsh and Hoak have assessed the incidence of venous thromboembolism in low-risk patients (younger than 40, uncomplicated surgery), moderate-risk patients (older than 40, undergoing general surgery, acute myocardial infarction, or leg fracture), and high-risk patients (hip and major knee surgery, previous venous thrombosis, surgery for extensive malignant disease) (Table 34.13). They recommend:

- Low-risk group: Early ambulation
- Moderate-risk group: Low-dose heparin (5000 U bid or intermittent pneumatic compression)
- High-risk group: Low-molecular-weight heparin, adjusted-dose heparin or moderate dose warfarin

BIBLIOGRAPHY

A Collaborative Study by the PIOPED investigators. Tissue plasminogen activator for the treatment of acute pulmonary embolism. Chest 1990;97:528–533.

Alpert JS. Mortality in patients treated for pulmonary embolism. JAMA 1976;236:1477–1480.

Alpert JS, Dalen JE. Epidemiology and natural history of venous thromboembolism. Prog Cardiovasc Dis 1994;36:417–422.

Anderson FA, et al. Physician practices in the prevention of venous thromboembolism. Ann Intern Med 1991;115:591–595.

Ansell JE. Oral anticoagulant therapy—50 years later. Arch Intern Med 1993;153:586–596.

Arnsen H et al. Streptokinase or heparin in the treatment of deep vein thrombosis: Follow-up results of a prospective study. Acta Med Scand 1982;11:65.

Ascer E, Gennaro M, Lorensen E, et al. Superior vena caval Greenfield filters: indications, techniques and results. J Vasc Surg 1996;23:498–503.

Ballew KA, Philbrick JT, Becker DM. Vena cava filter devices. Clin Chest Med 1995;16:295–305.

Becker DM, Philbrick JT, Bachhuber TL, et al. D-dimer testing and acute venous thromboembolism. A short cut to accurate diagnosis. Arch Intern Med 1996;156:939–946.

Becker RC, Ansell J. Antithrombotic therapy. An abbreviated reference for clinicians. Arch Intern Med 1995;155:149–161.

Bergqvist D, Jenpeg S, Johansen L, et al. Cost of long-term complications of deep venous thrombosis of the lower extremities: an analysis of a defined patient population in Sweden. Ann Intern Med 1997;126:454–457.

Beyth RJ et al. Long-term outcomes of deep-vein thrombosis. Arch Intern Med 1995;155:1031–1037.

Blum AG, Delfau F, Grignon B, et al. Spiral-computed tomography versus pulmonary angiography in the diagnosis of acute massive pulmonary embolism. Am J Cardiol 1994;74:96–98.

Brill-Edwards P, Ginsberg JS, Johnston M, et al. Establishing a therapeutic range for heparin. Ann Intern Med 1993;119:104–109.

Bussey HI et al. Reliance on prothrombin time ratios cause significant errors in anticoagulation therapy. Arch Intern Med 1992;152:278–282.

Caprini JA, Arcelus JI, Hoffman K, et al. Prevention of venous thromboembolism in North America: Results of a survey among general surgeons. J Vasc Surg 1994;20:751–758.

Carson JH, et al. Natural history of patients with pulmonary embolism. N Engl J Med 1992;326:1240–1245.

Carter CJ. The natural history and epidemiology of venous thrombosis. Prog Cardiovasc Dis 1994;36:423–438.

Clagett GP, et al. Prevention of venous thromboembolism. Chest 1992:102(Suppl4):391S–407S.

Clagett GP, Anderson FA, Heit J, et al. Prevention of venous thromboembolism. Fourth ACCP Consensus Conference on Antithrombotic Therapy. Chest 1995;108(Suppl):312S–334S.

Cole MS. Coumadin necrosis—a review of the literature. Surgery 1988;103:271–386.

Cornuz J, Pearson SD, Creager MA, et al. Importance of findings on the initial evaluation for cancer in patients with symptomatic, idiopathic deep venous thrombosis. Ann Intern Med 1996;125:785–793.

Come P, et al. Echocardiographic recognition of pulmonary

arterial disease and the determination of its cause. Am J Med 1988;84:384–394.

Comerota AJ. An overview of thrombolytic therapy for venous thromboembolism. In: Comerota AJ, ed. Thrombolytic therapy. Orlando, FL: Grune & Stratton, 1988:65–89.

Comerota AJ, et al. A strategy of aggressive regional therapy for acute iliofemoral venous thrombosis with contemporary venous thrombectomy or catheter-directed thrombolysis. J Vasc Surg 1994;20:244–254.

Coon W. Hemorrhagic complications of anticoagulant therapy. Arch Intern Med 1974;133:386–392.

Daily PO, et al. Current early results of pulmonary thromboendarterectomy for chronic pulmonary embolism. Eur J Cardiothorac Surg 1990;4:117–123.

Daily PO, et al. Risk factors for pulmonary thrombo-endarterectomy. J Thorac Cardiovasc Surg 1990;99:670–678.

Dalen JE, et al. Resolution rate of acute pulmonary embolism in man. N Engl J Med 1969;280:1194–1199.

Dalen JE. When can treatment be withheld in patients with suspected pulmonary embolism? Arch Intern Med 1993;153:1415–1418.

Dalen JE, Alpert JS. Natural history of pulmonary embolism. Prog Cardiovasc Dis 1975;17:259–269.

Elliot MS, et al. A comparative randomized trial of heparin vs. streptokinase in the treatment of acute proximal venous thrombosis: an interim report of a prospective trial. Br J Surg 1979;66:838.

Erdman WA, Peshock RM, Redman HC, et al. Pulmonary embolism: comparison of MR images with radionucleide and angiographic studies. Radiology 1994;190:499–508.

Fedullo PF, Auger WR, Channick RN, et al. Chronic thromboembolic pulmonary hypertension. Clin Chest Med 1995;16:353–374.

Finazzi G, Brancaccio V, Moia M, et al. Natural history and risk factors for thrombosis in 360 patients with antiphospholipid antibodies. A four-year prospective study from the Italian registry. Am J Med 1996;100:530–536.

Geerts WH, et al. A prospective study of venous thromboembolism after major trauma. N Engl J Med 1994;331:1601–1606.

Gefter WB, et al. Pulmonary thromboembolism: recent developments and diagnosis with CT and MR imaging. Radiology 1995;197:561–574.

Ginsberg JS. Management of venous thromboembolism. N Engl J Med 1996;335:1816–1828.

Ginsberg JS, Wells PS, Brill-Edwards P, et al. Antiphospholipid antibodies and venous thromboembolism. Blood 1995;86:3685–3691.

Gitter MJ, et al. Bleeding and thromboembolism during anticoagulant therapy: a population-based study in Rochester, Minnesota. Mayo Clin Proc 1995;70:725–733.

Goldberg RJ. Occult malignant neoplasm in patients with deep venous thrombosis. Arch Intern Med 1987;147:251–253.

Goldhaber SZ, Agnelli G, Levin MN. Reduced dose bolus alteplase vs conventional alteplase infusion for pulmonary embolism thrombolysis. Chest 1994;106:718.

Goldhaber SZ, Haire WD, Feldstein ML, et al. Alteplase versus heparin in acute pulmonary embolism: Randomized trial assessing right ventricular function and pulmonary perfusion. Lancet 1993;341:507–511.

Goldhaber SZ, et al. Recombinant tissue-type plasminogen activator vs. a novel dosing regimen of urokinase in acute pulmonary embolism: a randomized controlled multicenter trial. J Am Coll Cardiol 1992;20:24–30.

Goldhaber SZ, et al. Randomized control trial of tissue plasminogen activator and proximal deep venous thrombosis. Am J Med 1990;88:389–396.

Goldhaber SZ. Randomized controlled trial of recombinant tissue plasminogen activator vs. urokinase in the treatment of acute pulmonary embolism. Lancet 1988;1:293–298.

Goldhaber SZ. Pooled analysis of randomized trials of streptokinase and heparin in phlebographically documented acute deep venous thrombosis. Am J Med 1984;76:393–397.

Goldhaber SZ, et al. Quantitative plasma d-Dimer levels among patients undergoing pulmonary angiography for suspected pulmonary embolism. JAMA 1993;270:2819–2822.

Goodman LR, Curtin JJ, Mewissen MW, et al. Detection of pulmonary embolism in patients with unresolved clinical and scintigraphic diagnosis: helical CT versus angiography. Am J Radiol 1995;164:1369–1374.

Gray BH, Olin JW, Graor RA et al. Safety and efficacy of thrombolytic therapy for superior vena cava syndrome. Chest 1991;99:54–59.

Greenfield LJ et al. Long-term experience with trans-venous catheter pulmonary embolectomy. J Vasc Surg 1993;18:450–458.

Greenfield LJ. Twelve-year clinical experience with the Greenfield vena cava filter. Surgery 1988;104:706–712.

Harrison L, Johnston M, Massicotte MP, et al. Comparison of 5-mg and 10-mg loading doses in initiation of warfarin therapy. Ann Intern Med 1997;126:133–136.

Harvey RL, Roth EJ, Yarnold PR, et al. Deep vein thrombosis and stroke. The use of plasma D-dimer level as screening test in the rehabilitation setting. Stroke 1996;27:1516–1520.

Heijboer H, Buller HR, Lensing AWA, et al. A comparison of real-time compression ultrasonography with impedance plethysmography for the diagnosis of deep-vein thrombosis in symptomatic outpatients. N Engl J Med 1993;329: 1365–1369.

Hillarp A, Zoller B, Dahlback B. Activated protein C resistance as a basis for venous thrombosis. Am J Med 1996;101: 534–540.

Hirsch DR, Ingenito EP, Goldhaber SZ. Prevalence of deep venous thrombosis among patients in medical intensive care. JAMA 1995;274:335–337.

Hirsch DR, Mikkola KM, Marks PW. Pulmonary embolism and deep venous thrombosis during pregnancy or oral contraceptive use: Prevalence of Factor V Leiden. Am Heart J 1996; 131:1145–1148.

Hirsh J et al. The International Normalized Ratio. A guide to understanding and correcting its problems. Arch Intern Med 1994;154:282–288.

Hirsh J, Hoak J. Management of deep vein thrombosis and pulmonary embolism. A statement for health care professionals. From the Council on Thrombosis (in consultation with the Council on Cardiovascular Radiology), American Heart Association. Circulation 1996;93:2212–2245.

Hirsh J, Levine MN. Low molecular weight heparin. Blood 1992;79:1–17.

Hommes DW, et al. Subcutaneous heparin compared with continuous intravenous heparin administration in the initial treatment of deep vein thrombosis. A meta-analysis. Ann Intern Med 1992;116:279–284.

Hull RD, et al. A non-invasive strategy for the treatment of patients with suspected pulmonary embolism. Arch Intern Med 1994;154:289–297.

Hull RD, et al. Cost-effectiveness of pulmonary embolism diagnosis. Arch Intern Med 1996;156:68–72.

Hull RD, et al. Heparin for 5 days as compared with 10 days in the initial treatment of proximal deep venous thrombosis. N Engl J Med 1990;322:1260–1264.

Hull RD, et al. Low-probability lung scan findings: a need for change. Ann Intern Med 1991;114:142–143.

Hull RD, Raskob GE, Pineo GF, Brant RF. The low-probability lung scan. A need for change in nomenclature. Arch Intern Med 1995;155:1845–1851.

Imperial T, Speroff T. A meta-analysis of methods to prevent venous thromboembolism following total hip replacement. JAMA 1994;271:1780–1785.

Jaff M, Olin JW, Piedmonte M, et al. Heparin administration via nomogram versus standard approach in venous and arterial disorders. Vasc Med 1996;1:97–101.

Kakkar VV, et al. Low-molecular weight vs. standard heparin for prevention of venous thromboembolism after major abdominal surgery. Lancet 1993;341:259–265.

Kershaw B, White RH, Mungall D, et al. Computer-assisted dosing of heparin. In management with a pharmacy-based anticoagulation service. Arch Intern Med 1994;154: 1005–1011.

Konstantinides S, Geibel A, Kasper W. Role of cardiac ultrasound in the detection of pulmonary embolism. Semin Respir Crit Care Med 1996;17:39–49.

Konstantinides S, Geibel A, Olschewski M, et al. Association between thrombolytic treatment and the prognosis of hemodynamically stable patients with major pulmonary embolism. Results of a multicenter registry. Circulation 1997; 96: 882–888.

Koopman MMW, et al. Treatment of venous thrombosis with intravenous unfractionated heparin administered in the hospital as compared with subcutaneous low molecular weight heparin administered at home. N Engl J Med 1996;334:682–687.

Koster T, Rosendaal FR, Ronde HD, et al. Venous thrombosis due to poor anticoagulant response to activated protein C. Leiden thrombophilia study. Lancet 1993;342:1503–1506.

Leizorovicz A, et al. Comparison of efficacy and safety of low molecular weight heparin and unfractionated heparin in initial treatment of deep venous thrombosis. A meta-analysis. Br Med J 1994;309:299–304.

Levine MN. Thrombolytic therapy for venous thromboembolism. Complications and contraindications. Clin Chest Med 1995;16:321–328.

Levine M, et al. A comparison of low molecular weight heparin administered primarily at home with unfractionated heparin administered in the hospital for proximal deep-vein thrombosis. N Engl J Med 1996;334:677–681.

Levine MN. Hemorrhagic complications of long-term anticoagulant therapy. Chest 1989;95(Suppl):26S–36S.

Levine MN, et al. Optimal duration of oral anticoagulant therapy: A randomized trial comparing 4 weeks with 3 months of warfarin in patients with proximal deep vein thrombosis. Thromb Haemost 1995;74:606–611.

Levine MN, et al. Prevention of deep vein thrombosis after elective hip surgery. Ann Intern Med 1991;114:545–551.

Levine MN, et al. Prevention of deep venous thrombosis after elective hip surgery. A randomized trial comparing low molecular weight heparin with standard unfractionated heparin. Ann Intern Med 1991;114:545–551.

Lindblad B, et al. Incidence of venous thromboembolism verified by necropsy over 30 years. Br Med J 1991;302:709–711.

Lohr JM, James KV, Deschmukh RM, et al. Calf vein thrombi or not a benign finding. Am J Surg 1995;170:86–90.

Lualdi JC, Goldhaber SZ. Right ventricular dysfunction after acute pulmonary embolism: Pathophysiologic factors, detection and therapeutic implications. Am Heart J 1995;130: 1276–1282.

Machleder HI. Thrombolytic therapy and surgery for primary axillosubclavian vein thrombosis: Current approach. Semin Vasc Surg 1996;9:46–49.

Mandel H, Brenner B, Berant M, et al. Coexistence of hereditary homocysteinuria and Factor V Leiden-effect on thrombosis. N Engl J Med 1996;334:763–768.

Meier GH, Pollak JS, Rosenblatt M, et al. Initial experience with venous stents in exertional axillary-subclavian vein thrombosis. J Vasc Surg 1996;24:974–983.

Morgenthaler TI, Ryu JH. Clinical characteristics of fatal pulmonary embolism in a referral hospital. Mayo Clin Proc 1995; 70:417–422.

Moser KM, et al. Frequent asymptomatic pulmonary embolism in patients with deep venous thrombosis. JAMA 1994; 271:223–225.

Moser KM. Thromboendarterectomy for chronic major vessel thromboembolic pulmonary hypertension. Ann Intern Med 1987;107:560–565.

Nichols Heit JA. Activated protein C resistance and thrombosis. Mayo Clin Proc 1996;71:897–898.

Nicod P, Peterson K, Levine M, et al. Pulmonary angiography and severe chronic pulmonary hypertension. Ann Intern Med 1987;107:565–568.

Ofosu FA. Mechanisms of action of heparin: applications to the development of derivatives of heparin and heparinoids with anti-thrombotic properties. Semin Thromb Hemost 1988; 14:9–17.

Olin JW. Thromboembolic disease: under-diagnosed, under-treated, deadly. Cleve Clin J Med 1994;61:97–99.

Olin JW. Treatment of deep vein thrombosis and pulmonary emboli in patients with primary metastatic brain tumors. Anticoagulants or inferior vena cava filter? Arch Intern Med 1987; 147:2177–2179.

Olin JW, Fonseca CM. Axillary and subclavian deep vein thrombosis. In: Callow AD, Ernst CB, eds. Vascular surgery, theory and practice. Stamford, CT: Appleton-Lange, 1995: 1437–1452.

Pacouret G, Alison D, Dottier J, et al. Free-floating thrombus and embolic risk in patients with angiographically confirmed proximal venous thrombosis. A prospective study. Arch Intern Med 1997;157:305–308.

Perkins JM, Magee TR, Galand RB. Phlegmasia cerulea dolens and venous gangrene. J Surg 1996;83:19–23.

Peterson CE. Current concepts of warfarin therapy. Arch Intern Med 1986;146:581–584.

Petitti DB. Duration of warfarin anticoagulant therapy and the probabilities of recurrent thromboembolism in hemorrhage. Am J Med 1986;81:255–259.

Phillips MD. Interrelated risk factors for venous thromboembolism. Circulation 1997;95:1749–1751.

Piccoli A, Prandoni P, Goldhaber SZ. Epidemiologic characteristics, management and outcome of deep venous thrombosis in a tertiary-care hospital: The Brigham and Women's Hospital DVT Registry. Am Heart J 1996;132:1010–1014.

Prandoni P, Lensing AWA, Buller HR, et al. Deep-vein thrombosis in the incidence of subsequent symptomatic cancer. N Engl J Med 1992;327:1128–1133.

Prandoni P, Lensing A, Cogo A, et al. The long-term clinical course of deep venous thrombosis. Ann Intern Med 1996;125: 1–7.

Prandoni P, Polistena P, Bernardi E, et al. Upper-extremity deep venous thrombosis. Risk factors, diagnosis and complications. Arch Intern Med 1997;157:57–62.

Prins MH, Lensing AWA, Hirsh J. Idiopathic deep venous thrombosis. Is a search for malignant disease justified? Arch Intern Med 1994;134:1310–1312.

Pruszczyk P et al. Transesophageal echocardiography for definitive diagnosis of haemodynamically significant pulmonary embolism. Eur Heart J 1995;16:534–538.

Raschke RA, Reilly BM, Guidry JR, et al. The rate-based heparin dosing nomogram compared with ''standard care'' nomogram. A randomized controlled trial. Ann Intern Med 1993;119:874–881.

Remy-Jardin M, Remy J, Deschildre F, et al. Diagnosis of pulmonary embolism with spiral CT: comparison with pulmonary angiography and scintigraphy. Radiology 1996;200: 699–706.

Rich S. Pulmonary hypertension from chronic pulmonary thromboembolism. Ann Intern Med 1988;108:425–434.

Ridker PM, Glynn RJ, Miletich JP, et al. Age-specific incidence rates of venous thromboembolism among heterozygous carriers of Factor V Leiden mutation. Ann Intern Med 1997; 126:528–531.

Ridker PM, Hennekens CH, Selhub J, et al. Interrelation of hyperhomocyst(e)inemia, Factor V Leiden, and risk of future thromboembolism. Circulation 1997;95:1777–1782.

Ridker PM, Miletich JP, Stampfer MJ, et al. Factor V Leiden and risks of recurrent idiopathic venous thrombosis. Circulation 1995;92:2800–2802.

Rodgers LQ, et al. Streptokinase therapy for deep venous

thrombosis: a comprehensive review of the English literature. Am J Med 1990;88:235–240.

Rogers FB, Shakford SR, Ricci MA, et al. Routine prophylactic vena cava filter insertion in severely injured trauma patients decreases the incidence of pulmonary embolism. J Am Coll Surg 1995;180:641–647.

Rosove MH, Brewer PMC. Antiphospholipid thrombosis: clinical course after the first thrombotic event in 70 patients. Ann Intern Med 1992;117:303–308.

Rutherford RB. Pathogenesis and pathophysiology of post-thrombotic syndrome: clinical implications. Semin Vasc Surg 1996;9:21–25.

Schafer AI. Low molecular weight heparin-an opportunity for home treatment of venous thrombosis. N Engl J Med 1996; 344:724–725.

Schiebler ML, Holland GA, Hatabu H, et al. Suspected pulmonary embolism: prospective evaluation with pulmonary MR angiography. Radiology 1993;189:125–131.

Schulman S, et al. A comparison of six weeks with six months of oral anticoagulant therapy after a first episode of venous thromboembolism. N Engl J Med 1995;332:1661–1665.

Schulman S, Granqvist S, Holmostro M, et al. The duration of oral anticoagulant therapy after a second episode of venous thromboembolism. N Engl J Med 1997;336:393-398.

Semba CP, Dake MD. Iliofemoral deep venous thrombosis: aggressive therapy with catheter-directed thrombolysis. Radiology 1994;191:487–494.

Sharma GVRK, et al. Effect of thrombolytic therapy on pulmonary capillary blood volume in patients with pulmonary embolism. N Engl J Med 1980;303:842–845.

Simoni P, Prandoni P, Lensing AWA, et al. The risk of recurrent venous thromboembolism in patients with the AN Arg[506] Gln mutation in the gene for Factor V (Factor V Leiden). N Engl J Med 1997;336:399–403.

Slocum MM, Adams JG, Teel R, et al. Use of enoxaparin in patients with heparin-induced thrombocytopenia syndrome. J Vasc Surg 1996;23:839–843.

Sors H, Pacouret G, Azarian R, et al. Hemodynamic effects of bolus vs 2-h infusion of alteplase in acute massive pulmonary embolism. Chest 1994:106:712.

Stein PD, et al. Complications and validity of pulmonary angiography and acute pulmonary embolism. Circulation 1992; 85:462–468.

Stein PD, Gottschalk A. Critical review of ventilation/perfusion lung scans in acute pulmonary embolism. Prog Cardiovasc Dis 1994;37:13–24.

Stein PD, Henry JW. Prevalence of acute pulmonary embolism among patients in a general hospital and at autopsy. Chest 1995;108:978–981.

Stein PD, Hull RD, Raskob G. Risks for major bleeding from thrombolytic therapy in patients with acute pulmonary embolism. Ann Intern Med 1994;121:313.

Stewart JH, Olin JW, Graor RA. Thrombolytic therapy—a review. Cleve Clin J Med 1989;56:189-196, 290–296.

The PIOPED investigators. Value of ventilation-perfusion scan in acute pulmonary embolism. Results of the perspective investigation of pulmonary embolism diagnosis (PIOPED). JAMA 1990;263:2753–2759.

Thomas DP, Roberts HR. Hypercoagulability in venous and arterial thrombosis. Ann Intern Med 1997;126:638–644.

Toglia MR, Weg JG. Venous thromboembolism during pregnancy. N Engl J Med 1996;335:108–114.

Turpie AGG, et al. A randomized control trial of low molecular weight heparin (Enoxaparin) to prevent deep-vein thrombosis in patients undergoing elective hip surgery. N Engl J Med 1986;315:925–929.

Urokinase Pulmonary Embolism Trial. Circulation 1973; 47(Suppl2):1–108.

Urokinase Pulmonary Embolism Trial. Phase I results. A cooperative study. JAMA 1970;214:2163–2172.

Urokinase, Streptokinase Embolism Trial. Phase II results. A cooperative study. JAMA 1974;229:1606–1613.

Vandenbroucke JP, Koster T, Briet E, et al. The increased risk of venous thrombosis in oral-contraceptive users who are carriers of Factor V Leiden mutation. Lancet 1994;344: 1453–1457.

Warkentin TE, Kelton JG. A fourteen-year study of heparin-induced thrombocytopenia. Am J Med 1996;101:502–507.

Weinmann EE, Salzman EW. Deep-vein thrombosis. N Engl J Med 1994;331:1630–1641.

Wells PS, et al. A novel and rapid whole-blood assay for D-dimer in patients with clinically suspected deep vein thrombosis. Circulation 1995;91:2184–2187.

Wells PS, Lensing AWA, Davidson BL, et al. Accuracy of ultrasound for the diagnosis of venous thrombosis in asymptomatic patients after orthopedic surgery. A meta-analysis. Ann Intern Med 1995;122:47–53.

White RH et al. Diagnosis of deep vein thrombosis using duplex ultrasound. Ann Intern Med 1989;111:297–304.

Worsley DF, Alavi A. Comprehensive analysis of the results of PIOPED Study. J Nuc Med 1995;36:2380–2387.

Zeman RK, Silverman PM, Vieco PT, et al. CT angiography. J Radiol 1995;165:1079–1088.

SUGGESTED READINGS

Clagett GP, Anderson FA, Heit J, et al. Prevention of venous thromboembolism. Fourth ACCP Consensus Conference on Antithrombotic Therapy. Chest 1995;108(Suppl):312S–334S.

Ginsberg JS. Management of venous thromboembolism. N Engl J Med 1996;335:1816–1828.

Ginsberg JS, Wells PS, Brill-Edwards P, et al. Antiphospholipid antibodies and venous thromboembolism. Blood 1995; 86:3685–3691.

Hirsh J, Hoak J. Management of deep vein thrombosis and pulmonary embolism. A statement for health care professionals. From the Council on Thrombosis (in consultation with the Council on Cardiovascular Radiology), American Heart Association. Circulation 1996;93:2212–2245.

Levine M, et al. A comparison of low molecular weight heparin administered primarily at home with unfractionated heparin administered in the hospital for proximal deep-vein thrombosis. N Engl J Med 1996;334:677–681.

Olin JW, Fonseca CM. Axillary and subclavian deep vein thrombosis. In: Callow AD, Ernst CB, eds. Vascular surgery, theory and practice. Stamford, CT: Appleton-Lange, 1995: 1437–1452.

Raschke RA, Reilly BM, Guidry JR, et al. The rate-based heparin dosing nomogram compared with ''standard care'' nomogram. A randomized controlled trial. Ann Intern Med 1993;119:874–881.

The PIOPED investigators. Value of ventilation-perfusion scan in acute pulmonary embolism. Results of the perspective investigation of pulmonary embolism diagnosis (PIOPED). JAMA 1990;263:2753–2759.

Thomas DP, Roberts HR. Hypercoagulability in venous and arterial thrombosis. Ann Intern Med 1997;126:638–644.

Toglia MR, Weg JG. Venous thromboembolism during pregnancy. N Engl J Med 1996;335:108–114.

35

Lung Cancer

Alejandro C. Arroliga

As the leading cause of cancer death in the United States, lung cancer continues to be a major health hazard. At present, the lung cancer death rate is still rising. Although the death rate is expected to peak in the 1990s, it will remain very high over the next 2–3 decades.

In the United States, lung cancer is responsible for 28% of all deaths related to cancer and for 6% of all deaths. It continues to be the most common fatal malignancy in both genders. The American Cancer Society estimates that 171,500 cases of bronchogenic carcinoma will be newly diagnosed in 1998. The World Health Organization (WHO) estimated that there will be 2 million cases annually of bronchogenic carcinoma worldwide.

Bronchogenic carcinoma is very common in the minority population. Among African-Americans, bronchogenic carcinoma accounts for 25% of all cancer among males and 13% among females. This higher incidence of bronchogenic carcinoma and mortality is explained by socioeconomic factors; epidemiologic data suggest that the excess may be reduced when adjusted for education level and family income level of this population.

ETIOLOGY OF LUNG CANCER

Approximately 85% of all lung cancers are linked to smoking. The relationship between smoking and bronchogenic carcinoma has been appreciated since the 1950s. Smokers in general have 10–25 times the incidence of lung cancer than nonsmokers. When smokers quit, they experience a progressive decline in lung cancer risk; after 15 years of abstinence, the risk of developing lung cancer is near that of a life-long nonsmoker. Many factors are clearly related to high risk of developing bronchogenic carcinoma:

- Number of cigarettes smoked
- Duration in years of smoking
- Early age at initiation of smoking
- Depth of inhalation
- Tar and nicotine content in the cigarettes smoked

Smoking prevalence is highest in the group of individuals with incomes below poverty level. Smoking among women decreased from 33% in the 1970s to 25% in the 1990s, while smoking among men dropped from 43% to 28% in the same time period. Unfortunately, no decrease in smoking has been observed among those age 18–24, suggesting that the increased advertising and sales promotion by the tobacco industry is successfully reaching this age group. The prevalence of smoking among adolescents has remained unchanged (or even increased slightly) in the last few years. For example, in 1991, 28% of high school seniors had smoked within the previous 3 days. By 1993, the proportion had increased to 30%. Smoking prevalence among college freshman rose from 9% in 1985 to 13% in 1994. Every day, 3000 more young people become regular smokers. A person who has not started smoking as a teenager is unlikely to ever become a smoker. Therefore, it is important that our efforts should be directed at preventing young people from starting to smoke.

The carcinogenic effect of passive exposure—or second-hand smoke—has been determined lately. Second-hand smoking also increases the risk of bronchogenic carcinoma. The effect of passive smoking and lung cancer risk, under conditions of domestic exposure, increases a nonsmoker's low risk by about 30%. The significance of this lies not in the magnitude of the risk for any passive smoker exposed individually, which is quite small, but in the number of excess cancer deaths owing to the *frequency* of such environmental exposure in the general population. It is estimated that second-hand smoking from spouses of heavy smokers may explain 3000–5000 lung cancer deaths in the United States every year.

The carcinogenic substances in cigarette smoke are only partially understood. More than 40 carcinogens have been identified in cigarette smoke, including:

- Polycyclic aromatic hydrocarbons
- Nickel
- Vinyl chloride
- Aldehydes
- Catechols
- Peroxides
- Nitrosamines

There now is evidence that the formation of benzo (a) pyrene causes strong and selective adduct formation at guanine positions in codons 157, 248, and 273 of the P53 gene. This in turn appears to shape the P53 mutational spectrum in lung cancer, providing a direct etiologic link between a chemical carcinogen present in cigarette smoke and human cancer.

The use of filter-tipped, low-tar, and low-nicotine cigarettes does not reduce the risk of lung cancer because smokers increase the number of cigarettes smoked and the depth of inhalation with these cigarettes, resulting in an increased nicotine and carcinogen intake. In recent years, it has been suggested as well that the use of mentholated cigarettes actually increases the relative risk of lung cancer over nonmentholated cigarettes by 1.45 in men; in effect, this suggests that mentholation increases the lung-cancer-causing effect of cigarette smoking in men.

Other well-documented lung carcinogens include:

- Asbestos
- Ionizing radiation
- Chromium
- Nickel
- Mustard gas
- Vinyl chloride
- Arsenic
- Isopropyl oil
- Hydrocarbons
- Chloroethyl ether

Many of these materials have a carcinogenic effect that is additive or synergistic with cigarette smoke. For example, asbestos exposure in nonsmokers increases the incidence of bronchogenic cancer by 3–5 fold, but in smokers this risk may be increased 70–90 fold.

Radon gas, the decay product of uranium in the earth, has been recognized to be a carcinogen for many years. The interaction with cigarette smoking is synergistic. It is estimated that indoor and outdoor radon exposure in conjunction with past and current cigarette smoking may explain between 5–15,000 lung cancer deaths annually, or roughly 5%–10% of new lung cancer cases. The life-time risk of a nonsmoker is 1 in 357; if all radon was removed from all homes, this risk

would fall to 1 in 492. A life-long nonsmoker in a home with a high level of radon may have a life-time lung cancer risk of about 1 in 100; for a pack-a-day smoker, the risk rises to 1 in 14. With the removal of all radon from homes, the pack-a-day smoker's risk would drop to about 1 in 20.

Less well-established risk factors include:

- Air pollution
- Cigar and pipe smoking
- Lung scar
- Genetic determinants (such as elevated pulmonary cytochrome P450 enzymes)
- Vitamin A deficiency
- Vitamin E deficiency

PATHOPHYSIOLOGY OF LUNG CANCER

The four histopathological categories of bronchogenic carcinoma are:

- Nonsmall-cell lung cancers
  - Adenocarcinoma (30–35%)
  - Squamous-cell carcinoma (30–32%)
  - Large-cell carcinoma (15–20%)
- Small-cell carcinoma (20–25%)

During the mid-1980s, the rate of adenocarcinoma surpassed that of squamous cell carcinoma. All four major cell types have been associated with cigarette smoking.

The increased incidence of adenocarcinoma may be attributed partially to a more frequent appearance in women, changes in environmental exposures, and modification in the histologic calcification. Adenocarcinomas form acinar or glandular structures. Bronchoalveolar cell carcinoma, a subtype of adenocarcinoma, has unique histological and clinical presentations. Bronchoalveolar cell carcinoma might present as an isolated nodule but occurs in multicentric forms. The carcinoma arises from terminal bronchoalveolar regions and grows along alveolar walls, rather than invading the lung structure directly. Approximately 15% of all adenocarcinomas are subtyped as bronchoalveolar cell carcinoma.

Squamous cell carcinomas are composed of flattened or polygonal, stratified, epithelial cells that form intercellular bridges and elaborate keratin. The tumor tends to be bulky, usually an intrabronchial granular or polypoid mass that obstructs the lumen. Squamous cell carcinoma is the cell type more prone to cavitation, although in recent years higher incidence of cavitated adenocarcinoma has been reported.

Large cell carcinoma are composed of pleomorphic cells with variably enlarged nuclei and prominent nucleoli with abundant cytoplasm. The diagnosis of large cell carcinoma might be over estimated because tumors without clear differentiation often are classified as large cell tumors. Most of these tumors, similar to adenocarcinoma, are peripheral lesions unrelated to bronchi except for continuous growth. The metastatic pattern of large-cell carcinoma is similar to adenocarcinoma with cerebral metastases in half of the cases.

Squamous cell carcinoma, adenocarcinoma, and large-cell carcinoma belong to the clinical category of nonsmall-cell lung cancer. They are separated from the small-cell lung cancer group because the therapy is different. Small-cell lung cancer was felt to originate from the neuroectoderm, but actually may develop from a common pulmonary stem cell, with secondary differentiation into a cell type with neural characteristics. Approximately 80% of small-cell tumors are central in location and found mainly in a submucosal area. The small-cell tumor may spread into mediastinal lymph nodes without involving the respiratory tract.

CLINICAL PRESENTATION OF LUNG CANCER

In general, the clinical presentation of bronchogenic carcinoma depends on the cell type. Adenocarcinoma and large cell carcinoma tend to spread systemically relatively early in their course. Squamous cell carcinoma frequently invades locally prior to systemic spread. Small-cell lung cancer has a very aggressive behavior, with mediastinal and extra-thoracic spread. In the cases of mixed tumors, the behavior depends on the predominant cell type.

Approximately 15% of all patients are asymptomatic at the time of diagnosis; the tumor is found incidentally as a chest radiograph abnormality. As many as 40% of patients present with cough, while 70% to 80% develop cough during the course of the disease. A change in character of the cough in a smoker is a significant clinical manifestation and should trigger the search for a neoplasm. Streaky hemoptysis is present in 60% of the patients, and wheezing, dyspnea, stridor, obstructive pneumonitis, and vague chest pain are occasionally symptoms at the presentation. Bronchorrhea is an uncommon initial presentation of bronchoalveolar cell carcinoma; when it is present (20% of patients), it indicates extensive lung involvement.

Other signs and symptoms resulting from local tumor spread include:

- Hoarseness owing to involvement of the left recurrent laryngeal nerve, resulting in vocal cord paralysis
- Superior vena cava syndrome secondary to compression or invasion of the superior vena cava
- Pleural effusion owing to direct malignant invasion of the pleural space
- Mediastinal lymphatic obstruction or a parapneumonic effusion
- Esophageal obstruction
- Pericardial involvement
- Myocardial involvement
- Vertebral invasion
- In cases of superior sulcus tumors (Pancoast's tumors), direct invasion of the apex of the lung causing C7/T2 neuropathy and Horner's syndrome

Extra-thoracic manifestation of bronchogenic carcinoma may be because of direct tumor infiltration (metastasis) or to nonmetastatic complication known as paraneoplastic syndromes. Metastatic disease commonly involves:

- Thoracic lymph nodes
- Central nervous system (CNS)
- Liver
- Bone
- Adrenal glands
- Various areas of the lung

Bone and CNS involvement usually are symptomatic. Small-cell carcinoma predominantly involves bone marrow (up to 50% of the cases) with or without peripheral hematologic abnormalities.

Paraneoplastic syndromes occur between to 10–15% of patients with bronchogenic carcinoma. Paraneoplastic syndromes are manifestations of malignancies not caused by direct invasion of the tumor, infection, or side effects of the therapy of the primary tumor. The paraneoplastic syndromes most commonly present in bronchogenic carcinoma include:

- Hypercalcemia of malignancy
- Syndrome of inappropriate antidiuresis
- Ectopic Cushing's syndrome
- Paraneoplastic neurologic syndromes

Hypercalcemia of malignancy is predominantly associated with squamous cell carcinoma, although it may be caused by adenocarcinoma and large cell. Present in 15–20% of patients with advanced bronchogenic carcinoma, hypercalcemia is caused by the secretion of a protein called ''parathyroid hormone-related peptide'' by the tumor in 85% of the cases. The peptide, which has similar characteristics and function of the parathyroid hormone, increases the osteoclast activity with increased resorption of the bone. The management of hypercalcemia malignancy in patients with bronchogenic carcinoma include:

- Hydration
- Inhibition of bone resorption by administration of bisphosphonates
- Treatment of the malignancy

Inappropriate antidiuresis is caused by the ectopic secretion of arginine vasopressin. Atrial natriuretic factor and inappropriate thirst play an important role in the pathogenesis of this syndrome. Management of patients with inappropriate antidiuresis includes:

- Treatment of the small-cell carcinoma
- Water restriction
- Administration of demeclocycline and fludrocortisone

Ectopic Cushing's is caused by the secretion of proopiomelanocortin, a precursor of ACTH. Treatment of the ectopic Cushing's syndrome includes:

- Management of the tumor

- Administration of adrenal enzyme inhibitors like ketoconazole, metyrapone, and aminoglutethimide

Paraneoplastic neurologic syndromes, present in 1%–3% of patients with small-cell lung cancer, are more commonly associated with small-cell lung cancer. The most common of these fascinating disorders is the Eaton-Lambert syndrome. Other paraneoplastic neurologic disorders include subacute cerebellar degeneration, subacute sensory neuronopathy, and limbic encephalitis and polyneuropathy.

DIAGNOSIS OF LUNG CANCER

SCREENING

Mass screening of high-risk patients with serial chest radiographs and sputum cytology has showed a favorable impact on survival in patients with localized tumors. However, there has not been significant improvement in overall survival for lung cancer when all the patients entered into the studies were analyzed. Consequently, no consensus exists that high-risk patients should undergo yearly chest radiography or sputum cytology. Nevertheless, for the individual high-risk patient concerned about cancer, it may be reasonable to screen periodically, especially if the patient has multiple risk factors (such as a smoker who has been exposed to asbestos and radon). With significant airways disease, a yearly chest radiograph may be helpful.

DIAGNOSTIC STUDIES

Radiography

Most asymptomatic lung cancers are detected on plain chest radiographs. Lesions smaller than 5–6 mm in diameter are rarely noticed in the chest radiograph. In general, the radiographic appearance of a lesion will not distinguish between a benign or malignant process. The radiographic characteristic suggestive of a malignancy includes lobulation and margins that are shaggy and ill-defined. Adenocarcinoma usually presents as a peripheral lung mass and represents 40% of all peripheral lung tumors. At least 50% of the lesions are less than 4 cm.

Bronchoalveolar cell carcinoma presents as:

- A solitary nodule
- Numerous small unilateral or bilateral nodules
- A lobar or segmental unilateral or bilateral consolidation with or without air bronchograms

The majority of squamous cell carcinomas (65%) are centrally located and may cause:

- Partial or complete obstruction of the airways with radiographic changes of atelectasis
- Postobstructive pneumonia
- Lung abscess

- Bronchiectasis
- Mucoid impaction

When squamous cell carcinoma presents in a peripheral location, they usually cavitate and may resemble a lung abscess.

Large cell carcinoma is more frequently peripheral (72%) and tends to be sharply defined. The majority of lesions are more than 4 cm in diameter on presentation.

Small-cell lung cancer is a predominantly central lesion and presents as a hilar mass. The lesions almost never cavitate. Although the primary lesion does not tend to obstruct, the metastatic adenopathy will cause external compression of airways with a consequent atelectasis or postobstructive pneumonia. Small-cell lung cancer occasionally occurs peripherally.

Solitary Nodule Approximately 30% of all bronchogenic carcinomas present as a solitary nodule. Solitary pulmonary nodules are characterized by a single lesion up to 3 cm, surrounded by lung parenchyma. The number of nodules resulting from bronchogenic carcinoma will be approximately 55,000–111,000 per year.

In current medical practice, approximately 40–50% of solitary nodules are malignant. These malignancies are primarily bronchogenic carcinoma, but a small number (10%) are solitary metastatic deposits and approximately 2–3% are carcinoid tumors. Most of the malignant solitary nodules are large-cell carcinoma and adenocarcinoma. Small-cell carcinoma and squamous cell carcinoma rarely present as a solitary nodule. Benign nodules are almost all infectious granulomas. Other less common etiologies include hamartomas, other benign tumors, and noninfectious granulomas.

Establishing the etiology of solitary pulmonary nodules is a major clinical challenge. The goal in the management of a patient with a solitary pulmonary nodule is to identify malignant nodules that need surgery, while avoiding thoracotomy in those with benign nodules. Absence of growth in the size of the solitary pulmonary nodule for more than 24 months is considered to be a reliable sign of benignity. The presence of characteristic patterns of calcification, such as homogenous, popcorn, laminated and central calcifications, is considered to be evidence of benignity. If the solitary nodule is noncalcified and the pattern of growth in the last 2 years cannot be determined, the probability of cancer based on the clinical features (predictive variables) needs to be assessed. Important clinical features suggestive of malignancy include:

- Size of the nodule (> 3 cm)
- Age of the patient (patients under age 35 usually have benign nodules)
- Smoking history
- History of previous malignancy
- Radiological characteristics of the edge of the nodule
- Presence or absence of occult calcification determined by computerized tomography (CT)

The imaging techniques more commonly used in the evaluation of a solitary nodule include chest radiograph and CT. Obtaining previous chest radiographs is probably the most important diagnostic maneuver in the evaluation of a patient with a solitary nodule. As noted, a lesion that has remained stable in size for more than 2 years is more likely to be benign. Benign nodules, usually of infectious etiology, tend to grow very fast (i.e., faster than malignancies), with a doubling time of less than 21 days. CT allows better visualization of the nodule than the chest radiograph, provides better definition of the margins, and better helps detect calcifications and the presence of multiple lesions.

In addition to chest radiographs and CT, other imaging techniques that have been used in the evaluation of patients with solitary nodules include magnetic resonance imaging (MRI) and positron-emission tomography (PET). There is no role for MRI in the routine evaluation of the patient with a solitary pulmonary nodule. The PET scan uses uptake of 2 [F-18]-fluoro-2-deoxy-D-glucose (FDG) to measure uptake of glucose metabolism in the malignant tissue. Sensitivity of 95% and specificity of 80% has been reported in a group of patients with indeterminate nodules. Larger studies are needed of this new technique.

If the uncalcified nodule is still of undetermined etiology after all the above studies, and the probability of cancer is high, then a biopsy via transthoracic needle aspiration or thoracotomy is a reasonable choice, depending on the wishes of the patient. If the probability of cancer is high, immediate thoracotomy has the highest expected utility. However, in patients with low probability of cancer, a "wait and watch" strategy is favored.

Tissue Diagnosis

Currently available methods for tissue diagnosis of suspected lung cancer include:

* Sputum cytology
* Fiberoptic bronchoscopy
* Transthoracic needle aspiration
* Thoracotomy

Other techniques, potentially useful in selected cases, include:

* Thoracentesis (pleural biopsy)
* Pleuroscopy
* Mediastinoscopy

Sputum cytology is occasionally helpful in the diagnosis of central squamous and small-cell carcinomas. The results are variable and the interpretation may be technically difficult. A negative sputum cytology does not rule out the presence of bronchogenic carcinomas in the appropriate setting.

Bronchoscopy   Flexible fiberoptic bronchoscopy (FFB) is helpful in the diagnosis of central airway lesions. In this setting, FFB is diagnostic in 90% of the cases. In cases of peripheral lesions (tumor visible on chest radiograph but not on FFB), FFB has a diagnostic yield between 40–80% using transbronchial biopsy, brushings, and washings and biplanar fluoroscopy. This result is significantly lower than the yield in central lesions. The size of the lesion is the best determinant of diagnostic yield in peripheral lesions:

* Lesions < 2 cm diameter — 28–30% yield
* Lesions > 2 cm diameter — 64% yield
* Lesions > 4 cm diameter — 80% yield

Complications of bronchoscopy, which are infrequent (5%), include hemorrhage, pneumothorax, laryngospasm, and transient hypoxemia.

Transthoracic Needle Aspiration Biopsy   Transthoracic needle aspiration biopsy has been used to diagnose lung masses and mediastinal lesions. Needle aspiration, complements bronchoscopy in establishing the diagnosis of lung abnormalities. The diagnostic yield of percutaneous transthoracic needle aspiration is greater than 90% for peripheral lesions, but the prevalence of complication is increased, reportedly 25–30%. Up to 15% of patients require treatment with a chest tube to re-expand the lung.

It is important to emphasize that a negative result, unless it indicates a specific benign diagnosis, such as hamartoma, cannot be used to rule out carcinoma. If no contraindication exists (pulmonary and cardiac status no evidence of metastatic disease), one should proceed to thoracotomy.

STAGING

After tissue diagnosis, staging is important to assess the extent of local and distant disease. Accurate staging is crucial in the selection of therapy and for prognostic purposes. The TNM system is used to stage nonsmall-cell bronchogenic carcinoma. The TNM classification has been recently revised, and now more accurately reflects survival among homogenous groups:

* Resectable tumors
  * Stage IA (T1N0M0)
  * Stage IB (T2N0M0)
  * Stage IIA (T1N1M0)
  * Stage IIB (T2N1M0)
  * (T3N0M0)
  * Selected Stage IIIa (T3N1M0)
  * (T1-3N2M0)
* Unresectable tumors
  * Stage IIIb (any T, N3, M0)
  * Stage IV (any T, any N, M1)

Small-cell lung cancer generally is not included in the TNM classification because the majority of these tumors are in advanced stage at the time of the diagnosis. Small-cell lung cancer has 2 stages:

* Limited disease (implies that the tumor is confined within a radiation port)

- Extensive disease (implies disseminated disease beyond a radiation port)

Examination of the hilar and mediastinal areas is a key step in the staging process; CT scan of the chest is useful in this situation because it offers significant advantages compared with standard chest radiograph. When a lymph node is enlarged on CT (greater than 2 cm), histologic examination is needed before assuming tumor involvement. Transbronchial needle aspiration, transthoracic needle aspiration, and mediastinoscopy are some of the techniques that have been used to sample mediastinal lymph nodes. Mediastinoscopy remains the standard for the purpose of mediastinal staging in non-small-cell carcinoma patients. CT scan of the chest and MRI of the chest are of value in detecting chest wall or pleural involvement in patients with lung cancer. MRI has been found to be helpful, especially for patients who have superior sulcus tumors, for delineating vascular and neural invasion, and for patients with tumor invasion of the pericardium and heart.

COMPLICATIONS OF LUNG CANCER

The majority of lung cancers metastasize to the liver, CNS, bone, adrenal glands, and supraclavicular lymph nodes. The detection of extrapulmonary metastases begins with a thorough history and physical examination. Suspicious symptoms include:

- Weight loss
- Anorexia
- Neurologic symptoms
- Localized bone pain

Laboratory data, including liver function tests, alkaline phosphatase, and calcium, are necessary and will indicate the need for further workup.

Frequently used imaging techniques include CT scan of the chest, which includes liver and adrenal glands and bone and liver-spleen scans. CT scan of the CNS is probably only justified in patients with adenocarcinoma. Patients with other types of nonsmall-cell lung cancer do not need a routine CT scan of the head unless there is clinical suspicion of CNS involvement.

In small-cell lung cancer, extrathoracic staging is particularly important. In these patients, routine scans of bone, liver-spleen, and the head are necessary to detect tumor spread. Bone marrow aspiration and biopsy often are used to detect tumor at this site. However, in patients with obvious metastases, examination of the bone marrow is not necessary.

TREATMENT OF LUNG CANCER

NONSMALL-CELL LUNG CANCER

The three major treatment modalities for a patient with non-small-cell lung cancer are:

- Surgical resection
- Radiation therapy
- Chemotherapy

Surgical resection is the treatment of choice because it offers the best prospect of long-term survival. Unfortunately, only one-third of patients have resectable disease at the time of diagnosis. The overall 5-year survival for all stages of surgically resected lung cancer is in the range of 40%:

- Stage I — 55%
- Stage II — 29%
- Stage IIIa — 26%

The majority of patients with nonsmall-cell lung cancer present with locally advanced (Stage IIIb) or metastatic (Stage IV) disease that is not curable with surgery.

All patients with nonsmall-cell lung cancer should be evaluated for potential resection as initial therapy. Surgical procedures include pneumonectomy, lobectomy, segmentectomy, wedge resection, and sleeve bronchoplasty. Lobectomy is the surgical procedure of choice for patients with Stage I and some Stage II lung cancer. Evaluation of pulmonary reserve must be done using pulmonary function tests in patients undergoing resection for lung surgery. Preoperative FEV_1 greater than 2 liters or greater than 80% of predicted indicates a good lung reserve and the patient may tolerate up to a pneumonectomy. Patients who have an FEV_1 less than 80% of predicted need a quantitative perfusion scan in order to predict the postoperative lung function. A postoperative predicted FEV_1 of less than 40% of predicted, postoperative predicted DLCO less than 40% and presence of significant dyspnea suggests potential for high morbidity and mortality in patients undergoing lung resection.

Nonsmall-cell lung cancers are relatively unresponsive to chemotherapy. On the other hand, radiation therapy is effective in decreasing the size of local tumors in patients with nonsmall- and small-cell lung cancer. Radiation therapy is very useful as a palliative measure, especially in patients who have obstruction of airways, compression of vital chest structures by the tumors, pain or hemoptysis. Radiation therapy may be curative in fewer than 15% of patients with Stage I nonsmall-cell lung cancer.

SMALL-CELL LUNG CANCER

Treatment of small-cell carcinoma remains nonsurgical in the vast majority of patients because of the high frequency of the metastases at the time of diagnosis. In most cases, small-cell lung cancer is sensitive to both chemotherapy and radiation therapy. The agents most commonly used for patients with small-cell lung cancer include:

- Cisplatin
- Etoposide
- Vincristine

- Doxorubicin
- Cyclophosphamide

The majority of patients with limited disease have complete response to chemotherapy. However, only 15% to 20% of these patients with limited disease survive 3 years. Thoracic radiation is used in combination with chemotherapy to control local recurrence in patients with limited disease. Elective cranial irradiation has been used in complete responders to chemotherapy to treat occult brain metastasis.

In the uncommon patient with small-cell lung cancer that presents with an isolated lung nodule, surgical resection is considered to be the treatment of choice, followed by adjuvant chemotherapy, with a cure rate of up to 50%.

Patients with extensive diseases are treated with chemotherapy. The survival rate is 5% at 3 years.

PREVENTION OF LUNG CANCER

The most effective way to prevent lung cancer is to prevent smoking. Popularity of smoking by white males has already shown some decline. Unfortunately, smoking in women and minority ethnic groups is still very high. *Every physician has the duty of advising every single patient about quitting the smoking habits.*

Other modalities of prevention, such as chemotherapy prevention for lung cancer using beta-carotene and vitamin A, have not shown significant benefit in reducing the incidence of bronchogenic carcinoma.

SUGGESTED READINGS

Beckett W. Epidemiology and etiology of lung cancer. Clin Chest Med 1993;14:1:1–5.

Johnson BE. Management of small-cell lung cancer. Clin Chest Med 1993;14:1:173–187.

Lillington GA, Caskey CI. Evaluation and management of solitary and multiple pulmonary nodules. Clin Chest Med 1993;14:1:111–119.

Mountain CF. Lung cancer staging classification. Clin Chest Med 1993;14:1:43–53.

Patel AM, Peters SG. Clinical manifestations of lung cancer. Mayo Clin Proc 1993; 68:273–277.

Patel AM, Davila DG, Peters SG. Paraneoplastic syndromes associated with lung cancer. Mayo Clin Proc 1993;68: 278–287.

Shaw EG, Bonner JA, Foote RL, et al. Role of radiation therapy in the management of lung cancer. Mayo Clin Proc 1993; 68:593–602.

Shields TW. Surgical therapy for carcinoma of the lung. Clin Chest Med 1993;14(1):121–147.

White CS, Templeton PA. Radiologic manifestations of bronchogenic cancer. Clin Chest Med 1993;14(1):55–67.

C·H·A·P·T·E·R

36

Obstructive Lung Disease: Asthma and COPD

Mani S. Kavuru

Bronchial asthma and COPD represent major causes of morbidity in the United States. Asthma affects 3–5% of the U.S. population, while perhaps an additional 10 million to 15 million Americans are afflicted with COPD. Although asthma is not a leading cause of death, it is responsible for about 1% of all visits to physicians and results in about 500,000 hospital admissions per year. COPD was the fourth leading cause of death in the United States in 1991, with about 160,000 deaths. Therefore, both of these disorders are quite common and pose a significant burden on health-care resources, as well as in human suffering. It is essential for the general internist, as well as the pulmonary subspecialist, to be very familiar with the nuances of management. History, physical examination, and simple ancillary studies (such as a chest radiograph and spirogram) are usually adequate to establish a diagnosis of asthma or COPD and initiate proper management.

Chronic airflow obstruction is a feature of asthma, chronic bronchitis, emphysema, cystic fibrosis, and other bronchiectatic syndromes. The discussion here will be limited to the typical adult patient with asthma and cigarette smoking-related COPD. It is most essential to distinguish patients with bronchial asthma from the usual adult smoker with COPD, since the prognosis and emphasis on certain types of management are quite different.

ASTHMA

Asthma is a chronic, episodic disease of the airways with protean manifestations and is best viewed as a syndrome. Important features of this syndrome include:

- Episodic symptoms
- Airflow obstruction with a reversible component
- Bronchial hyperresponsiveness to a variety of nonspecific and specific stimuli

- Airway inflammation
- A tendency toward atopic and allergic inheritable disease

All of these features need not be present. Although there is some overlap in features between asthma and COPD, it is important to understand the distinctions of these conditions:

- Asthma typically occurs in younger individuals who are nonsmokers.
- The asthmatic's baseline level of functioning, exercise tolerance, and spirometric parameters are usually better preserved between episodes than individuals with COPD.
- The presence of extrinsic triggers, seasonal variability, family history, allergic rhinitis, and positive skin test results or atopy may be helpful in solidifying an initial diagnosis of asthma.
- Physiologically, asthmatics have a normal diffusing capacity, whereas patients with emphysema have a diffusing capacity reduced in proportion to the severity of airflow obstruction.

ETIOLOGY OF ASTHMA

Epidemiology of Asthma

During the past decade, a 35% increase in the morbidity and mortality from asthma (5000 deaths per year) has occurred, despite an increasing understanding of the pathogenesis of the disease. The evolving consensus from a number of retrospective studies is that there are several risk factors that contribute to fatal asthma:

- Patients with prior serious asthma, requiring emergency

room visits or mechanical ventilation, are at the greatest risk.

- Factors that interfere with compliance and access to medical care are important. In the United States, the mortality rate from asthma for blacks is three times that for whites.
- Inadequate objective assessment of asthma severity by pulmonary function testing or peak-flow measurements appears to be frequently noted in patients who die of asthma.
- Inadequate treatment with either inhaled or systemic corticosteroid is also a frequently described finding.

Therefore, underdiagnosis or underestimation of asthma severity is an important contributing factor in asthma-related fatality. Despite these recent trends, asthma remains a relatively infrequent cause of death.

Much controversy surrounds the potential role of β-agonist aerosols in the increasing asthma mortality. The hypothesis exists that excessive or continuous use of beta adrenergic bronchodilators can actually worsen asthma, perhaps contributing to morbidity and mortality. Overall, the exact contribution of β-agonists to the recent mortality trend remains unknown, but there is sufficient concern that if patients require increasing number of puffs of β-agonist aerosols, this is usually a marker for more effective anti-inflammatory therapy. β-agonist aerosols remain a critical part of the regimen for acute emergency room management of bronchial asthma. For chronic maintenance therapy, the need for restricted use remains unknown.

Pathogenesis of Asthma

In recent years, the central role of airway inflammation in the pathogenesis of asthma has been established. The mechanism by which airway inflammation is related to bronchial reactivity remains unclear. A classic model is that of an allergic asthmatic challenged with an inhaled antigen to which the patient is sensitive. This challenge may result in a biphasic decline in respiratory function. The early asthmatic response (EAR) may occur within minutes and resolve within 2 hours. The EAR is thought to be related to the release of preformed mediators (perhaps from mast cells) and is abolished by pretreatment with β-agonists (but not corticosteroids). A late asthmatic response (LAR) usually occurs within 6–8 hours and may last for 24 hours or longer. The LAR is classically associated with airway hyperreactivity and can be inhibited by pretreatment with corticosteroids (but not β-agonists). Cromoglycates may block both responses.

The current paradigm is that asthma is not simply bronchospasm but involves a complex cascade of inflammatory events that involves cellular, epithelial, neurogenic, and various biochemical mediators. In addition to the mast cell and eosinophil, the T-lymphocyte (T_{H2}) has been added as an important regulator of inflammation. The T_{H2} lymphocytes appear to mediate allergic inflammation in atopic asthmatics

by a cytokine profile that involves IL-4 (which directs B-lymphocytes to synthesize IgE) and IL-5 (which is essential for the maturation of eosinophils), along with IL-3 and GM-CSF. Products of arachidonic acid metabolism have also been implicated in airway inflammation and have been the target of pharmacologic antagonism. Prostaglandins are generated by the cyclooxygenation of arachidonic acid, and leukotrienes are generated by the lipoxygenation of arachidonic acid. The proinflammatory agents include all of the leukotrienes and prostaglandins PGD_2, PGF_{2A}, and thromboxane. Prostaglandins PGE_2 and PGI_2 (prostacyclin) are felt to be protective and produce bronchodilation.

CLINICAL PRESENTATION OF ASTHMA

The history and physical examination are important for several reasons:

- Confirm a diagnosis and exclude mimics such as upper airway obstruction, congestive heart failure.
- Assess the severity of airflow obstruction and the need for admission to a hospital.
- Identify factors that might place a patient at particular risk for poor outcome.
- Identify comorbid diseases that may complicate the management, such as sinusitis, gastroesophageal reflux, avoidable external triggers.

The cardinal symptoms of asthma include:

- Episodic dyspnea
- Chest tightness
- Wheezing
- Cough

Some patients may present with atypical symptoms, such as cough alone (''cough-equivalent asthma'') or only dyspnea on exertion. It is essential to specifically inquire about nocturnal symptoms, since this is often ignored.

The most objective indicator of asthma severity is the measurement of airflow obstruction by spirometry or peak expiratory flow. Both the FEV_1 and PEF yield comparable results. The National Asthma Education Prevention Program (NAEPP) in its Expert Panel Report II (Spring 1997) recently set forward the grading of asthma severity based on frequency of symptoms, the peak flows, and the need for inhaled β-agonists into four categories:

- Mild-intermittent
- Mild-persistent
- Moderate-persistent
- Severe

Hyperinflation, the most common finding on a chest radiograph, has no diagnostic or therapeutic value. A chest radiograph should not be obtained unless complications of pneumonia, pneumothorax, or an endobronchial lesion are suspected. The correlation of severity of acute asthma and arterial blood gases is poor. Mild-to-moderate asthma is typically associated with respiratory alkalosis and mild hypoxemia on the basis of V/Q mismatching. Severe hypoxemia is quite uncommon. Normocapnia and hypercapnia do imply severe airflow obstruction, with FEV_1 usually less than 25% predicted. Recent data suggest that hypercapnia in the setting of acute asthma does not necessarily mandate intubation or suggest a poor prognosis.

Numerous parameters from the physical examination and airflow measurement, either separately or as a composite score, have been evaluated to assess the severity of acute asthma and the need for hospital admission. It is true that physical findings such as pulsus paradoxus (inspiratory decline in systolic blood pressure > 12 mm Hg), accessory muscle use including sternocleidomastoid muscle retraction, respiratory rate > 30, and heart rate > 130 bpm are generally associated with more severe airflow obstruction. However, none of these signs alone or in combination is specific or sensitive.

Spirometry in an asthmatic typically shows obstructive airways disease with reduced expiratory flows that improve with bronchodilator therapy. Typically, there is an improvement in either FEV_1 or FVC with acute administration of inhaled bronchodilator (12% and 200 mL). However, the absence of a bronchodilator response by no means excludes asthma. The shape of the flow-volume loop may provide insight into the nature and location of airway obstruction. With disorders that cause upper-airway obstruction (UAO), there is classically a plateau in either limb of the flow-volume loop during periods of maximal flow. Specifically, the loop shows flattening of the inspiratory limb with variable extrathoracic UAO, likely caused by a lesion involving the glottic or subglottic area. Flattening of the expiratory limb is seen with variable intrathoracic UAO such as a mid or distal tracheal lesion. A fixed UAO produces a ''box like'' flattening of both inspiratory and expiratory limbs. In patients with atypical chest symptoms of unclear etiology (cough or dyspnea alone), a variety of challenge tests may help to identify the presence of airway hyperreactivity. By far the most commonly used agents are methacholine or histamine, which give comparable results. Exercise, cold air, and isocapnic hyperventilation—other approaches that require complex equipment—have a lower sensitivity. In a patient with known asthma, there is no indication for a challenge procedure. The methacholine challenge test is very sensitive, but it is nonspecific and can occur in a variety of other conditions, including COPD.

TREATMENT OF ASTHMA

The National Asthma Education Prevention Program (NAEPP) Expert Panel Report II provides an excellent algorithmic framework for the management of bronchial asthma. The general goals of asthma therapy include:

- Maintain normal activity levels, including exercise.
- Maintain near normal pulmonary function tests.
- Prevent chronic and troublesome symptoms or recurrent exacerbations of asthma.

- Avoid adverse effects from asthma medications.

Overall, asthma treatment has four key components:

1. Measure lung function both initially and during periodic evaluation including home peak expiratory flow monitoring.
2. Educate patients.
3. Avoid asthma triggers by controlling the environment.
4. Treat the condition pharmacologically.

The pharmacologic treatment for asthma can be classified as:

- Symptomatic therapy (''relievers'') with bronchodilators (β-agonists, theophylline)
- Anti-inflammatory therapy (''controllers'') with corticosteroids, cromolyn, nedocromil, antileukotrienes

The therapy is further classified as acute versus chronic maintenance therapy. The NAEPP outlines detailed guidelines for stepwise management with these agents. For the mildest asthma (mild-intermittent), the guidelines recommend as-needed use of 1–2 puffs of a beta-2 aerosol. Cromolyn may alternatively be used prior to exposure to a variety of triggers, such as exercise or allergen.

For all asthmatics with ''persistent'' asthma (symptoms more than one to two times per week), the mainstay of maintenance therapy is inhaled corticosteroids. These agents should be used in adequate doses to fully control the symptoms. Numerous studies have shown that inhaled steroid therapy provides an effective symptomatic control of chronic asthma, as well as reversal of a number of parameters of airway inflammation.

The efficacy of inhaled steroid therapy is dependent upon the daily dosage, dosing frequency, delivery system, and duration of therapy. It is generally felt that inhaled steroids should be introduced soon after a diagnosis of asthma has been made and used at the lowest dose for long periods of time. Recent data suggest that these agents probably do not cure asthma in the sense that symptoms promptly return if these agents are stopped. These agents clearly reduce airway hyperreactivity (unlike oral corticosteroids). In general, with the use of low-dose inhaled corticosteroid therapy (less than 1000 mcg/day), systemic complications appear to be negligible. Oral pharyngeal complications of inhaled steroid therapy, such as candidiasis, dysphonia, and hoarseness, are usually mild. Use of a spacer device and routine rinsing of the mouth helps to minimize these side effects. Data suggest that systemic effects may occur with the use of higher dosages (> 1200 mcg/day) of inhaled corticosteroids. Definitely, certain biochemical parameters of HPA axis (24-hour urinary free cortisol, AM serum cortisol, and ACTH stimulation test) and bone metabolism (serum osteocalcin and urinary hydroxyproline) may be affected. However, the clinical importance of these effects in terms of bone growth, likelihood for osteoporosis, or fractures is not known.

A minority of patients continue to have troublesome asthma symptoms, with frequent exacerbations requiring hospital stays, despite maximal conventional therapy. The literature suggests that this is a small subset, perhaps less than 10–15% of all asthmatics. The reversible factors that contribute to the subset of ''steroid-dependent asthma'' include:

- Patient noncompliance
- Poor self-management strategies by the patient
- Inadequate control of allergen burden at home
- Suboptimal inhaler technique
- Suboptimal pharmacotherapy prescription by the physician

There is ongoing research about the possibility of relative ''steroid resistance'' in a subset of these difficult-to-control asthmatics. Many factors—including steroid metabolism, steroid receptor subtypes, and a variety of intracellular factors—are being studied. It appears that steroid metabolism and steroid receptors are unlikely to be an explanation.

The placebo arm of a number of studies has clearly shown that a compulsive traditional management plan, with frequent follow-up (perhaps in an asthma center), can reduce the need for oral steroids by 40–50% in ''steroid-dependent'' asthma. The literature is replete with numerous studies demonstrating the efficacy of alternative anti-inflammatory therapies that provide a steroid-sparing effect in these individuals. Gold salts, methotrexate, cyclosporin, colchicine, troleandomycin (TAO), chloroquine, intravenous gammaglobulin, and dapsone are some of the agents that have been investigated. Overall, no alternative anti-inflammatory agent has been proved to be superior to inhaled corticosteroids in the treatment of asthma, and the use of these therapies should be restricted to clinical trials only.

COPD

Most adult patients with COPD exhibit features of both chronic bronchitis and emphysema:

- Chronic bronchitis is usually clinically defined (based on Ciba Guest Symposium report in 1959) as chronic cough with sputum production occurring on most days for at least 3 months of the year for at least 2 successive years.
- Emphysema is anatomically defined as an abnormal permanent enlargement of the air spaces distal to the terminal bronchiole, accompanied by destruction of their walls, and without obvious fibrosis.

There are several different anatomic types of emphysema, the most common being the typical smoking-related centriacinar emphysema. This centriacinar emphysema (synonyms are centrilobular or proximal acinar) involves dilatation of the air space between the terminal bronchiole and the first- and second-generation respiratory bronchiole. The other major type of emphysema, panacinar or panlobular emphysema, is usually seen in association with the inherited alpha 1-antitrypsin deficiency.

ETIOLOGY OF COPD

Epidemiology of COPD

Overall, smoking is the single most important risk factor for COPD. In the general nonsmoking population, the forced expiratory volume in the first second (FEV_1) percent predicted follows a unimodal distribution. Among cigarette smokers, the distribution is shifted leftward to lower FEV_1 values. A longitudinal study from East Boston with a 10-year follow up, suggested that asymptomatic nonsmoking males showed a prolonged period of either slow growth or plateau phase between ages 23 and 35. Age-related decline in lung function began after this period and occurred at a rate of 20–30 ml/yr. Though most heavy smokers have a slightly reduced FEV_1, only 10–15% have a significant chronic obstructive airflow limitation (i.e., $FEV_1 < 65\%$). In nonsusceptible smokers, the decline in FEV_1 is similar to that of nonsmokers. In the small subset of susceptible smokers, there is an accelerated decline in FEV_1 of approximately 70–150 ml/yr.

The IPPB trial group followed a cohort of 985 patients with established COPD who had a postbronchodilator FEV_1 of around 40% for a 3-year period. They noted an average mortality of 23% over the 3-year period and found the postbronchodilator FEV_1 and the patient's age as the most accurate predictors of death. There is also a slightly increased risk with an elevated resting heart rate, untreated hypoxemia, and hypercapnia. Respiratory tract infections do not influence the overall course of the disease. Early evidence suggests that increased baseline airway hyperresponsiveness may imply a better prognosis. This remains controversial and is contrary to the so-called Dutch hypothesis, which holds that in patients with increased bronchodilator responsiveness, there is an accelerated FEV_1 decline with time.

Pathogenesis of COPD

There is overwhelming evidence now to suggest that cigarette smoking is causally related to emphysema. The exact component in smoke that is responsible for this process is unknown. The lung destruction in emphysema is generally explained by the protease-antiprotease hypothesis. It is felt that in a normal nonsmoking individual, there is a fine balance between elastolytic enzymes (i.e., neutrophil elastase) and endogenous agents that inhibit their activity (i.e., alpha 1-antitrypsin). It appears that cigarette smoke affects both arms of this balance to produce severe lung destruction by a so-called two-hit concept. Most adult smokers with severe emphysema have serum alpha 1-antitrypsin levels within normal limits. The alpha 1-antitrypsin deficient form of emphysema should be suspected in a small minority (2–3%) of adult patients who present with the following features:

- Early-onset emphysema ($<$ age 50)
- Emphysema with minimal smoking history
- Predominantly basilar bullous emphysema

- Family history of emphysema, liver disease, or panniculitis
- Emphysema occurring with liver disease.

The diagnosis of alpha 1-antitrypsin deficiency is made by measuring the serum alpha 1-antitrypsin level followed by Pi typing for confirmation. The threshold level for emphysema ($<$ 80 mg/dl or 11 micromolar) is usually seen only in patients with PiZZ phenotype (homozygotes). In addition to cigarette smoking and alpha 1-antitrypsin deficiency, there are a number of rare causes for COPD: hypocomplementemic urticarial vasculitis syndrome (HUVs), intravenous methylphenidate (Ritalin) abuse, Ehlers-Danlos or Marfan's syndrome, Salla disease, alpha 1-antichymotrypsin deficiency, HIV-related emphysema, systemic necrotizing vasculitis.

CLINICAL PRESENTATION OF COPD

The cardinal symptoms of COPD include:

- Dyspnea
- Cough with or without sputum production and wheezing

Symptoms are usually chronic (i.e., at least 3–5 years) and slowly progressive. Patients may give a history of a variable course with occasional acute exacerbations interspersed with periods of stable or slowly progressive illness. However, the variability in the symptoms is not nearly as dramatic as in young patients with typical asthma, where the periods between acute exacerbations are quite symptom free.

Physical examination is tailored to establish whether a patient has an acute exacerbation of his illness, and whether there is a concomitant illness contributing to symptoms. Although some patients exhibit the classic body habitus of either a ''pink puffer'' (type A) or a ''blue bloater'' (type B), most adult patients with COPD exhibit features of both. The lung examination is most remarkable for a decrease in the intensity of breath sounds, prolonged expiratory phase, and occasional scattered wheezes on forced expiration. Rales are usually not present. Heart sounds are usually distant and difficult to appreciate. The presence of right ventricular strain or failure can be ascertained by a loud pulmonic component of the second heart sound, a right ventricular heave, elevated neck veins, a pulsatile liver, and edema in the lower extremities. Clubbing of the fingers is not usually present in smoking-related COPD, and its presence should strongly suggest a complicating illness such as lung cancer, pulmonary fibrosis, chronic infection, or liver disease.

Though the chest roentgenogram may offer clues supporting a diagnosis of obstructive airways disease, its primary importance is in excluding important concomitant diseases, such as pulmonary nodules, congestive heart failure, or pulmonary fibrosis.

Pulmonary function testing is essential to establish a diagnosis of COPD. The typical spirometric abnormalities in COPD consist of a reduction in the forced expiratory volume in one second (FEV_1) and in the ratio of the FEV_1 to the forced vital capacity (FVC). The single breath diffusing capacity (DLCO) is usually reduced in emphysema and has a good correlation with the extent of anatomic destruction in emphysema.

Many patients with COPD have a significant response to acute administration of inhaled bronchodilators (an increase in FEV_1 of 12% and 200 ml). Clearly, the presence of bronchodilator response itself is not adequate to distinguish asthma from COPD. Also, methacholine provocation test may be positive in over 60% of patients with COPD, and therefore this also does not distinguish COPD from emphysema. There is no indication for this challenge test in patients with known COPD.

TREATMENT OF COPD

Management of stable COPD will be considered separately from treatment during acute exacerbations. The critical interventions that have been shown to prolong survival and affect the natural history of the underlying disease are oxygen therapy for the chronically hypoxemic patient and perhaps smoking cessation. All other management strategies have less compelling data to suggest long-term measurable benefit, either in terms of survival or other criteria.

The commonly used therapy for stable COPD include prevention (smoking cessation, annual flu vaccination, and Pneumovax every 6–10 years), supplemental oxygen if indicated, inhaled bronchodilators, and in a small subset, theophylline preparations and inhaled or systemic corticosteroids. Recent data suggest that a comprehensive pulmonary rehabilitation program improves exercise tolerance and symptoms, though it probably does not improve FEV_1 or survival.

A current database showing survival advantage for supplemental oxygen therapy in chronically hypoxemic patients is largely based on two landmark studies, the Nocturnal Oxygen Therapy trial (NOTT) and the British Medical Research Council (MRC). Both studies included patients with severe but stable COPD and resting hypoxemia. Combined results from these studies suggest that continuous oxygen therapy for 24 hours and/or 12 hours confers a definite survival benefit. Other significant findings included improvement in quality of life and neuropsychiatric function, exercise tolerance, reduction in secondary polycythemia, and pulmonary artery pressure in selected groups of patients. Although the exact mechanism for the survival benefit is unknown, it is probably through improving pulmonary vascular resistance. Patients with a resting room air $P_aO_2 < 55$ or a S_pO_2 by pulse oximetry $< 88\%$ should be given supplemental oxygen. These criteria should be checked during a period of clinical stability rather than during an acute exacerbation. In patients with P_aO_2 between 55–59, additional clinical features of chronic hypoxemia and end organ damage should be present.

The three main bronchodilators that are currently available are:

- Anticholinergic agents
- Beta 2-selective adrenergic agents
- Theophylline preparations

There are a variety of studies that document the efficacy of each of these agents in the management of stable COPD, either alone or in combination. It appears that patients with COPD have a significantly increased cholinergic bronchomotor tone. A multicenter study suggested that ipratropium showed a superior bronchodilator effect than metaproterenol in patients with severe COPD. Also, a recent randomized trial suggests that theophylline improves respiratory function and dyspnea in patients with severe COPD.

Numerous studies have examined the role of oral corticosteroid therapy in patients with stable COPD. A recent meta-analysis by Callahan surveyed 33 original studies of oral corticosteroid use in the literature and selected 15 studies that met some preselected criteria of study quality. They concluded that stable COPD patients receiving steroids have a 20% or greater improvement in baseline FEV_1 in approximately 10% of the time more often than similar patients receiving placebo alone. Unfortunately, there are no satisfactory clinical predictors for response. In general, steroid use in these patients should be considered as an empirical trial, patient response should be objectively assessed, and benefits should be weighed against the well-known side effects of corticosteroids.

The role of inhaled corticosteriods in patients with stable COPD is unknown and is a source of some ongoing studies (Lung Health Study II). It is reasonable to say that a major difference between asthma and COPD is that inhaled corticosteroids are the mainstay of therapy for asthma but have a limited role in COPD. Mucokinetic agents, such as organic iodides, have not been shown to have objective benefit in COPD. Alpha 1-antitrypsin augmentation therapy is used in nonsmoking younger patients with severe alpha 1-antitrypsin deficiency and associated emphysema. Efficacy for this therapy is unproven, although it is assumed that increasing the serum concentration of the enzyme decreases the rate of decline of FEV_1. Human-pooled alpha 1-antitrypsin is administered by intravenous infusion weekly, biweekly, or monthly. The recommended weekly dose is 60 mg/kg and monthly dose is 250 mg/kg.

Acute exacerbations of COPD are often managed in a hospital setting with aggressive aerosolized and intravenous pharmacotherapy, with the agents discussed above. Repeated inhaled β-agonists (either nebulized or by MDI) are preferred over anticholinergics, since the onset of action is more rapid. Systemic corticosteroids are usually given during acute exacerbations of COPD (either outpatient setting or in the hospital), and there are some data to support this practice. The efficacy of antibiotic therapy for exacerbations of COPD is a topic of several studies with some controversy. In general, patients with a change in sputum, fever, and new infiltrate are optimal candidates for antibiotics. There is probably no need for a routine sputum culture. The vast majority of patients with COPD exacerbation can be successfully managed with this therapy alone.

Perhaps 5–10% of COPD patients either fail this therapy or initially present with acute respiratory failure requiring intensive care and perhaps 20–60% require mechanical ventilation. Most of the experience with respiratory failure in COPD has been with endotracheal intubation and positive pressure ventilation. There is extensive literature about the ICU management of COPD patients and is beyond the scope of this discussion. Previously, the prognosis for patients with acute respiratory failure secondary to COPD exacerbation alone, without complicating illness, was felt to be quite favorable. Recent studies suggest that exacerbation of COPD with admission to an ICU has a hospital mortality of 24%. For patients 65 and older, 1-year mortality is 30–59%. In patients with COPD exacerbation and hypercapnia (P_aCO_2 50 mm Hg), 1- and 2-year mortality rates are 43% and 49%. An episode of acute respiratory failure caused by an exacerbation of COPD appears not to significantly alter the overall prognosis of the disease, which is largely dictated by the FEV_1 and age. There have been several recent studies regarding noninvasive mechanical ventilation (mostly with positive pressure ventilation) for both stable COPD and acute exacerbation of COPD. In an appropriate setting with expertise, this remains an alternative to endotracheal intubation.

Finally, a variety of surgical techniques have been applied to a very small subset of patients with end-stage COPD. There has been recent interest in lung-volume reduction surgery in patients with diffuse emphysema wherein surgical resection of the most severely affected lung tissue is carried out. Preliminary data suggest that this surgery can increase the elastic recoil of the lung and provide short-term improvement in dyspnea and exercise tolerance. Similarly, lung transplantation is also a viable treatment modality in a carefully selected subset of patients with end-stage COPD. In general, patients should meet the following criteria:

- Younger than 55–60 years
- Expected survival from their underlying COPD of less than 12–18 months
- Absence of underlying malignancy or systemic illness
- Off chronic steroid therapy
- Not in acute respiratory failure

Several clinical centers around the United States have performed this procedure successfully. The long-term outcome of these surgical treatments for diffuse emphysema remains unknown.

REVIEW EXERCISES

QUESTIONS

1. Which of the following is the most important variable to correct in patients with severe COPD (either acute or chronic)?

   a. P_aCO_2
   b. pH
   c. Hypoxemia
   d. Pulmonary hypertension
   e. Cardiac output

2. Which one of the following has been shown to increase survival in patients with severe COPD?

   a. ICU care and mechanical ventilation
   b. Systemic steroids during acute exacerbations
   c. Long-term oxygen therapy
   d. Smoking cessation
   e. Chronic therapy with bronchodilators

3. All of the following are "pro-inflammatory" mediators (i.e., promote bronchospasm) in patients with asthma except

   a. PGI_2 (prostacyclin) and PGE_2
   b. Leukotrienes (C4, D4, E4)
   c. PGF_{2a}, PGD_2
   d. Thromboxane
   e. Histamine

4. Recent increase in asthma mortality may be owing to all of the following except:

   a. Toxicity related to excessive use of inhaled β-agonists
   b. Change in the natural history of asthma
   c. Poor patient education, noncompliance
   d. Physicians not following practice guidelines (i.e., inadequate use of inhaled steroids)
   e. Toxicity related to diluents in metered dose inhalers (i.e., chlorofluorocarbons or CFCs)

5. Which one of the following statements does not belong with the other choices?

   a. Bilateral vocal cord paralysis
   b. Postextubation stridor
   c. Factitious (or functional) asthma
   d. Variable "extrathoracic" upper airway obstruction
   e. Flattening of the expiratory limb of flow-volume loop

Answers

1. c, hypoxemia

   The overriding concern should be to improve tissue oxygen delivery. Though supplemental oxygen may contribute to hypercapnia (mostly by affecting V/Q mismatching rather than suppression of hypoxic drive), correcting hypoxemia (P_aO_2 60, S_aO_2 90%) is critical. The mechanism whereby chronic oxygen improves survival is probably by reducing pulmonary hypertension. The best way to reduce PA pressure is to correct hypoxemia.

2. c, long-term oxygen therapy

   All of these are reasonable therapies for COPD, but only ambulatory home oxygen for > 12 hours/day has been unequivocally shown to improve survival (in appropriate candidates who have baseline hypoxemia). In the NOTT study, survival in the continuous oxygen group was 75% versus 54% in the control group at 36 months (oxygen 12 hours/day).

3. a, PGI_2 (prostacyclin) and PGE_2

   The answer to this question requires a review of the arachidonic acid metabolism. This examination question lends itself to a matching-type format as well. There is currently intense research to block the pro-inflammatory effects of some of these lipid mediators. Leukotrienes (products of lipoxygenase) are uniformly pro-inflammatory. Prostaglandins (products of cyclooxygenase) are more heterogeneous, with PGE_2 and PGI_2 being considered protective.

4. e, toxicity related to diluents in metered dose inhalers (i.e., chlorofluorocarbons or CFCs)

   There has been an upward trend in asthma deaths worldwide over the past decade. Many theories have been put forward, but there is no widespread consensus. However, there is little or no evidence that CFCs play a role in this. The issue with CFCs, which are important as propellants in MDIs, is that they are known to be harmful to the ozone layer of the atmosphere.

5. e, flattening of the expiratory limb of flow-volume loop

   With variable extrathoracic upper airway obstruction (i.e., bilateral vocal cord paralysis, postextubation stridor, functional vocal cord adduction), the flow-volume loop would show flattening of the inspiratory limb.

SUGGESTED READINGS

ASTHMA

Barnes PJ. A new approach to the treatment of asthma. N Engl J Med 1989;321:1517–1527.

Barnes PJ. New drugs for asthma. Eur Resp J 1992;5: 1126–1136.

Djukanovic R, Roche WR, Wilson JW, et al. Mucosal inflammation in asthma. Am Rev Respir Dis 1990;142:434–457.

McFadden ER. Dosages of corticosteroids in asthma. Am Rev Respir Dis 1993;147:1306–1310.

National Asthma Education and Prevention Program Expert Panel Report II: Guidelines for the diagnosis and management of asthma. National Institutes of Health, Spring 1997 (in press).

Weiss KB, Gergen PJ, Hodgson TA. An economic evaluation of asthma in the United States. N Engl J Med 1992;326: 862–866.

COPD

Anthonisen NR, Connett JE, Kiley JP, et al. Effects of smoking intervention and the use of an inhaled anticholinergic bronchodilator on the rate of decline of FEV_1: the Lung Health Study. JAMA 1994;272:1497–1505.

ATS statement: standards for the diagnosis and care of patients with chronic obstructive pulmonary disease. Am Respir Crit Care Med 1995;152:S78–S121.

Connors AF, Dawson NV, Thomas C, et al. Outcomes following acute exacerbation of severe chronic obstructive pulmonary disease. Am J Respir Crit Care Med 1996;154:959–967.

Hill NS. Noninvasive ventilation: does it work, for whom, and how? Am Rev Respir Dis 1993;147:1050–1055.

Kotlke TE, Battista RN, DeFriese GH, et al. Attributes of successful smoking cessation interventions in medical practice: a meta-analysis of 39 controlled trials. JAMA 1988;259: 2882–2889.

Ries AL, Kaplan RM, Limberg TM, et al. Effects of pulmonary rehabilitation on physiologic and psychological outcomes in patients with chronic obstructive pulmonary disease. Ann Intern Med 1995;122:823–832.

Rutten-van Molken M, van Doorslaer E, Jansen M, et al. Costs and effects of inhaled corticosteroids and bronchodilators in asthma and COPD. Am J Respir Crit Care Med 1995;151: 975–982.

Saint S, Bent S, Vittinghoff E, et al. Antibiotics in chronic obstructive pulmonary disease exacerbations: a meta-analysis. JAMA 1995;273:957–960.

Tarpy SP, Celli BR. Long-term oxygen therapy. N Engl J Med 1995;333:710–714.

Thompson WH, Nielson CP, Carvalho P, et al. Controlled trial of oral prednisone in outpatients with acute COPD exacerbation. Am J Respir Crit Care Med 1996;154:407–412.

Weinmann GG, Hyatt R. Evaluation and research in lung volume reduction surgery. Am J Respir Crit Care Med 1996;154: 1913–1918.

Note added in proof:
Data over the past ten years suggest that the cysteinyl leukotrienes are involved in the pathogenesis of asthma. Three agents that antagonize the leukotriene pathway have been approved for use as maintenance therapy for mild persistent asthma. Zileuton is a synthesis inhibitor that blocks the 5-lipoxygenase enzyme. Zafirlukast and montelukast are selective, competitive receptor antagonists at the LTD_4 and LTE_4 level. Early clinical trials suggest these agents have beneficial effects in mild to moderate asthma compared to placebo. The exact place for anti-leukotrienes in the chronic maintenance therapy for asthma remains to be established. The EPR-II indicates a possible role for these agents in the initial therapy for mild persistent asthma as an alternative to inhaled corticosteroids. Also, EPR-II indicates a possible role for these agents as adjunctive therapy (in addition to inhaled steroids) for added asthma control at any level of severity for persistent asthma.

These agents have effects on early and late asthma response. Therefore, they act as a bronchodilator within 1–3 hours after administration as well as an anti-inflammatory agent with response over 2–4 weeks. The magnitude of increase in FEV1 at 4 weeks is about 14% above the placebo. There are no published studies directly comparing currently available inhaled corticosteroids to the anti-leukotrienes. It is likely that the inhaled steroids have more potent effects, especially in patients with moderate-severe disease. The anti-leukotrienes do facilitate a reduction in the need for inhaled beta agonists and inhaled corticosteroids, thereby minimizing certain side effects. Also, these oral agents may improve compliance compared to the metered dose inhalers. Antileukotrienes may be particularly beneficial as the drug of choice in a small sub set of patients with aspirin-sensitive asthma. (O'Byrne PM, Israel E, Drazen JM. Antileukotrienes in the treatment of asthma. Ann Intern Med 1997;127:472–480.)

37

Interstitial Lung Disease

Eugene J. Sullivan

The term interstitial lung disease (ILD) refers to a heterogeneous group of disorders. Thus, ILD is a category of disease rather than a specific diagnosis. They are generally progressive inflammatory/scarring processes that affect the interstitium to a greater extent than the airways or air spaces. In general these diseases are considered together because of their common clinical, radiographic, and physiologic picture. Because of these similarities, the term ILD is quite clinically useful and relevant. However, one must keep in mind that within this category there exist many diverse diseases with unique clinical characteristics, causes, treatments, and prognoses.

Figure 37.1 illustrates the distinction made between the pulmonary parenchymal interstitium as opposed to the conducting airways and airspaces (alveoli).

While the term *interstitial lung disease* refers to the fact that most of these diseases primarily involve the interstitium, many published lists and discussions regarding ILD also include diseases that involve other portions of the pulmonary parenchyma, such as chronic alveolar filling disorders (e.g., pulmonary alveolar lipoproteinosis), inflammatory lesions of the airways (e.g., broncholitis obliterans with organizing pneumonia, constrictive broncholitis), and inflammatory diseases primarily involving the blood vessels of the lung (various vasculitides). Some of these diseases, while pathologically distinct, may result in similar radiographic or physiologic abnormalities and thus are commonly grouped together with the other truly interstitial lung diseases.

ETIOLOGY OF INTERSTITIAL LUNG DISEASE

The interstitial lung diseases (ILD) are thus quite numerous and varied and may be difficult to organize into a usable con-

ceptual framework. When evaluating a patient with interstitial lung disease of uncertain etiology, it is helpful to consider diseases in the following categories; examples are given of specific types within each category.

Occupational ILD
  Asbestosis
  Silicosis
  Coal workers' pneumoconiosis

Drug-related ILD
  Radiation therapy
  Anti-inflammatory agents (e.g., methotrexate, gold)
  Amiodarone
  Chemotherapeutic agents (e.g., bleomycin, BCNU)
  Nitrofurantoin

Connective tissue disease-associated ILD
  Rheumatoid arthritis
  Scleroderma
  Polymyositis/dermatomyositis
  Sjögren's syndrome
  Systemic lupus erythematosus

"Allergic" or hypersensitivity reaction ILD
  Pigeon fancier's lung
  Farmer's lung
  Humidifier lung

Idiopathic and unclassified entities
  Idiopathic pulmonary fibrosis
  Sarcoidosis
  Lymphangioleiomyomatosis
  Eosinophilic granuloma (histiocytosis X)
  Bronchiolitis
  Chronic eosinophilic pneumonitis
  Pulmonary alveolar lipoproteinosis
  Various vasculitides

Figure 37.1. Conducting airways gas exchange in alveoli.

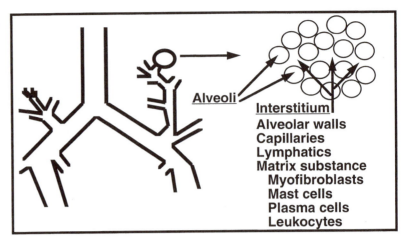

Acute interstitial pneumonitis
Neurofibromatosis
Tuberous sclerosis
Amyloidosis
Inflammatory bowel disease
Hepatic cirrhosis

While the final category, idiopathic and unclassified entities, turns out to include a fairly large number of diseases, this way of approaching interstitial lung diseases helps to guide the proper history and physical examination. If you consider each of these categories you will ask the right questions and be alert to the relevant signs.

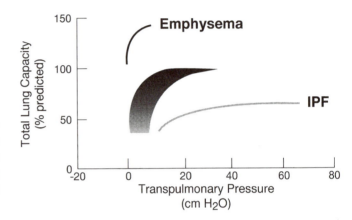

Figure 37.2. Pressure-volume curve of pulmonary compliance.

PULMONARY PHYSIOLOGY IN INTERSTITIAL LUNG DISEASE

In general, these diseases result in restrictive pulmonary physiology characterized by a reduced FEV_1 and FVC. The FEV_1/FVC ratio remains normal or in fact may be supranormal. The lung volumes are reduced, and the diffusing capacity is reduced. The diffusing capacity may improve somewhat when corrected for lung volume but tends not to return to the normal range. The pressure-volume curve, in which transpulmonary pressure is plotted against lung volume, is a test that can be performed in most pulmonary function laboratories (Fig. 37.2). However, it is not commonly performed as a matter of routine procedure because it requires the placement of an esophageal balloon with which to measure intrathoracic pressures. The pressure-volume curve demonstrates the increased elastic recoil that is seen with these restrictive lung diseases. At any particular lung volume, the transpulmonary pressure is markedly increased, reflecting the "stiffness" of these patients' lungs. This is exactly the opposite of what occurs in emphysema, in which destruction of pulmonary parenchyma leads to a loss of elastic recoil. Thus, in emphysema, the lung volumes are generally elevated, and at any particular lung volume, the transpulmonary pressure is much smaller than expected.

This concept of opposing effects on elastic recoil forces

raises the subject of a common pitfall in the diagnosis and management of interstitial lung disease. In a patient with increased interstitial markings on chest radiograph who is a heavy smoker, one must keep in mind the possibility that two disease entities, emphysema and interstitial lung disease, are present. Because of the opposing physiologic effects of the interstitial lung disease and the emphysema, the severity of the overall disease may be underestimated based solely on spirometry and lung volumes. This is because the elastic properties of the lung (its "stiffness") greatly influence both the dynamic flow rates and the measured lung volumes. Thus, a patient who is severely disabled from a combination of emphysema and idiopathic pulmonary fibrosis may have preserved spirometry and lung volumes. In such a patient, however, the diffusing capacity is usually quite low, and this should be a clue to this possibility.

DIAGNOSIS OF INTERSTITIAL LUNG DISEASE

HISTORY

Given the wide variety of diseases and exposures that can be associated with interstitial lung disease, the history is critically important in the evaluation of a patient with ILD. The history should include questions regarding symptoms such as cough and dyspnea, or symptoms of connective tissue disease. The description of the onset of these symptoms, their duration, and the general cadence of the illness may also help narrow the diagnostic possibilities. Clearly, these patients should be asked about significant occupational exposure such as asbestos, silica, or carcinogens. One must also investigate environmental exposures looking for possible antigenic sources, which could lead to chronic hypersensitivity pneumonitis. This includes questions related to mold or mildew in the home environment, pets (especially birds), and hobbies. In addition, it is important to take a careful medication history looking for agents that may be associated with drug-induced lung disease.

PHYSICAL EXAMINATION

The physical examination in patients with interstitial lung disease is fairly nonspecific. One tends to find crackles on examination of the chest. Clubbing and signs of cor pulmonale are late signs in interstitial lung disease. One must also look for signs of connective tissue disease, including skin rash, joint changes, hair loss, or muscle weakness.

RADIOGRAPHY

The chest radiograph in ILD is also generally nonspecific. Diffuse reticular or reticulonodular opacities may be seen in association with reduced lung volumes. These findings may be subtle at first and progress gradually. It is not uncommon for the radiologist to read ''chronic'' changes only. This is sometimes taken to mean that these chronic changes are not significant. However, despite the fact that the chest radiograph changes with many of the interstitial lung diseases are ''chronic'' and slowly progressive, these diseases may be quite serious and merit further evaluation. Another common pitfall in the analysis of chest radiographs in patients with ILD is the assumption that the decreased lung volumes resulted because ''the patient didn't take a deep breath.'' In general, routine chest films are taken after deep inspiration. Occasionally miscommunication between the technician and the patient may result in a film being taken anywhere in the respiratory cycle. However, if radiograph reports on a particular patient consistently comment on poor inspiration, one must consider the possibility that a restrictive lung disease is present, leading to small lung volumes despite appropriate inspiratory effort.

Although in general chest radiographs in the interstitial lung diseases are nonspecific, particular patterns or associated findings seen on the radiograph may be helpful in narrowing the diagnostic possibilities. For example, asbestos-related lung disease may be associated with pleural plaques or pleural effusions in addition to the reticulonodular infiltrates and reduced lung volumes. In general, the reticulonodular infiltrates in asbestosis are seen in a lower zone distribution.

The distribution of chest radiograph abnormalities may suggest certain diagnoses. Diseases that tend to involve predominately the upper lung zones include silicosis, chronic hypersensitivity pneumonitis, sarcoidosis, eosinophilic granuloma (also known as histiocytosis X), and ankylosing spondylitis. Diseases that tend to have a lower zone distribution include idiopathic pulmonary fibrosis, asbestosis, and the interstitial lung diseases associated with various connective tissue diseases. A disease that classically has a peripheral distribution is chronic eosinophilic pneumonia. The chest radiograph in chronic eosinophilic pneumonia is said to appear as a ''radiographic negative of congestive heart failure.'' When reticular or reticulonodular infiltrates demonstrate straight borders and are present within the ports of prior radiation therapy, radiation pneumonitis is a likely diagnosis.

The character of the infiltrates may also suggest certain disease entities. Cystic changes may be seen in lymphangioleiomyomatosis, in eosinophilic granuloma, and also in the later stages of lung diseases of various etiologies, so-called end-stage honeycombing. The presence of Kerley B lines should suggest the possibility of lymphagitic carcinoma or chronic interstitial edema. Nodular infiltrates are seen in sarcoidosis, silicosis, coal workers' pneumoconiosis, bronchiolitis obliterans, miliary distributions of various infections, and carcinoma.

Other aspects of the chest radiograph may also help to suggest certain diagnoses. While most of the interstitial lung diseases are associated with decreased lung volumes, several may result in the remarkable combination of diffuse reticular infiltrates along with normal or increased lung volumes. These include lymphangioleiomyomatosis, eosinophilic granuloma, chronic hypersensitivity pneumonitis, and sarcoidosis. In this setting, one must also consider the possibility that two disease processes are present, namely any interstitial lung disease along with significant smoking-related emphysema. The presence of a pneumothorax should raise the possibility of eosinophilic granuloma or lymphangioleiomyomatosis or tuberous sclerosis-related lung disease. The presence of a pleural effusion should raise the possibility of rheumatoid arthritis, asbestosis, carcinoma, or lymphangioleiomyomatosis. Likewise, pleural plaques are an indication of asbestos exposure and raise the possibility of asbestosis. Hilar adenopathy may be seen in sarcoidosis, silicosis, and carcinoma.

One must keep in mind that a small fraction of patients with interstitial lung disease will indeed have a normal chest radiograph. This has particularly been reported in chronic hypersensitivity pneumonitis. The use of high-resolution CT scanning has been increasing in the evaluation of patients with interstitial lung disease. High-resolution CT can be quite helpful regarding documentation of the extent of disease and in guiding subsequent open lung biopsy. Occasionally, certain high-resolution CT findings can suggest a specific diagnosis, such as in eosinophilic granuloma, lymphangioleiomyomatosis, or pulmonary alveolar lipoproteinosis. While exact correlations between high-resolution CT scan appearance and both pathologic findings and response to therapy are lacking, in general patients with more so-called ground glass opacities tend to respond better to therapy than those with extensive honeycomb lung.

LABORATORY AND OTHER STUDIES

Physiologic evaluation of the patient with interstitial lung disease should include full pulmonary function testing and arterial blood gases. Occasionally, physiologic findings may yield clues to the diagnosis. In addition, this testing will allow an estimate of the current disease severity and provide a baseline for future decision making. While not commonly performed, exercise testing is very useful in the evaluation and treatment of patients with interstitial lung disease. Exercise testing may reveal more impairment than is expected by the pulmonary function testing. In addition, it is a good measure of overall disease severity and is possibly the best parameter available to follow disease progression or response to therapy.

BRONCHOSCOPY

In general, bronchoscopy is most useful in its ability to help to rule out infection. Occasionally, the bronchoalveolar lavage may be diagnostic, as may be the case in pulmonary alveolar lipoproteinosis, lymphangitic carcinoma, and eosinophilic granuloma. The transbronchial biopsy specimens obtained through bronchoscopy are in general too small to make definitive diagnoses of most of the interstitial lung diseases. However, one may be able to obtain a diagnosis in patients with sarcoidosis or lymphangitic carcinoma with transbronchial biopsy specimens.

OPEN-LUNG BIOPSY

There is much controversy regarding the necessity of open-lung biopsy in patients with various interstitial lung diseases. Some believe, for instance, that the diagnosis of idiopathic pulmonary fibrosis may be reliably made based on clinical, physiologic, and radiographic findings without the necessity of open-lung biopsy; this remains to be established. I believe it is quite often desirable to pursue an open-lung biopsy in these patients, given the fact that the diagnosis may provide significant prognostic information and the treatments proposed may entail significant side effects. The newer thoracoscopic approach is generally quite well tolerated, even in fairly significantly impaired patients. The specific location for the lung biopsy should be discussed ahead of time with the surgeon. It is best to biopsy two or three locations in the lung and avoid areas of the lung that appear to exhibit end-stage honeycombing on CT scan, as this is a nonspecific pathologic finding. It is better to biopsy those areas which seem to be involved with ground glass opacities or even those areas that appear normal on the high-resolution CT scan, as these areas may give the most diagnostic information to the pathologist.

SPECIFIC ILD ENTITIES

IDIOPATHIC PULMONARY FIBROSIS

- Progressive inflammation and fibrosis of the lung parenchyma
- Incidence is approximately 5–25 per 100,000
- Onset is usually between the ages of 40 and 70
- Clinical presentation:
  - Progressive dyspnea on exertion
  - Cough
  - Bilateral velcro rales
  - Diffuse reticulonodular infiltrate on chest radiograph
  - Restrictive pulmonary physiology with decreased diffusing capacity for carbon monoxide (DLCO)
- The pathology is the usual interstitial pneumonitis (UIP)
- Treatments (none proven to prolong survival):
  - Corticosteroids
  - Cytotoxic agents (Cytoxan, Azathioprine)
- Colchicine
  (questionable)
- Prognosis
  - Approximately 20% objective response
  - Approximately 40% objective or subjective
  - "Responders" tend to live longer
  - Overall approximately 50% 5-year survival

SARCOIDOSIS

- Multisystem granulomatous disorder of unknown etiology
- Commonly presents as asymptomatic chest radiograph finding
- ACE level lacks sensitivity/specificity to be diagnostic but may be helpful in following response to treatment
- Transbronchial biopsy will be diagnostic in 85–90% of patients with parenchymal abnormalities (50–60% if only hilar adenopathy)
- Chronic beryllium disease can mimic sarcoidosis
- Treatment is probably indicated for symptoms, progressive pulmonary function test (PFT) abnormalities, hypercalcemia, or significant extrathoracic involvement (e.g., eye, central nervous system, or cardiac)

Radiographic Stages of Sarcoidosis

Stage 0—Normal chest radiograph
Stage 1—Hilar lymphadenopathy
Stage 2—Hilar lymphadenopathy and parenchymal infiltrate
Stage 3—Parenchymal infiltrates without adenopathy

Common Sites of Sarcoidosis Involvement

- Hilar adenopathy
- Pulmonary parenchyma
- Skin (erythema nodosum, lupus pernio)

- Ocular
- Cardiac (arrhythmias, congestive heart failure)
- Central nervous system (facial nerve palsy, cranial mass, seizures)
- Hepatic granulomas often present, usually not end stage liver disease (ESLD)
- Bone
- Parotid or lacrimal glands
- Renal impairment more likely in hypercalcemia

ASBESTOSIS

Asbestos-related lung disease is a term that can be used to encompass all of the pulmonary complications of asbestos exposure including pleural processes and rounded atelectasis (see below).

Asbestosis indicates pulmonary parenchymal fibrosis. The diagnostic criteria are:

- Dyspnea
- Persistent crackles on examination
- Restrictive lung disease
- Characteristic chest radiograph abnormalities
- Sufficient asbestos exposure

Asbestos exposure alone increases the risk of lung cancer only minimally (1.5–3 times). Asbestos and cigarette smoking act synergistically, however, as risk factors.

Pleural Manifestations of Asbestos Exposure

The characteristics of *benign asbestos pleural effusion* (BAPE) are as follows:

- May be asymptomatic or acute chest pain, fever, dyspnea
- Generally briefer lag time after initial exposure (under 15 yrs)
- Exudative, often bloody
- Spontaneous resolution with recurrences

The characteristics of *rounded atelectasis* are:

- Pleural-based parenchymal mass
- Often mistaken for carcinoma
- Characteristic CT appearance

SILICOSIS

Silicosis is a lung disease attributed to the inhalation of silicon dioxide or silica. The diagnosis is usually based on a characteristic chest radiograph with a history of exposure.

Those in the following occupations are most frequently affected:

- Mining
- Tunneling
- Quarrying
- Foundry
- Sandblasting
- Ceramics
- Stone work

Types of Silicosis

Following are the characteristics of *acute silicosis*:

- High-level fine dust exposure over weeks to months
- Chest radiograph shows airspace disease, which may progress to ARDS
- Pathology resembles alveolar lipoproteinosis

Following are characteristics of *accelerated silicosis* occurring after 5–15 years of exposure:

- Chest radiograph shows upper zone reticulonodular
- Pulmonary function impairment, which may progress to respiratory failure
- Pathology shows nodules with interstitial fibrosis

Following are the characteristics of *chronic silicosis* (chronic lower level exposure over decades):

- Pulmonary function abnormalities may or may not be present and may not progress
- Pathology shows silicotic nodules in upper lobes and hila

Complications and Associations of Silicosis

Progressive massive fibrosis (PMF) may occur with consolidation of silicotic nodules into upper lobe masses, which progress despite cessation of exposure. Tuberculosis superinfection may occur in all three types of silicosis, may be difficult to treat, and may occur with atypical mycobacteria. Underlying rheumatoid arthritis may increase the risk of developing silicosis in exposed individuals; scleroderma is associated with silica exposure. It is unclear whether silicosis is a risk factor for lung cancer.

Drug-Induced ILD

There are a myriad of offending agents. Some are well established, some only case reports. Drug-induced ILD may be acute, subacute, or chronic. Multiple histologic patterns include the following:

- Lymphoplasmacytic pneumonitis
- Eosinophilic infiltration
- Granulomatous inflammation
- PAP-like lesion
- Bronchiolocentric or vascular inflammation

The diagnosis is based on suspicion and is often difficult to prove.

The following drugs may induce ILD:

- Methotrexate
  - ILD may develop anytime
  - Interstitial pneumonitis, may have granulomas
  - Occasionally peripheral eosinophilia and hilar lymphadenopathy occur
  - ILD usually reversible with discontinuation of drug with or without steroids
  - ILD may not recur with subsequent rechallenge
- Bleomycin
  - Most common chemotherapy-related pulmonary toxicity
  - Risk factors: age over 70, more than 450 units total dose, prior thoracic radiation therapy, subsequent exposure to high FIO_2
  - Chest radiograph usually shows mixed interstitial and alveolar infiltrates
  - Nodules on chest radiograph may falsely suggest metastatic disease
- Radiation Pneumonitis
  - Acute:
    - 1–6 months after radiation therapy
    - Cough, dyspnea, fever, chest pain
    - Treatment: usually steroids if significant
  - Chronic:
    - Progressive fibrosis in areas of radiation
    - No correlation with presence/severity of prior acute injury
    - Symptoms depend on extent of lung involved
    - Treatment: may use steroids, although they are of uncertain benefit
- Nitrofurantoin
  - Acute (more common):
    - Occurs hours to days after initiation
    - Fever, dyspnea, cough, leukocytosis, with or without eosinophilia
    - Chest radiograph shows mixed interstitial/alveolar signs with or without effusion
    - Treatment is to discontinue the drug
  - Chronic:
    - No connection with acute
    - Symptoms and chest radiograph may mimic IPF
    - Treatment is to discontinue the drug, probably steroids
- Amiodarone
  - Histology: foamy alveolar macrophages; lamellar inclusions
  - Insidious cough and dyspnea (occasionally more acute)
  - Usually occurs with dose more than 400 mg every day for more than 1 month (cases have been reported with only 200 mg every day)
  - Chest radiograph is variable, with mixed interstitial/alveolar signs, focal or diffuse
  - CT scan shows infiltrates more dense than soft tissue (iodinated)
  - Treatment is to discontinue the drug, with or without steroids

CONNECTIVE TISSUE DISEASE-ASSOCIATED ILD

Characteristics of ILD associated with rheumatoid arthritis:

- Rheumatoid arthritis is more common in women, but the associated ILD is more common in men.
- Joint involvement may limit the patient's activity; therefore, more severe lung disease may be present by the time symptoms from the lung disease appear.
- Lung disease may occasionally predate joint symptoms.
- Severity of lung disease is not correlated with severity of joint symptoms.
- Pathology: usual interstitial pneumonitis most common. Bronchiolitis is also seen.

Characteristics of ILD associated with lupus:

- Acute lupus pneumonitis
  - Acute dyspnea, cough, fever
  - May be presenting manifestation of lupus (50%)
  - May be recurrent
- Chronic ILD
  - Uncommon
  - Progressive dyspnea and cough
  - Pathology: the usual interstitial pneumonitis

Characteristics of ILD associated with scleroderma:

- ILD, pulmonary hypertension, or both
- Incidence of ILD appears to be fairly high
- Poor correlation between severity of pulmonary and cutaneous manifestations

Characteristics of ILD associated with polymyositis/dermatomyositis:

- No correlation with severity of muscle disease
- Pathologies: bronchiolitis obliterans with organizing pneumonia (BOOP), usual interstitial pneumonitis, diffuse alveolar damage
- Jo-1 antibody may identify subset of polymyositis/dermatomyositis (PM/DM) patients with ILD

Characteristics of ILD associated with Sjögren's syndrome:

- Pathology often involves lymphocytes: lymphocytic interstitial pneumonitis (LIP), pseudolymphoma, or lymphoma. Others include the usual interstitial pneumonitis, BOOP, constrictive bronchiolitis.
- Airway disease is also common: proximal airway drying resulting in chronic cough, mucus plugs.

TREATMENT OF INTERSTITIAL LUNG DISEASE

The treatment of patients with ILD depends upon the specific disease entity. Many of these diseases, particularly the most common entities such as IPF and connective tissue disease-associated ILD, are characterized by progressive inflammation and fibrosis. For this reason, anti-inflammatory agents are commonly employed. The most frequently used agent is prednisone or another corticosteroid preparation. In general, fairly high doses (e.g., 40–60 mg per day) are used. In certain instances, such as with patients with strict contraindications to the use of steroids or when there is disease progression despite the use of prednisone, cytotoxic agents are often employed. Such agents would include cyclophosphamide or azathioprine. Recent reports have raised the possibility that colchicine may be effective in the treatment of IPF. Some of the ILDs are not felt to respond to anti-inflammatories and have unique treatments. Examples of these would include lymphangioleiomyomatosis, which is usually treated with hormonal manipulation (such as medroxyprogesterone), or pulmonary alveolar lipoproteinosis, which is treated with whole lung lavage.

Other general treatment measures usually include supplemental oxygen therapy, physical and occupational therapy, and removal from any etiologic exposure that can be identified. Lung transplantation is an emerging option for patients with end-stage ILD of various types.

PROGNOSIS OF INTERSTITIAL LUNG DISEASE

As with therapy, the prognosis of ILD depends greatly on the specific disease entity. Many of these diseases are characterized by slowly progressive loss of lung function over months to years. The pace of the decline may be slowed by treatment, but for many diseases progression occurs despite treatment. For instance, while some patients with IPF may seem to respond to therapy with subjective and/or objective improvements, the disease is almost uniformly fatal, with death occurring after a mean interval of 3–5 years after diagnosis. Likewise, ILD associated with connective tissue disease tends to have a poor prognosis. The clinical course of patients with chronic hypersensitivity pneumonitis is more variable. In general, the disease is more responsive to steroids acutely and the disease may stabilize, especially if the patient is removed from the exposure.

The interstitial lung diseases are a broad category of lung diseases. They tend to share common clinical, radiographic, and physiologic features but have many unique characteristics. Arriving at a specific diagnosis may be challenging and requires careful evaluation and often lung biopsy. Treatment often entails anti-inflammatory therapy such as corticosteroids or cytotoxic agents.

REVIEW EXERCISES

QUESTIONS

1. Which of the following chest x-ray findings is inconsistent with the diagnosis of asbestosis?

   a. Presence of pleural plaques
   b. Presence of pleural effusion
   c. Reticulonodular infiltrates
   d. Upper lobe predominance
   e. Reduced lung volumes

2. Which one of the following statements regarding idiopathic pulmonary fibrosis (IPF) is incorrect:

   a. IPF most commonly affects patients in their 6th and 7th decades of life.
   b. There is a familial variety of IPF.
   c. The histology of IPF is indistinguishable from that seen in rheumatoid arthritis.
   d. Clubbing is a late finding in IPF.
   e. Corticosteroids are the only proven effective therapy for IPF.

3. Which one of the following statements is incorrect?

   a. Obtaining an occupational history is imperative prior to diagnosing a patient with sarcoidosis.
   b. Elevated serum ACE level is not diagnostic.
   c. Sarcoidosis can involve any organ system.
   d. The presence of sarcoid granulomas in the pulmonary parenchyma is an indication for treatment.
   e. The most common presentation is an asymptomatic chest radiograph abnormality.

4. Which one of the following statements is incorrect?

   a. Benign asbestos pleural effusion (BAPE) is one of the earliest manifestations of asbestos exposure.
   b. Pleural thickening in a patient with asbestos exposure indicates asbestosis.
   c. Pleural plaques almost never result in symptoms or physiologic impairment.
   d. Mesothelioma may develop in patients with brief, low-level exposure to asbestos.
   e. Rounded atelectasis is a benign manifestation of asbestos exposure that can be mistaken for a malignancy.

5. Which one of the following statements is incorrect?

   a. There are three patterns of silicosis: acute, accelerated, and chronic (classic).
   b. Silicosis shows a predominantly lower zone distribution on the chest radiograph.
   c. Progressive massive fibrosis (PMF) is a complication of silicosis.
   d. There is an increased incidence of tuberculosis in patients with silicosis.
   e. There is an increased incidence of rheumatoid arthritis and scleroderma in patients with silicosis.

6. Which one of the following statements is incorrect?

   a. Methotrexate pulmonary toxicity may not recur upon reinitiation of the drug.
   b. Bleomycin pulmonary toxicity can he prevented by using supplemental oxygen after administration.
   c. Radiation pneumonitis may mimic infectious pneumonia (cough, fever, CP, dyspnea).
   d. Nitrofurantoin pulmonary toxicity may mimic IPF.
   e. Pneumonitis owing to amiodarone may appear more dense than surrounding soft tissue on a CT scan.

7. Which one of the following statements is incorrect?

   a. Interstitial lung disease is more common in men with rheumatoid arthritis than in women with rheumatoid arthritis.
   b. Fifty percent of patients presenting with acute lupus pneumonitis will have had no prior history of lupus.
   c. There is a good correlation between the severity of the cutaneous and pulmonary manifestations of scleroderma.
   d. Jo-1 antibody is associated with the presence of ILD in patients with polymyositis.
   e. ILD associated with Sjögren's syndrome often involves lymphocytic infiltration.

Answers

1. d.

Asbestosis is characterized by the presence of reticulonodular infiltrates in a lower zone distribution. As the disease progresses, there is often volume loss in the lower lobes. The presence of pleural disease, while not sufficient to make the diagnosis of true asbestosis, may be seen in patients with asbestos exposure and is therefore not inconsistent with the diagnosis of asbestosis.

2. e.

Answers a through d are all correct. This question is meant to emphasize the fact that while corticosteroid treatment may result in subjective or objective improvements, it has not been proven that this improves survival.

3. d

Making a histologic diagnosis of sarcoidosis is not considered sufficient reason to treat with steroids. Commonly accepted indications for treatment include significant symptoms or progressive loss of lung function. Involvement of critical extrapulmonary organs may also prompt treatment.

4. b

This question is meant to emphasize the fact that the term *asbestosis* should be reserved for patients with evidence of pulmonary parenchymal scarring. Pleural disease does not merit the diagnosis of asbestosis.

5. b

The distribution of abnormalities on the chest radiograph may be helpful in narrowing the differential diagnosis. Silicosis is associated with x-ray changes in the upper lobes.

6. b

The administration of supplemental oxygen is a risk factor for the development of bleomycin pulmonary toxicity.

7. c

As with many of the connective tissue disease associated interstitial lung diseases, there is no real correlation between the severity of the ILD and the extrapulmonary manifestations.

SUGGESTED READINGS

Graham WGB. Silicosis. Clin Chest Med 1992;13(2): 253–267.

Kaltreider HB. Hypersensitivity pneumonitis. Western J Med 1993;159:570–578.

Meier-Sydow J, Weiss SM, Buhl R, et al. Idiopathic pulmonary fibrosis: current clinical concepts and challenges in management. Semin Respir Crit Care Med 1994;15:77–96.

Mossman BT, Gee JB. Asbestos-related diseases. N Engl J Med 1989;320:1721–1730.

Muller NL, Miller RR. Computed tomography of chronic diffuse infiltrative lung disease. Am Rev Respir Dis 1990;142: 1206–1215.

Rosenow EC, Martin WJ. Drug-induced interstitial lung disease. In: Schwarz MI, King TE, eds. Interstitial lung disease. 2nd ed. St. Louis: CV Mosby , 1993.

Schwarz MI. Clinical overview of interstitial lung disease. In: Schwarz MI, King TE, eds. Interstitial lung disease. 2nd ed. St. Louis: CV Mosby, 1993.

Sharma OP. Sarcoidosis. Disease-A-Month 1990;36(9): 469–535.

C•H•A•P•T•E•R

38

Pleural Diseases

Atul C. Mehta and Herbert P. Wiedemann

A pleural effusion is among the most frequently encountered problems in chest medicine. One estimate places the annual incidence of pleural effusion in the United States at approximately 1 million individuals.

Accumulation of pleural fluid is not a specific disease but rather a reflection of underlying pathology. Pleural effusion may result from many different pulmonary or systemic diseases. The task facing the contemporary clinician is little different from that outlined by Osler in 1892:

In the diagnosis of pleuritic effusion, the first question is, ''Does a fluid exudate exist?'' The second, ''What is its nature?''

DIAGNOSIS OF PLEURAL EFFUSION

Clinical symptoms (dyspnea or pleuritic pain) or signs (diminished breath sounds and dullness to percussion) may suggest the presence of a pleural effusion. However, chest radiographic techniques are important in confirming the presence of pleural effusion and in detecting associated abnormalities that may provide important information regarding etiology (Fig. 38.1).

IMAGING STUDIES

Conventional Chest Radiograph

The standard posteroanterior (PA) and lateral chest radiographs remain the most important techniques for the initial diagnosis of pleural effusion (Fig. 38.1). The distribution of free pleural fluid around the normal lung is primarily influenced by gravity and lung elastic recoil, and to a lesser extent by ''capillary attraction'' between the pleural surfaces (which

creates the meniscus-shaped upper border). Fluid first gravitates to the inferior portion of the hemithorax and lies between the hemidiaphragm and the inferior surface of the lung. Small fluid collections are best appreciated by inspection of the posterior costophrenic angle on the lateral radiograph. Larger fluid collections completely obscure the hemidiaphragm on both projections and assume a very typical appearance. Most fluid collects around the lateral, anterior, and posterior thoracic wall; less fluid collects along the mediastinal surface of the lung, since there is relatively less elastic recoil in this region (lung is fixed at the hilum and pulmonary ligament).

Occasionally, relatively large pleural effusions may remain confined to the infrapulmonary location (the ''subpulmonic effusion''). Such effusions may give the radiographic appearance of elevation of the hemidiaphragm. When a subpulmonic effusion occurs on the left side, its presence is suggested by separation of the ''pseudohemidiaphragm'' from the gastric bubble. A lateral decubitus roentgenogram is extremely valuable in the detection of subpulmonic effusions.

Lateral decubitus films are also useful in distinguishing ''free'' pleural fluid from the ''loculated'' pleural effusion (fluid confined by fibrous pleural adhesions). Pleural effusions might be overlooked on supine or semi-erect roentgenograms (e.g., portable radiograph obtained in the ICU), since the only abnormality may be a vague increase in radiographic density over the hemithorax.

The lateral decubitus roentgenogram can detect effusions as small as 15 ml. The standard PA and lateral roentgenogram can detect roughly 250 ml. The ''moderate'' pleural effusion (1000 ml) extends upward about one-third or one-half of the hemithorax, typically obscuring the hemidiaphragm.

Other Radiographic Techniques

Ultrasound   Thoracic ultrasound is a rapid and safe technique to define and localize pleural fluid. A major advantage

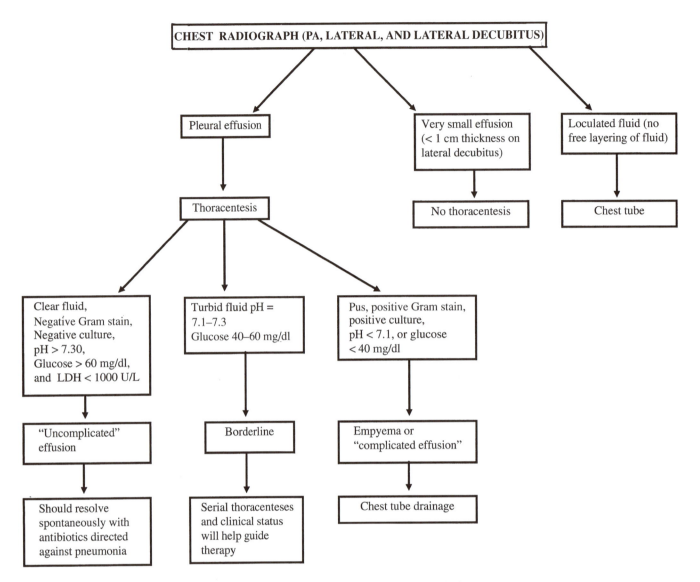

Figure 38.1. Approach to parapneumonic effusion.

over conventional roentgenograms is the ability of ultrasound to differentiate solid components (e.g., tumor or fibrous peel) from liquid components of a pleural process. Ultrasound is also valuable in detecting subpulmonic or subphrenic pathology and differentiating these abnormalities (evaluating the relationship of radiographic densities to the diaphragm). A major use of ultrasound is to guide thoracentesis needles into small or loculated pleural effusions, thereby increasing the yield and safety of thoracentesis. Portable ultrasound units can be brought to the bedside of very ill patients.

Computed Tomography Computed tomographic (CT) examination of the thorax is a major advance in the evaluation of pleural disease. The cross-sectional tomographic image allows the evaluation of complex situations in which the anatomy cannot be fully assessed by plain films or ultrasound. For instance, CT scans are helpful in distinguishing empyema from lung abscess, in detecting pleural masses (mesothelioma, plaques), and in outlining loculated fluid collections.

LABORATORY STUDIES

Transudate Versus Exudate

Although the history, physical examination, and radiographic studies may provide important clues to the etiology of a pleural effusion, almost all cases should be evaluated through a diagnostic thoracentesis. After obtaining fluid, the first diagnostic step is to classify the effusion as a transudate or an exudate, using the protein and lactate dehydrogenase (LDH) values of serum and pleural fluid (Table 38.1). The following method is 99% accurate (Light, et al. Ann Intern Med 1972; 77:507–513).

Table 38.1.	Transudate and Exudate Classification				
	Fluid/ Serum Protein		*Fluid/ Serum LDH*		*Fluid LDH*
Transudate	< 0.5	and	< 0.6	and	< 200
Exudate	> 0.5	or	> 0.6	or	> 200

Previous methods, which used cut-off values for pleural fluid total protein (3.0 gm/100 ml) or specific gravity (1.016), are considerably less accurate (60%–90%).

In recent years, the combination of pleural fluid cholesterol of more than 45 mg/dl and LDH of more than 200 mg/dl has been found to be 98% specific and 99% sensitive in diagnosing exudative effusion. These indicators are likely to replace traditional parameters because they are more accurate and cost effective and do not require simultaneous measurement of serum values (Costa, et al. Chest 1995;108:1260).

Transudates Transudates are formed secondary to elevations in hydrostatic pressure or reductions in colloid osmotic pressure of the systemic or pulmonary circulations. Causes of transudates include:

- Congestive heart failure
- Nephrotic syndrome
- Cirrhosis with ascites
- Peritoneal dialysis
- Atelectasis (early)
- Urinothorax

Pleuropulmonary disease rarely exists, thus the importance of finding a transudate. Further analysis of the pleural fluid, or a pleural biopsy, is unlikely to provide positive information and probably can be avoided. A recent study by Peterman and Speicher (JAMA 1984;252:1051–1053) supports this approach: 83 transudates were evaluated with 725 further tests. Only nine of these follow-up tests were positive, and seven gave false positive results.

Nonetheless, it is important to maintain some wariness before dismissing a transudative effusion. The clinician needs to remain alert to the few instances in which a transudate may be associated with underlying lung disease. Early atelectasis may be associated with a transudate. Also, it is well documented, but often unappreciated, that some patients with malignant pleural effusions have transudative fluids (Sahn. Clin Chest Med 1985;6:113–125). Most of these patients have concomitant congestive heart failure, nephrotic syndrome, or the early stage of mediastinal lymph node involvement with malignancy.

Exudate Exudative effusions signal the presence of disease involving the lungs or pleura. Important or common causes of exudates include:

- Malignancy
- Infection
- Collagen vascular disease
- Parapneumonic effusion (pleural reaction to pneumonia)
- Pulmonary embolus
- Chylothorax (thoracic duct disruption)
- Uremia
- Asbestos exposure
- Thoracic lymphatic obstruction (e.g., lymphoma, radiation)
- Pancreatitis
- Empyema
- Tuberculosis (TB)
- Viral
- Yellow-nail syndrome
- Postcardiotomy syndrome
- Subdiaphragmatic abscess
- Esophageal rupture
- Atelectasis (chronic)
- Idiopathic

Exudative effusions should not be ignored, and attempts to establish the diagnosis should be undertaken. Additional studies of pleural fluid, such as cell count and differential, cytology, Gram stain, cultures, glucose, amylase, pH, ANA, and complement, may help establish the etiology. Pleural biopsy may sometimes help establish the cause of an exudative effusion. Biopsy specimens should be examined histologically (tumor, granuloma) and sent for culture (TB, fungal).

Usefulness of Some Specific Tests of Pleural Fluid

Glucose The pleural fluid glucose level of transudates and most exudates is similar to that of serum. There are few causes of a very low pleural fluid glucose (less than 25 mg/100 ml). Such a finding is seen with rheumatoid disease, TB, empyema, and tumors with extensive pleural involvement. Since the latter two conditions are usually obvious by the clinical setting or other pleural fluid findings, a low glucose may be an important first clue to TB or rheumatoid disease. It has been reported that an intravenous glucose infusion will raise the pleural fluid glucose in TB, but not rheumatoid disease.

Amylase A high pleural fluid amylase usually indicates pancreatitis or esophageal rupture. Iso-enzymes can be used to distinguish pancreatic amylase from salivary gland amylase; however, the clinical setting usually separates these two entities. Also, the fluid pH is low with esophageal rupture and normal in pancreatitis. About 10% of malignant effusions may have elevations of amylase.

pH The pH of the small amount of pleural fluid present in normal individuals is about 7.64. A low pleural fluid pH (pH less than 7.30) may be seen with infected parapneumonic effusions, frank empyema, malignancy, collagen-vascular disease, TB, esophageal rupture, and urinothorax (the only cause of a low pH transudative effusion). Effusions from other causes will almost always have a pH greater than 7.30. It is essential that pleural fluid for pH analysis be aspirated anaerobically and transported on ice. A falsely high pH will result if the fluid is exposed to room air and a falsely low pH will result if it is not kept on ice. The pH will be stable for 1 to 2 hours at 0°C. The major utility of pleural fluid pH is in the management of parapneumonic effusions, as popularized by R.W. Light (see later discussion of the management of parapneumonic effusions). However, the pH may provide no independent information in this regard beyond that which can be learned by measuring pleural fluid glucose (Potts, et al. Arch Intern Med 1978;138:1378–1380).

Diagnostic Aspects of Certain Exudative Effusions

Collagen-Vascular Disease   Systemic lupus erythematous (SLE) and rheumatoid disease are important causes of pleural effusion. Up to 75% of SLE patients will have pleural involvement during the course of their disease. Frequently, the effusion is the only radiographic abnormality in these patients. Lupus effusions are characteristically small to moderate in size but associated with significant pleuritic pain (pleurisy). Pleuritis may be an important first manifestation of SLE; in about 6% of patients, pleural effusion is an isolated first sign and in an additional 30% of patients there are only minor antecedent symptoms.

The pleural fluid ANA titer may be helpful in separating SLE effusions from effusions because of other etiologies, even in patients with known SLE. A pleural fluid ANA greater than 1:160 or a pleural fluid/serum ANA ratio greater than 1.0 indicates lupus pleuritis (Good, et al. Chest 1983;84:714–718). Although these criteria appear to be highly specific, they are not highly sensitive (some patients with SLE pleuritis will not fulfill them). The presence of LE cells in pleural effusions is highly specific for SLE or drug-induced lupus, and this finding has been reported to precede the appearance of LE cells or ANA in serum by several months in some patients. However, the finding of LE cells may not have a high sensitivity. The presence of a speckled staining pattern usually suggests an alternate diagnosis.

Pleural effusions occur in about 5% of rheumatoid arthritic patients. Unlike SLE, the effusions are often asymptomatic, may be quite large, and often persist for many months without change. Interestingly, rheumatoid effusions are more common in males, despite the fact that rheumatoid disease is more common in women. Usually, effusions occur in patients with high serum RF titers and rheumatoid nodules. Pleural fluid RF titers are not helpful since they may be elevated in pneumonia, TB, malignancy, and SLE. "Silent empyema" is a risk, especially in steroid-treated patients.

SLE and rheumatoid effusions may have low complement levels and high levels of immune complexes, but these findings are not completely specific (tumors, empyema).

Tuberculosis   The most common form of TB effusion is a "hypersensitivity" reaction that occurs in the postprimary phase of the initial infection. Other evidence of infection is usually lacking. Although these exudates usually resolve spontaneously, about 30% of patients will develop active disease within 5 years. The diagnosis is difficult and usually requires a pleural biopsy, in which the pleura is examined histologically for granulomas and AFB and cultured for TB. Pleural fluid analysis (AFB and culture) will be positive in only 20–25% of cases; pleural biopsies increase the yield to 55–80%.

Chylothorax   Disruption of the thoracic duct (trauma, surgery, tumor) leads to a chylothorax. The milky appearance is characteristic, but occasionally a chronic TB or rheumatoid effusion will have this appearance ("pseudochylothorax"). A true chylothorax has a high fat content (greater than 400 mg/100 ml), mostly triglycerides. The psuedochylothorax, in contrast, has low fat and high cholesterol levels. A pleural fluid triglyceride level above 110 mg/dl indicates a probable chylothorax, whereas a level below 50 mg/dl essentially rules out chylothorax. In borderline situations (pleural fluid triglyceride level between 50 and 100 mg/dl), lipoprotein electrophoreses of the pleural fluid is helpful; the finding of chylomicrons in the fluid establishes the diagnosis of chylothorax.

Urinothorax   Urinothorax is a relatively rare disorder in which urine collects in the pleural space because of ipsilateral urinary tract obstruction. The diagnostic triad is:

1. Transudate
2. Low pH (< 7.30)
3. Pleural fluid/serum creatinine ratio > 1.0

Malignancy   Pleural fluid cytology will be positive in 60–90% of patients with effusion secondary to involvement of the pleura by tumor, except for mesiothelioma, where its sensitivity is only 32%. Remember that bronchogenic cancer may cause effusion owing to atelectasis, pneumonia, or lymphatic obstruction without involving the pleura. Carcinoembryonic antigen (CEA) may help differentiate malignant from benign effusions in some cases, but the sensitivity and specificity of this test are not high enough to make it useful in routine evaluation. Mesothelioma appears to be the only cause of a very high hyaluronic acid level, although this finding may not be very sensitive. Immunocytometry recently proved helpful in the diagnosis of lymphoma in an idiopathic pleural effusion, in which conventional cytologic and histopathologic techniques were nondiagnostic (Kavuru, et al.).

Asbestos   The entity of "benign asbestos effusion" has been recognized recently, and its natural history better defined. These effusions are often bloody but are otherwise nonspecific exudates. The peak incidence is about 10–15 years after onset of asbestos exposure (somewhat earlier than the other pleural complications of asbestos). About one-third of patients are asymptomatic; the others may have pleuritic discomfort, mild fever, or dyspnea. The effusions persist for a mean of 4 months and then resolve spontaneously in most patients. A variable amount of pleural fibrosis often results. About one-third of patients may have recurrent effusion or persistent pleural pain. Few cases of mesothelioma have occurred in these patients and usually only after an interval of several years. Thus, benign asbestos pleurisy does not seem to be an indicator for increased risk of mesothelioma. Diagnosis of benign asbestos pleurisy is by history of asbestos exposure and exclusion of other causes.

Amyloidosis Amyloidosis can be accompanied by pleural effusion in up to 30% of patients. These effusions are usually transudative and are probably most often caused by congestive heart failure. However, a recent report suggests that amyloid deposition can be found on pleural biopsy specimens in a high percentage of these patients, suggesting that pleural biopsy may be a reasonably sensitive technique in the diagnosis of systemic amyloidosis (Kavuru, et al.).

Furthermore, some patients with pleural amyloidosis have otherwise unexplained exudative effusions, raising the possibility that amyloid deposits may play a causative role in pleural fluid formation in some patients.

AIDS Pleural effusion in hospitalized AIDS patients is not uncommon (27%). Bacterial infection (30%), pneumocystis carinii (15%), and TB (8%) are the most common causes. Kaposi's sarcoma and hypoalbuminemia are the most common noninfectious causes.

TREATMENT OF PLEURAL EFFUSIONS

THERAPEUTIC THORACENTESIS

When a pleural effusion is large enough to cause symptoms (usually dyspnea) and specific therapy of the underlying etiology is ineffective or too slow, a ''therapeutic'' thoracentesis is indicated. If fluid reaccumulates and symptoms recur, thoracentesis can be repeated two or three times. However, repetitive removal of large amounts of fluid over a short period of time is discouraged because of potential complications from protein loss and fluid shifts. More definitive therapy such as instillation of a pleural sclerosing agent is usually indicated when a symptomatic pleural effusion rapidly recurs after a few attempts at drainage with thoracentesis.

In general, no more than 1000–1500 ml of fluid should be removed at one time. Removal of more fluid risks the development of edema in the underlying lung (''re-expansion pulmonary edema'') or rapid fluid shift from the intravascular space into the pleural space (''post-thoracentesis shock''). Both of these phenomena appear to be related, in part, to creating excessive negative pleural pressures during thoracentesis. If desired, pleural fluid pressures can be directly measured periodically during thoracentesis, using an Abrams needle connected to a three-way valve and a manometer. Fluid can be safely withdrawn until a pressure of about −20 cm water is reached (measured in the eighth or ninth posterior intercostal space). This technique has allowed up to 4 L of effusion to be safely withdrawn at one time. However, since removal of 1–1.5 L usually is enough to provide at least temporary relief of dyspnea, measuring pleural fluid pressures during thoracentesis is generally unnecessary.

Dyspnea secondary to pleural fluid accumulation is probably more related to intrathoracic volume changes than to chemoreceptor input. Even in those instances when thoracentesis provides relief of dyspnea, there often is a temporary decrease in arterial oxygenation (pO_2). The magnitude and duration of hypoxia bears a rough correlation to the amount of fluid removed. Hypoxia may last 12 hours or more. Thus, if a large amount of fluid is removed, or the patient has a low baseline pO_2, supplemental nasal oxygen probably should be given for several hours following a thoracentesis.

TRANSUDATES

Pleural effusions secondary to heart failure, ascites, or nephrotic syndrome can usually be managed with appropriate medical therapy, such as diuretics and sodium restriction. Acutely, therapeutic thoracentesis will allow time for medical management. Rarely recurrent symptomatic pleural effusions complicate cirrhosis or nephrosis despite optimal medical therapy; doxycycline sclerosis of the pleural cavity (see below) will usually be successful.

EXUDATES

Parapneumonic Effusions

The management of parapneumonic effusions represents a particular challenge to the clinician. These exudative effusions often accompany bacterial pneumonias, but they usually spontaneously resolve with appropriate antimicrobial therapy of the pneumonia. A minority, probably a subset of those that become infected, will progress to empyema (frank pus in the pleural space) and subsequent loculation and fibrosis of the pleura. Treatment at this late stage may require several tube thoracostomies or even surgical decortication. These complications can usually be prevented by early and complete drainage of the pleural space with a single chest tube. However, indiscriminate universal application of tube thoracostomy would constitute unnecessary therapy for the majority of patients with parapneumonic effusions. Thus, the task is to intervene with tube thoracostomy selectively, but early enough to be definitive.

All parapneumonic effusions should be immediately evaluated by thoracentesis. An exception may be very small parapneumonic effusions (fluid layer seen on lateral decubitus chest film less than 1 cm in thickness), which rarely cause complications. The following findings are all indications for complete drainage of the pleural space:

- Presence of frank pus (admittedly a loosely defined term)
- Bacteria on Gram stain
- Evidence of loculation (by chest roentgenogram)

Thoracentesis may be adequate for complete pleural space drainage in some instances, but usually tube thoracostomy is required. Conversely, effusions that are sterile and not turbid in appearance do not require aggressive intervention. However, many parapneumonic effusions will be ''borderline,'' occupying a position between these extremes.

The use of fluid pH has been advocated as a means of evaluating these borderline effusions. Unfortunately, the literature does not support the use of a single ''cut-off'' pH value as a predictor. Furthermore, misinterpretation is possible if fluid specimens for pH analysis are not kept anaerobic and on ice. Nevertheless, a low pH (less than 7.0–7.2) usually indicates a fluid with high potential for loculation, while a high pH (greater than 7.3) suggests a very low risk for complications. In cases that are doubtful, serial evaluation of the pleural fluid may help guide therapy. All parameters (e.g., appearance, Gram stain, WBC count, glucose, protein, LDH, pH) should be evaluated on each thoracentesis. In this setting, a declining pH would argue for tube drainage. Pleural loculation can occur rapidly (less than 24 hours) with certain infections; serial evaluation should not be allowed to delay necessary therapy. At times, 2–3 thoracenteses should be used in the first day.

Finally, it is better to err on the side of early tube drainage rather than risk incomplete drainage of an infected parapneumonic effusion.

Malignant Effusions

A variety of malignancies can lead to pleural effusion, usually secondary to direct extension or metastases of the tumor to the pleura. Breast and lung cancer are the most frequent, but many others, including pancreas, colon, esophageal, and ovarian cancers, can also involve the pleura. Lymphomas, in contrast, frequently cause pleural effusion without direct involvement of the pleura, probably via central obstruction of lymphatics.

The first step in controlling malignant effusions is radiation therapy or systemic chemotherapy, if appropriate for the tumor. With lymphomas, the use of mediastinal radiation (1400–2600 rads) is usually effective, even when the chest roentgenogram shows no evidence of central lymph node involvement. Radiation therapy directed to the pleura usually is not appropriate therapy for malignant effusions because of unavoidable exposure of the lung parenchyma. Chemotherapy for carcinomas is usually not effective in controlling malignant effusions, except sometimes with breast, ovarian, or small-cell lung cancer.

Needle aspiration is an important early step to assess whether symptoms are relieved by fluid removal and to determine the rate of fluid reaccumulation. Most malignant effusions will recur rapidly within 3–4 days. Prolonged drainage by tube thoracostomy may be tried but will fail in at least 50% of cases.

Pleural Sclerosis

In patients with uncontrolled and symptomatic malignant effusions, pleural symphysis achieved by instillation of a ''sclerosing'' agent is indicated. Pleural sclerosis should be attempted only if the lung expands fully after fluid removal. Agents that can be instilled into the pleural cavity to achieve pleural sclerosis include:

- Doxycycline
- Talc slurry
- Bleomycin
- Quinacrine

We believe that these agents work by producing a chemical serositis that heals by fibrosis, rather than a direct antitumor effect. This is probably true even for most of the antineoplastic agents that have been employed. Regardless of what agent is used, proper technique is essential for success. The pleural cavity should be completely drained of fluid to avoid dilution of the sclerosing substance. More important, the visceral and parietal pleura need to be closely approximated, obliterating the pleural space, so that fibrotic healing achieves pleural symphysis, thus preventing recurrence of the effusion.

The ideal sclerosing agent would be readily available at low cost, have a low morbidity and toxicity, and be highly effective. Doxycycline appears to be the agent of first choice. With proper technique, doxycycline sclerosis is 80–90% effective:

1. Evacuate pleural cavity by tube thoracostomy at low suction (15–20 cm water).
2. Order a chest radiograph to verify position of tube, clearance of pleural fluid, and re-expansion of lung.
3. Premedicate with narcotic analgesic 30–60 minutes before sclerosis.
4. Instill 15–20 mg/kg of tetracycline hydrochloride in 80 ml of saline, combined with 20 cc of 1% lidocaine, into chest tube.
5. Flush tube with 20 ml of saline.
6. Clamp tube (no suction).
7. Put patient in prone, supine, right decubitus, left decubitus, and sitting position for 4–5 minutes each (20–25 minutes). Repeat each position for 30 minutes each (2 1/2 hours).
8. Unclamp tube and connect to low suction.
9. Continue until drainage <100–150 ml/day (may take 3 to 5 days).
10. Remove tube.

Side effects are mild. About one-third of patients will have a low-grade febrile response. Chest pain is unpredictable;

sometimes it is absent and at other times it is rather severe. However, the pain is self-limited, lasting 30–45 minutes. Generally, pain can be prevented by premedication with parenteral narcotics and concurrent administration of intracavitary lidocaine. Some have advocated giving the intracavitary lidocaine 30 minutes before instilling doxycycline, but this is probably unnecessary. The effectiveness of doxycycline sclerosis is not diminished by peripheral neutropenia, since a white cell inflammatory response is not necessary for its action. Tetracycline appears to produce a prompt destruction of the mesothelial cell-lining layer. The low pH of tetracycline solutions appears to be a factor but does not explain the entire effect.

Treatment failures usually are related to inability to approximate the pleural surfaces during doxycycline administration. This may be owing to atelectasis (central bronchial obstruction because of tumor) or owing to a ''trapped lung'' encased by either a fibrotic visceral pleura or massive tumor involvement. The latter circumstance may be suggested when a malignant effusion has a very low pH and glucose.

If doxycycline is contraindicated because of allergy or other reasons, bleomycin appears to be a good choice. Although experience with this agent is limited, instillation is well-tolerated and often effective. Systemic side effects have not been reported.

Talc is very effective in producing pleural symphysis. Traditionally, this agent has been introduced as a dry powder abrasive (talc poudrage) at open thoracotomy or insufflated through a chest tube. Since even the latter approach is usually done under general anesthesia, use of talc has been limited. However, a bedside technique using instillation of a talc saline suspension has been advocated. In this method, 10 gm of talc USP powder (previously gas sterilized and aerated) is suspended in 250 ml of sterile saline solution. This can be accomplished with a bulb syringe and sterile plastic cup. The suspension is administered with tube thoracostomy in a manner analogous to doxycycline sclerosis. Since instillation of talc may be painful, narcotic premedication should be given. Talc pleurodesis has rarely been associated with acute pneumonitis and ARDS.

Surgical Therapy

Parietal pleurectomy and, if necessary for trapped lung, decortication of the visceral pleura are both definitive procedures that give a 100% response rate. However, mortality is high (up to 5–10%) and morbidity may be great (air leaks after decortication). Thus, these procedures should be applied selectively. Surgery generally should be limited to instances in which sclerosis has failed or lung expansion is prevented by a thickened pleura. Important considerations before resorting to surgery include:

- Good condition of the underlying lung
- Low tumor burden outside the chest

- Expected long-term survival
- General medical condition good enough for major surgery

When a malignant cause for pleural effusion is discovered at thoracotomy, it is usually appropriate to attempt pleural abrasion, talc poudrage, or pleurectomy at that time.

CHYLOTHORAX

The accumulation of chyle in the pleural space is usually secondary to disruption of the thoracic duct by trauma (surgical or nonsurgical) or by malignancy. A congenital form also exists. Most ''idiopathic'' adult cases are thought to be caused by unrecognized mild trauma. Chylothorax is differentiated from pseudochylothorax by its high triglyceride and low cholesterol content.

Chylothorax may cause dyspnea; other local complications are rare. Chyle is bacteriostatic and infections rarely occur. Furthermore, chyle does not seem to be highly fibrogenic. The major problem is the nutritive and immunologic cost of the continuous loss of thoracic duct contents. Chyle is high in protein, electrolytes, fat, fat-soluble vitamins, and lymphocytes. Cell-mediated immunity assessed by skin tests and graft survival decreases at 3–6 weeks of continuous drainage. Furthermore, there is the theoretical problem of permanent loss of T-lymphocytes in adults who have little thymic activity. Before modern nutritional and surgical therapy, chylothorax had a 50% mortality.

The flow within the thoracic duct is highly dependent on diet, especially fat intake. Normal lymph flow is about 2.5 l/day (1.38 ml/kg/hr); in starvation, it may decrease to 300–500 ml. Dietary manipulation that decreases lymph flow rate is important for the healing of thoracic duct lesions and forms the rationale for conservative therapy. Of note, medium-chain triglycerides (MCT) are absorbed through the portal venous system, while long-chain triglycerides are carried via lymph. Thus, lymph flow is greatly reduced if dietary fat is limited to MCT.

Conservative Therapy

Initially, 2–3 thoracenteses are done to assess reaccumulation rate. If leakage continues tube thoracostomy drainage should be instituted. Concurrently, oral intake should be limited to a MCT diet (Portagen or MCT oil, both by Mead Johnson). If necessary, lymph flow is reduced further by use of venous hyperalimentation and avoidance of oral intake. Of course, this is much less convenient and carries risk of infection and other complications.

Chyle itself should not be reinfused intravenously because of the possibility of venous thrombosis or fatal anaphylaxis.

Pleural sclerosis is usually avoided since it may complicate subsequent surgical therapy if this proves necessary. If a patient is not a surgical candidate, pleural sclerosis may be attempted when dietary manipulation fails.

Surgical Therapy

Surgical therapy consists of ligation of the thoracic duct. Two general approaches are available. The duct can be ligated most easily via a right thoracotomy at the level of T8 to T10, where it usually exists as a single trunk. Alternatively, closure may be attempted directly at the leakage site. However, locating the site (despite use of dyes to stain the lymph) and sealing the leak may both be technically difficult. Furthermore, the duct will have to be ligated both above and below the leak because of rich anastomotic communications. With either choice, ligation of the thoracic duct has little adverse consequence, since lymph reaches the venous system by alternate channels.

Choice of Therapy

The major difficulty is deciding how long to try conservative therapy before resorting to surgery. There is no easy answer to this; each case must be individualized. A few generalizations may help. Congenital chylothorax in neonates usually responds well to conservative management. With chylothorax owing to malignancies, radiation or systemic chemotherapy may halt chyle leakage in up to two-thirds of lymphomas and one-half of carcinomas; furthermore, unless relatively long-term survival is expected, therapy should remain conservative. Traumatic chylothorax will eventually spontaneously cease in about 50% of cases; however, it is difficult to predict this outcome. In trauma and other causes of chylothorax, the rate of chyle loss should help guide therapy. If chyle loss is low (less than 0.25 ml/kg/hr), this would enable a longer trial of conservative therapy. If chyle loss is dramatic (more than 2 ml/kg/hr), then conservative therapy will likely be less effective and should be abandoned earlier. As a general rule, it is reasonable to try 1–4 weeks of conservative therapy before resorting to surgery.

EFFUSIONS OF INDETERMINATE ETIOLOGY

The etiology of some pleural effusions remains obscure even after thoracentesis and 2–3 closed pleural biopsies done on separate occasions. A careful general clinical examination including appropriate lab tests (PPD, ANA, and rheumatoid factor) or radiographs (CT of the thorax) may provide important clues. However, the cause often remains perplexing. At this point, the clinician is faced with a choice of observing the patient or proceeding with thoracoscopy or thoracotomy. A case for taking the conservative approach derives from the fact that many of these effusions (roughly one-half) will resolve spontaneously and no disease will be apparent on long-term follow-up. But that leaves the other half, who

will have carcinoma, mesothelioma, lymphoma, or other serious diseases.

If the patient looks well and has no fever, pain, or weight loss, then careful observation may be warranted. If there are indications of underlying disease, an aggressive diagnostic approach is warranted. There is some information in the literature to support the general soundness of this approach. It should be noted, finally, that even a negative exploratory thoracotomy does not rule out occult malignancy as a cause for pleural effusion.

OTHER EFFUSIONS

Moderate or large-sized hemothorax should be promptly and completely evacuated. Blood in the pleural space may lead to fibrin deposition, causing adhesions and limitation of lung expansion. Furthermore, as a practical point, tube thoracostomy will help evaluate the rate or recurrence of bleeding. Small hemothoraces usually resolve spontaneously without residua.

Treatment of pleural effusions associated with collagen vascular diseases is directed against the underlying disease. Lupus effusions usually are not large enough to cause symptoms; rather, pain from the pleuritis heralds the process. Appropriate analgesics or anti-inflammatory medications are given. Rheumatoid effusions may present with dyspnea and require therapeutic thoracentesis. Clinically "silent" empyemas may occur in rheumatoid patients on corticosteroids and require tube thoracostomy drainage.

Effusions owing to pulmonary thromboembolism or pancreatitis require no specific therapy for the effusion itself.

Asbestos

Asbestos exposure may lead to benign, often serosanguineous, exudative effusions. The diagnosis is difficult to make and usually must be presumptive based on history and ruling out other causes. These effusions will resolve spontaneously but often leave behind a thickened pleura. It is not known whether aggressive drainage of the effusion will prevent this sequela.

Tuberculous Effusions

Tuberculous effusions may occur early in the course of the infection, often as part of an otherwise occult process. Such tuberculous pleurisy is usually self-limited, clearing without treatment. However, up to one-half of untreated patients will subsequently develop active disease elsewhere within 5 years. Thus, antituberculous therapy with an appropriate drug regimen is indicated. Often therapy must be presumptive, pending results of pleural fluid and biopsy cultures. If the effusion is large and symptomatic, concurrent use of systemic corticosteroids may have a salutary effect. TB may also involve the pleura by direct spread from active disease of lung, lymph nodes, or bone. Frank tuberculous empyema requires chest tube drainage.

REVIEW EXERCISES

QUESTIONS

1. A 30-year-old African-American male presents with acute, excruciating, right-flank and lower chest pain, NV.

    Past medical history: 1 episode of hematuria 1 year ago
    Family history: Twin sister with sarcoid
    On examination: Patient in distress with pain, right flank tenderness and upper quadrant guarding.
    Right dullness and pleural rub
    CXR: Moderate right effusion
    KUB film: Not obtainable
    Pleural fluid: Appearance: amber, pH 6.9, LDH 40 IU/dl, protein 0.5 g/dl, hemoglotin +1.
    Following administration of adequate analgesia, the most appropriate action would be:

    a. Ultrasound of gallbladder and pancreas
    b. V/Q scan
    c. Closed pleural biopsy
    d. Urology consult
    e. Upper endoscopy

2. A 70-year-old male, with a history of IDDM, alcohol abuse, severe GERD, emphysema, and BPH requiring indwelling catheter and frequent courses of intravenous antibiotics, presents with high-grade fever, congestion, cough productive of thick, yellow, blood-tinged sputum and right pleuritic chest pain.

    On examination: Ill-looking M with RUL consolidation and right base dullness
    CXR.: Right upper lobe alveolar infiltrate with cavity and moderate right effusion
    LAB: Leukocytosis with left shift
    ABG: pH 7.32, PCO_2 52, PO_2 80 on 3 L FIO_2
    Pleural fluid: Thick, yellow purulent material; pH 7.82, glucose 30, LDH 1050

    The most appropriate immediate action would be:

    a. Urine culture and sensitivity, replace Foley
    b. Continuous broad spectrum positive/negative intravenous antibiotics
    c. Thoracic surgery consult for open thoracostomy
    d. Tube thoracostomy
    e. Stop antacid, order esophagogastroduodenoscopy

3. A 60-year-old white male presents with bilateral, vague, nonpleuritic chest pain and mild SOB; no fever, cough, night sweats.

    Past medical history: 15 months ago pt. had right effusion, resolved spontaneously, occ. bilateral wrist pain × 5 years, treated with aspirin. Annual PPD negative 3 months ago.

    On examination:Bibasilar dullness, hard nodule on the nose
    CXR: Bilateral moderate pleural effusion
    Pleural fluid: WBC 2000/cumm, P: 90%, pH 7.05, LDH 1000 IU/Lt, protein 4 g/dl, glucose 5 mg/dl

    Based on the most likely diagnosis, appropriate action would be:

    a. INH 300 mg, rifampin 600 mg, ethanbutol 900 mg/d
    b. Prednisone 40 mg/d
    c. Bilateral chest tube placement
    d. Intravenous ceflazidime and garamycine
    e. Close observation for spontaneous resolution of fluid

4. A 30-year-old female presents with slowly progressing SOB of 6 months. Past medical history: Pnemothoraces, one on either side, 4 weeks apart 1 year ago.

    On examination: Increased dullness left base, right basilar crackles, small ascites
    CXR: Hyperinflated lungs, vague interstitial changes and left effusion
    Pleural tap: Milky white fluid, triglycerides 200 mg/dl

    Most likely diagnosis is:

    a. Lymphoma
    b. Catamenial pneumothorax
    c. Gorham's syndrome
    d. Lymphangioleiomyomatosis
    e. Histiocytosis—X

5. A 63-year-old male in a wheelchair presents with crippling rheumatoid arthritis. The annual chest radiograph revealed moderate bilateral effusion. No chest pain, cough, SOB.

    CXR: Review of old radiograph: bilateral subpulmonic effusion × 5 years
    PPD: Negative
    Pleural fluid: Milky white shiny fluid, WBC 2000/CML, 90% L, glucose 16 mg/dl, LDH 1200 IU/dl, triglycerides 30 mg/dl, cholesterol 150 mg/dl, large amount of cholesterol crystals

    The most appropriate action would be:

    a. Start MCT diet
    b. Lymphangiogram
    c. Serology for W. Bancrofti infestation
    d. Bilateral pleuroparetoneal pump
    e. Conservative treatment

6. A 70-year-old male with history of CHF, on optimal Rx, underwent thoracentesis in ER for large right effusion using 16g spinal needle (3.5 l of serosanguinous fluid was removed uneventfully). Minutes following the procedure, the patient developed progressive SOB and needed 100% FIO_2. On examination: Tachypnea, right lung wheeze and basilar rales, BP 100/70, pulse 100/min

The most appropriate statement regarding the event would be:

a. Place large bore chest tube for tension pneumo.
b. Transfuse 2 units of pack cells for hemothorax.
c. Lasix 60 mg intravenously.
d. Intrapleural pressure monitoring could have avoided the event.
e. Check CPK and V/Q lung scan.

7. What is the most important mechanism for the relief of dyspnea after thoracentesis:

a. ↑ PaO_2
b. Placebo effect
c. ↑ Intrathoracic volume
d. ↑ FEV_1, FVC
e. ↑ Static lung compliance

Answers

1. d
2. d
   Proteus empyema, urea-splitting property leads to ammonia production and an increased pH.
3. b
4. d
5. e
6. d
7. c

SUGGESTED READINGS

GENERAL

Sahn SA. The pleura. Am Rev Respir Dis 1988;138:184–234.

Chretien J, Bignon J, Hirsch A, Huchon G, eds. The pleura in health and disease. Volume in: Lung Biology in Health and Disease. New York: Marcel Dekker, 1985.

Light RW, ed. Pleural diseases. (Clin Chest Med, Vol. 6, No. 1) Philadelphia: WB Saunders, 1985.

THORACENTESIS

Brandstetter RD, Cohen RP. Hypoxemia after thoracentesis: a predictable and treatable condition. JAMA 1979; 242: 1060–1061.

Brown NE, Zamel N, Aberman A. Changes in pulmonary mechanics and gas exchange following thoracentesis. Chest 1978;74:540–542.

Estenne M, Yernault J-C, Troyer A. Mechanism of relief of dyspnea after thoracentesis in patients with large pleural effusions. Am J Med 1983;74:813–819.

Sprung CL, Loewenherz JW, Baier H, et al. Evidence for increased permeability in reexpansion pulmonary edema. Am J Med 1981;71:497–500.

DIAGNOSTIC ASPECTS

Adelman M, Albelda SM, Gottlieb J, et al. Diagnostic utility of pleural fluid eosinophilia. Am J Med 1984;77:915–920.

Costa M, Quiroga T, Cruz E. Measurement of pleural fluid cholesterol and lactate dehydrogenase. Chest 1995;108: 1260–1063.

Good JT, Taryle DA, Maulitz RM, et al. The diagnostic value of pleural fluid pH. Chest 1980;78:55–59.

Hammersten JF, Honska WL, Limes BJ. Pleural fluid amylase in pancreatitis and other diseases. Am Rev Tuberc 1959;79: 606.

Hunder GG, McDuffie FC, Huston KA, et al. Pleural fluid complement, complement conversion, and immune complexes in immunologic and non-immunologic diseases. J Lab Clin Med 1977;90:971–980.

Jay SJ. Diagnostic procedures for pleural disease. Clin Chest Med 1985;6:33–48.

Klockars M, Pettersson T, Riska H, et al. Pleural fluid lysozyme in human disease. Arch Intern Med 1979;139:73–79.

Light RW, MacGregor MI, Ball WC, et al. Diagnostic significance of pleural fluid pH and pCO_2. Chest 1973;64:591–596.

Light RW, MacGregor MI, Luchsinger PC, et al. Pleural effusions: the diagnostic separation of transudates and exudates. Ann Intern Med 1972;77:507–513.

Peterman TA, Speicher CE. Evaluating pleural effusions: a two-stage laboratory approach. JAMA 1984;252:1051–1053.

Pettersson T, Riska H. Diagnostic value of total and differential leukocyte counts in pleural effusions. Acta Med Scand 1981;210:129–135.

PLEURAL BIOPSY

Mezies R, Charbonneau M. Thoracoscopy for the diagnosis of pleural disease. Ann Intern Med. 1991;114:271–276.

Poe RH, Israel RH, Utell MJ, et al. Sensitivity, specificity, and predictive values of closed pleural biopsy. Arch Intern Med 1984;144:325–328.

RADIOGRAPHIC EVALUATION

Pugatch RD, Spirn PW. Radiology of the pleura. Clin Chest Med 1985;6:17–32.

Ravin CE. Thoracentesis of loculated pleural effusions using grey scale ultrasonic guidance. Chest 1977;61:666–668.

PARAPNEUMONIC EFFUSIONS/EMPYEMA

Lew DP, Despont J-P, Perrin LH, et al. Demonstration of a local exhaustion of complement components and of an enzymatic degradation of immunoglobulins in pleural empyema: a possible factor favoring the persistence of local bacterial infections. Clin Exp Immunol 1980;42:506–514.

Light RW. Management of parapneumonic effusions. Arch Intern Med 1981;141:1339–1341.

Light RW, Girard WM, Jenkinson SG, et al. Parapneumonic effusions. Am J Med 1980;69:507–512.

Potts DE, Levin DC, Sahn SA. Pleural fluid pH in parapneumonic effusions. Chest 1976;70:328–331.

Potts DE, Taryle DA, Sahn SA. The glucose-pH relationship in parapneumonic effusions. Arch Intern Med 1978;138:1378–1380.

Varkey B, Rose HD, Kutty K, et al. Empyema thoracis during a ten-year period. Arch Intern Med 1981;141:1771–1776.

Wiedemann HP, Reynolds HY. Humoral immune defenses in bacterial infection of the pleural spaces. In: Chretien J, Bignon J, Hirsch A, Huchon G, eds. The pleura in health and disease. New York: Marcel Dekker, 1985:347–368.

MALIGNANT EFFUSIONS

Austin EH, Flye MW. The treatment of recurrent malignant pleural effusion. Ann Thorac Surg 1970;28:190–203.

Bitran JD, Brown C, Desser RK, et al. Intracavitary bleomycin for the control of malignant effusions. J Surg Oncol 1981;16:273–277.

Bouchama A, Chastre J, Gaudichet A, et al. Acute pneumonitis with bilateral pleural effusion after talc pleurodesis. Chest 1984;86:795–797.

Canto A, Ferrer G, Romagosa V, et al. Lung cancer and pleural effusion: clinical significance and study of pleural metastatic locations. Chest 1985;87:649–652.

Ceyhar BB, Demiralp E, Celirel T. Analysis of pleural effusions using flowcytometry. Respiration 1996;63:17–24.

Decker DA, Dines DA, Payne WAS, et al. Significance of a cytologically negative pleural effusion in bronchogenic carcinoma. Chest 1978;74:640–642.

Dewald GW, Hicks GA, Dines DE, et al. Cytogenetic diagnosis of malignant pleural effusions: culture methods to supplement direct preparations in diagnosis. Mayo Clin Proc 1982;57:488–494.

Gupta N, Opfell RW, Padova J, et al. Intrapleural bleomycin versus tetracycline for control of malignant pleural effusion: a randomized study. Proceed Am Assn Cancer Res, Am Soc Clin Onc 1980;23:C–189.

Heffner JE, Standerfer RJ, Torstveit J, et al. Clinical efficacy of doxycycline for pleurodesis. Chest 1994;105:1743–1747.

Kavuru MS, Tubbs R, Miller ML, et al. Immunocytometry in the diagnosis of lymphoma in an idiopathic pleural effusion. Am Rev Respir Dis 1992;145:209–211.

Leff A, Hopewell PC, Costello J. Pleural effusion from malignancy. Ann Intern Med 1978;88:532–537.

Livingston RB, McCracken JD, Trauth CJ, et al. Isolated pleural effusion in small cell lung carcinoma: favorable prognosis. Chest 1982;81:208–211.

Nystrom JS, Dyce B, Wada J, et al. Carcinoembryonic antigen titers on effusion fluid: a diagnostic tool? Arch Intern Med 1977;137:875–879.

Ostrowski MJ, Halsall GM. Intracavitary bleomycin in the management of malignant effusions: a multicenter study. Cancer Treat Rep 1982;66:1903–1907.

Prakash UBS, Reiman HM. Comparison of needle biopsy with cytologic analysis for the evaluation of pleural effusion: analysis of 414 cases. Mayo Clin Proc 1985;60:158–164.

Renshaw AA, Dean BR, Antman KH, et al. The role of cytologic evaluation of pleural fluid in the diagnosis of malignant mesothelioma. Chest 1997;111:106–109.

Rerger HW, Maher G. Decreased glucose concentration in malignant pleural effusions. Am Rev Respir Dis 1971;103: 427–429.

Rinaldo JE, Owens GR, Rogers RM. Adult respiratory distress syndrome following intrapleural instillation of talc. J Thorac Cardiovasc Surg 1983;85:523–526.

Rittgers RA, Loewenstein MS, Feinerman AE, et al. Carcinoembryonic antigen levels in benign and malignant pleural effusions. Ann Intern Med 1978;88:631–634.

Sahn SA. Malignant pleural effusions. Clin Chest Med 1985; 6:113–125.

Whitcomb ME, Schwarz MI. Pleural effusion complicating intensive mediastinal radiation therapy. Am Rev Respir Dis 1971;103:100–106.

COLLAGEN-VASCULAR DISEASES

Good JT, King TE, Antony VB, et al. Lupus pleuritis: clinical features and pleural fluid characteristics with special reference to pleural fluid antinuclear antibodies. Chest 1983;84: 714–718.

Halla JT, Schrohenloher RE, Volanakis JE. Immune complexes and other laboratory features of pleural effusions: a comparison of rheumatoid arthritis, systemic lupus erythematosus, and other diseases. Ann Intern Med 1980;92:748–752.

Hunder GG, McDuffie FC, Hepper NG. Pleural fluid complement in systemic lupus erythematosus and rheumatoid arthritis. Ann Intern Med 1972;76:357–363.

Khare V, Baetlige B, Larg S, et al. ANA in pleural fluid. Chest 1994;106; 866–871.

Pettersson T, Klockars M, Hellstrom P-E. Chemical and immunological features of pleural effusions: comparison between rheumatoid arthritis and other diseases. Thorax 1982; 37:354–361.

Sahn SA. Immunologic diseases of the pleura. Clin Chest Med 1985;6:83–102.

Sahn SA, Kaplan RL, Maulitz RM, et al. Rheumatoid pleurisy: Observations on the development of low pleural fluid pH and glucose level. Arch Intern Med 1980;140:1237–1238.

ASBESTOS

Epler GR, McLoud TC, Gaensler EA. Prevalence and incidence of benign asbestosis pleural effusion in a working population. JAMA 1982;247:617.

Robinson BWS, Musk AW. Benign asbestos pleural effusion: diagnosis and course. Thorax 1981;36:896–900.

ESOPHAGEAL RUPTURE

Bellman MH, Rajaratnam HN. Perforation of the esophagus with amylase-rich pleural effusion. Br J Dis Chest 1974;68: 18–22.

Dye RA, Laforet EG. Esophageal rupture: diagnosis of pleural fluid pH. Chest 1974;66:454–456.

Sherr HP, Light RW, Merson MH, et al. Origin of the pleural fluid amylase in esophageal rupture. Ann Intern Med 1972; 76:985–986.

URINOTHORAX

Miller KS, Wooten S, Sahn S. Urinothorax: a cause of low pH transudative pleural effusions. Am J Med 1988;85:448–449.

Stark DD, Shaves JG, Baron RL. Biochemical features of urinothorax. Arch Intern Med 1982;142:1509–1511.

CHYLOTHORAX

Sassoon CS, Light RW. Chylothorax and pseudochylothorax. Clin Chest Med 1985;6:163–171.

Teba L, Dedhia HV, Bowen R, et al. Chylothorax review. Crit Car Med 1985;13:49–52.

MISCELLANEOUS

Fine NL, Smith LRE, Sheedy PF. Frequency of pleural effusions in mycoplasma and viral pneumonias. N Engl J Med 1970;283:790–793.

George RB, Penn RL, Kinasewitz GT. Mycobacterial, fungal, actinomycotic, and nocardial infections of the pleura. Clin Chest Med 1985;6:63–75.

Hansen RM, Caya JG, Clowry LJ Jr., et al. Benign mesothelial proliferation with effusion: clinicopathologic entity that may mimic malignancy. Am J Med 1984;77:887–892.

Hiller E, Rosenow EC III, Olsen AM. Pulmonary manifestations of the yellow nail syndrome. Chest 1972;61:452–458.

Hughson WG, Friedman PJ, Feigin DS, et al. Postpartum pleural effusion: a common radiologic finding. Ann Intern Med 1982;97:856–858.

Weil PH, Margolis IB. Systematic approach to traumatic hemothorax. Am J Surg 1981;142:692–694.

Weiss JM, Spodick DH. Association of left pleural effusion

with pericardial disease. N Engl J Med 1983;308:696–697.

POSTCARDIAC INJURY

Stelzner TJ, King TE, Antony VB, et al. The pleuropulmonary manifestations of the postcardiac injury syndrome. Chest 1983;84:383–387.

PULMONARY EMBOLISM

Brown SE, Light RW. Pleural effusion associated with pulmonary embolization. Clin Chest Med 1985;6:77–81.

Bynum LJ, Wilson JE III. Characteristics of pleural effusions associated with pulmonary embolism. Arch Intern Med 1976;136:159–162.

INDETERMINATE EFFUSIONS

Black LF. Pleural effusions (editorial). Mayo Clin Proc 1981;56:210–212.

Canto A, Rivas J, Saumench J, et al. Points to consider when choosing a biopsy method in cases of pleurisy of unknown origin. Chest 1983;84:176–179.

Gunnels JJ. Perplexing pleural effusion. Chest 1978;74:390–393.

Ryan CJ, Rodgers RF, Unni KK, et al. The outcome of patients with pleural effusion of indeterminate cause at thoracotomy. Mayo Clin Proc 1981;56:145–149.

AMYLOIDOSIS

Kavuru MS, Adamo JP, Ahmad M, et al. Amyloidosis and pleural disease. Chest 1990;98:20–23.

AIDS

Joseph J, Strange C, Sahn SA. Pleural effusions in hospitalized patients with AIDS. Ann Intern Med 1993;118:856–859.

C•H•A•P•T•E•R

39

Selected Aspects of Critical Care Medicine for the Internist: Pulmonary Artery Catheterization and Noninvasive Blood Gas Monitoring*

Herbert P. Wiedemann

THE PULMONARY ARTERY CATHETER

Bedside catheterization of the pulmonary artery was introduced in 1970 by Swan and coworkers. The positioning of an inflatable balloon at the tip of the flexible catheter was an important adaptation that allows the catheter to be directed by blood flow, and thus fluoroscopy usually is not necessary for proper positioning. Some common indications for right heart catheterization in the intensive care unit or operating room are as follows (see Goldenheim & Kazemi, 1984):

1. To distinguish between noncardiogenic and cardiogenic pulmonary edema
2. Adult respiratory distress syndrome: to manage positive end expiratory pressure (PEEP) and volume therapy
3. Myocardial infarction complicated by:

   a. Hypotension unresponsive to volume challenge
   b. Hemodynamic instability requiring vasoactive drugs or mechanical assist devices
   c. Suspected cardiac tamponade (equalization of end-diastolic pressures)
   d. Suspected mitral regurgitation (giant ''v'' waves)
   e. Suspected ruptured interventricular septum (step-up in right heart oxygen saturation)

4. Unresponsive congestive heart failure
5. To resolve doubts about volume and cardiovascular status in complex illnesses (e.g., sepsis, pulmonary embolism)
6. Diagnosis and monitoring of pulmonary hypertension
7. Major cardiac surgery

PRIMARY PHYSIOLOGIC MEASUREMENTS AND CALCULATED DATA

The properly positioned balloon-tipped right heart catheter allows for three important direct measurements:

1. Cardiac output
2. Mixed venous arterial blood gases
3. Intravascular pressures:
   Right atrial pressure
   Right ventricular pressure
   Pulmonary artery pressure
   Pulmonary artery occlusion, or ''wedge,'' pressure

From these primary measurements, several important physiologic variables can be calculated. These include systemic and pulmonary vascular resistances, ventricular stroke work, and oxygen delivery. The equations for calculating these ''derived'' values are given in Table 39.1.

INSERTION SITES

The insertion sites are described in Table 39.2.

FLOW-DIRECTED PASSAGE AND NORMAL WAVEFORMS

The catheter should be advanced with continuous ECG and pressure monitoring.

The balloon of the standard 7 French catheter should be inflated with 1.3 to 1.5 cc of air to minimize complications and to ensure a proper ''proximal'' wedge position that helps avoid inaccurate thermodilution cardiac output and mixed venous PO_2 determinations.

During the catheter's passage through the chambers of the right heart and into the pulmonary artery, characteristic

---

* Reproduced with permission from the American College of Chest Physicians

Table 39.1. Physiologic Data Derived from Invasive Monitoring

a) Cardiac Index (liters/min/m²)

$$CI = \frac{CO}{BSA}$$

Normal Range: 2.4–4.4

b) Systemic Vascular Resistance (dyne.sec.cm⁻5)

$$SVR = \frac{MAP - CVP}{CO} \times 79.9$$

Normal Range: 900–1400

c) Pulmonary Vascular Resistance (dyne.sec.cm⁻5)

$$PVR = \frac{MPAP - PAWP}{CO} \times 79.9$$

Normal Range: 150–250

d) Stroke Volume (ml/beat)

$$SV = \frac{CI}{HR} \times 1000$$

Normal Range: 50–100

e) Stroke Volume Index (ml/min/m²)

$$SVI = \frac{SV}{BSA} = \frac{CI}{HR}$$

Normal Range: 30–65

f) Left Ventricular Stroke Work Index (gm.meters/m²)
LVSWI = SVI × (MAP − PAOP) × 0.0136

Normal Range: 43–61

g) Right Ventricular Stroke Work Index (gm.meters/m²)
RVSWI = SVI × (MPAP − CVP) × 0.0136

Normal Range: 7–12

h) Oxygen Content (ml/dl blood)
CaO_2 = Hgb × Arterial O_2 Saturation × 1.36 + (PO_2 × 0.003)

Normal: about 19.5

i) Arteriovenous Oxygen Content Difference (ml/dl)
$avDO_2 = CaO_2 - CvO_2$

Normal Range: 3–5

j) Oxygen Delivery (ml/min)
O_2 Delivery = CO × CaO_2 × 10

Normal Range: 800–1200

k) Oxygen Consumption (ml/min)
$VO_2 = CO \times (CaO_2 - CvO_2) \times 10$

Normal Range: 180–280

l) Pulmonary Shunt (veno-arterial admixture) (%)

$$Qs/Qt = \frac{CcO_2 - CaO_2}{CcO_2 - CvO_2}$$

Normal Range: < 3%–5%

BSA, Body Surface Area; CaO_2, Arterial Oxygen Content; CcO_2, Pulmonary Capillary Oxygen Content (assumed equal to alveolar PO_2); CI, Cardiac Index; CO, Cardiac Output; CvO_2, Mixed Venous Oxygen Content; CVP, Central Venous Pressure; HgB, Hemoglobin Concentration; HR, Heart Rate; LVSWI, Left Ventricular Stroke Work Index; MAP, Mean Arterial Pressure; MPAP, Mean Pulmonary Artery Pressure; PAWP, Pulmonary Artery Wedge Pressure; PVR, Pulmonary Vascular Resistance; Qs/Qt, Pulmonary Shunt; RVSWI, Right Ventricular Stroke Work Index; SV, Stroke Volume; SVI, Stroke Volume Index; SVR, Systemic Vascular Resistance; Modified from Sprung CL, ed. The pulmonary artery catheter: methodology and clinical applications. Baltimore: University Park Press, 1983.

waveforms and pressures are usually obtained. The clinician should remain alert for situations in which the usual waveforms may not be seen. Examples include right ventricular infarction (marked attenuation of usual right ventricular pressure generation) and severe mitral regurgitation (large ''v'' wave in wedge position may mimic pulmonary artery pressure waveform).

Normal values for the pressures are listed in Table 39.3.

Effect of Respiration and Mechanical Ventilation

Large variations in intrathoracic (pleural) pressure owing to labored spontaneous respiration (e.g., in patients with asthma) or mechanical ventilation (especially with PEEP) cause problems in interpreting measurements of vascular pressure. The influence of pleural pressure changes can be minimized

through the practice of measuring vascular pressures at end-expiration. In patients with rapid respirations, this may necessitate the use of a strip-chart recorder rather than digital readout systems. In patients receiving PEEP, pleural pressure will remain positive at end-expiration. The effect of this on interpretation of wedge pressure is discussed below.

COMPLICATIONS

Following are the complications of balloon flotation in right heart catheterization:

1. Arrhythmias
   a. Transient premature ventricular contractions (PVCs)
   b. Sustained ventricular tachycardia
   c. Ventricular fibrillation

Table 39.2.	Insertion Sites
Site	*Comments*
Subclavian Vein	Rapid and easy insertion, including hypotensive patients, but risk of pneumothorax or subclavian artery laceration. Site is immobile and easy to maintain.
Internal Jugular Vein	Generally easy insertion; less risk of pneumothorax, but carotid artery puncture may occur.
Antecubital Vein	Good for severely thrombocytopenic patients. Often requires cutdown. Passage into thorax may be difficult. Arm motion may cause migration of catheter tip.
Femoral Vein	Risk of deep vein thrombosis and subsequent embolism.

Table 39.3.	Normal Values	
Right Atrial Pressure		0–8 mm Hg
Right Ventricle		
Systolic		15–30 mm Hg
Diastolic		0–8 mm Hg
Pulmonary Artery		
Systolic		15–30 mm Hg
Mean		9–16 mm Hg
Diastolic		4–12 mm Hg
Pulmonary Artery Occlusion Pressure (PAOP), also called Pulmonary ''Wedge'' Pressure (PWP)		2–12 mm Hg

  d. Atrial fibrillation
  e. Atrial flutter

2. Right bundle branch block (RBBB)

3. Pulmonary infarction

4. Pulmonary artery rupture

5. Catheter-related infections

6. Balloon rupture

7. Catheter knotting

8. Endocardial damage
  a. Valve cusps
  b. Chordae tendineae
  c. Papillary muscles

9. Complications at insertion site
  a. Pneumothorax
  b. Arterial puncture
  c. Venous thrombosis or phlebitis
  d. Air embolism

Arrhythmias

Arrhythmias are most likely to occur during the initial passage through the right atrium and right ventricle. Ventricular tachycardia requiring therapy occurred in 1.5% of 500 consecutive insertions in one series. However, the risk is higher in patients with hypocalcemia, myocardial ischemia, hypotension, and hypokalemia. The most significant risk factors identified in one study were hypoxemia (PO_2 less than 60 mm Hg) and acidosis (pH less than 7.2). Prophylactic lidocaine during catheter insertion should be considered in high-risk patients.

Pulmonary artery catheterization is associated with a new RBBB in about 3% of catheterizations. In patients with pre-existing LBBB, therefore, the potential for developing complete heart block exists. However, two recently published investigations evaluated a total of 61 patients with pre-existing LBBB; in more than 100 catheterizations in these patients, no acute episodes of complete heart occurred. Therefore, routine temporary pacemaker insertion is not recommended in patients with LBBB prior to pulmonary artery catheterization, but appropriate equipment should be readily available.

Pulmonary Infarction

Although an early report (1974) found a 7.2% prevalence of infarction, subsequent experience in the 1980s and 1990s suggests a frequency of less than or equal to 1.3%. Avoidance of distal migration and ''persistent wedging'' of the catheter tip is important. Also, the now routine use of a continuous flush with a heparin solution has probably reduced the frequency of thrombus formation on the tip.

Pulmonary Artery Rupture

The frequency of pulmonary artery rupture is about 0.2%. Cardiopulmonary bypass surgery is a higher risk situation. One-half of cases are fatal. Hemoptysis is seen in some cases and provides an important early warning.

THERMODILUTION CARDIAC OUTPUT

Generally, there is a good correlation of thermodilution cardiac output measurements with those from Fick or dye dilution techniques.

The following method provides the best accuracy:

1. Average three separate measurements obtained a minute apart.
2. Inject the indicator solution at the same phase of respiration, preferably end-expiration.
3. Room temperature injectate provides adequate results in most patients, including those who are moderately hypothermic (32°C), but iced injectate is necessary in markedly hypothermic patients (< 30°C).

Measurements may be inaccurate in patients with tricuspid regurgitation (falsely low reading) or intracardiac shunts, or if the catheter position is too distal (falsely high reading).

MIXED VENOUS BLOOD SAMPLING

Mixed venous blood sampling is obtained by withdrawing blood from distal orifice of the catheter with the balloon deflated. Prior to sampling, 2.5 ml dead space of the 7 French catheter must be eliminated. A slow rate of blood withdrawal (less than 3 ml/min) is recommended in patients receiving high inspired oxygen or high levels of PEEP to avoid "contamination" with oxygenated capillary blood.

Measurement may be inaccurate with a tip placement that is too distal or if the patient has severe mitral regurgitation or a left-to-right cardiac shunt (this latter situation may cause an abnormal "step-up" in oxygenation of blood obtained serially from the right atrium, right ventricle, and pulmonary artery and may be a useful diagnostic test to detect left-to-right shunts).

Normal mixed venous oxygen tension is 36–42 mm Hg, and normal mixed venous oxygen saturation is about 75%. Note that in cases of sepsis or adult respiratory distress syndrome (ARDS), normal or stable mixed venous oxygenation may be found despite inadequate tissue oxygenation and/or large decreases in oxygen delivery.

Clinically, mixed venous oxygenation is used to monitor changes in cardiac output and to assess tissue oxygenation. In normal individuals and many patients, as oxygen delivery (cardiac output multiplied by arterial oxygen content) decreases, increased extraction of oxygen from circulating blood allows tissue oxygen consumption to remain stable (oxygen consumption is independent of oxygen delivery until a critically low level of delivery), but causes the mixed venous oxygen content to decrease. Thus, a decrease in cardiac output will be reflected by a corresponding decline in mixed venous oxygen. Furthermore, as mixed venous PO_2 approaches 27 to 30 mm Hg (normal: 39 mm Hg) blood lactate levels usually increase, indicating that tissue oxygenation is reaching a critically low level (see discussion of lactic acid below).

These interpretations of mixed venous oxygenation are most valid in patients with "simple" hemodynamic problems, such as isolated myocardial dysfunction. In more complex illnesses, including sepsis and the adult respiratory distress syndrome (ARDS), the interpretation of mixed venous oxygenation is much more complex. In sepsis, peripheral "shunting" of arterial blood past tissue beds may lead to maintenance of high mixed venous oxygen levels despite tissue oxygen deprivation indicated by high blood lactate levels. Furthermore, in some ARDS patients, oxygen consumption varies with oxygen delivery, even at normal or high cardiac outputs, suggesting an abnormal "supply dependency" of oxygen consumption. This phenomenon may be related in part to abnormalities in the systemic capillary circulation that prevent normal tissue oxygen extraction. The result is that mixed venous oxygenation remains high and relatively stable despite large, and presumably clinically important, decreases in cardiac output, oxygen delivery, and oxygen consumption. It is clear that solely monitoring mixed venous oxygenation in patients with sepsis or ARDS is inadequate. The clinician needs

to monitor several other parameters, including cardiac output, arterial oxygen saturation, and lactate levels in order to be informed about changes in hemodynamic states of these patients.

Pulmonary artery catheters that provide a continuous measurement of the mixed oxygen saturation through use of fiberoptic reflectance oximetry are currently available. Although the continuous monitoring of mixed venous oxygenation may provide a helpful "early warning system" for detecting adverse hemodynamic trends, its value in this regard may be limited to patients with pure cardiac disease, since reliance on stable mixed venous oxygenation may provide a false sense of security in patients with more complex illnesses.

Left-to-right intracardiac shunts will cause an elevated mixed venous oxygenation. This fact may be helpful in diagnosing atrial or ventricular septal defects; during passage of the catheter, blood samples will show an abnormal "step-up" in oxygen saturation as the tip is passed into the right atrium or right ventricle. An example of how this maneuver may provide important diagnostic information is a patient with myocardial infarction who develops sudden hemodynamic instability and a systolic murmur. The major diagnoses to be considered are acute ventricular septal defect or acute mitral valve insufficiency. These possibilities can be easily distinguished through an assessment of oxygen saturation in the chambers of the right heart (echocardiography is also useful).

It is important to remember that mixed venous oxygenation has an important influence on arterial oxygenation saturation when there is a high degree of shunt through the lungs (e.g., in ARDS). Although clinicians often reflexively attribute a decrease in PaO_2 to a worsening of lung function, such a decrease may in fact be because of nonrespiratory factors that cause a reduction in mixed venous oxygenation (e.g., anemia, increased oxygen consumption, or low cardiac output). If such factors are corrected, arterial oxygen saturation may improve even if the lung disease does not improve.

Measurement of serum lactic acid levels may be a helpful adjunct in assessing the adequacy of tissue perfusion and oxygenation. Lactic acid is the end-product of anaerobic metabolism but is also produced in small amounts in aerobic conditions. The normal serum lactate level is usually 2 mEq/L or less, but "stressed" patients in the ICU may have normal levels up to 4 mEq/L. The serum lactate level is used clinically as a marker for tissue ischemia. However, unresolved issues and concerns remain regarding the specificity and sensitivity of the serum lactate level used for this purpose.

The major concern regarding sensitivity is the probability that lactate from areas of regional hypoperfusion and tissue ischemia will be diluted and contribute little to the total venous pool. Thus, significant regional tissue ischemia may exist despite a normal serum lactate level. With regard to specificity, it is important to recognize that certain clinical disorders can be associated with an elevated serum lactate level without widespread organ ischemia (e.g., generalized seizures, thiamine deficiency, and respiratory alkalosis). Finally, although the lactate anion is cleared by the liver (where it is used for gluconeogenisis), liver failure alone does not seem to produce an increase in the serum lactate level. It appears that reduced hepatic clearance of lactate contributes to blood lactate accumulation only when hepatic blood flow is severely reduced (below 70% of control levels) or if hepatic venous PO_2 falls below 24 mm Hg. Thus, in most clinical circumstances (including liver failure and moderate shock), an elevated blood lactate level probably mostly reflects an increase in lactate production rather than reduced hepatic clearance.

PULMONARY ARTERY OCCLUSION PRESSURE ("WEDGE" PRESSURE)

The measurement of pulmonary artery wedge pressure is a major use of the pulmonary artery catheter. The wedge pressure allows the clinician to make an *indirect* assessment of the left ventricular preload and pulmonary capillary hydrostatic pressure.

Despite its value and importance, correct measurement and physiologic interpretation of wedge pressure are not always simple and straightforward.

A valid wedge position can be confirmed using four criteria:

1. The mean pulmonary artery wedge pressure should be lower than or equal to the pulmonary artery diastolic pressure and lower than the mean pulmonary artery pressure. (In cases of severe mitral regurgitation, the wedge pressure may transiently exceed the pulmonary artery diastolic pressure.)
2. A waveform characteristic of left atrial pressures should be seen. A "damped" waveform, straight line, or waveform deflections solely related to ventilatory pressures are not acceptable. The "wedge" waveform should disappear promptly with balloon deflation (giving a pulmonary artery tracing) and return rapidly after balloon reinflation.
3. A free-falling column of fluid or continuous flush excludes catheter obstruction.
4. Blood gas analysis of blood samples withdrawn from a presumed wedge position may be helpful. Blood withdrawn with the balloon inflated will reflect alveolar capillary gas pressures; often this blood is highly saturated with oxygen owing to the local high ventilation/perfusion (V/Q) relationship caused by balloon-induced blood stasis.

Adherence to criteria 1 to 3 should be checked frequently, but criterion 4 is usually not routinely assessed. Nevertheless, blood gas analysis of blood samples withdrawn from a presumed wedge position may be helpful at times. Despite theoretical concern that criterion 4 may not hold if the catheter tip lies in an area of lung with very low V/Q, recent experiments suggest that highly oxygenated blood is usually withdrawn from a true wedge position even in areas of radiographic infiltrates or in patients with large intrapulmonic shunts. Adherence to these criteria will help prevent incorrect wedge pressure readings, such as may occur if the tip of the catheter is not in a West zone 3 of the lung. Although the flow-directed catheter usually initially migrates to a zone 3 location, physiologic changes may occur during subsequent therapy that decrease the size of zone 3 (e.g., application of PEEP, diuresis).

What Does Wedge Pressure Measure?

Balloon occlusion of a branch of the pulmonary artery causes flow to cease between the catheter tip and the "junction point" at which pulmonary venous radicles served by the occluded artery join other radicles in which blood is still flowing toward the left atrium. Wedge pressure appears to reflect pulmonary venous pressure at this junction point. The junction point is probably located in a pulmonary vein about the same size as the occluded pulmonary artery. Thus, the usual wedge pressure (produced by occluding a lobar artery) correlates well with venous pressure at or near the left atrium. In short, wedge pressure approximates left atrial pressure (in the absence of mechanical disruption of the large pulmonary veins because of tumor, mediastinal fibrosis).

Relationship of Wedge Pressure to Left Ventricular Preload

According to the Frank-Starling principle, the strength of cardiac contraction is related directly to muscle fiber length at end-diastole, or preload. Preload is thus proportionate to end-diastolic ventricular volume. In contrast, the wedge measurement approximates pressure within the left atrium, which is usually close to the pressure within the left ventricle at end-diastole, or intracavitary left ventricular end-diastolic pressure ("filling pressure").

The relationship between preload (filling volume) and wedge pressure (filling pressure) depends on two factors: ventricular compliance and the transmural distending pressure (intracavitary pressure minus juxtacardiac pressure). Thus the clinician must make a mental adjustment for changes in juxtacardiac pressure (e.g., PEEP therapy) or ventricular compliance (e.g., ischemia, neurohumoral effects, or medications) when using wedge pressure to assess myocardial function.

In addition, mitral or aortic valve dysfunction will cause left atrial pressure (wedge pressure) to diverge from its usual close reflection of left ventricular end-diastolic pressure.

Relation of Wedge Pressure to Pulmonary Capillary Pressure

A major clinical use of the wedge pressure is that it provides a means of assessing pulmonary capillary pressure. This is important, for instance, in distinguishing cardiac pulmonary edema from ARDS (lung injury edema).

However, wedge pressure is not equal to pulmonary capillary pressure, even though the term "pulmonary capillary wedge pressure" is often incorrectly applied. As already discussed, wedge pressure approximates left atrial pressure. Pulmonary capillary pressure exceeds left atrial pressure by a variable degree, depending on the amount of vascular resistance in the pulmonary venous system. If marked resistance exists, high pulmonary capillary pressures may be present despite a normal wedge pressure. Pulmonary veno-occlusive disease is one example, although rare, in which this consideration is important. However, many common physiologic and pharmacologic alterations (e.g., hypoxia, serotonin, prostaglandins, or sympathetic stimulation) may also influence pulmonary venous resistance. Increased pulmonary venous resistance may therefore contribute to pulmonary edema in a central nervous system injury, hypovolemic shock, acute lung injury, infusion of vasoactive agents such as norepinephrine, and other clinical settings. In such cases, the wedge pressure may underestimate the degree to which elevated pulmonary capillary pressure is contributing to the development of pulmonary edema.

Future advances (e.g., analysis of pulmonary artery pressure decay curve following balloon inflation) may allow for more accurate assessment of pulmonary capillary pressure. Until then, the wedge pressure remains a valuable indirect assessment of pulmonary capillary pressure, but the clinician must remain alert to possible confounding situations.

HEMODYNAMIC PROFILES

The direct measurements and the calculated values obtained through right heart catheterization provide a "hemodynamic profile," which can be helpful in recognizing the underlying etiology in critically ill patients (Table 39.4).

GOAL-DIRECTED HEMODYNAMIC THERAPY?

It is frequently observed that patients who survive critical illness had cardiac index and oxygen delivery values that were higher than those seen in nonsurvivors and higher than normal. This has led to the hypothesis that "goal-directed" hemodynamic management of critically ill patients (to achieve, for example, a cardiac index greater than 4.5 and/or an oxygen delivery index of greater than 650) will result in improved survival. However, recent randomized trials (Yu, et al., 1993; Hayes, et al., 1994; Gattinoni, et al., 1995) indicate that hemodynamic therapy aimed at achieving supranormal values for

cardiac index and oxygen delivery (or normal values for mixed venous oxygenation) does not reduce morbidity or mortality in critically ill patients. Thus, current evidence suggests that patients who respond to critical illness with high cardiac output and oxygen delivery are more likely to survive than those who do not; however, manipulation of hemodynamics to raise cardiac index and oxygen delivery to supranormal target values does not appear to improve outcomes.

"SWAN SONG" FOR THE PULMONARY ARTERY CATHETER?

In a retrospective analysis, Connors and coworkers studied the association between the use of a pulmonary artery catheter (during the first 24 hours of intensive care) and clinical outcomes. A complex statistical method ("propensity scoring") was used to compare heterogenous populations. The authors concluded that use of the pulmonary artery catheter was associated with an increased 30-day mortality (odds ratio 1.24, 95% confidence interval 1.03–1.49), and an increased ICU length of stay (14.8 versus 13.0 days) and increased cost for the total hospital stay (median $30,5000 versus $20,600). The validity of these results depends highly on the ability of the "propensity score" to adequately adjust for the risk of adverse outcomes in heterogenous patient groups. In fact, the patients in whom pulmonary artery catheters were used were more severely ill as assessed by the APACHE III score (mean 61 versus 51, without Glasgow Coma Score; $P < 0.001$). The authors themselves appropriately acknowledge the limitations of their study, which was not prospective and randomized. Nevertheless, this study is thought provoking. For example, it has been pointed out that the period of time that data were collected for this study (1989–1994) corresponded to a time when many intensive care units had a policy of attempting to achieve "super normal" hemodynamic values in critically ill patients (Dobb, 1996). As reviewed above, subsequent clinical studies now suggest that such a global policy may actually worsen outcome in some patients.

Most experts feel that selective use of the pulmonary artery catheter by trained and knowledgeable clinicians in appropriately selected patients is not contraindicated. Future studies to help define appropriate guidelines for catheter insertion are warranted.

Table 39.4.   Representative Hemodynamic Profiles

Condition	SAP	SVR	CO	PAP	PAWP
LV Failure	N or ↓	↑	↓	↑	↑
Volume Depletion	↓	↑	N or ↓	↓	↓
Sepsis	↓	↓	↑	N or ↓	N or ↓
ARDS	Variable	Variable	Variable	↑	N or ↓
Pulmonary Embolism	N or ↓	N or ↑	N or ↓	↑	N or ↓

SAP, Systemic Arterial Pressure; SVR, Systemic Vascular Resistance; CO, Cardiac Output; PAP, Pulmonary Artery Pressure; PAWP, Pulmonary Artery "Wedge" Pressure

NONINVASIVE MONITORING OF GAS EXCHANGE

CAPNOGRAPHY

Capnography is the measurement of the carbon dioxide (CO_2) tension in expired gases. Capnographic analysis can be achieved by two physical methods: infrared spectroscopy and mass spectroscopy. The use of mass spectrometry has been limited somewhat by the expense and technical expertise required for its use. Within the last decade, technical advances have provided improved and portable infrared capnographic devices, generating renewed interest in the use of capnography in clinical medicine. Carbon dioxide analysis of expired gas can be achieved by so-called sidestream or mainstream systems. In sidestream capnographs, a thin sampling tube is attached to the patient's endotracheal tube or anesthetic mass connector. A major potential disadvantage of the sidestream system is the tendency for the sampling tubing to become blocked with water or secretions; a minor disadvantage of the sidestream systems is the lag time present between the actual expired gas flow and the subsequent gas analysis. Mainstream analyzers are connected directly to the expired gas circuit, usually at the end of the endotracheal tube. Recent design modifications have reduced the size and weight of these sensors and have made them more clinically practical.

Expired carbon dioxide tension can be displayed numerically (capnometer) or as a continuous waveform (capnograph). Since analysis and visual recognition of various waveform configurations provides helpful information, the capnograph is preferred. Following is the typical pattern:

1. In early exhalation, only a negligible CO_2 tension is measured, since this air is coming primarily from the anatomical dead space.
2. Shortly thereafter, alveolar gas starts to mix with dead space air, and a rapid rise in the recorded CO_2 tension is observed.
3. As the anatomical dead space is then cleared, only mixed alveolar gas is exhaled, and a plateau (the so-called alveolar plateau) is observed.
4. The CO_2 concentration at the end of this plateau is the end-tidal CO_2 tension ($P_{ET}CO_2$).
5. When inhalation is initiated, the CO_2 tension rapidly decreases back to the baseline of zero.

In patients with normal lungs, the end-tidal CO_2 usually closely approximates the arterial carbon dioxide tension ($PaCO_2$). Normally, the end-tidal CO_2 is slightly lower than $PaCO_2$ (generally within 1–4 mm Hg). In view of the close relationship between end-tidal CO_2 and $PaCO_2$ in patients with normal lungs, capnography can be used as a noninvasive and continuous estimate of $PaCO_2$ (providing obvious advantages over intermittent arterial blood gas sampling). However, it is extremely important to recognize that increases in physiologic dead space (for example, as in COPD, pulmonary embolism, or shock) will cause end-tidal CO_2 to diverge from, and

significantly underestimate, $PaCO_2$. This limits the usefulness of capnography as a noninvasive monitor of arterial $PaCO_2$ in patients with significant cardiopulmonary disease. Established and potential uses of capnography include:

- Monitoring ventilatory status during general anesthesia
- Esophageal intubation: Quick confirmation of appropriate endotracheal intubation is sometimes difficult. Capnography is a rapid and practical technique for the detection of inadvertent esophageal intubation. When the esophagus is intubated, the CO_2 tension of the "expired" gas quickly falls to very low values.
- Venous gas embolism: Venous gas embolism is an uncommon but potentially serious complication of neurological or gynecological surgery. Air embolism causes a sudden reduction in the end-tidal CO_2 by increasing dead space ventilation and possibly by decreasing cardiac output as well. As reviewed by Morley, a recent study by Bedford and colleagues found that air embolism during neurosurgery resulted in a mean fall in $P_{ET}CO_2$ of approximately 8.5 mm Hg.
- Cardiopulmonary resuscitation: Cardiac arrest is associated with a marked drop in $P_{ET}CO_2$, presumably because only small amounts of carbon dioxide are presented to the lungs when the cardiac output is extremely low or absent. Recent studies indicate that the development of adequate cardiac output during successful cardiopulmonary resuscitation is associated with a dramatic rise in $P_{ET}CO_2$ and may be one of the earliest and most reliable indicators of adequate resuscitation.
- During mechanical ventilation: Capnography may be a valuable technique for monitoring the status of patients undergoing mechanical ventilation. For example, in patients undergoing IMV ventilation, capnographic monitoring can easily help identify lack of synchrony between a patient's spontaneous respiration and the ventilator-delivered breaths. Another purported value of capnography is the use of the $PaCO_2$–$P_{ET}CO_2$ gradient to titrate PEEP therapy in patients with ARDS. Some studies suggest that when the optimum level of PEEP is exceeded, this is reflected by a relatively abrupt increase in the $PaCO_2$–$P_{ET}CO_2$ gradient owing to worsening of ventilation perfusion matching (secondary to an increase in physiologic shunt because of "overdistention" of many gas exchange units). However, the usefulness of capnography for this purpose remains investigational, and at the current time titration of PEEP therapy should not be undertaken using capnographic criteria alone.
- Weaning from mechanical ventilation: Capnography may be helpful in the detection of altered breathing patterns and hypoventilation that may accompany unsuccessful attempts at weaning from mechanical ventilation.

TRANSCUTANEOUS OXYGEN AND CARBON DIOXIDE

Heated skin probes can measure the concentration of oxygen or carbon dioxide that diffuses from the capillaries through the skin. At relatively normal cardiac outputs, the transcutaneous PO_2 ($PtcO_2$) is a reliable trend monitor of the PaO_2, although the $PtcO_2$ will average only about 80% of the PaO_2 (a $PtcO_2$ value of 80 mm Hg corresponds to a PaO_2 of 100 mm Hg). However, at moderate levels of hypoperfusion (cardiac index between 1.5 and 2.2 $1/min/m^2$), even when not associated with frank hypotension, the $PtcO_2$ averages only about 50% of the PaO_2. This represents an important limitation of transcutaneous monitoring, since such patients may not be easily distinguished without invasive monitoring of the cardiac output. And finally, in cases of cardiogenic shock (cardiac index less than 1.5 $1/min/m^2$), changes in $PtcO_2$ actually reflect changes in the cardiac output (or tissue oxygen delivery), rather than the PaO_2. The physiologic interpretation of the $PtcO_2$ value, therefore, is relatively well established. In patients with normal cardiac output and cutaneous blood flow, the $PtcO_2$ reflects PaO_2. However, in low flow states, the $PtcO_2$ diverges from PaO_2 and reflects tissue oxygen delivery instead. This represents both a problem and an opportunity. The problem is that monitoring of the $PtcO_2$ alone may be inadequate in many clinical situations, since a decreasing $PtcO_2$ may reflect either pulmonary decompensation (decreasing PaO_2) or hemodynamic failure (decreasing cardiac output). A separate, independent measurement of respiratory or cardiac function may be necessary to properly interpret the change in $PtcO_2$. On the other hand, $PtcO_2$ can detect overall decreases in tissue oxygen delivery that are otherwise difficult to assess noninvasively.

Several practical considerations limit the use of transcutaneous monitors. The heated electrodes may produce mild erythema, need to be moved frequently, have a fairly long initial equilibration time (about 5 minutes), and take time to fully respond to subsequent changes (about 1 minute). Conjunctival monitors are available that have much shorter equilibration and response times.

The transcutaneous PCO_2 is usually about 5 to 20 mmmHg higher than $PaCO_2$. The transcutaneous PCO_2 measurement is less sensitive to changes in hemodynamic status than transcutaneous PO_2 and responds faster to changes in arterial gas tension.

Because of the practical and theoretical limitations, transcutaneous monitoring has not achieved widespread use as a noninvasive technique to monitor arterial blood gases in adult intensive care unit patients. As mentioned, this technology may have greater potential in the noninvasive assessment of tissue oxygenation in patients with hypoperfusion.

PULSE OXIMETRY

The use of pulse oximetry has grown remarkably since its introduction a few years ago. The ability to measure noninvasively such an important parameter as arterial O_2 saturation with a portable and simple device has had a predictably profound impact on clinical medicine. In Severinghaus' judgment, "pulse oximetry is arguably the most significant technological advance ever made in monitoring the well being and safety of patients during anesthesia, recovery and critical care" (Severinghaus, 1987).

Unlike the earlier nonpulse transmission oximeters, pulse oximeters are designed to detect and measure only the pulsatile change in light transmission through living tissue; arterial saturation can be calculated, since the change in light transmission is owing solely to the change in intervening blood volume. Therefore, the absorption of light by venous blood, skin pigments, tissue, and bone is automatically eliminated from consideration. Since pulse oximetry "observes" only arterial blood, only two wavelengths of light are required to calculate arterial oxygen saturation, since blood is usually composed of only two major light absorbers, oxygenated hemoglobin (HbO_2) and deoxyhemoglobin (reduced hemoglobin or RHb). (Beer's Law states that only "n" wavelengths are required to identify and distinguish among "n" different absorbers of light.) The two wavelengths most commonly used in pulse oximeters are approximately 660 nm in the red region and approximately 940 nm in the near infrared region. These wavelengths are chosen because the HbO_2 and the RHb extinction curves are distinct and inverted from each other at these two different wavelengths. Thus, any change in the hemoglobin saturation will produce a large change in the ratio of absorptions at these two wavelengths, allowing for a calculation of oxygen saturation.

It is generally accepted that pulse oximetry is accurate within $\pm 3\%$–4% (95% confidence) in a wide range of clinical circumstances, including the critically ill. However, it is worth pointing out that even a relatively small degree of inaccuracy in the saturation measurement can have a large impact on the assumed corresponding PaO_2. For example, a measured saturation of 95% ($\pm 4\%$) could be associated with a true PaO_2 value from 60 mm Hg (91% saturation) to 160 mm Hg (99% saturation).

Pulse oximetry measurements are not significantly affected by skin pigmentation or jaundice. However, patients with significant amounts of carboxyhemoglobin (COHb) or methemoglobin (MetHb) will have a spurious oximeter reading, since these hemoglobin forms have significant absorption at 600 nm and/or 940 nm. Because of its absorption profile, COHb is viewed by the pulse oximeter as though it was mostly HbO_2, although some of it is attributed to RHb. Thus, the pulse oximeter reports approximately the sum of HbO_2 + COHb as HbO_2. It is important for the clinician to be aware of this; in a patient with significant carbon monoxide poisoning, for example, the pulse oximeter will significantly overestimate the true arterial oxygen saturation. The presence of methemoglobinemia has a different effect. Increasing amounts of methemoglobinemia deviate the pulse oximeter toward a reading of 85%, causing an underestimation if true oxygen saturation is higher than this and an overestimation if true oxygen saturation is less than 85%. Intravenously administered dyes such as methylene blue, indigo carmine, and indocynin green have significant absorption at 660 nm and produce spuriously low pulse oximeter measurements.

ARTERIAL BLOOD GASES — TEMPERATURE CORRECTION?

It has long been recognized that pH and PCO_2 change with temperature both in vivo and in vitro. Although at normal body temperature (37°C) the normal pH is about 7.4 and the normal PCO_2 is about 40 mm Hg, at 30°C, for example, the same blood sample will have a pH of 7.50 and PCO_2 of approximately 30 mm Hg. Because blood gas samples are measured in the laboratory at a standard temperature of 37°C, it is necessary to "temperature correct" the measurement to

ascertain what the actual values are in a given patient at his or her body temperature. However, reporting of these temperature-corrected values is potentially confusing and clinically hazardous, if it is incorrectly assumed that the ideal physiologic pH is 7.40, regardless of temperature. In fact, relatively recent theoretical arguments and clinical experience suggest that the physiologically appropriate pH (and PCO_2) varies according to temperature and apparently in the same direction and magnitude as the temperature-induced changes themselves. Thus, the clinician will arrive at the correct acid-base interpretation by using the values measured at 37°C and ignoring both the patient's temperature and the temperature-corrected values. Alternatively, the temperature-corrected values could be compared against temperature-specific "normal ranges," but this method lacks the simplicity (especially when comparing serial values in a patient whose body temperature is changing) of simply using the uncorrected measurements.

REVIEW EXERCISES

QUESTIONS

1. Through the use of a balloon-tipped artery catheter (Swan-Ganz catheter) and a peripheral artery catheter, all of the following can be measured or calculated, except:

    a. Cardiac output
    b. Left ventricular filling pressure
    c. Left ventricular preload
    d. Systemic vascular resistance
    e. Oxygen consumption

2. Which of the following parameters would be most helpful in distinguishing cardiogenic pulmonary edema from noncardiogenic pulmonary edema (e.g., adult respiratory distress syndrome)?

    a. Cardiac output
    b. Pulmonary artery pressure
    c. Systemic vascular resistance
    d. Mixed venous oxygen saturation
    e. Pulmonary artery occlusion ("wedge") pressure

3. An ARDS patient receiving mechanical ventilation (with PEEP = 20 cm) is hypotensive and oliguric. The "wedge" pressure at end-expiration is 8 mm Hg. The cardiac index, 2.0 liters/min/m²; FiO_2, .9; ABGs, 7.40/40/60. Which of the following is the most reasonable initial therapy?

    a. Start nitroprusside infusion
    b. Start dobutamine infusion

    c. Reduce PEEP
    d. Start volume infusion
    e. Obtain blood cultures and start antibiotics

4. Following are the hemodynamic data for a patient:

	Pressure	O_2 saturation %
Radial artery	98/80	96%
SVC	12	96%
Right atrium	11 (mean)	61%
Right ventricle	57/8	89%
Pulmonary artery	54/22	85%
"Wedge"	24 (mean)	
	V wave = 46	

    What are the most likely diagnoses?

    a. Pulmonary embolism and patent foramen ovale
    b. Right ventricular infarction and tricuspid regurgitation
    c. Mitral regurgitation and intraventricular septal defect
    d. Mitral regurgitation and cardiac tamponade
    e. Left ventricular failure and patent foramen ovale

5. An arterial blood gas measurement reveals PaO_2, 60 mm Hg; HbO_2, 70%; COHb, 20%. A simultaneous pulse oximetry reading is most likely to be approximately:

    a. 50
    b. 60
    c. 70
    d. 90
    e. 100

Answers

1. c

2. e

3. d

4. c

5. d

SUGGESTED READINGS

Wiedemann HP, Matthay MA, Matthay RA. Cardiovascular-pulmonary monitoring in the intensive care unit (Parts 1 & 2). Chest 1984;85:537–549, 656–668.

This review article concentrates in detail on the pulmonary artery (Swan-Ganz) catheter. The topics discussed include indications, complications, insertion, and normal waveforms. In addition, guidelines for the proper acquisition and interpretation of thermodilation cardiac output, mixed venous oxygenation, and intravascular pressures (including "wedge" pressure) are provided.

Iberti TJ, Fisher EP, Leibowitz AB, et al. A multicenter study of physician's knowledge of the pulmonary artery catheter. JAMA 1990;264:2928–2932.

A 31-question multiple-choice examination was given to 496 physicians in 13 medical facilities. The mean test score was 67% correct. The authors argue that use of the Swan-Ganz should be restricted to physicians with documented competency.

Connors AF, McCaffree DR, Gray BA. Evaluation of right-heart catheterization in the critically ill patient without acute myocardial infarction. N Engl J Med 1983;308:263–67.

Sixty-two critically ill patients (without myocardial infarction), whose clinical condition was deteriorating rapidly or who did not respond to initial therapeutic trials, received right-heart catheterization. Before the procedure, physicians were asked to predict (high, low, or normal) various hemodynamic parameters (cardiac output, wedge pressure, etc.) based upon clinical information (such as physical examination, chest radiograph). The accuracy of predictions was about 44%. Furthermore, in 48% of cases the information obtained by catheterization prompted a change in therapy.

Gigarroa RG, Lange RA, Williams RH, et al. Underestimation of cardiac output by thermodilution in patients with tricuspid regurgitation. Am J Med 1989;86:417–420.

In 17 patients with tricuspid regurgitation (severity distribution: 12 patients had 2 + TR, 4 patients had 3 + TR, one patient had 4 + TR), the thermodilution cardiac output was consistently lower than Fick or indocyanine green determinations (4.22 ± 1.45 versus 4.99 ± 1.67).

Shellock FG, Riedinger MS, Bateman TM, et al. Thermodilution cardiac output determination in hypothermic postcardiac surgery patients: Room vs. ice temperature injectate. Crit Care Med 1983;11:668–670.

The room temperature injectate method is acceptable even in moderately hypothermic (32.7 ± 1.2° C) patients.

Hasan FM, Weiss WB, Braman SS, et al. Influence of lung injury on pulmonary wedge-left atrial pressure correlation during positive end-expiratory pressure ventilation. Am Rev Respir Dis 1985;131-246–250.

West zone 3 conditions are better preserved in areas of lung injury, compared with normal lung regions, during ventilation with positive end-expiratory pressure (PEEP). Thus, areas of abnormal lung on the chest radiograph do not need to be avoided during flotation of the Swan-Ganz catheter in order to lessen the possibility of obtaining invalid wedge measurements.

Sprung CL, Elser B, Schein RMH, et al. Risk of right bundle-branch block and complete heart block during pulmonary artery catheterization. Crit Care Med 1989;17:1–3.

In 279 pulmonary artery catheterizations, 8 (3%) were associated with the development of new RBBB. None of 14 patients with existing LBBB developed complete heart block. The results indicate that RBBB is a rare complication of right heart catheterization and doesn't seem to occur at higher frequency in those patients with pre-existing LBBB. Therefore, routine prophylactic pacemaker insertion is probably not warranted in patients with pre-existing LBBB.

Morris D, Mulvihill D, Lew WYW. Risk of developing complete heart block during bedside pulmonary artery catheterization in patients with left bundle-branch block. Arch Intern Med 1987; 147:2005–2010.

In 82 pulmonary artery catheterizations performed in 47 patients with LBBB, there were no episodes of complete heart block that appeared to be related to the catheterization in patients with either old LBBB (more than 1 month in duration) or indeterminate age LBBB. In 2 of the 9 patients with new LBBB, complete heart block occurred 1 day after catheter insertion, but in the context of unstable recurrent ventricular tachycardia. Routine temporary pacemaker insertion is not recommended in patients with LBBB prior to pulmonary artery catheterization.

Wiedemann HP, McCarthy K. Noninvasive monitoring of oxygen and carbon dioxide. Clin Chest Med 1989;10: 239–254.

This article reviews pulse oximetry, transcutaneous oxygen and carbon dioxide measurements, capnography, and respiratory-inductive plethysmography.

Sanders AB, Kern KB, Ott CW, et al. End-tidal carbon dioxide monitoring during cardiopulmonary resuscitation: A prognostic indicator for survival. JAMA 1989;262:1344–1351.

Falk JL, Rackow EC, Weil MH. End-tidal carbon dioxide concentration during cardiopulmonary resuscitation. N Engl J Med 1988;318:607–611.

The above two articles demonstrate how the sudden increase in end-tidal carbon ioxide that is associated with restoration of adequate circulation can be used to clinical advantage.

Morley TF. Capnography in the intensive care unit. J Intens Care Med 1990;5:209–223.

This is a comprehensive and clear overview of capnography.

Hoffman RA, Krieger BP, Kramer MR, et al. End-tidal carbon dioxide in critically ill patients during changes in mechanical ventilation. Am Rev Respir Dis 1989; 140:1265–1268.

In critically ill patients undergoing alterations in ventilator settings (frequency and tidal volume), measurements of $P_{ET}CO_2$ did not reliably reflect changes in $PaCO_2$, owing to variations in the $PaCO_2$–$P_{ET}CO_2$ gradient.

Carlon GC, Ray C, Miodownik S, et al. Capnography in mechanically ventilated patients. Crit Care Med 1988; 16: 550–556.

This article reviews the clinical role and technical problems of CO_2 waveform analysis in the mechanically ventilated patient. Several illustrative waveform patterns are provided.

Rahn H, Reeves RB, Howell BJ. Hydrogen ion regulation, temperature evolution. Am Rev Resp Dis 1975;112:165–172.

This article provides an in-depth discussion regarding acid-base regulation in relation to body temperature. Physiologically, the ''normal'' extracellular pH (about 7.40 at 37°C) bears a constant relationship (a difference of about 0.6 to 0.8 pH units) with intracellular neutrality, the value of which varies according to temperature. Thus, ''normal blood pH'' varies according to temperature. Rather than memorizing or looking up normal values for each temperature, one can solve the problem simply by using ''uncorrected'' pH and PCO_2 values measured at 37°C and interpreting them in the usual manner (normal pH = 7.40) without regard to the patient's temperature.

Ream AK, Reitz BA, Silverberg G. Temperature correction of PCO_2 and pH in estimating acid-base status: an example of the emperor's new clothes? Anesthesiology 1982;56:41–44.

This article explains the rationale for not ''temperature correcting'' the values for PCO_2 and pH obtained by standard analysis of arterial blood gases at 37°C.

Collee GG, Lynch KE, Hill RD, et al. Bedside measurement of pulmonary capillary pressure in patients with acute respiratory failure. Anesthesiology 1987;66:614–620.

Wedge pressure does not accurately reflect true pulmonary capillary pressure in many ARDS patients. The use of the ''pressure decay curve'' technique may provide a more accurate measurement of pulmonary capillary pressure.

Shoemaker WC, Appel PL, Kram HP, et al. Prospective trial of supranormal values of survivors as therapeutic goals in high-risk surgical patients. Chest 1988;94:1176–1186.

Boyd O, Grounds RM, Bennett ED. A randomized clinical trial of the effect of deliberate perioperative increase of oxygen delivery on mortality in high-risk surgical patients. JAMA 1993;270:2699–2707.

The above two studies of surgical patients purport to show a decrease in mortality when supranormal levels of cardiac index and oxygen delivery are achieved.

Yu M, Levy MM, Smith P, et al. Effect of maximizing oxygen delivery on morbidity and mortality rates in critically ill patients: a prospective, randomized, controlled study. Crit Care Med 1993;21:830–838.

Hayes MA, Timmins AC, Yau EHS, et al. Elevation of systemic oxygen delivery in the treatment of critically ill patients. N Engl J Med 1994;330:1717–1720.

Gattinoni L, Brazzi L, Pelosi P, et al. A trial of goal-oriented hemodynamic therapy in critically ill patients. N Engl J Med 1995;333:1025–1032.

The above three studies all show that hemodynamic therapy aimed at achieving supranormal values for the cardiac index and oxygen delivery (and in one study, normal mixed venous oxygenation, as well) fails to lead to improved survival in mixed groups of critically ill patients.

Connors AF, Speroff T, Dawson NV, et al. The effectiveness of right heart catheterization in the initial care of critically ill patients. JAMA 1996;276:889–897.

In a retrospective analysis, the association between the use of a pulmonary artery catheter (during the first 24 hours of intensive care) and clinical outcomes was examined. After complex statistical methods (''propensity scoring'') were used to compare heterogenous populations, the authors found that catheter use was associated with increased 30-day mortality, increased ICU stay, and increased costs. The validity of these findings is extremely dependent on the ability of the propensity score to correct for risk of adverse outcomes in the two populations. The authors acknowledged the limitations of this study, which was not randomized and prospective.

Dobb GJ. The pulmonary artery catheter: Too soon for its swan song? Intensive Care World 1996;13:139–140.

This is an editorial perspective on the Connors article above. The author states what appears to be an emerging consensus; that is, catheterization is unlikely to be harmful if done by trained and knowledgeable clinicians in carefully selected patients. Future studies to help define the appropriate guidelines for catheter insertion are warranted.

Goldenheim PD, Kazemi H. Cardiopulmonary monitoring of critically ill patients. N Engl J Med 1984; 311:717–720, 776–780.

Severinghaus, JW. History, status, and future of pulse oximetry. Adv Exp Med Biol 1987;220:3–8.

40

......

Board Simulation: Pulmonary Medicine

James K. Stoller

......

CASES 1–5

Patient Information

Patient profile 1:

    55-year-old man with history of multiple trauma, ARDS, and prolonged intubation.

Patient profile 2:

    65-year-old man with long-standing rheumatoid arthritis and cricoarytenoid involvement.

Patient profile 3:

    40-year-old woman with painful ears, saddle nose deformity, and arthralgias.

Patient profile 4:

    45-year-old woman with ''factitious asthma'' presenting as stridor.

Patient profile 5:

    30-year-old man with relapsing polychondritis and expiratory wheezing.

QUESTIONS

    Match the patient profiles described above to the correct patterns of the flow-volume loop shown in Figure 40.1.

1. Pattern for patient 1: _____

2. Pattern for patient 2: _____

3. Pattern for patient 3: _____

4. Pattern for patient 4: _____

5. Pattern for patient 5: _____

Discussion and Answer Explanations

1. In patient profile 1, the patient is a 55-year-old male with a history of multiple trauma, ARDS, and prolonged intubation. This is the first of the cases calling upon the reader to recognize an upper airway lesion and to match this with the appropriate pattern of the flow-volume loop. In this first case, the patient described has fixed laryngotracheal obstruction resulting from prolonged intubation complicating adult respiratory distress syndrome. Overall, the frequency of clinically significant upper airway obstruction following prolonged intubation is 5–15%, though controversy still exists regarding whether the risk of laryngeal injury rises as the duration of intubation lengthens. In upper airway obstruction following prolonged intubation, upper airway obstruction may result from several different lesions, including vocal cord stricture (especially at the posterior glottic chink) and tracheal stenosis, either at the site of the tracheostomy stoma or at the site of the cuff on the endotracheal tube. Because upper airway obstruction complicating prolonged intubation usually consists of granulation tissue, the airway obstruction is usually characterized by fixed upper airway obstruction, as demonstrated by pattern 4 in Figure 40.1. This pattern shows flattening of both the expiratory and inspiratory limbs of the flow-volume loop. In contrast, a fixed lesion is constant and shows airflow limitation both on inspiration and expiration. In this terminology, ''extrathoracic'' denotes a position along the airway cephalad of the thoracic inlet and ''intrathoracic'' denotes an airway lesion caudal to the thoracic inlet as far down the main carina.

    Recognizing the patterns of an abnormal flow-volume loop can be helpful in determining the presence

Figure 40.1.   Patterns of the flow-volume loop.

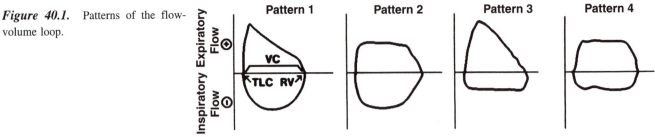

and position of upper airway obstruction. In understanding the flow-volume loop, it is important to recognize that positive flow (i.e., above the horizontal line) denotes expiration, and negative flow (below the horizontal, Fig. 40.1, pattern 1) denotes the inspiratory limb.

The flow-volume loop is a different way of graphically presenting the information gathered in a spirogram or volume-time tracing. Specifically, in determining the flow rate (i.e., in liters per second), the slope of the volume-time tracing is taken. The first derivative of volume with respect to time represents flow. The flow rate or slope of the volume-time tracing is then plotted against the volume (which is on the vertical axis of the volume-time tracing) but is transposed to become the horizontal axis of a flow-volume loop. Thus, the expiratory limb of the flow-volume loop is an algebraic transformation of the volume-time tracing. However, the inspiratory limb of the flow-volume loop is not depicted on a volume-time tracing (which is confined to expiration). To obtain the inspiratory component, the patient must inspire from residual volume to total lung capacity. In addition to the normal flow-volume loop (Fig. 40.1, pattern 1), three characteristic deviations from the normal flow-volume loop suggest various forms of upper airway obstruction (Fig. 40.1, patterns 2, 3, 4).

Pattern 2 represents dynamic intrathoracic upper airway obstruction, pattern 3 represents dynamic extrathoracic upper airway obstruction, and pattern 4 represents fixed upper airway obstruction. The descriptor ''dynamic'' denotes that the airway lesion is floppy or malacic, and so the degree of airway blockage will be affected by the transmural pressure gradient (across the airway wall). To understand these three variant patterns of the flow-volume loop, one must consider the pressure gradient across the airway walls during inspiration and expiration (Figs. 40.2 and 40.3). During inspiration, intrapleural pressure is negative, so atmospheric gas flows into the lung across a gradient from higher to lower pressures. The situation reverses during exhalation. During exhalation, as intrapleural pressure becomes more positive relative to atmospheric pressure, gas leaves the lung and moves to the outside atmosphere, which is now lower in pressure. With this in mind, it stands to reason that any fixed obstruction to

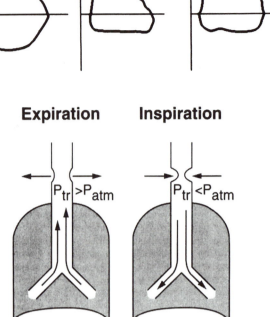

Figure 40.2.   Effect of expiration and inspiration on dynamic or nonfixed extrathoracic airway obstruction. **Left.** During forced expiration, intratracheal pressure (P_{tr}) exceeds the pressure around the airway (P_{atm}) or atmospheric pressure), lessening the obstruction. **Right.** During forced inspiration, when pressure around that airway is greater, the obstruction worsens. (Adapted from Kryger MH, Bode F, Antic R, et al. Diagnosis of obstruction of the upper and central airways. Am J Med 1976;61:85–93.)

airflow in the upper airway will produce a decrease in flows during both inspiration and expiration, causing flow to decrease in both limbs of the flow-volume tracing (Fig. 40.1, pattern 4). Thus, as in the patient profile, flow is decreased both during expiration and inspiration, giving rise to the characteristic flattening of both the inspiratory and expiratory limbs. In contrast to the situation with fixed airway obstruction, ''dynamic'' airflow can occur in the upper airway. To better understand how dynamic airflow obstruction affects the shape of the flow-volume loop, it is important to recognize that dynamic airflow obstruction can occur in the extrathoracic upper airway (e.g., caudal to the thoracic inlet). As shown in Figure 40.1, pattern 3, dynamic extrathoracic upper airway obstruction is characterized by flattening of the inspiratory limb of the flow-volume loop with preservation of a normal expiratory limb. Examples of such conditions might include tracheomalacia of the extrathoracic upper airway or vocal cord paralysis. In contrast, dynamic intrathoracic obstruction produces flattening of only the

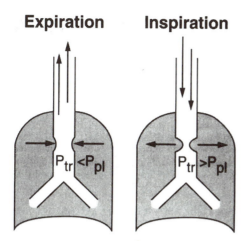

Expiration Inspiration

$P_{tr} < P_{pl}$ $P_{tr} > P_{pl}$

Figure 40.3. Effects of expiration and inspiration on dynamic or nonfixed intrathoracic airway obstruction. **Left.** During forced expiration, pressure exerted around the airway (P_{pl}, or pleural pressure) may exceed intratracheal pressure (P_{tr}), worsening the obstruction. **Right.** During forced inspiration, intratracheal pressure is greater, relieving the obstruction. (Adapted from Kryger MH, Bode F, Antic R, et al. Diagnosis of obstruction of the upper and central airways. Am J Med 1976;61:85–93.)

expiratory limb of the flow-volume loop (Fig. 40.1, pattern 3). Examples of conditions that cause dynamic intrathoracic upper airway obstruction include tracheomalacia of the intrathoracic airway or tumors that straddle the main carina. Figures 40.2 and 40.3 graphically review the pathophysiology of dynamic upper airway obstruction.

2. Patient profile 2 presents a 65-year-old male with long-standing rheumatoid arthritis and cricoarytenoid involvement. The best answer is Figure 40.1, pattern 4, denoting fixed extrathoracic upper airway obstruction. This case demonstrates the consequences of arthritis or ankylosis of the cricoarytenoids, which can cause upper airway obstruction in patients with rheumatoid arthritis. In a series by Lawry, et al. (Arthritis Rheum 1984;27: 873–882), the prevalence of inspiratory difficulty was 29% among 45 patients with rheumatoid arthritis.

3. Patient profile 3 regards a 41-year-old female with painful ears, saddle nose deformity, and arthralgias. This profile describes the scenario of upper airway involvement in relapsing polychondritis, clinical features of which include recurrent inflammation primarily affecting the nose, respiratory tract, ears, and joints. Notably, 25% of patients with relapsing polychondritis present with respiratory tract complaints, and 50% of patients have respiratory tract symptoms at some time over the course of their illness. Laryngotracheal involvement is responsible for 10% of deaths by pneumonia or by upper airway compromise in patients with relapsing polychondritis. The spectrum of upper airway lesions may include acute inflammation, fibrosis,

or dissolution of cartilage and malacia. As a result, the flow-volume loop abnormalities may include fixed upper airway obstruction, as well as dynamic intrathoracic or extrathoracic obstruction. As such, the correct answer in this case may be patterns 2, 3, or 4 in Figure 40.1, all of which are possible. In the absence of more defining symptoms such as inspiratory stridor (which would suggest dynamic extrathoracic upper airway obstruction) or expiratory wheezing (which might favor dynamic intrathoracic upper airway obstruction), any of the abnormal patterns is an acceptable answer.

4. Patient profile 4 presents a 45-year-old woman with "factitious asthma" presenting as stridor. The correct pattern is 3 in Figure 40.1, characterized by flattening of the inspiratory limb only. The cause of "factitious asthma" is vocal cord dysfunction. A spectrum of functional vocal cord problems has been observed including paradoxic inspiratory closure and paradoxic expiratory closure. As noted above, paradoxic inspiratory closure would be more likely to present as stridor and to be characterized by flattening of the inspiratory limb of the flow-volume loop.

5. Finally, patient profile 5 presents a 30-year-old male with relapsing polychondritis and expiratory wheezing. The correct flow-volume loop abnormality is Figure 40.1, pattern 2. In this case, unlike patient profile 2, the presence of expiratory wheezing should suggest the presence of intrathoracic upper airway obstruction.

CASES 6–10

Patient Information

Patient profile 6:
    25-year-old with von Recklinghausen's disease.
Patient profile 7:
    62-year-old man 2 days post-CABG.
Patient profile 8:
    35-year-old obese man with nocturnal cough.
Patient profile 9:
    45-year-old woman with a cirrhotic child.
Patient profile 10:
    60-year-old man 1–2 pack per day smoker.

QUESTIONS

Match each appropriate patient above to the best pulmonary function test profile in Table 40.1. Note that each pulmonary function test profile may be used once, more than once, or not at all.

6. Results for patient 6: _____

7. Results for patient 7: _____

Table 40.1. Pulmonary Function Test Results

	FEV_1 % Pred	FVC % pred	↓ FVC (sit to supine)	TLC % pred	DLCO % pred
1.	60%	78%	19%	73%	83%
2.	50%	52%	11%	65%	60%
3.	84%	91%	8%	90%	90%
4.	52%	81%	12%	105%	70%
5.	45%	55%	27%	70%	55%

8. Results for patient 8: _____

9. Results for patient 9: _____

10. Results for patient 10: _____

Discussion and Answer Explanations

6. Patient profile 6 presents a 25-year-old with von Recklinghausen's disease. The most appropriate pulmonary function test profile is number 2, demonstrating pulmonary restriction characterized by a total lung capacity of 65% predicted, a proportionate decline in the diffusing capacity (60% predicted), and proportionate decreases in both FEV_1 and FVC, such that the FEV_1/FVC is preserved. Also, the change in forced vital capacity going from sitting to supine is normal, i.e., under 20%. This pulmonary function profile is characteristic of extra-thoracic pulmonary restriction, such as might be seen by the kyphoscoliosis that accompanies von Recklinghausen's disease in up to 20% of patients. Notably, in approximately 5% of affected individuals, the kyphoscoliosis is clinically significant. The sine qua non of restrictive lung disease is decreased total lung capacity. In this case, the proportionate decrease in the diffusing capacity suggests extrathoracic disease rather than a parenchymal restrictive lung disease, e.g., interstitial lung disease.

7. Patient profile 7 presents a 62-year-old man 2 days after coronary artery bypass graft surgery. The most appropriate pulmonary function test result profile is number 5. As in previous cases, this is a pattern depicting extrathoracic pulmonary restriction with decreased total lung capacity. However, unlike the former case, the decrease in the forced vital capacity on moving from sitting to supine posture exceeds the normal upper boundary of 20%. In this case, the cause is bilateral diaphragmatic paralysis causing an accentuated decline in the forced vital capacity on lying down, as the diaphragm is pushed into the chest by the abdominal contents. This case demonstrates the phenomenon of ''frostbitten'' phrenic nerves, which may complicate coronary artery bypass graft surgery (as a result of bathing the phrenic(s) in cold

cardioplegia solution) in up to 5% of cases. Unilateral diaphragmatic paralysis is more common than bilateral diaphragmatic paralysis, and unilateral paralysis is usually clinically not apparent. However, when both phrenic nerves are affected, the patient exhibits marked orthopnea accompanied by the decline in forced vital capacity as noted above.

8. Patient profile 8 presents a 35-year-old obese man with nocturnal cough. Pulmonary function profile 1 is the best choice and indicates a pattern of airflow obstruction (i.e., a disproportionate decrease in FEV_1 compared with FVC). In this case, the patient's obesity likely accounts for the mild restrictive lung disease (TLC 73% of predicted, below the 80% predicted that is the lower limit of normal). In fact, this case presents combined restrictive and obstructive lung disease, the differential diagnosis of which includes asthma with obesity as well as eosinophilic granuloma of lung (histiocytosis X), sarcoidosis, lymphangioleiomyomatosis, and congestive heart failure. In this case, the patient's nocturnal cough is a manifestation of asthma. In fact, nocturnal symptoms accompany asthma in up to one-third of patients and may frequently dominate the clinical presentation. Management strategies may include the use of long-acting theophylline preparations or long-acting inhaled beta agonists, e.g., salmeterol.

9. Patient profile 9 is that of a 45-year-old woman with a cirrhotic child. The case is meant to prompt consideration of severe (e.g., PI* ZZ homozygous) alpha 1-antitrypsin deficiency. In this regard, the best pulmonary function profile is number 4, demonstrating a pattern of airflow obstruction with a suggestion of alveolar-capillary unit loss demonstrated by the mild decrease in the diffusing capacity. Overall, this pattern suggests lung parenchymal loss consistent with emphysema rather than asthma alone. Alpha 1-antitrypsin deficiency is an autosomal codominant condition. The major pulmonary manifestation is emphysema, but individuals with the Z allele may also develop cirrhosis and hepatoma, related to inadequate secretion of Z protein from the hepatocyte.

    This case also invites consideration of the causes of a decreased diffusing capacity for carbon monoxide. The diffusing capacity (or DLCO) is a measurement of gas transfer across the alveolar-capillary units, which may be decreased when there is loss of pulmonary vasculature (e.g., pulmonary vascular disease or lung resection) or loss of lung parenchyma (as may be seen in emphysema or interstitial lung disease). Because uptake of carbon monoxide by erythrocytes requires adequate red blood cells with hemoglobin avid for carbon monoxide, the diffusing capacity will also be decreased in the face of anemia or prior carbon monoxide poisoning (which creates a back pressure that decreases further uptake of carbon monoxide by red blood cells).

Pulmonary features that should lead to consideration of severe alpha 1-antitrypsin deficiency include emphysema at an early age (e.g., under 50 years old), emphysema in the absence of antecedent smoking, emphysema with a positive family history of lung and/or liver disease, and/or radiographic changes showing basilar hyperlucency (in contrast to the more apical distribution of emphysema changes in "garden variety" emphysema unrelated to alpha 1-antitrypsin deficiency).

10. Patient profile 10 presents a 60-year-old man who smokes 1–2 packs per day. Pulmonary function profile 3 is considered the best choice, though profile 4 (characteristic of emphysema) would be acceptable. Pulmonary function profile 3 represents normal lung function, emphasizing that although cigarette smoking can cause an accelerated decline in FEV_1, most cigarette smokers escape accelerated airflow obstruction. In fact, "susceptible smokers" with accelerated airflow decline are said to make up approximately 10–15% of all smokers. Even in "susceptible smokers," cessation of cigarette smoking slows the rate of decline of lung function to that of nonsmokers, though recovery of lost lung function after smoking cessation is uncommon.

CASES 11–15

Patient Information

Patient profile 11:
    70-year-old man with fasciculations and upper motor neuron disease.
Patient profile 12:
    50-year-old man with dyspnea and panniculitis.
Patient profile 13:
    48-year-old heavy smoker with acute confusion.
Patient profile 14:
    45-year-old woman with neck trauma.
Patient profile 15:
    25-year-old man 3 weeks after a ski accident and tibial fracture.

QUESTIONS

Match the five patient profiles above with the appropriate room air arterial blood gas pattern in Table 40.2. As before, each arterial blood gas pattern in Table 40.2 may be used once, more than once, or not at all.

11. Pattern for patient 11: _____

12. Pattern for patient 12: _____

13. Pattern for patient 13: _____

14. Pattern for patient 14: _____

15. Pattern for patient 15: _____

Discussion and Answer Explanations

11. Patient profile 11 presents a 70-year-old male with fasciculations and upper motor neuron disease. The clinical scenario is intended to elicit the diagnosis of amyotrophic lateral sclerosis, a degenerative disease of the motor neurons which is slowly progressive and is associated with extrathoracic pulmonary restriction as well as blood gases reflecting hypoventilation and/or the effect of V/Q mismatch. In this instance, the most appropriate blood gas pattern would be profile 3 or 5. Profile 3 represents a pattern of pure hypoventilation which may be seen with neuromuscular disease such as amyotrophic lateral sclerosis. Alternately, patient profile 5 represents hypoxemia with hypocapnia (i.e., chronic respiratory alkalosis). In arterial blood gas profile 5, the alveolar-arterial oxygen gradient is widened, consistent with ventilation/perfusion mismatch or anatomic shunt.

    In interpreting room air arterial blood gases, calculation of the alveolar-arterial oxygen gradient is helpful. Table 40.3 depicts this calculation. Normal values of the alveolar-arterial oxygen gradient are age-dependent, as depicted in Figure 40.4. A useful mnemonic for the mean-age specific alveolar-arterial oxygen gradient is (age/4 + 4), with the upper limit

Table 40.2. Room Air Arterial Blood Gases

	PaO_2 (mm Hg)	$PaCO_2$ (mm Hg)	pH
1.	50	65	7.30
2.	60	60	7.20
3.	50	65	7.37
4.	85	28	7.51
5.	65	35	7.42

Table 40.3. Alveolar-Arterial Oxygen Gradient ($AaDO_2$)

1. Calculate the alveolar oxygen tension (P_AO_2)
    $P_AO_2 = (P_B - 47) FIO_2 - [(PaCO_2)/(Resp Quotient)]$,
    P_B = Barometric pressure, e.g., 760 mm Hg
    $PaCO_2$ = arterial CO_2 tension
    Resp Quotient = Respiratory quotient (moles CO_2 produced per mole of O_2 consumed, usually 0.8)
2. Subtract P_aO_2 (arterial oxygen tension)
3. $AaDO_2 = P_AO_2 - P_aO_2$

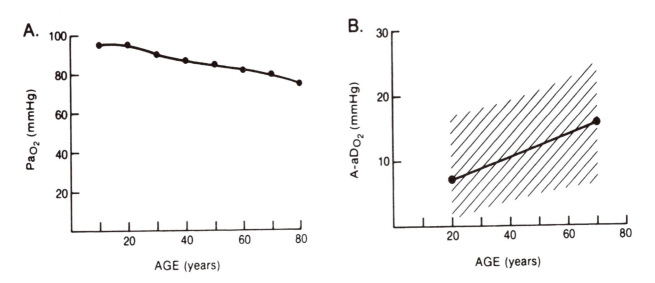

Figure 40.4. **A.** Variations of arterial oxygen tension (PaO_2) with age. **B.** Variations of alveolar-arterial oxygen gradient ($A - aDO_2$) with age; mean values for $A - aDO_2 = 2.5 + 0.21 \times$ age; bold line indicates mean values, shaded area $+$ 2 standard deviations. (From Tisi G. Pulmonary physiology in clinical medicine. Baltimore: Williams & Wilkins, 1980:78.)

value of the age-specific alveolar-arterial oxygen gradient roughly calculated by the equation (age/4 + 4) + 10 mm Hg. Calculation of the alveolar-arterial oxygen gradient is useful in approaching the differential diagnosis of hypoxemia. Six causes of hypoxemia should be remembered: anatomic shunt, ventilation-perfusion mismatch, diffusion impairment, hypoventilation, inhaling a decreased inspired oxygen fraction, and diffusion-perfusion impairment (e.g., seen in the hepatopulmonary syndrome). Of these six causes, diffusion-perfusion impairment is uncommon and is confined to patients with hypoxemia caused by the hepatopulmonary syndrome. Hypoxemia relating to inhaling decreased inspired oxygen fractions occurs only when the patient is exposed to high altitude or when a hypoxic gas mixture is breathed at sea level. Among the other four causes of hypoxemia (anatomic shunt, ventilation-perfusion mismatch, diffusion impairment, and hypoventilation), the age-specific alveolar-arterial oxygen gradient is increased for all causes except hypoventilation, where the alveolar-arterial oxygen gradient is normal. Using a rule of thumb equation (Table 40.3) for calculating the room air alveolar-arterial oxygen gradient: $149 - [PaO_2 + PaCO_2 (1.25)]$, the alveolar-arterial oxygen gradient in blood gas profile 3 is $149 - [50 + 65 (1.25)]$, or 18 mm Hg, which is normal for a 70-year-old male. Therefore, for a 70-year-old, arterial blood gas profile 3 indicates hypoventilation, which might accompany neuromuscular disease like amyotrophic lateral sclerosis. In contrast, the value of the room air alveolar-room arterial oxygen gradient for blood gas profile 5 is 40 mm Hg, which is elevated even for a

70-year-old. Such a profile might be seen in neuromuscular disease in which atelectasis is causing ventilation/perfusion mismatch, resulting in hypoxemia without hypoventilation.

12. Patient profile 12 presents a 50-year-old man with dyspnea and panniculitis. The case is meant to suggest alpha 1-antitrypsin deficiency characterized by panniculitis and emphysema. Arterial blood gas profile 5 is considered the best answer, indicating hypoxemia with chronic respiratory alkalosis on the basis of long-standing ventilation/perfusion mismatch.

13. Profile 13 presents a 48-year-old heavy smoker with acute confusion. The history of heavy smoking is meant to suggest severe chronic obstructive lung disease. Such a patient might demonstrate chronic hypoxemia with chronic hypercapnia and compensated respiratory acidosis. However, the presence of acute confusion suggests an acute worsening of respiratory acidosis, as best demonstrated by the arterial blood gas profile 1.

14. Patient profile 14 presents a 45-year-old female with neck trauma. One should consider spinal cord injury above the level of C3, resulting in acute hypoventilation. The expected arterial blood gas profile is that of hypoventilation with acute respiratory acidosis, best represented by arterial blood gas profile 2. In this case, a pH of 7.20 indicates acute respiratory acidosis and the room air alveolar-arterial oxygen gradient is 14 mm Hg, again demonstrating hypoventilation.

15. Patient profile 15 presents a 25-year-old male who is 3 weeks after a ski accident and a tibial fracture. The clinical setting should suggest the possibility of an

acute pulmonary embolism. An acute respiratory alkalosis with a widened alveolar-arterial oxygen gradient would be expected and is best demonstrated by arterial blood gas profile 4. In this case, the alveolar-arterial oxygen gradient is 29 mm Hg, which is above normal for a 25-year-old male. This case serves as a reminder that patients with acute pulmonary emboli may not demonstrate hypoxemia but that the alveolar-arterial oxygen gradient is usually (but not uniformly) elevated.

SUGGESTED READINGS

Aboussouan LS, Stoller JK. Diagnosis and management of upper airway obstruction. Clin Chest Med 1994;15:35–53.

Kryger MH, Bode F, Antic R, et al. Diagnosis of obstruction of the upper and central airways. Am J Med 1976;61:85–93.

McFarlane MJ, Imperiale TF. Use of the alveolar-arterial oxygen gradient in the diagnosis of pulmonary embolism. Am J Med 1994;96:57–62.

Miller RD, Hyatt RE. Obstructing lesions of the larynx and trachea: clinical and physiologic characteristics. Mayo Clin Proc 1969;44:145–161.

Stein PD, Goldhaber SZ, Henry JW. Alveolar-arterial oxygen gradient in the assessment of acute pulmonary embolism. Chest 1995;107:139–143.

Stoller JK. Spirometry: a key diagnostic test in pulmonary medicine. Cleve Clin J Med 1992;59:75–78.

Endocrinology

Thyroid Disorders

Charles Faiman

Thyroid hormone secretion is regulated by the hypothalamo-pituitary-thyroid axis (Fig. 41.1). Characteristics include:

- Approximately 25% of the circulating T_3 is derived from direct secretion by the thyroid gland; the remainder comes from peripheral conversion.
- Reverse T_3 (rT_3), which is biologically inert, is produced instead of active T_3 in the sick euthyroid state and in the fetus.
- Circulating thyroid hormones are mainly bound to proteins:
  - TBG (thyroxine-binding globulin) binds both T_4 and T_3
  - Prealbumin (TBPA, also called transthyretin) binds only T_4
  - Albumin binds both T_4 and T_3
  - 99.97% of T_4 and 99.7% of T_3 are bound
  - The free hormone is active

Thyroid Function Tests

Thyroid function tests include:

- TSH (sensitive/ultrasensitive), the best single indicator of thyroid function
- Total T_4
- T_4U or T_3RU (estimates of binding)
- FTI (free thyroxine index), adjusted for serum protein binding
- Free T_4
- Total T_3
- Free T_3

Factors that alter binding or binding capacity result in alterations in total T_4 and total T_3:

- Changes in TBG influence both T_4 and T_3 values
- Changes in TBPA influence T_4 values only

Conditions associated with TBG excess:

- Pregnancy
- Drugs (estrogen, tamoxifen, heroin, methadone, perphenazine)
- Acute hepatitis
- Chronic active hepatitis
- Acute intermittent porphyria
- Hereditary

Conditions associated with TBG deficiency include:

- Androgens
- Acromegaly
- Hypoproteinemia
- Nephrotic syndrome
- Chronic liver disease
- Glucocorticoids (large doses)
- Hereditary

Measurement of the binding proteins by a T_4U test or T_3RU test and calculation of the FTI will help to correct for the effect of changes in the binding proteins on thyroid hormone levels. Newer assays of free T_4 are at least equal to the FTI and in some cases better. Free T_4 by equilibrium dialysis remains the gold standard, but it is too expensive for routine clinical use.

Remember:

- A high T_4U test (or low T_3RU test) indicates that thyroid hormone binding sites are present in excess, which can be owing to:
  - Excessive binding protein (see above)
  - Diminished occupancy (hypothyroidism)

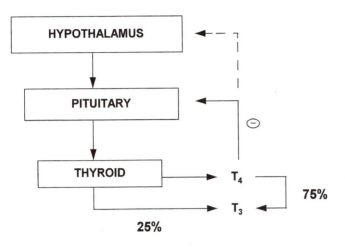

Figure 41.1. Hypothalamo-pituitary-thyroid axis.

- A low T_4U (or high T_3RU test) indicates that thyroid hormone binding sites are deficient owing to:
  - Diminished binding protein (see above)
  - Excessive occupancy (hyperthyroidism)
  - Drugs or conditions (e.g., sick euthyroidism) that interfere with thyroid hormone-protein binding

Thyroid function tests are readily interpretable in ambulatory individuals, but are often not helpful or confusing in the hospitalized sick patient.

TESTS FOR HYPOTHYROIDISM

Thyroid function tests for diagnosing hypothyroidism include:

- TSH (normal 0.4–5.5 μU/ml)
  - >15–20 μU/ml, diagnostic (caveats: newborn or recovery phase of sick euthyroidism)
  - 5.5–15 μU/ml, borderline or subclinical hypothyroidism (may be normal for geriatric population), assess for goiter; order T_4, FTI, or free T_4; order thyroid microsomal antibodies (TMA); decide on replacement therapy versus observation
  - Beware that normal (or low) values can be seen with pituitary (2°) or hypothalamic (3°) hypothyroidism
- FTI or FT_4
  - May also be used as primary test
  - Less-discriminating
- T_3
  - Of no value
- RAIU
  - Not indicated and may even mislead
- TMA
  - As a cause for hypothyroidism/goiter

TESTS FOR HYPERTHYROIDISM

Thyroid function tests for diagnosing hyperthyroidism include:

- TSH (normal 0.4–5.5 μU/ml)
  - Suppressed <0.02–0.1 μU/ml (depends on assay sensitivity)
  - 0.1–0.4 μU/ml, consider:
    - Early autonomy
    - Slight over-replacement
    - Drugs (e.g., steroids, dopamine)
    - Pregnancy (first trimester)
- FTI or FT_4
  - Helpful particularly if TSH low
- T_3 (if TSH suppressed and FTI or FT_4 normal)
  - Think of early hyperthyroidism or thyroid extract treatment

TESTS FOR EUTHYROID SICK SYNDROME

Thyroid function tests for diagnosing euthyroid sick syndrome include:

- T_4 – N or ↓
- T_4U – ↓ or N
- T_3RU – ↑ or N
- FT_4 – N or ↓
- T_3 – ↓
- rT_3 – ↑
- TSH–N or ↓ (↑ in recovery phase)

Response to TRH is normal or blunted (TRH testing is of little or no value with the advent of sensitive TSH assays, except as a test for pituitary function [TSH and prolactin reserve]).

There is no more vexing problem in the interpretation of thyroid function tests than the euthyroid sick syndrome. The above is a guide but does not represent an absolute. Overlap in test results is common, and frequently there are confounding factors. Therefore, clinical acumen is critical. Since isolated TSH deficiency is uncommon (isolated 2° hypothyroidism), look for other signs of hypopituitarism. However, gonadotropins may also be suppressed during the acute stress/starvation state. The new tests of free T_4 have similar problems to the FTI in this syndrome. The changes in thyroid function tests reflect severity of illness. Mortality is inversely proportional to total T_4 in euthyroid MICU patients. However, T_4 treatment of patients with severe nonthyroidal illness and low T_4 does not help and could possibly harm.

Factors inhibiting T_4 to T_3 conversion include:

- Systemic illness (acute or chronic)
- Caloric deprivation (fasting, anorexia nervosa, or protein-calorie malnutrition)
- Surgery
- Newborn
- Aging
- Drugs (glucocorticoids, propranolol [high doses], amiodarone, propylthiouracil)
- Contrast media (ipodate, iopanoic acid)

Euthyroid hypothyroxinemia is characterized by:

- Decreased TBG production
  - Severe systemic illness
  - Glucocorticoids
  - Androgens
  - Familial X-linked (many variants)
- Excessive TBG loss
  - Protein-losing enteropathy
  - Nephrosis
  - Jejuno-ileal bypass
- Inhibition of protein binding
  - Systemic illness (free fatty acids and tissue factor)
  - Dilantin (in vitro, possibly not in vivo)
  - Salicylates
  - Furosemide
  - Fenclofanac
- Exogenous T_3 administration

Euthyroid hyperthyroxinemia is characterized by:

- Binding protein abnormalities [excess binding to TBG, TBPA, or albumin (rare to T_4 antibodies)]
- Transient hyperthyroxinemia of acute medical or psychiatric illness
- Decreased peripheral conversion of T_4 to T_3, especially by propranolol or amiodarone
- Amphetamine ingestion
- Tissue resistance to thyroid hormone

OTHER THYROID TESTS

Other diagnostic thyroid tests include:

- TMA (thyroid microsomal antibodies), also called thyroid peroxidase (TPO) antibodies
- Thyroglobulin antibodies
- TRAB (thyroid receptor antibodies), stimulating (TSI) and receptor binding
- Thyroglobulin
- Serum or urinary iodide
- Radioactive iodine uptake (RAI uptake or RAIU)
- Thyroid scan (RAI or pertechnetate)
- Thyroid ultrasound
- Fine-needle biopsy

Measurement of serum thyroglobulin (Tg, the protein that is iodinated to make T_4 and T_3) can reveal the following:

- Elevated Tg levels reflect increased secretory activity by or damage to the thyroid.
- Low Tg levels indicate a paucity of thyroid tissue or suppressed activity.

The test is useful in the diagnosis of thyrotoxicosis factitia. As the highest Tg levels are seen in metastatic differentiated nonmedullary thyroid carcinoma, the test is useful in following patients with thyroid cancer. (See "Thyroid Nod-

ules and Cancer" below.) Beware of artifacts caused by the presence of antithyroglobulin antibodies.

Measurement of serum thyroid antibodies provides additional information:

- Antimicrosomal (peroxidase) antibodies and antithyroglobulin antibodies are occasionally of use in the management of hypothyroidism and in screening for the polyglandular autoimmune syndrome.
- TSH receptor stimulating antibodies, the cause of thyrotoxicosis in Graves' disease, may help predict remission of the disease following treatment with antithyroid drugs.

Thyroid scanning and radioactive iodine uptake (RAIU) is less helpful:

- Patients with hypothyroidism can have low, "normal," or high RAIU.
- Patients with hyperthyroidism can have low, "normal," or high RAIU.

The RAIU is clinically useful only in the differential diagnosis of hyperthyroidism, in the calculation of radioiodine dosage, and in concert with a scan, in the management of thyroid carcinoma. Note that RAIU gives you a number; a scan gives you a picture.

SCREENING FOR THYROID DYSFUNCTION

NEONATAL SCREENING

Screening programs, usually based upon heel-prick blood TSH assays, are mandatory in most states in the United States and in most developed countries. Prevention of cretinism (1:4000 live births) is far more cost-effective than original PKU screening programs.

Problems encountered include:

- Location, institution, and maintenance of therapy in neonates with abnormal test results
- Need for new strategies to help differentiate the physiological neonatal TSH surge from pathological primary hypothyroidism (not a problem when studies done on or after 3 days of life)
- Rare cases of hypothalamic-pituitary hypothyroidism missed unless a simultaneous T_4 assay is performed

ADULT SCREENING

Who should be screened? Keep in mind that to screen for a disease assumes that detecting the disease is beneficial to the patient and that screening itself is not harmful to those without the disease. Even in hypothyroidism, where therapy is easy, the costs of screening a large population are not trivial. Therefore, screening should be performed only in populations with a reasonably high prevalence of thyroid dysfunction, such as women over the age of 40 and patients admitted to specialized geriatric units. There is little reason to screen the general population either in the ambulatory setting or upon hospitalization. The issue of treatment of subclinical thyroid disease is controversial.

How should screening be done? High-sensitivity TSH screening is probably the most effective way to screen ambulatory populations because it has superior test characteristics, because 1° hypothyroidism is the most common form of abnormal thyroid function (far more common than 2° hypothyroidism), and because 1° hyperthyroidism is far more common than 2° hyperthyroidism.

In outpatients, the sensitivity and specificity of FT_4 and FTI are approximately 90% in the diagnosis of hyperthyroidism, while the sensitivity and specificity of the high sensitivity TSH assay are about 99%. The operating characteristics of these tests are far worse in hospitalized patients in whom the specificity of the TSH assay is particularly low.

Hypothyroidism

Hypothyroidism is the clinical disorder that results from insufficient thyroid hormone action.

ETIOLOGY OF HYPOTHYROIDISM

Hypothyroidism is a common disease, more prevalent in women (1%–2% prevalence) than in men (0.1% prevalence). In one large study from England, 25%–30% of patients were iatrogenic. Hypothyroidism is particularly common in the elderly. Congenital hypothyroidism occurs in one of every 4000 newborns.

The causes of hypothyroidism can be subdivided into three groupings (common causes are italicized):

- *Primary (thyroid cause)*
  - Agenesis
  - Destruction of gland
    - *Surgical removal*
    - *Irradiation* (therapeutic radioactive iodine for thyrotoxicosis or external irradiation therapy for nonthyroid malignant disease of the neck)
    - *Autoimmune disease* (Hashimoto's)
    - *Idiopathic atrophy* (possibly following autoimmune disease)
    - Replacement by cancer or other infiltrative process
  - Inhibition of synthesis and release of thyroid hormone
    - Iodine deficiency
    - Excess iodide in susceptible individuals
    - Antithyroid drugs
    - Lithium
    - Inherited enzyme defects

- Transient
  - After surgery or therapeutic radioactive iodine
  - Postpartum
  - In the course of thyroiditis
- Secondary to pituitary or hypothalamic disease
- Resistance to thyroid hormones

CLINICAL PRESENTATION OF HYPOTHYROIDISM

Clinical presentation depends upon the pathogenesis—sudden onset (e.g., following thyroidectomy) versus gradual decline (e.g., owing to idiopathic atrophy). In the former, the clinical onset relates to the serum half-life of T_4 (1 week) and occurs in a matter of weeks. In the latter, decreases in thyroid hormone levels may take place over years. In addition, the clinical picture depends on the age of the patient. Since thyroid hormone is essential for brain development, a neonatal onset will have different manifestations from an adult onset. (Sometimes it is helpful to read lay literature rather than medical literature. One of the best descriptions of hypothyroidism is in a wonderful novel, *The Citadel*, by A.J. Cronin.)

Symptoms include:

- Constitutional symptoms (weakness, fatigue, lethargy, and sleepiness)
- Mental slowness
- Cold intolerance
- Muscle aches
- Paresthesias (especially carpal tunnel syndrome)
- Diminished sweating
- Hoarseness
- Weight gain
- Constipation
- Hair loss
- Menstrual dysfunction (usually heavy, frequent menses, rarely amenorrhea and galactorrhea)

Signs include:

- Dry, coarse, cold skin
- Edema of eyelids
- Puffy hands and swelling of feet (myxedema)
- Coarse hair and hair loss
- Thick tongue
- Slow speech
- Hoarse voice
- Slow movements
- Pseudomyotonia (delayed relaxation phase of deep tendon reflexes)
- Sallow and pale complexion

Note that many of these features are common in normal aging.

Myxedema coma represents the end stage of hypothyroidism or the combination of severe hypothyroidism, plus one or more complicating factors. The pathophysiology involves:

- Respiratory failure
- Decreased cardiac output
- Anemia
- Hypothermia
- Hypoglycemia
- Hyponatremia
- Thyroid hormone deficiency

Respiratory dysfunction plays an important role in the development of most cases of myxedema coma. Hypothyroidism affects the respiratory system at all levels, from the respiratory center to peripheral oxygen delivery. Respiratory center depression is manifest by impaired responses to hypercapnia and hypoxia and results in hypoventilation and a diminished ability to respond to acute hypoxemia-producing insults.

DIAGNOSIS OF HYPOTHYROIDISM

Laboratory study manifestations include:

- Increased serum creatine phosphokinase (CPK) and cholesterol
- Decreased serum sodium
- ECG (low voltage)

Primary hypothyroidism caused by Hashimoto's thyroiditis is associated with other autoimmune diseases; for example, autoimmune adrenal insufficiency and the polyglandular autoimmune syndrome.

Questions to answer in the diagnosis include:

- Is the patient hypothyroid?
- If the patient is hypothyroid, what is the cause? Is it primary or secondary?

The latter has important implications for therapy. (See above for details.)

TREATMENT OF HYPOTHYROIDISM

Treatment is two-pronged:

- Administer thyroid hormone
- Treat the underlying disease

The causes of secondary and tertiary hypothyroidism—that is, hypothyroidism because of pituitary or hypothalamic insufficiency—often require therapy directed at both the cause and the effects of thyroid hormone deficiency. The causes of primary hypothyroidism (i.e., diseases directly affecting the thyroid gland) do not as a general rule require treatment directed at the cause. Rather, the key in treatment is therapy directed toward amelioration of the effects of thyroid hormone deficiency.

The treatment of hypothyroidism is simple: Administer thyroid hormone. Levothyroxine ($L-T_4$) is the preparation of choice. Its advantages include:

- The patient given T_4 develops a substantial peripheral pool of T_4, which turns over more slowly than does T_3 and provides a buffer against lapses in the ingestion of medication.
- The pool of T_4 acts as a continuous source of T_3, thereby maintaining a stable T_3 serum concentration.

When first diagnosed, hypothyroidism is usually of long duration and seldom requires rapid reversal. Therefore, the restoration of a normal metabolic state may be undertaken gradually. The untreated hypothyroid patient is very sensitive to small doses of thyroid hormone. In the hypothyroid patient with long-standing hypothyroidism, high-dose T_4 may precipitate a myocardial infarction or congestive heart failure.

In secondary hypothyroidism, it is important to treat adrenal insufficiency, if present, prior to thyroid replacement.

On the other hand, there is no untoward risk of initiating therapy with full replacement doses of $L-T_4$ in most younger adult patients with hypothyroidism (estimated at 1.6 $\mu g/kg$ body weight). In the pediatric age group, requirements are considerably higher. Monitoring therapy is best accomplished by means of the high-sensitivity TSH assay, with the aim of restoration to the normal range. Because of the inherent lag of TSH in the system, no dose adjustments based on the TSH value should be made for a minimum 6-week interval. However, on clinical grounds, small dose adjustments working toward total replacement can be made safely at 2-week intervals in the elderly and in those with a precarious cardiac status.

In hypothalamic-pituitary hypothyroidism, TSH determinations are of no value. Monitoring is best accomplished using a FTI or FT_4 assay. If hyperthyroxinemia develops, use the T_3 RIA to determine whether overtreatment has occurred (values should be <130–140 ng/dl [normal 80–170 ng/dl]). Overtreatment may result in accelerated osteopenia.

The following additional considerations should be noted in patients on $L-T_4$ therapy:

- Use the same brand-name drug (avoid generics).
- Monitor compliance/dosage requirements at 6–12-month intervals.
- Beware of concomitant use of medications that may interfere with absorption (soybean [infant formula], cholestyramine, sucralfate [polyaluminum hydroxide], antacids [aluminum hydroxide], or iron) or with metabolism (anticonvulsants [phenytoin or carbamazepine] or rifampin). The effects of anticonvulsants are complex; TSH values remain the best guide (except in hypothalamic-pituitary hypothyroidism).

Hyperthyroidism

Hyperthyroidism is a common clinical condition.

ETIOLOGY OF HYPERTHYROIDISM

As with most thyroid disorders, hyperthyroidism is much more common in women than men. A cross-sectional study of autoimmune thyroid disease in an English community revealed a prevalence of established hyperthyroidism of 2% in women and an annual incidence of 3/1000 women.

The causes of hyperthyroidism can be subdivided into three groupings (common causes are italicized):

- Primary thyroid overproduction (RAIU elevated or high normal, unless iodide pool expanded, such as, recent radiocontrast, Jod-Basedow [iodide-induced hyperthyroidism])
  - *Graves' disease*
  - *Toxic multinodular goiter*
  - *Toxic adenoma*
  - Thyroid carcinoma (metastatic)
  - HCG-mediated
    - Trophoblastic disease
    - Hyperemesis gravidarum
  - Fetal/neonatal
  - TSH-mediated
    - Pituitary adenoma
    - Pituitary thyroid hormone resistance
  - Iodide excess
  - Intrinsic TSH receptor abnormality
- Thyroid damage (RAIU low)
  - Subacute (painful, de Quervain's) thyroiditis
  - Painless and postpartum thyroiditis
  - Amiodarone (clinical significance uncertain)
- Nonthyroidal disease (RAIU low)
  - Exogenous hormone use (excessive dose; factitious use) [common]
  - Accidental exposure (laced hamburgers)
  - Struma ovarii (theoretical)

CLINICAL PRESENTATION OF HYPERTHYROIDISM

Symptoms include:

- Nervousness
- Fatigue
- Weakness
- Palpitations
- Heat intolerance
- Increased sweating
- Dyspnea
- Hyperdefecation
- Insomnia
- Poor concentration
- Infrequent, scanty menses

Signs include:

- Weight loss
- Proximal myopathy
- Tachycardia, arrhythmias
- Warm, moist skin
- Tremor

- Eye conditions (stare, lid lag, and lid retraction)
- Emotional liability
- Hyperactive deep tendon reflexes

A thyroid storm, which represents the extreme form of hyperthyroidism, includes:

- Exaggerated typical signs
- Exaggerated typical symptoms
- Fever
- Changes in neurologic function (delirium)

DIAGNOSIS OF HYPERTHYROIDISM

A biochemical diagnosis of suppressed TSH and elevated circulating T_4 and/or T_3 requires an RAI-uptake test (a thyroid scan may also prove useful) in order to confirm the diagnosis and aid in the treatment plan. Contraindications to the use of RAI in testing or therapy include:

- Pregnancy
- Lactation
- Iodide (nonradioactive) overload
- Intercurrent illness/therapy (which precludes waiting for the test to be done)

A positive TRAB test can be helpful in such situations.

GRAVES' DISEASE

Robert Graves published a report in 1835 of three patients with cardiac palpitations and goiter. One of the three patients also had exophthalmos. This is now recognized as the most common cause of noniatrogenic hyperthyroidism in the United States. There are three major manifestations of the disease:

- Hyperthyroidism with diffuse goiter
- Ophthalmopathy (eye disease)
- Dermopathy (pretibial myxedema)

There are several lines of evidence to support the role of hereditary factors in the development of Graves' disease in the children and siblings of patients with Graves'. The presence of certain Human Leukocyte Antigens (HLA) is associated with an increased incidence of Graves'; in particular, the HLA-DR-3 antigen in Caucasians may confer a 4-fold risk for the development of the disease. There is also an increased incidence in patients with Graves' disease and their family members of other autoimmune disorders (e.g., Hashimoto's thyroiditis, pernicious anemia, myasthenia gravis, and Addison's disease). The disease occurs most frequently between the ages of 20 and 40 and it has a marked female sex preponderance (approximately 3–8:l). Therapy may consist of ^{131}I, antithyroid drugs or, rarely, surgery (see below). Symptomatic treatment with beta blockers is also very useful.

Hyperthyroidism with Diffuse Goiter

The thyrotoxicosis and goiter of Graves' disease result from stimulation of the gland by autoantibodies (immunoglobulins of the IgG class). These autoantibodies are polyclonal and collectively are referred to as thyroid-stimulating immunoglobulins (TSI). The antigen to which these are directed is the TSH receptor, or a region adjacent to it, on the plasma membrane. Binding of these immunoglobulins to the TSH receptor mimics the action of TSH, stimulating adenyl cyclase, thereby initiating a chain of reactions that leads to thyroid growth, increased vascularity, and hypersecretion of hormone.

Ophthalmopathy

The ophthalmopathy (eye disease) of Graves' disease is probably present to some degree in most patients, although only about one-third to one-half of patients will have obvious symptoms or signs of eye disease. Symptoms include:

* Pain
* Lacrimation
* Photophobia
* Blurred vision
* Double vision

    Signs include:

* Periorbital edema
* Lid edema
* Lid lag
* Chemosis
* Ophthalmoplegia
* Proptosis
* Corneal ulcerations
* Optic neuropathy

Dermopathy

Infiltrative dermopathy (skin disease) occurs in only about 1% of patients with Graves' disease. The pretibial myxedema (most common site) is a consequence of accumulation of acid mucopolysaccharides and lymphocytes, and the presentation is quite variable. The etiology is not known.

AUTOIMMUNE THYROID DISEASE

Autoimmune thyroid disease can be viewed as a spectrum of diseases in individuals and in their family members (Fig. 41.2). The clinical presentation of the disorder, according to this view, is dependent upon the morphologic state of the gland and the mixture of circulating antibodies at any particular point in time. The antibodies include:

* Microsomal (TMA;TPO)
* Tg
* Thyroid-damaging

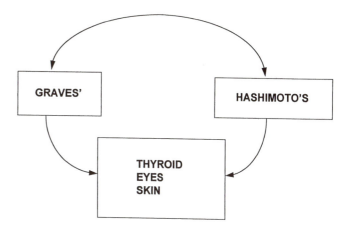

Figure 41.2. Spectrum of autoimmune thyroid disease.

* Receptor-binding [stimulating (TSI), blocking, binding]
* Growth-promoting (may be independent from stimulating)

    Thus, Graves' disease may "burn out" to become hypothyroidism, receptor-blocking antibodies may result in transient hypothyroidism, giving way to Graves' hyperthyroidism when TSI prevails, and different family members may have different presentations.

TOXIC MULTINODULAR GOITER (PLUMMER'S DISEASE)

Toxic multinodular goiter (TMNG) is a disorder in which hyperthyroidism arises in a multinodular goiter, usually of long-standing duration. The development of this type of goiter probably starts with the appearance of local areas of autonomous thyroid hyperplasia within individual follicles, followed by their continued replication and growth. The process is accompanied by areas of involution so functional and anatomic heterogeneity ("nodules") appear. If the autonomous regions grow and function sufficiently, hyperthyroidism ensues. Because this process is a slow one, the typical age of appearance of hyperthyroidism tends to be older than with Graves' disease, usually past age 50. Therapy may consist of ^{131}I (high, multiple doses may be required) or occasionally surgery; antithyroid drugs may be used but therapy will have to be permanent.

TOXIC ADENOMA

The toxic adenoma, considered to be a true benign tumor of the thyroid gland, is a far less common cause of thyrotoxicosis than either Graves' disease or TMNG. Adenomatous tissue develops in the thyroid, which secretes thyroid hormone autonomously, without stimulation by TSH or other thyroid stimulators. This condition tends to occur in patients in their 30s and 40s, somewhat younger than those with TMNG. A single palpable nodule is found on physical examination; a radioactive iodine scan will reveal uptake of the isotope only in the adenoma, resulting in a "hot nodule." (The excess circulating thyroid hormone suppresses TSH secretion, and the nonautonomous areas of the thyroid gland, therefore, neither take up iodine nor produce thyroid hormone.) Therapy usually consists of ^{131}I or surgery.

IODIDE-INDUCED THYROTOXICOSIS (JOD-BASEDOW PHENOMENON)

Jod-Basedow phenomenon refers to iodide-induced hyperthyroidism. (Jod is German for iodine and von Basedow was one of the early describers of thyrotoxicosis.) This condition occurs most commonly in patients with underlying thyroid disease residing in areas of iodide deficiency who subsequently receive a load of exogenous iodide (e.g., iodide-containing contrast dye). The pathogenesis, though unclear, is thought to be due to overproduction of thyroid hormone by autonomously functioning thyroid tissue when presented with excess substrate (iodide). This is the only form of thyrotoxicosis in which there is ongoing overproduction of thyroid hormone by the thyroid gland associated with a low RAIU. This occurs because the radioactive isotopic iodide is diluted out by large quantities of circulating stable iodide, and therefore, only a small quantity of the radioisotope is taken up by the gland. Therapy consists of removing the source of iodide. Occasionally, surgery will be necessary (especially in amiodarone-induced hyperthyroidism).

SUBACUTE THYROIDITIS (DE QUERVAIN'S, GRANULOMATOUS THYROIDITIS)

Subacute thyroiditis is a painful inflammatory process involving the thyroid gland that results in elevation of the serum concentration of thyroid hormone into the thyrotoxic range. There is often a history of a preceding viral illness, and a number of different viruses have been shown to be associated. The inflammation in the thyroid gland results in destruction of the follicular epithelium, with discharge of large amounts of preformed thyroid hormone into the circulation. Histologically, there is infiltration of the interstitial areas with histiocytes and lymphocytes, which often appear to congregate into "giant cells." The characteristic feature of subacute thyroiditis is a painful, tender, mildly enlarged thyroid gland. Systemic manifestations, such as fever, fatigue, and malaise, are also common. Half of the patients will experience symptoms of hyperthyroidism. Laboratory abnormalities include a very high erythrocyte sedimentation rate and a very low RAIU (the damaged follicles are unable to concentrate iodine). Moreover, the suppressed TSH resulting from the release of excessive amounts of preformed thyroid hormone (the thyroid gland usually has a month's supply of thyroid hormone stored) leads to inactivity even of the undisrupted thyroid follicles. The course of subacute thyroiditis is self-limited with complete recovery being the general rule. Therapy is primarily supportive and directed toward relief of symptoms (aspirin and β-

blockers). Occasionally glucocorticoids are necessary, but relapses may occur when the glucocorticoids are stopped.

PAINLESS THYROIDITIS

Painless thyroiditis is another inflammatory condition of the thyroid in which preformed thyroid hormone is discharged from damaged follicles into the circulation. The association in a majority of cases with high titers of antimicrosomal antibodies suggests an autoimmune pathogenesis. Painless thyroiditis occurs most commonly in postpartum women. The course is quite similar to that of subacute thyroiditis, except for the absence of pain and thyroidal tenderness. The RAIU is similarly low, although the erythrocyte sedimentation rate is usually normal. Therapy is primarily supportive.

TREATMENT OF THYROTOXICOSIS

RADIOACTIVE IODINE

^{131}I administration results in thyroid damage by two different mechanisms:

- Acute radiation thyroiditis
- Chronic gradual thyroid atrophy

Acute cell death leads to an inflammatory response, with infiltration by granulocytes and mononuclear cells. The eventual result is progressive atrophy associated with an obliterative endarteritis and interstitial fibrosis that occurs over a period of years. The usual dose of ^{131}I for treatment of Graves' disease results in delivery of 7,000–10,000 rads to the thyroid bed. Treatment for TMNG or toxic adenoma generally requires higher doses of ^{131}I. Therapy with ^{131}I is safe, with the only major side effect being the frequent development of hypothyroidism in patients with Graves' disease. Post-treatment hypothyroidism has been thought to be quite uncommon with TMNG or toxic adenoma.

In the latter two conditions, after destruction of autonomously functioning tissue, follicles that were previously suppressed and thus did not take up the radioiodine, resume normal function. A recent study suggests, however, that eventual hypothyrodism may be seen in as many as 30% of ^{131}I-treated solitary toxic adenoma patients (see Goldstein & Hart, 1983). Fears that ^{131}I therapy is a risk factor for thyroid or other neoplasms have proved unfounded. The gonadal radiation exposure following a standard dose of ^{131}I is less than 3 rads (about the same as for an intravenous pyelogram or a barium enema) and thus does not pose a risk for an increased incidence of genetic defects in offspring of treated patients. Since iodine crosses the placenta and is also excreted in breast milk, ^{131}I therapy is absolutely contraindicated in pregnant women or breast-feeding mothers, since destruction of the fetal or neonatal thyroid gland may be the consequence. One disadvantage of this form of therapy is that amelioration of the thyrotoxicosis may take up to 3 months or longer. Therefore, for patients who are very symptomatic, treatment both before and after radioiodine therapy may be necessary using other agents (e.g., antithyroid drugs or beta blockers). [131]I therapy is not effective in treating those conditions in which thyrotoxicosis is not a consequence of overproduction of thyroid hormone by the thyroid gland (e.g., subacute thyroiditis).

ANTITHYROID DRUGS (PROPYLTHIOURACIL OR METHIMAZOLE)

The mechanism of action of antithyroid drugs is inhibition of biosynthesis of thyroid hormone by blocking iodine oxidation, organification, and iodotyrosine coupling, all reactions that are catalyzed by thyroid peroxidase. An additional mechanism of action unique to propylthiouracil (PTU) is the inhibition of peripheral conversion of T_4 to T_3. This particular effect is useful in patients who are very thyrotoxic. In addition to their antithyroid effects, both drugs have immunosuppressive activity and thus may ameliorate the underlying pathogenetic process in Graves' disease. Since these drugs inhibit thyroid autoantibody production, their use in Graves' disease for a 12-month period is associated with long-term remission in about 30–40% of cases.

These drugs do not alter the underlying pathogenetic process in TMNG or toxic adenoma, and therefore, life-long term therapy would be required for these conditions. Some improvement in symptoms is usually apparent after 1–2 weeks of therapy and is substantial after 4–6 weeks of treatment. This fairly rapid onset of action makes antithyroid drug therapy particularly useful for toxic patients prior to definitive treatment with ^{131}I or surgery.

Adverse drug reactions occur in as many as 5–10% of patients treated with antithyroid medication. The commonest side effect is a rash, occurring in 3–5% of patients.

The most serious side effect, agranulocytosis (complete absence of circulating granulocytes), is seen in 0.5% of patients. It occurs abruptly, and though reversible with cessation of the drug, may result in serious illness on even death, especially in older patients. *Patients must be cautioned* to discontinue the drug and report for a white blood count immediately upon the advent of a severe sore throat and/or fever. Monitoring white blood counts in anticipation is of no value and is not recommended.

SURGERY

Surgical removal of abnormally functioning thyroid tissue is usually definitive, although there may be 10% of patients with Graves' disease in whom thyrotoxicosis recurs following subtotal thyroidectomy. The prevalence of postoperative hypothyroidism (up to 40%) and other surgical complications (vocal cord paralysis owing to recurrent laryngeal nerve damage or permanent hypoparathyroidism) makes surgery less-than-ideal as a form of therapy and rarely the first choice—although in expert hands surgical complications are minimal.

BETA-BLOCKING AGENTS

Many of the symptoms and signs of thyrotoxicosis are similar to those of excessive beta-adrenergic stimulation. These mani-festations are ameliorated when pharmacologic agents, which block the beta receptor, are used (e.g., propranolol). These agents, therefore, are very useful in treating some of the symptoms of thyrotoxicosis until definitive therapy of the underlying cause is effective or a transient pathogenetic process resolves (e.g., subacute thyroiditis). Caution must be exercised in patients with a history of asthma or in the presence of cardiac failure.

Thyroiditis

ACUTE SUPPURATIVE THYROIDITIS

Bacterial infection of the thyroid is rare. It presents with pain, fever and other signs of infection.

SUBACUTE THYROIDITIS

A cause of thyrotoxicosis (see above).

HASHIMOTO'S THYROIDITIS

Hashimoto's (lymphocytic) thyroiditis, an autoimmune disorder, is a common cause of goiter (enlarged thyroid) and hypothyroidism. It is more frequent in women and may run in families.

It is associated with autoimmune disorders involving other endocrine glands—such as Addison's disease (adrenal insufficiency) and insulin-dependent diabetes mellitus—and involving other systems—such as rheumatoid arthritis. The pathogenesis involves cell-mediated immunity. In addition, thyroid autoantibodies against thyroglobulin and the microsome (thyroid peroxidase enzyme) are found, although their significance in vivo is not clear.

In Hashimoto's, the titer of antimicrosomal antibodies is usually $> 1:400$. Pathologically, diffuse lymphocytic infiltration with germinal centers, fibrosis, and obliteration of the thyroid follicles are observed. Abnormalities in thyroid hormone biosynthesis include an organification defect demonstrable by perchlorate discharge of radioiodine. Abnormal iodoproteins may be released. As long as there are intact follicles, iodine trapping is preserved.

This disorder frequently produces a goiter and some patients develop hypothyroidism. Some patients with Graves' disease may have histologic features of Hashimoto's thyroiditis, giving rise to the basically meaningless term "Hashitoxicosis" (see autoimmune thyroid disease above).

PAINLESS THYROIDITIS

Painless thyroiditis most commonly occurs postpartum. It may have a typical three-phase course—hyperthyroidism, hypothyroidism, then a return to the euthyroid state—or it can present with hypo- or hyperthyroidism alone. Women with antimicrosomal antibodies are more likely to get this disease: Some clinicians advocate measuring TMA in pregnancy, especially in the presence of goiter, and monitoring thyroid status routinely in the puerperium. For now, I see no compelling evidence to support such a practice.

Drugs and Thyroid Dysfunction

LITHIUM

Lithium causes primary hypothyroidism. Also, lithium therapy has been associated with hyperthyroidism and hypercalcemia, and it can cause nephrogenic diabetes insipidus.

AMIODARONE

Amioidarone causes both hypothyroidism and hyperthyroidism. The former is more common in individuals with antimicrosomal antibodies. The latter probably has more than one cause: iodine-induced thyrotoxicosis and drug-induced thyroid damage.

Therapy of the hypothyroidism should include cautious thyroid hormone replacement; patients on amiodarone have significant heart disease. Therapy of the hyperthyroidism may be difficult. Antithyroid drugs are often ineffective. The combination of high dose PTU and potassium perchlorate (not routinely available) has been effective in some patients. Sometimes surgery is necessary.

Thyroid Nodules and Cancer

THYROID NODULES

Thyroid nodules occur commonly and may be single or multiple. Most are benign. The major issue for the clinician is to determine which nodules are likely to be malignant and require surgical removal. Most thyroid nodules are ''cold'' on thyroid scans, so this procedure is not very helpful.

Clinical features raising the likelihood of malignancy include:

- Male sex
- Family history (especially of multiple endocrine neoplasia Type II, which includes medullary thyroid carcinoma)
- History of radiation treatment to the head and neck, especially in childhood or adolescence
- Hoarseness or vocal cord paralysis
- A single nodule or a dominant nodule in a multinodular gland
- Lymphadenopathy

Diagnostic techniques include:

- Fine-needle biopsy
  - Most cost effective
  - Various techniques
  - Need experienced cytologist
- Ultrasound
  - Beware the incidental nodule(s)
- RAI scan
  - Limited value
- CXR
- Thyroglobulin

The best diagnostic approach involves fine-needle-aspiration biopsy, which has excellent sensitivity and specificity. There are some limitations, especially in the diagnosis of follicular neoplasms, since cytologic differentiation between adenoma and carcinoma cannot be done with any certainty. Such lesions should be removed.

THYROID CANCER

The major types of thyroid cancer are:

- Primary
  - Papillary
  - Follicular
  - Anaplastic
  - Medullary [sporadic, familial, multiple endocrine neoplasia (MEN) Type II]
  - Hürthle cell
  - Mixed
- Secondary
- Lymphoma

Papillary and follicular cancers—which tend to be relatively slow growing—account for the vast majority of cases. Papillary tends to metastasize to lymph nodes, while follicular tends to have earlier hematogenous spread, primarily to lung and bone.

Anaplastic cancer, which presents with a rapidly growing mass, has a dismal prognosis.

Medullary cancer is a tumor of C-cells and is associated with calcitonin production. It can be sporadic, familial, or as part of MEN Type II. Family members should be screened.

Thyroid lymphoma appears to be increasing in frequency. It may occur in a gland involved with Hashimoto's thyroiditis.

Treatment of the common cancers (papillary or follicular) usually includes surgery (near-total thyroidectomy is recommended, although some centers recommend more conservative surgery), ablative ^{131}I therapy, and L-thyroxine suppression of TSH. Serial serum thyroglobulin determinations are of value in monitoring disease eradication or recurrence.

ACKNOWLEDGMENT

The author is grateful to David C. Aron, MD, Professor of Medicine, Case Western Reserve University, for allowing me to make liberal use of his 1994 teaching syllabus.

REVIEW EXERCISES

QUESTIONS

1. A patient being screened for intermittent diarrhea has a T_4 (total) value of 19.6 μg/dl (normal 5.0–10.5). There are no other features of hyperthyroidism; no goiter is present. A T_4 uptake (T_4U) test is elevated at 2.01 (normal 0.8–1.20), whereas the T_3 resin uptake (T_3RU) test is subnormal at 15% (normal 25%–35%). The free thyroxine index (FTI) is calculated to be 9.8 (normal 5.0–10.5). What single test would be most helpful in delineating the patient's thyroid status:

   a. TSH
   b. Thyroid receptor antibodies
   c. Serum T_3
   d. Serum free T_4 by equilibrium dialysis
   e. None of the above

2. The serum TSH test result is 3.0 μU/ml (normal 0.4–5.5). There are no drugs or hepatic disease to explain the findings. What is the best working diagnosis?

   a. Antibodies against circulating T_3
   b. Hereditary increase in TBG production (X-linked)
   c. Hereditary increase in transthyretin (TBPA) production
   d. All of the above
   e. None of the above

3. A patient with primary hypothyroidism has been stable (normal TSH) on replacement L-thyroxine (L-T_4; dose 1.6 μg/kg B.W.) for a number of years. On annual follow-up, the following lab tests are obtained: T_4 14.1 μg/dl (normal 5.0–10.5); TSH 23.4 μU/ml (normal 0.4–5.5). She saw a gastroenterologist 6 months previously for NSAID-related gastritis and takes an iron preparation and occasional antacids. The most likely diagnosis is:

   a. Malabsorption of L-T_4 owing to concomitant use of antacids and iron
   b. Progressive loss of endogenous thyroid function
   c. Development of thyroid hormone resistance
   d. Poor compliance this past year with attempt to "catch-up" with excessive L-T_4 intake recently
   e. None of the above

4. The development of Graves' hyperthyroidism following the presence of Hashimoto's hypothyroidism is best explained by:

   a. The finding of histopathological changes of Hashimoto's thyroiditis in Graves' thyroid glands.
   b. Graves' hyperthyroidism is a natural phase of Hashimoto's disease.
   c. The two disorders are part of the spectrum of autoimmune thyroid disease, the clinical manifestations of which are dependent upon the mixture of circulating polyclonal antibodies and the morphologic state of the gland at a particular point in time.
   d. All of the above
   e. None of the above

5. You are asked to see a 75-year-old white man who was admitted to the psychiatric ward with a diagnosis of delirium. The history obtained from the wife revealed that he was well until 6 months prior to admission. He has had a 30-pound weight loss with a poor appetite since that time. There was no history of any medication, recent investigations involving radio-contrast media, goiter, or neck discomfort. There is no family history of thyroid disease. On physical examination, he is afebrile; he looks cachectic but is not pigmented; there are no features of infiltrative eye changes; the thyroid gland is prolapsed but may be just palpable on swallowing. The pulse rate is irregular at 120 beats per minute. The ECG shows atrial fibrillation. The serum T_4 is 19.7 μg/dl (normal 5.0–10.5) with a serum TSH <0.02 μU/ml (normal 0.4–5.5).

   Part 1. The next step in diagnosis is to order:
   a. Serum T_3
   b. 24-hour RAI uptake
   c. 24-hour RAI uptake and scan
   d. Thyroid stimulating antibodies
   e. Thyroid microsomal (thyroid peroxidase [TPO]) antibodies

   Part 2. Management should include all of the following except:
   a. β-blockers
   b. Digoxin
   c. Coumadin
   d. Propylthiouracil
   e. Stress doses of glucocorticoids

Answers

1. a

The aim of the question is to help gain understanding of the role of free (nonprotein-bound) thyroid hormone in regulating TSH secretion. The hypothalamo-pituitary unit ''reads'' the free hormone level, not the total hormone level, which is subject to changes owing to alterations in protein binding ([TBG, transthyretin, albumin] and/or conditions which may interfere with binding).

In practice, FTI can be calculated from total T_4 and an estimate of protein binding (T_4U or T_3RU; T_4U measures binding directly, whereas T_3RU provides an index of unbound hormone). Automated free T_4 assays are replacing these more indirect indices; the gold standard, free T_4 by equilibrium dialysis, is available in some reference labs, but is rarely needed.

Thus, serum TSH in this patient should provide the best indicator of thyroid function status and is independent from thyroid hormone protein binding abnormalities.

2. b

The aim of the question is to explore thyroid hormone binding in more detail. The major normal thyroid hormone binding proteins are TBG and TBPA. Certain drugs and conditions can alter levels and/or binding capacity. Antibodies against T_4 and/or T_3 rarely occur in patients who commonly have Hashimoto's thyroiditis (haptenic autoantigen). Hereditary increases in TBG (binds both T_4 and T_3) or transthyretin (binds T_4 only) occur uncommonly. The increases in thyroid hormone binding capacity in this patient are reflected by both the T_4U (high) and the T_3RU (low) tests. Antibodies against T_3 would be expected to lower the T_3RU test results but not affect the T_4U test; increased TBPA levels would result in increased T_4U values but not affect T_3RU values (since T_3 does not bind to the TBPA ligand).

3. d

The aim of this question is to help understand the time lag in the hypothalamo-pituitary-thyroid axis. Although TSH secretion may be acutely altered with stress, illness or drugs, the major regulation is based on the integrated thyroid hormone exposure over the preceding 2–5 weeks. Although iron preparations and aluminum-containing compounds can interfere with T_4 absorption, the elevated serum T_4 level argues against this notion. Similarly, progressive loss of thyroid function would be expected to lead to low or low-normal T_4 values. Although acquired thyroid hormone resistance may occur hypothetically, there are no clinical descriptions of such disorders. The correct answer is not a rare occurrence: Patients often wish to ''please'' their health care provider, even if it means not being ''perfectly honest'' on occasion.

4. c

The aim of this question is to gain understanding of the concept that the correct answer helps to explain this, as well as a number of other clinical conditions. (See Autoimmune Thyroid Disease above.)

5.

Overview: The aim of the question is to reinforce the clinical presentation of elderly patients with thyrotoxicosis and their management. Although weight loss despite a generous appetite is characteristic in the younger adult, anorexia is not an uncommon finding in the elderly. Cachexia in an ''apathetic'' patient should be watched for. (Concomitant Addison's disease in a patient with known thyroid autoimmunity is a ''distractor'' in the current-case presentation; the lack of pigmentation was intended to get the reader back on focus.) A cardiac dysrhythmia (usually atrial fibrillation) $\pm$ congestive heart failure may be the major feature(s). The most common cause of hyperthyroidism in this age group is toxic multinodular goiter (sometimes iodide-induced), but the absence of a goiter may be seen in up to 25% of elderly patients (5% in young adults).

Part 1:

c

Serum T_3 may be of academic interest (and occasionally a higher T_4/T_3 ratio may help to discriminate thyroiditis or toxic multinodular goiter from Graves' hyperthyroidism) but is generally reserved for cases in which total T_4 and free T_4 values are normal. Thyroid stimulating antibodies are of minor value in ruling out Graves' disease (usually a positive family history is obtained), but this diagnosis can be inferred from an elevated RAI uptake and diffuse scan. Thyroid microsomal antibodies are a less expensive but less specific surrogate for Graves' disease. The RAI uptake is necessary to discriminate thyroid hyperfunction (autonomous nodule(s), receptor antibody, TSH or HCG driven) from subacute or silent thyroiditis, iatrogenic, or factitious causes. (Recent exposure to radiocontrast media or iodine-containing drugs or pregnancy (not in males) may preclude its use, however.) A scan is of particular value when the clinician is unsure of the size and nature of the thyroid gland.

Part 2:

e

β-blockers and propylthiouracil are helpful as primary therapy for hyperthyroidism in the elderly. Propylthiouracil (PTU) is initiated only after the diagnosis is confirmed by a RAI uptake (and scan, if necessary). RAI therapy may cause a transient worsening (radiation thyroiditis) of the hyperthyroidism and is often postponed in the elderly until euthyroidism is attained (and antithyroid medication transiently withdrawn for 2–3 days prior to ^{131}I treatment). Digoxin is helpful to control the heart rate in atrial fibrillation. Coumadin is indicated in preventing embolic consequences of atrial fibrillation. The only drug not indicated without more data (the patient was not in ''thyroid storm'') is the glucocorticoid.

BIBLIOGRAPHY

American Association of Clinical Endocrinologists Clinical Practice Guidelines for the Evaluation and Treatment of Hyperthyroidism and Hypothyroidism (1995).

Barbot N, Calmettes C, Schuffenecker I, et al. Pentagastrin stimulation test and early diagnosis of medullary thyroid carcinoma using an immunoradiometric assay of calcitonin: comparison with genetic screening in hereditary medullary thyroid carcinoma. J Clin Endocrinol Metab 1994;78:114–120.

Borst GC, Eil C, Burman KD. Euthyroid hyperthyroxinemia. Ann Intern Med 1983;98:366–378.

Borst GC. Euthyroid hyperthyroxinemia. Ann Intern Med 1983;98:366–378.

Brent GA, Hershman JM. Thyroxine therapy in patients with severe nonthyroidal illnesses and low serum thyroxine concentration. J Clin Endocrinol Metab 1986;63:1–8.

Burrow GN, Fisher DA, Larsen PR. Mechanisms of disease: maternal and fetal thyroid function. N Engl J Med 1994;331:1072–1078.

Campbell NRC, Hasinoff BB, Stalts H, et al. Ferrous sulfate reduces thyroxine efficacy in patients with hypothyroidism. Ann Intern Med 1992;117:1010–1013.

Cavalieri RR, Gerard SK. Unusual types of thyrotoxicosis. Adv Int Med 1991;36:271–286.

Char DH. The ophthalmopathy of Graves disease. Med Clin North Am 1991;75:97–119.

Cooper DS. Antithyroid drugs. N Engl J Med 1984;311:1353–1362.

Cooper DS. Subclinical hypothyroidism. Adv in Endocrinol Metab 1991;2:77–88.

de los Santos ET, Starich GH, Mazzaferri EL. Sensitivity, specificity, and cost-effectiveness of the sensitive thyrotropin assay in the diagnosis of thyroid disease in ambulatory patients. Arch Int Med 1989;149:526–532.

DeGroot LJ. Long-term impact of initial and surgical therapy on papillary and follicular thyroid cancer. Am J Med 1994;97:499–500.

Docter R, Krenning EP, de Jong M, et al. The sick euthyroid syndrome: changes in thyroid hormone serum parameters and hormone metabolism. Clin Endocrinol 1993;39:499–518.

Dolan JG. Hyperthyroidism and hypothyroidism. In: Panzer RJ, Black ER, Griner PF, eds. Diagnostic strategies for common medical problems. Philadelphia: American College of Physicians, 1991:375–384.

Doria R, Jekel JF, Cooper DL. Thyroid lymphoma: the case for combined modality therapy. Cancer 1994;73:200–206.

Farrar JJ, Toth AD. Iodine-131 treatment of hyperthyroidism: current issues. Clin Endocrinol 1991;35:207–212.

Fisher DA. Screening for congenital hypothyroidism. Trends Endocrinol Metab 1991;2:129–133.

Gharib H, Goellner JR. Fine-needle aspiration biopsy of the thyroid: an appraisal. Ann Intern Med 1993;118:282–289.

Goldstein R, Hart IR. Follow-up of solitary autonomous thyroid nodules treated with [131]I. N Engl J Med 1983;309:1473–1476.

Hamburger JI. The various presentations of thyroiditis: diagnostic considerations. Ann Intern Med 1986;104:219–224.

Helfand M, Crapo LM. Monitoring therapy in patients taking levothyroxine. Ann Intern Med 1990;113:450–454.

Helfand M, Crapo LM. Screening for thyroid disease. Ann Intern Med 1990;112:840–849 (see letters to the editor: Ann Intern Med 1990;113:896–897).

Klein I, Levey GS. Unusual manifestations of hypothyroidism. Arch Intern Med 1984;144:123–128.

Lazarus JH, Othman S. Thyroid disease in relation to pregnancy. Clin Endocrinol 1991;34:91–98.

Ledger GA, Khosla S, Lindor NM, et al. Genetic testing in the diagnosis and management of multiple endocrine neoplasia type II. Ann Intern Med 1995;122:118–124.

Liel Y, Sperber AD, Shang S. Nonspecific intestinal adsorption of levothyroxine by aluminum hydroxide. Am J Med 1994;97:363–365.

Lips CJM, Landsvater RM, Höppener JWM, et al. Clinical screening as compared with DNA analysis in families with multiple endocrine neoplasia type 2A. N Engl J Med 1994;331:828–835.

Mandel SJ, Larsen PR, Seeley EW, et al. Increased need for thyroxine during pregnancy in women with primary hypothyroidism. N Engl J Med 1990;323:91–95.

Mandel SJ, Brent GA, Larsen PR. Levothyroxine therapy in patients with thyroid disease. Ann Intern Med 1993;119:492–502.

Mazzaferri EL. Long-term impact of initial surgical and medical therapy on papillary and follicular thyroid cancer. Am J Med 1994;97:418–428.

Mazzaferri EL. Management of a solitary thyroid nodule. N Engl J Med 1993;328:553–559.

McDougall IR. Graves disease: current concepts. Med Clin North Am 1991;75:79–95.

Mendel CM. The free hormone hypothesis; a physiologically

based mathematical model. Endocrinol Rev 1989;10: 232–274.

Mulligan DC, McHenry CR, Kinney W, et al. Amiodarone-induced thyrotoxicosis: clinical presentation and expanded indications for thyroidectomy. Surgery 1993;114:1114–1119.

Ozata M, Suzuki S, Miyamoto T, et al. Serum thyroglobulin in the follow-up of patients with treated differentiated thyroid cancer. J Clin Endocrinol Metab 1994;79:98–105.

Pineda JD, Lee T, Ain K, et al. Iodine-131 therapy for thyroid cancer patients with elevated thyroglobulin and negative diagnostic scan. J Clin Endocrinol Metab 1995; 80:1488–1492.

Refetoff S, Lever EG. The value of serum thyroglobulin measurement in clinical practice. JAMA 1983;250:2352–2357.

Rosenbaum D, Davies TF. The clinical use of thyroid autoantibodies. The Endocrinologist 1992;2:55–62.

Ross DS. Subclinical thyrotoxicosis. Adv in Endocrinol Metab 1991;2:89–105.

Schectman JM, Pawlson LG. The cost-effectiveness of three thyroid function testing strategies for suspicion of hypothyroidism in a primary care-setting. J Gen Intern Med 1990;5: 9–15.

Sherman SI, Tielens ET, Ladenson PW. Sucralfate causes malabsorption of L-thyroxine. Am J Med 1994;96:531–535.

Slag MF, Morley JE, Elson MK, et al. Hypothyroxinemia in critically ill patients as a predictor of high mortality. JAMA 1981;245:43–45.

Stagnaro-Green A. Postpartum thyroiditis: prevalence, etiology, and clinical importance. Thyroid Today 1993;16:1–11.

Surks MI, Sievert R. Drugs and thyroid function. N Engl J Med 1995;333:1688–1694.

Surks MI, Smith PJ. Multiple effects of 5,5′-diphenylhydantoin on the thyroid hormone system. Endocrinol Rev 1984;5: 514–524.

Surks MI, Chopra IJ. Mariash CN, et al. American Thyroid Association guidelines for use of laboratory tests in thyroid disorders. JAMA 1990:263:1529–1532.

Tachman ML, Guthrie GP Jr. Hypothyroidism: diversity of presentation. Endocrinol Rev 1984;5:456–465.

Van Middlesworth L. Effects of radiation on the thyroid gland. Adv Int Med 1989;34:265–284.

Weetman AP, McGregor AM. Autoimmune thyroid disease: further developments in our understanding. Endocrinol Rev 1994;15:788–830.

Weiss RE, Refetoff S. Thyroid hormone resistance. Ann Rev Med 1992;43:363–375

Woeber KA. Thyrotoxicosis and the heart. N Engl J Med 1992;327:94–98.

Wong TK, Hershman JM. Changes in thyroid function in nonthyroidal illness. Trends Endocrinol Metab 1992;3:8–11.

Yassa R, Saunders A, Nastase C, et al. Lithium-induced thyroid disorders: a prevalence study. J Clin Psychiatry 1988;49: 14–16.

42

Androgenic and Reproductive Disorders

Adi E. Mehta

FEMALE REPRODUCTIVE DISORDERS

ANDROGENIC DISORDERS: ANATOMY AND PHYSIOLOGY

Androgenic Sources

The ovaries and adrenal glands are the source of androgens in females. These may be secreted, in small amounts, as biologically active androgens or serve as precursor compounds for conversion to active androgens in the periphery. Both glands produce the hormones in response to their tropic hormones (LH and ACTH, respectively), but the androgens cannot act as powerful negative feedback control hormones for the pituitary. Thus, their secretion is not self-controlled.

The major products of adrenal secretion are dehydro-epi-androsterone sulfate (DHEAS), DHA, and androstenedione. The major ovarian secretory product is androstenedione. About half the circulating levels of testosterone in women is secreted from both glandular sources, while the rest is made by peripheral conversion of 17-ketosteroids in the liver, skin, and adipose tissue.

Transport in Serum

The bulk of active androgen (and estradiol, E_2) is tightly bound in the circulation to sex-hormone binding globulin (SHBG), of hepatic origin. Lesser binding to albumin also occurs. Thus, only small amounts of free (unbound) sex steroids are present. SHBG production by the liver is influenced by the androgen/estrogen balance, as well as by thyroid hormone. Estrogen and thyroid hormone stimulate SHBG production. Androgen is inhibitory.

BIOLOGIC ACTIVITY OF ANDROGENS

The major biologically active androgen in most target tissues is dihydrotestosterone (DHT), which is formed by the conversion of testosterone (T) under the influence of 5 alpha reductase present in skin and external genitalia. The effect of androgen on target tissues is thought to be mediated by the ratio of free T/free E_2 in the circulation. Thus, simple measurements of total T and/or E_2 may be misleading.

The SHBG multiplier effect can be summarized:

- Hepatic SHBG production is influenced by the androgen/estrogen status.
- Binding kinetics for T and E_2 to this protein are different. (As SHBG concentration falls under an androgenic influence, there is a greater increment in unbound T compared with unbound E_2.)
- Androgen excess begets androgen excess.

CLINICAL PRESENTATION OF ANDROGENIC DISORDERS

The clinical presentation of androgenic disorders in women is relatively classical and restrictive in focus. The most common presentation is with a complaint of hirsutism, possibly with acne and irregular and infrequent menses. Obesity is not an uncommon associated finding in such individuals.

SPECIFIC ANDROGENIC DISORDERS

Polycystic Ovary Syndrome (PCOS)

The 1990 NIH consensus criteria defines PCOS as the invariable presence of chronic oligo/anovulation associated with hyperandrogenism (i.e., signs of androgen excess, such as acne, alopecia, or hirsutism, even without clearly elevated serum androgen levels) in the absence of other known causes of androgen excess, such as congenital adrenal hyperplasia (CAH), tumor, or hyperprolactinemia. While there may be associated abnormal ovarian morphology, abnormal gonadotropins, or abnormal insulin regulation, they do not have to be invariably present to make the diagnosis.

Pathophysiology of PCOS   The pathophysiology of PCOS is unclear, but there are numerous theories. Most point to the establishment of a vicious cycle of events, possibly initiated by the presence of two phenomena normally occurring in puberty that, in the predisposed individual, sets this cycle in motion:

- An early increase in LH and androgen levels
- Insulin resistance

 Predispositions to PCOS include:

- A family history of NIDDM
- Maternal gestational DM
- Borderline adrenal hyperplasia accentuated by the pubertal adrenarche
- Occult-hypothyroidism
- Childhood obesity

In the PCOS-predisposed individual, LH and androgen levels are higher, while in the normal individual, ovulating cycles decrease LH and attenuate the insulin resistance of puberty; in PCOS-predisposed individuals, this does not occur. Thus, PCOS is sometimes termed ''hyperpuberty.''

Clinical PCOS frequently presents as hirsutism (70–75%), oligomenorrhea (50%), and resulting infertility. Obesity and insulin resistance leading to diabetes may be present (30–40%).

Biochemically, an elevation of LH values is frequent (up to 75%), and some schools emphasize an elevated LH/FSH ratio (more than 2:1 or 3:1). Androgens, especially ovarian androgens, are elevated, and adrenal androgens (DHEA) may have up to a two-fold increase.

Metabolic Consequences of PCOS   To summarize the metablic consequences of PCOS:

- Insulin resistance is present in a large percentage of women with PCOS.
- Insulin resistance can be present in nonobese women with PCOS, as well as in obese women with PCOS, although a percentage of lean women with PCOS are not insulin resistant.
- The insulin resistance is more manifest peripherally than in the liver.
- Insulin potentiates LH-stimulated androgen production from the theca and stroma of the ovary.
- The ovary is not resistant to insulin in the face of the peripheral muscle and adipose tissue insulin resistance.

- Acanthosis nigrincans, a marker of insulin resistance, can be seen. This may fade with reduction of circulating androgens.
- An increased waist-to-hip ratio is commonly associated with the elevated androgens.
- There are later associations with hyperlipidemia, and hypertension, as well as NIDDM (the so-called syndrome X of Reaven), all of which predispose to premature cardiac disease.
- There is an increased risk of endometrial and breast cancer.

The proposed theoretical basis of PCOS appears below:

```
Adrenal Function
(peripubertal)
    ⇓
Androstenedione            ⇐  ⇐  ⇐
    ⇓                          ⇑
(peripheral conversion) ⇐ ⇐ ⇐ ⇐ ⇐ ⇐Excess fat tissue
    ⇓                          ⇑                    ⇓
Estrone                                     Insulin resistance
    ⇓                          ⇑                    ⇓
Disturbed feedback of                       Hyperinsulinemia
HPA axis
    ⇓                          ⇑                    ⇓
Disturbed LH        ⇒Ovarian Androgens  Increased IGF-I action
pulsatility                      ↖                ⇓?
(LH/FSH ratio)                        Dysregulated cytochrome
                                      P450 17
```

The late consequences of acne/hirsutism/PCO and relative subfecundity include:

- Infertility
- Hyperlipidemia
- Hypertension
- Late development of NIDDM
- Increased risk of endometrial and breast cancer
- Cardiovascular disease

Hirsutism

Hirsutism—excess terminal (sexual) hair in a woman—is characterized by two types of hair:

- Vellous (small in diameter, soft in texture, and nonmedullated)
- Terminal (large in diameter, coarse, medullated)

Usually found in sex-hormone-sensitive skin, terminal hair is androgen-dependent for growth.

Etiology of Hirsutism   Causes of hirsutism—and virilization—include:

- Genetic-racial-atavistic (e.g., Mediterranean women)
- Iatrogenic
  - Drugs
    - Hormones (''pill,'' anabolics)
    - Diphenylhydantoin
    - Hexachlorobenzene

- Diazoxide
- Cyclosporine
- Minoxidil (nonsteroid drugs cause hypertrichosis)
- Adrenal conditions
  - Congenital adrenal hyperplasia (note adult-onset variant)
  - Benign and malignant tumors
  - Cushing's syndrome
  - Prolactin or growth hormone excess
- Ovarian conditions
  - ''Idiopathic hirsutism''
  - Polycystic ovary syndrome (PCOS) (Stein-Leventhal)
  - Stromal hyperthecosis (likely a more severe variant of PCOS)
  - Virilizing neoplasms
  - Ovarian steroidogenic block
  - Hermaphroditism
  - HCG-related
- Peripheral androgen overproduction
  - Obesity
  - Other

Diagnosis of Hirsutism and Virilization In diagnosing hirsutism and virilization, attempt to answer the following questions:

1. Is hirsutism present? Is it because of androgen excess?

   a. Hypertrichosis: Nonsexual excessive hair growth (i.e., ethnic, in malnutrition, owing to nonsteroid drugs); not associated with virilism.
   b. Hirsutism: Excessive sexual hair (pubic, axillary, abdominal, chest and facial) coarse and pigmented.

2. What is the degree of virilism?

   a. Acne and hirsutism are the earliest (and frequently the only) signs of excessive circulating androgen(s).
   b. Anovulation and oligomenorrhea-amenorrhea manifest relatively early in ovarian conditions but tend to appear later in adrenal disorders.
   c. Frontal balding, clitoromegaly, low-pitched voice, and increased muscularity indicate marked androgenic stimulation.

3. What are the points of importance for differential diagnosis?

   a. Onset
      – Peripubertal: Usually benign
      — Pre- or late-postpubertal: More ominous
   b. Progression
      — Slow or static: Benign
      — Progressive: Malignant
   c. Family history: Positive points to benign
   d. Libido enhancement of recent onset: Inauspicious
   e. Medication

   f. Menstrual regularity: Uncommon in face of excess androgen

4. What is the source of androgen?

   a. Rule out exogenous sources.
   b. Rule out neoplasia:
      — Sudden onset and rapid progression (suggests a neoplasm)
      — Abdominal or pelvic masses
      — High androgen levels (i.e., 17-ketosteroids, DHEAS, testosterone)
   c. Cushing's disease: Very rare among obese, hirsute women (adult-onset CAH may be common).
   d. Other functional syndromes may have an ovarian or adrenal origin. (At present, these cannot be distinguished by dynamic stimulation or suppression tests. Indeed, having ruled out organic disease, definition of the precise source has little practical significance.)

5. Laboratory tests:
   — Serum DHEAS and/or urinary (24-hour) 17-ketosteroids (17-KS) (useful to rule out adrenal neoplasms)
   — Serum T– into the normal male range (> 8 nmol/L) in ovarian (or adrenal) neoplasms
      — Mild to moderately elevated in most cases PCOS
      — Normal or borderline high (slightly > 2 nmol/L) in ''idiopathic hirsutism''
   — 17-OH-progesterone (may pick up an occasional adult CAH case)
   — Index of free T or T/SHBG ratios where available (often elevated, even when total T levels are normal)
   — Other steroids (e.g., androstenedione or metabolites)
   — 5-androstanediol glucuronide (of questionable additional benefit)
   — Serum prolactin (elevations may be associated with PCOS)
   — Thyroid function tests (hirsutism may be seen in primary hypothyroidism)
   — Anatomic studies generally not indicated

Treatment of Hirsutism Treatment regimen includes:

- Treat organic disease
- Medical therapy
  - Glucocorticoids
  - Estrogen/progestin (BCP)
  - Antiandrogens
    - Cyproterone acetate and estrogen (BCP)
      - Spironolactone
      - Flutamide
      - Finasteride
      - Cimetidine

- GnRH analogues
- Ketoconazole
- Local application of steroids
  - Progesterone
  - Cyproterone
  - Spironolactone
- Local depilation
- Ovulation induction (if the major complaint is infertility)
- Reassurance and support: patience and perserverance (8–14 months to clinical effect)

AMENORRHEA

Amenorrhea is the absolute lack of menses for more than 3 months in a woman with previously regular cycles (secondary amenorrhea) or no menses by age 16 (primary amenorrhea).

DIAGNOSIS OF AMENORRHEA

Classification of Amenorrhea

It is important to ascertain whether this is primary or secondary amenorrhea and whether it is anatomic, owing to hormonal/functional hormone dysregulation, or because of other endocrine or systemic illnesses. The classification breakdown for amenorrhea includes:

- Anatomic
  - Primary
    - Congenital uterine absence
    - Cryptomenorrhea
  - Secondary
    - Asherman's syndrome
    - Iatrogenic
    - Hysterectomy/oopherectomy
- Chromosomal
  - XO/XO mosaic (Turner's syndrome)
  - XY androgen insensitivity
- Hormonal/functional (could be primary but more frequently secondary)
  - Pregnancy
  - Prolactin excess
  - Androgen excess
  - Weight loss
  - Excessive exercise
  - Anorexia nervosa
  - Excessive weight gain
  - Emotional stress
  - Hypopituitarism
  - Ovarian failure
- Others illnesses (usually secondary amenorrhea, occasionally primary)
  - Other endocrine diseases
    - Hyper/hypothyroidism
    - Adrenal disease
    - Diabetes mellitus
- Chronic systemic illnesses
  - Crohn's
  - Ulcerative colitis
  - Rheumatoid arthritis

Laboratory Studies

After ruling out pregnancy as a cause for the amenorrhea, an evaluation of gonadotropin, estrogen, androgens, prolactin, and thyrotropin, general chemistry, and a complete blood count are usually required. In primary amenorrhea or amenorrhea occurring after only a few irregular cycles in young individuals, a karyotype is also indicated.

TREATMENT FOR AMENORRHEA

Treatment is groomed to the individual patient's requirements and may include simple gonadal steroid replacement, correcting the underlying etiological disorder, if possible, psychiatric or psychosocial support, and re-establishment of puberty with exogenous medications or hormones or the newer reproductive technologies. It is important to remember that the presence of the Y chromosome in a phenotypic female requires the operative removal of the gonads, because they are considered precancerous.

PREMATURE OVARIAN FAILURE

Growing evidence in the literature indicates that premature ovarian failure (POF) is multifactorial and encompasses a spectrum of clinical presentations, including:

- Permanent hypergonadotropic amenorrhea
- The apparent presence of a prematurely early perimenopausal state
- A condition waxing and waning from normogonadotropic menstrual cycles
- Hypergonadotropic amenorrhea

ETIOLOGY OF PREMATURE OVARIAN FAILURE

Normal Menopause

The mean age at menopause in North America, 52, appears to be unrelated to the age of menarche or to parity, ethnic extraction, nutrition, or environmental factors. Menopause, owing to ovarian failure and the virtual absence of primordial follicles in the ovary, is characterized by low estradiol levels, amenorrhea, and sustained elevation of gonadotropin levels. The final cessation of menses may be preceded by 2–10 years of progressively irregular cycles with prolonged intermenstrual intervals. During this time, gonadotropins, particularly FSH, may be variably elevated, but estradiol levels are usually normal, ovulation is sporadic, and hot flashes are common.

Studies indicate a correlation between the size of the residual follicular stock and the preservation of more normal menstrual function at this stage. Although the primary cause of cessation of menstrual function is no doubt because of the disappearance of ovarian follicles, the nature of pituitary-ovarian interrelationships and a change in the ovarian milieu may help to explain the apparent gonadotropin resistance and relative infertility at this stage.

Premature Menopause

Since less than 2% of women reach menopause prior to age 40, this is the currently accepted cut off for the definition of prematurity. The etiology of POF is outlined in Table 42.1.

Classification of POF based upon the presence or absence of follicles on an ovarian biopsy (at a particular time point) may be overly simplistic, since factors that govern the number of endowed ova, the rate of follicular atresia, the changes in ovarian steroid and peptide hormone production, and the intraovarian milieu as a function of age remain poorly understood.

Table 42.1. Etiological Classification of Premature Ovarian Failure

1) CHROMOSOMAL
   - X Linked: Turner syndrome and variants
                  Familial long arm X deletion
                  Triple X syndrome
   - Autosomal: Trisomy 13
                  Trisomy 18
2) ENZYMATIC DEFECTS
   - 17 α-hydroxylase deficiency
   - Galactosemia
3) GONADOTROPIN APPARATUS DEFECTS
   - Abnormal gonadotropin molecules
   - Abnormal gonadotropin receptors
4) INFECTION
   - Tuberculosis
   - Mumps
   - Others
5) IATROGENIC
   - Surgery
   - Chemotherapy
   - Irradiation
6) VASCULAR
   - Torsion/hemorrhage
7) IMMUNOLOGIC
   - Deficiency   - Ataxia telangiectasia
                   - DiGeorge's syndrome
   - Autoimmune   - Oophoritis
8) IDIOPATHIC
   - With follicles   - Resistant ovary syndrome
   - Afollicular

Autoimmune Oophoritis

Circulating antibodies against some ovarian component (including gonadotropin receptors) define the condition of autoimmune oophoritis in patients presenting with primary or secondary hypoestrogenic, hypergonadotropic amenorrhea, and the biopsy-proven presence of ovarian follicles. This occurs in 15%–40% of such patients. Follicular lymphocytic infiltration, often transient, may also be found in ovarian biopsy specimens, particularly during the early evolution of the condition.

Variables such as the type of antigen used, assay technic, and the time of testing in relationship to disease onset appear to be of critical importance in the detection of this disorder. This concept should not seem surprising, in light of identical issues that apply to the prototypic autoimmune glandular disease, Hashimoto's thyroiditis. In this condition, the antibody mix is heterogenous (organ damaging, antienzyme, growth-promoting, receptor-agonist, receptor-blocking), the antibody mix is not fixed in proportion with time (the response varies with the antibody mix and the state of the thyroid gland at a particular time, so transient or permanent hypofunction of the thyroid gland may occur), and the antibodies may disappear after organ death.

The coexistence of autoimmune POF in patients with Addison's disease may be as frequent as 25% and may relate to the presence of antibodies directed against common steroidogenic enzymes shared by the two organs. The association of POF with hypothyroidism is less frequent, but more so than is the general population. As with Type 1 diabetes mellitus and Hashimoto's thyroiditis, there is an HLA-DR3 association with autoimmune oophoritis.

Idiopathic Premature Ovarian Failure and the Resistant Ovary Syndrome

A significant proportion of women with POF—in whom circulating autoantibodies are either not detected or not looked for, and for whom no other cause has been identified—are defined as having idiopathic POF. If ovarian follicles are present, the term "resistant ovary syndrome" has been used to define the condition. The presence or absence of follicles in patients presenting with POF is pivotal, not only for establishing a diagnosis but also in delineating therapeutic options.

DIAGNOSIS OF PREMATURE OVARIAN FAILURE

The patient history and physical examination may help to establish the diagnosis. Documentation requires the presence of hypoestrogenemic hypergonadotropism, especially on more than on one occasion. A karyotype is mandatory in primary amenorrhea and can be of help in secondary amenorrhea, as well. Searching for antibodies may be helpful; a positive finding opens up a number of therapeutic options. Testing is generally not available, however, and the procedures have not been standardized.

Establishing the presence or absence of primordial follicles in the ovary is crucial. The gold standard has been a full thickness biopsy of the ovary to look for primordial follicles. The results are qualitative, however, and presume appropriate representation in the specimen obtained—the major disadvantage of such biopsies. Moreover, the ensuing potential risk of adhesions and mechanical infertility is added to the already existing infertile state. Thus, attempts have been made to use the noninvasive transvaginal ultrasound to document the presence of follicles. The data are still preliminary as to the usefulness and accuracy of such an evaluation.

TREATMENT OF PREMATURE OVARIAN FAILURE

The impetus to find methods to treat POF has been obtunded or lost in the 1990s by the availability of successful egg donation, in vitro fertilization (IVF), and embryo-transfer programs. However, in those individuals desiring biological offspring, the whole question of our ability to better differentiate the heterogenous group of POF patients is crucial if successful (and presumably less costly) treatment programs are to evolve.

- The group with no primordial follicles, if clearly defined, are really untreatable except by donor IVF techniques.
- The group with immunologic abnormalities and discernible primordial follicles might benefit from such therapies as high-dose glucocorticoids and/or plasmapheresis.
- Others might benefit from megadoses of exogenous gonadotropins or short-term down-regulation by estrogen.

Estrogens might also act by ameliorating the autoimmune process. Such regimens have been variably reported to yield successful pregnancies. A more recent approach has been the ''down-regulation'' by gonadotropin releasing hormone agonists followed by attempts at ovulation induction with exogenous gonadotropins.

Overall, the success with therapeutic intervention has been remarkably small, and most schools of thought feel that such attempts are futile. The easy, safe, and highly successful egg donation/IVF programs have, therefore, mainly replaced all such endeavors.

Male Endocrine Disorders

MALE HYPOGONADISM

Male hypogonadism is defined as the failure to produce testosterone and/or sperm.

ETIOLOGY OF MALE HYPOGONADISM

Hypogonadism is usually classified as primary or secondary:

- Primary
  - Genetic disease
    - Klinefelter's syndrome
    - Androgen-resistance syndrome
    - Steroidogenic enzyme defects
    - Congenital anorchia
  - Infection
  - Iatrogenic
    - Drugs
    - Chemotherapy
    - Radiation
    - Vasectomy
  - Toxin
    - Mercury
    - Cadmium
- Secondary
  - Endocrine
    - Pubertal delay
    - Hypopituitarism
    - Hypothalamic
      - Kallmann's syndrome
    - Hyperprolactinemia
    - Adrenal gland dysfunction
    - Thyroid gland dysfunction
  - Systemic Illness
    - Malnutrition
    - Weight loss
    - Anorexia nervosa
    - Cancer
    - Drug abuse

SPECIFIC HYPOGONADISM CONDITIONS

Klinefelter's Syndrome

Klinefelter's syndrome is a chromosomal disorder characterized by the presence of one or two extra X chromosomes:

- XXY or XXXY
  - 1:500 male births
  - Variable androgen deficiency
  - On average taller with disproportionate lower segment growth
  - Small testes
  - Azoospermia
  - Gynecomastia
  - Hypergonadotropic hypogonadism

Uncommon Testicular Disorders

Table 42.2 presents uncommon testicular disorders.

Table 42.2.   Uncommon Testicular Disorders

Testicular Disorder	Association/Cause

Hypogonadotropic hypogonadism	Craniofacial anomalies
	    Congenital deafness
	    Intellectual impairment
	    Cerebellar ataxia
	    Laurence-Moon-Biedl syndrome
	    Prader-Willi syndrome
	    Hemochromatosis
	    Anorexia nervosa
	    Excessive exercise

Primary hypogonadism	Myotonic dystrophy
	    Noonan's syndrome
	    Reifenstein's syndrome
	    Androgen receptor defects

Absent vasa deferentia	Cystic fibrosis
Zero motility (cilial defects)	Kartagener's syndrome
Varicocele	Renal carcinoma Renal malformations

Testicular infarction/orchitis	Polyarteritis nodosa
	Hemophilia
	    Sickle cell anemia
	    Brucellosis
	    Gonorrhea

CLINICAL PRESENTATION OF MALE HYPOGONADISM

Peripubertally, hypogonadism presents as an absence of secondary sex characteristics:

- Small testes
- Penis indicating a lack of development
- Eunuchoid proportions (arm span > 5 cm longer than height)

    Postpubertally, the cardinal features are:

- Decreased libido
- Impotence
- Loss of secondary sexual hair
- Wrinkled skin
- Testicular atrophy
- Little change in penile size

DIAGNOSIS OF MALE HYPOGONADISM

In investigation, a check for gonadotropins, prolactin, and testosterone is needed. If hypogonadotropic with or without hyperprolactinemia, do a standard evaluation to rule out hypothalamic or pituitary abnormality. If hypergonadotropic, do a karyotype.

TREATMENT OF MALE HYPOGONADISM

Treatment of male hypogonadism is usually geared to replacement. In hypogonadotropic individuals, fertility may be stimulated by the use of gonadotropins.

IMPOTENCE

ETIOLOGY OF IMPOTENCE

The etiology of impotence lends itself to a unique description:

I nflammatory

M echanical

P sychological

O cclusive-vascular

T raumatic/operative

E ndurance-related

N eurologic

C hemical

E ndocrine

Up to 35% (in one study) of patients with impotence have an endocrine cause—usually an easy diagnosis to make and relatively easy and gratifying to treat. Common endocrine causes include:

- Hypogonadotropic hypogonadism — Kallmann's
- Hypergonadotropic hypogonadism — Kleinfelter's
- Hyperprolactinemia
- Diabetes mellitus

In hyperprolactinemia, the impotence is thought to be by two mechanisms:

- Direct feedback of prolactin on the GnRH neurons in the hypothalamus by the ultra-short-loop feedback (the major operative mechanism), whereby GnRh pulsatility, and thus LH pulsatility, is dampened, slowed and thereby made significantly dysfunctional. Consequently, there is no stimulation of the testes and hypogonadotropic hypogonadism ensues.
- Direct effect on the "libidigenous" center by prolactin, and resultant decreased sexual interest and drive. Thus testosterone supplementation alone is not always or totally effective in restoring libido and potency and normoprolactinemia is usually required for the full effect of testosterone to be manifested.

Diabetes mellitus is probably the most common cause of impotence. While the age of the patient is a factor (older men are more likely to develop impotence than younger men), the duration of diabetes is also an important variable in the tendency to develop impotence. The longer the duration of diabetes, the higher the incidence of impotence. Etiologically, the impotence of diabetes is caused by the combination of vasculopathy and neuropathy, the relative contribution of each being variable in any one patient. Psychogenic factors may play a significant role early in the disorder—the expectation and fear of failing after one failure commonly worsens the problem initially, and the decreased sensation of orgasm and ejaculation because of neuropathy and retrograde ejaculation takes its toll. Actual hormonal deficiency secondary to diabetes is very rare.

DIAGNOSIS OF IMPOTENCE

Clinical aspects to be considered in the evaluation of impotence include an evaluation of hormonal function, both by history (libido, hair growth, gynecomastia, previous fertility, and history of alcohol or drug abuse) and by physical examination (hair distribution, body habitus, testes size, prostate size, visual fundii and fields, evidence of other endocrinopathy, and evidence of other illnesses).

In the investigation of impotence, in addition to an evaluation of testosterone, gonadotropin, and prolactin, it is important to evaluate vascular integrity by Doppler flow studies and neurogenic integrity by the snap gauge test or the more cumbersome nocturnal penile tumescence evaluation. There is no place for an OGTT in the evaluation of impotence.

TREATMENT OF IMPOTENCE

The goal of treatment is to find the underlying cause, if possible. Otherwise, replacement of testosterone, if needed, and/or the provision of intracavernous injections of papaverine, or PGE$_2$, or the prescription of external or internal prosthetic devices may be of help.

GYNECOMASTIA

Gynecomastia is defined as palpable glandular tissue below the areola.

PATHOGENESIS OF GYNECOMASTIA

Gynecomastia is owing to either increased estrogen or decreased androgens. Estrogens stimulate breast tissue; androgens inhibit breast tissue. Thus, the ratio of estrogen to androgen determines the degree of stimulation. More important, in the absence of androgens, it requires very small concentrations, even below those measurable by conventional assays, to stimulate mammary growth. Estrogen, in the male, is derived from peripheral conversion of precursors like androstenedione and testosterone. LH and HCG stimulate estradiol secretion by the testes.

DIAGNOSIS OF GYNECOMASTIA

The evaluation of gynecomastia usually demands a methodologic search to establish:

- Presence
- Associations
- Speed of development
- Progression
- Systemic illnesses
- Associated drugs
- Genital abnormalities

Physical Examination

The physical examination must rule out a malignancy with a good detailed examination, including a detailed testicular examination and a mammogram if the index of suspicion is high.

Laboratory Studies

Laboratory evaluation may be unnecessary in asymptomatic nontender gynecomastia. If the physical evaluation reveals pain, rapid growth, or a large size, laboratory evaluation should include testosterone, LH, HCG, DHEAS, or urinary 17-ketosteroids, as well as estradiol, prolactin, thyroid, and liver functions.

Differential Diagnosis

The differential diagnosis of gynecomastia includes:

- Physiologic
  - Newborn
  - Pubertal
  - Aging
- Pathologic
  - Increased estrogens
    - Tumors
      - Adrenal
      - Testes (Leydig cell tumors)
      - Choriocarcinoma
      - Ectopic gonadotropin
      - Ectopic placental-like hormone
    - Cirrhosis
    - Hyperthyroidism
  - Decreased androgen effect
    - Hypogonadism
      - Klinefelter's
      - Mumps
      - Cytotoxic chemotherapy
      - Irradiation
    - Androgen insensitivity
    - Refeeding
    - Chronic renal failure/dialysis
- Pharmacologic
  - Estrogens
  - Aromalizable androgens
  - HCG
  - Antiandrogens

- Psychotropics—phenothiazines
- Methyldopa
- Reserpium
  - Spironolactone
  - Cimetidine
  - Ketoconazole
  - Cyproterone
  - Flutamide
  - Estrogenlike
    - Digitalis
    - Marijuana
  - Others
    - Central nervous system (CNS) acting
    - Miscellaneous
- Idiopathic
- Pseudogynecomastia (mimics appearance of normal breast)
  - Lipomastia (adipose-related)
  - Neoplasm

Specific observation on the differential diagnosis of gynecomastia include:

- Neonatal: 60–90% of newborns have gynecomastia. Likely secondary to placental estrogen exposure. Regresses over weeks.
- Pubertal: 50–70% of pubertal boys have unilateral or bilateral gynecomastia. Thought to be secondary to the preponderance of estrogen production over testosterone, and the earlier achievement of normal adult values of estrogen. Regresses in most.
- Aging: 4% of elderly men may have gynecomastia at autopsy. Likely secondary to a decrease in testosterone with aging, while estradiol is still maintained possibly by increased peripheral conversion.
- Tumors, whether de novo producing estrogen or its precursors (adrenal or Leydig cell testicular tumors), or producing hormones such as HCG, which stimulate the testes to produce estrogen, cause gynecomastia.
- Gynecomastia in cirrhosis is thought to occur because of two mechanisms:

- Increased peripheral conversion owing to decreased clearance of androstenedione
- An alcohol-mediated suppression of testosterone production by suppression of the hypothalamo-pituitary axis
- Hyperthyroidism induces sex-hormone-binding globulins, thereby increasing the level of total testosterone and estradiol. Free testosterone remains normal, but free estradiol is increased because of the increased androstenedione available for peripheral conversion.
- Gynecomastia associated with hypogonadism is secondary to the increased estradiol/testosterone ratio.
- Refeeding seems to induce a "second puberty," and the mechanism of gynecomastia is the same as that seen in pubertal gynecomastia. This is also thought to be one of the factors that cause gynecomastia in chronic renal failure or dialysis.

TREATMENT OF GYNECOMASTIA

The treatment is usually to address the underlying cause, if any (which generally helps to resolve the problem), and to reassure the patient, if the cause is likely physiological or residual. If no obvious etiology is found, follow-up and observation are all that is indicated. It must be remembered that resolution of the problem may still leave a mass of fibrous tissue.

Treatment regimen may include:

- Androgen (testosterone), danazol, or antiestrogens, although medical treatments are not frequently used
- Prevention by radiation prior to estrogen treatment has been advocated by a few
- Surgery and a reduction mammoplasty remains the most appropriate treatment of significant psychologically damaging gynecomastia, although the words of NuHall are very appropriate and bear keeping in mind: "In the absence of pain, rapid change in size, eccentric, or hard breast mass or testicular mass, no further evaluation of gynecomastia in men is necessary."

REVIEW EXERCISES

1. Match the hormone profile, taken in the morning, to the disease in these women with acne and hirsutism:

   1. ACTH 22, cortisol 35, DHEAS 5.6, testosterone 75, TSH 0.5, T_4 6.4.
   2. ACTH 22, cortisol 19, DHEAS 3.6, testosterone 72, TSH 3.4, T_4 6.4.
   3. ACTH < 5, cortisol 5, DHEAS 0.9, testosterone 12, TSH 0.6, T_4 6.4.
   4. ACTH 38, cortisol 14, DHEAS 5.6, testosterone 78, TSH 0.9, T_4 7.3.
   5. ACTH < 5, cortisol 42, DHEAS 9.8, testosterone 112, TSH 0.5, T_4 7.8.
   6. ACTH 16, cortisol 21, DHEAS 2.5, testosterone 66, TSH 9.8, T_4 6.2.

   Diseases:
   a. Primary hypothyroidism
   b. Exogenous steroids
   c. Polycystic ovary disease
   d. Adrenal carcinoma
   e. Congenital adrenal hyperplasia
   f. Cushing's disease

2. Match the disease scenario with the hormone profile:

   1. A 21-year-old woman with primary amenorrhea and no sense of smell
   2. A 19-year-old woman with short stature, primary amenorrhea and webbed neck
   3. A 24-year-old woman with schizophrenia on treatment presenting with amenorrhea
   4. A 23-year-old with postpill amenorrhea
   5. A 26-year-old with headaches, visual blurring and amenorrhea

   Hormone profile
   a. LH < 2, FSH < 2, prolactin 683
   b. LH < 2, FSH < 2, prolactin 68
   c. LH < 2.0, FSH < 2.0, prolactin 6
   d. LH 2.3, FSH 3.1, prolactin 18
   e. LH 23, FSH 47, prolactin 8

3. Match the hormonal profile to the case presented:

   1. A 26-year-old, tall young man with gynecomastia, microphallus, and small, soft testes (< 3 cc)
   2. A 24-year-old, tall young man with widely spread teeth, goiter, skin tags, microphallus, and small, normal-sized testes (6–7 cc)
   3. A 19-year-old, tall young man with bilateral inguinal hernia and an empty scrotum
   4. A 25-year-old, tall young man with a history of pubertal mumps orchitis, a normal-size penis, and normal testes (8–10 cc)
   5. A 22-year-old, tall young man with microphallus, small testes (4–5 cc), and no sense of smell

   Hormonal profile:
   a. LH < 2, FSH < 2, testosterone 25, prolactin 7, growth hormone 11
   b. LH < 2, FSH 2.3, testosterone 48, prolactin 38, growth hormone 18
   c. LH 3.8, FSH 23, testosterone 389, prolactin 7, growth hormone 0.9
   d. LH 13.6, FSH 13.8, testosterone 176, prolactin 9, growth hormone 0.6
   e. LH 76, FSH 95, testosterone 92, prolactin 12, growth hormone 1.6

4. Impotence is commonly seen in:

   a. Diabetes mellitus
   b. Congenital adrenal hyperplasia
   c. Schizophrenia that is well controlled
   d. Androgen insensitivity syndrome
   e. a and c only
   f. b and d only
   g. All of the above

5. Gynecomastia is commonly seen in:

   a. An XY individual with bilateral inguinal scars and a total lack of secondary sexual hair
   b. An XY individual with well-treated and controlled salt losing congenital adrenal hyperplasia
   c. An XY individual with spider nevii, asterixis, and ascites
   d. An XY individual who is the timid member of a gay couple
   e. a and c only
   f. b and d only
   g. All of the above

6. A 27-year-old Italian woman presents for evaluation of hirsutism and a 2-year history of irregular heavy menses. Menarche was at age 13, and her periods were always irregular, except when she was on birth-control pills (age 18–24). Thelarche and adenarche were normal. She noted the onset of significant acne at age 17, for which she was treated with antibiotics and accutane. Accutane had to be discontinued because of severe hypertriglyceridemia. At about the same time, she noted the development of hirsutism, which has slowly progressed. She had been trying to become pregnant for the past 3 years.

   On examination: Weight, 170 pounds; height, 5 feet, 3 inches. She has hyperpigmentation of the neck and axillary folds, a small goiter, and hirsutism on the chin, upper lip, and side of her face, as well as periareolar and periumbilical coarse dark terminal hair. Blood pressure is 120/82. Waist/hip ratio is 0.95 and no striae. Liver edge is palpable 1 cm below the costal margin.

Part 1: The differential diagnosis in our signal case would include:
a. Genetic hirsutism
b. Adult onset congenital adrenal hyperplasia
c. Polycystic ovarian disease
d. Cushing's syndrome
e. a, b, and c
f. a and c
g. All of the above

Part 2: In our case, the appropriate laboratory tests include:
a. Serum DHEAS/testosterone/free testosterone
b. Serum TSH/prolactin
c. Serum 17 hydroprogesterone
d. Gonadotropins and estradiol
e. a, b, and c only
f. All of the above
e. Laboratory tests
—Serum DHEAS and/or urinary (24-hour) 17-keto-steroids (17-KS) (useful to rule out adrenal neoplasms)
—Serum T — into the normal male range (> 8)

7. A 26-year-old woman presents for evaluation of amenorrhea of 6 months' duration. She had a normal menarche at age 12 and normal puberty. Her menses had become progressively lighter over the past 2–3 years and occurred 4–9 weeks apart prior to amenorrhea. She has been under a significant amount of stress in the past 2 years, completing her medical degree, competing on the university gymnastic team, and experiencing a long-term relationship break-up. She has never taken the birth-control pill and has never been pregnant. She denies galactorrhea, has had a 15-pound weight loss, has no hirsutism, acne, or headache. She was diagnosed with Hashimoto's hypothyroidism at age 16, for which she is on L-thyroxine with a normal serum TSH over the years.

In our case, laboratory evaluation showed an FSH of 4 IU/L, an LH of 2 IU/L, and a prolactin of 12 mg/ml with a serum TSH of 10.8 uU/ml, testosterone 42 ng/dl, and DHEAS 3.3 ng/ml. The rest of the biochemistry was normal. Which of the following would not be in the differential diagnosis:

a. Functional amenorrhea secondary to stress, weight loss and exercise
b. Hypothyroidism
c. PCO
d. Premature ovarian failure

8. A 26-year-old male presents with primary infertility. He has been married for 4 years and has been trying to father a child for 3 years. He has no difficulty with sexual function. Past and family history are unremarkable, and he is on no medications and does not smoke, drink, or take any street drugs. He is 6 feet, 2 inches (the tallest in his family), weighs 264 pounds, has an arm span of 80 inches, and has a pubis-to-heel length of 39 inches. He has bilateral gynecomastia, a 2 ½-inch penis partially embedded in the mons, bilateral small, soft testes, and sparse, but present, secondary sexual hair growth. His testosterone value is 210 ng/dl (N $>$ 220 ng/dl) and he is azoospermic.

Part 1: Your diagnosis:
a. Klinefelter's syndrome
b. Congenital hypoorchia
c. Postsubclinical mumps orchitis
d. Kallmann's syndrome
e. Pubertal hyperprolactinemia

Part 2: In our signal case, does our young man with primary infertility, no sexual dysfunction, and azoospermia with small testes but nearly low normal testosterone need treatment with testosterone?

9. A 52-year-old man presents with a complaint of impotence. He reports progressively increasing difficulty—first with maintaining and later with achieving an erection. He is an attorney, married for 24 years, has 4 children, the youngest age 16, and has no verbalized stress. He was found to have hypertension about 6 years before and suffered an MI 4 years earlier. He has been controlled on beta blockers and a thiazide diuretic, has no angina and no arrhythmias, and has well-controlled blood pressure. He has no other symptoms of note. He has family history of diabetes, hyperlipidemia, hypertension, and heart disease. He does not smoke and only drinks socially.

Examination shows: weight, 180 pounds, height, 5 feet, 9 inches. Blood pressure is 135/84 and pulse is 68/minute and regular, with an occasional extrasystole. Liver is palpable 1 cm below the costal margin with a span of 17 cm. There are no bruits. Bilateral lipomastia is noted. Genital examination reveals a normal penis and testicles that measure 4.5 $\times$ 3.1 cm bilaterally. There is a small varicocele on the right side. The prostate is mildly enlarged with an intact median groove. Fundi and fields are normal.

Part 1: Laboratory evaluation required would include:
a. Gonadotropins, testosterone, and thyroid function tests
b. Testosterone, prolactin, TSH
c. Liver, kidney, electrolyte, glucose panel
d. OGTT
e. a and c only
f. b and c only
g. b, c, and d

Part 2: Further evaluations needed are:

a. A snap gauge
b. Nocturnal penile tumescence study
c. MRI of the head
d. a and c only
e. All of the above
f. None of the above

Part 3: The treatment option in our case is:

a. Testosterone shots
b. Bromocryptine
c. Intravenous injection of papaverine
d. Discontinue inderal and thiazides
e. Penile prosthesis placement
f. Reassurance and support with no treatment

Answers

1. 1-f, 2-c, 3-b, 4-e, 5-d, 6-a
2. 1-c, 2-e, 3-b, 4-d, 5-a
3. 1-e, 2-b, 3-d, 4-c, 5-a
4. e
5. e
6. Part 1: e
   No clinical evidence given for Cushing's.
   Part 2: e
   Gonadotropins and estradiol are no clinical help.
7. d
   Gonadotropins indicate that this is impossible.

8. Part 1: a
   Part 2: Yes.
   The patient needs treatment to stop continued stimula-tion of testes, which synthesizes estradiol and contributes to gynecomastia.

9. Part 1: f
   Part 2: d
   A snap gauge will give almost the same information as noctural penile tumescence evaluation.
   Part 3: d
   If possible, these should be changed to other medica-tions to see if they are contributing to the problem.

SUGGESTED READINGS

MALE

Braunstein GD. Gynecomastia. N Engl J Med 1993;328:490.

Glass AR. Gynecomastia. Endocrinol Metab Clin North Amer 1994;23(4):825–827.

Krane RJ, Goldstein L, Saenz De Tejada I. Impotence. N Engl J Med 1989;321:1648–1659.

FEMALE

Barbieri RL. Hyperandrogenic disorders. Clin Obstet Gynecol 1990;33:640–659.

Barnes R, Rosenfeld RL. The polycystic ovary syndrome: pathogenesis and treatment. Ann Intern Med 1989;110:386–399.

Biffignandi P, Massucchetti D, Molinatti GM. Female hirsu-tism: pathophysiological considerations and therapeutic im-plications. Endocrinol Rev 1984;5:498–513.

Brodie BL, Wentz AC. Late onset congenital adrenalhyperpla-sia: a gynecologist's perspective. Fertil Steril 1987;48:175–188.

Lobo RA. Hirsutism in polycystic ovary syndrome: current concepts. Clin Obstet Gynecol 1991;36:817–826.

McKenna TJ. Pathogenesis and treatment of polycystic ovary-syndrome. N Engl J Med 1988;318:558–562.

Rittmaster RS, Loriaux DL. Hirsutism. Ann Intern Med 1987;106:96–107.

Yen SSC. The polycystic ovary syndrome. Clin Endocrinol (Oxf) 1980;12:177–207.

MENSTRUAL DISORDERS

Dalkin AC, Marshall JC. Medical therapy of hyperprolactin-emia. Endocrinol Metab Clin North Amer 1989;18:259–276.

Reindollar RH, Novak M, Tho SP, et al. Adult-onset amenor-rhea: a study of 262 patients. Am J Obstet Gynecol 1986;155:531–543.

PREMATURE OVARIAN FAILURE

Mehta AE, Matwijiw L, Lyons EA, et al. Noninvasive diagno-sis of resistant ovary syndrome by ultrasonography. Fertil Steril 1992;57:56–61.

Diabetes Mellitus: Control and Complications

S. Sethu K. Reddy

Diabetes mellitus (DM) affects more than 7 million individuals in the United States. (As many as 8 million others may not be aware they have diabetes.) Diabetes is a complex metabolic condition with major health and social ramifications. In recent years, many advances have been made that have increased the ability to achieve optimal metabolic control of diabetes, while a wealth of accumulated data show that improved control does delay the long-term complications of the disease.

ETIOLOGY OF DIABETES

TYPES OF DIABETES

Quite broadly, diabetes can be classified as follows:

- Type 1, insulin-dependent diabetes mellitus (IDDM)
- Type 2, noninsulin-dependent diabetes mellitus (NIDDM)
- Gestational
- Other
  - Pancreatic disease, hormonal disease, drugs
  - Rare genetic forms, insulin-receptor abnormalities
- Impaired glucose tolerance (IGT)

In North America, most individuals with diabetes will have either Type 1 DM or Type 2 DM. Both of these conditions display a tremendous interaction between gene and environment (see Table 43.1).

Type 1 Diabetes

There appears to be positive correlation with the incidence of Type 1 DM and the distance away from the equator. Finland has the highest incidence, with southern European countries having a lower incidence, and with Mediterranean countries having even lower incidence. Whether this is related to the different genetic background or the environment alone is unknown. No male-female differences are known. Type 1 DM, predominantly striking those below age 30, is associated with absolute insulin deficiency owing to chronic autoimmune destruction of pancreatic β-cells. These individuals need insulin for daily existence.

In genetically susceptible individuals, this autoimmune process, which can be detected by the presence of antibodies to various components of the β-cells (e.g., insulin, glutamic acid decarboxylase, phosphotyrosin, phosphatase), results in gradual deterioration of insulin production. During this phase (which may be longer than 10 years), there may be no evidence of hyperglycemia; at a later time, a critical event such as surgery or a viral illness may result in acute deterioration of pancreatic function, resulting in acute severe hyperglycemia.

The presence of a gene(s) within the major histocompatibility complex is essential to the development of Type 1. More than 90% of Caucasians with Type 1 DM express either HLA-DR3 or HLA-DR4. However, 40% of the nondiabetic population also express one of these alleles. This genetic linkage has been further enhanced by studies showing 96% of patients with Type 1 DM to be homozygous for amino acid nonaspartate/nonaspartate at position 57 of the DQ-β-chain. Despite such great progress in understanding the genetic susceptibility to Type 1 DM, the approximate 60% discordance of Type 1 DM in identical twins suggests an important role for environmental factors. These environmental factors may be nutritional components, such as cow's milk, viral infections, or chemical toxins.

Having a first-degree relative with Type 1 diabetes increases one's risk of Type 1 DM 10-fold. However, 95% of these individuals will not develop Type 1 DM.

As Type 1 DM is an autoimmune disease, the prevention of Type 1 DM has focused on immune intervention. Various

Table 43.1.　Features of Type 1 DM vs. Type 2 Diabetes

	Type 1 Diabetes	Type 2 Diabetes
Prevalence (%)	0.4	6.6
Incidence in U.S. per year	15,000	500,000
Ketosis prone	+ + + +	+
Anti-islet cell Ab	+ + +	−
Anti-GAD Ab	+ + + +	−
Prevalence of other autoimmune conditions	+ + +	−
Usual age of onset	< 30 yrs.	> 40 yrs.
Prevalence of obesity	+	+ + +
Family history	+	+ + +
HLA linkage	DR3, DR4 DQβ- polymorphism	−
Insulin secretion	Absent	Abnormal
Insulin resistance	−	+ + +

immunosuppressives and immunomodulators have been tested in multicenter trials. Some early studies from Australia and the United States (using azathioprine with or without prednisone in subjects with recent-onset Type 1 DM) were favorable, but further study has been abandoned in favor of safer immunotherapies.

Cyclosporine A has been evaluated in two large and two small double-blinded, placebo-controlled studies and also in later open studies. In recent-onset Type 1 DM subjects, insulin-free remission rates of 18–24% at 12 months were observed, but no remissions were evident at 24 months, despite continued cyclosporine therapy.

Intensive insulin therapy has also been demonstrated to preserve pancreatic insulin secretion in new-onset Type 1 DM patients, and a pilot study at the Joslin Diabetes Center in Boston showed that repeated courses of intravenous insulin therapy to a small group of prediabetics significantly delayed the onset of Type 1 DM in about 2.5 years of follow-up. Other potential interventions include induction of tolerance to islet cells by oral antigens (including insulin itself), avoidance of cow's milk in infancy, newer immunomodulatory agents, and free radical scavengers.

Type 2 Diabetes

Type 2 diabetes accounts for about 85% of the diabetic population. Type 2 DM is presently believed to be the result of many years of insulin resistance, leading to disordered pancreatic insulin secretion, which in turn leads to fasting hyperglycemia. Quite often, weight gain (particularly central obesity), physical inactivity, and a high-fat diet exaggerate the insulin resistance and may accelerate the development of

Type 2 diabetes. Individuals with Type 2 DM may require insulin therapy for improved control of glucose levels but are then labeled as "insulin-requiring Type 2 DM." In most westernized countries, the risk of developing Type 2 DM continues to increase with age, resulting in close to 30% prevalence of Type 2 DM in the geriatric population. In many of the aboriginal communities, incidence of Type 2 tends to peak before age 50.

Genetic risk of Type 2 DM can be illustrated by the differences in the risk of developing Type 2 DM related to the familial prevalence of Type 2 DM. If both parents have Type 2 DM, offspring have a 50% chance of developing Type 2 DM, while with only one parent with Type 2 DM, the risk drops to 20%. If an identical twin has Type 2 DM, the risk is estimated to be more than 90%.

There are striking differences in the prevalence of Type 2 DM among different ethnic groups. The Pima Indians of the Southwestern United States, for example, have greater than 30% prevalence of Type 2 DM, while Americans of European ancestry have approximately a 5% prevalence.

Environment, however, is equally important in the development of Type 2 DM. Within an ethnic group, the prevalence of Type 2 DM varies depending on the presence of obesity, physical inactivity, dietary composition and on whether living conditions are urban or rural. Studies of Japanese Americans, aboriginals of North America, Asian immigrants to Europe, Mexican-Americans, and natives of the South Pacific have confirmed the importance of the above risk factors.

Obesity (particularly central obesity) and elevated insulin/glucose ratios have generally been considered to be important risk factors. It should be noted that a family history of Type 2 DM connotes a higher-than-usual risk of developing Type 2 DM in the obese, as well.

Physical activity may also be important. Bjorntorp, et al. have shown that physically trained, insulin-resistant obese subjects could decrease their plasma insulin values by almost 50% without decreasing body fat. Helmrich, et al., in a cohort of 5990 males, studied lifestyle habits and health aspects in 1962 and again in 1976. A total of 202 men developed diabetes during the 14 years. The incidence rate of diabetes decreased by 41% in patients doing the highest level of physical activity (> 3500 kcal/week) compared with those with the lowest level (< 500 kcal/week). This effect was independent of other risk factors. A high BMI (> 26) was the strongest predictor of Type 2 DM. Such data are certainly encouraging for the design of preventive programs for Type 2 diabetes.

Although not confirmed universally, excess dietary fat may result in insulin resistance, dyslipidemias, and glucose intolerance. Other behavioral factors related to diet and stress remain to be clarified.

Molecular defects in the insulin receptor, glucose transporters, and the insulin gene have been reported in different diabetes syndromes, but none appears to cause the common form of Type 2 DM. Recently, interest has grown in the glucokinase gene, with abnormalities reported in maturity onset diabetes of the young.

Secondary Diabetes

Other conditions that damage the pancreas may also cause diabetes, including:

- Chronic pancreatitis
- Cystic fibrosis
- Hemochromatosis
- Pancreatectomy

Conditions associated with elevated counter-regulatory hormones—pheochromocytoma, acromegaly, and Cushing's syndrome—may also precipitate diabetes. Drugs such as glucocorticoids, thiazide diuretics, phenytoin, α-interferon, pantamidine, and diazoxide may cause hyperglycemia.

COSTS OF DIABETES: MORBIDITY

The prognosis for an individual with Type 2 diabetes may be affected by:

- The inherent background morbidity pattern of the nondiabetic in his/her population
- Competing risks
- The pattern of risk factors
- The quality and quantity of available health care
- The possible differences in etiology of that patient's Type 2 diabetes

More than 10 studies have documented an excess mortality in Type 2 diabetes; several studies have estimated a 5–10-year loss in life expectancy in patients older than 40. Diabetes is the leading cause of blindness in adults 25–74 years old in Europe and North America. Women appear to be predisposed to retinopathy, and blacks appear to be at more risk than whites. Diabetes is also the leading cause of end-stage renal disease, which also has major implications on the patient's quality of life. Diabetes, which may also have an adverse effect on productivity, leads to a greater use of health-care resources. The life expectancy of children with Type 1 DM is about 75% of that of nondiabetics.

The direct and indirect costs of diabetes are extremely high. In the United States alone, it has been estimated that care of diabetes costs more than $20 billion per year, or approximately $3,000 per individual with diabetes. Patients with diabetes require two to three times the cost of health care of individuals without diabetes.

DIAGNOSIS OF DIABETES

SCREENING

Individuals with the following characteristics should be screened for diabetes:

- Increased number of risk factors
- Obesity
- Family history of Type 2 diabetes

- History of gestational diabetes/giving birth to infant > 9 pounds
- Hypertension
- Cardiovascular disease
- Belonging to a high-risk ethnic group
- Increasing age (> age 45)

Screening should be accomplished with a fasting plasma glucose. The use of the Oral Glucose Tolerance Test (OGTT), insulin, and C-peptide levels cannot be recommended, except for research trials. Additional research is needed to assess the reliability of glycated hemoglobin measurements in diagnosing diabetes mellitus. Screening on a population basis cannot be recommended.

Screening for Type 1 diabetes cannot be recommended at present because of the high cost of testing and the lack of clearly defined management of an individual who may be positive on testing.

ORAL GLUCOSE TOLERANCE TEST (OGTT)

The OGTT is a useful tool when appropriately used, but it is often overused and rarely leads to a change in management decisions.

The subject needs to fast for 8 hours (abstaining from caffeine and nicotine) prior to receiving 75 grams of glucose (for adults) or 1.75 grams/kg (for children). The total volume is between 250 to 300 ml, and should be ingested over 5 minutes. The patient should not be malnourished and should have eaten at least 150 grams of carbohydrate per day for at least 3 days prior to the test. Patients should be ambulatory and not be acutely ill. The formal OGTT in a pregnant individual requires a 100 gram glucose load and is extended to 3 hours. Remember that the plasma glucose values are about 15% higher than whole blood glucose values. The discussion below uses plasma glucose values.

Interpretation of the OGTT

In mid-1997, the diagnostic criteria for diabetes mellitus were revised and accepted by the National Institutes of Health, the Center for Disease Control and Prevention, and the American Diabetes Association. For most individuals with diabetes mellitus, the designation should be either Type 1 or Type 2 diabetes. The classification should be based on an etiological basis, rather than on the type of treatment.

Two fasting plasma glucose levels greater than 126 mg/dl (7 mM) indicates presence of diabetes mellitus. If the 2-hour postprandial value is greater than 200 mg/dl, then the patient is deemed to have diabetes mellitus (Table 43.2).

Fasting glucose levels between 110–126 mg/dl indicate impaired fasting glucose tolerance. During an oral glucose tolerance test, 2-hour postprandial glucose levels between 140–200 mg/dl indicate impaired glucose tolerance. Of patients with OGT, 1%–5% will develop diabetes per year.

Table 43.2.   Interpretation of OGTT

	Normal	*Impaired Glucose Tolerance*	*Diabetes Mellitus*	*Diabetes Mellitus*	*DM (Pregnancy)*
Fasting (mg/dl)	< 126	< 126	> 126 (Cancel test)	< 126	< 105
0.5, 1.0 or 1.5 hrs. PC (mg/dl) 2.0 hours PC (mg/dl) 3.0 hours PC (mg/dl)	< 140	140–200		> 200	≥ 190 ≥ 165 ≥ 145

However, 50% of patients with IGT will have a normal glucose tolerance test if repeated in 6 months.

Variables Affecting the OGTT

Reproducibility of the OGTT results is notoriously poor. Several studies have shown that repeat testing of the same individual may result in blood sugars that vary by 18–27 mg/dl. There is no doubt this variability is caused by changes in nutritional status, weight, medications, use of caffeine/nicotine and the normal physiological variability of glucose metabolism. Thus, some advocate that at least two OGTTs are needed to properly classify a patient.

In addition, as one ages, the prevalence of glucose intolerance increases dramatically. In the geriatric population, up to 30% may have DM. Aging is associated with delayed absorption of glucose, but, more important, is also associated with delayed glucose-induced insulin secretion and insulin resistance at the level of the liver and skeletal muscle. The major disturbance appears to be insulin-mediated glucose uptake. It is also worthy to note that as one ages, although the total weight may not change, the weight distribution may be altered to that of a central obesity pattern. Such a pattern has been linked to insulin resistance and related disorders.

Careful medical history must always be performed in assessing the risk of DM, including the use of the following medications, which adversely affect glucose tolerance:

- Diazoxide
- Furosemide
- Thiazides
- Glucocorticoids, oral contraceptives
- Adrenaline
- Isoproterenol
- Nicotinic acid
- Phenytoin

If necessary, these medications may need to be withdrawn (if possible).

IGT refers to intermediate glucose levels between normal and diabetic individuals. It can only be determined by an OGTT. IGT replaces previous terms such as borderline diabetes, prediabetes, and chemical diabetes. The clinical significance of IGT is controversial and the subject of much research.

However, it is widely felt that an individual with IGT may be at a higher risk of developing diabetes and/or cardiovascular disease.

Other Potential Uses of the OGTT

Reactive Hypoglycemia   It has become common practice to perform a 5-hour, prolonged OGTT in patients who appear to have apparent hypoglycemic symptoms postprandially. Several studies have shown significant inconsistencies between symptoms and the presence of hypoglycemia. Other studies have confirmed the inadequacies of the OGTT in the workup of hypoglycemia.

Pregnancy   Gestational diabetes is characterized by a diabetic state first detected during a pregnancy. The prevalence of gestational diabetes has varied from 0.15% to 12.3%, depending again on the study group and the set of diagnostic criteria. The WHO Expert Committee on Diabetes Mellitus recommended that the diagnostic procedures should be the same for both pregnant and nonpregnant adults. Whether gestational diabetes should be diagnosed and managed is highly controversial. In North America, gestational diabetes has been reported to be associated with higher frequency of metabolic abnormalities, higher birth weights, and increased morbidity and mortality. In the United States, the relative risk of perinatal mortality of gestational diabetic women as compared with normal control women was 2.2.

The U.S. Preventive Services Task Force, the Second International Workshop Conference on Gestational Diabetes Mellitus, and the American Diabetes Association recommend screening all pregnant women with a 50-gram OGTT at 24–28 weeks. If the 1-hour postload glucose level is > 140 mg/dl, then a 3-hour, 100 gram glucose tolerance test should be performed. This diagnostic algorithm seems to be the most cost-effective in North America. The formal OGTT during pregnancy uses a 100-gram glucose load. Two of the three PC glucose levels need to be met or exceeded to make the diagnosis of gestational diabetes.

Acromegaly   Growth Hormone (GH) secretion is suppressed by a rise in blood glucose Consequently, the gold-standard diagnostic test for acromegaly is detection of unsuppressed GH levels during an OGTT.

Patients with Apparent Complications of Diabetes Rarely, patients will present with retinopathy, neuropathy, or nephropathy that is suggestive of diabetic complications but may have equivocal plasma glucose levels. In such situations, an OGTT can be performed to definitively confirm or refute the diagnosis of DM.

Epidemiological Research In the study of the natural history of DM, the OGTT is an invaluable tool. The OGTT has been used in many population-based studies to determine the prevalence of diabetes and associated risk factors.

TREATMENT OF DIABETES
DIETARY MANAGEMENT

Dietary management is the cornerstone of diabetes care and should be used in conjunction with exercise to promote a healthy lifestyle. This will then hopefully lead to maintenance of lower or ideal body weight, decreased insulin resistance, and improved control of hyperglycemia, dyslipidemia, and hypertension.

Individuals with diabetes should be referred to a registered dietitian for detailed and practical advice. The physician can help greatly by inquiring about the patient's lifestyle and by imparting good nutritional principles. Having three balanced meals per day, enjoying a variety of foods, and spacing meals 4–6 hours apart will be helpful. Including high fiber and low fat in food choices, as well as moderating intake of simple sugars, will further the overall goals of reducing complications of diabetes. Dietary instructions will often depend upon the ''state'' of the patient. The rigor of the lifestyle changes will depend upon:

- Age
- Comorbid conditions (such as pregnancy or renal failure)
- Activity levels
- Target metabolic goals (Table 43.3)

A maintenance diet is approximately 25 kcal/kg of ideal body weight. The simplest way to calculate the ideal body weight is to use Body Mass Index (BMI) Formula [BMI = weight(kg) / height(m^2)]. An optimal BMI is less than 25. A BMI of more than 27 would be considered obesity. One kilogram of weight loss is = 7500 to 8000 kcal; thus, reducing energy intake by 500–1000 kcal per day should result in 0.5 to 1 kg of weight loss per week.

Alcohol should be consumed in moderation only, and salt intake should be restricted in patients with hypertension or nephropathy. Artificial sweeteners, aspartame, cyclamates, acesulfame K, and lactulose can be consumed and are safe in the amounts used in most diets. (Often, patients focus only on the sugar component and do not realize that although they are eating a low-sugar food, they may be taking in excess fat.) The focus of a ''diabetic diet'' has shifted away from pure avoidance of sugars to a more complete, healthy, risk-reduction nutrition plan. The American Diabetes Association's dietary recommendation allows a diabetic to ingest up to 10% of their daily energy intake from simple carbohydrates.

A fat substitute now available (Olestra™) consists of a sucrose core with six to eight fatty acids, making the molecule too large to be absorbed. There has been concern related to GI side effects and possible decrease in absorption of fat-soluble vitamins. Presently, the FDA has approved its use in snack foods only. Used judiciously, this may allow many patients with diabetes to meet their nutritional goals in fat reduction.

EXERCISE

Potential Benefits and Risks of Exercise

Exercise has many effects—psychosocial, cardiovascular, and metabolic—that may benefit the patient with diabetes. The benefits of exercise include:

- Improving the quality of life and sense of well-being
- Enhancing work capacity

Table 43.3. Summary of Nutritional Recommendations

Nutrient Type	Recommended Intake	Sources
Carbohydrates	50–55% of total daily energy intake Mainly complex carbohydrates, high in fiber	Bread, cereals, fruits Vegetables Milk Cakes, muffins
Protein	60.8 gm/kg of ideal body weight	Meat, fish, poultry Legumes, tofu, cheese, milk

Fat/Cholesterol	Up to 30% of total daily energy intake
	
	Less than 10% saturated
	10% polyunsaturated
	> 10% monounsaturated
		Saturated fat:
		  butter, dairy products, animal fats
		Margarine
		Cholesterol:
		  animal products, egg yolk, organ meats, milk

- Ameliorating cardiovascular risk factors, such as hypertension and obesity
- Favorably altering the lipid profile
- Reducing serum triglyceride levels
- Raising high-density lipoprotein (HDL)-cholesterol levels (To cause significant changes in HDL-cholesterol levels, moderate to heavy exercise, equivalent to running 4 to 8 miles per day, is required.)
- Achieving ideal body weight (Interestingly, improvements in insulin sensitivity may be evident, independent of the weight loss.)

There is a myth that exercise alone will normalize metabolic control. In Type 1 diabetes, exercise has not been shown to significantly improve glycemic control. It is, however, a useful adjunct to nutritional and pharmacological therapy. Exercise plays an important role in the management of Type 2 diabetes (Type 2 DM).

In the fasting state, skeletal muscles obtain energy from fat, while in the fed state, glycogen is first consumed, followed by anaerobic glycolysis. This process would be most important during a short burst of exercise, but as the exercise continues, glucose uptake rises to almost 20 times the basal rate. With prolonged exercise, free fatty acids become the major substrate for muscle energy production.

Insulin levels are usually lower during exercise, allowing more glycogenolysis, but the insulin is more effective at stimulating peripheral glucose uptake.

Acute Effect

In the well-controlled diabetic, exercise may lower glucose levels, since the patient is well-insulinized and hepatic glucose production is suppressed. The poorly controlled patient, however, is under-insulinized, and hepatic glucose production in response to the stress hormones is unchecked and skeletal muscle glucose uptake is diminished. This results in an increase in glucose levels and may even lead to ketosis. Prolonged strenuous exercise (exceeding 80% of your maximal capacity) may also lead to elevation of blood sugars.

Delayed Effect

Muscle glycogen stores are depleted after 40–60 minutes of moderate-intensity exercise; postexercise, glucose flux across muscle increases significantly, which may lead to delayed hypoglycemia!

Risks of Exercise

As with any therapeutic maneuver, there are potential risks of exercise as well. The action of hypoglycemic medications, including sulfonylureas and insulin, may be enhanced with resultant hypoglycemia. Since the patient with diabetes is more likely to have heart disease, symptomatic and asymptomatic, the risk of arrhythmias or ischemic episodes is also

increased. In elderly individuals, antigravity exercise may aggravate degenerative joint disease or more likely lead to soft-tissue injuries. In patients with active retinopathy, strenuous exercise may precipitate intraocular hemorrhage or retinal detachment.

Relative Contraindications to Exercise

Before one proceeds to begin an exercise program, the patient and physician must be aware of some relative contraindications:

- Poor metabolic control
- Significant micro- or macrovascular disease
- Severe peripheral neuropathy
- Hypoglycemic unawareness
- Cardiac autonomic neuropathy

One should correct these problems as much as possible before proceeding to develop an individualized and safe exercise program.

Practical Tips

The type of exercise remains the choice of the patient, but improvement in insulin sensitivity and reduction in cardiovascular risk is evident after relatively mild training. Although aerobic exercise is preferred, resistance exercise in selected groups is safe and also improves glucose control. Exercise sessions should last for about 20–40 minutes, and systolic blood pressures during exercise should be kept below 180–200 mm Hg. One should exercise at least three times weekly.

Planning and foresight is essential. The ability and willingness to self-monitor blood glucose is also crucial. In general, it is better to exercise after meals. One must check blood glucose pre- and postexercise and have a source of carbohydrate readily available. Dehydration should be avoided. Depending on the time of exercise, reduction in either the intermediate-acting insulin (NPH or Lente) or short-acting insulin (Regular) will be necessary. It is preferable to use the abdomen for insulin injections since absorption of insulin in this area is least affected by exercise.

STANDARDS FOR GLUCOSE CONTROL

It is necessary to determine whether an individual's blood sugar control is inadequate on dietary/exercise therapy and whether pharmacological therapy should be initiated. Since the diagnosis of diabetes rests on a fasting blood sugar greater than 126 mg/dl, the goal should be a fasting glucose less than 80–120 mg/dl. An acceptable hemoglobin A_{1c} target would be less than 7% (normal range of 4.0–6.0%). These criteria could also be used with regard to later initiation of insulin therapy. In fact, the current ADA recommendations suggest the goals shown in Table 43.4.

ORAL AGENTS

Sulfonylureas

The sulfonylureas are derived from sulfonamides; thus, there is about a 15 % chance of allergy to a sulfonylurea if the patient has a history of allergy to sulfonamides. The sulfonylureas chiefly increase insulin secretion in response to glucose by inhibiting potassium efflux from pancreatic beta cells, which results in depolarization of the cell membrane. Prolonged therapy leads to increased insulin sensitivity, but the mechanisms for this are poorly understood. It is well known that hyperglycemia will exacerbate insulin resistance; conversely, normalization of glucose levels will reduce the degree of insulin resistance. Direct effects of sulfonylureas on insulin receptors are still the point of much debate. Sulfonylureas are also known to inhibit hepatic glucose production (see Table 43.5).

The newer extended-release preparations and glimepiride appear not to raise fasting insulin levels and thus have lower incidences of hypoglycemia. Potency is a relative variable and is reflected by the actual dosage size of the medications.

Approximately one-third of Type 2 diabetics do not respond to sulfonylureas initially (''primary failure'') and of those who respond, 5–10%/year have ''secondary failure.'' Many of the primary failures may be owing to use of the drugs in inappropriate patients.

The characteristics of a responder include:

- > 40 years of age
- < 5 years duration of diabetes
- Body weight (110%–160% IBW)
- No previous insulin therapy or good control with < 40 u/day
- Fasting plasma glucose < 180 mg/dl

An older obese patient with mild elevation of blood sugars would be the ideal patient. Secondary failure may be related to decreasing pancreatic function but is often caused by noncompliance with lifestyle changes.

Adverse Side Effects of Sulfonylureas   Fewer than 2% of patients taking sulfonylureas will discontinue therapy because of side effects. There is 1–3 % prevalence of GI side effects and less than 0.1% prevalence of hematologic and dermatologic side effects. Patients should be warned of a possible disulfiramlike reaction if alcohol is ingested (this is observed more frequently with chlorpropamide than with other agents). Chlorpropamide can also cause SIADH with symptomatic hyponatremia.

The risk of severe hypoglycemia is about 0.22 per 1000 patient-years compared with 100 per 1000 patient-years for insulin. Prolonged hypoglycemia with glyburide or chlorpropamide may be caused by these drugs' metabolites, which also have a hypoglycemic effect. Gliclazide's metabolites have no hypoglycemic effect. The risk factors for sulfonylurea-induced hypoglycemia include:

- > age 60
- Poor renal function (creatinine > 250 umol/L)
- Poor nutrition
- Interaction with drugs such as insulin, alcohol, salicylates, phenylbutazone, sulfonamides, warfarin, allopurinol, and beta-blockers

Biguanides

The only biguanide available is metformin. Metformin is not bound to plasma proteins and is solely eliminated via the renal route. Exhibiting a half-life is 2–4 hours, metformin is given

---

Table 43.4.   Targets of Glycemic Control

	Goals	Action if:
Premeal glucose (mg/dl)	80–120	< 80 or > 140
Bed-time glucose (mg/dl)	100–140	< 100 or > 160
HbA$_{1c}$ (N = 4%–6%)	< 7%	> 8%

Table 43.5.   Sulfonylureas

Sulfonylureas	Relative Potency	Duration of Action (hr)	Dose Range (mg/day)	Risk of Hypoglycemia
Tolbutamide	1	6–10	500–3000	< 1%
Chlorpropamide	6	24–72	100–500	4%–6%
Glyburide	150	18–24	1.25–20	4%–6%
Glyburide (extended release)	300	24	12	< 4%
Glipizide	75	12–24	2.5–40	5%
Glipizide (extended release)	150	24	5–20	< 4%
Glimepiride	300	24	1–8	< 1.7%

with meals (500–1000 mg) up to three times a day, to a maximum dosage of 2500 mg/day. Metformin does not cause hypoglycemia—thus its mechanism of action is not by enhancing pancreatic insulin secretion. It may be increasing insulin sensitivity or affecting glucose metabolism directly. Metformin also can have an anorexiant effect, which may be beneficial to obese Type 2 diabetics. It also has been shown to lower plasma triglyceride levels.

Typically, metformin has been used in patients who have "failed" on sulfonylureas; one may also use metformin as a first-line medication. It can be combined with sulfonylureas or insulin. Its chief side effects are gastrointestinal (up to 20% of patients), but these can be minimized by starting at a low dose and gradually increasing it as tolerance develops. These side effects would include dyspepsia, anorexia, diarrhoea, and an unpleasant metallic taste. Lactic acidosis is potentially a major side effect, thus metformin should be avoided in patients with cirrhosis, alcoholism, heart failure, and/or renal failure. In more than 20 years of use in Canada and Europe, not one case of lactic acidosis has been reported when metformin was used appropriately.

The FDA recommends that individuals with creatinine values greater than 1.5 mg/dl (1.4 mg/dl for women) should not receive metformin.

Acarbose

Acarbose is a pseudotetrasaccharide that inhibits α-glucosidases in the brush border of the small intestine. These enzymes are responsible for digestion of starch, dextrins, maltose, and sucrose into monosaccharides, which can then be absorbed. Acarbose reduces postprandial hyperglycemia and is currently approved for use in patients with Type 2 DM. Side effects may include flatulence and diarrhea. It can be safely combined with other oral agents. It may also have a role in reducing postprandial hyperglycemia in those taking insulin therapy. Starting dose is 25 mg once daily, gradually increasing to three times a day; the dose may be increased to 50 mg three times a day with meals. The expectation is that HbA_{1c} may be reduced by an absolute level of about 0.75% to 1.0% (N = 4–6%). However, in patients with higher levels of HbA_{1c}, the effect of acarbose may be larger.

Troglitazone

Troglitazone is the first product available from the family of compounds known as insulin sensitizers (thiazolidenediones). It increases insulin sensitivity in the liver, skeletal muscle, and fat. It has no effect on insulin secretion. The dose range is 200 to 600 mg once daily.

Troglitazone modestly reduces fasting and postmeal sugar levels in obese Type 2 DM individuals. In individuals with insulin resistance or impaired glucose tolerance, troglitazone has been shown to be very effective. It does appear to have moderating effects on VLDL-triglyceride levels and on blood pressure levels.

Troglitazone seems to be well tolerated. It may increase some liver enzymes, which is reversible. There are some other minor side effects of troglitazone.

Troglitazone may be quite effective in early diabetes or in treating impaired glucose tolerance. With concern about hyperinsulinemia and associated macrovascular risk, troglitazone may also be used to reduce one's dose of insulin. Initially, troglitazone was recommended for those with Type 2 diabetes who take more than 35 units of insulin per day and have uncontrolled diabetes (HbA_{1c} greater than 8.5%). Recently, it has been approved as a single-agent therapy for Type 2 diabetes. Additional recommendations include periodic monitoring of liver enzymes to screen for any hepatotoxocity.

Therapy with Several Oral Agents

There is certainly no benefit of prescribing two sulfonylureas at the same time and certainly a greater chance of side effects. However, a sulfonylurea can be combined with metformin, resulting in improved glucose control and delay of insulin therapy. One normally adds another oral agent if the patient is already taking maximal doses of the initial oral agent. At this stage in the patient's diabetes, it would be prudent to advise the patient of the need for insulin therapy in the near future. The potential of hypoglycemic episodes increases with use of multiple medications and thus may best be initially supervised by a specialist.

INSULIN THERAPY

All patients beginning insulin therapy should be started on human insulin preparations. Patients receiving insulin temporarily (e.g., intercurrent illness, operation, or pregnancy) should also be prescribed human insulin preparations (see Table 43.6).

Fast-Acting Insulin Analog (Lispro Insulin)

This insulin analog is 100% homologous with human insulin with respect to amino acid composition and 95% homologous

Table 43.6.   Commonly Used Insulin Preparations

Type of Insulin	Onset (hrs)	Peak (hrs)	Duration (hrs)
Rapid			
Lispro	0.25	1	3–4
Short			
Regular	0.5	2–4	5–7
Intermediate			
NPH	1–2	6–12	14–24
Lente	1–2	6–12	18–24
Long			
Ultra-lente	4–6	18–24	32–36

with respect to amino acid sequence. Two amino acids, lysine and proline in the C-terminal of the B-chain of insulin, have been transposed, leading to the following characteristics of lispro:

- Dissociates very rapidly after subcutaneous injection into monomers and thus begins to work within 15 minutes of injection
- Acts for 3–4 hours only
- Half-life does not seem to be affected by increases in dose (as happens with regular insulin)
- Can be mixed with other insulins, such as NPH or Lente or Ultra-lente
- Unit for unit offers the same potency of regular insulin but with quite different onset and duration

Lispro insulin has been extensively studied in both Type 1 DM, as well as Type 2 DM individuals. It is accepted easily by patients because of convenience of not having to take insulin injections 30–45 minutes prior to a meal. Nocturnal hypoglycemic events are less common and postprandial glucoses are significantly lower than with the use of regular insulin. There is no increase in antibody response to lispro insulin. There does not appear to be any difference in HbA$_{1c}$ values between patients treated with regular insulin and those treated with lispro insulin.

Some modifications with respect to timing of intermediate acting insulins in combination with lispro insulin may have to be made. Early trials using lispro insulin in insulin pump therapy have been very positive.

There are special premixed insulin preparations (e.g., 30% regular/70% NPH and 50% regular/50% NPH), which may be useful for those with very stable diabetes or for those who might have difficulties with mixing insulins manually. The above time frames are quite variable and can fluctuate by 20–30% between individuals and even within the same individual. Factors that decrease or delay the action of insulin injections include:

- Higher dose of insulin
- Higher glucose levels preinjection
- Site of absorption: (thigh > arm > abdomen)
- Cooler temperature of skin
- Sedentary (versus exercise)
- Hepatic and renal degradation
- High titers of anti-insulin antibodies (rarely)

Side effects of insulin include hypoglycemia and lipohypertrophy. Allergic phenomena include both local and systemic skin reactions and lipoatrophy.

Dosage regimens may start simply and can increase in complexity, depending on the patient's target goals and his or her motivation. More intensive regimens require more frequent self-monitoring of blood glucose. Blood sugar monitoring caveats include:

- Morning sugar reflects the evening intermediate insulin dose.

- Lunch sugar reflects the morning regular insulin dose.
- Supper/dinner sugar reflects morning intermediate insulin dose.
- Bed-time sugar reflects the presupper regular insulin dose.
- Most individuals will require two injections per day.

The use of sulfonylureas in combination with insulin therapy in Type 2 diabetics has become popular recently, but published clinical data has been equivocal. Insulin therapy is thought to ''rest the pancreatic β-cells'' and lead to sulfonylurea responsiveness. Thus combination therapy might initially lead to smoother and better glucose control, but there is not likely to be any long-term benefit. A recent study by Yki-Jarvinen, et al. reported that there were no differences in glucose control between combination therapy and insulin therapy alone, but in patients treated with oral agents and evening NPH insulin, there was less hyperinsulinemia and less weight gain. Some consider hyperinsulinemia a risk factor for development of atherosclerosis and hypertension and thus favor combination therapy on a theoretical basis. If hyperinsulinemia is indeed a biologically significant risk factor, then combination therapy may be preferred in the future. This is certainly not recommended as a usual approach and should be initiated or supervised by a specialist.

Initiating Insulin

Most patients begin with approximately 0.3 to 0.5 units per kg of insulin per day. Typically 2/3 of insulin is given in AM and 1/3 given in PM. If both intermediate and rapid-acting insulins are needed, typically 2/3 is intermediate while 1/3 is regular. Insulin regimens:

- Phase I
  - AM intermediate only or
  - HS intermediate only or
  - HS ultralente only or
  - HS intermediate + oral agents during the day
- Phase II
  - Intermediate insulin two times a day (before breakfast and supper) or
  - Intermediate insulin two times a day (before breakfast and hs)
- Phase III
  - Add regular insulin before breakfast + supper
- Phase IV
  - Regular before meals and hs + hs intermediate or
  - Regular before meals and hs + hs long-acting or
  - Insulin pump therapy

Oral agents are safe and effective in the management of Type 2 diabetes, if patients for therapy are chosen wisely and are followed judiciously. One may begin with either a sulfonylurea or a biguanide; both types of oral agents may be prescribed later if blood glucose control is still unacceptable.

COMPLICATIONS OF DIABETES

GENERAL MECHANISMS

The chronic hyperglycemia to which individuals with diabetes are exposed is paramount in the etiology of diabetic complications. Hyperglycemia may play a role via several mechanisms:

- Nonenzymatic glycosylation of protein structures, leading to altered blood vessel function
- Conversion of glucose to sorbitol via intracellular aldose reductase enzyme, which leads to accumulation of sorbitol, which in turn can have several deleterious effects on cellular function
- Adversely affecting coagulability, platelet function, atherogenic potential of lipoproteins and increased susceptibility to free oxygen radical induced damage

Diabetes Control and Complications Trial

Results of the Diabetes Control and Complications Trial (DCCT), a historic study designed to test whether chronic hyperglycemia is related to development of complications in Type 1 DM, clearly demonstrated that intensive treatment of individuals with Type 1 DM delays the onset and progression of long-term complications in patients without complications and in those patients with early complications. More than 1400 individuals with Type 1 DM (between the ages of 13 and 39 years) were entered into the study, and more than 99% of them completed it. Half of the subjects were enrolled in a standard treatment program (twice-daily insulin injections), while the others were intensively treated (multiple daily insulin injections or insulin pump therapy). The standard treatment group's goals were to remain clinically well and symptom-free, while the goal of the intensive treatment group was normalization of blood sugar levels.

Intensive therapy included:

- More-frequent doses of insulin per day
- Self-adjustment of insulin according to meal content, exercise activity, and sugar levels
- Frequent dietary instructions and monthly clinic visits

This regimen required a great deal of commitment from both the volunteer subjects and the Diabetes Health Care Teams.

Intensive therapy resulted in a substantially lower HbA_{1c} than standard therapy. Intensive therapy reduced clinically meaningful eye changes by 34–76% and reduced the first appearance of any eye changes by 27%. Evidence of kidney complications was reduced by 35%. Evidence of nerve damage was reduced by 60%. Subjects in the intensively treated group were three times more likely to have severe low blood sugar reactions. However, intensive therapy did not worsen their quality of life.

Wang Analysis

A meta-analysis by Wang, et al. included 16 studies of patients with Type 1 diabetes and concluded that long-term intensive glycemic control significantly reduced risks of progression of diabetic retinopathy and nephropathy. Patients with the following characteristics may not be good candidates for intensive therapy:

- Unable to follow the intensive treatment
- Younger than age 13
- Elderly and have established severe complications
- Significant heart disease
- Hypoglycemic unawareness
- Repeated severe hypoglycemia (more than 2 episodes in previous 2 years)
- End-stage complications

Kumamoto Study

The Kumamoto Study compared the incidence and progression of microvascular complications in 110 Japanese patients with Type 2 DM treated with intensive insulin therapy with that of conventionally treated patients with Type 2 DM. The intensively treated group had a HbA_{1c} of 7.1%, while the conventionally treated group had a mean HbA_{1c} of 9.4%. Reductions in the progression of retinopathy and nephropathy, similar to the rates observed in the DCCT trial, were observed in the intensively treated group. Thus, intensive therapy appears to be beneficial to patients with Type 2 diabetes, as well.

Wisconsin Epidemiological Study of Diabetic Retinopathy

The Wisconsin Epidemiological Study of Diabetic Retinopathy (WESDR), a population-based study with a longitudinal follow-up of 2990 subjects with diabetes, revealed a significant relationship between baseline glycated hemoglobin and all aspects of retinopathy, microalbuminuria, and gross proteinuria. In both the Type 1 and Type 2 diabetic groups, the study showed a similar relationship between glycosylated hemoglobin and lower extremity amputation, as well as all-cause mortality.

Smoking

Despite the background of public strategies to educate society about the hazards of smoking and to reduce tobacco consumption, many individuals with DM smoke. The 1988 Behavioral Risk Factor Surveillance System in the United States reported that prevalence of smoking in the diabetic population was the same as in the general population. It was also noted that young African-Americans with diabetes (ages 18–34) who had not completed high school had higher rates of smoking compared with the controls.

Considering the overall health of individuals with diabetes, cigarette smoking is an important cause of further increase in complications of diabetes and in diabetes-associated morbidity and mortality. There have been several prospective cohort studies that have lent support to this conclusion. Yudkin calculated that smoking cessation would prolong life by 3 years in a man with diabetes, while aspirin and antihypertensive therapy would prolong life by 1 year only.

MICROVASCULAR COMPLICATIONS

Retinopathy

Diabetes is responsible for 8% of blindness in the United States and is the leading cause of blindness in the 20–64 age range. The most common form of retinopathy is nonproliferative (background) retinopathy, which consists of microaneurysms, intraretinal hemorrhages, and/or exudates. Infarction of the nerve layer of the retina may occur, causing cotton-wool exudates. This ischemia is thought to play a role in the eventual proliferation of new, friable vessels from the retina into the vitreous. This latter phase is termed proliferative retinopathy and is associated with vitreous hemorrhages, retinal scarring, and potential retinal detachment. Altered expression of various local growth factors within the retina are thought to mediate the vascular changes in the retina. Macular edema is also more prevalent in those with diabetes, and may occur with or without proliferative retinopathy. Referral to an ophthalmologist should be done at the time of diagnosis of Type 2 DM, while referral to an ophthalmologist should be made 5 years after diagnosis of Type 1 DM, if the patient is asymptomatic.

The most important risk factors for retinopathy include:

- Duration of diabetes
- Glycemic control
- Hypertension

Depending on the stage of retinopathy, management includes:

- Appropriate frequency of funduscopic examination (more during pregnancy)
- Improved control of hyperglycemia and hypertension
- Early laser treatment
- Vitrectomy

Nephropathy

Renal failure is a major cause of mortality in patients with diabetes. In the United States, approximately one in three patients on dialysis has diabetes. Whereas retinopathy eventually occurs in almost all patients with diabetes, clinical nephropathy develops in about 40% of individuals with Type 1 DM and in less than 20% of those with Type 2 DM. The most important risk factors for nephropathy include:

- Duration of diabetes
- Glycemic control
- Hypertension
- Smoking
- Hypercholesterolemia

Recent prospective studies lend support to the hypothesis that smoking accelerates nephropathy in patients with diabetes. In a clinic-based prospective study by Chase and colleagues, the odds ratio of developing significant albuminuria was 2.2 times higher in smokers. Most other studies also confirm this finding. Recent interest has focused on polymorphism of various genes linked to hypertension, such as the angiotensin converting enzyme (ACE) gene. Proteinuria, which is 15 times more frequent in diabetics compared with nondiabetics, worsens the prognosis and is a prognostic factor with respect to renal failure and macrovascular disease.

In 1996, the National Kidney Foundation recommended that all diabetics ages 12–70 have their urine tested for albumin at least annually. Ideally, the individual should be metabolically stable. Heavy exercise, urinary tract infection, acute febrile illness, and heart failure may transiently increase urinary albumin excretion. NSAIDs and ACE inhibitors should be avoided during screening.

A 24-hour or overnight (8–12-hour timed) collection is the most sensitive screening method. Albumin excretion rates greater than 30 mg/24 hours or above 20 μg/min are indicative of diabetic nephropathy when confirmed on at least two urine samples. Since timed-collections are often impractical, the recommendation of using albumin/creatinine ratio was made. A urinary albumin/creatinine ratio of 30–300 mg/g indicates the presence of microalbuminuria. Various national guidelines have recommended testing for microalbuminuria at the time of diagnosis of Type 2 DM and 5 years after diagnosis of Type 1 DM (see Table 43.7).

In most circumstances, the blood pressure should be lower than 140/90 mm Hg, but in the presence of microalbuminuria, the blood pressure should be 130/85 mm Hg or lower. The first measures should be to improve blood glucose control, quit smoking, achieve an optimal body weight, and to follow the proper lifestyle. Subsequently, ACE-inhibitors, calcium channel blockers and alpha-blockers may be used. In the presence of microalbuminuria, the use of ACE-inhibitors is generally favored. Recent trials have shown that use of captopril can reduce the need for dialysis and delay adverse outcomes.

Neuropathy

Neuropathy, one of the most common complications of diabetes, can affect the sensory, motor, and autonomic nervous systems. Some patients develop painful symptoms or paresthesiae. For peripheral painful neuropathy, tricyclics, diphenylhydantoin, and carbamazepine have been used, but newer agents that are potentially helpful are available, including topical capsaicin, mexilitene, and GABApentin.

Hypoglycemic unawareness is a sign of autonomic dysfunction and is often present in individuals with Type 1 DM for more than 15 years. At this point, intensive control of diabetes is dangerous, and one should set appropriately higher targets for blood glucose control.

Symptoms of postural hypertension are associated with a

Table 43.7. Natural History of Diabetic Nephropathy

Stage	Renal Pathology	Albumin Excretion	GFR	Management
Diagnosis	Normal or renal hypertrophy	None	Increased	1. Improved glucose control
3–15 years	1. Basement membrane thickening 2. Increased mesangial matrix 3. Glomerulosclerosis	Microalbuminuria (30–300 mg/24 hrs.)	Normal	1. As above 2. Monitor and treat hypertension
Incipient nephropathy	Advancing glomerulosclerosis	Macroalbuminuria	Normal	1 & 2 and 3. Protein restriction
Nephrotic syndrome	Progression	> 1.5 g/24 hrs.	Normal or decreased	1 & 2 & 3 and 4. Diuretic therapy
End-stage renal disease	Loss of tubular function		Progressively decreasing	1, 2, 3, 4 and management of renal failure

poor prognosis in those with diabetes. Traditionally, levophed and/or 9-β fludrocortisone (Florinef) have been used. Patients may also respond to low doses of beta-blockers. For associated nocturnal diarrhea, once infectious causes have been ruled out, clonidine or bile acid sequestrants may be helpful.

Autonomic dysfunction may affect the GI system, or GU system, resulting in constipation, gastroparesis, diabetic diarrhea, erectile dysfunction and/or a neurogenic bladder.

It is crucial to always consider causes other than diabetes in the etiology of any neuropathy.

MACROVASCULAR COMPLICATIONS

Atherosclerotic vascular disease is a major cause of morbidity and mortality in patients with DM. For Type 1 diabetic patients, greater than one-third of the mortality is owing to cardiac and cerebral vascular disease; for Type 2 diabetic patients, two-thirds of the mortality is because of large vessel disease (macrovascular disease).

In the classic Whitehall study, there was clearly increased mortality from coronary heart disease in glucose-intolerant individuals and diabetics. Age and blood pressure were the most strongly related risk factors related to subsequent death from coronary heart disease. Various other epidemiological studies have implicated cigarette smoking, dyslipidemias, and hyperinsulinemia as important corisk factors in DM. Other factors associated with development of macrovascular disease are high fibrinogen levels and the presence of cataracts.

Clinical Presentation

Not only the incidence but extent of atherosclerosis is greater in diabetics, as confirmed by pathological and angiographic studies. Within any artery the disease may be diffuse as well. Although infarct size may not differ from that of nondiabetics,

post-MI complications occur more frequently in the diabetic population. In a prospective study, Oswald, et al. showed that the patient's metabolic control prior to the MI had an impact on early mortality (23% mortality with normal HbA$_{1c}$, 33% mortality with HbA$_{1c}$ of 7.5–8.5%, and 63% mortality with Hb greater than 8.5%). There is also greater late-mortality post-MI. These and above features are no doubt owing to coexisting changes in the hearts of diabetic patients (such as cardiomyopathy, autonomic neuropathy and more diffuse atherosclerotic disease).

Females with diabetes tend to be at a relatively higher risk. The Framingham study reported that the average adjusted incidence of intermittent claudication was 12.6 per 1000 for diabetic men and 8.4 per 1000 for diabetic women, compared with 3.3 per 1000 and 1.3 per 1000 for nondiabetic men and women, respectively. One potential reason for the absence of protection versus atherosclerotic disease in diabetic women is the markedly different lipid profiles evident in these patients. Quite often, they exhibit elevated triglycerides and lower HDL-cholesterol levels.

Coronary Bypass Surgery

Although coronary bypass surgery is efficacious in diabetics with coronary heart disease (diabetic patients must pass the same criteria as nondiabetics), many studies have shown that diabetics will have more associated risk factors, poorer left ventricular function, and a poorer long-term prognosis. The Bypass Angioplasty Revascularization Investigation (BARI Study) of 1829 patients needing a first revascularization reported that in a subgroup of 353 drug-treated diabetics, the 5-year mortality rate with CABG was 19% compared with 35% for angioplasty. The 5-year mortality for the remainder of the subjects was 9%. The mortality was not due to acute complications of the procedures.

There is compelling evidence for the role of hyperglycemia in accelerating atherosclerosis, but there is well-documented evidence that individuals with impaired glucose tolerance but without DM (as defined by national and international guidelines) have much higher rates of cardiovascular disease (CVD). This would imply that individuals with impaired glucose tolerance of any degree are at increased risk of CVD.

Also, the duration of Type 2 diabetes does not correlate very highly with the incidence of cardiovascular disease. This latter observation may be because of a lack of early diagnosis of DM in asymptomatic individuals.

The risk of CVD in a particular patient will also depend upon his or her ethnic origin. For example, Japanese have a lower prevalence of atherosclerosis, which is evident when one compares Japanese diabetics with those from North America. On the other hand, Japanese who have migrated to Hawaii have a higher incidence of CVD than those still living in Japan, underscoring the tremendous interplay between inherited and environmental factors.

PREGNANCY

Pregnancy complicated by pre-existing diabetes has a 10–20-fold increase in risk of congenital malformations. These include neural tube defects and cardiac defects. Excellent control after conception leads to a dramatic decrease in complications but still a 2–3-fold increase in congenital malformations. It is highly advisable that excellent metabolic control be instituted prior to pregnancy. The metabolic complications of the fetus, such as perinatal death, hypoglycemia, hypocalcemia, respiratory distress syndrome, and jaundice, are reduced in prevalence to levels observed in normal pregnancies. There is sufficient animal data demonstrating toxic effects of ketones to CNS development that ketosis should be actively prevented.

The ''White'' classification of diabetic pregnancies has been useful in predicting outcomes. Unfavorable variables include:

- Increasing age
- Increasing duration of diabetes
- Presence of retinopathy
- Nephropathy
- Heart disease

Gestational diabetes occurs in approximately 2–3% of pregnancies, and its treatment is controversial. In North America, all pregnant individuals are recommended to be screened for diabetes between the 24th and 28th weeks, according to guidelines outlined above in the OGTT discussion. By definition, the woman should not have diabetes postpartum. There is no increase in congenital malformations, but there does appear to be an increase in macrosomia and neonatal hypoglycemia. The management is usually with diet and exercise and insulin, if necessary. Oral agents are not used. There is some preliminary evidence that the infants of diabetic mothers may later develop insulin resistance.

HYPOGLYCEMIA

Diabetes-Associated Hypoglycemia

Diabetes-associated hypoglycemia is often caused by a mismatch of caloric intake to insulin peaks. Physicians need to take a careful history, being particularly attentive to:

- Late or missed meals
- Exercise
- Excessive insulin or sulfonylureas
- Hypoglycemic unawareness
- Gastroparesis
- Use of alcohol or sedatives
- Renal or hepatic impairment
- Coincidental hypoadrenalism or hypopituitarism

Nondiabetes-Associated Hypoglycemia

The symptoms may be either adrenergic or neuroglycopenic, with the adrenergic signs occurring earlier at glucose levels less then 50 mg/dl. Clinically, one needs to distinguish between fasting and reactive hypoglycemia. Fasting hypoglycemia infers a pathological cause, while reactive hypoglycemia tends to be a functional, benign phenomenon.

The gold standard test is the 72-hour fast to measure serial glucose and insulin levels. At the time of hypoglycemia or symptoms, a C-peptide level is also drawn. This is critical in ruling out exogenous insulin as a cause. Sulfonylureas may increase C-peptide levels and thus should be screened for in a 24-hour urine.

The liver is of prime importance in the etiology of hypoglycemia. Thus, GH or cortisol deficiencies, severe malnutrition, excessive alcohol, and liver failure can be associated with reduced hepatic glucose output. Sulfonylureas, quinine, pentamidine, disopyramide or MAO inhibitors may increase insulin levels. Rarely anti-insulin receptor Ab or anti-insulin Ab may be linked to hypoglycemia. A thorough history and physical examination can rule out many of the above causes.

An insulinoma is favored in the presence of fasting symptoms, accompanied by an insulin/glucose ratio of > 0.3 mU/L/mg/dl; elevated C-peptide levels are very supportive. Insulinomas should be localized preoperatively with use of CT-angiography of the pancreas and occasionally with the help of selective transhepatic catheterization of pancreatic veins or intraoperative ultrasound of the pancreas. Less than 10% are multiple and associated with MEN-I syndrome.

REVIEW EXERCISES

QUESTIONS

1. Fred Paulesco, a 55-year-old businessman, comes to your office complaining of fatigue. He denies any weight change. He has nocturia X 1–2. His 75-year-old mother is a diabetic. His father died at age 60 of premature heart disease. Fred has history of hypertension treated with hydrochlorthiazide 50 mg/day. Physical examination revealed him to be 50% above his ideal body weight with a blood pressure of 135/90. The rest of the examination is unremarkable. Laboratory evaluation revealed his fasting plasma glucose to be 120 mg/dl, Na = 143 meq/L, K = 3.1 meq/ml, Cl = 100 meq/L, bicarbonate = 26 meq/L. BUN = 12 mg/dl and creatinine = 1.1 mg/dl. Hemoglobin A1c = 6.0% (N = 4–6%). Which of the following is false:

   a. With a normal HbA_{1c}, he is unlikely to have diabetes.
   b. An oral glucose tolerance test is not indicated.
   c. Risk factors for diabetes include his family history, obesity, hypertension, and hypokalemia.
   d. His hypokalemia should be corrected prior to retesting his plasma glucose level.
   e. He would benefit from weight reduction, increased exercise, and improved dietary habits.

2. Fred returns to your office 6 months later, having missed several return appointments. Despite following your lifestyle prescription, he continues to be fatigued, has experienced a 10-pound weight loss, and presents with polydipsia, polyuria, and blurred vision. He has been monitoring his capillary blood sugars, and they have been consistently above 250 mg/dl. You make the diagnosis of DM. You examine him more closely. Which of the following feature(s) favor Type 1 (Type 1 DM):

   a. Presence of vitiligo
   b. Obesity and age of 55 years
   c. Negative for islet cell antibodies
   d. Family history of diabetes
   e. C-peptide levels at upper limit of normal

3. The dietitian is on holiday, and you have to counsel the patient regarding nutrition. Which of the following recommendations would you not make:

   a. Avoid all sweet foods.
   b. Encourage 50% carbohydrate, less than 30% fat and 20% protein.
   c. No need for vanadium or chromium supplements.
   d. Increase fiber intake and decrease amount of saturated fat.
   e. Space your caloric intake over the whole day.

4. Fred is interested in increasing his physical activity. He wonders how exercise will affect his diabetes. Which of the following is false:

   a. Exercise may acutely increase his blood sugar levels.
   b. Exercise may acutely decrease his blood sugar levels.
   c. Exercise may not benefit his glucose control if he has Type 2 DM.
   d. Exercise may not benefit his glucose control if he has Type 1 DM.
   e. Exercise will have to be individualized according to his previous habits and to the presence of any diabetic complications.

5. Fred's sister, Charlotte, who is visiting from out of town, is also known to have Type 2 DM and hypertension. She is treated with glyburide 10 mg two times a day and her fasting blood sugars are averaging 160 mg/dl and her HbA_{1c} is 8.8% (N = 4%–6%). She seeks your counsel. Physical examination is unremarkable except for moderate obesity. Lab work: fasting glucose = 200 mg/dl, BUN = 25 mg/dl, creatinine = 1.9 mg/dl, electrolytes are normal. Liver enzymes are normal. Which of the following would be reasonable recommendations in addition to improving her dietary habits and exercise regimen:

   a. Decrease glyburide to 5 mg two times a day.
   b. Add metformin 500 mg two times a day after meals.
   c. Add acarbose 25 mg three times a day.
   d. Add troglitazone 600 mg every day.

6. Five years later, on a clinic visit, Fred is noted to have microalbuminuria. Your review indicates he has Type 2 DM, a BP of 140/90 and a HbA_{1c} of 9.0%. He is being treated with an ACE-inhibitor and maximal doses of glyburide. Which of the following options would be your management:

   a. Intensify your antihypertensive regimen.
   b. Intensify glucose control only.
   c. Begin insulin injection therapy.
   d. Aim to lower blood pressure and blood sugars.

7. Ten years later, Fred is noted have orthostatic hypotension. There are no signs or symptoms of heart failure or respiratory distress. Sitting blood pressure is 130/75. He is afebrile. Which of these is not compatible with his presentation:

a. Insomnia
b. Constipation
c. Supine blood pressure of 150/95
d. Gastroparesis
e. Persistent resting sinus tachycardia

Answers

1. a
    A normal HbA_{1c} does not exclude diabetes mellitus.
2. a
    Vitiligo is an autoimmune condition and more likely to occur with Type 1 DM.
3. a
    Some simple sugars are allowed (up to 15% total calories), provided the overall dietary intake is appropriate.
4. c
    Exercise is very important for controlling Type 2 DM.

5. c
    One would not reduce glyburide dose. With an elevated creatinine, one would not prescribe metformin.
    Troglitazone could be used but should be started at 200 mg/day.
6. d
    Both glycemic control and blood pressure are key factors in the development of diabetic nephropathy.
7. e
    All are symptoms/signs of autonomic neuropathy except insomnia.

SUGGESTED READINGS

The Diabetes Control and Complications Trial Research Group. The effect of intensive treatment of diabetes on the development and progression of long-term complications in insulin-dependent DM. N Engl J Med 1993;329:977–986.

JE Gerich. Oral hypoglycemic agents. N Engl J Med 1989; 321;1231–1245.

Okhubo Y, Kishikawa H, Araki E, et al. Intensive insulin therapy prevents the progression of diabetic microvascular complications in Japanese patients with non-insulin dependent diabetes mellitus: a randomized prospective 6-year study. Diabetes Res Clin Pract 1995;28:103–117.

The physician's guide to Type 2 diabetes: diagnosis and treatment. American Diabetes Association, 1996.

Becker K, ed. Principles and practice of endocrinology and metabolism. 2nd ed. Philadelphia: JB Lippincott, 1995.

Zinman B. Physiologic replacement of insulin. N Engl J Med 1989;321:363–370.

The Expert Committee on the Diagnosis and Classification of Diabetes Mellitus. Report. Diabetes Care 1997;20: 1183–1197.

44

Adrenal Disorders

Rossana D. Danese

ANATOMY AND PHYSIOLOGY OF THE ADRENAL GLAND

The adrenal gland consists of the medulla and the cortex, which is further divided into the zona reticularis, the zona fasciculata, and the zona glomerulosa (Fig. 44.1). The medulla produces catecholamines, norepinephrine, and epinephrine. The zonae fasciculata and reticularis produce cortisol and androgens (mainly DHEAs), while aldosterone is the product of the zona glomerulosa. The lack of cortisol and androgen production by the zona glomerulosa is a result of the absence of 17 hydroxylase.

The zonae reticularis and fasciculata are under the control of ACTH released by the pituitary gland in response to hypothalamic CRH. CRH, in turn, is regulated by cortisol negative feedback, stress, and a circadian rhythm. Besides increasing the synthesis of cortisol, ACTH is trophic for the adrenal gland, so that a lack of ACTH results in atrophy of the zonae fasciculata and reticularis. Although ACTH has some effect on aldosterone production, the zona glomerulosa is predominantly under the control of renin. Understanding the anatomy and physiology of the adrenal gland is crucial to understanding its hypofunction and hyperfunction.

Adrenal Insufficiency

ETIOLOGY OF ADRENAL INSUFFICIENCY

Clinical adrenal insufficiency (AI) results from the hypofunction of part or all of the adrenal cortex. This may be due to destruction of the adrenal gland itself (Addison's disease, primary AI), or a lack of ACTH (secondary AI), or CRH.

The most common cause of Addison's disease is autoimmune destruction of the adrenal gland (~ 80%). In adults, this is often seen in association with other autoimmune diseases, including Hashimoto's thyroiditis or Graves' disease and Type I diabetes mellitus. This is known as Type II autoimmune polyglandular syndrome. (Type I autoimmune polyglandular syndrome, more commonly seen in children, consists of Addison's disease, hypoparathyroidism, and mucocutaneous candidiasis.) Other clues to the presence of autoimmune AI include:

- Chromosomal disorders (Down, Klinefelter's, and Turner's syndromes)
- Alopecia
- Vitiligo
- Other autoimmune disorders (pernicious anemia, chronic active hepatitis, myasthenia gravis, primary hypogonadism)

Besides autoimmune disease, other causes of primary AI in the adult include:

- Infection
  - Mycobacterial
  - Fungal
  - Viral
- Hemorrhage/infarction
  - Anticoagulants/coagulopathy
  - Sepsis
  - Thrombosis
- Metastatic cancer
  - Breast
  - Lung

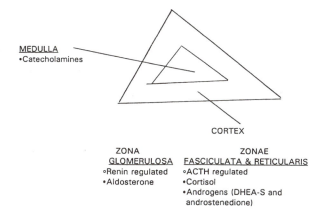

Figure 44.1. The adrenal gland.

- GI
- Lymphoma
- Infiltrative disorders
  - Amyloidosis
  - Sarcoidosis
  - Hemochromatosis
- Adrenoleukodystrophy/adrenomyeloneuropathy
  - Affects young men (X-linked) — abnormal accumulation of very-long chainfatty acids in adrenal cortex, brain, testes and liver
  - Adrenal insufficiency and CNS demyelination

Currently, AIDS is the most common cause of infectious adrenal destruction, while the antiphospholipid syndrome (lupus anticoagulant) is being increasingly recognized as a cause of adrenal hemorrhage.

Secondary adrenal insufficiency is a result of adrenal gland atrophy from ACTH deficiency. This most often results from:

- Pituitary corticotroph atrophy owing to previous exogenous glucocorticoid
- Hypopituitarism

CLINICAL PRESENTATION OF ADRENAL INSUFFICIENCY

The underlying etiology of the adrenal insufficiency determines the clinical presentation (Table 44.1). Under the regulation of ACTH, cortisol and the adrenal androgens are lost in both primary and secondary AI. Aldosterone production, predominantly under regulation by renin, remains intact in secondary AI. Therefore, hyperkalemia and profound dehydration with orthostatic hypotension are seen in primary adrenal insufficiency only. Likewise, hyperpigmentation of the skin or mucus membranes (owing to increased ACTH) is seen in primary AI only. Consequently, the absence of hyperkalemia and/or hyperpigmentation does not exclude AI.

Table 44.1. Adrenal Insufficiency Signs and Symptoms

	Primary AI	*Secondary AI*
Cortisol Deficiency		
Anorexia/nausea/vomiting		
Weight loss/fatigue		
Myalgias/arthralgias	Yes	Yes
Hypotension		
Hyponatremia		
Androgen Deficiency		
Loss of axillary & pubic hair (usually female only)	Yes	Yes
Aldosterone Deficiency		
Hyperkalemia		
Orthostasis	Yes	No
ACTH Excess		
Hyperpigmentation	Yes	No

In addition to hyponatremia and hyperkalemia, lab abnormalities in adrenal insufficiency may include:

- Hypoglycemia
- Hypercalcemia
- Eosinophilia
- Lymphocytosis

DIAGNOSIS OF ADRENAL INSUFFICIENCY

The diagnosis of adrenal insufficiency is made by demonstrating diminished responsiveness of the hypothalamic-pituitary-adrenal (HPA) axis to stimulation. A morning cortisol less than 3 μg/dl (assuming normal cortisol binding globulin) can be sufficient to make the diagnosis; however, the cortrosyn stimulation test (CST) is usually required. Cortrosyn (synthetic ACTH), 250 μg intramuscularly or intravenously, is administered after a baseline cortisol and the cortisol response at 30 and 60 minutes measured. A rise in the cortisol level to $\geq$ 18 μg/dl is a normal response. If an abnormal response is obtained, an ACTH level then determines primary (high ACTH) versus secondary disease (normal or low ACTH).

In secondary AI, the CST is not always abnormal, however. Adequate ACTH may be present to prevent adrenal gland atrophy (thereby resulting in a response to the supraphysiologic dose of ACTH used in the CST), but the HPA axis may not be able to respond to stress. In patients with suspected secondary AI and a normal CST, the insulin tolerance test or the metyrapone test can be used to make the diagnosis. These tests evaluate the integrity of the HPA axis by its response to hypoglycemia and inhibited cortisol synthesis, respectively.

TREATMENT OF ADRENAL INSUFFICIENCY

Treatment summary:

- Hydrocortisone 30 mg =
- Prednisone 7.5 mg =
- Dexamethasone 0.75 mg

The treatment of adrenal insufficiency is replacement of the deficient hormones. Cortisol—usually given as Cortef 20 mg in the morning and 10 mg in the evening or prednisone 5–7.5 mg daily—provides dramatic relief of symptoms. However, to prevent Cushing's syndrome, the smallest dose needed to control the patient's symptoms should be used. For a minor illness, the glucocorticoid dose should be doubled for as short a time as needed. For a major stress, 200–400 mg/24 hrs of parenteral hydrocortisone is given initially then rapidly tapered. Aldosterone replacement is required in primary AI only and is given as fludrocortisone 0.05–0.2 mg daily. The dose is usually adjusted according to the blood pressure and potassium level. The adrenal androgens are not replaced.

In undiagnosed patients with suspected adrenal crisis, dexamethasone, 2–4 mg intravenously or intramuscularly, should be given along with saline and glucose. Dexamethasone will not interfere with establishing the diagnosis by cross-reacting with cortisol in its assay. The CST should then be done as soon as possible.

In the management of secondary adrenal insufficiency caused by previous exogenous steroids, glucocorticoids with short half-lives (usually cortisone) should be given as larger doses in the morning and smaller doses in the evening. The PM doses are gradually tapered, as symptoms permit, to allow overnight hypothalamic/pituitary ''desuppression'' and a rise in ACTH. This leads to return of adrenal gland function; once a morning cortisol reaches 10 μg/dl, replacement glucocorticoid can generally be discontinued. Stress glucocorticoids, however, should be given until a CST is normal. Recovery of the HPA axis from glucocorticoid suppression generally requires 6–12 months.

Hypoaldosteronism

Hypoaldosteronism is the result of decreased aldosterone production by the zona glomerulosa of the adrenal cortex. In the adult, primary hypoaldosteronism is caused by destruction of the adrenal gland, as in Addison's disease, and therefore renin levels are elevated. Chronic heparin use and critical illness have also been associated with hyperreninemic hypoaldosteronism.

Secondary hypoaldosteronism results from a deficiency of renin action. In the adult, hyporeninemic hypoaldosteronism should be suspected in:

- Elderly patients with renal insufficiency (frequently owing to diabetes mellitus, pyelonephritis, or gout)

- Use of NSAIDs and β-blockers
- Autonomic insufficiency
- AIDS

The symptoms and signs of mineralocorticoid deficiency include hyperkalemia and metabolic acidosis. Blood pressures may be low, normal, or high. Sodium may be normal or low. If necessary, the diagnosis may be established by low renin and aldosterone levels that fail to rise with standing or volume depletion with diuretics. Treatment involves mineralocorticoid replacement with fludrocortisone, 0.05–0.2 mg daily, basing dose adjustments on blood pressure and potassium levels. Patients with hypertension or congestive heart failure are treated with loop diuretics.

Cushing's Syndrome

ETIOLOGY OF CUSHING'S SYNDROME

Cushing's syndrome is a result of glucocorticoid excess. Endogenously, this may be caused by increased ACTH secretion by the pituitary gland (Cushing's disease) or ectopically, or to increased cortisol secretion by an adrenal adenoma or carcinoma. The most common cause of Cushing's syndrome, however, is the exogenous administration of glucocorticoids.

CLINICAL PRESENTATION OF CUSHING'S SYNDROME

Clinical features appear in Table 44.2. With respect to specificity for Cushing's syndrome, thinning of skin, purple striae,

Table 44.2. Signs and Symptoms of Cushing's Syndrome

Clinical Feature	Approximate Prevalence (%)
Obesity	
General	80–95
Truncal	45–80
Hypertension	75–90
Menstrual disorders	75–95
Osteopenia	75–85
Facial plethora	70–90
Hirsutism	70–80
Impotence/decreased libido	65–95
Neuropsychiatric symptoms	60–95
Striae	50–70
Glucose intolerance	40–90
Weakness	30–90
Bruising	30–70
Kidney stones	15–20
Headache	10–50

and bruising are the best clinical signs. Hypokalemia, edema, and hyperpigmentation are more commonly seen in ectopic ACTH, where ACTH and cortisol levels tend to be much higher.

DIAGNOSIS OF CUSHING'S SYNDROME

The diagnosis of Cushing's syndrome revolves around the inability to suppress the HPA axis. Two screening tests are employed:

- 24-hour urine collection for free cortisol and creatinine (UFC)
- Overnight dexamethasone suppression test (ODST) — dexamethasone 1 mg is given at 11 PM and a serum cortisol drawn the following morning — cortisol < 5 μg/dl is a normal (or negative) response

The 24-hour UFC is more specific but is also more cumbersome. The value may be elevated in depression, acute illness, and alcoholism. The 1 mg ODST is easy to perform but has several false positive and negative responses. Causes of a false positive test include increased cortisol binding globulin (high circulating estogen) depression, acute illness, and alcoholism. Drugs that increase the metabolism of dexamethasone (rifampin, phenobarbital, and phenytoin) may also result in a false positive-response. False-negative tests may be seen in Cushing's disease or cyclical intermittent Cushing's syndrome.

DIFFERENTIAL DIAGNOSIS

If an abnormal result is obtained by either the 24-hour UFC or the 1 mg ODST, the pseudo-Cushing's state of alcoholism or endogenous depression should first be sought by a careful history, physical examination, and lab evaluation. Repeat UFC with alcohol abstention should be normal. If necessary, the low-dose DST may document true hypercortisolism. Dexamethasone, 0.5 mg orally every 6 hours, is administered for 48 hours, while 24-hour urine for free cortisol and 17-hydroxysteroids (17-OHCS) is collected before and on the second day of dexamethasone. Failure to suppress 24-hour urine 17-OHCS to less than 4 mg/24 hrs or UFC to < 25 mg/24 hrs suggests pathologic hypercortisolism, though pseudo-Cushing's states can occasionally not suppress. (Currently, the urinary 17-OHCS are not as essential since the advent of availability of UFCs but UFCs are not as well standardized.) Once true Cushing's syndrome has been documented, an ACTH level separates ACTH-dependent from ACTH-independent disease:

- ACTH-dependent hypercortisolism
  - Cushing's disease
  - Ectopic ACTH
  - Ectopic CRH
- ACTH-independent hypercortisolism
  - Adrenal adenoma

- Adrenal carcinoma
- Nodular adrenal hyperplasia
- Exogenous glucocorticoids

A normal or elevated ACTH suggests Cushing's disease or ectopic ACTH; these can be differentiated by the high-dose (8 mg) ODST. If a morning cortisol dose suppresses by 50% in response to 8 mg dexamethasone the evening prior, the diagnosis is presumed to be Cushing's disease. However, the specificity is not 100%; occult bronchial carcinoids with ACTH secretion especially can suppress in response to high-dose dexamethasone.

MRI is not definitive for distinguishing pituitary from nonpituitary tumors since ~ 50% of Cushing's disease patients have occult pituitary adenomas. Furthermore, up to 10% of patients with ectopic ACTH may have a false positive pituitary scan (the pituitary "incidentaloma"). Inferior petrosal sinus sampling (enhanced with corticotropin-releasing hormone) may be necessary; an elevated sinus to peripheral ACTH gradient suggests Cushing's disease.

TREATMENT OF CUSHING'S DISEASE

It should be apparent that the diagnostic workup of Cushing's syndrome can have many pitfalls. False-positive screening tests, pseudo-Cushing's states, modest specificity of the high-dose DST, and pituitary imaging can all lead to an erroneous diagnosis. It is important to correctly diagnose Cushing's disease, since the most appropriate treatment is transphenoidal pituitary adenomectomy by an experienced neurosurgeon (although XRT, ketoconazole, or bilateral adrenalectomy may be needed in some cases). Resection or chemotherapy of the underlying tumor is the treatment for adrenal neoplasia and ectopic ACTH.

Hyperaldosteronism

Excess aldosterone results in hyperaldosteronism with hypertension, hypokalemia, and metabolic alkalosis. This may be associated with Cushing's syndrome, particularly in patients with adrenal carcinoma. Isolated primary hyperaldosteronism (elevated aldosterone, suppressed plasma renin activity [PRA]) accounts for 1–2% of patients with hypertension; the presence of spontaneous hypokalemia or K + < 3.0 mEq/L on diuretics should prompt an evaluation.

Once hypokalemia is corrected and interfering drugs discontinued (most antihypertensives except α-adrenergic blockers), the aldosterone (ng/dl) to PRA (ng/ml/hr) ratio is a simple screening test. A ratio greater than 20 is quite sensitive, but not specific. The saline suppression test (administer 2L normal saline over 4 hours with aldosterone and PRA measured pre- and post; normal patients suppress aldosterone to < 5 ng/dl) confirms the diagnosis. A persistently elevated aldosterone-to-PRA ratio after captopril can also be used to confirm the diagnosis.

The next step is to differentiate adrenal adenoma from hyperplasia; this can be done by CT, measurement of 18-OH corticosterone, or bilateral adrenal vein catheterization. Spironolactone, an aldosterone antagonist, is the treatment of choice for patients with hyperplasia, small adenomas, or contraindications to surgery.

Other Mineralocorticoid Excess Syndromes

The pathogenesis of several mineralocorticoid excess syndromes has recently been elucidated. Dexamethasone-suppressible hyperaldosteronism is an entity that should be suspected in a young patient with elevated aldosterone, suppressed renin, and a family history of such. Through the development of a hybrid gene, the enzyme responsible for the final steps of aldosterone production becomes regulated by ACTH. Treatment with dexamethasone suppresses ACTH and subsequently excess aldosterone production.

In patients with suppressed PRA and low aldosterone, a mineralocorticoid other than aldosterone is present. In the syndrome of apparent mineralocorticoid excess, seen in young adults, the mineralocorticoid has recently been identified as cortisol (which normally has little mineralocorticoid effect). Normally cortisol is inactivated to cortisone in the renal tubular cell by 11-β hydroxysteroid dehydrogenase. Deficiency of this enzyme allows cortisol to bind the mineralocorticoid receptor, resulting in hypertension, hypokalemia, and suppressed PRA. Licorice (glycyrrhizic acid) is now known to inhibit 11-β hydroxysteroid dehydrogenase, explaining licorice-induced hypermineralocorticoidism.

Excess sodium itself serves to suppress PRA and cause hypertension in Liddle's syndrome. In this familial syndrome, constitutive activation of the kidney's epithelial sodium channel results in increased sodium resorption and potassium excretion independent of any mineralocorticoid. Spironolactone is therefore ineffective; triamterene is the treatment of choice.

Pheochromocytoma

CLINICAL PRESENTATION OF PHEOCHROMOCYTOMA

Pheochromocytomas arise predominantly in the adrenal medulla, where catecholamines are secreted. These tumors account for approximately 0.1% of hypertensive patients. They should be especially suspected in MEN 2A and 2B (where disease is frequently bilateral):

- MEN 2A
  - Pheochromocytoma
  - Medullary thyroid CA
  - Hyperparathyroidism
- MEN 2B
  - Pheochromocytoma

- Medullary thyroid CA
- Mucosal neuromas
- Marfanoid habitus

The neuroectodermal syndromes also have an increased incidence of pheochromocytoma:

- Neurofibromatosis
  - Neurofibromas
  - Café-Au-Lait spots
- Cerebelloretinal hemangioblastosis
  - Renal cell cancer
  - Retinal angiomata
  - CNS hemangioblastomas
- Tuberous sclerosis
  - Seizures
  - Mental deficiency
  - Adenoma sebaceum

The triad of headaches, palpitations, and diaphoresis in the presence of hypertension is classic for pheochromocytoma. Other signs and symptoms include:

- Postural hypotension
- Tachycardia
- Weight loss
- Pallor
- Hyperglycemia
- Anxiety
- Nausea/vomiting
- Constipation
- Tremulousness

More frequently recognized are "silent" pheochromocytomas. Cocaine abuse may be mistaken for pheochromocytoma.

DIAGNOSIS OF PHEOCHROMOCYTOMA

Screening for pheochromocytoma consists of a 24-hour urine collection for catecholamines and catecholamine metabolites [metanephrines and vanillymandelic acid (VMA)]. Plasma catecholamines may also be useful; plasma norepinephrine greater than 2000 pg/ml is quite specific for pheochromocytoma. Borderline or indeterminate results require further testing. The clonidine suppression test is used to confirm the diagnosis in patients with indeterminate urine or plasma studies. (Clonidine 0.3 mg is administered by mouth, and plasma-catecholamines are measured pre- and 3 hours post; a normal response is plasma norepinephrine less than 500 pg/ml or a 50% decrease from baseline.) The glucagon-stimulation test may also be used; an increase in blood pressure and plasma catecholamines strongly suggests pheochromocytoma. However, the sensitivity is limited, and the test may be potentially dangerous (hypertensive crisis). Chromogranin A, a neuropeptide secreted with the catecholamines, is reasonably sensitive for pheochromocytoma, but of poor specificity (elevated with even minor degrees of renal insufficiency).

Once the diagnosis is biochemically established, radiographic localization is indicated. Although CT is the initial choice, MRI may be especially useful since pheochromocytomas are markedly hyperintense (white) on T2 weighted images. Scanning with MIBG (^{131}I meta-iodobenzyl-guanidine) is most specific and particularly useful for extra-adrenal pheos (10%) and malignant metastatic pheos (10%). Treatment of a pheochromocytoma is resection of the tumor after appropriate operative preparation (volume loading and adrenergic receptor blockade).

Incidentally Discovered Adrenal Mass

DIFFERENTIAL DIAGNOSIS OF AN INCIDENTALLY DISCOVERED ADRENAL MASS

Incidental adrenal masses are common, detected on approximately 2% of all abdominal CT scans. The differential diagnosis includes:

- Functioning and nonfunctioning adenomas
- Functioning and nonfunctioning carcinomas
- Pheochromocytomas
- Metastases from other tumors (especially malignant melanoma, lung, breast and gastrointestinal cancer)
- Myelolipomas
- Cysts
- Focal enlargement in hyperplastic glands (e.g., Cushing's disease, congenital adrenal hyperplasia)

The management of the incidentaloma is controversial; clinical judgment is required. The patient should first be clinically evaluated for evidence of adrenal hormone production (cortisol, androgens, aldosterone, catecholamines). If the tumor appears to be nonfunctional clinically, most endocrinologists would still screen biochemically for pheochromocytoma because of the associated morbidity and mortality. Several authors also recommend dexamethasone suppression testing to exclude preclinical Cushing's syndrome (PCS). These patients will not have the classic signs or symptoms of hypercortisolism but will have evidence of hypothalamic-pituitary-adrenal axis dysfunction, such as loss of diurnal rhythm. The long-term implications of PCS are unknown and the optimal management therefore controversial, but at minimum, these patients require identification prior to adrenal surgery since they can develop postoperative adrenal insufficiency.

Despite an absence of hormone excess, nonfunctional tumors greater than 4–6 cm should probably be resected owing to an increased risk of malignancy; nonfunctional tumors less than 4–6 cm can be further evaluated radiographically to determine likelihood of benign disease. The attenuation value, obtained from a noncontrast CT scan, is a measure of the tumor's lipid content. A value less than 10 Hounsfield units is quite specific for adenoma. Masses of indeterminate attenuation value (10–20 HU) can be further classified by opposed-phase MRI. Masses inconsistent with adenoma by CT or MRI require repeated follow-up CT scanning to assess growth or fine-needle aspiration biopsy.

REVIEW EXERCISES

QUESTIONS

1. A 40-year-old white female with a history of severe asthma and Hashimoto's thyroiditis presents with 2 months of fatigue, anorexia, nausea, weight loss, and myalgia. Her examination is remarkable only for blood pressure 98/60 and pulse 98 without orthostasis. She is not hyperpigmented. Labs reveal Na 130, K 4.5, Cl 105, and HCO$_3$ 24. A cortrosyn stimulation test shows T = 0' (cortisol 5.8 μg/dl) and T = 60' (cortisol 13.2 μg/dl). Which of the following is correct:

   a. The most likely cause of her adrenal insufficiency is Addison's disease.
   b. The most likely cause of her adrenal insufficiency is prior exogenous corticosteroid use.
   c. She does not have adrenal insufficiency since her cortrosyn stimulation test is normal.
   d. She will require treatment with prednisone 7.5 mg daily and Florinef 0.1 mg daily.

2. A 37-year-old female presents to you for evaluation of weight gain and hirsutism for several years. Her OB/GYN has her on oral contraceptives for oligomenorrhea. She has noted easy bruisability but no muscle weakness. On examination, she weighs 240 pounds with central obesity. Her blood pressure is 144/92. She has significant facial hair, mild acne, multiple thin whitish striae on her abdomen, and a small buffalo hump. Her proximal muscle strength is normal. Chemistries are remarkable for a random glucose of 183 mg/dl and a potassium of 3.9 mEq/L. Her OB/GYN sends you a morning cortisol (drawn the morning after an 11 PM dose of 1 mg dexamethasone) of 6.2 μg/dl and a random ACTH of 25 pg/ml. Which of the following would you do next:

   a. Obtain an MRI of the pituitary
   b. Obtain a CT scan of the adrenals
   c. Obtain a 24-hour urine free cortisol
   d. Perform a high-dose (8 mg) dexamethasone suppression test

3. A 63-year-old woman you follow for hypertension, osteoarthritis, gout, recurrent DVT, and a 10-year history of type II diabetes mellitus develops a potassium of 6.2 mEq/L. Her serum aldosterone is 1.8 ng/dl. Which of the following is false:

   a. β-blockers and NSAIDs may be contributing to the hyperkalemia.
   b. An ACE-inhibitor may be contributing to the hyperkalemia.
   c. Long-term heparin may be contributing to hypoaldosteronism.
   d. Prednisone will likely be required as treatment.
   e. Florinef will likely be required as treatment.

4. A 52-year old-female is referred to you by her urologist for a 3 cm right adrenal mass detected on an abdominal CT. Her weight has been stable and she has generally felt well. She has not noted hirsutism, acne, proximal myopathy, or easy bruisability, but she has felt depressed lately. She has also had diaphoresis and occasional headaches, but no palpitations. Her last menstrual period was 6 months earlier. She has a history of diabetes mellitus × 2 years, well controlled by diet. Her last mammogram 8 months earlier was negative. She smokes 1 pack of cigarettes daily. On examination, blood pressure 135/85, pulse 95, weight 174 pounds. There is no buffalo hump or supraclavicular fat and no abdominal striae. She is not hirsute. Proximal muscle strength is normal. There are no breast masses. Stool is negative for occult blood. Labs reveal normal CBC and chemistry profile. Which of the following would you do next:

   a. 24-hour urine-free cortisol
   b. Aldosterone/PRA ratio
   c. Serum DHEAS and androstenedione
   d. 24-hour urine for catecholamines and metanephrines
   e. All of the above

Answers

1. b

This case illustrates the differences between primary and secondary adrenal insufficiency in clinical presentation and treatment. In secondary adrenal insufficiency, the renin aldosterone axis is intact, therefore hyperkalemia and metabolic acidosis are not seen and fludrocortisone is not required for treatment.

2. c

This case illustrates the evaluation of Cushing's syndrome. Generally, the 24-hour UFC is the best screening test; the 1 mg Overnight Dexamethasone Suppression Test is easier to perform but has more false-positives, including increased cortisol binding globulin owing to oral contraceptives. Radiographic imaging is not indicated until the diagnosis is established biochemically.

3. d

This case illustrates several conditions associated with hypoaldosteronism.

4. d

This case illustrates workup of an incidental adrenal mass. Biochemical testing should be influenced by clinical findings. If no evidence of hormone production is apparent by history and physical, biochemical screening for pheochromocytoma should nonetheless be done.

SUGGESTED READINGS

Bravo EL. Primary aldosteronism. Issues in diagnosis and management. Endocrinol Metab Clin North Amer 1994;23:271–283.

Byny RL. Withdrawal from glucocorticoid therapy. N Engl J Med 1975;1:30–32.

Grinspoon SK, Biller BM. Clinical review 62: laboratory assessment of adrenal insufficiency. J Clin Endocrinol Metab 1994;79:923–931.

Gross MD, et al. Clinical review 50: clinically silent adrenal masses. J Clin Endocrinol Metab 1993;77(4):885–888.

Kong MF, Jeff CW. Eighty-six cases of Addison's disease. Clin Endocrinol 1994;41:757–61.

Orth DN. Cushing's syndrome. N Engl J Med 1995;332:791–803.

Pituitary Disorders and Ectopic Hormone Syndromes

S. Sethu K. Reddy

ANATOMY AND PHYSIOLOGY OF THE PITUITARY GLAND

The pituitary gland is divided into two lobes:

- Anterior (developed from Rathke's pouch)
- Posterior (developed as a diverticulum growing downward from the base of the hypothalamus)

The median eminence is an intensely vascular component at the baseline of the hypothalamus that forms the floor of the third ventricle. The pituitary stalk arises from the median eminence. The hypothalamus extends anteriorly to the optic chiasm and posteriorly to the mammillary bodies. It was hypothesized in the 1930s that releasing hormones traveled from the hypothalamus to the pituitary via the hypothalamic-pituitary portal system, but it was not until the mid-1960s that these releasing hormones were isolated and identified (see Table 45.1).

The first releasing hormone to be identified (by two separate laboratories of Guillemin and Schally in 1969) was the thyrotropin releasing hormone (TRH). In subsequent years, other releasing hormones were identified. Of note, prolactin is under tonic inhibitory influence, with dopamine acting as a prolactin release-inhibiting factor. Also, growth-hormone releasing hormone (GHRH) was first isolated as an ectopic hormone arising from a pancreatic islet cell tumor causing acromegaly.

The pituitary gland weighs from 500–1000 mg and sits in the sella turcica, immediately behind the sphenoid sinus. It has anterior and posterior bony walls, as well as a bony floor. Above is a layer of dura (diaphragma sella) and then the optic chiasma, hypothalamus, and the third ventricle. Laterally on each side is the cavernous sinus inclusive of the internal carotid artery and components of the III to VI cranial nerves. The chiasma may be anterior to the sella (15%), above the sella (80%), or perhaps behind the sella (5%). Impingement of the chiasma and/or its branches by pituitary pathology may result in visual defects in one or both eyes and in temporal or homonymous hemianopsia.

Pituitary Tumors

Pituitary tumors may present with either hypofunction or hyperfunction, as well as symptoms directly related to mass effect of the tumor. Since the advent of CT-scanning, microadenomas have been arbitrarily designated to be less than 10 mm in diameter, while macroadenomas are greater than 10 mm in diameter. They are invariably benign, with no sex predilection. Pituitary adenomas may rarely be associated with parathyroid and pancreatic hyperplasia/neoplasia as part of the MEN I syndrome (multiple endocrine neoplasia, type I). Pituitary carcinomas are rare, but metastases from other solid malignancies can occur more frequently (see Table 45.2).

More than 50% of pituitary adenomas are prolactinomas, while 10–15% are GH producing, 10–15% are ACTH producing, and less than 5% secrete gonadotrophins or TSH. Less than 20% appear to be nonfunctioning. With progressive invasion of the anterior pituitary, hormonal deficiency can develop, usually affecting GH first, followed in sequence by LH, FSH, TSH, ACTH, and prolactin.

HYPOPITUITARISM

Isolated deficiencies of various anterior pituitary hormones have been described. The deficiency state may be caused by hormone deficiency or by resistance to the hormones at the receptor level. Pituitary tumors are the most common cause of hypopituitarism, but other etiologies must also be considered.

Table 45.1.   Pituitary Hormones: Hypothalamic Hormones and Other Regulatory Factors

Pituitary Hormones		Hypothalamic Hormones	Other Regulatory Factors
Thyrotropin (TSH)	+	TRH	Pit-1
	−		T_4, T_3, dopamine
Adrenocorticotrophin (ACTH)	+	CRH	ADH, adrenalin
	−		Cortisol
Luteinizing Hormone (LH)	+	LHRH	Estrogen
	−		Progesterone, testosterone
Follicular Stimulating H. (FSH)	+	LHRH	Activin, estrogen
	−		Inhibin, follistatin, testosterone
Growth Hormone (GH)	+	GHRH	Estrogens, T_4, Pit-1
	−	Somatostatin	
Prolactin	+	PRF	TRH, Pit-1, estrogen, serotonin, VIP
	−	Dopamine	GAP

Table 45.2.   Clinical Manifestations of Pituitary Tumors

Mass Effects	Endocrine Effects	
	Hyperpituitarism	Hypopituitarism
Headaches	PRL-hyperprolactinemia	GH-short stature in children
	GH-acromegaly	?silent in adults
Chiasmal syndrome	ACTH-Cushing's disease	LH/FSH-hypogonadism
	Nelson's syndrome	PRL-failure of postpartum lactation
Hypothalamic syndrome	TSH-hyperthyroidism	ACTH-hypocortisolism
Disturbance of thirst, appetite, satiety,	LH/FSH-gonadal dysfunction	TSH-hypothyroidism
sleep and temp. regulation	or silent α-subunit secretion	
Diabetes insipidus		
SIADH		
Obstructive hydrocephalus		
Frontal lobe dysfunction		
Cranial III, IV, V, and VI dysfunction		
Diplopia, facial pain		
Temporal lobe dysfunction		
Nasopharyngeal mass		
CSF rhinorrhea		

ACQUIRED

Almost any of the midline cleft syndromes can present with hypothalamic hypopituitarism. A recent MRI study of 35 patients with ''idiopathic'' GH deficiency found that more than 40% had an anatomical defect in the neurohypophysis, suggesting that these patients had variants of the midline cleft syndrome.

Irradiation of the brain can result in hypothalamic dysfunction in about 65% of treated subjects, with a wide spectrum of clinical presentation of any of the hypopituitarism. It should be noted that the hypopituitarism is usually delayed for 2 to 10 years.

The diagnosis of empty-sella syndrome is made increas-ingly, with the prevalence of CT and MRI scanners. Most patients have no pituitary dysfunction, but a wide spectrum of pituitary deficiencies have been described in adults (< 35%) and in children (> 75%). Coexisting tumors can occur. Primary empty sellas are often associated with benign intracranial hypertension, while secondary empty sellas may result from previous surgery or irradiation, or infarction of pre-existing tumor. Management is usually with reassurance and hormone replacement if necessary. Surgery is only necessary if visual field defects occur or if there is CSF rhinorrhea.

Pituitary apoplexy is an emergency resulting from hemorrhagic infarction of the pituitary, usually associated with a pre-existing pituitary tumor. The patient can present with a variety of altered sensoria, severe headache, stiff neck, and fever. Any evidence of sudden visual field defects, oculomotor palsies, hypothalamic compression, or coma should lead to immediate surgery. Surprisingly, patients may be quite hypotensive with sudden decrease in ACTH, and thus they should all be treated with intravenous corticosteroids.

Sheehan's syndrome is hypopituitarism resulting from pituitary ischemia secondary to postpartum hemorrhage and hypotension. There is history of failure to lactate postpartum, failure to resume menses, cold intolerance, and/or fatigue. Some women may have an acute crisis within 30 days postpartum and mimic apoplexy. There is often subclinical central diabetes insipidus.

Perhaps more common than Sheehan's syndrome is lymphocytic hypophysitis, an autoimmune disease often presenting in women during or after pregnancy. There may be slight pituitary enlargement. Prolactin levels may be slightly elevated and diabetes insipidus may be present. Prognosis varies, but some may recover fully, while others may need selective hormone replacement.

GENETIC

Two families have been described in which a mutation of a Pit-1 gene results in a protein that binds poorly to the 5' flanking region of prolactin, GH, and TSH-β genes. This results in deficiency of prolactin, GH, and TSH. Kallmann's syndrome is associated with hypogonadotropic hypogonadism and anosmia, as well as occasionally cerebellar ataxia, nerve deafness, color blindness, and cleft lip and palate.

Recently, a gene defect on the X chromosome (KALIG-1), resulting in loss of an adhesion molecule that regulates the migration of olfactory and GnRH neurons and other neuronal tissue in the brain, has been described. This resulted in an X-linked form of Kallmann's syndrome. In most patients with idiopathic GnRH deficiency, the defect is not in the GnRH gene but in the secretory process of GnRH. Growth hormone is not necessary for in utero growth, and thus any deficiency is detected toward the end of year one.

Isolated GH deficiency is thought to be on a genetic basis in about 5–30% of patients, but few structural defects in GH gene or in GHRH gene have been identified. Isolated TSH deficiency is rare, but a few families with mutations in the TSH β subunit gene have been described. Isolated ACTH deficiency has been described more often, but not as a result of a genetic defect. Most cases appear to be due to specific lymphocytic hypophysitis.

Receptor defects for TSH, prolactin, and GNRH have not been described. Mutations in GH receptor have been described (Laron-type dwarfism), in which GH fails to induce IGF-1 synthesis. Of note, about 50% of circulating GH is bound to a binding protein, which is a byproduct of GH receptor cleavage. Measuring this binding protein can indicate the status of the GH receptor. Children insensitive to GH typically have

delayed motor development, bone maturation, and tooth eruption, in addition to short stature. These individuals should respond to IGF-1 injections. An autosomal recessive form of ACTH resistance has been described with clinical presentation of cortisol deficiency and normal aldosterone levels.

PROLACTINOMA

Prolactin is secreted by lactotropes, which are 1/10th as prevalent as somatotropes (GH secreting cells) (see Table 45.3.). The pituitary content of prolactin is approximately 100 μg but can increase 10- to 20-fold during pregnancy and lactation. Although breast tissue is the most important target organ for prolactin, prolactin receptors have been identified in a variety of tissues including:

- Liver
- Kidney
- Ovaries
- Testes
- Prostate
- Seminal vesicles

In breast tissue, prolactin increases synthesis of casein and β-lactalbumin.

Dopamine is the major inhibitor of prolactin secretion, and any mechanisms that interrupt dopamine transport from the hypothalamus or reduce dopamine activity in the pituitary can lead to elevated levels of prolactin (PRL). A gonadotrophin releasing hormone associated peptide (GAP), a 56-amino acid precursor for GnRH, has been shown to inhibit prolactin secretion. Estrogens, TRH, and serotonin also increase prolactin levels. H_2 receptors inhibit PRL secretion, while H_1 receptors stimulate PRL secretion.

Except for pregnancy and postpartum states, the above physiological states are generally associated with prolactin levels less than 50 ng/ml, while pharmacological causes result in prolactin levels less than 100–150 ng/ml. Hypothyroidism, pituitary stalk section, renal failure, or hypothalamic causes also result in prolactin levels less than 100–150 ng/ml. Prolactin levels greater than 150 ng/ml usually indicate a pituitary adenoma. A careful history and examination and assessment of the prolactin level will rule out most of the above diagnoses. Despite above clinical caveats, one should rule out a sellar lesion in those with any significant PRL elevation.

PROLACTINOMAS

Women usually present with amenorrhea and/or galactorrhea. Men often present with larger prolactinomas and hypogonadism. Careful case-cohort studies have found no evidence that oral contraceptives induce or exacerbate prolactinomas. The prolactin level usually correlates well with the size of the tumor. TRH-testing should result in poor prolactin response (less than a 100% rise) but is now rarely necessary in the diagnostic workup. An MRI-scan of the pituitary is perhaps

Table 45.3.   Differential Diagnosis of Hyperprolactinemia

Physiological	*Pathological*	*Pharmacological*
Pregnancy	Prolactinoma	TRH
Postpartum	Acromegaly (25% frequency)	Psychotropic medications
Newborn	Hypothalamic disorders	Phenothiazines
Stress	"Chiari-Frommel"	Reserpine
Hypoglycemia	Craniopharyngioma	Alphamethyl dopa
Sleep	Metastatic disease	Estrogen therapy
Postprandial	Pituitary stalk section or	Metoclopramide
Hypoglycemia	compression	Cimetidine (esp. IV)
Intercourse	Hypothyroidism	Opiates
Nipple stimulation	Renal failure	
	Liver disease	
	Chest wall trauma (burns, shingles)	

the most sensitive radiographic technique for detecting pituitary microadenomas.

Since surgical resection is not curative (less than 40% of time) and often results in a recurrence of the tumor, medical therapy with long-acting dopamine agonists is now the first-line treatment. Bromocriptine, pergolide, and cabergoline are potent inhibitors of prolactin secretion and often result in shrinkage of the tumor. Medical therapy controls the tumor but rarely causes permanent regression of it. Usually within 2 weeks after discontinuation of the medication, prolactin levels again rise. It would be reasonable to try a "drug holiday" after several years of therapy, however. These medications, especially bromocriptine, are best given at night with gradually increasing doses to minimize nausea, headaches, and postural symptoms.

Medical therapy during pregnancy often stirs debate about continuation of bromocriptine. Tumor-related complications are only seen in about 15% of pregnancies, and for women with microadenomas, in only 5% of patients. A sensible approach would be to stop bromocriptine when pregnancy begins and then follow the clinical status with prolactin levels and visual fields. If there is any significant worsening of the tumor, bromocriptine could be reinstituted.

Men with prolactinomas may often need exogenous testosterone, as well as bromocriptine.

Surgery, typically, trans-sphenoidal resection, is reserved for patients refractory to medical therapy or for those with large tumors having a mass effect. The main advantage of surgery is avoidance of chronic medical therapy. Larger tumors are less likely to be cured, however, and there is risk of hypopituitarism, as well as recurrence of tumor. For those in whom surgery may be high risk, radiotherapy with either conventional or proton beams is a useful adjunct. Some patients with a microadenoma may be followed. Less than 5% would be expected to progress.

ACROMEGALY

The classic and well-known clinical features of acromegaly include:

- Prevalence of 3–4 cases per million
- Mean age at diagnosis is 40 (male) and 45 (female)
- Tumors more aggressive in young
- Coarsening of facial features
- Prominent jaw, frontal sinus, broadening of hands, feet
- Hyperhidrosis
- Macroglossia
- Signs of hypopituitarism
- Diabetes mellitus (10–25%)
- Skin tags (must screen for colonic polyps)
- Hypertension (25–30%), cardiomyopathy (50–80%)
- Carpal tunnel syndrome
- Sleep apnea (5%)

Acromegaly is usually caused by a GH-secreting tumor and rarely by ectopic GHRH secretion by a carcinoid tumor or an islet-cell tumor. Diagnosis is confirmed by failure to suppress GH to less than 2 ng/ml within 2 hours of an oral glucose tolerance test and by elevated IGF-I levels. Measurement of IGF-I may actually be the more precise and cost-effective screening test.

Recently, a *gsp* mutation in a Gs_α subunit in GH cells, leading to continuous Gh secretion, has been shown to cause acromegaly. This mutation results in uncoupling of the GHRH receptor and adenyl cyclase. Occasionally, the pituitary adenomas may be monoclonal, expressing GH and prolactin or biclonal expressing GH and prolactin separately. Ectopic GH secretion has been documented in extracts of lung adenocarcinoma, breast cancer, and ovarian cancer; none of these conditions has been reported to cause acromegaly. Only one pancreatic tumor has been shown to secrete GH and cause acromegaly. Ectopic GHRH secretion has been widely reported in carcinoids, pancreatic islet-cell tumors, small-cell lung cancer, adrenal adenoma, and pheochromocytomas.

It is noteworthy that although 50% of carcinoids may be associated with elevated GH levels, rarely do they cause acromegaly. It is difficult to distinguish (clinically or biochemically), the GH-secreting pituitary adenoma from an ectopic, GHRH-secreting tumor. If GHRH levels exceed 300 ng/liter then one should suspect an ectopic tumor.

Management usually includes surgical resection, followed by irradiation, if necessary. Bromocriptine is only effective in about 10% of individuals and must be used in high doses. Octreotide, a long-acting analog of somatostatin, can lower GH and IGF-I levels in up to two-thirds of patients and shrink the tumor in about one-third of patients. Side effects include malabsorption and cholelithiasis, and the response is present only as long the therapy is administered. Many of these patients display a paradoxical GH response to TRH, and thus TRH testing could be used in follow-up to document remission/relapse. Those patients over age 50 or with symptoms of acromegaly for more than 10 years or with increased numbers of skin tags should be screened regularly at 2–3-year intervals by colonoscopy. Overall there is a 3–8-fold increase in risk of colon cancer and 2–3-fold increase in other malignant tumors.

CUSHING'S DISEASE

ACTH-secreting adenomas are usually microadenomas causing excess cortisol production, resulting in:

- Central obesity
- Muscle loss with proximal muscle weakness
- Thinning of skin and connective tissue
- Osteopenia
- Ease of bruising
- Glucose intolerance
- Hypertension

Androgen production is also stimulated, resulting in hirsutism and menstrual abnormalities. Depression and/or panic attacks are also commonly observed. Chronic ACTH elevation leads to bilateral hyperplasia of adrenal cortices. After Cushing's syndrome is established with unequivocal 24-hour urinary-free cortisols, the ACTH dependence is documented by elevated/inappropriate ACTH levels. Occasionally ectopic ACTH syndrome may cause Cushing's syndrome, but this can be differentiated by:

- More rapid course
- Much higher levels of ACTH
- Unresponsiveness to CRH
- More prominent hypokalemia
- Hyperpigmentation

Most tumors associated with ectopic ACTH syndrome are carcinomas and have a poor prognosis. Some benign tumors,

however, such as carcinoids or islet-cell tumors, have been shown to cause ectopic ACTH syndrome and are difficult to differentiate from pituitary causes of Cushing's syndrome. This difficulty is exaggerated by radiological investigations of the sella that are often negative or unhelpful.

First course of management would be trans-sphenoidal resection, followed by radiotherapy 6–12 months later, if necessary. About 20% of patients remain uncured after surgery. Postoperatively, the HPA axis hypofunction is usually not seen but normalizes over several months. Conventional megavoltage therapy or ''Photon Knife'' (computer-assisted stereotactic linear accelerator) or ''Gamma Knife'' (with ^{60}Co) may be used. Patients unresponsive to these therapies may then be offered medical or surgical adrenalectomy. Mitotane is perhaps the most effective adrenolytic agent. Other medications (such as aminoglutethimide, ketoconazole, or metyrapone) are useful as temporizing agents only.

NONFUNCTIONING OR GLYCOPROTEIN-SECRETING TUMORS

These tumors are usually clinically silent because of their inefficiency in actual secretion of these hormones and the lack of a clinically recognizable syndrome. These features lead to the clinical presentation of neurologic symptoms, primarily:

- Visual defects
- Headaches
- Large macroadenomas

Patients, of course, can present with varying degrees of hypopituitarism. Rarely, a TSH adenoma may cause hyperthyroidism, an FSH adenoma may cause amenorrhea in women, and an LH adenoma may cause precocious puberty in a boy. Diagnosis is confirmed by either measurement of intact glycoprotein hormones and their subunits (α- and β-subunits). The α-subunit levels tend to be elevated inappropriately compared with the intact hormone itself. There may be a supranormal response of FSH, LH, or LH-β to TRH injection.

The standard treatment is trans-sphenoidal surgery, especially if visual impairment is present. Surgery is rarely curative, and radiotherapy is needed as adjunctive therapy. Octreotide therapy may be helpful in reducing hormone secretion but has not been shown to reduce tumor size. Dopamine agonists, such as bromocriptine, have been used in high doses, but clinical responses (i.e., changes in tumor size, visual symptoms) have not been poor. GnRH agonists, which normally inhibit GnRH secretion, have been able to reduce secretion of FSH and LH by the tumors but not tumor size.

PITUITARY INCIDENTALOMAS

Autopsy studies suggest that about 10–20% of normal individuals may harbor incidental pituitary microadenomas that pathologically are similar in distribution to those that present clinically. From CT scans and MRI imaging studies, the incidence of pituitary microadenomas > 3 mm is 4–20% in normal individuals. The differential diagnosis may include:

- Cysts
- Infarcts
- Aneurysm of the internal carotid artery
- CNS tumors
- Granulomatous disease
- Metastatic cancer

Unless clinical presentation warrants, however, further testing is rarely warranted. Yearly scanning to follow the size of the lesion is sufficient in most cases. The clinical decision will depend upon the natural history of the microadenoma.

Multiple Endocrine Neoplasia (MEN) Syndromes

There are several types of Multiple Endocrine Neoplasia (MEN) syndromes:

- MEN I
- MEN IIa
- MEN IIb

MEN I syndrome, which may involve pituitary tumors, is inherited as an autosomal dominant trait and usually manifests in the fourth to fifth decades. Not only are multiple glands involved, but also each gland is likely to be widely affected. Thus, patients with MEN I, which affects parathyroid glands (80–90%), the pancreas (80%) and the pituitary (65%), will often have parathyroid hyperplasia or multiple parathyroid adenomas. Also, the pancreas may have multicentric islet-cell tumors secreting a variety of pancreatic hormones. Carcinoid tumors are also associated with MEN I and MEN II.

The hyperparathyroidism is similar to usual primary hyperparathyroidism clinically and biochemically. About 28% of patients with hyperparathyroidism may have MEN I.

Gastrinoma (Zollinger-Ellison syndrome) is the most common pancreatic tumor (70%), followed by insulinoma; this tumor usually presents after hyperparathyroidism. The pancreatic tumor may secrete gastrin, insulin, vasoactive intestinal peptide (VIP) (Werner-Morrison syndrome), serotonin, glucagon, somatostatin, pancreatic polypeptide, or GHRH.

The pituitary tumors occur in a similar distribution as isolated pituitary adenomas.

From molecular biological studies, it appears that a mutation at the q13 locus in chromosome 11 results in loss of a tumor suppressor product. If the q13 locus is lost from both chromosomes 11, this leads to homozygous deficiency of the suppressor protein. This suppressor protein has been termed menin and has recently been isolated. Until the utility of measuring this protein levels has been tested, clinical management must include genetic counseling, careful gathering of family history, and screening first-order relatives. Screening with calcium, prolactin, and glucose levels at 1–2-year intervals beginning at age 15 would be reasonable.

For MEN II (medullary cancer of thyroid, hyperparathyroidism, and pheochromocytomas), MEN IIb (medullary cancer of thyroid, pheochromocytoma, and mucosal neuromas) and familial medullary cancer of thyroid, a mutation of the RET proto-oncogene appears to be strongly correlated with the presence of disease. This has largely supplanted calcium injection/pentagastrin stimulation of calcitonin levels as a screening test.

Ectopic Hormone Production

BIOLOGY

All somatocytes in the body have the genetic material encoding all protein structures of the human body. It is therefore expected that altered regulation of a cell frequently could lead to production of a protein. As the tools for detecting polypeptide hormones improve, cells previously unexpected to secrete certain hormones have clearly been demonstrated to do so. Many of these cells produce these "ectopic" hormones for autocrine or paracrine purposes.

Findings in the 1980s of peptides similar to insulin and other hormones being synthesized by unicellular organisms have broadened the view of origin of endocrine cells. Traditionally, endocrine cells were thought to originate from the neural crest, but it seems more likely that both neural cells and endocrine cells originate directly from unicellular organisms. *From the clinician's viewpoint, ectopic hormone production occurs at a site not usually necessary for normal clinical function.*

It is highly unlikely that ectopic production of steroid hormones can occur, since it is necessary to have a number of synthetic enzymes present in order to produce the final hormone. Thus polypeptide hormones are the usual ectopic products. A TATA regulatory box, which regulates the translation of DNA to mRNA, is upstream for any polypeptide gene. A number of transcription factors can interact with this regulatory region to increase the synthesis of the appropriate mRNA. The tumors that synthesize ectopic hormones often translate the mRNA inefficiently or the mRNA is translated into an alternate reading frame. The resulting shorter mRNAs may result in peptides that are immunologically reactive but functionally inactive. The peptides may not even be able to be secreted. Also, as for ACTH, the initial translation product is often a pre-pro-peptide, which must then undergo several post-translational cleavages to result in a biologically active hormone. The clinical relevance of all these phenomena is that many tumors synthesize peptide hormones or fragments

Table 45.4. Ectopic Hormone Syndromes

Hormone	Reported Tumors
ACTH, lipotrophin (β-MSH, endorphins, enkephalins)	Oat-cell cancer of lung, thymoma, islet-cell tumor, bronchial carcinoid, ovarian tumors, pheochromocytomas, medullary cell cancer
GHRH	Carcinoid, islet-cell tumors
HCG-B subunit	Adenocancer of pancreas, malignant islet-cell tumors
GnRH	Choriocarcinoma, hepatoblastomas, adenocancer, malignant islet-cell tumors, breast cancer, melanoma
ADH (vasopressin)	Oat-cell cancer, pancreatic adenocancer
Erythropoietin	Renal cell cancer, cerebellar hemangioblastoma, pheochromocytoma, hepatoma, uterine fibroids
Serotonin/5-OH tryptophan	Non-β-islet-cell tumors, oat-cell cancer, pancreatic adenocancer

of peptide hormones but only occasionally cause the clinically evident syndrome of hormone excess (see Table 45.4).

To confirm a true ectopic hormone syndrome, five criteria ideally should be fulfilled:

1. Association of tumor with the clinical endocrine syndrome
2. Following removal of tumor, return of endocrine status to normal
3. Persistence of endocrine abnormality after removal of the primary gland normally responsible for that hormone
4. A-V gradient of hormone across the tumor
5. Demonstration of the appropriate mRNA and peptide in the tumor cells

Realistically, criteria 3 and 4 are either impractical or difficult to observe.

Recognized as early as in 1928, ectopic ACTH syndrome is the most frequent and best-studied of the ectopic-hormone syndromes. Many cases were reported in the early 1960s by Liddle and others. Most of these cases were those of lung malignancies. Ectopic ACTH syndrome usually presents as a rapid-onset syndrome (within 6 months), associated with profound muscle weakness, hyperpigmentation, hypertension, and hypokalemia and edema. These features were typical when the primary tumor was a malignant pulmonary cancer. When slower-growing tumors such as carcinoid or islet-cell tumors present with Cushing's syndrome, however, the patient's symptoms are difficult to differentiate from the usual Cushing's disease of pituitary origin. Hirsutism is reported by 70% of female patients with ectopic Cushing's, in addition to

findings suggestive of adrenal hyperandrogenism. Men, however, have glucocorticoid-induced Leydig cell suppression. The prominent hypokalemia has been attributed to high levels of 11-deoxycorticosterone (11-DOC), as well as increased levels of cortisol, and corticosterone. The hyperpigmentation is thought to be from the cosecretion of β-MSH, one of the by-products of ACTH synthesis.

Plasma ACTH levels tend to be higher than levels observed in pituitary Cushing's, but there can be some overlap. CRH stimulation may not lead to further rise in ACTH in those with ectopic ACTH syndrome. These patients also fail to suppress their cortisol levels during the high-dose dexamethasone (8 mg/day) test.

ACTH originates from pre-pro-opiomelanocortin, which is cleaved to pro-opiomelanocortin (POMC). Further cleavage results in pro-ACTH and β-lipotropin. Pro-ACTH is processed to pro-γMSH and ACTH, while β-LPH is processed to γ-Lipotropin and β-endorphin.

Localization of the tumor is not difficult for the classic ectopic ACTH syndrome, but for the more benign tumors that cause ectopic ACTH syndrome, many investigations may be necessary:

- MRI scanning of the chest may be more sensitive than CT for bronchial carcinoids.
- Ultrasonography, CT, and MRI have been used to investigate the abdomen, as well.
- Selective venous sampling for ACTH has not been helpful.
- Pancreatic tumours are best seen with ultrasound and CT.
- Endoscopic ultrasonography may be even more sensitive for pancreatic lesions.
- Some preliminary studies have found ^{125}I-octreotide scanning useful in localizing some of these tumors.

Management would ideally be surgical resection of the tumor, but occasionally, with nonresectable tumors, or metastatic disease or an occult cause, one may have to use other anticancer modalities or use antiadrenal medications. Octreotide may inhibit ectopic ACTH secretion. Aminoglutethimide in doses of 0.5 to 2.0 g/day and/or metyrapone in doses of 500–4000 mg/day have been used. Ketoconazole, which interferes with cytochrome P-450 enzymes and interferes with adrenal and gonadal steroidogenesis, has also been used in doses of 200–600 mg/day. Mitotane, which is used in the treatment of adrenal cancer, has not been used often because of its severe side effects. It often takes several months of therapy to normalize the cortisol levels. The investigational glucocorticoid antagonist RU-486 is a promising therapy that appears to have few side effects. One difficulty is that one cannot rely on cortisol measurements to follow the effect of RU-486. Bilateral surgical adrenalectomy with adjunct sellar irradiation could also become an option in the event of failure of other options.

Table 45.5. Common ADH-Related Syndromes

Clinical Presentation	Thirst	ADH Secretion	ADH Action	Diagnosis
Polyuria/Polydipsia	N	↓	N	Central DI
Polyuria/Polydipsia	N	N	↓	Nephrogenic DI
Polyuria/Polydipsia	↑	N	N	1° Polydipsia
↑ Na+	↓	N	N	Hypodipsia
↓ Na+	↓	↑	N	SIADH

Posterior Pituitary

The posterior pituitary acts as a repository for antidiuretic hormone (ADH, vasopressin) and oxytocin. Clinically, disorders of ADH are most relevant (see Table 45.5).

Antidiuretic hormone secretion is regulated by serum osmolality, as well as plasma volume. Small increments in serum osmolality > 290 mosm/kg leads to prompt secretion of ADH. However, more than a 10% plasma volume decrease will override any osmolar stimulus (e.g., a severely dehydrated individual can thus be hyponatremic). Pain, nicotine, and caffeine can increase ADH secretion. ADH is a potent vasoconstrictor, whereas desmopressin (DDAVP) is an ADH analogue with pure antidiuretic action.

If Na^+ < 143 mEq/L, conduct a dehydration test. If urine osmolarity (OSM) < 300 mosm/L and Na^+ >143 mEq/L, then a test dose of DDAVP should be given. This should lead to greater than 50% increase in urine osmolarity. If Na^+ >143 mEq/L, proceed to a DDAVP test. If the urine osm is < 360 mosm/L during dehydration but the Na^+ fails to rise above 143 mEq/L, then suspect a surreptitious cause. There are many causes of diabetes insipidus:

- Central DI
  - Familial
  - Idiopathic
  - Accidental/surgical trauma
  - Granulomatous disease
    - Sarcoid, TB, histiocytosis
  - Tumors
    - Craniopharyngioma
    - Pituitary tumors
    - Metastatic Cancer
  - Infectious
  - Meningitis, encephalitis
  - Vascular
    - Aneurysms
    - Sheehan's syndrome
  - Drugs
    - Alcohol, dilantin

- Nephrogenic DI
  - Renal medullary osmotic gradient
    - Psychogenic polydipsia
      - Low-protein diet
    - Furosemide therapy
  - Disruption of counter-current system
    - Sickle-cell nephropathy
    - Many forms of interstitial nephropathy
    - Analgesic
    - Hypokalemia
  - Disrupted adenyl cyclase system
    - Lithium
    - Demeclocycline
    - Familial nephrogenic DI
    - Hypercalcemia
    - Familial amyloidosis

It is important to distinguish between central and nephrogenic diabetes insipidus and psychogenic polydipsia.

Summary of workup for diabetes insipidus:

- Dehydration, followed by observing response to DDAVP injection
- Normal: No further increase in urine osm (< 5%) since urine should already be maximally concentrated
- Central DI: Greater than 50% rise in urine osm
- Nephrogenic DI: No rise in urine osm

N.B. patients with psychogenic polydipsia have a diluted medullary concentrating gradient and may develop a partial nephrogenic DI.

The posterior pituitary enhances on MRI with gadolinium and is a "good assay" of ADH reserve. Other pituitary / hypothalamic lesions can also be ruled out. Partial DI may be treated with chlorpropamide or thiazides, while complete central DI needs to be treated with DDAVP-nasal spray. A tablet form of DDAVP is now available for clinical use.

REVIEW EXERCISES

QUESTIONS

1. **Part I**

A 25-year-old shoe salesman, Harvey Dulait, complained of frontal headaches for 6 months. Four months ago, his primary-care physician diagnosed him to be hypothyroid with a total T4 of 3 ug/dL and a TSH of 0.41 mIU/mL (N = 0.4-5.5). He had also been complaining of some loss of energy and dry skin. What other history would one want to obtain:

a. Change in body hair distribution and fat distribution
b. Symptoms of erectile dysfunction
c. Visual field disturbances
d. Symptoms of polydipsia
e. All of the above

Part II

MRI of the sella turcica revealed a 2 cm mass. Visual fields by confrontation appeared normal, but by Goldmann perimetry showed bilateral superior-temporal defects to the color red. Laboratory studies:
BUN, Cr, electrolytes are normal.

Testosterone	30 ng/dL (200–1000)
LH	2 mIU/mL (<1–7)
FSH	1.5 mIU/mL (2–10)
Morning cortisol	4.5 ug/dL (3.4–26.9)
Prolactin	400 ng/mL (< 15)

Which of the following is false:

a. Patient has secondary hypogonadism.
b. Patient is likely to have cortisol deficiency.
c. Patient's GH reserve is probably normal.
d. Patient has a prolactinoma.

2. Match the case scenario with the most compatible laboratory findings (each laboratory result is used only once):

Case Scenarios

1. 25-year-old chronic schizophrenic woman with galactorrhea.

2. 25-year-old male with impotence, galactorrhea, and visual field defect.

3. 18-year-old male with delayed puberty, anosmia and appropriate bone density.

4. 45-year-old fireman with worsening diabetes control, coarsening features, and skin tags.

5. 40-year-old homemaker with headaches, normal menses, no visual field defect, CT-head suggests an empty sella.

Laboratory Results

A. Low testosterone, low LH and FSH, prolactin of 15 ng/mL

B. Elevated IGF-I levels

C. Normal TSH and prolactin response to TRH
Normal LH and FSH response to LHRH
Normal cortisol and GH response to insulin-induced hypoglycemia

D. Normal T4, TSH, prolactin of 50 ng/mL

E. Normal T4, TSH, prolactin of 200 ng/mL

Answers

1. Part I: e

The low T_4 with an inappropriate TSH level in an individual who is clinically hypothyroid should prompt a search for pituitary dysfunctions.

Part II: c

In the presence of pituitary tumors, the pituitary sequentially loses the ability to secrete GH, LH, FSH, TSH, and ACTH. This patient has secondary hypogonadism, hypothyroidism, and likely hypoadrenalism. It is almost certain that GH secretion is abnormally low.

2. 1 d

This patient likely has drug-induced hyperprolactinemia.

2 e

Men with prolactinomas often present with gradual onset of symptoms.

3 a

This patient likely has Kallman's syndrome.

4 b

This scenario describes acromegaly.

5 c

This patient has an empty-sella syndrome, which is often associated with normal pituitary function.

SUGGESTED READINGS

Bichet DG. Diabetes insipidus and vasopressin. In: Moore WT, Eastman RC, eds. Diagnostic endocrinology. Toronto: BC Decker, 1990:111–124.

Eastman RC, Sainz de la Pena M, Moore WT, et al. Acromegaly, hyperprolactinemia, gonadotrophin-secreting tumors and hypopituitarism. In: Moore WT, Eastman RC, eds. Diagnostic endocrinology. Toronto: BC Decker, 1990:33–53.

Melmed S. Acromegaly. N Engl J Med. 1990;322:966–977.

Molitch ME. Pathologic hyperprolactinemia. Endocrinol Metab Clin North Amer 1992;21:877–901.

Orth DN, Kovacs WJ, Debold CR. The adrenal cortex. In: Wilson JD, Foster DW, eds. Williams' textbook of endocrinology. 8th ed. Philadelphia: WB Saunders, 1992:536–562.

Vance ML. Hypopituitarism. N Engl J Med 1994;330:1651–1662.

Metabolic Bone Disease and Calcium Disorders

Angelo A. Licata

The degree of patient's symptomatology from hypercalcemia is directly dependent upon two major factors:

- The duration of the hypercalcemic process
- The rapidity of its development

The more chronic and slowly progressive the rise in serum calcium, the less likely a patient will be aware of it. If it persists occultly for years, the typical scenario seen in parathyroid disease becomes manifest. If the hypercalcemic process arises within weeks to months and does so in a fairly rapid course, symptoms develop that are generally of a neurological or musculoskeletal nature. Diagnosis of hypercalcemia is seprated by 2 major areas; parathyroid and nonparathyroid. These areas are discussed below.

CLINICAL PRESENTATION OF HYPERCALCEMIA

Symptoms of hyperparathyroid hypercalcemia have taken on a vastly different presentation over the last 2–3 decades:

- Asymptomatic   47%
- Symptomatic   53%
  - Bone pain   6%
  - Renal stones (colic) 21%
  - Gastritis (ulcer)   13%
  - Pancreatitis   2%
  - Mental changes   20%
  - Weakness   7%

Most cases of hyperparathyroidism are asymptomatic. Detecting abnormalities in serum calcium by routine chemical assays now identifies patients many years before symptoms arise. Historical descriptions of hyperparathyroidism, however, emphasize symptoms such as osteitis fibrosa cystica (bone pain and arthralgias), renal-stone disease, gastric ulcers, pancreatitis, decreased mental status and weakness.

The unique presentation of hyperparathyroidism may not be the clinical presentation of other causes of hypercalcemia.

Abrupt onset of lethargy, confusion, fatigue, and even outright coma is often the presentation of many patients whose calcium rises abruptly. These cases occur so rapidly that renal-stone disease may not have time to develop. However, there may be manifestations of bowel dysfunction—such as pain or constipation and generalized muscular weakness. The older patient is more likely to be overcome by these symptoms; younger individuals tolerate higher levels of hypercalcemia with fewer symptoms.

DIAGNOSIS OF HYPERCALCEMIA

Textbook descriptions of hypercalcemia list extensive causes of this condition:

- Primary hyperparathyroidism
- Cancer (e.g., PTH-related protein [PTHrp], ectopic vitamin D, bone metastases)
- Endocrine disorders (e.g., thyrotoxicosis, VIP, Addison's disease, pheochromocytoma)
- Granulomatous diseases
- Drugs (e.g., thiazides, lithium, antiestrogens, vitamins A and D)
- Familial hypocalciuric hypercalcemia
- Parenteral nutrition
- Immobilization
- Milk-alkali syndrome
- Acute and chronic renal insufficiency

A workable approach to this diagnosis separates the causes into two major areas:

- Parathyroid
- Nonparathyroid

- Vitamin D (endo-/exogenous)
- Malignant (metastatic/humoral)

Nonparathyroid causes of hypercalcemia are caused by vitamin D-mediated processes or malignant processes. Intoxication with exogenous vitamin D is seen now because of its use in treatment for osteoporosis.

Endogenous hypervitaminosis D arises from granulomatous diseases, such as sarcoidosis, but granuloma located in any part of the body may cause this form of hypercalcemia.

Malignant diseases also produce hypercalcemia. Some malignant diseases, such as breast cancer, cause skeletal destruction. Others, such as myeloma and epidermal (squamous) tumors, make chemical substances (humoral substances) that increase bone metabolism and its destruction. Myeloma tumors release interleukins and cytokines within the bone marrow from plasma cells that stimulate osteoclastic activity and ultimately bone turnover and calcium loss. Squamous or epidermal tumors produce parathyroid hormone-related protein (PTHrP). This substance, which increases bone loss and renal tubular reabsorption of calcium, is distinct from true parathyroid hormone.

LABORATORY STUDIES: PARATHYROID HORMONE ASSAY

The recent introduction of the intact parathyroid hormone assay, which uses sophisticated chemical techniques, has virtually eliminated problems noted in the past trying to differentiate parathyroid disease from other forms of hypercalcemia (e.g., ectopic) that might be caused by parathyroid hormone-related protein. This new assay clearly differentiates hyperparathyroidism and other disorders. The normal range is 10–65 pg/mL PTH for a serum calcium of 8.5–10.5 mg/dL. Increased values beyond the normal reference interval in combination with a high calcium value are diagnostic of the disorder. Nonparathyroid hormone-mediated causes of hypercalcemia should have no measurable intact parathyroid hormone.

DIFFERENTIAL DIAGNOSIS

The workup of hypercalcemia can be accomplished simply by using the algorithm shown in Figure 46.1. The measurement of parathyroid hormone immediately indicates parathyroid or nonparathyroid problems. Primary hyperparathyroidism is differentiated from other causes by measurable or increased values. If no measurable hormone is found, vitamin D intoxication or a malignancy is probably present. The serum phosphorus level can sometimes help make the distinc-

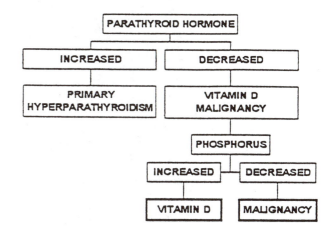

Figure 46.1. Diagnostic algorithm for hypercalcemia.

tion between these processes: When the serum phosphorus level is elevated or high normal, a vitamin D-mediated process is suspect (if renal function is normal). In some cases of metastatic disease to bone, one might see an elevation in serum phosphorus also, but this should not be a diagnostic difficulty because the history, physical, and radiological examinations help differentiate the two diseases. When the phosphorus level is low, a humoral agent from a cancer is often suspect, the most common being parathyroid hormone-related protein.

For purposes of board examinations, the algorithm in Figure 46.1 can be quite useful to quickly focus one's thinking—although the algorithm may oversimplify. Various permutations and combinations of secondary diseases can very well cloud the reality of which this diagram speaks.

TREATMENT OF HYPERCALCEMIA

Treatment of hypercalcemia is directed toward:

- Acute symptoms
- Long-term control of the underlying process

Treatment of acute symptoms begins with saline hydration to increase the excretion of sodium and calcium in the urine. Adequate hydration is mandatory to avert declining renal function and reabsorption of calcium. Loop diuretics (i.e., furosemide) have been considered first-line therapy in the past, but this is probably not the major approach taken today. Intravenous doses of biphosphonates, such as pamidronate (60–90 mg intravenous) or etidronate (7.5 mg/kg), are used to control the hypercalcemic process (pamidronate being more efficacious than etidronate). Use of a diuretic agent in hypercalcemia might be risky if the patient has not been sufficiently hydrated. Worsening dehydration in the face of diuretic use can actually promote worsening hypercalcemia, renal shutdown, and even death.

Table 46.1. Long-Term Control of Hypercalcemia	
Cause	*Treatment*
Parathyroid disease	Surgery
	No curative medication
Vitamin D related	Steroids
Malignancy	Control symptoms
	Chemotherapy for underlying tumor
	Steroids

Steroid use in treatment of hypercalcemia is helpful for specific disorders, such as vitamin D and myeloma, but is ineffective in parathyroid disease.

Injectable calcitonin has been used in the past for control of the hypercalcemia with a moderate degree of success. The doses range from 7–10 units per kilogram body weight per day. The side effects from administration of this drug—including nausea and vomiting—limit its usefulness.

Nasal spray calcitonin and oral bisphosphonates are not efficacious.

Long-term control of hypercalcemia is directed at eradicating the underlying disease (Table 46.1).

Parathyroid surgery is curative in almost all cases in which the parathyroid is the cause. Steroid therapy is curative for problems of vitamin D intoxication and certain tumors. Other forms of chemotherapy for cancer may offer long-term control of the hypercalcemic process. However, for malignancy-related hypercalcemia, weekly or monthly administration of an intravenous bisphosphonate is useful when the underlying disease cannot be completely eradicated.

Oral phosphates (i.e., neutrophos) do not work well over the long term. Intestinal side effects limit the necessary dose and tolerability.

Hypocalcemia and Osteomalacia

PATHOPHYSIOLOGY OF HYPOCALCEMIA AND OSTEOMALACIA

Osteomalacia is the hallmark of poor skeletal mineralization owing to hypocalcemia and/or hypophosphatemia. Symptoms range from subtle and obscure complaints to overt bone pain with palpation or movement and muscle weakness. Overt fractures and pseudofractures are the sign of insufficient mineralization. Osteomalacia and hypocalcemia arise from vitamin D deficiency or phosphate depletion, with the following causes:

- Vitamin D deficiency
  - Dietary lack
  - Deprivation of sunlight
  - Malabsorption
  - Increased catabolism
  - Decreased formation metabolites of vitamin D
- Phosphate depletion
  - Vitamin D deficiency
  - Renal tubular disorders
  - Oncogenic
  - Secondary hyperparathyroidism

Endogenous vitamin D arises from ultraviolet light irradiation of epidermal cholesterol. Deprivation of sunlight causes deficiency, but dietary sources of vitamin D will substitute for endogenous forms. In situations in which there is a dietary lack of this vitamin or abnormalities in the GI tract preventing absorption, deficiency may arise. Any gastrointestinal disease that alters absorption can lower serum vitamin D. Likewise, increased catabolism of vitamin D will produce a relative deficiency of vitamin D. (This occurs when drugs stimulate liver mitochondrial cytochrome P450 and increase the catabolism of the vitamin D.) Likewise, renal failure will decrease the serum concentration of bioactive vitamin D (1,25-dihydroxyvitamin D).

Phosphorus depletion—an uncommon cause of osteomalacia—may be an isolated finding or may be combined with hypocalcemia. Vitamin D deficiency causes hypophosphatemia and hypocalcemia. Renal tubular disorders cause a primary phosphorus leak or a widespread abnormality, such as noted in the Fanconi syndrome. In either case, correction of the phosphorus leak is very difficult. Rare mesenchymal tumors also cause osteomalacia because they block production of active vitamin D. Surgical removal of these tumors reverses the process.

Secondary hyperparathyroidism because of prolonged hypocalcemia also causes hypophosphatemia.

DIAGNOSIS OF HYPOCALCEMIA AND OSTEOMALACIA

LABORATORY STUDIES

The primary findings of osteomalacia include:

- Hypocalcemia
- Hypophosphatemia
- Hyperphosphatasia (defined as increased alkaline phosphatase)

Increased alkaline phosphatase is not invariably present in all cases. The degree to which it is elevated is directly proportional to the underlying changes in bone metabolism. Secondary findings include decreased urinary calcium and phosphorus; however, urinary phosphorus increases in renal tubular leak and secondary hyperparathyroidism. Other laboratory findings arise from the underlying diseases.

To summarize the osteomalacia laboratory data:

- Primary findings
  - Decreased calcium and/or phosphorus
  - Variable increase in alkaline phosphatase
- Secondary findings
  - Decreased urinary calcium/phosphorus
  - Increased parathyroid hormone
  - Other disease specific changes

DIFFERENTIAL DIAGNOSIS

Figure 46.2 contains a useful clinical algorithm with which to establish the general categories of hypocalcemia. The presence of hypocalcemia prompts the evaluation of albumin first. Decreased serum albumin causes a corresponding decrease in total serum calcium. Every gram of albumin binds 0.8 mg calcium, hence a given serum calcium must first be corrected for serum albumin. (Serum ionized calcium does not respond to changes in serum albumin.) If serum albumin is normal, then the presence of hypocalcemia is real. The ambient phosphorus level thereafter serves to differentiate the causes of hypocalcemia quite nicely. With normal phosphatemia or hypophosphatemia, intestinal disease is probable. Suitable workup is therefore undertaken in that respect. In the presence of increased phosphorus, parathyroid disease or renal disease is the main cause. Serum creatinine differentiates these two possibilities. In renal disease, the level is elevated, and in parathyroid disease, it is normal.

Hypoparathyroidism is a very rare phenomenon:

- Primary hypoparathyroidism—clearly the most rare of the disorders—generally arises early in life. It is associated with either an autoimmune phenomenon of other endocrine glands or embryological atresia of the parathyroid gland.
- Secondary hypoparathyroidism is more common. Postoperative hypoparathyroidism may occur after neck surgery for parathyroid, thyroid, or malignant diseases.
- Acute hypoparathyroidism is unusual.
- Some patients develop hypoparathyroidism years after neck surgery.
- Infiltrated diseases of the parathyroid gland are rare.

There are a number of subtypes of ''apparent'' hypoparathyroidism that are even more rare. In pseudohypoparathyroidism, for example, there is appropriate secretion of parathyroid hormone, but the activity of this hormone does not occur because of dysfunction in the target organ receptor for the hormone. Another form of apparent hypoparathyroidism arises in intestinal dysfunction, magnesium malabsorption, and deficiency. A low magnesium level causes poor synthesis and secretion of parathyroid hormone, poor activity of the hormone at its receptor sites, and poor production of vitamin D. True hypoparathyroidism would not cause osteomalacia or bone disease, but in pseudohypoparathyroidism, in which there are defective receptors in the kidneys, one may actually see normal receptors in the bone that do respond to parathyroid hormone and cause osteitis.

TREATMENT OF HYPOCALCEMIA AND OSTEOMALACIA

Treatment options include:

- Correct the underlying disease
- Calcium supplementation
  - Empirical (i.e., 2.0 g elemental Ca)
  - Tablet or liquid preparations
  - Meal timing
- Vitamin D supplements
  - Calciferol, calderal, calcitriol

Attention to the underlying disease process causing abnormalities in the vitamin D and phosphorus is primary. Calcium supplementation is used if the dietary sources are limited. Dairy products are essential because they provide 80% of daily calcium. The minimum daily requirement in men and premenopausal women is 1000 mg elemental calcium. In its absence, calcium supplements are needed. Most supplements are carbonate salt. These provide more calcium per tablet (40% by weight) than other calcium supplements. The carbonate salt may not be absorbed in patients with achlorhydria or other intestinal diseases. The citrate salt has a theoretical advantage because it is absorbed more efficiently in patients with normal physiology. There are no data showing how effective it might be in situations in which intestinal dysfunction occurs.

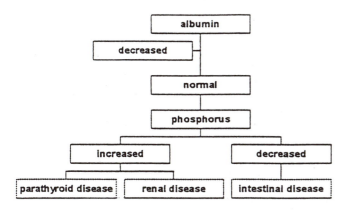

Figure 46.2. Diagnostic algorithm for hypocalcemia.

Another consideration is the use of liquid calcium supplement. Liquids may be more easily absorbed than tablets. In general, generic brands of calcium might be as readily bioavailable as brand names. However, this may not always be the situation. Studies have indicated that the dissolution or breakdown of calcium tablets in an ounce or two of household vinegar is a good sign of the relative bioavailability in the stomach.

Vitamin D supplementation for patients who are vitamin D deficient or who may need assistance in the absorption of calcium is the next consideration. The cheaper forms of the vitamin are generally the cholecalciferol or ergocalciferol derivatives, precursors to the 25- and 1,25-hydroxyl derivatives. These vitamins are available in 50,000 unit doses per capsule. In profound hypocalcemia from hypoparathyroidism, for example, the number of units daily may range from 50,000 to 500,000. In simple cases of hypocalcemia and osteomalacia, the dose may be as small as 50,000 a week. The most potent vitamin D forms, the 25-hydroxy D (calderol) and 1,25-dihydroxyvitamin D (calcitriol) are more expensive, but they are safer to use. If there is evidence of hypercalcemia, discontinuation of the vitamin restores eucalcemia within days. In patients who cannot absorb oral medications, the use of injectable vitamin D is mandatory. Ergo-calciferol is generally the vitamin used, although an injectable form of calcitriol is used for dialysis patients and may be given intravenously.

Osteoporosis

PATHOPHYSIOLOGY OF OSTEOPOROSIS

Osteoporosis is a multifactorial disease that ultimately leads to insufficiency of skeletal strength and increased susceptibility to fracture from relatively minor or nontraumatic causes. It is histologically manifested by thinning, perforation, and breakage of trabecular plates within the interior of the bone and a subsequent lack of compression strength.

Epidemiologically, the disorder is broken down as follows:

* Primary disorder
  * Type I
  * Type II
* Secondary disorders
  * A variety of problems (i.e., drugs, cancer)

Type I form occurs from high bone turnover secondary to estrogen deficiency at the time of menopause; the latter arises later in life from a host of factors that result from prior menopausal bone loss and insufficient osteoblastic or bone formation properties. Attendant abnormalities include decreased calcium absorption, vitamin D metabolism, and increased parathyroid hormone levels.

Secondary causes of osteoporosis run the gamut of many diseases. The reference list covers these topics in greater depth.

Pathophysiology of osteoporosis can be categorized into four major headings:

* Genetic
* Nutritional
* Hormonal
* Lifestyle

GENETIC IMPACT

There is a genetic component to the disorder, as it occurs in families. Of all risk factors spoken about in the literature, the most robust clinically is that of the prior history of osteoporosis in the family. This fact alone will often pinpoint individuals in the family—both men and women—whose parents have had osteoporosis and who themselves have evidence of bone deficiency (osteopenia) without evidence of clinical fracturing. Epidemiological studies clearly indicate that the daughters of osteoporotic patients have osteopenia, even in their early years. The daughters of patients without osteoporosis have normal bone mass for age.

Racial differences, too, are noted clearly. More often osteoporosis is present in Caucasian and Asian women than in African-Americans. However, this does not imply that the African-American woman cannot get osteoporosis from secondary causes.

NUTRITIONAL IMPACT

The major nutritional factor involved in osteoporosis is that of calcium sufficiency. The debate still rages whether calcium is a causal or promoting factor. Deficiency of dairy products in the diet will lead to insufficiency of calcium, since most of our nutrient source comes from the dairy elements. Most people require 1000 mg of elemental calcium a day. More may be required in the postmenopausal woman because of a relative inability to efficiently absorb calcium. The generally recommended dose is 1500 mg or more.

The effects of calcium on the skeleton are directly related to the age of the individual. There is a degree of bone loss attributable to the aging process, the exact details of which are not well understood. This degree of loss is small in nature (about 0.1% yearly). It tends to arise after the age of 30 and in the later years of life, usually about 10 or more years postmenopause. Calcium is helpful to control bone metabolism due to the aging process.

The time immediately around menopause and 5–10 years beyond is a point when calcium supplementation cannot control the turnover of bone. This time period is associated with a high degree of bone loss from osteoclastic activity secondary to estrogen deficiency.

Overuse of other substances in the diet, such as alcohol and tobacco, has a negative influence on bone metabolism and must be a consideration in osteoporosis. Most individuals do not develop nephrolithiasis when the calcium content is increased in the diet. The body regulates its absorption of calcium to the point where hypercalciuria and stone disease generally will not occur. However, if there is a pre-existing problem with hypercalciuria or history of renal stones in a patient or in the family, this is a sign to evaluate for the presence of hypercalciuria before supplementation and, more important, after supplementation is started. This simple test can uncover potential problems before they lead to stone disease.

HORMONAL IMPACT

Hormonal factors have long been known to be an associated problem in osteoporosis. The postmenopausal woman with her loss of estrogen has an increased production of osteoclasts and secondary increased bone turnover and loss. This is the reason why estrogen and antiosteoclastic drugs are the most useful treatment in women at this point in time and why calcium alone is not sufficient. During menopause, the rates of loss of bone might be 10 to 20 times higher than the rate caused by the aging process.

Pubertal development of estrogen also should be considered. Estrogen is a major stimulant of bone growth in the teenage girl. Any aberrations in growth at this time will ultimately lead to insufficiency of the amount of bone a child will have in adult life. Adolescent development directly determines the peak bone mass each individual will have. Inability to attain this during adolescence leads to a less than maximally calcified adult skeleton.

LIFESTYLE IMPACT

One's lifestyle or exercise pattern, too, is intimately related to the overall strength of the skeleton. Increasing muscle mass and strength concurrently increases skeletal mass. The dilemma clinicians face is the amount and types of exercise that are needed to promote a healthy skeleton. In premenopausal women, especially, too little, as well as too much exercise, is risky. Too much exercise causes amenorrhea and bone weakening. Exercise maximizes peak bone mass during adolescence, helps maintain adult bone mass, and attenuates loss because of the aging process.

DIAGNOSIS OF OSTEOPOROSIS

The diagnosis of osteoporosis in its early asymptomatic stage was a challenge until the introduction of dual-energy x-ray absorptiometry (DEXA) instruments for measurement of bone density. Diagnosis was formerly done by exclusion, since there were no diagnostic biochemical tests or noninvasive measurements of bone density.

Early osteoporosis produces no symptoms; finding it obviously is a challenge. The presence of osteopenia noted on radiographs usually indicates a loss of at least 20–30% of bone mass, which represents about 10 years of silent osteoporosis. Most cases of asymptomatic disease will have no abnormal biochemical test. The new bone markers that have been promoted commercially do not diagnose osteoporosis; they are only markers of alterations in bone metabolism.

Bone densitometry is the single most important factor in the prediction of fractures in patients who have osteoporosis. These tests (which cost from $75 to $200) are performed either at the initiation of a diagnostic workup or initiation of therapy and then repeated 1 or 2 years later to assess therapy. The usual considerations for its use include:

- Family history
- Atraumatic fractures
- Steroid use
- Back pain
- Monitor therapy
- Decision point for hormone-replacement therapy

These measurements concentrate on the rapidly turning over trabecular bone in the spine or femoral head and neck that is lost earliest. Bone density measurements at these sites more than 2.5 standard deviations below peak mass are classified as osteoporosis by World Health Organization guidelines. (At these levels, the fracture risk shows a 2–300% rise.) Values between −1.0 and −2.5 standard deviations below peak bone mass are classified as osteopenic, an intermediate zone that has relatively poor prognostic significance regarding fracture. Fracture risk is dramatically increased with deficits in density over two standard deviations below peak bone mass. By the time a patient develops fractures, back pain, height loss, and kyphosis, there is little challenge in diagnosing osteoporosis because this is the hallmark of the disease that has occurred unchecked for years.

TREATMENT FOR OSTEOPOROSIS

Therapy for established osteoporosis includes:

- Calcium supplementation with or without vitamin D
- Exercise
- Skeletal pharmacological agents
  - Antiresorptives (e.g., estrogen, calcitonin, and bisphosphonates)
  - Stimulators (e.g., fluoride and parathyroid hormone)

Stimulators of bone growth are not yet well established in the pharmacological treatment of osteoporosis. Although there is evidence that sodium fluoride increases bone mass, an inappropriate dose may very well lead to poor and weak bone that usually fractures despite the increment in mass. For this reason, fluoride is not a widely used drug in the general treatment of osteoporosis but is reserved for use by specialists. Parathyroid hormone at low doses is anabolic for the skeleton. Investigative efforts are underway in its use for bone growth.

All therapies used to date are antiresorptive in nature; they work against osteoclasts and reduce bone turnover and loss:

- Estrogen controls the local production of bone marrow cytokines that stimulate osteoclastic bone resorption, thus its use in menopause is more potent than that of calcium supplementation.
- Calcitonin is another antiosteoclastic drug that has, up until recently, been available only as an injection. (It is now available as a nasal spray. The spray dosage is one puff per day, representing about 200 units of calcitonin.)
- The bisphosphonate drugs hold a major place in the treatment of osteoporosis and will do so for the foreseeable future. These potent antiresorbers effect osteoclastic function, decrease bone turnover, and actually increase bone mass to varying degrees depending on the individual biphosphonate.
- The recently approved bisphosphonate alendronate (Fosamax) increases bone density in the spine and hip and prevents vertebral fractures when given at a daily dose of 10 mg. Recent data suggest that lower doses may actually prevent the progression or development of osteoporosis in much the same fashion as estrogen has done.

THERAPY FOR PREVENTION

Estrogen therapy in the prevention of osteoporosis has been used for more than 20 years. In women with an intact uterus, it is combined with a progestin agent to stop development of endometrial hyperplasia and reduce the risk of endometrial cancer. The usual daily doses of estrogen are 0.625 mg conjugated estrogen or its equivalent. Corresponding doses of progestin are between 2.5 mg and 5 mg. These may be given cyclically or daily. Cyclical use produces menses to varying degrees. Daily combined use prevents menses but affords the bone protective effect. The influence of the progestin on lipid and cardiovascular function is only beginning to be understood. Women with a prior hysterectomy generally do not use the progestin. However, some believe it has skeletal benefit. Some women complain of premenstrual symptoms from progestins, which limits its use.

Estrogen patches are also used to provide replacement therapy. Although they have not been available as long as the oral agents, there is evidence suggesting that they too may be useful agents to prevent osteoporosis. Clinical evidence shows significant impact on hip fractures with use of estrogen. Long-term use of estrogen therapy is mandatory since discontinuation abruptly will lead to bone loss as would have been the case had it not been used. Additional benefits of the use of estrogen include beneficial effects on the vascular system, the heart, and lipoprotein profiles. Estrogen increases HDL cholesterol and lowers LDL cholesterol because of the increased clearance of LDL through hepatic uptake. Although estrogen patches have similar effects upon menopausal symptoms in the skeleton, they may not have as many effects upon lipoprotein profiles.

The controversy of breast cancer and the use of estrogen continues. There is yet no definitive evidence completely excluding the possibility of an effect of estrogen on breast cancer, nor is there any conclusive evidence indicating that it causes it. The antiestrogen drugs that are used in the treatment of breast cancer have served as a model for the development of other forms of antiestrogen drugs that may substitute for estrogen in the treatment of menopausal problems. These agents have antiestrogen effects on the uterus and breasts, but estrogenlike effects upon the heart, blood vessels, lipid profiles, and bone. Low dose alendronate (5 mg daily) can substitute for estrogen. Likewise the new drug, raloxifene, will prevent bone loss.

Paget's Disease of Bone

Paget's disease of bone is a common finding in the general population. It is most often found incidentally during routine radiographs for other purposes. It may be present in as many as 3–5% of the population older than 50. Generally, an asymptomatic finding without clinical significance, Paget's disease is often monostotic. With spread of the disorder, bone deformity and pain may arise. Most common, the pelvic, femoral, cranial, and vertebral bones are affected, although any and all bones may be involved.

In the absence of significant clinical findings, most patients will not seek any medical care. Only after pain develops and skeletal deformity arises do most patients seek assistance. Cranial nerve involvement may arise when skeletal deformity of the vault occurs. More common, cranial nerve 8 is involved, although all cranial nerves might be troubled in very severe cases. Higher incidence of fractures arises because the skeletal structure, although looking more massive, is actually architecturally weaker. Osteosarcoma is an extraordinarily rare complication.

Biochemical evaluation of the disorder usually shows the presence of increased alkaline phosphatase with normal calcium and phosphorus levels. With immobilization, hypercalcemia may arise, although this is not an invariable finding.

Treatment of the disorder is generally directed toward the control of pain and the underlying pagetic process. Unfortunately, most patients are seen considerably far along the course of the disorder, so anatomical skeletal deformities are beyond treatment with the usual antiresorptive drugs. Generally, calcitonin and the bisphosphonates are the first-line therapy. Any tolerable and effective analgesic may be used to control pain, although control of the underlying pagetic process may completely eradicate the pain that brings the patient to the physician's office.

REVIEW EXERCISES

QUESTIONS

1. A 35-year-old man presents with a 10 year history of renal-stone disease and diffuse arthralgias. He is otherwise healthy and uses no vitamins, minerals or drugs.

- Review of systems normal
- Tibial radiograph showed a lesion at the midshaft
- Serum data
  - Calcium, 11.8 mg/dL (8.5–10.5)
  - Phosphorus, 2.9 mg/dL (2.5–4.5)
  - Creatinine, 1.0 mg/dL (0.5–1.3)
  - Intact PTH, 87.0 pg/ mL (10–65)
  - Calcitriol, 52.0 pg/mL (13–60)

All of the following are true except:

a. Treatment with pamidronate (Aredia) is not necessary.
b. Adenomectomy is curative is most cases.
c. Recurrence is unlikely.
d. The chronicity of the problem argues for the presence of an ectopic disorder.
e. Steroids will not control the problem.

2. A 53-year-old woman presents with generalized pain, muscle weakness, and weight loss. She uses estrogen and progestin for menopausal symptoms and has lost 30 pounds over 3–5 years. Her bowel habits may be more frequent. She shows diffuse pain in all bones on examination. Her gait is painful and her muscles are tender to touch.

- Baseline data
  - Hemoglobin, 10.3 g/dL
  - Calcium, 5.2 mg/dL
  - Phosphorus, 2.8 mg/dL
  - Albumin, 3.5 g/ dL
  - Creatinine, 1.0 mg/dL
  - Alkaline phosphatase, 226 IU/L

- Other data
  - iPTH 206 pg/mL (10–65)
  - Calcitriol 35 pg/mL (15–52)
  - Urine calcium 3 mg/d (100–300)

She is given calcium and vitamin D. The urine calcium rises to 15 mg/d. She calls and says she has bruises on her arms an legs.

All the following are true except:

a. She may have celiac disease.
b. She requires surgery for the hyperparathyroidism.
c. Her serum carotene is likely elevated.
d. Increased calcium and vitamin orally may be the only therapy needed.
e. Increased osteoid should be found.

3. A spinal deformity is noted on the radiograph of 73-year-old woman who was seen for back pain and spinal compression fracture. She was previously healthy except for cholecystectomy. She is a heavy tobacco and perhaps alcohol user and was on a golf outing when the incident occurred. She is being treated with calcium and analgesics.

- Radiograph of spine showed fracture at L2
- Examination: An emaciated woman in severe pain noted in lumbar region
- Data
  - Calcium, 8.6 mg/dL
  - Alkaline phosphatase, 100 IU/L
  - Protein ,6.0 g/dL
  - Hemoglobin, 10 g
  - Sed rate, 100 mm/hr

You decide to:

a. Continue analgesics
b. Start estrogen and extra calcium
c. Evaluate the problem further
d. Start Fosamax
e. Start calcitonin and physical therapy

Answers

1. d

The chronicity of the renal stone disease combined with the increased serum calcium, decreased phosphorus, increased parathyroid hormone, and high normal calcitriol (1,25-dihydroxyvitamin D) is typical of hyperparathyroidism. The radiograph finding of a brown tumor or cyst typifies the bone disease (osteitis fibrosa cystica) of hyperparathyroidism. The best treatment is parathyroidectomy of the offending adenoma. Hyperplasia is an unusual finding in most cases.

2. b

Her examination is significant for muscle tenderness and bone pain. Biochemical data show hypocalcemia, hypophosphatemia, hypoalbuminemia, hyperphosphatasia, and anemia. She has secondary hyperparathyroidism, very low levels of urinary calcium, and normal vitamin D (calcitriol). She is given more calcium and vitamin D, but the urinary calcium increases little. She notes bruising on her arms and legs, suggesting clotting abnormalities from vitamin deficiency.

3. c

A diagnosis of osteoporosis was made. When the patient was originally seen, she was quite ill appearing. Her laboratory tests showed anemia and increased sedimentation rate. Serum calcium was low normal, and alkaline phosphatase was high normal. The best response to the question is to evaluate the problem further. None of the answers deals with the critical issue of the abnormal tests. Primary osteoporosis is not associated with any chemical abnormality. The elevated sedimentation rate and the anemia are harbingers of other problems. Starting her on analgesics to temporize and control some of her discomfort might be reasonable, but clearly more needs to be done. The use of estrogen and calcium or Fosamax or physical therapy and calcitonin is a long-term solution to the problem if it proves to be primary osteoporosis. In this particular case, the patient's disorder was much more ominous than evidenced by the compression deformity on radiograph; the compression deformity was the result of an erosive tumor rather than primary osteoporosis.

SUGGESTED READINGS

Belizekian JP. Management of acute hypercalcemia. N Engl J Med 1992;326:1196–1203.

Bourke E, Delaney B. Assessment of hypocalcemia and hypercalcemia. Clin Lab Med 1993;13:157–181.

Consensus Development Conference. Prophylaxis and treatment of osteoporosis. Am J Med 1991;90:107–119.

Dilmas PD, ed. Osteoporosis: who should be treated? Am J Med 1995;98(Suppl 2A).

Edelson G, Kleerekoper M. Hypercalcemic crisis. Med Clin North Am 1995;79:79–92.

Johnston CC, Slemenda CW, Melton LJ. Clinical use of bone densitometry. N Engl J Med 1991;324:1105–1109.

Lang P, Steiger P, Faulker K, et al. Osteoporosis: current techniques and recent developments in quantitative bone densitometry. Radiol Clin North Am 1991;29:49–76.

Marcus R. Laboratory diagnosis of primary hyperparathyroidism. Endocrinol Metab Clin North Amer 1989;18:647–658.

Mundy GR. Incidence and pathophysiology of hypercalcemia. Calcified Tissue Intl 1990;165(Suppl 2):3–10.

NIH Conference. Diagnosis and management of asymptomatic primary hyperparathyroidism: consensus development conference statement. Ann Intern Med 1991;114:593–597.

Osteoporosis: epidemiology, screening, diagnosis, treatment and prevention. Am J Managed Care 1996;2(Suppl 1).

Riggs BL. Overview of osteoporosis. Western J Med 1991; 154:63–77.

Board Simulation: Endocrinology

S. Sethu K. Reddy

QUESTIONS

1. A 40-year-old Type 1 diabetic patient has a blood pressure of 150/95, a pulse of 96, HgbA$_{1c}$ of 10%, and elevated triglycerides. Which class of antihypertensive agents should be avoided in this patient?

   a. ACE-inhibitors
   b. Angiotensin II receptor blockers
   c. Calcium channel blockers
   d. Alpha-adrenergic blockers
   e. Beta-blockers

2. A 40-year-old Type 1 diabetic patient has a blood pressure of 150/95, a pulse of 96, HgbA$_{1c}$ of 10%, and elevated triglycerides. Which class of antihypertensive agents would most consistently help lower triglycerides in this patient?

   a. ACE-inhibitors
   b. Angiotensin II receptor blockers
   c. Calcium channel blockers
   d. Alpha-adrenergic blockers
   e. Beta-blockers

3. A 37-year-old white male with Type 1 diabetes mellitus has a blood pressure of 140/90, HgbA$_{1c}$ of 8.6%, urinary albumin excretion rate of 45 microgm/min (N = < 30), and normal electrolytes. Which of the following should be started to treat his blood pressure?

   a. Clonidine 0.1 mg at bedtime
   b. Captopril 12.5 mg three times a day
   c. Propranolol 20 mg three times a day

   d. Doxazosin 1 mg twice a day
   e. Diltiazem 60 mg three times a day

4. A 40-year-old white male with a 27-year history of Type 1 diabetes mellitus on a four-times-a-day insulin regimen complains of nausea, diarrhea, and postprandial hypoglycemia. Which of the following laboratory tests may help to establish a diagnosis?

   a. Gastric emptying study
   b. Serum electrolytes
   c. Cortrosyn stimulation test
   d. All of the above
   e. None of above

5. Figure 47.1 shows what type of diabetic retinopathy?

   a. None
   b. Background with macular edema
   c. Preproliferative with cotton wool exudates
   d. Preproliferative with hard exudates
   e. Proliferative diabetic retinopathy

6. A 45-year-old white female with Type 2 diabetes mellitus presents with a skin rash (Fig. 47.2). Which of the following should be done?

   a. Refer to dermatology for a biopsy.
   b. Check a HgbA$_{1c}$ and treat as appropriate.
   c. Start Flagyl 250 mg three times a day.
   d. Start prednisone 40 mg daily and taper over 10 days.
   e. Hospitalize patient for intravenous antibiotics.

7. Which is the most likely lipid profile associated

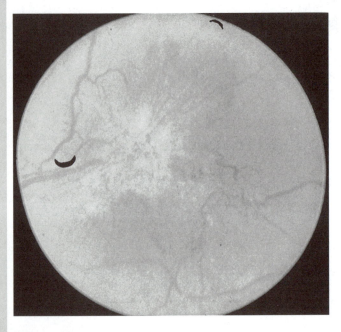

Figure 47.1. Diabetic retinopathy for the patient in question 5 (see color plate).

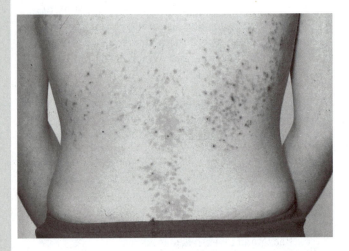

Figure 47.2. Skin rash in the patient in question 6 (see color plate).

with the situation in Question 6? (All values are mg/dl.)

	TC	TG	HDL-C	LDL-C
A.	200	100	40	140
B.	3000	10,000	13	45
C.	450	100	40	390
D.	225	540	25	110
E.	500	480	35	385

8. A drug from which of the following drug classes would be the best to treat the associated lipid disorder?

   a. HMG CoA reductase inhibitor

   b. Niacin
   c. Bile acid sequestrant
   d. Fibric acid derivative
   e. Probucol

9. A patient is referred to you with the following thyroid indices: T_4 = 15.5 μg/dl (4–10.8), TSH = 5 uIU/mL (0.4–5.0). Which of the following situations is least compatible with this profile?

   a. Thyroid hormone resistance
   b. Symptoms of hyperthyroidism and a TSH adenoma
   c. Patient is on oral contraceptives
   d. Patient has acute hepatitis
   e. Patient has subacute thyroiditis with symptoms of hyperthyroidism for the past 4 weeks

10. A 25-year-old woman presents with classic symptoms of hyperthyroidism, an elevated T_4, and a suppressed TSH. Which of the following best confirms the diagnosis of Graves' disease?

    a. Increased RAIU by the thyroid
    b. Stare and lid lag
    c. Pretibial myxedema
    d. Positive antimicrosomal (anti-TPO) antibodies
    e. Family history of Graves' disease

11. A woman with Graves' disease has been treated with propylthiouracil (PTU) 100 mg three times a day for the past 2 months. Her symptoms have abated, her pulse is 72/min, and she has gained 5 pounds in weight. Her T_4 is 11.0 μg/dL(4–10.8) and TSH <0.03 μIU/mL (0.4–5.0). What do you do now?

    a. Increase the PTU until TSH returns to normal.
    b. Reassure her that her weight gain will stop.
    c. Add propranolol to regimen.
    d. Stop the PTU.
    e. Do not make any changes and reassess in 6–8 weeks.

12. You are asked to see a patient in the ICU for pneumonia after gastrointestinal surgery. His T_4 is 3.9 μg/dL (4–10.8), and his TSH is 2.5 μIU/mL (0.4–5.0). Which of the following is false?

    a. He should be started on cytomel to rapidly correct the problem until the pneumonia resolves.
    b. He should have thyroid function tests in 2 to 3 months.
    c. His T_3 will be low.
    d. His free T_4 will be normal.
    e. A RAIU and scan of thyroid are of no value.

13. A 50-year-old woman with a 5-year history of menopausal symptoms is evaluated for osteoporosis prevention. She has a family history of breast cancer and refuses hormonal replacement therapy. She has a 20-year history of hyperprolactinemia treated with

bromocryptine with good success. Her spinal bone density has declined from 1.12g/cm² to 0.92g/cm² in 5 years. Options for her care include all of the following except:

a. Daily etidronate
b. Alendronate
c. Calcium
d. Etidronate cyclically
e. Calcitonin (intranasal)

14. An 85-year-old man is admitted for hypercalcemia. He is comatose and anuric. Calcium, 15.1 mg/dL; Phos., 2.0 mg/dL; Creat., 6.0 mg/dL; CO_2, 18 meq/L; Alkaline Phosphatase, 184 IU/L; intact PTH, 110 mg/ml. He has been ill for 6 months and has lost 30 pounds. He has a 20-year history of renal stones. Therapy may include all of the following except:

a. Furosemide
b. Prednisone
c. Saline hydration
d. Intravenous pamidronate

15. A 73-year-old woman has severe pain with walking. She had a history of ovarian cancer many years ago treated with a total abdominal hysterectomy and postoperative radiation. Her weight has gradually declined about 30 pounds but has remained stable for 5 years. Her legs hurt with movement. A bone scan shows multiple hot spots in the ribs and right femur. Her ESR is 5 mm/hr; alk-ptase, 550 IU/L; creatinine, 0.8 mg/dL; calcium, 7.5 mg/dL. Which of the following is most likely to be correct?

a. Bone biopsy, osteomalacia; PTH, low; phos, high
b. Bone biopsy, metastatic cancer; PTH, normal; phos, normal
c. Bone biopsy, osteoporosis; PTH, normal; phos, low
d. PTH, high; 25-hydroxy D, low; urine calcium, low
e. Bone biopsy, osteomalacia; PTH, high; carotene, high

16. A 35-year-old woman has epilepsy since her teens for which she has been treated with a variety of anticonvulsants. Recently, she developed rib and spinal fractures with a seizure. Her menstrual periods are irregular. She has been on oral contraceptive agents. Serum Ca^{++}, 8.6 mg/dL; Phos, 3.0 mg/dL; alk ptase, 110 IU/L. Her bone density is more than 2 SD below her age norms. Which is the best option to offer her?

a. Cyclical editronate, repeat bone mineral densitometry (BMD) in 6 months
b. Daily alendronate, repeat BMD in 6 months
c. Vitamin D and calcium, repeat BMD in 1–2 years
d. Calcium, repeat BMD in 1–2 years
e. Nasal calcitonin, repeat BMD in 1 year

17. A 55 year-old man has a 20-year history of hypoparathyroidism following thyroidectomy. He has been eucalcemic with daily calcium lactate and 150,000 units ergocalciferol. Until recently efforts to self-wean from these drugs caused mild tetany. One year ago, he discontinued his calcium and vitamin D without developing tetany. His only other medical problem is use of cigarettes. His weight has decreased 5 pounds, but he has no other complaints. His calcium is 10.0 mg/dL, Phos is 3.1 mg/dL. You order a chest radiograph. Which of the following additional tests would you not order initially?

a. TB skin test
b. Serum electrolytes and osmolality
c. PTH-related peptide
d. ACE level
e. Colonoscopy

18. Which of the following patients would be likely to require treatment with fludrocortisone?

a. A 23-year-old female with Hashimoto's thyroiditis and Type 1 DM who is having recurrent hypoglycemia despite decreasing doses of insulin
b. A 63-year-old man with bitemporal hemianopsia who presents with decreased libido, impotence, cold intolerance and anorexia/nausea
c. A 34-year-old hyperkalemic, pregnant woman with lupus anticoagulant on chronic heparin, but no evidence of adrenal hemorrhage on CT
d. Two of the above
e. All of the above

19. A 35-year-old male presents with muscle weakness. He has hypertension treated with hydrochlorthiazide. His family history is positive for early onset hypertension. His lab evaluation shows: K^+, 2.9 mEq/L; HCO_3, 34 mEq/L. Further evaluation shows suppressed plasma renin activity and low aldosterone. Which of the following is least likely?

a. Cushing's syndrome
b. Liddle's syndrome
c. Licorice ingestion
d. An adenoma of the zona glomerulosa
e. Renal artery stenosis

20. A 22-year-old woman has headaches. An MRI suggests a 3 mm pituitary nodule. She has no symptoms of hormone excess or deficiency. Her serum prolactin level is 16 ng/ml (N< 15). Appropriate management would be?

a. Bromocriptine 1.25 mg orally at bedtime
b. Refer to radiotherapist
c. Referral to a neurosurgeon
d. Continued observation of prolactin levels
e. Repeat MRI in 1 month

21. A 40-year-old man presents with a history of headaches, impotence, and difficulty with his vision. Which of the following defects rules out a pituitary tumor as the cause of his symptoms?

    a. Homonymous hemianopsia
    b. Unilateral visual loss
    c. Bitemporal hemianopsia
    d. None of the above
    e. a and b only

22. Which of the following case scenarios is least likely to be associated with elevated prolactin levels?

    a. A 25-year-old woman with chronic schizophrenia
    b. A 45-year-old woman with reflux esophagitis on cisapride
    c. A 50-year-old man with peptic ulcer disease and heart burn on metaclopramide
    d. A 53-year-old woman with shingles along T_5
    e. A 42-year-old woman with cold intolerance and a goiter

23. The wife of a patient whom you are following for his recent history of hyperparathyroidism and a gastrinoma contacts you. She is concerned about their children, who are ages 20 and 25 years. How would you perform annual screening in these adult children?

    a. Calcitonin
    b. Calcium
    c. Prolactin
    d. Glucose
    e. Gastrin

24. A 30-year-old woman has a 3-month history of polyuria. Her serum glucose is 95 mg/dL. After fluid restriction, her urine osmolality is 500 mOsm/kg and her plasma osmolality is 295 mOsm/kg. After a test dose of DDAVP, her urine osmolality rises to 750 mOsm/kg. The likely diagnosis is:

    a. Psychogenic polydipsia
    b. Complete central diabetes insipidus
    c. Nephrogenic diabetes insipidus
    d. Partial central diabetes insipidus
    e. No diabetes insipidus

25. A 54-year-old nonsmoker presents with hyperpigmentation. Which of the following scenarios is least compatible with this?

    a. History of left adrenalectomy for a benign nodule
    b. Recently emigrated from the Far East, with a positive PPD
    c. History of previous Cushing's syndrome treated with bilateral adrenalectomy
    d. Chest radiograph showing a new RUL lesion

26. A 30-year-old accountant with a recent diagnosis of prolactinoma complains of impotence as his main problem. He is wondering how such a small tumor can cause this. The best explanation for his symptoms is?

    a. Prolactin has a deleterious effect on the testes and reduces testosterone production.
    b. Prolactin decreases adrenal androgens.
    c. Prolactin inhibits GnRH secretion.
    d. Prolactin by its effect on salt and water excretion has direct vascular effects on penile blood flow.
    e. Prolactin increases conversion of testosterone to estradiol.

27. A 19-year-old woman with primary amenorrhea associated with short stature and a webbed neck is most likely to have which of the following laboratory profiles?

	LH (mIU/ml)	FSH (mIU/ml)	PROLACTIN (ng/ml)
a.	< 2	< 2	683
b.	< 2	< 2	68
c.	< 2	< 2	6
d.	2.3	3.1	18
e.	23	47	8

28. An 18-year-old postpubertal woman presents with primary amenorrhea and galactorrhea. Her initial laboratory evaluation should include?

    a. Serum prolactin, thyroid function tests
    b. β-HCG, serum prolactin, thyroid function tests
    c. Serum prolactin, MRI of pituitary
    d. Growth hormone, thyroid function tests, gonadotrophins
    e. β-HCG, mammogram

29. A 33-year-old woman presents with a 5-month history of secondary amenorrhea and galactorrhea. Her initial laboratory evaluation should include:

    a. Serum prolactin, thyroid function tests
    b. β-HCG, serum prolactin, thyroid function tests
    c. Serum prolactin, MRI of pituitary
    d. Growth hormone, thyroid function tests, gonadotrophins
    e. β-HCG, mammogram

30. A 46-year-old woman has had Type 1 diabetes mellitus for 3 years. Her self-monitoring blood glucose meter has been calibrated recently. She has no signs or symptoms of hypoglycemia. She is taking N30u in the morning and N10u before supper. Her lab results are: glucose, 170mg/dL; HgbA$_{1c}$, 8.9% (N = 4%–6%). Her SMBG record is very neat and shows: B: 95–130; L: 100–136; S: 100–130; hs: 90–117. How would you manage her diabetes at present?

    a. Monitor sugars less often and have patient return in 6 months.
    b. Continue present treatment.
    c. Disregard her SMBG records; review her diet,

lifestyle, and insulin regimen; and aim for improved glucose control.

   d. Book an eye clinic appointment and review in 6 months.

   e. Have patient purchase a new meter.

31. A 39-year-old white female has a 4-year history of episodic weakness and hunger relieved by food, especially at night and in morning. The symptoms are increasing in frequency, and she has gained 100 pounds. She had a capillary glucose of 30 mg/dL during one episode. She has a family history of hypothyroidism; she is G2P2 (gravida 2, para 2). On physical examination, she weighs 220 pounds and is 5 feet, 4 inches tall; otherwise, the examination is negative. The most useful test would be:

   a. Insulin antibodies

   b. Insulin tolerance test

   c. OGTT with glucose/insulin /C-peptide levels

   d. 72-hour fast with glucose/insulin/C-peptide levels

   e. ACTH-stimulation test

32. A 24-year-old white male with a 6-year history of Type 1 diabetes mellitus is brought to the emergency room in a coma, febrile, and stuporous. Pulse is 120/min, blood pressure is 100/50, RR is 20/min, and breath is "fruity." Lab results are plasma glu, 527 mg/dL; Na, 130 mEq/L; K, 3.6mEq/L; Cl, 95mEq/L; Bicarb, 14mEq/L; BUN, 30 mg/dL; Cr, 1.4 mg/dL; Ca, 9.8 mg/dL; Phos, 1.0 mg/dL; ABGs; pH, 7.18; pO_2, 85 mm Hg; pCO_2, 24 mm Hg.

   Which of the following is least essential in your management?

   a. KCl replacement

   b. Intravenous normal saline at 500–1000 mL/hr

   c. Potassium phosphate replacement

   d. Chest radiograph

   e. Intravenous regular insulin

33. A patient is taking 20 units of NPH, 10 units of regular in the morning. His average/typical capillary sugars on self-testing are:
Breakfast: 150mg%
Lunch: 110mg%
Supper: 180mg%
Bedtime: 145mg%
The best initial adjustment would be:

   a. Add some regular insulin at supper.

   b. Increase morning NPH insulin.

   c. Increase morning NPH and regular insulin.

   d. Add some regular insulin at supper and some NPH insulin at bedtime.

   e. Add NPH insulin at supper.

34. A 36-year-old man with Type 1 diabetes mellitus for 15 years presents with brittle DM. He has a history of proliferative retinopathy and recent diagnosis of

hypertension being treated with captopril. Routine labs show: HgbA$_{1c}$ of 7% (4%–6%); BUN, 25mg/dL; Cr, 1.4 mg/dL; Na, 135; K, 6.0; Cl, 104; Bicarb, 28; ECG, Normal. What is your best option?

   a. ACTH stimulation test

   b. Begin kayexalate

   c. Admit for ECG monitoring

   d. Change to a different antihypertensive drug

   e. Doppler study of renal arteries

35. Which of these XY individuals' scenarios are least compatible with presence of gynecomastia?

   a. Bilateral inguinal scars and absence of secondary sexual hair

   b. Well-controlled salt-losing congenital adrenal hyperplasia

   c. Spider-nevi, asterixis, and ascites

   d. A competitive body builder

   e. Hyperaldosteronism treated with spironolactone

36. A 19-year-old woman has primary amenorrhea. Which of the following is false in your evaluation?

   a. A karyotype is essential.

   b. Asherman's syndrome is a possibility.

   c. Prolactin and FSH levels would be helpful.

   d. A pregnancy test is necessary.

   e. The patient could be an XY male.

37. A 21-year-old woman has irregular menses, increasing facial hair, and acne. Which of the following is not indicated in your initial approach?

   a. Determine onset and progression of her symptoms

   b. order an ultrasound of the ovaries

   c. A high LH/FSH ratio might point to polycystic ovary syndrome

   d. An ACTH stimulation test might give the diagnosis

   e. Assure her that you will be able to improve her symptoms and signs in the next 6–9 months

38. A 36-year-old white female has a 3 cm thyroid nodule detected on routine physical examination. Which of the following is the best initial approach to her management?

   a. TSH and fine-needle aspiration biopsy

   b. TSH, radioactive iodine uptake and scan

   c. TSH and thyroglobulin

   d. Radioactive iodine uptake and scan

   e. Referral to surgeon for removal

39. A 55-year-old white male comes for evaluation of episodic hypertension. His family history reveals a brother who had "neck surgery" and takes cortisone. Which of the following is the most appropriate screening test panel for this multiple endocrine neoplasia (MEN)?

   a. Thyroglobulin, catecholamines

b. Test patient and his brother for "ret" protooncogene mutation

c. Calcitonin, calcium, catecholamines

d. Prolactin, calcitonin, calcium, gastrin

e. Catecholamines, prolactin, insulin

Answers

1. e

Of all the listed antihypertensive agents, the beta-blockers are the only agents that may raise serum triglyceride levels. Some of the newer beta-blockers with intrinsic sympathomimetic activity (ISA) may be less likely to affect serum triglyceride levels. If the patient also has hypoglycemic unawareness, beta-blockers should be avoided.

2. d

ACE-inhibitors, angiotensin II receptor blockers, and calcium channel blockers would be relatively neutral, whereas alpha adrenergic blockers have been shown to lower triglyceride levels and raise HDL cholesterol levels. Beta-blockers, of course, would be the least favored (see Question 1.).

3. b

In an individual with Type 1 diabetes, hypertension, and microalbuminuria, the use of ACE-inhibitors is favored because of their additional effect on intraglomerular hypertension. It should be noted, however, that any method of lowering blood pressure will lead to improvement in albumin excretion rates. Of course, improvement in glucose control is also crucial.

4. d

Individuals with Type 1 diabetes are more likely to develop another autoimmune disorder, including Addison's disease. Chronic diabetes may also cause autonomic neuropathy, and if the gastrointestinal system is involved, the patient may develop constipation initially and symptoms of gastroparesis, widely fluctuating blood sugars, and/or diarrhea.

5. e

Fig. 47.1 shows fronds of new blood vessels. These vessels are more friable and more likely to bleed. It is thought retinal hypoxia and resulting local secretion of growth factors result in the neovascularization. Early laser therapy may preserve vision and reduce the degree of subsequent neovascularization.

6. b

This individual has eruptive xanthoma that may be related to severe hypertriglyceridemia secondary to uncontrolled diabetes. There is no need for antibiotics, hospitalization, or a skin biopsy. Prednisone would not alleviate the rash and may actually worsen the hypertriglyceridemia.

7. b

In an individual with eruptive xanthoma, the serum triglycerides are usually greater than 1000 mg/dl. Remember that most laboratories report a calculated LDL cholesterol level, and triglyceride levels greater than 450–500 mg/dl invalidate Friedwald's formula.

8. d

Such dyslipidemias are best treated by a low-fat diet intended to maintain an ideal body weight and by improved glycemic control. If the mixed dyslipidemia (with much higher triglyceride levels) is still present, then a fibric acid derivative such as gemfibrozil is indicated. Other potential choices include niacin or atorvastatin, if the degree of mixed dyslipidemia is more modest.

9. e

If the individual is euthyroid, one must consider thyroid hormone resistance as well as causes of increased thyroid binding globulin levels such as oral contraceptive use or acute hepatitis. If the individual is hyperthyroid, it is possible that a TSH adenoma may be the cause, since the level of TSH is inappropriate for primary hyperthyroidism. With subacute thyroiditis, if the patient has elevated levels of thyroid hormone, the TSH should be suppressed below the normal range.

10. c

Increased radioactive iodide uptake only suggests increased thyroid activity, and a stare and lid lag may be observed in cases of hyperthyroidism of any cause. Antimicrosomal antibodies are nonspecific, and a family history of Graves' disease is suggestive but not confirmatory. Pretibial myxedema develops only in patients with Graves' disease. These patients also invariably have proptosis.

11. e

In the management of hyperthyroidism, as one normalizes the thyroid hormone levels, the TSH may remain suppressed, sometimes for more than 6 months. Therefore the TSH is not a good indicator for adjustment of therapy during initial treatment. This individual has clearly improved and is becoming euthyroid. One would not increase PTU, add propranolol, or stop PTU. Weight gain is a common problem during the treatment of hyperthyroidism, and the patient should be adequately informed of such a possibility.

12. a

This is a case of sick euthyroid syndrome. Although the low T_4 and T_3 levels are signs of poor prognosis, there is no value of thyroid replacement. Free T_4 levels, especially if checked by equilibrium dialysis method, will be normal. A RAIU and scan are never of value in the diagnostic workup of hypothyroidism.

13. a

All of the suggested agents are useful in the management of osteoporosis except daily etidronate. Daily etidronate may cause osteomalacia. Calcium alone will help reduce age-related osteoporosis but not menopause-related osteoporosis. In combination with other agents, however, calcium supplementation is helpful.

14. b

This patient appears to have severe hyperparathyroidism, which is unlikely to respond to glucocorticoids. The current standard therapy for treating severe hypercalcemia is adequate hydration followed by intravenous pamidronate.

15. d

This patient most likely has hypocalcemia related to osteomalacia secondary to vitamin D deficiency. This leads to increased PTH secretion. Malabsorption is the likely cause, and thus carotene levels may be expected to be low.

16. c

This patient has osteomalacia, probably secondary to presumed phenytoin therapy, and thus would most likely benefit from vitamin D and calcium therapy.

17. e

Since this patient does not require vitamin D and calcium therapy for his chronic hypoparathyroidism, one must be suspicious of another source of Vitamin D. Sarcoidosis, tuberculosis, or a malignancy must be considered. All of the investigations would be helpful except colonoscopy.

18. d

The first answer choice describes a patient with possible Addison's disease, and the third choice describes an individual with possible isolated hypoaldosteronism. Both these individuals may benefit from fludrocortisone therapy. The second choice describes a man with hypopituitarism, and thus mineralocorticoid supplementation is not necessary.

19. e

Renal artery stenosis is associated with increased plasma renin activity. The other causes are associated with decreased plasma renin activity.

20. d

This patient likely has nonfunctioning pituitary microadenoma. There is no need for therapy at present. The prolactin elevation is trivial and should just be followed.

21. d

A pituitary tumor may cause any of the described visual field defects, depending on whether the tumor impinges on the optic nerve, optic chiasm, or the optic tract.

22. b

All of the scenarios may be associated with elevated prolactin levels except answer choice b. Cisapride is not known to cause hyperprolactinemia.

23. b

The patient appears to have MEN 1, and thus hypercalcemia is most likely to precede other manifestations of this syndrome.

24. d

The patient appears to partially concentrate her urine with water deprivation and then has a further response to DDAVP. This suggests partial central diabetes insipidus.

25. a

A left adrenalectomy should not result in elevated ACTH

levels and hyperpigmentation. Immigrants from the Far East are more likely to have tuberculosis and thus more likely to have bilateral adrenalitis. The scenario in answer choice c describes Nelson's syndrome, in which an individual with an ACTH adenoma is treated with bilateral adrenalectomy, resulting in very high levels of ACTH and severe hyperpigmentation. Lung malignancies, in particular small cell Ca, are associated with ectopic ACTH syndrome and hyperpigmentation.

26. c

Prolactin does not have a direct effect on androgen production and in humans has no effect on salt and water balance. It is thought to inhibit GnRH secretion.

27. e

This scenario describes Turner's syndrome in which primary ovarian failure is associated with elevated gonadotrophins.

28. b

Any amenorrheic patient should always have the β-HCG checked to rule out pregnancy. Checking the prolactin and thyroid hormone levels is reasonable.

29. b

See explanation for Question 28.

30. c

It is important to rely on the HbA_{1c} as well as the self-monitoring blood glucose record to assess glycemic control. Often patients report only the better glucose levels. When one observes discordant results, one should look for alternative explanations. In this situation, the HbA_{1c} is more reliable, and thus the patient's control needs to be reassessed and therapy intensified.

31. d

This patient appears to have fasting hypoglycemia, and the gold standard test is still a prolonged fast with measure of glucose, insulin, and C-peptide levels. Many physicians check the C-peptide basally and again if patient develops hypoglycemia (plasma glucose less than 50 mg/dl). One should never rely on capillary blood glucose levels, and it is always important to document Whipple's triad.

32. c

In a case of diabetic ketoacidosis, fluids, insulin, avoiding hypokalemia, and ruling out a possible inciting cause are lifesaving. Even though the patient is probably depleted of phosphate, phosphate replacement as IV potassium phosphate is not beneficial.

33. b

The highest glucose levels occur at supper, which reflect the morning NPH effect. The first step would be to increase the morning NPH insulin dose and reassess the patient in a few days. Reducing the presupper glucose levels may have further salutary effects on later glucose levels.

34. d

In this scenario, a patient with chronic diabetes presents with hyperkalemia while on an ACE inhibitor. The potassium level is not critical, and the next step would be to change to another class of antihypertensive agents.

35. b

Hypogonadism, chronic liver disease, and the use of anabolic steroids and aldactone could cause gynecomastia. Salt-losing congenital adrenal hyperplasia is not linked to gynecomastia.

36. b

Asherman's syndrome describes secondary amenorrhea due to uterine scarring.

37. b

The presence or absence of cystic changes in the ovaries is not necessary to make a diagnosis of polycystic ovary syndrome. A rapid onset of symptoms or severe symptoms, often associated with extremely high androgen levels, would suggest a possible adrenal or ovarian tumor.

38. a

One should confirm a euthyroid status, and then a fine needle aspiration biopsy is indicated. If the biopsy reveals obvious suspicious cells or increased numbers of follicular cells, one would proceed to surgical exploration.

39. b

For a possible MEN II, screening for a mutation in the ''ret'' protooncogene has become the gold standard. If there is linkage in the family and an asymptomatic family member screens ''positive'' for the mutation, that individual should have a thyroidectomy since chances of medullary cancer are extremely high.

ACKNOWLEDGMENT

Questions were contributed by members of the Department of Endocrinology (Drs. BJ Hoogwerf, R Danese, C Faiman, AE Mehta, A Licata, and S Reddy), Cleveland Clinic Foundation.

Nephrology and Hypertension

Acute Renal Failure

Joseph V. Nally

Acute renal failure (ARF) is a rapid decrease in renal function characterized by progressive azotemia (best measured by serum creatinine), which may be accompanied by oliguria. It is important to distinguish the three major causes of ARF:

- Prerenal azotemia
- Postrenal azotemia or obstruction of the urinary tract
- Renal parenchymal disease

Distinguishing among the three basic categories of ARF is a challenging clinical exercise. The importance of differentiating the major causes of ARF must be stressed, as it affects the initial evaluation and management of the ARF patient. Since nearly 75% of all hospital-acquired acute renal failure is secondary to acute tubular necrosis (ATN), special emphasis will be placed on ATN.

PRERENAL AZOTEMIA

Prerenal azotemia is caused by transient renal hypoperfusion that may induce both azotemia and urinary sodium avidity. Prerenal azotemia may be encountered in both the volume-depleted and volume-overloaded patient (Table 48.1). True volume depletion may result from renal or extrarenal losses. In the volume-overloaded patient—with edematous states such as cirrhosis, nephrosis, and congestive heart failure—prerenal azotemia may exist as the kidney perceives that the vascular tree is ''underfilled,'' resulting in renal hypoperfusion. In addition, prerenal azotemia may exist owing to high-grade bilateral renal artery stenosis.

The pathophysiology of prerenal azotemia relates to the reduction in renal blood flow. Renal hypoperfusion stimulates both the sympathetic nervous system and renin-angiotensin system to cause renal vasoconstriction and sodium avidity. Furthermore, hypotension is a powerful stimulus to the release

of an antidiuretic hormone, which mediates water reabsorption. Hence, urine production is characterized by low volume, decreased concentration of urinary sodium, and increased urinary excretion of creatinine with a high-urine osmolality. Microscopy of the urinary sediment is usually bland. In essence, ''prerenal azotemia is a good kidney looking at a bad world.''

Therapy for prerenal azotemia is directed at optimizing volume status with isotonic fluids. In patients with the edematous disorders who have prerenal azotemia, special efforts are directed at treating the underlying disease states (i.e., heart failure, cirrhosis), and optimizing systemic hemodynamics and renal perfusion.

POSTRENAL AZOTEMIA

Obstruction of the urinary tract may cause ARF. To be the cause of azotemia, urinary tract obstruction must involve the outflow tract of both normal kidneys unless pre-existing renal dysfunction is present, in which case the obstruction may involve only a single kidney. Patients with acute urinary tract obstruction may present with hematuria, flank or abdominal pain, or signs of uremia. A high index of suspicion for urinary tract obstruction should exist in patients with prior abdominal or pelvic surgery, neoplasia, or radiation therapy. Although oligo-anuria suggests complete obstruction, partial obstruction may exist in the presence of adequate urinary output. Oligo-anuria is a powerful diagnostic clue that suggests:

- Urinary tract obstruction
- Severe ATN with cortical necrosis
- Bilateral vascular occlusion

Lesions that may cause obstruction can be either intrinsic or extrinsic to the genitourinary tract (Table 48.2). If urinary tract obstruction is a diagnostic consideration,

Table 48.1. Prerenal Acute Renal Failure

A. Cardiac causes: Primary decrease in cardiac output
  1. Acute disorders: Myocardial infarction, trauma, arrhythmias, malignant hypertension, tamponade, acute valvular disease (e.g., endocarditis)
  2. Chronic disorders: Valvular diseases, chronic myocardiopathies (ischemic heart disease, hypertensive heart disease)
B. Volume depletion
  1. Gastrointestinal losses: Vomiting, diarrhea, fistulae
  2. Renal: Salt-wasting disorders, overdiuresis
C. Redistribution of extracellular fluid
  1. Hypoalbuminemic states: Nephrotic syndrome, advanced liver disease, malnutrition
  2. Physical causes: Peritonitis, burns, crush injury
  3. Peripheral vasodilatation: Sepsis, antihypertensive agents
  4. Renal artery stenosis (bilateral)

Table 48.2. Postrenal Acute Renal Failure

A. Ureteral and pelvic
  1. Intrinsic obstruction
      Blood clots
      Stones
      Sloughed papillae
      Fungus balls
  2. Extrinsic obstruction
      Malignancy
      Retroperitoneal fibrosis
      Iatrogenic: Inadvertent ligation
B. Bladder
    Stones
    Blood clots
    Prostatic hypertrophy or malignancy
    Bladder carcinoma
    Neuropathic
C. Urethral
    Strictures
    Phimosis

the renal ultrasound is sensitive and specific ($\geq$90–95%) in confirming the diagnosis of hydronephrosis. This test may be operator-dependent, so the experience of the radiologist is crucial. False negative tests may be seen with periureteral metastatic disease or retroperitoneal fibrosis. Abdominal CT or retrograde pyelography may be helpful in this circumstance. Remember, if urinary tract obstruction is a diagnostic consideration, renal ultrasound should be obtained, as obstruction represents a potentially reversible cause of ARF.

RENAL PARENCHYMAL DISEASE

The major causes of ARF owing to renal parenchymal disease include:

- Acute glomerulonephritis
- Acute interstitial nephritis (AIN)
- Acute tubular necrosis (ATN)

Since ATN is by far the most common cause of ARF developing in the hospital setting, special emphasis will be given to that condition.

SPECIFIC CONDITIONS OF RENAL PARENCHYMAL DISEASE

Acute Glomerulonephritis

The importance of the urinalysis in the evaluation of patients with ARF cannot be overemphasized: Physicians must develop skill and expertise in interpreting the microscopic findings of the urinalysis. In cases of ARF owing to renal parenchymal disease, such skills are critical. The presence of proteinuria, hematuria, and red blood cell casts are pathognomonic of glomerulonephritis. The differential diagnosis of rapidly progressive glomerulonephritis is beyond the scope of this review (see Chapter 49, Parenchymal Renal Disease: Assessment and Treatment.) Evaluation usually includes a renal biopsy, as well as a detailed serologic evaluation for the presence of systemic vasculitis, collagen vascular disease, and infectious processes. Specific therapies tailored to the disease entity diagnosed after this thorough evaluation may be life-saving.

Acute Interstitial Nephritis (AIN)

The diagnosis of ARF owing to AIN may also be suggested upon microscopy of the urinalysis by the presence of sterile pyuria, white blood cell casts, and eosinophiluria on Hansel's stain. The AIN may be secondary to a variety of drugs, including penicillin, methicillin, cephalosporin, furosemide, and thiazide diuretics. The clinical syndrome may be quite variable, although it is likely to involve an abnormal urinary sediment (proteinuria and pyuria), eosinophilia/eosinophiluria, and fever. Skin rash is seen in approximately 25% of cases. The specific diagnosis of AIN as a cause of ARF should lead to the discontinuation of possibly offending medications. If the renal insufficiency does not resolve in days to weeks, a renal biopsy may confirm the diagnosis of AIN. In selected cases, a trial of steroid therapy may hasten recovery of renal function.

Acute Tubular Necrosis (ATN)

Incidence and Etiology of ATN   Overall, ARF may affect 2–5% of patients in a tertiary care hospital, and nearly 75% of all hospital-acquired ARF is secondary to ATN. From an early comprehensive review of nearly 2200 cases of hospital-acquired ATN, the etiology of the problem appeared to be:

- Surgery, 43%
- Trauma, 9%
- Medicine, 26%
- Pregnancy, 13%
- Nephrotoxins, 9%

Renal hypoperfusion and renal ischemia are the most common causes of ATN, although nephrotoxic insults from various agents are being recognized with increasing frequency. As shown in Table 48.3, the incidence of ARF in the intensive care unit and following extensive vascular surgery, such as aortic aneurysm repair or coronary artery bypass grafting, is significant. Since ''volume is the primal scream of the kidney,'' renal ischemia is the leading cause of ARF in this population. Agents (either endogenous or exogenous) that may be toxic to the kidney are summarized in Tables 48.4 and 48.5.

Table 48.4 lists endogenous nephrotoxic products. Pigment nephropathy may be suspected in the appropriate clinical situation where the following discrepancies exist:

- Hematuria by dipstick
- The absence of red blood cells on urinary microscopy

The combination of renal hypoperfusion and the nephrotoxic insult of myoglobin or hemoglobin on the proximal tubule may result in ATN. Early recognition of this disorder is crucial, as a forced alkaline diuresis is indicated to minimize nephrotoxicity. Similarly the tumor lysis syndrome may be suspected in the appropriate clinical setting, when marked hyperuricemia/hyperurocosuria and crystalluria are recognized. A forced alkaline diuresis may limit nephrotoxicity and is usually recommended prophylactically before an aggressive chemotherapy regimen.

Table 48.4. ARF Related to Endogenous Nephrotoxic Products

Pigment nephropathy
  Myoglobin
  Hemoglobin[a]
  Methemoglobin[a]
Intrarenal crystal deposition
  Uric acid
  Calcium
  Oxalate
Tumor-specific syndromes
  Tumor lysis syndrome
  Plasma cell dyscrasias (e.g., myeloma kidney)

[a] Questionable direct nephrotoxic effect

The list of potential exogenous nephrotoxic agents is exhaustive (see Table 45.5). Simply stated, a patient who develops ATN while receiving medications should have each medication reviewed for the possibility of nephrotoxicity. Commonly seen nephrotoxins in the hospitalized patient include:

- Radiographic contrast material
- Antibiotics (especially aminoglycosides and amphotericin B)
- Chemotherapeutic agents
- Nonsteroidal antiinflammatory drugs
- ACE-inhibitor drugs

More recently, potential nephrotoxicity of newer agents, such as acyclovir, recombinant IL-2, interferon, and selected chemotherapeutic agents, are being appreciated.

Pathophysiology of ATN Several pathogenic mechanisms have been proposed to account for the abnormalities noted in ARF secondary to ATN. Of note, there are two significant dichotomies regarding the renal physiology and pathology of ATN:

- The first dichotomy is a striking reduction in glomerular filtration rate (GFR) in oliguric ARF that is accompanied by a more modest fall in renal plasma flow. This dichotomy of GFR and renal plasma flow reductions suggests a contribution, at least in part, to an intense afferent arteriole vasoconstriction.
- The second dichotomy relates to the pathology of ATN. The distribution of the tubular necrosis appears patchy and the degree of necrosis does not correlate clinically with the level of renal dysfunction. These observations may be reconciled by understanding the pathologic location of early ATN. In general, the renal cortex is well-perfused and well-oxygenated. However, the cortico-medullary junction is much less well-oxygenated, and oxygen demand and oxygen supply are nearly equal under basal conditions. Following a

Table 48.3. Frequency of ARF in Different Clinical Settings

	Percentage Mild ARF ($S_{Cr} < 3$ mg/dL)	Percentage Severe ARF ($S_{Cr} > 5$ mg/dL)
Open heart surgery	5–20	2–5
Abdominal aortic aneurysm resection		
Emergency	30–50	15–25
Elective	5–10	2–5
Severe trauma	10–20	1–5
Neonatal ICU admission	17	6
Aminoglycoside drug administration	5–20	1–2
Admission to general medical/surgical unit	4–10	1–2

Table 48.5.	Causes of Exogenous Toxic Acute Renal Failure

Antibiotics
  Aminoglycosides
  Cephalosporin
  Sulfonamide, co-trimoxazol
  Tetracyclines
  Amphotericin B
  Polymyxin, colistin
  Bacitracin
  Pentamidine
  Vancomycin
  Acyclovir
  Foscarnet

Anesthetic Agents
  Methoxyflurane
  Enflurane

Contrast Media
  Diatrizoate
  Iothalamate
  Bunamiodyl
  Iopanoic acid

Antiulcer Regimens
  Cimetidine
  Excess of milk-alkali

Analgesics
  Nonsteroidal anti-inflammatory drugs (NSAIDs)

Diuretics
  Mercurials
  Ticrynafen
  Others

Chemotherapeutic and Immunosuppressive Agents
  Cis-platinum
  Carboplatin
  Ifosfamide
  Methotrexate
  Mitomycin
  5 azacytidine
  Nitrosourea
  Phicamycin
  Cyclosporin A and tacrolimus (FK506)
  D penicillamide
  Recombinant IL-1
  Interferon alpha or gamma 1 B

Organic Solvents
  Glycols (ethylene glycol, diethylene glycol)
  Halogenated hydrocarbons (CCl_4, tetra- and trichloroethylene)
  Aromatic hydrocarbons (toluene)
  Aliphatic-aromatic hydrocarbons (Vaseline, kerosene, turpentine, paraphenylene diamine)

Heavy Metals

Poisons
  Insecticides (chlordane)
  Herbicides (paraquat, diquat)
  Rodenticide (elemental P)
  Mushroom
  Snake bites[a]
  Stings[a]
  Bacterial toxins[a]

Chemicals[a]
  Aniline
  Hexol
  Cresol
  Chlorates
  Potassium bromate

Recreational Drugs[b]
  Heroin
  Amphetamines

Miscellaneous
  Dextrans
  EDTA
  Radiation
  Silicone
  Epsilon-amino captroic acid[a]
  ACE-inhibitors

[a] Direct toxicity or indirect systemic effects (shock, intravascular hemolysis, or coagulation)
[b] Slow onset of renal failure, unless associated with rhabdomyolysis

hypotensive or hypoxic insult, oxygen demand exceeds supply and ATN develops in the energy-rich, thick ascending limb of Henle in the corticomedullary junction. This imbalance may account for the patchy nature seen pathologically on a renal cross-sectional biopsy.

Both ischemic and toxic insults may result in identical clinical syndromes associated with azotemia. The pathophysiologic mechanisms postulated for acute renal failure include:

- Tubular backleak of glomerular filtrate
- Tubular obstruction owing to debris/casts
- Vascular theories invoking afferent arteriolar vasoconstriction (i.e., the renin-angiotensin system)
- Diminished permeability of the glomerular membrane

Disorders of intracellular adenosine triphosphate and calcium metabolism; membrane and phospholipase abnormalities; abnormalities of tubular cell polarity and cytoskeletal function; and generation of free radical oxygen species and proteases may all be significant in the tubular damage of ATN.

Diagnosis of ATN   The tools available to the clinician include:

- A thorough history and physical examination to assess volume status, potential nephrotoxic insults, and evidence of systemic disease
- Urine output
- Urinalysis
- Urine electrolytes
- Radiologic/renal ultrasound evaluation

The schema for evaluating the patient with ARF is outlined in Table 48.6. The urine output may be a clue to the diagnosis of ARF. The presence of marked oligo-anuria might suggest urinary tract obstruction, renovascular occlusion, or cortical necrosis. In contrast, nonoliguric ARF is being recognized with increased frequency, and careful monitoring of serum creatinine in patients at risk is of paramount importance.

Examination of the urinalysis is fundamental to the evaluation of the patient with acute renal failure. The simple urinalysis may distinguish the cause of ARF among the various possibilities. Table 48.7 highlights the various urinary abnormalities associated with the clinical diagnoses. For example, proteinuria, hematuria, and red blood cell casts are pathognomonic of glomerulonephritis. The classic sediment for ATN includes pigmented (''muddy brown'') granular casts and renal tubular epithelial cells, which may be seen in nearly 80% of cases of oliguric ARF.

Determination of urinary chemistries may be helpful in determining the etiology of the acute renal failure. The urine

---

Table 48.6.   Diagnosis of Acute Renal Failure

Step I
History and Physical Examination
↓

Prerenal	*Renal*	*Postrenal*
Volume depletion; congestive heart failure; severe liver disease or other edematous states	ATN AIN AGN	Palpable bladder or hydronephrotic kidneys; enlarged prostate; abnormal pelvic examination; large residual bladder urine volume; history of renal calculi

Step II
Urine Sediment
↓

Eosinophils ↓ Suspect AIN	RBC casts ↓ Glomerulonephritis or vasculitis	No abnormalities ↓ Suspect prerenal or postrenal azotemia	Renal tubular epithelial cells and ''muddy-brown'' casts ↓ Suspect ATN

Step III
Urinary Indices
↓

Urinary $[Na^+] < 20$ mEq/L	Urinary $[Na^+] > 40$ mEq/L
Urine: plasma creatinine ratio (U/P Cr) > 30	Urine: Plasma creatinine ratio (U/P Cr) < 20
Renal failure index ((U_{Na}/ U/P Cr) < 1	Renal failure index (U Na/U/P Cr) > 1
Fractional excretion of sodium < 1	U Osm < 400
U Osm > 500	Confirm ATN or obstruction
Confirm prerenal azotemia or glomerulonephritis	↓

Step IV
↓

Correct prerenal or postrenal factors	Urine volume < 500 mL/day	Optional trial of furosemide and dopamine to convert oliguric to nonoliguric ARF

Table 48.7. ARF Urinary Sediment				
Bland or Scant Findings	*Granular Casts*	*RBCs, RBC Casts*	*Epithelial and White Blood Cells, WBC Casts*	*Crystalluria*
Vasculitides: Preglomerular vasculitis Hemolytic-uremic syndrome Scleroderma	*ATN:* Pigmented Coarsely granular Casts common	*Glomerulonephritis:* RPGN Small vessel vasculitis	*Eosinophiluria Present:* Acute interstitial nephritis likely	*Uric Acid:* Tumor lysis syndrome
Renovascular Diseases: Arterial thrombosis or emboli Prerenal azotemia		*Interstitial Nephritis:* Rarely seen *ATN:* Rarely seen	*Eosinophiluria Absent:* Acute interstitial nephritis still possible *Pyelonephritis:* Severe, with abscesses	*Calcium Oxalate:* Penthrane toxicity Glycol
Postrenal azotemia				

sodium, creatinine, and osmolality should be measured and either the fractional excretion of sodium (FE_{Na}) or renal failure index (RFI) should be calculated, using the following equation:

$$FE_{Na} = \frac{\dfrac{U_{Na}V}{P_{Na}}}{\dfrac{U_{creat}V}{P_{creat}}} \times 100\% \text{ or RFI} = \frac{U_{Na} \times P_{creat}}{U_{creat}}$$

Note that a low fractional excretion of sodium (or renal failure index) may be associated with either prerenal azotemia or acute glomerulonephritis. These entities could be separated clinically by examination of the urinalysis. Conditions associated with prerenal azotemia would have a bland urinalysis; whereas, proteinuria, red blood cells, and RBC casts would be seen with acute GN. Both ATN and obstruction may have an increased fractional excretion of sodium or renal failure index. Here again the urinalysis would be key. ATN would have a classic sediment with pigmented coarsely granular casts, but the urinalysis seen in obstruction is often bland.

Radiologic evaluation in ARF might include:

- Renal ultrasound
- KUB
- Retrograde urography

The value of the renal ultrasound in the evaluation of possible urinary tract obstruction was discussed earlier. Such studies as the intravenous pyelogram (IVP) or abdominal CT, which employ contrast material, should be avoided because of potential nephrotoxicity.

Stages of ATN The oliguric phase usually begins less than 24 hours after the inciting incident and may last for 1 to 3 weeks. Urine volume averages 150–300 cc/day. The oliguric phase may be prolonged in the elderly. During this phase, the clinician must be alert for the expected complications, with special emphasis on metabolic consequences, gastrointestinal bleeding, and infection.

The diuretic phase is characterized by a progressive increase in urine volume—a harbinger of renal recovery. However, the serum creatinine may continue to rise for another 24 to 48 hours before it reaches a plateau and falls. Severe polyuria during this phase is seen less frequently now. Careful management during this phase is crucial, as up to 25% of deaths with ARF may occur in this phase, usually related to fluid and electrolyte abnormalities, as well as infection. Finally, the recovery phase ensues. Renal function returns to near baseline, but abnormalities of urinary concentration and dilution may persist for weeks or months.

Treatment of ATN During the initial evaluation, it is imperative to search for reversible causes, such as volume depletion, obstruction, and vascular occlusion. During the initial stages, a trial of parenteral hydration with isotonic fluids may correct ARF secondary to prerenal causes. In early established ARF secondary to ATN, a trial of a loop diuretic with or without "renal dose" dopamine may be warranted. Pharmacologic intervention to convert oliguric ATN to nonoliguric ATN is a salutary clinical goal. In general, increases in urinary volume make it easier to deal with problems of volume overload, hyperkalemia, and metabolic acidosis. Increases in urine volume may also provide room for supplemental TPN in the critically ill patient. Morbidity, need for dialysis, and mortality may be less in the nonoliguric form of ATN. Unfortunately, there are very few prospective, randomized trials that have adequately tested this hypothesis (see Cosentino, 1995). In particular, the data available for "renal dose" dopamine therapy in oliguric ARF are surprisingly scant. In fact, the only such prospective trial is reported in ARF caused by malaria. If considered, a trial of "renal dose" dopamine should be used after a clinical challenge of parenteral hydration and a loop diuretic agent. If unsuccessful, dopamine should be ta-

Table 48.8. Check List of Conservative Measures in the Management of ARF

Fluid balance
- ▶ Careful monitoring of intake/output and weights
- ▶ Fluid restriction

Electrolytes and acid-base balance
- ▶ Prevent and treat hyperkalemia
- ▶ Avoid hyponatremia
- ▶ Keep serum bicarbonate > 15 mEq/L
- ▶ Minimize hyperphosphatemia
- ▶ Treat hypocalcemia only if symptomatic or if intravenous bicarbonate is required

Uremia-nutrition
- ▶ Restrict protein (0.5 g/kg/day) but maintain caloric intake; consider forms of nutritional support
- ▶ Carbohydrate intake at least 100 gm/day to minimize ketosis and endogenous protein catabolism

Drugs
- ▶ Review all medications
- ▶ Stop magnesium-containing medications
- ▶ Adjust dosage for renal failure; readjust with improvement of GFR

pered off within 24 hours. More recently, a prospective, randomized with atrial natriuretic peptide (ANP) in patients with ATN (oliguric and nonoliguric) has been reported. Overall, there was no established benefit on morbidity and mortality with ANP. In a subset of patients with oliguric ATN, clinical improvement was seen with ANP infusion. Further studies in such a select population are currently underway.

Once the clinical diagnosis of ATN is made, conservative medical management is in order (Table 48.8). This would include attempts to minimize further renal parenchymal injury, ensure provision of nutrition, maintenance of metabolic balance, and promote recovery of renal function. Optimizing the patient's volume status is imperative, particularly in patients with oliguric ARF. Protein restriction and maintenance of essential amino acids and carbohydrate intake may limit catabolism and help maintain nitrogen balance. Dietary phosphorous and potassium may be restricted. Medications should be adjusted for the level of renal dysfunction.

Dialysis (either hemodialysis or peritoneal dialysis) may be instituted when clinically indicated. The indications for acute dialysis would include:

- Volume overload
- Severe hyperkalemia
- Severe, uncorrectable metabolic acidosis
- Pericarditis
- Selected poisonings
- Uremic symptomatology

Intermittent hemodialysis provides a rapid treatment of hyperkalemia and volume overload. However, newer dialytic

techniques such as the use of bicarbonate dialysis and controlled ultrafiltration may allow better treatment tolerance in the hemodynamically unstable patient.

Prognosis of ATN The prognosis of ATN is dependent upon the underlying primary disease that resulted in the ARF, as well as any complications that arise during the bout of ARF (e.g., infection, cardiovascular, gastrointestinal bleeding, or CNS). The mortality rate for patients with ATN is nearly 50%. This pessimistic outlook has changed very little in the last three decades, despite the advent of effective dialysis. Mortality rates remain high today despite effective control of uremia, since we are caring for an older, sicker population with severe concomitant illnesses. Mortality rates have been recently quantified as high as 75% in several series in the ICU population. Higher mortality rates are seen in elderly patients and in patients with respiratory failure, multiorgan failure with severe forms of oliguric ATN, pre-existing chronic diseases and systemic hypotension. Leading causes of death include bronchopulmonary infections, sepsis, cardiovascular disease, and bleeding disorders. Of patients who survive ATN, nearly half will have a complete recovery of renal function, and a majority of the remainder have an incomplete recovery (Fig. 48.1). Only approximately 5% of all ARF patients require chronic maintenance dialysis. In short, with ARF "you either die or you get better."

Prevention of ATN Since the management of ATN is primarily one of conservative care and support, special attention should be focused on the prevention of ARF. Patients at high risk (i.e., patients with preexisting azotemia, the elderly, volume-depleted individuals) warrant careful clinical consideration of the relative risks and benefits of diagnostic or therapeutic interventions that have a potential for nephrotoxicity. This is especially true for patients at risk undergoing cardiac catheterization or other diagnostic studies requiring intravenous contrast material. Two recent studies deserve comment:

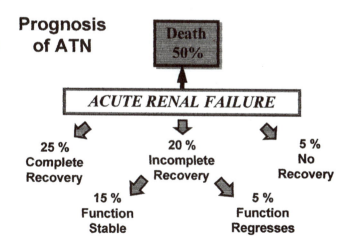

Figure 48.1. Prognosis of ATN.

- A study by Solomon and coworkers published in the New England Journal of Medicine confirmed that prestudy intravenous hydration with saline was critical in lessening the nephrotoxic effect for patients with pre-existing azotemia. The addition of either a loop diuretic or mannitol did not improve outcome.
- Rudnick et al. published a prospective, randomized trial of nearly 1200 well-hydrated patients undergoing cardiac catheterization to examine the effects of the newer non-ionic contrast material. Patients were stratified for the presence or absence of azotemia (serum creatinine ≥ 1.5 %) or diabetes mellitus. In patients without azotemia (with or without diabetes mellitus), the incidence of contrast-induced renal dysfunction was low (i.e., $< 1\%–2\%$) with either the ionic or nonionic contrast material. In contrast, those with pre-existing azotemia had a 50% reduction in contrast-associated renal dysfunction with the non-ionic material.

These data suggest that in azotemic patients who require cardiac angiography, a protocol of intravenous hydration and use of a nonionic contrast material appear warranted.

SUGGESTED READINGS

Allgren RL, Marbury TC, Rahman SN, et al. Anaritide in acute tubular necrosis. N Engl J Med 1997;336:828–871.

Brezis M, Rosen S, Epstein FH. Acute renal failure. In: Brenner BM, Rector FC, eds. The kidney. 3rd ed. Philadelphia: WB Saunders, 1986:735–799.

Cooper K, Bennett WM. Nephrotoxicity of common drugs used in clinical practice. Arch Intern Med 1987;147:1213–1218.

Cosentino F. Drugs for the prevention and treatment of acute renal failure. Cleve Clin J Med 1995;62:248–253.

Denton MD, Chertow GM, Brady HR. "Renal-dose" dopamine for the treatment of acute renal failure: scientific rationale, experimental studies and clinical trials. Kidney Int 1996;50:4–14.

Lake EW, Humes HD. Acute renal failure including cortical necrosis. In: Glassock RJ, Massry SG, eds. Textbook of Nephrology. 3rd ed. Baltimore: Williams & Wilkins, 1995:984–1003.

Miller TR, Anderson RJ, Linas SL, et al. Urinary diagnostic indices in acute renal failure. A prospective study. Ann Intern Med 1978;89:45–50.

Rudnick MR, Goldfarb S, Wexler L, et al. Nephrotoxicity of ionic and nonionic contrast media in 1196 patients: a randomized trial. The Iohexol Cooperative Study. Kidney Int 1995;47:254–261.

Solomon R, Werner C, Mann D, et al. Effects of saline, mannitol, and furosemide to prevent acute decreases in renal function induced by radiocontrast agents. N Engl J Med 1994;331:1416–1420.

Thadhani R, Pascual M, Bonventre JV. Acute renal failure. N Engl J Med 1996;334:1448–1460.

49

Approach to Patients with Parenchymal Renal Disease

Gerald B. Appel

Parenchymal renal diseases affect millions of people in the United States and worldwide. In 1990, more than 200,000 people in the United States were in end-stage renal disease (ESRD) programs largely as a result of renal involvement by parenchymal diseases. One form of glomerular damage alone, diabetic glomerulophropathy, is said to affect almost 14 million people in the United States and costs the government billions of dollars annually. Worldwide glomerular disease associated with infectious agents, such as malaria and schistosomiasis, and interstitial diseases, such as chronic bacterial pyelonephritis, are a major health problem.

The mechanisms of both glomerular and tubulointerstitial injury are quite varied. In glomerular disease, while certain common mechanisms may underlie the hematuria and proteinuria leakage (e.g., loss of the glomerular charge barrier), the nature of the processes initiating this damage differ. Immune-mediated renal injury is a major pathogenetic mechanism of glomerular damage. In diabetic nephropathy and amyloidosis, other mechanisms clearly are at work. In tubulointerstitial disease, the primary insult may be immunologic (e.g., drug-induced AIN), toxic-metabolic (e.g., analgesics, oxalate), or vascular (e.g., sickle cell disease and atheroemboli) in nature. The end result is damage to tubules and interstitial space of the kidney with eventual interstitial scarring and fibrosis.

THE GLOMERULOPATHIES

Each glomerulus, the basic filtering unit of the kidney, consists of a tuft of anastomosing capillaries formed by the branchings of the afferent arteriole. There are approximately 1 million glomeruli, which make up about 5% of the kidney weight and provide almost 2 square meters of glomerular capillary filtering surface. Each glomerulus consists of a combination of cellular elements (the endothelial cells, mesangial cells, visceral and parietal epithelial cells) and extracellular matrix (the glomerular basement membrane and mesangial matrix). The endothelial cells lining the lumens of the glomerular capillaries have a highly fenestrated cytoplasm attached to the internal aspect of the glomerular basement membrane.

The glomerulus possesses a variety of histocompatibility antigens, may express Fc and C3b receptors allowing the adhesion of macrophages and complement activation, and may produce and secrete numerous vasoactive substances including AHF-f actor VIII, thrombin receptors, prostacyclin, and heparin-like growth factors. They may contribute to the synthesis and maintenance of the glomerular basement membrane (GBM).

The mesangium or central stalk region of the glomerulus is composed of both matrix and cells. The mesangium is important for mechanical support of the glomerulus, transport of molecules out of the capillary loops, and the contractile nature of the glomerular capillaries. The mesangial matrix consists predominantly of Type IV collagen, fibronectin, laminen, and proteoglycans. The mesangial cells consist of two types: contractile cells with actin-myosin filaments and bone-marrow derived phagocytic monocytes. Mesangial cells may proliferate and/or produce many vasoactive substances including prostaglandins, oxygen radicals, and platelet-derived growth factor.

The GBM is composed of a central dense layer (lamina densa) and outer and inner more lucent layers (laminae rara interna and externa). The GBM is chemically composed of Type IV collagen and a variety of proteins including entactin, laminen, and fibronectin. The GBM is highly negatively charged, in part owing to the regular, ordered latticelike distribution within the lamina densa of viscous anionic charged proteoglycans molecules, of which the most important is heparan sulfate. The GBM provides both a size and charge selective barrier to the passage of circulating macromolecules.

The visceral epithelial cells contain numerous extensions called foot processes or podocytes, which interdigitate with the foot processes of neighboring visceral epithelial cells and are tightly bound to the lamina rara externa of the GBM. The filtration slit pores, the spaces between adjoining foot processes, are bridged by a slit diaphragm, which may be one of the barriers to the passage of circulating macromolecules. The visceral epithelial cells are coated with a highly anionic layer of sialoprotein and are important in the synthesis of many of the components of the GBM. The parietal epithelial cells are simple flat cells that line Bowman's capsule and are contiguous with the cuboidal epithelium lining the proximal tubule.

HISTOPATHOLOGIC TERMS

Understanding renal histopathology requires knowledge of only a few terms. When referring to the entire kidney, if all glomeruli are involved, a process is called "diffuse" or "generalized." If only some glomeruli are involved, it is called "focal." When referring to the individual glomerulus, a process is "global" if the whole glomerular tuft is involved and "segmental" if only part of the glomerulus is involved. The terms "proliferative," "sclerosing," and "necrotizing" are often used (e.g., focal and segmental sclerosing glomerulonephritis, diffuse global proliferative lupus nephritis). Extracapillary proliferation or crescent formation is caused by the accumulations of macrophages, fibroblasts, proliferating epithelial cells, and fibrin within Bowman's space. In general, this term conveys a serious prognosis to any form of glomerular damage.

CLINICAL MANIFESTATIONS OF GLOMERULAR DISEASES

Several findings are common to many glomerular diseases and focus the differential diagnosis of unknown parenchymal renal diseases toward a glomerular origin. They include the findings of erythrocyte casts and/or dysmorphic erythrocytes in the urinary sediment and the presence of large amounts of albuminuria. In normal humans, the urinary excretion of albumin is less than 50 mg daily. While increases in urinary protein excretion may come from the filtration of abnormal circulating proteins, such as light chains in multiple myeloma, or from the deficient proximal tubular reabsorption of normal filtered small molecular weight, such as beta 2-microglobulin, the most common cause of proteinuria and in specific albuminuria is glomerular injury. Proteinuria associated with glomerular disease may range from several hundred milligrams daily to more than 30 g per day. In some disease with heavy proteinuria, such as minimal change nephrotic syndrome, albumin is the predominant protein found in the urine. In these diseases the proteinuria is said to be highly "selective." In other glomerular diseases, such as focal segmental glomerulosclerosis (FSGS) and diabetes, the proteinuria, although still largely composed of albumin, contains many larger weight molecular proteins, as well, and is said to be "nonselective" proteinuria. The associated clinical manifestations will be influenced largely by the amount of the proteinuria. When proteinuria exceeds 3 to 3.5 g/daily, patients commonly develop hypoalbuminemia, hyperlipidemia, edema, and other manifestations described as the nephrotic syndrome.

Although a small number of erythrocytes may appear in the urine of normal individuals, urinary excretion of greater than 500 to 1000 erythrocytes per ml defines abnormal hematuria. While hematuria is common in many glomerular diseases, it is not, of course, specific for glomerular pathology. However, erythrocytes that pass through gaps in the GBM and must traverse the osmotic changes imposed as they pass down the tubules become deformed. These dysmorphic erythrocytes can easily be seen with a phase contrast microscope and are highly suggestive of glomerular pathology. Likewise, red blood cell casts that form when erythrocytes pass the glomerular capillary barrier and become enmeshed in a proteinaceous matrix in the tubules are highly suggestive of glomerular disease.

THE NEPHROTIC SYNDROME

The nephrotic syndrome is classically defined by proteinuria in amounts greater than 3–3.5 grams daily accompanied by hypoalbuminemia, edema, and hyperlipidemia. In clinical practice, many nephrologists refer to "nephrotic range" proteinuria regardless of whether their patients have the other manifestations of the full syndrome, since the latter are consequences of the proteinuria. Nephrotic proteinuria, regardless of the inciting disease, is always predominantly because of albuminuria.

Hypoalbuminemia is in part a consequence of urinary protein loss. It is also owing to the catabolism of filtered albumin by the proximal tubule, as well as caused by redistribution of albumin within the body. This redistribution accounts for, in part, the inexact relationship between urinary protein levels and the level of the serum albumin and other secondary consequences of heavy albuminuria. The salt and volume retention in the nephrotic syndrome can occur through at least two different major mechanisms. In the classic theory, proteinuria leads to hypoalbuminemia, a low plasma oncotic pressure, and intravascular volume depletion. Subsequent underperfusion of the kidney stimulates the priming of sodium retentive hormonal systems as the renin-angiotensin-aldosterone axis causes increased renal sodium and volume retention. In the peripheral capillaries with normal hydrostatic pressures and decreased oncotic pressure, the Starling forces lead to transcapillary fluid leakage and edema. Evidence to support this theory comes from studies documenting the low oncotic pressure and intravascular volume of some nephrotic patients and the stimulated renin angiotensin-aldosterone axis in these individuals. In some patients, however, the intravascular volume has been measured and found to be increased along with suppression of the renin-angiotensin-aldosterone axis. In an animal model of unilateral proteinuria, created by unilateral infusion of the aminonucleoside puromycin, there is evidence for primary renal sodium retention at a distal nephron site, perhaps owing to altered responsiveness to hormones, such as atrial natriuretic factor. Here, only the proteinuric kidney retains sodium and volume, and this occurs at a time when the animal is not yet hypoalbuminenic. Thus, local factors within the kidney may account for the volume retention of the nephrotic patient, as well.

As recently as a decade ago investigators disagreed as to the pattern and significance of the hyperlipidemia noted in nephrotic patients. In the past, both epidemiologic and histopathologic studies failed to clarify whether nephrotic patients have an increased risk of atherosclerotic cardiovascular disease. A recent epidemiologic study has strongly supported an increased risk of atherosclerotic complications in the nephrotic syndrome. Moreover, many nephrotic patients have additional risk factors besides hyperlipidemia for cardiovascular disease, including hypertension, smoking, and left ventricular hypertrophy. Studies of the pattern of hyperlipidemia have generally agreed that the majority of patients will have elevated levels of total and low-density lipoprotein (LDL) cholesterol. Moreover, recent studies suggest that most patients have low or normal high-density lipoprotein (HDL) cholesterol levels and that the ratio of total or LDL cholesterol to HDL cholesterol is elevated. Recent trials with a number of antihyperlipidemic medications suggest that treatment of the hyperlipidemia of the nephrotic syndrome may be both safe and effective for favorably altering lipoprotein levels. Bile acid binding resins, probucol, gemfibrozil, and most recently the HMG-CoA reductase inhibitors have all been successfully used.

The initial evaluation of the nephrotic patient includes a variety of simple laboratory tests to define whether the patient has primary or idiopathic nephrotic syndrome or a secondary cause (e.g., fasting blood sugar (FBS), anti-nuclear antibody (ANA), serum complement). Once secondary causes have been excluded, treatment of the adult nephrotic patient often requires a renal biopsy to define the pattern of glomerular involvement. The vast majority of children with idiopathic nephrotic syndrome have the minimal change pattern and are responsive to corticosteroid therapy. While there has been some controversy over whether a similar course of "blind" steroid treatment would be reasonable in adults, most nephrologists prefer to biopsy the patient first, since the majority of adults will not have the minimal change pattern. In adults, the nephrotic syndrome is one of the most common conditions coming to renal biopsy. In virtually every study defining the role of the renal biopsy, patients with heavy proteinuria were the most likely group to benefit in terms of a change from the prebiopsy diagnosis and in terms of changes in prognosis and therapy. Selected groups of nephrotic patients, such as elderly nephrotic patients, will also have a slightly different spectrum of disease, but once again, the renal biopsy is the best guide to treatment and prognosis.

Minimal Change Disease

Minimal change disease, also known as "Nil" disease and as part of the older entity of "lipoid nephrosis," is the most common pattern of idiopathic nephrotic syndrome in children and makes up nearly 20% of cases of idiopathic nephrotic syndrome in adults. Patients typically present with periorbital and peripheral edema related to the proteinuria. Although the onset of the disease is coincident with upper respiratory infections and allergies in some adults, most have no precipitating event. Proteinuria is usually well into the nephrotic range, with values less than 3.0 g daily being uncommon. In children, the proteinuria is highly selective, whereas in adults, selectivity of proteinuria is a less reliable finding in patients with minimal change disease. Additional findings in adults are hypertension in 30% and microscopic hematuria. However, active urinary sediment with erythrocyte casts is not found. Many patients will have mild to moderate azotemia that may be related to intravascular volume depletion.

In true minimal change disease, the histopathology typically reveals no glomerular abnormalities in the light microscopy (hence the acronym "nil" disease for "nothing in light microscopy"). The tubules may show lipid droplet accumulation from absorbed lipoproteins (hence the older term "lipoid nephrosis"). Immunofluorescence staining in true minimal change disease shows no deposits, and electron microscopy also shows an absence of immune type deposits. The glomerular basement membrane is normal in size and contour, and effacement or "fusion" of the visceral epithelial foot processes is noted along virtually the entire distribution of every capillary loop.

The course of minimal change nephrotic syndrome in both children and adults is often one of relapses and responses to additional treatment. From 90% to 95% of children will experience a remission of the nephrotic syndrome when treated with corticosteroids for 8 weeks. Regimens have generally been 1 mg/kg/day prednisone, or a similar dose for the first month, followed by every other day therapy, or alternate day treatment from the start. In adults, the response rate is somewhat lower, with 75–85% of patients responding to regimens of daily (60 mg/day) or alternate day (120 mg/every other day) prednisone therapy.

The time to clinical response may be slower in adults, and they should not be considered to be steroid resistant until they have failed to respond to 16 weeks of treatment. Tapering of the steroid dose should begin 1 to several weeks after complete remission and should continue gradually over 1–2 months. Both children and adults are likely to have a relapse of their minimal change disease once steroids have been discontinued. Approximately 50% of children and 30% of adults will relapse by 1 year, with the number increasing to almost 80%, and 50% by 5 years. Most clinicians will treat the first relapse in a similar fashion to the initial nephrotic syndrome.

Those patients who relapse a third time or who become dependent upon steroids (unable to decrease the prednisone dose beyond a certain level without proteinuria recurring) are usually treated with a short course of an alkylating agent. Both chlorambucil and cyclophosphamide up to 2–3 mg/kg day have been used successfully. Up to 50% of patients who are so treated have a prolonged remission of the nephrotic syndrome (at least 5 years). The response rate is lower in steroid-dependent patients. Both drugs have well-recognized toxicity (e.g., marrow suppression, risk of infection, gonadal toxicity), and should be used for a minimal time period (8 weeks) to avoid cumulative toxicity. An alternative to an alkylating agent is the use of low-dose cyclosporine (4–6 mg/kg/day), but this carries the risk of nephrotoxicity and a high potential relapse rate.

Focal Segmental Glomerulosclerosis

Approximately 15–20% of adults with idiopathic nephrotic syndrome will have focal segmental glomerulosclerosis (FSGS) that is noted at biopsy. This is a histologic diagnosis, and the focal segmental glomerulosclerosis may be either idiopathic or secondary to a number of different causes (e.g., heroin nephropathy, HIV nephropathy, sickle cell nephropathy, reflux nephropathy, lesions associated with single or remnant kidneys, and the healed phase of focal glomerulonephritis, among other causes).

Patients with idiopathic FSGS typically present with either asymptomatic proteinuria or edema. Although the nephrotic syndrome is present at the patient's presentation, the 24-hour urinary protein excretion may vary from less than 1 g/D to levels as high as 20–30 g/D. Proteinuria is typically nonselective. Hypertension is found in 30%–50% and microscopic hematuria in 25–75% of these patients. Glomerular filtration rate (GFR) is decreased at presentation in 20–30% of patients. Complement levels and other serologic tests are normal in FSGS.

The histologic diagnosis of FSGS depends on identifying only some of the glomeruli (focal) areas of glomerulosclerosis restricted to only some part of the glomerular tufts (segmental lesions). By immunofluorescence staining, IgM and C3 are commonly found in the areas of glomerular sclerosis and are felt to result from entrapment of immunoglobulin and complement components rather than true immune complex deposition. Using electron microscopy, fusion or effacement of foot processes are found to some extent in all of the glomeruli, even those unaffected by areas of segmental sclerosis, and there are no electron dense immune deposits. In biopsies taken early in the course of FSGS when the GFR is preserved, there will be few glomeruli with segmental sclerosing lesions and almost no global glomerulosclerosis. As renal function declines, repeat biopsies will show many glomeruli with segmental or global sclerosis.

Although quite variable, the course of unresponsive FSCS is usually one of progressive proteinuria and declining GFR. Patients with asymptomatic proteinuria typically develop the nephrotic syndrome over time. Only a minority of patients experience a spontaneous remission of proteinuria. Eventually, most patients develop ESRD 5–20 years from presentation. Children and adults experience the same decline in GFR

over time. The influence of treatment is debated. Some patients with the collapsing variant (or so-called malignant FSGS) will have a more rapid course to ESRD in 2–3 years. Idiopathic FSCS may recur in the transplanted kidney and is then manifested by the occurrence of severe proteinuria and the nephrotic syndrome. Patients who present with more severe degrees or proteinuria and a more rapid course to renal failure are at greater risk for recurrence in the transplant.

The therapy of FSGS is controversial. There are few randomized, controlled trials on which to base judgments, and newer studies with promising results remain uncontrolled. In general, patients with a sustained remission of their nephrotic syndrome are unlikely to progress to ESRD, while those with unremitting nephrotic syndrome are likely to progress. In older studies, only 10–35% of patients appeared to respond to a course of corticosteroids or other immunosuppressives with a complete remission of proteinuria, and the relapse rate after treatment was high. Thus, many clinicians considered FSGS to be a nonresponsive lesion and did not advocate treatment. Recent studies using more intensive and more prolonged immunosuppressive regimens with steroids and cytotoxics have achieved up to a 60% remission rate with preservation of long-term renal function. A number of recent trials have also used low-dose cyclosporine (4–6 mg/kg/day for 2–6 months) to treat FSGS patients. Even patients who have been unresponsive to steroids and cytotoxics may respond to this therapy. Unfortunately, some patients will experience increased renal damage from the cyclosporine, and many patients will relapse when therapy is stopped.

At the present time, the best regimen for FSGS is unclear. Many clinicians do not treat patients with subnephrotic levels of proteinuria and little damage on their renal biopsies. Others treat patients with ACE inhibitors to reduce proteinuria and its side effects but not the specific glomerular lesion. Finally, some treat with a prolonged course of corticosteroids or other immunosuppressive medication in the hopes of inducing a remission of the nephrotic syndrome and preventing eventual ESRD.

Membranous Nephropathy

Membranous nephropathy is the most common pattern of idiopathic nephrotic syndrome in white Americans. It typically presents with the onset of proteinuria leading to periorbital and pedal edema. Hypertension and microhematuria are not infrequent findings, but the renal function and the GFR are usually normal at presentation. Membranous nephropathy is the most common pattern of the nephrotic syndrome to be associated with thrombotic events and especially renal vein thrombosis. The presence of sudden flank pain, deterioration of renal function, or symptoms of pulmonary emboli in a patient with membranous nephropathy should prompt an investigation for renal vein thrombosis. Certain elderly patients with membranous nephropathy may have an underlying carcinoma as an occult cause of their renal lesion.

There has been considerable debate about the variable

natural history of this disease. In general, most large series show that renal survival is over 75% at 10 years. There is also a spontaneous remission rate that varies from 20%–30% of patients. Both the slow progression and spontaneous remission rate have confounded clinical treatment trials. Both a retrospective study and a controlled clinical trial suggested that short-term corticosteroid therapy led to a reduction in the number of patients progressing to renal insufficiency. Another study found that prolonged therapy with corticosteroids led to not only preservation of renal function but remissions of the nephrotic syndrome. These studies have been criticized: two of them lacked a control group, and the controlled trial had an extremely rapid rate of progression of the control group toward renal insufficiency, conferring a favorable advantage upon those patients receiving corticosteroids.

Two recent studies have shown no benefit of corticosteroid regimens for the course of membranous nephropathy in terms of reduction of proteinuria or preservation of renal function. Recent trials with cytotoxic agents have given promising results. A controlled trial of pulse methylprednisolone followed by oral prednisone for 1 month alternating with 1 month of oral chlorambucil has led to a greater number of total remissions and better preservation of renal function. Recent controlled studies with corticosteroids have shown similar beneficial results.

At present, it is unclear whether this or another regimen will become widely accepted. Until further controlled trials are done, most clinicians treat only those types of patients who in retrospective studies have had the highest rate of progression to renal failure (males, older patients, those with greater degrees of proteinuria). Whether to use corticosteroids or cytotoxics or a combination of therapies depends on the clinician's preference.

ACUTE GLOMERULONEPHRITIS

IgA Nephropathy

IgA nephropathy was originally thought to be an uncommon and benign form of glomerulopathy (Berger's disease). It is now recognized as the most frequent form of idiopathic glomerulonephritis worldwide (making up 15–40% of primary glomerulonephritides in parts of Europe, Asia, and Japan) that clearly can progress to ESRD. In geographic areas where renal biopsies are commonly performed for milder urinary findings, a higher incidence of IgA has been noted. In the United States, some centers report that IgA nephropathy makes up nearly 20% of all primary glomerulopathies. Although males outnumber females and the peak occurrence is in the second to third decade of life, it can occur in patients of both sexes and all ages.

The diagnosis of IgA nephropathy is established by the finding of glomerular immunoglobulin A deposits either as the dominant or codominant immunoglobulin on immunofluorescence microscopy. In addition to IgA, deposits of C3 and

IgG are found in many patients. The light microscopic picture may vary from minimal change to mesangial proliferation to crescenteric glomerulonephritis. The most common picture is mesangial hypercellularity, often in a focal and segmental distribution. By electron microscopy, electron dense deposits are typically found in the mesangial and paramesangial areas. The pathogenesis of IgA nephropathy is unknown. While the predominant antibody appears to be composed of polymeric IgA1 originating in the secretory-mucosal system, the antigen to which it is directed is unknown in the vast majority of cases. Environmental antigens such as viral or other pathogens and diet-related antigens have been proposed but unproved. Which factors subsequent to the deposition of immune complexes containing IgA lead to the inflammatory and sclerosing glomerular features of the disease are also unknown.

IgA nephropathy often presents with one of two syndromes: asymptomatic microscopic hematuria and/or proteinuria (most common in adults) or episodic gross hematuria following upper respiratory and other infections or exercise (most common in children). The course of IgA nephropathy is variable, with some patients showing no decline in GFR over decades and others developing the nephrotic syndrome, hypertension, and renal failure. Patients who present without episodes of gross hematuria are more likely to have severe proteinuria, hypertension, and renal insufficiency. Hypertension is present in 20–50% of all patients. Increased serum IgA levels, noted in one-third to one-half of cases, do not correlate with the course of the disease. A newer test analyzing IgA serum fibronectin aggregates has proved promising for diagnosis, but as of yet, there are insufficient data to evaluate the value of such serum levels as predictors of the course of the disease.

Factors predictive of a poor outcome in IgA nephropathy have included:

- Older age at onset
- Absence of gross hematuria
- Hypertension
- Persistent and severe proteinuria
- Males
- Reduced GFR and elevated serum creatinine
- Certain histologic features on renal biopsy including severe proliferation and sclerosis, severe tubulo-interstitial damage, and extracapillary glomerular proliferation (i.e., crescent formation)

Renal survival is estimated at 85–90% at 10 years and 75–80% at 20 years. A significant percent of patients transplanted will have a morphologic recurrence in the allograft, but graft loss owing to the disease is uncommon.

Since the pathogenesis of IgA nephropathy is thought to involve abnormal antigenic stimulation of mucosal IgA production and subsequent immune complex deposition in the glomeruli, treatment has been directed at these sites. Efforts to prevent antigenic stimulation or entry have included the use of broad spectrum antibiotics (e.g., doxycycline), tonsillectomy, and dietary manipulations to eliminate certain dietary antigens (e.g., gluten). With few exceptions, these attempts have not been successful. The benefit of glucocorticoids and other immunosuppressives is far from clear for those IgA nephropathy patients with fixed significant proteinuria, severe proliferative lesions, and a decreased GFR. Uncontrolled trials of alternate day corticosteroids have suggested benefit, but ongoing prospective randomized trials are only now underway to define the value of this therapy. Other efforts at immunosuppression have included combinations of cyclophosphamide, dipyridamole, and warfarin, which may have had beneficial effects in some patients when chronically administered for years, and immunosuppression with cytotoxics and pulse solumedrol for patients with crescenteric lesions. At least one recent trial with omega fish oils has shown improved renal survival and decreased proteinuria in IgA nephropathy, but two smaller trials showed no beneficial effect of treatment. With no clearly proven therapy, many physicians chose not to treat the lesion of IgA nephropathy or only to treat those patients at highest risk for progression to renal failure.

Idiopathic Membranoproliferative Glomerulonephritis

Membranoproliferative or mesangiocapillary glomerulonephritis (MPGN) is an uncommon glomerular disease that may present in three histologic forms based on the glomerular ultrastructure (Types I, II, and III MPGN). In biopsied series, it makes up only a small percent of glomerular disease cases.

By light microscopy, the lesions of Types I, II, and III MPGN include diffuse mesangial proliferation with infiltration of the glomerular tuft by mononuclear cells. There is exaggeration of the lobular pattern of the glomerular tufts and thickening of the peripheral capillary wall characterized by reduplication of the basement membrane, resulting in a double contour or ''tram track'' appearance. This is most prominent in Type I MPGN. By IF, there is diffuse granular deposits of C3 along the GBM and often IgG, IgA, and IgM. Electron microscopy clearly distinguishes the three patterns of MPGN. Type I has subendothelial and mesangial deposits with interposition of the mesangial cells and/or mononuclear phagocytes along the GBM. Type II has a broad dense intramembranous deposits along the GBM, Bowman's capsule, and tubular basement membranes. Type III has subepithelial deposits and intramembranous deposits in addition to subendothelial and mesangial deposits.

The pathogenesis of the idiopathic form of this type of glomerulonephritis is by definition unknown. By light microscopy, similar patterns of glomerular damage have been seen in association with certain infectious agents (hepatitis), autoimmune disease (SLE), and disease of intraglomerular coagulation. All of these stimuli have been proposed to incite the glomerular mesangial cells to grow out along the capillary wall and split the GBM. Type II MPGN, dense deposit disease, has been called an autoimmune disorder with an autoantibody (an IgG, C3 nephrotic factor) directed against C3bBb, the alternate pathway C3 convertase. By preventing degradation

of the enzyme, there is increased activation and consumption of complement noted in dense deposit disease.

Although MPGN may present with asymptomatic microhematuria and proteinuria in some patients, most patients present with the nephrotic syndrome. Other patients may present with an acute nephritic picture with active urinary sediment, renal insufficiency, and hypertension. Presenting findings that correlate with a poor prognosis include hypertension, a reduced GFR, and the nephrotic syndrome. Hypocomplementemia or its persistence does not necessarily indicate a poor prognosis. Glomerular crescent formation and severe tubulointerstitial changes have been correlated with a poor prognosis. Most studies have found similar results for the various patterns of MPGN and have treated them as one disease entity. Attempts to treat MPGN have included the use of corticosteroids and other immunosuppressive medications, anticoagulants, and antiplatelet agents to minimize glomerular damage from coagulation, and NSAIDs. No therapy has been proved to be effective in adults with MPGN. In children, long-term corticosteroids lead to greater remissions of the nephrotic syndrome and preservation of renal function.

It appears that patients with bad prognostic features and/or a progressive course may benefit from either alternate day steroids or perhaps from more vigorous regimens of immunosuppression. These regimens will have to be maintained for extended periods of time to prove successful in the treatment of MPGN.

Rapidly Progressive Glomerulonephritis

RPGN comprises a group of glomerulonephritides that have in common progression to renal failure in a matter of weeks to months from diagnosis and the presence of extensive extracapillary proliferation, i.e., crescent formation, in a large percent of the glomeruli. RPGN includes renal diseases with different etiologies, pathogeneses, and clinical presentations. Patients with RPGN have been divided into three patterns defined by immunologic pathogenesis:

- Type I, with anti-GBM disease
- Type II, with immune complex deposition (e.g., SLE, poststreptococcal)
- Type III, without immune deposits or anti-GBM antibodies, so-called pauci-immune

Many of the last patients fall into the category of ANCA positive RPGN. In the past, with the exception of postinfectious RPGN, prognosis was generally poor for most patients, regardless of pathogenesis. This prognosis has dramatically changed for some patterns of RPGN.

Anti-GBM Disease Anti-GBM disease is caused by circulating antibodies that are directed against the noncollagenous domain of type 4 collagen and that damage the GBM. This leads to an inflammatory response, breaks in the GBM, and the formation of a proliferative and often crescenteric glomerulonephritis. If the anti-GBM antibodies cross-react with and cause damage to the basement membrane of pulmonary capillaries, the patient will develop pulmonary hemorrhage and hemoptysis. The association of anti-GBM antibody mediated damage to the kidneys and lungs is called Goodpasture's syndrome. The disease most commonly affects young adults, and males are far more commonly affected than females. The presentation is with a nephritic picture with hypertension, edema, hematuria, and active urinary sediment, and reduced renal function. Renal function may deteriorate from normal to levels requiring dialysis in a matter of days or weeks. Patients with pulmonary involvement may have life-threatening hemoptysis, as well. The course of the disease once it has progressed to renal failure is usually one of permanent renal dysfunction. If treatment is started early in the course of the disease, patients may regain considerable kidney function.

The pathology of anti-GBM disease shows a proliferative glomerulonephritis, often with severe extracapillary involvement of Bowman's space by crescent formation. By IF, there is linear deposition of immunoglobulin along the GBM. Electron microscopy does not show any electron dense deposits.

The treatment of Type I RPGN mediated by anti-GBM antibodies is unproved, with no significant controlled trials of this least common form of crescenteric GM. For patients with pulmonary hemorrhage and thus Goodpasture's syndrome, high-dose oral or intravenous corticosteroids have been used successfully to halt the pulmonary bleeding. They have usually not proved effective in treating the renal lesions. Intensive therapy to reduce the production of anti-GBM antibodies (immunosuppressives agents such as cyclophosphamide or azathioprine and corticosteroids) combined with plasmapheresis to remove circulating anti-GBM antibodies has proved effective therapy for the renal lesion in many cases. Therapy is most effective in patients who have less extensive crescent formation and who have a preserved GFR. However, some patients with advanced renal failure even requiring dialysis have responded to this form of treatment. Clearly, Type I RPGN is the most resistant pattern to any form of therapeutic intervention, and rapid intensive therapy is necessary to prevent irreversible renal damage.

Immune Complex RPGN   Type II RPGN associated with immune complex mediated damage to the glomeruli may occur with a spectrum of diseases from primary glomerulopathies such as IgA nephropathy and MPGN to postinfectious GM, to systemic lupus erythematosus. The therapy of IgA nephropathy and MPGN is discussed above. Most cases of postinfectious GM resolve with successful treatment of the underlying infection. Here, the potential hazards of immunosuppressive treatment and the limited data available on its benefit should prompt caution in the use of this therapeutic option. The treatment of severe SLE is described in a later section.

Pauci-Immune RPGN and Vasculitis-Associated RPGN
Pauci-immune Type III RPGN includes patients with and without evidence of systemic vasculitis. A large retrospective analysis from the Mayo Clinic found no difference in prognosis between the patients with small artery or medium-sized artery involvement by vasculitis with focal segmental necrotizing GN (polyarteritislike) and those with the necrotizing GM alone (RPGN). Patients often present with progressive renal failure and a nephritic picture with hematuria, oliguria, and hypertension. Many patients will have circulating antibodies directed against neutrophil cytoplasmic antigens (ANCA). Patients who are P-ANCA positive more often have a clinical picture akin to polyarteritis (with arthritis, skin involvement with leukocytoclastic angiitis, constitutional and systemic signs), whereas those who are C-ANCA positive more likely have granulomatous disease associated with their glomerulonephritis (akin to Wegener's granulomatosis). There is considerable overlap between these groups. As in all forms of RPGN, renal function may deteriorate rapidly. An elevated serum creatinine level and the presence of hypertension are risk factors for poor renal outcome. In a study by Falk et al. of the course of ANCA-associated glomerulonephritis and systemic vasculitis, no difference in renal or patient survival was noted between patients with isolated renal disease and those with systemic involvement. In the earlier literature the response rate to any treatment for this disease was in the 20%–25% range. Subsequent reports on the use of oral cyclophosphamide in addition to corticosteroids in disease such as Wegener's granulomatosis and polyarteritis nodosa have shown markedly improved survival rates. For example, in the NIH series of 158 patients with Wegener's granulomatosis, more than 90% experienced marked improvement and 75% experienced a complete remission rate. These excellent results includes some patients with crescentic GM, and only 11% of these patients eventually required dialysis. More recently, using steroids plus cytotoxic agents, successful results have been reported even in oliguric patients and in those who are already dialysis-dependent.

It is clear that pauci-immune RPGN has the most favorable response rate of all patterns of RPGN. It responds well to a number of different immunosuppressive regimens, including pulse steroids and cyclophosphamide given orally or intravenously. The therapeutic regimen of choice and the optimal duration of therapy will have to be determined in controlled trials.

GLOMERULAR INVOLVEMENT IN SYSTEMIC DISEASES

Systemic Lupus Erythematosus

Renal involvement greatly influences the course and choice of treatment of lupus patients. The incidence of clinically detectable renal disease varies from 15% to 75% of patients with SLE. Histologic evidence of renal involvement in SLE is found in the vast majority of biopsies when studied by LM, IF, and EM even in the absence of clinical renal disease.

The WHO classification of LN has been used successfully

for both clinical and research activities. It has the advantages of using LM, IF, and EM to classify each biopsy rather than only one form of microscopy; of separating the milder mesangial forms of LN from the true focal and diffuse proliferative forms; and of using well-defined criteria allowing different groups to compare results. The WHO classes correlate well with the clinical picture of the patients at biopsy. They also help define the clinical course of the patient and provide a guide to therapy.

Patients with WHO Class I (normal) biopsies are extremely rare. Such biopsies are found only in patients without clinical renal findings very early in the course of their disease. Patients with WHO Class II (mesangial involvement) biopsies usually have only mild clinical renal disease. They are virtually never nephrotic but may have active serology. They have an excellent long-term prognosis and require no treatment directed at their renal lesions. Patients with WHO Class III lesions (focal proliferative LN) have more active sediment changes, increased proteinuria, and often active serology. About one-fourth are nephrotic, and some transform or evolve into a class IV pattern. Patients with WHO Class IV (diffuse proliferative) LN have the most severe renal involvement, with active sediment, hypertension, heavy proteinuria, frequent nephrotic syndrome, and often a reduction of glomerular filtration rate. They have the worst prognosis. Patients with WHO Class V (membranous) LN are often older at presentation, and some present with the nephrotic syndrome before fulfilling the ARA criteria for SLE. They are typically nephrotic with inactive serology. Although their short-term prognosis is good, they can progress to renal failure over many years. Membranous LN is the only pattern commonly associated with renal vein thrombosis.

In general, all patients with Class IV lesions on biopsy deserve vigorous therapy for their LN. Many Class III patients (especially those with active necrotizing lesions and large amounts of subendothelial deposits) also would benefit from such therapy. The optimal therapy for Class V patients is less clear, with some clinicians treating all membranous LN patients vigorously and others reserving such therapy for those with serologic activity or more severe nephrotic syndrome. Vigorous therapy of LN may include intravenous pulse steroids, plasmapheresis, oral azathioprine or cyclophosphamide, intravenous cyclophosphamide, and cyclosporine. Intravenous pulse methylprednisolone is most effective in patients with a recent decline in GFR, with diffuse proliferative lesions, and with greater serologic activity. It is clearly not effective in all patients, and recent studies at the NIH have shown it to be less effective than intravenous cyclophosphamide in preventing long-term renal failure in patients with severe LN. Plasmapheresis has been reported to be successful in some anecdotal cases. It has recently proved unsuccessful in a major clinical controlled trial of more than 80 patients with severe LN. Patients treated with steroids-cytotoxics and plasmapheresis had no improvement in clinical activity or in renal or patient survival when compared with a control group at a mean follow-up at 80 weeks.

Recently, a series of well-performed studies by the group at NIH has reviewed the results of patients randomized to one of five treatment protocols: oral prednisone, oral azathioprine, oral cytoxan, oral azathioprine plus oral cytoxan, and every third month intravenous cytoxan. Patients treated with any of the cytotoxic agents fared better than those with steroid treatment. Extended long-term follow-up shows the azathioprine group to be no different from the prednisone groups. Intravenous cytoxan appeared to be a most effective form of therapy for preventing progressive renal failure. The side effects were no worse in the cytotoxic treatment group than the steroid group and were lowest in the intravenous cytoxan group.

Currently, a regimen of once monthly intravenous cytoxan therapy has been used for Class IV LN. We and others have found this regimen of monthly intravenous cytoxan therapy with rapid steroid taper to give good short-term results with rapid resolution of serologic and clinical abnormalities, decreases in proteinuria, and remissions of the nephrotic syndrome, and stabilization of serum creatinine levels. A recent trial from the NIH has found similar efficacy for this regimen.

Initial trials with cyclosporine in more than 100 SLE patients have been promising. Yet owing to poor patient selection, poor study design, or concurrent therapy, conclusions about this form of therapy remain speculative.

Many patients with LN (40–75%) will produce autoantibodies against certain phospholipids. These may be detected by assays against cardiolipin (anticardiolipin antibodies), by interference with coagulation systems (lupus anticoagulant), or by biologic false-positive tests for syphilis (VDRL). These patients are predisposed to recurrent venous and arterial thromboses, spontaneous abortions, neurologic disorders from focal ischemia, and thrombocytopenia. A high titer of IgG anticardiolipin antibody by ELISA correlates best with the risk of thrombotic events. Some patients have renal thrombotic microangiopathy with evidence of coagulation in their glomeruli and arterioles. These patients with anticardiolipin antibodies may require treatment with anticoagulation and or antiplatelet agents, as well as with immunosuppressive medications.

Amyloidosis

Amyloidosis is a generic term for a group of diseases in which there is extracellular deposition of one of a number of insoluble fibrillar proteins in a characteristic beta-pleated sheet configuration. Although the proteins may be very different, all have this configurational structure on radiograph diffraction, leading to the defining tintorial properties such as Congo red binding with apple-green birefringence on polarization microscopy. They also have amyloid P component (AP), a glycoprotein composed of 10 identical subunits each of molecular weight 25,000 D. One of the two most common forms of amyloidosis is primary amyloidosis, now called AL amyloidosis, owing to a plasma cell dyscrasia with overproduction of a monoclonal immunoglobulin light chain. Twenty percent of

AL amyloid patients have overt myeloma, and while approximately 10–15% of myeloma patients have AL amyloidosis. AL fibrils are derived predominantly from the variable portion of the light chain. It is unclear why certain light chains deposit in a fibrillar configuration as in amyloid. Two-thirds to four-fifths of patients with AL amyloid who have a monoclonal protein have overproduction of a lambda light chain. So far, however, amino acid sequencing of amyloid fibrils has not shown any unique property to account for the characteristic structural changes that produce fibrils.

Secondary amyloidosis (AA amyloidosis) is associated with high circulating levels and the deposition of the nonimmunoglobulin serum amyloid A protein (SAA)—a 12 KD high-density lipoprotein apoprotein synthesized by hepotocytes as an acute phase reactant in disease states. AA amyloid occurs in chronic infections and inflammatory states including rheumatoid arthritis, ankylosing spondylitis, tuberculosis osteomyelitis, and intravenous drug abuse. It presents with proteinuria and the nephrotic syndrome and progresses to renal insufficiency and renal failure in the majority of cases. Other forms of amyloid are caused by deposition of other proteins (e.g., prealbumin, beta-2 microglobulin).

Amyloid deposits are predominantly found within the glomeruli often appearing as amorphous, eosinophilic extracellular nodules. They also may be found deposited in the tubular basement membranes, the interstitium, and the vessels. They stain positively with Congo red and under polarized light display apple-green birefringence. Under electron microscopy amyloid appears as nonbranching rigid fibrils 8–10 mm in diameter.

Although almost 80% of patients with AL amyloid have renal disease, amyloidosis is a disease with multisystem involvement and thus patients may present with symptoms referable to other organ involvement, as well as renal symptoms. Diagnosis may be made from organ biopsy, gingival biopsy, rectal biopsy, or fat pad biopsy. Regardless of the type of biopsy, tissue documentation is required to establish the diagnosis. Extrarenal symptoms include cardiac symptoms, peripheral neuropathy, and macroglossia. The most common renal manifestations are proteinuria owing to albuminuria and renal insufficiency found in almost half of patients. Approximately 25% of patients with AL amyloid present with the nephrotic syndrome, and this is the major manifestation of the disease process in up to half of patients. Amyloid is rarely found in association with light chain cast nephropathy.

There is no specific effective therapy for renal amyloidosis. In patients with AL amyloidosis, both chemotherapy directed at the abnormal clone of B cells (e.g., melphalan and prednisone) and colchicine have been shown to have beneficial results. In a study at the Mayo clinic, Kyle et al. found that of 100 primary amyloid patients treated with either melphalan/prednisone or colchicine, the chemotherapy treatment was superior. However, some patients with primary amyloid have responded with complete remissions of their nephrotic syndrome with either regimen. In the majority of cases, the amyloid has been progressive, and organ system involvement continues. Survival times of 1 or 2 years are typical for treated patients with AL amyloid. Dialysis with either hemodialysis or peritoneal dialysis and transplantation have been effective in small numbers of patients with primary amyloid and ESRD.

HIV Nephropathy

More than 200,000 cases of AIDS have been recorded in the United States, with more than 40,000 deaths from this disease. Some cities such as New York have reported more than 10,000 cases of AIDS, and up to 500,000 people in the New York metropolitan area have been reported to be infected with the virus. Many studies have found populations of intravenous drug abusers (IVDA) to have a 60–85% carriage rate for HIV. Infection with this virus has been associated with a number of patterns of renal disease, including acute renal failure and a unique form of glomerulopathy now called HIV nephropathy.

The course of patients with acute renal failure and AIDS has been described by a number of investigators. Rao et al. at Downstate Medical Center have described the course of 23 such patients, and Valeri et al. reviewed 88 episodes of acute renal failure in 449 AIDS patients at Bellevue Hospital in New York City. The most common precipitating factors for acute renal failure in both studies included medications (pentamidine, aminoglycosides, TMP-SMX, NSAIDs) and pyrexia and dehydration superimposed on sepsis-hypotension-respiratory failure. In Rao's study, all six patients with mild renal failure regained renal function. Of those 17 with severe renal failure (serum creatinine > 6 mg/dl), 8 of the 11 who did not undergo dialysis died in renal failure, while 5 of the remaining 6 who were dialyzed regained renal function. Some survived for many months (up to 24 months) after recovery of function. Thus, dialysis support is indicated for AIDS patients with acute renal failure.

Several histologic patterns of glomerulopathy have been seen in patients with AIDS or HIV infection. These include minimal change pattern, mesangial hyperplasia, glomerulopathies associated with immune complex deposition and/or IgA deposition, and most important, HIV nephropathy. HIV nephropathy is a unique pattern of glomerulopathy in HIV-infected patients, characterized by heavy proteinuria and rapid progression to renal failure, and characteristic USG and renal biopsy findings. HIV nephropathy is a better term than AIDS nephropathy, since this glomerulopathy may occur in patients with AIDS or ARC or in asymptomatic HIV carriers. While HIV nephropathy has a prevalence of only 3–7% of unselected autopsy series, it is by far the most common lesion found in HIV-infected patients undergoing renal biopsy. For example, of 37 consecutive renal biopsies in HIV-infected patients at Columbia-Presbyterian Medical Center, 30 proved to be HIV nephropathy. The classic clinical features of HIV nephropathy include a strong predilection for blacks, heavy proteinuria usually with the nephrotic syndrome, renal insufficiency and a rapid progression to ESRD, and large echogenic kidneys by USG.

The course of HIV nephropathy is usually a rapid progression to renal failure. In an early study Rao et al. found the mean time from diagnosis to uremia was 3–4 months for AIDS nephropathy patients with a Ccr > 60 cc/min. It was 43.7 months for heroin nephropathy patients with a similar Ccr, and even for heroin nephropathy patients with a Ccr < 20 cc/min at diagnosis, the time to uremia was still 7 months. In a more recent study, Rao followed 59 AIDS patients with HIV nephropathy. Ten were lost to follow-up, 2 died without uremia, and 43 progressed to uremia. Of these, 43 patients progressing to ESRD, 12 were not dialyzed and all died, 31 were dialyzed, and 26 died with 3 months of initiating dialysis. Thus, this group was skeptical about the benefits of providing dialysis support to the population with HIV nephropathy and overt AIDS. In our study of 26 patients with HIV nephropathy, the stage of involvement with their HIV infection proved to be the most important prognostic feature in their survival. Seropositive HIV patients without AIDS but with HIV nephropathy can have prolonged survival on dialysis for years!

An important question is whether this entity of HIV nephropathy is truly different from the older entity of heroin nephropathy. Heroin nephropathy refers to a form of glomerulopathy, usually focal segmental glomerulosclerosis, that occurs in intravenous drug users. It presents with proteinuria and often the nephrotic syndrome and renal insufficiency. Its etiology is unclear but is almost certainly not immune complex mediated. Clinical and histologic data would suggest that HIV nephropathy and heroin nephropathy are distinct entities (Table 49.1).

The pathology of HIV nephropathy shows several features distinct from classic focal segmental glomerulosclerosis or heroin nephropathy. On light microscopy, diffuse global glomerular sclerosis and collapse are common, with striking visceral epithelial cell hypertrophy with large cytoplasmic vacuoles and resorption droplets. There are also severe tubulointerstitial changes with interstitial inflammation, edema, microcystic dilatation of tubules, and severe tubular degenerative changes. On electron microscopy, tubuloreticular inclusions (TRI) are prevalent in the glomerular endothelium. While these TRI may only be a marker for the presence of a severe viral infection, their presence in a patient with classic light microscopic changes of HIV nephropathy makes the diagnosis quite certain.

The optimal treatment of HIV nephropathy remains unclear. So far, there is no convincing evidence that treatment with AZT or other agents will delay the appearance of AIDS or prevent the progression of renal disease in HIV nephropathy. Trials with other antiretroviral agents and with corticosteroids and other immunosuppressives are all underway. Obviously any immunosuppressive medication has the potential for significant harm in this population. At present, we recommend therapy with AZT for patients with HIV nephropathy and consider other modalities experimental. Dialysis and support seem appropriate for patients with HIV nephropathy without the full-blown AIDS syndrome. Once AIDS has developed, whether dialysis support will prolong useful life is open to debate.

INTERSTITIAL NEPHRITIS

DRUG-INDUCED ACUTE INTERSTITIAL NEPHRITIS

In recent years, it has become clear that all acute interstitial nephritides (AINs) are not caused by bacterial invasion of the kidney. Among the causes of AIN that have been defined, drug-induced AIN has a prominent role. The distinct clinical picture, histopathologic pattern, and clinical course of this form of acute renal failure (ARF) have been defined. Drug-induced AIN is now recognized as a common and reversible form of ARF. Since much of the knowledge of drug-induced AIN comes from the study of patients receiving β-lactam antibiotics of the penicillin or cephalosporin classes, this review focuses on this prototype group of drugs. The clinical picture, histopathologic pattern, and course of these patients can then be contrasted with those of patients suffering AIN in association with other medications. Recent data using monoclonal antibodies to study the cellular infiltrates in these diseases will also be reviewed.

Drug-induced AIN may be defined as a pattern of ARF causally related to drug therapy, with a probable immunologic pathogenesis, in which the renal histology reveals predominantly edema and interstitial infiltrates of mononuclear cells and eosinophils without marked fibrosis and with only patchy tubular damage. In general, glomerular and vascular changes are not prominent. Well more than 50 medications have been associated with AIN, and the list of offending drugs grows each year. Table 49.2 lists some of the drugs currently known to be associated with AIN.

Penicillin-Associated AIN

Despite the numerous incriminating drugs, the beta-lactam antibiotics, the penicillins and cephalosporins remain among the foremost offenders. Table 49.3 is a review of 155 individual episodes of AIN caused by these antibiotics. All agents of the beta-lactam group are capable of producing this lesion. Why methicillin is the number one offender is less clear. The cause does not appear related to the extent of serum protein binding, the route of excretion by renal tubular secretion, or

Table 49.1. HIV Nephropathy vs. Heroin Nephropathy		
	HIV	*Heroin*
Epidemiology	⅓–½ IVDA	All IVDA
Pathology	LM-collapsing FS and GS	Classic FSGS
Progression	Rapid to ESRD	Moderate

Table 49.2. Drugs Associated with Acute Interstitial Nephritis

Beta-Lactam Antibiotics	*Nonsteroidal Antiinflammatory Agents*
Methicillin	Fenoprofen
Penicillin G	Indomethacin
Ampicillin	Naproxen
Flucloxicillin	Ibuprofen
Oxacillin	Benoxaprofen
Nafcillin	Phenazone
Carbenicillin	Mefanamic Acid
Amoxicillin	Tolmetin
Mezlocillin	Diflunisal
Cephalothin	Zomepirac
Cephalexin	Piroxicam
Cephradine	Diclofenac
Cephaloridine	Ketoprofen
Cefoxtaxime	Suprofen
Cefoxitin	*Others*
Cefaclor	Phenindione
Other Antibiotics	Glafenin
Sulfonamides	Diphenylhydantoin
Trimethoprim-	Cimetidine
Sulfamethoxazole	Sulfinpyrazone
Rifampin	Allopurinol
Polymyxin Sulfate	Aspirin
Ethambutol	Carbamazepine
Vancomycin	Clofibrate
Chloramphenicol	Azathioprine
Gentamicin	Phenylpropanolamin
Isoniazid	Aldomet
Minocycline	Phenobarbital
Para-aminosalicylic acid	Leukocyte A Interferon
Ciprofloxacin	Floctafenin
Norfloxacin	Haldol
Piromidic acid	Coumadin
Erthyromycin	Tofranil
Spiramycin	Diazepam
Diuretics	Sodium valproate
Thiazides	Chlorprothixene
Furosemide	Captopril
Chlorthalidone	Propranolol
Ticrynafen	Amphetamines
Triamterene	Doxepin
	Quinine

lection. The dose of the beta-lactam antibiotic has usually not been excessive; however, the duration of therapy is often prolonged, with more than three-fourths of patients receiving more than 10 days of therapy and more than one-third receiving more than 20 days of therapy. The clinical features of penicillin-associated AIN include the hypersensitivity triad of rash (43%), secondary fever (77%), and eosinophilia (80%) (Table 49.4). However, fewer than one-third of patients have the complete triad at diagnosis, and one must not wait for this full picture to make a presumptive diagnosis of drug-related AIN. Of the urinary findings, mild proteinuria and pyuria are common but not specific. Nephrotic range proteinuria and RBC casts are uncommon in this nonglomerular disease and can usually be explained by incidental concomitant glomerular pathology. Hematuria is a cardinal feature of penicillin-associated AIN, being present in more than 90% of cases and being macroscopic in one-third. Urinary eosinophiluria on Wright or Hansel stain of the urinary sediment is often present. Although its significance (sensitivity and specificity) remains unclear at present, a recent study suggests eosino-

Table 49.3. β-Lactam Agents Causing Acute Interstitial Nephritis

Drug	*Number of Episodes*[a]
Methicillin	100
Penicillin	12
Ampicillin	8
Nafcillin	3
Oxacillin	4
Carbenicillin	2
Amoxicillin	1
Cephalothin	11
Cephalexin	2
Cephradine	1
Cefotaxime	1
Multiple Agents	10
	Total = 155

[a] Two patients had 2 distinct episodes with different agents.

Table 49.4. Clinical Features of 153 Patients with β-lactam–related Acute Interstitial Nephritis

Rash	43%
Fever	77%
Eosinophilia	80%
Triad (R + F + E)	31%
Hematuria	91%
Gross Hematuria	33%
Eosinophiluria	?%

the type of infections being treated by methicillin, since none of these features is unique to methicillin among the beta-lactam antibiotics.

Penicillin-induced AIN occurs in all decades of life. Although males predominate by a 3:1 ratio, this predominance may be owing to a higher percentage of males requiring antistaphylococcal drugs such as methicillin than a true sex predi-

philuria of more than 5% of the total urinary leukocytes to be strongly suggestive of AIN. Eosinophiluria has also been noted in rapidly progressive glomerulonephritis, cystitis, and prostatitis. Of interest, there is no good correlation between the degree of eosinophilia in the peripheral blood and the degree of eosinophiluria. Regardless of clinical presentation, most patients have nonoliguric renal failure and never have less than 400 cc of urine volume per day. Recently, Gallium scanning has been suggested as a screening test to distinguish drug-induced AIN from renal failure owing to acute tubular necrosis.

The histopathology in more than 70 cases of penicillin-associated AIN has shown patchy tubular damage, interstitial edema, and infiltrates of mononuclear cells and often eosinophils. IF may rarely show linear deposits of immunoglobulins, complement, and drug hapten along the TBMs. Of the 40 cases with IF reported, only 11 clearly had the presence of immunoglobulins and/or complement along the TBMs or within the interstitium. EM has only rarely shown electron dense deposits along the TBMs.

While the pathogenesis of penicillin-associated AIN remains to be defined, there is good evidence for an allergic-immunologic mechanism of renal damage. The small number of afflicted patients despite the extensive use of these drugs; recurrences on rechallenge with another beta-lactam drug; the hypersensitivity features of rash, fever, and eosinophilia; and the histopathologic findings in many cases all support an allergic-immunologic mechanism. The first step may be binding of drug hapten to kidney structural protein, either tubular or interstitial. Subsequently, a humoral response with development of anti-TBM antibodies to combined drug hapten and kidney protein may damage the kidney. In most cases, there is no evidence for such a response (negative IF staining, normal serum complement, lack of circulating anti-TBM or anti-drug antibodies), and a cell-mediated cytotoxic reaction may be the cause of ultimate renal damage. As recently elucidated by Nielson, the pathogenesis may actually be far more complex.

Therapy for penicillin-associated AIN includes prompt discontinuation of the drug and avoidance of rechallenge with other beta-lactam agents, which may lead to a recrudescence or hypersensitivity symptoms and renal failure. Dialysis and good supportive care are crucial, since most patients recover good renal function. The use of corticosteroids is controversial. Anecdotal reports of dramatic reversal of renal failure and two partially controlled studies support their use, but rigorous proof of their benefit is lacking and the hazards of steroid therapy in such a population are well recognized. The use of other immunosuppressive agents remains unproved and has been reported in isolated cases only. Their use should be individualized until further data become available.

Other Antimicrobial Agents Causing AIN

Sulfonamides have long been known to produce ARF through a mechanism other than intratubular crystallization and obstruction. AIN has been well documented in several cases. Of special concern, the widely used antimicrobial combination of trimethoprim-sulfamethoxazole can produce this form of renal damage. Rifampin is associated with a unique pattern of ARF. In more than 60 patients receiving either intermittent or discontinuous therapy, on rechallenge with rifampin, there was a sudden onset of fever, flank pain, hematuria, and ARF. Histopathology ranges from classic AIN to a picture indistinguishable from acute tubular necrosis. Clearly it is wise to avoid the intermittent or discontinuous use of this drug. A recent study documents two new unusual features of rifampin-related AIN: its occurrence during continuous therapy and nephrotic range proteinuria. A number of other antimicrobials producing AIN infrequently or in a less well-documented fashion are listed in Table 49.2.

Diuretics

Diuretics including the thiazides and chlorthalidone, furosemide, and ticrynafen have all been well documented to cause AIN. This is a rare occurrence, usually in patients with prior renal disease (the nephrotic syndrome, hypertension), and patients present with the classic hypersensitivity features of rash, fever, and eosinophilia. The AIN responds readily to discontinuing the drug and corticosteroid therapy.

Nonsteroidal Anti-Inflammatory Drugs (NSAIDs)

The NSAIDs may produce salt and water retention, decreased renal blood flow and GFR, and hyperkalemia associated with hyporenin hypoaldosteronism, perhaps all caused by inhibition of prostaglandins. They also can cause AIN with a number of unique features. The population developing AIN is usually older (50–80 years old) despite many young patients receiving these drugs. Patients typically have a prolonged exposure to the drugs (months to years) before developing AIN. The hypersensitivity features of rash, fever, and eosinophilia are rare, as are hematuria and eosinophiluria. This is true even when AIN with interstitial eosinophilia is found on renal biopsy. Perhaps the peripheral hypersensitivity features of the disease are modified by the analgesic-antipyretic nature of these drugs. Finally, AIN caused by the NSAIDs has frequently been associated with "minimal change" nephrotic syndrome (NS). The drug-induced nature of this lesion is clear: "minimal change" is the exclusive pattern of NS reported (despite comprising less than 20% of idiopathic NS in this age group; its onset coincides with the onset of ARF from AIN; the NS and AIN remit several weeks after discontinuing the NSAID regardless of whether steroid therapy is given. Why the AIN of the NSAIDs should uniquely be associated with the minimal change NS is not known.

Recently, using monoclonal antibodies to analyze the interstitial inflammatory infiltrates in cases of AIN associated with use of NSAIDs, a predominance of T lymphocytes over B lymphocytes has been noted. Among the T cell subsets, the cytotoxic-suppressor cell population has outnumbered the helper-inducer T cell population (T4/T8 ratio <1). We have found similar results in our recent studies of patients with AIN caused by NSAIDs. However, the percentage of each cell subtype has not been statistically different from that in patients with AIN owing to beta-lactam drugs (T4/T8 ratio 1). Although a role for cell-mediated reactions is suggested by this data, the exact mechanism(s) of tissue injury remain to be defined.

Other Drugs Associated with AIN

Two drugs not used in the United states, the analgesic glafenin and the anticoagulant phenidone, have been associated with numerous cases of well-documented AIN. The widely used drug cimetidine has caused this pattern of renal failure, as has the uricosuric, antiplatelet agent sulfinpyrazone recently used in postmyocardial infarct patients. Virtually no area of medical therapy is free from medications that can cause AIN. Greater awareness of the clinical picture and course of AIN will surely lead to an increasing number of incriminating medications and yet also to appropriate intervention for this reversible form of ARF.

DRUG-INDUCED CHRONIC INTERSTITIAL NEPHRITIS (CIN)

The use of certain medications has been associated with the development of chronic renal insufficiency and chronic interstitial damage. In general, the relationship between the drug use and the renal lesions has often been more difficult to define than with drug-induced AIN. This is related in part to the slower disease process and its insidious nature and to the complexity of the medication regimens of many of the patients developing such lesions. Several important groups of medications indicted as causing CIN include the analgesics, phenacetin, acetaminophen, and aspirin; lithium; and the antineoplastic chemotherapeutic agents, cisplatinum, methyl-CCNU, and BCNU.

Analgesic agents have been extensively used in over-the-counter preparations in recent decades, and concern about their nephrotoxic potential has generated considerable attention and controversy. The incidence of analgesic nephropathy varies greatly among countries and even within regions of one country. In general, those countries with a higher per capita consumption of phenacetin and other analgesic compounds have had a higher incidence of analgesic nephropathy. Recent studies have documented analgesic nephropathy as the cause of end stage renal disease (ESRD) in more than 16% of patients in West Germany, 18% of ESRD patients in Belgium, and 13% of all ESRD patients in Australia. In the United States, reports vary from an incidence of more than 10% in the Southeast to a low of only a few percent elsewhere. The exact nature of the offending analgesic or combinations of analgesics remains to be defined. Dubach's well-controlled study of more than 600 middle-aged Swiss working women clearly documented a higher incidence of renal insufficiency,

as well as an increased mortality, owing to urinary tract disease and cardiovascular disease in a phenacetin-consuming population. A recent retrospective case-controlled study in North Carolina also found significantly more renal disease in consumers of analgesics than in the control population. The risk of renal disease was increased with daily consumption of phenacetin and acetaminophen, but not with the daily use of aspirin. This study confirms the risk of renal damage with phenacetin (which has been removed from most analgesic preparations in the United States), but raises the strong possibility that acetaminophen, the major metabolite of phenacetin, is also nephrotoxic.

The characteristic patient who develops analgesic nephropathy is a middle-aged female (females out number males 4 : 1) with chronic headaches or arthritic problems who has consumed large amounts of phenacetin, acetaminophen, and/ or aspirin-containing compounds on a daily basis for many years. The ingestion of at least 1 g or more daily of the analgesics longer than 2–3 years is thought to be the minimum dose-time requirement to produce clinical analgesic nephropathy. Systemic symptoms such as malaise, weight loss, emotional-psychiatric disorders, anemia, and peptic ulcer disease may be related in part to the syndrome or analgesic nephropathy and in part to the population that uses these medications excessively. Diagnosis is often difficult, since most patients do not consider these over-the-counter preparations to be medications and to have potential side effects. Renal findings are related to chronic interstitial disease and may include nocturia and polyuria, sterile pyuria, urinary tract infections, acidification defects, a predisposition to volume depletion, renal colic and hematuria, and hypertension. Renal insufficiency may be present in asymptomatic patients and is often progressive if analgesic consumption is continued. The finding of papillary necrosis on IVP, USG, or CAT scan is helpful in establishing the diagnosis.

The mechanisms of chronic renal insufficiency and interstitial damage produced by analgesics are unclear. Acetaminophen, a major metabolite of phenacetin, can accumulate in the renal medulla. Here, it may be oxidized into reactive intermediates that can cause cell necrosis especially when reduced glutathione has bean depleted. By decreasing renal blood flow through prostaglandin inhibition, some analgesics such as aspirin can further decrease the oxygen supply to the medulla, leading to lower concentrations of the protective reduced glutathione. This may account for the potential increased toxicity of analgesic compounds containing both phenactein and aspirin or their metabolites. While the NSAIDs have rarely been reported to produce CIN in the past, it is unclear if this incidence will increase now that ibuprofen is available as an over-the-counter medication.

Lithium salts, widely used to treat affective disorders, have been associated with a number of renal abnormalities, most prominently a nephrogenic diabetes insipidus-polyuria syndrome. While reductions in the GFR and chronic interstitial nephritis have been attributed to lithium use, the relationship is not clearly established. Although some studies have found that a small percentage of lithium-treated patients have an abnormal plasma creatinine, most studies have not confirmed this when the lithium-treated subjects are compared with normal subjects or psychiatric populations not receiving lithium. In a composite review of studies covering almost 500 patients receiving lithium, only 15% had a reduced creatinine clearance. Likewise, in studies using EDTA clearances in more than 500 patients, the GFR was found to be reduced in only 17%. In those patients with a reduced GFR, the reduction was mild, with most patients having a GFR of 60–75 cc/min. Clearly, even the renal dysfunction of these patients cannot all be attributed to lithium use, since psychiatric patient populations not receiving lithium have been noted to have reduced GFR, as well as chronic changes on their renal biopsies, when compared with normal subjects. Many studies have also failed to document a positive correlation between duration of lithium treatment and the reduction in GFR. However, in studies with longer durations of treatment (6.5 to 10 years), a positive correlation has been noted. There are only a few prospective studies examining the effects of lithium on reduction in GFR, and although no significant change in GFR has been noted, the duration of follow-up has been short.

Lithium has been noted to produce lesions in the distal nephron including cytoplasmic swelling with accumulation of glycogen deposits, dilated tubules, and microcyst formation in the kidneys of many species of experimental animals. Renal histologic studies of patients receiving lithium have noted tubular dilatation, microcyst formation, tubular atrophy, and cortical and medullary interstitial fibrosis. Such changes have been noted in both patients with a normal or decreased CFR. Most studies have documented a significant positive correlation between the duration of lithium administration and the degree of tubulointerstitial damage. In some studies the renal biopsies of lithium-treated patients with a normal GFR have shown focal interstitial fibrotic changes. Such changes have been described in some studies as greater and in other studies as no greater than those changes found in control subjects

untreated with lithium. Thus, in one study of almost 50 patients treated with lithium for 5 years, there was no difference in interstitial fibrosis when compared with 32 control patients with affective disorders never treated with lithium. Thus, it is unclear if lithium is the causative agent of the renal histologic damage in those patients.

Overall, prolonged use of lithium for many years is probably associated with some degree or decline in the GFR and interstitial damage. The damage is usually mild to moderate and appears to occur only after prolonged use of lithium. The contribution to renal disease of other psychotropic medications or of other factors associated with the affective disorders or these patients remains to be defined.

Cisplatinum, an antineoplastic agent widely used to treat a variety of carcinomas and germ cell tumors, may cause both acute renal failure and less frequently chronic renal insufficiency. In those patients suffering chronic renal damage, interstitial fibrosis and chronic inflammatory changes have been noted on renal biopsy. The nitrosourea compounds methyl-CCNU and BCNU can both produce dose-related nephrotoxicity and chronic interstitial nephritis. Renal biopsies from patients suffering renal damage after receiving these medications have shown severe tubular atrophy, glomerulosclerosis, and interstitial fibrosis with chronic inflammatory infiltrates. In some patients, the chronic tubulointerstitial damage has led to end stage renal disease.

Cyclosporine, a potent immunosuppressive agent now widely used in transplantation, can cause not only acute renal damage but also chronic tubulointerstitial fibrosis. This is often associated with drug-related microvascular damage to the arterioles of the kidney. Cyclosporine can produce a chronic form of tubulointerstitial damage in a bandlike pattern within the kidney, so-called striped fibrosis. This has been seen in both transplant populations and patients without prior renal disease taking this immunosuppressive medicine for autoimmune conditions. It is usually associated with a decreased GFR and renal insufficiency.

Hallmarks of Essential and Secondary Hypertension

Martin J. Schreiber, Jr.

The most recent National Health and Nutrition Examination Survey (NHANES III) reported that only 24% of patients with hypertension had their blood pressure (BP) controlled to less than 140/90 mm Hg, and that only 53% were receiving antihypertensive therapy. Furthermore, 35% were unaware they even had hypertension (1). Evidence is emerging that hypertension not only is being untreated (2), but that prevention, timely initiation of treatment, selection of medication, and level of control based on risk stratification have not been emphasized enough.

Treatment recommendations from the fifth Joint National Committee on Detection, Evaluation and Treatment of High Blood Pressure (JNC-V) generated significant discussion because of the emphasis on diuretics and β-blockers as initial treatment selections (3–6). This report also stressed, however, that the following variables should be considered during selection of antihypertensive agents and determination of subsequent treatment goals:

- Comorbidities for cardiac events (7)
- Prevention of diabetic complications (8–10)
- Prevention of target organ disease (i.e., progressive azotemia)
- Age (11)
- Race (e.g., black, white, Hispanic, and so on) (12)
- Specific clinical situations (e.g., pregnancy, benign prostatic hyperplasia, migraines, tachyarrhythmias) (13)

The upcoming report of the sixth Joint National Committee most likely will emphasize prevention of hypertension, reassess the starting point for hypertensive treatment, define more clearly the steps in selecting initial drug treatment, explain how to structure a treatment regimen to achieve target BPs, and reemphasize the importance of selecting drugs on the basis of clinical situations and comorbid conditions.

In patients with clinical clues for secondary hypertension or those demonstrating patterns of resistant hypertension, appropriate additional evaluations should be performed. Because systolic BP is a more reliable predictor than diastolic BP of cardiovascular morbidity and mortality, as well as of all-cause mortality, controlling the systolic BP is a primary goal of antihypertensive intervention (4). The actual target BP may be reexamined in the future, with consideration of race, cardiovascular status, age, renal disease, and so on becoming important determinants of the optimal level. We now may be moving from a population-based "safe range" to an individualized "optimal range."

ETIOLOGY AND EPIDEMIOLOGY

Based on the JNC-V, hypertension is classified into four different categories:

- Optimal
- Normal
- High-normal
- Hypertension

Figure 50.1 promotes the concept of optimal BP control. To combat complacency when treating mild hypertension, the optimal category emphasizes the importance of such treatment, especially in patients with comorbid risk or a strong family history of vascular or renal events. Results of epidemiologic studies have demonstrated that the optimal BP is less than 120/80 mm Hg, and those of the Treatment of Mild Hypertension Study (TOMHS) supported the concept of "the lower, the better" (14). If systolic/diastolic BPs fall into different categories, the higher value should determine the treatment category.

Hypertension is further divided into four different stages depending on the severity of BP elevations. Each stage of

Figure 50.1. A new classification system for high blood pressure. (Adapted with permission from The Joint National Committee. The fifth report of the Joint National Committee on detection, evaluation, and treatment of high blood pressure. Arch Intern Med 1993; 153:154–183.)

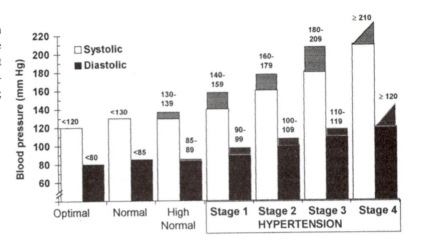

hypertension is associated with an increased risk for cardiovascular disease and renal disease (15). The greater the elevation, the greater the risk over time. More than one set of readings is essential for a true estimate of BP.

Typical BP readings in hypertensive patients show a marked fall in BP during the early hours of sleep and a marked rise before awakening. A relationship may exist between this early rise and an increased risk for cardiovascular events. Those individuals who do not experience a lower BP during sleep have an increased risk for left ventricular hypertrophy.

Approximately 50% of whites and 60% of blacks have either systolic or diastolic hypertension (16, 17). In individuals older than 60 years, a diastolic pressure of more than 95 mm Hg carries an increased risk for cardiovascular events. In this age group, the prevalence of diastolic hypertension tends to decrease over time. Men older than 65 years as well as both men and women older than 85 years may benefit from somewhat higher BP levels compared with younger age groups. Patients with isolated systolic hypertension have three to four times more strokes and myocardial infarctions than those with a normal systolic BP.

An association between hypertension, lipid abnormalities, and glucose intolerance with upper-body obesity is increasingly recognized, and this constellation of risk factors has been termed the ''insulin-resistant syndrome'' (18). Resistance to the actions of insulin on glucose utilization and peripheral muscle is the primary effect. There also is a compensatory increase in insulin levels. As demonstrated by Haffner et al. (19), hyperinsulinemia is a metabolic precursor of hypertension (Fig. 50.2). The San Antonio Heart Study followed 1039 patients for 7 years. Initially, these patients were nonhypertensive and nondiabetic. During the observation period, however, almost 10% became hypertensive, and elevated insulin levels predicted the development of hypertension. This phenomenon also can be seen in patients with hypertension who are not obese. Physiologically, hyperinsulinemia can result in volume retention, sympathetic overactivity, and vascular hypertrophy, and insulin sensitivity may be affected by the specific antihypertensive agent used (i.e., pro-

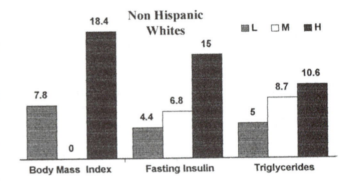

Figure 50.2. Metabolic precursors of hypertension (San Antonio Heart Study). Univariate relation of incidence of hypertension to body mass index, insulin level, and triglyceride values. L = low, <25.2; M = medium, 25.2–29.6; H = high, ≥29.6. (Adapted with permission from Haffner SM, Miettinen H, Gaskill SP, et al. Metabolic precursors of hypertension. The San Antonio Heart Study. Arch Intern Med 1996;156:1994–2001.)

pranolol decreases insulin sensitivity, prazosin and doxazosin increase sensitivity).

DIAGNOSIS AND TREATMENT

Initial evaluation of a patient with hypertension includes a history, physician examination, baseline serum chemistries, urinalysis, and electrocardiography for those 30 years and older (Table 50.1). For routine evaluation, 24-hour ambulatory BP monitoring (20), echocardiography, plasma renin level, and aldosterone activity are not recommended. The first examination should include two or more BP readings to establish whether patients with elevated BPs consistently measure as >140 / ≥90 mm Hg.

Proper patient positioning, the use of appropriate equipment, and standardized technique should be used when measuring BP. Disappearance of the ''tapping'' sound (i.e., Korotkoff phase V) is more reliable than the phase IV

Table 50.1.   Initial Laboratory and Radiographic Assessment of Patients with Hypertension

Standard	Special Situations
Baseline serum chemistries[a]	24-hour ambulatory BP monitoring
Electrocardiography if older than 30 years	Echocardiography
Urinalysis	Carotid ultrasonography
	Plasma renin level
	Plasma aldosterone level

[a] Blood urea nitrogen, serum creatinine, serum potassium, serum glucose, uric acid, total cholesterol, high- and low-density lipoprotein, serum calcium.

"muffling" of the sound. Especially in elderly patients with very calcified and rigid arteries, the bladder may not be able to fully collapse the brachial artery, thus producing falsely high readings, or "pseudohypertension." Those elderly patients with rigid vessels and little other evidence of vascular disease at fundoscopy may benefit from the Osler maneuver to diagnose pseudohypertension caused by rigid vessels.

Home BP monitoring is helpful for the diagnosis of "white coat" hypertension, response to treatment, and long-term follow-up of borderline hypertension readings in the office. Evidence of target organ damage and concomitant risk factors should be managed aggressively. Ambulatory BP recording also can be helpful in diagnosing apparent drug resistance, nocturnal hypotension, labile, or episodic hypertension (21, 22).

DIAGNOSIS AND TREATMENT OF SECONDARY HYPERTENSION

Less than 5% of the 50 million U.S. patients with hypertension have a curable cause, such as renovascular disease, Cushing's syndrome, pheochromocytoma, primary aldosteronism, coarctation of the aorta, or other nonendocrine causes (Table 50.2). Specific clinical or laboratory clues may help in the diagnosis of secondary hypertension (Table 50.3). The younger (i.e., <30 years) or older (i.e., >55 years) the patient at the time of onset, and the more severe the hypertension (diastolic >125 mm Hg), then the greater the possibility for a secondary cause of the hypertension. Specific clues from the patient history or physical examination can help in initiating a workup for secondary hypertension. Therefore, several features of a patient's presentation should trigger a response to inappropriate hypertension and signal an evaluation for secondary causes, including:

- Age of onset < 30 or > 55 years
- Actual BP >180/120 mm Hg
- Grade III fundoscopic changes (i.e., hemorrhages), with or without an elevated serum creatinine level
- Left ventricular hypertrophy

A poor response to an effective drug regimen also should alert physicians to the possibility of secondary hypertension. Several features may be indicative of other causes, including unprovoked hypokalemia, abdominal bruit, family history of renal disease, and labile BP with sweating, tremor, and tachycardia.

11β-Hydroxylase Deficiency

11β-hydroxylase deficiency (23) presents in females as virilization and in males as precocious puberty and advanced masculinity (i.e., androgen excess). The diagnosis is made on the basis of an increased plasma level of 11-deoxycortisol, increased urinary levels of tetrahydro-S and 17-kerosteroids, dexamethasone inhibition of adrenocorticotropic hormone (ACTH) secretion. Treatment involves dexamethasone, 0.50 to 0.75 mg/day, to control BP and ketosteroids.

17α-Hydroxylase Deficiency

17α-Hydroxylase deficiency (24) presents in females as an absence of secondary sex characteristics and in males as a failure of normal masculine genitalia to develop (i.e.,androgen and estrogen deficiency). The diagnosis is made on the basis of elevated levels of deoxycorticosterone and corticosterone, decreased androgen production, and dexamethasone inhibition of ACTH secretion. Treatment involves dexamethasone, 0.50 to 0.75 mg/day, to control BP and ketosteroids.

Cushing's Syndrome

Cushing's syndrome (25) presents as truncal obesity, "moon" facies, ecchymoses, muscular atrophy, striae, and glucose in-

Table 50.2.   Etiologies for Secondary Hypertension

Renal
  Renal artery stenosis
  Renal parenchymal
  Obstruction
  Polycystic kidney disease
Other
  Preeclampsia
  Acute intermittent porphyria
  Thyroid (hyper-, hypo-)
  Drugs
  Hypercalcemia
Endocrine
  Cushing's syndrome
  Adrenogenital syndrome
  Pheochromocytoma
  Adrenal and adrenal-like
  Acromegaly
  Liddle syndrome, Gordon syndrome
Coarctation of the aorta

Table 50.3. Clues to the Diagnosis of Secondary Hypertension

Pheochromocytoma
   Headache
   Sweating
   Paroxysmal hypertension
   Weight loss
   Palpitations
Renovascular hypertension
   Age < 30 or > 60 years
   Diastolic BP, > 120 mm Hg
   Grade III/IV fundoscopic changes
   Recent onset or exacerbation of hypertension
   Systolic-diastolic bruit in epigastrium
   Evidence of extra renal arteriosclerosis obliterans
Coarctation
   Absent, delayed pulsations in the lower extremity
   Cold feet
   Diminished femoral pulses
   Leg claudication
Cushing's syndrome
   Truncal obesity
   ''Moon'' facies
   Ecchymoses
   Prominent striae
   Glucose intolerance
Primary aldosteronism
   Inappropriate kaliuresis (serum potassium, <3.5 mEq/L, U_kV, >30 mEq/L)
   Refractory hypertension
   Muscle spasms
   Metabolic alkalosis
Adrenogenital syndrome
   11 β-2 hydroxylase
      Virilization
      Female
      Precocious puberty
      Advanced masculinity
   17 α-hydroxylase deficiency
      Absence of secondary sex characteristics
      Failure of normal masculine development

tolerance. The diagnosis is made on the basis of increased 24-hour urinary free cortisol (i.e., >100 mg) and an overnight dexamethasone suppression test (1 mg dexamethasone at midnight, check 8:00 AM plasma cortisol). If the plasma cortisol level is more than 7 mg/dL, proceed with a prolonged dexamethasone suppression test of 0.5 mg dexamethasone every 6 hours for 2 days and followed by 2 mg every 6 hours for 2 days. Results are interpreted as follows:

- *Cushing's disease:* Failure to suppress on low-dose, suppressed to < 50% by high-dose dexamethasone; ACTH level is normal to elevated.

- *Adrenal tumor:* Lack of suppression with low- or high-dose dexamethasone.
- *Ectopic ACTH syndrome:* Elevated ACTH levels with no suppression (i.e., > 200 pg/mL).

Adrenal adenoma or carcinoma require a surgical resection. For ectopic ACTH, identify the location of the tumor and remove it. For a pituitary abnormality, consider transphenoidal microsurgery. Prevent postoperative hypoadrenalism following selective adenomectomy with preoperative glucocorticoid therapy

Primary Aldosteronism

Primary aldosteronism (26–29) presents as spontaneous hypokalemia (serum potassium, <3.5 mEq/L), diuretic hypokalemia (serum potassium, <3.0 mEq/L), difficulty achieving a normal potassium level with oral potassium supplements, refractory hypertension, muscle spasms, weakness, metabolic alkalosis, and development of multiple renal cysts. The serum potassium level is normal in 7 to 38% of patients.

Table 50.4 reviews the laboratory assessment for hypertension and hypokalemia (i.e., <3.5 mEq/L). To summarize:

- Plasma renin activity (PRA), <1 ng/m per hour
- Plasma aldosterone/renin ratio, >20
- 24-hour urine potassium level, >30 mEq/day with hypokalemia (serum potassium, <3.5 mEq/L)
- 24-hour sodium, creatinine, cortisol (discontinue diuretics) on a high-sodium diet (urine sodium (U_{NA}), ≥250 mEq per 24 hours)
- Saline loading, 2 L of normal saline over 4 hours (25 mL/kg [0.9% saline]), or 5 days of salt (1 tsp/day) added to a normal dietary intake
- Urinary aldosterone excretion rate, >14.0 μg in 24 hours with a 24-hour urine sodium >250 mEq.
- Thin-cut, 3-mm computed tomography (CT) of adrenal gland to identify adenoma

Table 50.4. Laboratory Workup of Hypertension and Hypokalemia[a] with Kaliuresis[b]

Serum electrolytes
Serum creatinine, urea
Plasma aldosterone (PA), cortisol, PRA
24-hour urinary sodium, potassium, creatinine, aldosterone, and free cortisol
High-salt diet (U_{NA}, ≥ 250 mEq per 24 hrs)[c]
   Normal PA (with PRA ≤ 1.0 ng/mL)
   High PA with normal/high PRA
   Normal PA and PRA with spontaneous hypokalemia

PRA, plasma renin activity.
[a] Serum potassium, <3.5 mEq/L.
[b] K_V, >20 mEq per 24 hours.
[c] Plasma aldosterone, 22 ng/dL; PRA, 0.7 pg/mL; urinary aldosterone, 14 μg per 24 hours.

Note that Liddle syndrome involves hypertension, hypokalemic alkalosis, and muscle weakness. In children, this syndrome can result in growth retardation, failure to thrive, or both. Aldosterone and renin levels are suppressed. This syndrome responds to triamterene, but not to spironolactone.

For adrenal adenoma, treatment involves spironolactone and surgical resection after 6 months of BP and potassium control. For bilateral adrenal hyperplasia, treatment involves potassium-sparing diuretics (spironolactone [100–200 mg/day], triamterene [10–20 mg/day], or ameloride [10–20 mg/day]).

Pheochromocytoma

Pheochromocytoma (30, 31) presents with hypertension; (persistent 50%, paroxysmal, 50%); episodic palpitations; headaches; sweating; orthostatic hypertension; weight loss; and glucose intolerance. Ninety percent of pheochromocytomas arise in chromaffin cells of an adrenal gland. Solitary lesions are more common on the right. Five percent of lesions are bilateral, and 10% are extra-adrenal (e.g., cardiac, bladder walls). Most arise within the abdomen and a few in the chest and neck. From 3 to 14% of pheochromocytomas are malignant. Multiple endocrine neoplasia (MEN) type II consists of medullary carcinomas of the thyroid, pheochromocytomas, and parathyroid abnormalities.

Diagnosis is made on the basis of the following 24-hour urinary measurements:

* Metanephrines, ≥1.8 mg
* Norepinephrine plus epinephrine, >200 μg
* Norepinephrine, ≥170 μg
* Vanillylmandelic (VMA) ≥ 11 mg

Other measurements include a plasma catecholamine level of more than 2000 pg/mL; if 400 to 2000 pg/mL, proceed with clonidine suppression test (i.e., failure to suppress by 50% or more 3 hours after a 0.3-mg clonidine tablet). CT is used for localization, and ^{131}I-meta-iodobenzylguanidine (MIBG) scanning or selected arteriography may be indicated for patients in whom standard tests do not localize the tumor.

Interfering drugs include calcium channel blockers, angiotensin-converting enzyme (ACE) inhibitors, bromocryptine, methyldopa, α-blockers, and labetalol (Table 50.5).

Table 50.5. Medications that Interfere with the Biochemical Diagnosis of Pheochromocytoma[a]

Metanephrine	Catecholamines	VMA
↓ Methylglucamine	↓ α-Agonists	↓ Methyldopa
	↓ ACE inhibitors	↓ Monoamine oxidase inhibitor
	↓ bromocriptine	
↑ Sotalol	↑ α₁-Blockers	↑ Naldixic acid
	↑ β-Blockers	↑ Anileridine
	↑ Labetalol	

[a] **Variable changes:** phenothiazines, L-dopa, tricyclic antidepressants.

Treatment involves surgical resection. Cholelithiasis may occur in approximately 30% of cases. α-adrenergic receptor blockade (e.g., phenoxybenzamine or doxazosin, prazosin, phentolamine) should be used preoperatively until the patient is normotensive for 5 to 7 days. With arrhythmias, α-adrenergic blockade may be necessary to expand intracellular volume. Ten percent of patients may experience reoccurrence.

Coarctation of the Aorta

Coarctation of the aorta presents with cold feet, leg claudication, and diminished femoral pulses (2–3/6 systolic ejection mumur in the posterior left infrascapular area).

Diagnosis is made on the basis of an abnormal chest radiograph with a three-sign (i.e., proximal aorta, coarctated segment with poststenotic dilatation, and indentation of the aortic knob). Arteriography delineates the abnormality.

Treatment is surgical repair or angioplasty with prophylactic β-blockade.

Renovascular Hypertension

There are two main categories of renovascular hypertension (4, 32): atherosclerosis, and fibrous disease (unilateral and bilateral). Clinical clues include abrupt onset of hypertension before age 30 or after age 55, diastolic pressure of greater than 120 mm Hg, grade 3 or 4 fundoscopic changes, triple drug failure, evidence of diffuse vascular disease, epigastric bruit, and azotemia induced by therapy with ACE inhibitors.

Noninvasive diagnostic tests include the captopril plasma renin activity test, BP, and PRA both before and 1 hour after captopril challenge (25–50 mg orally). Specific diagnostic techniques (Table 50.6) include:

Table 50.6. Screening Tests for Renovascular Hypertension

Test	Sensitivity (%)	Specificity (%)
Intravenous pyelography	~75	~85
Routine renal flow scan	80–85	~75–85
Captopril renogram[a]	93	95
PRA	50–80	~84
Captopril-stimulated PRA[b]	74	89
Duplex ultrasonography	84	97
Intravenous digital subtraction angiography	88	90

Adapted with permission from Mann SJ, Pickering TG. Detection of renovascular hypertension. State of the art:1992 Ann Intern Med 1992;117: 845–853.
PRA, plasma renin activity.
[a] Give 50 mg crushed captopril by mouth and DTPA 1 hour later. A positive test is: peak activity ≥ 11 minutes and glomerular filtration rate < 1.5.
[b] Measure PRA, administer 50 mg of captopril, and recheck PRA after 1 hour. A positive test is an increase renin by 10 μg/L per hour and increase in renin by 150%, or 400% if for a baseline < 3 μg/L per hour.

- Captopril renography, either [^{99m}TC]-DTPA, ^{99m}Tc-[MAG3], or [^{131}I]-OIH (orthoiodohippurate) with captopril (25–50 mg). A decrease in function or perfusion is observed on these nuclear scans if significant stenosis is present.
- Duplex Doppler ultrasonography (renal-aortic flow velocity ratio, $\geq$3.5).
- Angiography, which is the "gold standard."
- Digital subtraction angiography (DSA), which uses varying quantities of contrast by route (i.e., more for intra-aortic, less for intravenous). Results are not consistent in obese patients
- Renal vein renin lateralization is $\geq$1.5 times the contralateral renin vein value.

Intervention with surgery or percutaneous transluminal angioplasty (PTCA) with or without stent is reserved for patients whose BP is not adequately controlled by pharmacologic treatment (33). Approximately 30% of patients with fibrous dysplasia have branch-vessel disease, which increases the difficulty of PTCA and often necessitates surgical renal revascularization.

HYPERTENSIVE TREATMENT APPROACHES

Nonpharmacologic Therapy

Nonpharmacologic therapy is achieved by lifestyle modifications, including (34):

- Dietary sodium restriction ($\leq$5 g of NaCl per day)
- Weight reduction
- Aerobic exercise

Insulin resistance, as manifested by increased levels of plasma insulin, triglycerides, LDL, and increased waist-to-hip ratio (i.e., insulin resistance), warrants nonpharmacologic intervention coupled with pharmacologic treatment. Calcium supplementation may be helpful in decreasing BP during pregnancy and in avoiding toxemia. Moderate salt restriction (100 mmol/day, or approximately 2.4 g) should be tried in all individuals with elevated BP. Individual variation in response to salt restriction cannot be predicted. An adequate dietary intake of magnesium should be maintained, but at present, omega-3 fatty acids cannot be recommended to lower BP.

Pharmacologic Therapy

Drug therapy initially is indicated in addition to lifestyle modifications when the diastolic BP is consistently greater than 100 mm Hg or the systolic BP is greater than 160 mm Hg (stage 2–4) if the lifestyle modifications fail to bring the diastolic BP to less than 90 mm Hg within 3 to 6 months. In patients without target organ disease or a family history of cardiovascular and cerebrovascular events, it is unclear whether those with a diastolic BP of 90 to 95 mm Hg or a systolic BP of 140 to 150 mm Hg should be treated. Most authors agree that drug therapy is indicated for patients with

Table 50.7. Indications for Drug Treatment for Hypertension

Classification	Target Organ Damage[a]		Other Major Risk Factors	
	+	−	+	−
High normal[b]	No	No	No	No
Stage 1[c]	Yes[d]	?	Yes[d]	?
Stages 2–4[e]	Yes	Yes	Yes	Yes

Adapted with permission from Gifford RW Jr. What's new in treatment of hypertension? Cleve Clin J Med 1997;64:143–150.
[a] Cardiac, cerebrovascular, peripheral vascular, renal, retinopathy.
[b] Systolic BP, 130–139 mm Hg; Diastolic BP, 85–89 mm Hg.
[c] Systolic BP, 140–150 mm Hg; Diastolic BP, 90–95 mm Hg.
[d] After trial of lifestyle modification.
[e] Systolic BP, >160 mm Hg; Diastolic BP, >100 mm Hg.

a diastolic BP of 90 to 95 mm Hg if target organ damage exists or there is a family history of significant vascular events (Table 50.7) (35). The benefits of treating isolated systolic hypertension have not been demonstrated in a controlled trial, yet increases in pulse pressure (i.e., systolic BP—diastolic BP), which commonly occur in patients with isolated systolic hypertension, may adversely affect coronary filling, increase myocardial work, and produce an increased risk for cardiovascular events. Potentially, the wider the pulse pressure, the greater the enthusiasm for treatment.

The major antihypertensive agents are listed in Table 50.8. The JNC-V suggested that in patients without contraindications to diuretics and β-blockers and without indications for specific alternative drugs, diuretics or β-blockers should be the preferred initial therapy, because they have been shown in large, randomized, prospective trials to reduce cardiovascular morbidity and mortality. Other drug classes have not undergone this level of scrutiny. Seemingly lower doses of diuretics (i.e., 12.5–25.0 mg of chlorthalidone hydrochlorothiazide) and use of potassium-sparing diuretics have decreased the metabolic concerns and risks for hypokalemic cardiovascular events (36). Several new pharmacologic agents (i.e., angiotensin II type AT-1 receptor blockers, calcium antagonists, T-channel blockers, and so on) have been approved by the U.S. Food and Drug Administration (FDA) and, most likely, will gain increasing application over the next several years. Specific drug classes demonstrated to be more effective in certain clinical settings are shown in Table 50.9.

Several novel approaches to consistent reduction of BP are being pursued (37). These newer antihypertensive drug categories now under development are listed in Table 50.10. Neutral endopeptidase inhibitors prevent degradation of atrial natriuretic peptide, thus resulting in natruresis and vasodilation. Renin inhibitors block the action of renin on angiotensinogen, thus preventing formation of angiotensin 1. Endothelin inhibitors potentially block the vasoconstrictor action of endothelin at its specific receptor site, and potassium

Table 50.8.   Antihypertensive Agents

Drug Category	*Clinical Indications*	*Comments*
Neuroeffector adrenergic inhibitors		
Guanadrel sulfate (Hylorel), guanethidine (Ismelin), rauwolfia alkaloids (generic), reserpine (generic)	Alternate agent in limited situations	Can cause orthostatic hypotension Contraindicated in pregnancy, depression, and patients with diabetic autonomic neuropathy Pseudotolerance
Direct vasodilators		
Hydralazine (Apresoline), minoxidil (Loniten)	Eclampsia (hydralazine) Severe hypertension (minoxidil)	''Lupus syndrome'' with hydralazine
Calcium antagonists		
Benzothiazepine derivative: diltiazem (cardizem SR, Cardizem CD, Dilacor, Tiazac)	Elderly patient Angina pectoris and hypertension	Avoid in heart failure with systolic dysfunction Can increase levels of cyclosporine Can worsen esophageal reflux Can cause gingival hypertrophy
Diphenylalkylamine derivative: verapamil (Calan, Isoptin, Calan SR, Isoptin SR, Verelan, Covera HS)		
Dihydropyridines: amlodipine (Norvasc), felodipine (Plendil), isradipine (Dynacirc), nicardipine (Cardene, Cardene XL), nifedipine (Procardia XL, Adalat CC), nisoldipine (Sular)		Short-acting preparations of nifedipine associated with an increased risk of myocardial infarction and cancer Avoid nondihydropyridines in Wolff-Parkinson-White syndrome, sick sinus syndrome, more than first-degree block
T-type calcium channel ion influx inhibitor		
Mibefradil dihydrochloride (Posicor)	Chronic stable angina pectoris	Contraindicated with sick sinus syndrome
ACE inhibitors		
Benazepril (Lotensin), captopril (Capoten), enalapril (Vasotec), fosinopril (Monopril), lisinopril (Zestril, Prinivil), moexipril (Univasc), quinapril (Accupril), ramipril (Altace), trandolapril (Mavik)	Congestive heart failure due to systolic dysfunction Type I diabetes mellitus with nephropathy	Contraindicated in pregnancy Can cause reversible acute renal failure in patients with bilateral renal artery stenosis or unilateral disease in a solitary kidney May cause significant hypotension with high renin or dehydration Hyperkalemia with renal failure, potassium sparing diuretics or NSAIDs Can cause angioedema (rare)
Angiotensin II receptor (type AT_1) antagonist		
Losartan (Cozaar)	Congestive heart failure due to systolic dysfunction	May cause less cough than ACE inhibitors, otherwise the same side effects as ACE inhibitors.

(continued)

Table 50.8. *(continued)*

Drug Category	*Clinical Indications*	*Comments*
Thiazide/related diuretics Bendroflumethazide (Naturetin), chlorothiazide (Diuril), chlorthalidone (Hygroton, Thalitone), hydrochlorothiazide (Hydro-DIURIL, Esidrix, Oretic), hydroflumethiazide (Diucardin), indapamide (Lozol) methylclothiazide (Enduron), metolazone (Zaroxolyn), polythiazide (Renese), trichlormethiazide (Naqua)	Patients with uncomplicated hypertension unless contraindicated: Black Obese Congestive heart failure Resistant BP on two nondiuretic drugs	Avoid in uncontrolled gout, asymmetric septal hypertrophy, preeclampsia, eclampsia Ineffective with GFR <20 mL/min Decreases urinary calcium May increase lithium levels
Loop diuretics Bumetanide (Bumex), ethacrynic acid (Edecrin), furosemide (Lasix), torsemide (Demadex)	Effective when GFR <30 mL/min Resistant high BP with edema despite thiazide	Increases urinary calcium excretion Except for torsemide (Demadex), administer b.i.d. for BP control
Potassium-sparing diuretics Amiloride (Midamor), spironolactone (Aldactone), triamterene (Dyrenium), hydrochlorothiazide and triamterine (Maxzide)	Hypokalemia (hyperaldo, nonaldo)	Avoid in chronic renal failure Hyperkalemia with ACE inhibitors, potassium supplements, angiotensin II (type AT_1) receptor blockers Triamterene may result in renal calculi
α_1-Adrenergic-blocking agents Nonselective Phentolamine (Regitine), phenoxybenzamine (Dibenzyline)	Nonselective agents used in patients with pheochromocytoma	Orthostatic hypotension, "first-dose" syncope
Selective Prazosin (Minipres), terazosin (Hytrin), doxazosin (Cardura)	Hypertension and benign prostatic hypertrophy Low HDL	"Selective" agents may relieve prostate symptoms, "first-dose" syncope
Centrally acting α_2-adrenergic agonists Clonidine (Catapres), clonidine TTS (Catapres TTS patch), guanabenz (Wytensin), guanafacine (Tenex), methyldopa (Aldomet)	Elderly patients Preeclampsia (Aldomet) In conjunction with other agents	Rebound hypertension may occur with abrupt withdrawal Methyldopa (Aldomet) interferes with urinary catecholamine levels Dry mouth Orthostatic hypotension
β-Adrenergic-blocking agents Cardioselective with ISA Acebutolol (Sectral)	Agents of choice in patients with uncomplicated hypertension Hyperadrenergic, hyperkinetic circulation	Avoid in asthma, COPD, heartblock Avoid abrupt discontinuation
Cardioselective without ISA Atenolol (Tenormin), betaxolol (Kerlone), bisoprolol (Zebeta), esmolol (Brevibloc) metoprolol (Lopressor, Toprol XL)		Use *non-ISA, non-α-blocking agents:* Cardioprotective Status post–myocardial infarction Angina Idiopathic hypertrophic subacute stenosis

Table 50.8. *(continued)*

Drug Category	Clinical Indications	Comments
Noncardioselective without ISA		
Noncardioselective with ISA		
Carteolol (Cartol), penbutolol (Levatol), dindolol (Vishen)		*Do not use* in cases of greater than first-degree block, sick sinus syndrome, or acute left ventricular failure
Labetalol (Normodyne, Trandate), nadolol, propranolol (Inderal and Inederal LA), timolol (Blocadren)		Labetalol can be given intravenously, conversion to oral may have different pharmacologic effect versus intravenous

Adapted with permission from Gifford RW Jr. Treatment of patients with systemic arterial hypertension. In: Hurst's the heart. 9th ed. New York: McGraw Hill, 1997.

COPD, chronic obstructive pulmonary disease; *GFR*, glomerular filtration rate; *HDL*, high-density lipoprotein; *ISA*, intrinsic sympathomimetic activity; *NSAIDs*, nonsteroidal anti-inflammatory drugs.

Table 50.9. Matching Antihypertensive Agents to Clinical Situations

Clinical Setting	Preferred Antihypertensive Agent(s)
Congestive heart failure (systolic dysfunction) (53)	ACE inhibitors (67)
Type I diabetes mellitus	ACE inhibitors (26, 68–70)
Postinfarction (71)	Non-ISA β-blockers[a]
Atrial fibrilization (control ventricular rate)	Non-ISA β-blocker Verapamil Diltiazem
Prostate hyperplasia (72)	α_1-Blocker
Irritable bowel with diarrhea	Long-acting verapamil

[a] For example, atenolol, betaxolol, bisoprolol, metoprolol, nadolol, propranolol, and timolol.

channel openers hypopolarize cells, thus altering calcium flux and resulting in vascular smooth muscle relaxation (38).

TREATMENT CONTROVERSIES

Safety of Short-Acting Calcium Antagonists (39)

Both Furberg et al. (40) and Psaty et al. (41) have raised concerns about the safety of short-acting antagonists (e.g., nifedipine), and the FDA has issued a warning concerning use of short-acting nifedipine. In particular, use of the 10-mg nifedipine capsule, whether orally or sublingually, to control

Table 50.10. Future Therapeutic Categories for Antihypertensive Drug Development

Imidazole receptor–preferring agents
Neutral endopeptidase inhibitors
Angiotensin II receptor blockers
Combined neutral endopeptidase inhibitors and ACE inhibitors
Renin inhibitors
Endothelin receptor antagonists
Nitric oxide sythetase inducers
Potassium-channel openers
Renomedullary vasodepressor lipid

Adapted with permission from Sullivan JM. A 1996 update on antihypertensive agents. Curr Opin Cardiol 1996;11:496–500.

severe hypertension should be avoided. Short-acting forms of nifedipine and diltiazem have never been approved for the treatment of hypertension. There are significant differences among the various calcium channel blockers and within the 1,4-dihydropyridine agents. Calcium channel blockers act at different regions of the calcium channel, and they have different tissue selectivity and different final hemodynamic effects. In addition, an increased risk of gastrointestinal hemorrhage and cancer with calcium channel blockade deserves further study (42, 43). No increase in coronary risks among patients on long-acting formulations has been reported.

Medication-Specific Left Ventricular Hypertrophy Effect

Whether drug-induced regression can improve the prognosis of hypertensive left ventricular hypertrophy independent of the antihypertensive effect remains unclear. Experimental studies have demonstrated normalization of hypertensive myocardium and coronary remodeling with ACE inhibitors and calcium antagonists (44–46). ACE inhibitors may be the most effective drug therapy in reducing left ventricular hypertrophy, but a clinical correlate warrants further definition.

Intracranial Pathology and Hypertension

Treatment of patients with hypertension and intracranial pathology warrants special consideration as to the effect of drugs on cerebral blood flow, autoregulation, and intracranial pressure (47). Both α_1- and β_1-blockade decreases arterial BP, with little effect on intracranial pressure. Direct vasodilators and calcium channel blockers are limited by cerebrovascular dilatation and increased intracranial pressure. ACE inhibitors also may increase intracranial pressure. For most hypertensive emergencies, nitroprusside remains the drug of choice. Newer agents hopefully will produce fewer effects on intracranial hemodynamics.

Microalbuminuria and Target BP Level

The usefulness of microalbuminuria as a strong predictor of mortality in patients with type 2 diabetes has undergone significant discussion, though it has been correlated in patients with benign essential hypertension (48–50). Whether microalbuminuria may define patients who warrant significantly lower decreases in their BP during therapy than needed in the general population remains unanswered.

Endothelial Factors and Hypertension

Endothelium-derived vasoactive factors may play an important role in hypertension. The role of nitric oxide (NO) in hypertension seems to vary depending on the disease stage and the model studied (51). NO-cyclic guanosine monophosphate systems cause smooth muscle relaxation in vessels. In human hypertension, pharmacologic experiments have demonstrated an impaired NO vasodilatory mechanism that responds to BP elevations. Endothelins are potent vasoconstrictor polypeptides and are produced by endothelial cells. Endothelin-1 causes profound vasoconstriction by activation of endothelin$_A$ and endothelin$_B$ receptors. Their levels are normal in most patients with hypertension, but local activity may be defective.

"J-Curve" and Mortality (52)

Several reports suggest that a decrease in diastolic BP to less than 85 to 90 mm Hg may be associated with a paradoxic increase in coronary mortality among patients with evidence of ischemic heart disease (53). The J-curve is a retrospective observation in nonrandomized clinical trials. It remains unclear whether the J-curve truly exists and, if so, if it applies only to diastolic or also to systolic BP.

Table 50.11. Trough/Peak Characteristics and Drug Effectiveness

Optimal BP control equals 24-hour effectiveness
Agents should maintain effect beyond dosing interval
BP load[a] determines hypertensive heart disease
High trough-to-peak ratio[b] is associated with low BP load
Drug classes, specific agents, and concentrations have varying trough-to-peak ratios

[a] Percentage of BP > 140/90 mm Hg while awake.
[b] Percentage of BP > 120/80 mm Hg while asleep.

Table 50.12. Individual Therapeutic Trough-to-Peak Ratios for Diastolic BP Calculated from 24-Hour BP Monitoring

Drug	Dosage Range (mg)	Trough-to-Peak (%)
Captopril	12.5–100 b.i.d.	0–40
Benazepril	5–40 q.i.d.	10–40
Perindopril	4–8 q.i.d.	30
Quinapril	20–40 q.i.d.	30–40
Ramipril	10–40 q.i.d.	40–50
Lisinopril	10–80 q.i.d.	40–70[a]
Enalapril	5–20 q.i.d.	50–80[a]
Trandolapril	2 q.i.d.	80–100[a]

Adapted with permission from Zannad F. Trandolapril: how does it differ from other angiotensin converting enzyme inhibitors? Drugs 1993;46(Suppl 2): 172–182.
[a] Agents with ratios < 50% may provide a better 24-hour BP profile.

Trough-to-Peak Ratio and Drug Dosing

Chronic pressure overload can induce myocardial and vascular damage (18, 54–56). BP load refers to the percent of BP measurements exceeding 140/90 mm Hg while awake and 120/80 mm Hg while asleep. As Table 50.11 indicates, newer drugs should be developed to provide more consistent control of BP, and older drugs should be classified according to their 24-hour level of control. Drugs with a low trough-to-peak ratio should have an increased BP load, which can be calculated using the integrated area under the BP curve. Antihypertensive medication should have a dosing interval essentially constant with the trough-to-peak ratio (Table 50.12).

COMPLICATIONS

HYPERTENSIVE EMERGENCIES

Hypertensive encephalopathy and accelerated malignant hypertension most commonly occur in individuals with essential hypertension (57, 58). The acceleration in BP elevation may occur with cessation of medications, during pregnancy, or in patients taking monamine oxidase inhibitors who ingest tyramine-containing foods (e.g., red wine, ripened cheese). Both cocaine and phenopranolamine also cause accelerated hypertension. Patients presenting with abnormal renal function may experience a temporary worsening with improved BP control.

Several conditions may mimic a hypertensive emergency and should be considered at initial presentation. These include central nervous system abnormalities, subarachnoid hemorrhage, head injury, brain tumor, postictal seizure, lupus encephalitis, nonprescribed drug ingestion, hypercalcemia, and intermittent porphyria. The goal of initial treatment is to achieve a *partial* reduction in diastolic BP, to a safer, noncritical level but not to the point of normalcy. Hypertensive crises are classified as either urgencies or emergencies. Urgent BP reduction consists of lowering the BP over several to 24 hours rather than an immediate need for decrease to a safe zone; 160 to 170/100 to 110 mm Hg is a reasonable reduction with vasodilating drugs and adrenergic inhibitors.

RESISTANT HYPERTENSION

Patients who have taken two or more medications for longer than 6 months without achieving a reduction in diastolic or systolic BP of 10% or more, or the target reduction, or both can be classified as having resistant hypertension (59, 60). Patients with resistant hypertension who are compliant on adequate treatment regimens comprise approximately 1 to 3% of the hypertensive population; this percentage increases dramatically if noncompliance and suboptimal therapy are responsible for "apparent" resistance. Of the 436 patients treated at the Yale Hypertension Clinic, 91 (21%) had resistant hypertension, which most commonly was attributable to suboptimal treatment (Fig. 50.3) (61). There are several reasons for suboptimal response to therapy, including:

- Nonadherence
- Drug doses either too small or in inappropriate combinations

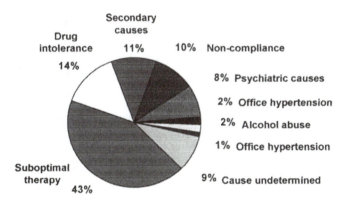

Figure 50.3. Etiologies for refractory hypertension. (Adapted with permission from Yakovlevitch M, Black HR. Resistant hypertension in a tertiary care clinic. Arch Intern Med 1991;151: 1786–1792.)

Table 50.13. Hemodynamic Workup in Resistant Hypertension

Medication analysis
Blood volume
 Plasma volume
 Hematocrit (%)
Systemic hemodynamics
 BP supine, head-up tilt
 Cardiac index, ejection fraction
 Distribution blood volume
 Left ventricular relaxation/ejection rate (%)

- Rapid inactivation
- Volume overload (e.g., inadequate diuretic therapy, increased sodium intake, >150 mEq per 24-hour urine collection)
- Progressive renal insufficiency
- Associated conditions (e.g., chronic renal failure, excess alcohol intake < 30 mL/day, increasing obesity, and so on)
- Secondary hypertension

In this study, 7% demonstrated renovascular disease, and 5% were diagnosed with hyperaldosteronism.

For patients with continued difficulty in hypertension control in whom no secondary cause is identified, further hemodynamic evaluation is warranted (Table 50.13). This approach examines the physiologic basis for hypertension, so that antihypertensive agents can be matched to the inciting mechanism.

Medications that may interfere with drug effectiveness include nonsteroidal anti-inflammatory drugs, oral contraceptives, cocaine, diet pills (i.e., sympathomimetics), nasal sprays, phenylpropanolamine, licorice, psychotropic agents, and topical fluorinated steroids.

HYPERTENSION AND PREGNANCY

Hypertension complicates between 5 and 10% of all pregnancies. Preeclampsia is the leading cause of maternal and fetal morbidity (62–64). Several different types of hypertension can occur during pregnancy, including:

- Preeclampsia, eclampsia
- Chronic hypertension
- Chronic hypertension with preeclampsia
- Hypertension

In addition, hypertension during pregnancy occurs more frequently in young patients, in those with multiple pregnancies or a hydatidocele, or in those with diabetes mellitus.

Mean BP decreases occur early during pregnancy (i.e., 10–15 mm Hg or less). A decrease in total peripheral resistance is a main feature of this decrease in BP during pregnancy. Major reasons for lowering of the total peripheral resistance are vasodilatory effects of prostaglandins, the vascular refractoriness to thromboxane A_2, and increase in ureteral placental blood flow.

Hypertension during pregnancy rapidly disappears after the pregnancy is complete, but the incidence of hypertension increases as term approaches. The syndrome has a hereditary tendency. This type of hypertension occurs almost exclusively during the first pregnancy, and nulliparous females are six to eight times more susceptible than multiparous females.

Hypertension during pregnancy should be treated when the diastolic BP is greater than 105 mm Hg. The most commonly used medications include methyldopa and hydralazine. β-Blockers have been used as well. Calcium channel blockers are under investigation, but ACE inhibitors are contraindicated.

Preeclampsia is characterized by increasing urinary protein excretion, edema, abnormal liver function tests, coagulation abnormalities, and thrombocytopenia. Preeclampsia may progress to eclampsia (e.g., severe headache, hyperreflexia, epigastric pain, visual disturbances).

The syndrome of hemolysis, elevated liver enzymes, and low platelet counts (i.e., thrombocytopenia), or HELLP syndrome, is another disorder in pregnancy, and it constitutes a medical emergency. Overall, patients deteriorate very rapidly. Treatment is termination of the pregnancy, even if hypertension and renal dysfunction are minimal.

Calcium supplementation is currently under evaluation as a preventive strategy for preeclampsia. Uteroplacental blood flow is reduced in preeclampsia, and subsequent short-term lowering of BP may adversely affect placental profusion further. Magnesium sulfate may perpetuate the effects of calcium channel blockade. Diuretics should be avoided.

Women with chronic hypertension have an increased risk of developing superimposed preeclampsia, which increases fetal morbidity and mortality. Excessive reductions in BP should be avoided. β-Blockers given early during therapy may be associated with low-birth-weight babies. ACE inhibitors also may cause acute renal failure in neonates.

REFERENCES

1. Burt VL, Whelton P, Roccella EJ, et al. Prevalence of hypertension in the U.S. adult population. Results from the Third National Health and Nutrition Examination Survey, 1988–1991. Hypertension 1995;25:305–313.

2. Gifford RW Jr. What's new in treatment of hypertension? Cleve Clin J Med 1997;64:143–150.

3. The Joint National Committee. The fifth report of the Joint National Committee on detection, evaluation, and treatment of high blood pressure (JNCV). Arch Intern Med 1993;153:154–183.

4. National High Blood Pressure Education Program (NHBPEP) Working Group. 1995 update of the working group reports on chronic renal failure and renovascular hypertension. Arch Intern Med 1996;156:1938–1947.

5. Dollery C. Hypertension trial results: consensus and conflicts. J Hum Hypertens 1995;9:403–408.

6. Alderman MH. Which antihypertensive drugs first—and why! JAMA 1992;267:2786–2787.

7. Kannel WB. Cardioprotection and antihypertensive therapy: the key importance of addressing the associated coronary risk factors (the Framingham experience). Am J Cardiol 1996;77(Suppl):6B–11B.

8. Cziraky MJ, Mehra IV, Wilson MD, et al. Current issues in treating the hypertensive patient with diabetes: focus on diabetic nephropathy. Ann Pharmacother 1996;30:791–801.

9. Rett K, Wicklmayr M, Standl E. Hypertension in the non-insulin-dependent diabetes mellitus syndrome: a critical review of therapeutic intervention. J Hypertens 1995;13(Suppl):S81–S85.

10. Skyler JS, Marks JB, Schneiderman N. Hypertension in patients with diabetes mellitus. Am J Hypertens 1995;8(Suppl):100S–105S.

11. Kaplan NM. Hypertension in the elderly. Ann Med Rev 1995;46:27–35.

12. LaPalio LR. Hypertension in the elderly. Am Fam Phys 1995;52:1161–1165.

13. Ramirez AG. Hypertension in Hispanic Americans: overview of the population. Pub Health Rep 1996;111(Suppl 2):25–26.

14. Neaton JD, Grimm RH Jr, Prineas RJ, et al. Treatment of Mild Hypertension Study. Final results. JAMA 1993;270:713–724.

15. Collins R, Peto R, MacMahon S, et al. Blood pressure, stroke, and coronary heart disease. Part 2. Short-term reductions in blood pressure: overview of randomised drug trials in their epidemiological context. Lancet 1990;335:827–838.

16. Lackland DT, Keil JE. Epidemiology of hypertension in African Americans. Semin Nephrol 1996;16:63–70.

17. Saunders E. Hypertension in minorities: blacks. Am J Hypertens 1995;8(Suppl):115S–119S.

18. Weidmann P, Bohlen L, de Courten M. Insulin resistance and hyperinsulinemia in hypertension. J Hypertens 1995;13(Suppl):S65–S72.

19. Haffner SM, Miettinen H, Gaskill SP, et al. Metabolic precursors of hypertension. The San Antonio Heart Study. Arch Intern Med 1996;156:1994–2001.

20. Prasad N, MacFadyen RJ, MacDonald TM. Ambulatory blood pressure monitoring in hypertension. Q J Med 1996;89:95–102.

21. Pickering T. Recommendations for the use of home (self) and ambulatory blood pressure monitoring. American Society of Hypertension Ad Hoc Panel. Am J Hypertens 1996;9:1–11.

22. Appel LJ, Stason WB. Ambulatory blood pressure monitoring and blood pressure self-measurement in the diagnosis and management of hypertension. Ann Intern Med 1993;118:867–882.

23. Gomez-Sanchez CE, Gomez-Sanchez EP, Yamakita N. Endocrine causes of hypertension. Semin Nephrol 1995; 15:106–115.

24. Mantero F, Palermo M, Petrelli MD, et al. Apparent mineralocorticoid excess: type I and type II. Steroids 1996; 61:193–196.

25. Whitworth JA, Brown MA, Kelly JJ, et al. Mechanisms of cortisol-induced hypertension in humans. Steroids 1995;60:76–80.

26. Bravo EL, Tarazi RC, Dustan HP, et al. The changing clinical spectrum of primary aldosteronism. Am J Med 1983;74:641–51.

27. Irony I, Kater CE, Biglieri EG, et al. Correctable subsets of primary aldosteronism. Primary adrenal hyperplasia and renin responsive adenoma. Am J Hypertens 1990;3: 576–82.

28. Steigerwalt SP. Unraveling the causes of hypertension and hypokalemia. Hosp Pract 1974;30:67–71.

29. Bravo EL. Primary aldosteronism. Issues in diagnosis and management. Endocrinol Metab Clin North Am 1994;23: 271–283.

30. Bravo EL. Evolving concepts in the pathophysiology, diagnoses, and treatment of pheochromocytoma. Endocrin Rev 1994;15:356–358.

31. Bravo EL, Gifford RW, Jr. Current concepts. Pheochromocytoma: diagnosis, localization and management. N Engl J Med 1984;311:1298–1303.

32. Jensen G. Renovascular hypertension. New diagnostic and therapeutic procedures. Scand J Urol Nephrol Suppl 1995;170:1–78.

33. Salvetti A, Arzilli F, Parrucci M, et al. Renal artery stenosis in the nineties: screening dilemmas. Contrib Nephrol 1996;119:45–53.

34. Gavras H, Gavras I. Modern approaches to initiating antihypertensive therapy. Cardiol Clin North Am 1995;13: 593–598.

35. Barron HV, Amidon TM. Options in antihypertensive drug therapy. Help in choosing from among the many agents. Postgrad Med 1996;100:89–94.

36. Hoes AW, Grobbee DE. Diuretics and risk of sudden death in hypertension—evidence and potential implications. Clin Exp Med 1996;18:523–535.

37. Reid JL. New therapeutic agents for hypertension. Br J Clin Pharmacol 1996;42:37–41.

38. Sullivan JM. A 1996 update on antihypertensive agents. Curr Opin Cardiol 1996;11:496–500.

39. Grossman E, Messerli FH, Grodzicki T, et al. Should a moratorium be placed on sublingual nifedipine capsules given for hypertensive emergencies and pseudoemergencies? JAMA 1996;276:1328–1331.

40. Furberg CD, Psaty BM, Meyer JV. Nifedipine. Dose-related increase in mortality in patients with coronary heart disease. Circulation 1995;92:1326–1331.

41. Psaty BM, Heckbert SR, Koepsell TD, et al. The risk of myocardial infarction associated with antihypertensive drug therapies. JAMA 1995;274:620–625.

42. Pahor M, Guralnik JM, Furberg CD, et al. Risk of gastrointestinal haemorrhage with calcium antagonists in hypertensive persons over 67 years old. Lancet 1996;347: 1061–1065.

43. Pahor M, Guralnik JM, Salive ME, et al. Do calcium channel blockers increase the risk of cancer? Am J Hypertens 1996;9:695–699.

44. Otterstad JE, Smiseth O, Kjeldsen SE. Hypertensive left ventricular hypertrophy: pathophysiology, assessment and treatment. Blood Press 1996;5:5–15.

45. Cruickshank JM, Lewis J, Moore V, et al. Reversibility of left ventricular hypertrophy by differing types of antihypertensive therapy. J Hum Hypertens 1992;6:85–90.

46. Dahlof B, Pennert K, Hansson L. Reversal of left ventricular hypertrophy in hypertensive patients. A meta-analysis of 109 treatment studies. Am J Hypertension 1992;5: 95–110.

47. Tietjen CS, Hurn PD, Ulatowski JA, et al. Treatment modalities for hypertensive patients with intracranial pathology: options and risks. Crit Care Med 1996;24:311–322.

48. Bigazzi R, Bianchi S. Microalbuminuria as a marker of cardiovascular and renal disease in essential hypertension. Nephrol Dial Transplant 1995;10(Suppl 6):10–14.

49. Weir MR. Differing effects of antihypertensive agents on urinary albumin excretion. Am J Nephrol 1996;16: 237–245.

50. Bar J, Hod M, Erman A, et al. Microalbuminuria: prognostic and therapeutic implications in diabetic and hypertensive pregnancy. Diabetes Med 1995;12:649–656.

51. Haynes WG. Endothelins as regulators of vascular tone in man. Clin Sci 1995;88:509–517.

52. Farnett L, Mulrow CD, Linn WD, et al. The J-curve phenomenon and the treatment of hypertension. Is there a point beyond which pressure reduction is dangerous? JAMA 1991;265:489–495.

53. ACC/AHA Task Force on Practice Guidelines. ACC/AHA guidelines for the evaluation and management of heart failure. Report of the American College of Cardiology/American Heart Association Task Force on Practice Guidelines. Circulation 1995;92:2764–2784.

54. Morgan T, Anderson A. How important is 24-hour control of blood pressure? Drug Safety 1996;15:243–248.

55. Elliott HL, Meredith PA. Trough:peak ratio: clinically useful or practically irrelevant? J Hypertens 1995;13: 279–283.

56. White WB. Relevance of the trough-to-peak ratio to the 24 h blood pressure load. Am J Hypertension 1996; 9(Suppl):91S–96S,108S.

57. Murphy C. Hypertensive emergencies. Emerg Med Clin North Am 1995;13:973–1007.

58. Abdelwahab W, Frishman W, Landau A. Management of hypertensive urgencies and emergencies. J Clin Pharmacol 1995;35:747–762.

59. Kaplan NM. Southwestern Internal Medicine Conference: difficult-to-treat hypertension. Am J Med Sci 1995; 309:339–346.

60. McAlister FA, Lewanczuk RZ, Teo KK. Resistant hypertension: an overview. Can J Cardiol 1996;12:822–828.

61. Yakovlevitch M, Black HR. Resistant hypertension in a tertiary care clinic. Arch Intern Med 1991;151:1786–1792.

62. Gallery ED. Hypertension in pregnancy. Practical management recommendations. Drugs 1995;49:555–562.

63. Zamorski MA, Green LA. Preeclampsia and hypertensive disorders of pregnancy. Am Fam Phys 1996;53:1595–1610.

64. Walker JJ. Care of the patient with severe pregnancy induced hypertension. Eur J Obstet Gynecol Reprod Biol 1996;65:127–135.

65. Mann SJ, Pickering TG. Detection of renovascular hypertension. State of the art: 1992. Ann Intern Med 1992;117:845–853.

66. Gifford RW Jr. Treatment of patients with systemic arterial hypertension. In: Hurst's the heart. 9th ed. New York: McGraw-Hill, 1997.

67. Leonetti G, Cuspidi C. Choosing the right ACE inhibitor. A guide to selection. Drugs 1995;49:516–535.

68. Consensus Development Conference Panel. CONSENSUS PANEL Statement on the treatment of hypertension in diabetes. Diabetes Care 1993;16:1394–1401.

69. O'Hare JP. Practical problems in the management of hypertension in the diabetic patient. J Diabetes Complication 1996;10:146–148.

70. Leese GP, Savage MW, Chattington PD, et al. The diabetic patient with hypertension. Postgrad Med J 1996;72:263–268.

71. Meredith PA. Implications of the links between hypertension and myocardial infarction for choice of drug therapy in patients with hypertension. Am Heart J 1996;132:222–228.

72. Kaplan SA, Kaplan NM. Alpha-blockade: monotherapy for hypertension and benign prostatic hyperplasia. Urology 1996;48:541–550.

73. Zannad F. Trandolapril: how does it differ from other angiotensin converting enzyme inhibitors? Drugs 1993; 46(Suppl 2):172–182.

Critical Fluid and Electrolytic Abnormalities in Clinical Practice

Marc A. Pohl

SODIUM

There are approximately 3500 mEq of sodium in the body of a 70-kg adult male. About one-fifth of this total body sodium is chemically bound in bone and thought to be metabolically unavailable for exchange among the body fluid compartments. The remainder of the total body sodium, about 40 mEq/kg of body weight, is biologically active and comes into equilibrium with radioactive sodium within 24 hours. Most of the total body exchangeable sodium resides in the extracellular fluid compartment (about 2000 mEq) at a concentration of approximately 135–145 mEq/L. Thus, sodium is principally a cation of the extracellular fluid compartment.

There is only a small amount of sodium within cells, i.e., allocated to the intracellular fluid volume compartment, approximately 10 mEq/kg of intracellular water (in muscle). It appears that the great discrepancy between the extracellular fluid volume sodium concentration (135–145 mEq/L) and the intracellular fluid volume sodium concentration (10 mEq/L) does not result from an absolute impermeability of cell membranes to sodium. Rather, sodium is continuously diffusing into cells from the extracellular fluids and is continuously being extruded to maintain its low intracellular concentration. This extrusion of sodium ions from within the cells to the extracellular fluid volume compartment appears to be the major transport activity of cells. Since this process requires that sodium be transported out of the cell against both an electrical and a chemical concentration gradient, work must be performed in maintaining the external (ECF) position of sodium. The energy for this process derives from the metabolism within cells, but it also is important in preserving cell volume. An impaired cellular metabolism appears to disrupt the active extrusion of sodium from cells, allowing sodium to continually leak into the cell from the extracellular fluid and thus allows sodium to accumulate within the cells. This leads to depolarization of the cell membrane potential so that chloride also accumulates in the cell, and as a net gain of intracellular solute occurs, cellular swelling ensues. This cellular swelling may have important consequences in clinical conditions of ischemia to kidney tissue cells, heart muscle cells, and brain cells.

Since the sodium ion is the major ion in the extracellular fluid volume compartment, the extracellular fluid volume is a function of sodium content in this compartment. Thus, external sodium balance is the most important regulator of the extracellular fluid volume and hence, of the plasma volume. Deficits in total body sodium are often clinically reflected by a reduction in the extracellular fluid volume, which, if critical enough, leads to serious hemodynamic compromise. Marked excess in total body sodium content is usually manifested by an expansion of the extracellular fluid volume compartment, often resulting in congestion in the central circulation and/or edema.

SODIUM EXCESS STATES

I. Increased extracellular fluid volume with increased plasma volume
   A. Nonsuppressable afferent stimulus
      1. Primary hyperaldosteronism
   B. Renal resistance to natriuretic forces
      1. Oliguric acute renal failure
      2. Severe chronic renal failure
      3. Acute glomerulonephritis (nephritic syndrome)
II. Increased extracellular fluid volume with decreased effective (arterial) plasma volume and reduced renal blood flow
   A. Cardiac
      1. Congestive heart failure
      2. Constrictive pericarditis

Principles of Volume Regulation

A. Extracellular fluid volume is a function of sodium content and not sodium concentration.
B. Sodium balance is regulated by urinary sodium excretion.
C. Urinary sodium excretion is a function of effective intravascular plasma volume.

Loss of One Liter Saline	Type of Change	Loss of One Liter H_2O
− 150 mEq	Change in Na content	0
− 1000 mL	Change in TB H_2O	− 1000 mEq/L
0	Change in P_{osm}	+ 2.5% (7.5 mOsm/L)
− 1000 mL	Change in ECF volume	− 333 mL
− 250 mL	Change in plasma volume	− 83 mL

B. Decompensated liver diseases with venous outflow obstruction
C. Nephrotic syndrome
D. Pre-eclampsia
E. Hypothyroidism
F. Vascular
 1. Great vein obstruction
 2. Arteriovenous fistulas
G. Vasodilator drugs
H. Idiopathic edema

The normal daily nutritional sodium requirement is met by the average daily diet, and is generally in the range of 75–250 mEq/day. This variance in daily sodium intake is conditioned by dietary habit and taste in seasoning one's food. Although there is a small loss of sodium in the form of sweat and desquamated epithelium (12–20 mEq/day) in normal people, for all practical purposes the urinary sodium excretion is a reflection of the daily dietary sodium intake. Thus, there is no normal value for urinary sodium excretion since the urinary sodium excretion varies directly with the dietary intake of sodium.

Osmotic and Volume Effects with Additions of NaCl, H_2O, or Isotonic Saline

	3% NaCl	H_2O	Isotonic Saline
Plasma osmolality	↑	↓	0
Plasma Na	↑	↓	0
ECF volume	↑	↑	↑
Urine Na	↑	↑	↑
Urine osmolality	↑	↓	0
ICF volume	↓	↑	0

The serum sodium concentration is the ratio of sodium in mEq to body water in liters. Thus, the serum sodium concentration is regulated primarily by water balance and not by the total amount of sodium in the body. A low serum sodium concentration (hyponatremia) may be present in the face of a deficit in total body sodium (e.g., salt and water depletion from gastrointestinal fluid losses) or in the presence of an overabundance of total body sodium content (e.g., edematous states such as ascites and congestive heart failure).

RELATION OF PLASMA SODIUM TO PLASMA OSMOLALITY

$P_{osm} = 2 \times P_{Na} + glucose/18 + BUN/2.8$
$Effective\ P_{osm} = 2 \times P_{na}$

POTASSIUM

The body of a 70-kg male contains about 3200 mEq of potassium or approximately 45–50 mEq/kg of body weight. In the female, because of a smaller body cell mass in proportion to body weight, the normal potassium content is about 35–40 mEq/kg, or about 2300–2500 mEq of total body potassium for females. Only a small amount of potassium is present in the extracellular fluid volume compartment (50–70 mEq), and the majority of the total body potassium resides within the cells, where this intracellular potassium forms the major cation of intracellular water, at a concentration of approximately 150 mEq/L. Most of the total body potassium resides within muscle cells. Total body potassium declines with age as body cell mass diminishes. In the healthy adult, the serum potassium concentration (reflecting the concentration of potassium in the extracellular fluid volume compartment) ranges between 3.5 and 5.0 mEq/L.

The normal daily dietary potassium requirements are met by the average diet. Daily potassium intake in food is generally in the range of 40–100 mEq, almost all of which is excreted in the urine with a small component excreted in the stool. Accordingly, 24-hour urinary potassium excretion reflects the dietary potassium intake.

The plasma potassium concentration is not a reliable index for estimating total body potassium. Indeed, the serum potassium concentration may be drastically elevated in the presence of marked total body potassium deficits. Several factors affect the distribution of potassium between the intracellular and the extracellular fluid volume compartments, including extracellular fluid pH, extracellular fluid osmolality, drugs (e.g., succinylcholine), and cellular catabolic rate and/or cellular necrosis. For example, metabolic acidosis with a resulting fall in blood pH (acidemia) is commonly associated with an elevated serum potassium concentration, reflecting a redistribution of potassium from the intracellular to the extracellular fluid volume compartment, rather than an increase in total body potassium content. Conversely, metabolic alkalosis with an increase in blood pH (alkalemia) is often associated with a low serum potassium concentration, again owing to a redistribution of potassium between the extracellular and intracellular fluid volume compartments. Thus, acidosis is usually associated with hyperkalemia and alkalosis is usually associated with hypokalemia, and in neither situation is the serum potassium concentration a reflection of the body's potassium content. On the other hand, most patients with metabolic acidosis have moderate deficits of total body potassium, and patients with significant metabolic alkalosis have moderate-to-large total body potassium deficits.

Since neuromuscular excitability is determined largely by the concentration of potassium in the extracellular fluid, both hypokalemia and hyperkalemia are of critical clinical importance. Concentrations of the serum potassium greater than 7 mEq/L are extremely dangerous, and values of 10–12 mEq/L are usually fatal, the cause of death being cardiac arrhythmia or arrest. Hence, hyperkalemia of this magnitude is always a medical emergency.

Deficits in total body potassium are often observed in conjunction with a reduced serum potassium concentration (hypokalemia). The more common causes of hypokalemia with a reduction in total body potassium content include losses of potassium from the gastrointestinal tract, such as in vomiting, nasogastric suction, and diarrhea. Occasionally, a very low dietary potassium intake (e.g., anorexia nervosa) may cause significant hypokalemia. Renal losses of potassium, with consequent hypokalemia, are typically seen in patients taking diuretics, and in patients with renal tubular acidosis and mineralocorticoid excess or hyperadrenocorticism. In nearly all clinical conditions associated with hypokalemia and total body potassium deficits, the potassium replacement should be in the form of potassium chloride. This is because most of these clinical situations of hypokalemia and total body potassium deficit occur in conjunction with metabolic alkalosis and administration of chloride appears to be necessary for correction of metabolic alkalosis.

CHLORIDE

The total body chloride in man is approximately 2000 mEq for a 70-kg man or about 3 mEq/kg body weight. The figure for women is slightly less, about 27 mEq/kg. Although there is some chloride in the intracellular fluid volume compartment, most of the body chloride resides in the extracellular fluid volume compartment, at a concentration of 95–105 mEq/L. The dietary intake of chloride is usually somewhat in excess of dietary sodium and virtually the % dietary chloride intake is excreted in the urine. Changes in chloride ion concentration in the plasma generally move in the same direction as the concentration of sodium in the plasma, and any deviation from the normal sodium/chloride ratio of not quite 3/2 in the plasma is usually caused by excessive chloride loss from the gastrointestinal tract. Thus, hypochloremia (a reduced plasma chloride concentration) is usually seen in conjunction with hyponatremia (e.g., chloride loss from the gastrointestinal tract, as a result of diuretic usage with a loss of chloride in excess of sodium, and sometimes following administration of adrenal steroids). Hyperchloremia (an increased plasma chloride concentration) is usually seen in combination with hypernatremia, normal anion gap metabolic acidoses (e.g., ureterosigmoidostomies, renal tubular acidosis, diarrhea, mild-to-moderate chronic renal failure), and iatrogenically, with excessive administration of ammonium chloride or hydrochloric acid.

HYPONATREMIA

INTRODUCTION AND PHYSIOLOGY

The range of the serum sodium concentration in most clinical laboratories is from 135–145 mEq/L. The serum sodium concentration is the ratio of total body sodium in milliequivalents to total body water in liters. Hyponatremia is present when the serum sodium concentration falls below 135 mEq/L.

Although total body sodium balance determines the extracellular fluid volume, sodium balance per se does not determine the serum sodium concentration. Indeed, a decrease in the serum sodium concentration (hyponatremia) or an increase in the serum sodium concentration (hypernatremia) can exist in the face of either deficit or excess of total body sodium. The patient with cirrhosis and ascites is typically hyponatremic despite an obvious excess of total body sodium. The patient with profound diarrhea or excessive gastrointestinal fluid losses is often hyponatremic in the face of total body sodium deficit. Thus, the tonicity of the body fluids, usually indicated by the serum sodium concentration, may vary independently of the extracellular fluid volume.

Aberrations in the serum sodium concentration reflect abnormalities in water balance. For this discussion, hyponatremia indicates a ''positive water balance'' (water intake exceeds water excretion). This situation usually develops secondary to an abnormality in water excretion by the kidney. With this concept at hand, nearly all types of hyponatremia are "dilutional," rendering the term "dilutional hyponatremia" of little differential diagnostic value.

In the normal subject, hyponatremia (or hypotonicity) is prevented by the renal excretion of water excess. The physiological requirements for the elimination of excess water are:

1. Capacity to inhibit ADH secretion by the neurohypophysis in response to hypotonicity
2. Normal intrinsic renal diluting mechanisms:
   a. adequate delivery of salt containing fluid to the distal diluting sites of the nephron
   b. intact salt transport at the diluting sites in the distal nephron
   c. impermeability of the distal nephron to water in the absence of ADH

Since hyponatremia is prevented in normal subjects by the excretion of water excess, the critical question to ask in any patient with hyponatremia is: "Why is the excess water not excreted?" Further, in most situations of hyponatremia, the urinary osmolality will be relatively high (i.e., the urine is "inappropriately" concentrated), reflecting the inability of the patient to excrete free water. Thus, hyponatremia is a disorder of urinary dilution and reflects the aforementioned problem in maintaining "free water" balance.

APPROACH TO THE DIAGNOSIS OF HYPONATREMIC SYNDROMES

In evaluating the patient with hyponatremia, one initially attempts to exclude causes of factitious hyponatremia such as hyperlipidemia and hyperproteinemia. In these two conditions, although the serum or plasma sodium concentration may be factitiously low, the sodium concentration of plasma water is normal. With severe hyperlipidemia, the serum will appear lactescent; factitious hyponatremia in conjunction with severe hyperproteinemia is usually observed when the plasma protein concentration is in excess of 12–15 gm/dL. In these two conditions, the plasma sodium concentration is low, but the plasma osmolality is normal.

In patients with marked hyperglycemia or hypermannitolemia, water moves from the intracellular to the extracellular fluid compartment, resulting in a reduction of the plasma sodium concentration. In contrast to hyperlipidemia and hyperproteinemia, the low plasma sodium concentration associated with hyperglycemia or hypermannitolemia is a true reflection of the extracellular fluid sodium concentration. In these latter two conditions, the serum sodium concentration is low and the plasma osmolality may be normal or elevated. In other situations of true hyponatremia (to be discussed), the serum osmolality, as well as the serum sodium concentration, is de-

pressed. Thus, hyponatremia usually means hypotonicity of the body fluids.

After excluding factitious hyponatremia, hyperglycemia and hypermannitolemia, it is worthwhile to consider several causes of hyponatremia related to drugs such as morphine, barbiturates, anesthesia, clofibrate, cyclophosphamide, vincristine, oxytocin, and chlorpropamide. Endocrine disorders such as Addison's disease and myxedema may be associated with hyponatremia and should be excluded. Acute water intoxication in an individual with normal renal function is an extremely rare entity and would be expected to occur only when maximal renal water output (about 25 liters/day) is exceeded by an unusually large water intake (e.g., psychogenic polydipsia). Most clinical situations of acute water intoxication develop in patients with chronic renal failure and a marked reduction of glomerular filtration rate, since these patients have an inability to maximally dilute their urine and are more susceptible to developing severe hyponatremia after receiving an acute water load (e.g., hypotonic intravenous solutions, psychogenic polydipsia).

With the above clinical situations eliminated, a useful approach to the patient with hyponatremia makes use of an attempt to place the hyponatremic patient into one of three broad categories:

I. Hyponatremia with hypovolemia (inadequate circulation)
   A. With renal salt retention (urinary sodium concentration <10–15 mEq/L)
      1. G.I. losses
      2. Profuse sweating
   B. With urinary sodium wasting (urinary sodium >20 mEq/L)
      1. Adrenal insufficiency
      2. Diuretics
      3. Renal salt wasting as in chronic renal failure or distal renal tubular acidosis
II. Hyponatremia with edema (urinary sodium concentration usually <10 mEq/L)
   A. Congestive heart failure
   B. Hepatic cirrhosis with ascites
   C. Nephrotic syndrome
III. Hyponatremia without evidence of hypovolemia or edema
   A. Syndrome of inappropriate secretin of anti-diuretic hormone (SIADH)
   B. Reset osmostat
   C. Drugs (as mentioned above)

The physical examination easily differentiates patients in Category I from patients in Category II, and patients who are euvolemic (Category III) can usually be differentiated from those patients who are either hypovolemic (Category I) or edematous (Category II).

Diagnostic Approach to Hyponatremia

Step 1. Measure Serum Osmolality

Normal (280–285 mOsm)	Low (<280 mOsm)	Elevated (>285 mOsm)
Step 1A: Measure blood sugar, lipids, protein	↓	Step 1B: Measure blood sugar
Isotonic hyponatremia		*Hypertonic hyponatremia*
1. Pseudohyponatremia	↓	1. Hyperglycemia
• Hyperlipidemia		2. Hypertonic infusions
• Hyperproteinemia	↓	• Glucose
2. Isotonic infusion		• Mannitol
• Glucose	↓	• Glycine
• Mannitol		
• Glycine		

Step 2. Clinically Assess the Extracellular Fluid Volume

Tachycardia, hypotension, poor skin tugor	Edema	Normal pulse, blood pressure, skin turgor, no edema

Hypovolemic Hypotonic Hyponatremia					**Hypervolemic Hypotonic Hyponatremia**					**Isovolemic Hypotonic Hyponatremia**				
Causes	BUN/Cr	Uric Acid	Urinary Osm	Na	Causes	BUN/Cr	Uric Acid	Urinary Osm	Na	Causes	BUN/Cr	Uric Acid	Urinary Osm	Na
GI losses	↑↑/↑	↑	↑↑	↓↓	CHF	↑↑/↑	↑	↓	↓	H₂O intox.	↓/↓	↓	↑(↓)	↓
Skin losses	↑↑/↑	↑	↑↑	↓↓	Liver damage	↑↑/↑	↑	↑	↑↓	Renal failure	↑↑/↑↑	↑	ISO	↑
Lung losses	↑↑/↑	↑	↑↑	↓↓	Nephrosis	↑↑/↑ (↑↑/↑↑)	↑	↑ (ISO ↑)	↓	K⁺ loss	↑/↑(N)		↑	↑↓
3rd space	↑↑/↑	↑	↑↑	↓↓						SIADH	↓/↓	↓↓	↑	↑
Renal losses										Reset osmostat	N	N	V	V
Diuretics	↑↑/↑	↑	ISO ↑											
Renal damage	↑↑/↑↑	↑	ISO ↑											
Partial urinary tract obstruction	↑↑/↑	↑	ISO ↑(↓)											
Adrenal insufficiency	↑↑	↑	↑	↑										

Arrows indicate direction of change. Single and double arrows define the magnitude of change. ISO, isotonic; N, normal; V, variable.
Narins et al. Diagnostic strategies in disorders of fluid, electrolyte and acid-base homeostasis. Am J Med 1982, 72:496–519.

SYNDROME OF SIADH

Any discussion of hyponatremia would be incomplete without some comment about the syndrome of inappropriate secretion of ADH (SIADH). This relatively rare condition is characterized by: (1) hyponatremia with corresponding hypo-osmolality of the serum and extracellular fluids; (2) continued renal excretion of sodium; (3) absence of clinical evidence of fluid volume depletion or edema; (4) normal renal function; (5) normal adrenal function; (6) an osmolality of the urine which is greater than that appropriate for the concomitant osmolality of the plasma, or, a urine that is less than maximally dilute. Also, many patients with SIADH have a low or low/normal serum uric acid level. Disorders in which there is a syndrome probably resulting from inappropriate secretion or aberrant production of ADH (SIADH) include malignant tumors such as carcinoma of the lung, duodenum, and pancreas; CNS tu-berculosis, purulent bacterial meningitis, acute intermittent porphyria, and subdural hemorrhage; pulmonary disorders such as tuberculosis, pulmonary abscess, aspergillosis and viral and bacterial pneumonias; and finally, idiopathic SIADH. Over the last several years, the long-term ambulatory management of patients with SIADH has become easier with the use of demeclocycline in dosages from 600–900 mg daily. In addition, the patient should be warned against excessive water intake.

TREATMENT OF HYPONATREMIA

As a general principle, treat the underlying basis for the clinical disorder:

I. If there is a contracted extracellular fluid volume, give sodium and water (e.g., normal saline).

II. If an edematous state exists, restrict sodium and water.
III. If SIADH, restrict water (or treat with demeclocycline).

For patients with moderate hyponatremia (e.g., SNa<125–135 mEq/L), one should discontinue the responsible factor (e.g., drug or diuretic), and restrict fluids to allow correction of the hyponatremia through losses of excess water via the skin and mucous membranes.

Finally, if severe life-threatening hyponatremia is present (SNa,<110–115 mEq/L), and especially if obtundation, coma, or seizures exists: (1) give enough NaCl to raise the serum sodium concentration to about 120 mEq/L; (2) use isotonic saline, or 3% NaCl; (3) administer diuretic and replace urinary electrolyte losses; (4) restrict free water; (5) allow occasional use of drugs such as demeclocycline. In recent years, much discussion has been generated about the speed (rate) of correction of hyponatremia, the osmotic demyelinization syndrome, and central pontine myelinosis (CPM). Several points should be emphasized regarding the rate of correction of severe hyponatremia:

- Severe acute hyponatremia may be associated with considerable morbidity, including seizures, coma, irreversible neurologic abnormalities, and death.
- This is most likely to occur with water administration to postoperative patients or thiazide-induced hyponatremia.
- Rapid initial treatment is both safe (since the cerebral adaptation is not complete) and may be life saving.
- The plasma sodium concentration should be raised by 1.5 to 2 mEq/L per hour for the first 4 to 6 hours, but to no more than 20 mEq/L per day.
- Overly rapid correction may lead to central pontine myelinolysis, particularly if plasma sodium is raised to more than 25 mEq/L per day to above 140 mEq/L.
- Plasma sodium concentration should be raised in asymptomatic patients at a maximum rate of 0.5 mEq/L per hour.
- Too rapid correction is most likely to occur with hypertonic saline or after correction of hypovolemia with isotonic saline.

HYPERNATREMIA

Hypernatremia is defined as a serum sodium concentration greater than 145 mEq/L. Hypernatremia may exist in the presence of a decrease in total body sodium, an increase in total body sodium, or even in the face of a normal total body sodium. Again, hypernatremia tells us simply something about the ratio of total body sodium in milliequivalents to total body water in liters.

Almost always, hyponatremia is a sign of either relative or absolute water deficiency. Since normal osmoregulation closely fixes body osmolality (and hence the serum sodium concentration) between 280 and 295 (serum sodium concentration between 135–145 mEq/L), hypertonicity always

means inadequate water intake. The serum sodium concentration is rarely increased by virtue of administration of excess sodium per se unless a large amount of sodium salt is given as an exogenous solute. Hypernatremia is prevented in normal people by the thirst mechanism:

1. Slight increase in serum tonicity leads to turning on of thirst, which in turn increases water intake, voluntarily (obviously, this chain of events would not take place if the patient were comatose, did not have access to water, could not express to someone that she or he was thirsty, or if she or he were not carefully administered to by paramedical personnel).
2. If the thirst mechanism remains intact, the tonicity of the body fluids is protected, but at the expense of marked polydipsia and polyuria.

The clinical circumstances associated with hypernatremia are listed below:

- Unconscious or confused patients who receive insufficient fluids
- Osmotic diuresis
  - Uncontrolled diabetes mellitus
  - Tube feedings
- Loss of both thirst and neurohypophyseal function — rare
- Water-wasting conditions (if not enough water provided)
  - True diabetes insipidus
  - Nephrogenic diabetes insipidus
- In infants, especially given NaCl-containing fluids
- Rapid infusion of hypertonic saline — unusual
- Hyperaldosteronism or Cushing's syndrome

TREATMENT OF HYPERNATREMIA

1. Provide sufficient water
2. Reduce solute intake in order to decrease obligatory water losses
3. If diabetes insipidus:
   a) provide sufficient water
   b) chlorothiazide
   c) chlorpropamide
   d) pitressin

HYPOKALEMIA

The normal range for serum potassium concentrations in most laboratories is from 3.5–5.0 mEq/L. Thus a serum potassium concentration of <3.5 mEq/L is generally regarded as ''hypokalemia.''

I. Causes of hypokalemia
   A. Gastrointestinal losses
      1. Vomiting, nasogastric suction, intestinal fistulas
      2. Diarrhea

3. Villous adenoma
4. Laxative abuse
B. Low dietary potassium intake (anorexia nervosa)
C. Tumors
1. Primary aldosteronism
2. Cushing's syndrome
3. Insulinoma
D. Renal losses
1. Secondary aldosteronism (cirrhosis, congestive heart failure, accelerated hypertension)
2. Alkalosis — metabolic or respiratory
3. Diuretics
4. Renal tubular acidosis
E. Familial periodic paralysis
II. Symptoms of hypokalemia
A. Muscular — fatigue, hypotonicity of muscles, paralysis, apnea
B. Myocardial
1. Ectopic beats — atrial, nodal, ventricular
2. Tachycardia — atrial, nodal, ventricular
C. Mental — confusion, agitation

III. Electrocardiographic changes in hypokalemia
A. Diagnostic when the serum potassium drops below 2.5 mEq/L
1. Wide T wave, with flattening or inversion of the T wave
2. Prolonged Q-T interval
3. Prominent U wave

IV. Diagnostic considerations in establishing the cause of hypokalemia
A. Causes of Hypokalemia: ''Rule of Thumb''

Serum K (mEq/L)	*Urinary K (mEq/24 hrs)*	*Cause*
3.0	>30	Renal
3.0	<30	Extra-renal

B. Etiology of Hypokalemia
1. Cellular shift
2. Dietary deficiency
3. Nonrenal loss
4. Renal loss
C. Nonrenal potassium loss
1. Vomiting
2. GI suction
3. Biliary fistula
4. Diarrhea
5. Rectal Tumors
6. Laxatives
D. Hypokalemia without hypertension
1. Drugs — diuretics, amphotericin
2. Renal tubular acidoses, Fanconi
3. Bartter's syndrome (J.G. hyperplasia)
4. Welt's syndrome
5. Hypomagnesemia
6. Hypercalcemia
7. Periodic paralysis

E. Hypokalemia with hypertension
1. Elevated Renin*
a. Renovascular hypertension
b. Malignant hypertension
c. Renin secreting tumors
d. Birth control pills
2. Depressed Renin
a. Variable aldosterone
1) Cushing's syndrome
2) ACTH-producing tumors
b. Elevated aldosterone
1) Adenoma
2) Hyperplasia
c. Decreased aldosterone—Licorice, doca & corticosterone excess, CAH (11, 17 hydroxylase deficiency), pseudoaldosteronism

*Diuretic therapy in subjects with essential hypertension can present this way.

HYPERKALEMIA

Since the normal serum potassium concentration is generally in the range of 3.5–5.0 mEq/L, hyperkalemia is generally defined as a serum potassium concentration > 5.0 mEq/L.

I. Causes of hyperkalemia
A. Factitious
1. Laboratory error
2. Pseudo-hyperkalemia — in vitro hemolysis, thrombocytosis, leukocytosis
B. Acidosis — each decrease of 0.1 pH unit generally produces an increase in serum potassium of 0.5 mEq/L
C. Increased input
1. Exogenous — diet, drugs, (KCI, K-penicillin, infusions of potassium chloride at a rate > 50 mEq/hr), salt substitutes, low sodium diet
2. Endogenous — hemolysis, GI bleed, catabolic states
D. Inadequate distal delivery of Na (e.g., severe sodium depletion)
E. Renal failure
1. Acute renal failure
2. Chronic renal failure with oliguria
F. Impaired renin-angiotensin-aldosterone axis
1. Addison's disease
2. Enzyme deficiency
3. Primary hypoaldosteronism
4. Primary hyporeninism
5. Angiotensin deficiency or insensitivity
6. Other

G. Primary renal tubular secretory defect
   1. SLE
   2. Post renal transplantation
   3. Congenital — children of short stature
H. Inhibition of tubular secretion
   1. Aldactone, triamterene, amiloride
I. Hyperkalemic periodic paralysis
II. Electrocardiographic changes in hyperkalemia
   A. 6.5–7.5 mEq/L: tall, peaked or tented T waves with narrow-based T waves
   B. 7.5–8.0 mEq/L:
      1. Loss of P waves
      2. Widening of QRS complexes
   C. > 8.0 mEq/L:
      1. Biphasic QRS complexes
      2. Idioventricular rhythm
      3. Terminal sine wave

III. Treatment of severe or moderate hyperkalemia

Treatment of Acute Hyperkalemia

Treatment	Onset	Duration
Calcium infusion	5 minutes	1 to 2 hours
Glucose and insulin	15 to 30 mintues	1 to 4 hours
Sodium bicarbonate	15 to 60 mintues	1 to 4 hours
Hypertonic saline	30 to 60 mintues	2 to 6 hours
Cation exchange resins:		
Rectal	30 to 90 mintues	Indefinite (repeat)
Oral	2 to 12 hours	Indefinite (repeat)
Dialysis	2 to 8 hours	Indefinite (repeat)

APPROACH TO THE PATIENT WITH HYPERKALEMIA

1. History and examination exclude:
   - K administration
   - K-sparing diuretics
   - Volume contraction
   - Acute ↓ GFR
   - Obstructive uropathy
2. Measure PRA and plasma aldosterone
   - Plasma aldosterone/plasma K ratio > 2 excludes hypo-aldosteronism
3. If necessary, stimulate K secretion by increasing Na delivery with $NaHCO_3$, diamox, or Na_2SO_4
4. Hyperchloremic, hyperkalemic metabolic acidosis

DIAGNOSIS OF HYPERKALEMIC CONDITIONS

P_{aldo}/P_k <2 = True selective aldosterone deficiency

P_{aldo}/P_k >3 = Aldosterone resistance or tubular insensitivity to aldosterone

P_{aldo}/P_k >3 = Normal (no hypokalemia)

FEATURES OF ISOLATED HYPOALDOSTERONISM

1. Hyperkalemia—may be episodic
2. Hyperchloremic metabolic acidosis—may be episodic
3. Middle age—elderly
4. Diabetes mellitus—common
5. Cardiovascular and renal disease—common
6. PRA—low

DRUGS THAT MAY UNMASK HYPOALDOSTERONISM

1. Beta-blockers
2. PG inhibitors
3. Heparin (long term)
4. ACE inhibition (especially if refractory CHF)

CAUSES OF HYPERCHLOREMIC—HYPERKALEMIC METABOLIC ACIDOSIS

1. KCl
2. K-sparing drugs
3. Isolated hypoaldosteronism
4. Addison's disease
5. Obstructive uropathy
6. C.D. defects

TREATMENT OF HYPERKALEMIA

1. Stop K salts and K-sparing drugs
2. Correct ECF contraction
3. If patient has S_k >6.0 mEq/L, persistently, secondary to selective hypoaldosteronism:
   - Florinef 0.1 mg qd or bid
4. If patient has tubular defect for K secretion:
   - Use kayexalate
5. $NaHCO_3$ for patients with ↑ S_k and metabolic acidosis
6. In extreme cases, consider salt, diuretic, and florinef

Hyperkalemic Syndrome

Normal Total Body K$^+$	*Excessive Total Body K$^+$*
Pseudohyperkalemia	Excessive intake:
Hemolysis of drawn blood	K$^+$ penicillin (1.7 mEq/10^6 units)
Tourniquet-induced ischemia	Salt substitutes (10 to 14 mEq/g)
High leukocyte count ($>5 \times 10^5$ mm^3)	Stored blood
High platelet count ($>7.5 \times 10^5$ mm^3)	Low salt diet is K$^+$ rich
Redistributional	Defects in renin-aldosterone-renal axis
Acidosis (inorganic > organic)	Renin-substrate deficiency
Hormonal	Liver failure
Insulin deficiency	Glucocorticoid deficiency
Alpha-adrenergic agonists	Hyporeninemia
Beta-adrenergic blockers	Aging
Aldosterone deficiency	Extracellular fluid expansion
Tissue necrosis	Diabetes mellitus
Familial periodic paralysis	Interstitial nephritis
Drugs and toxins	Hydronephrosis
Digital poisoning	Drugs and toxins
Succinylcholine	Nonsteroidal antiinflammatory drugs (NSAIDs)
Arginine, lysine	Beta-blockers
THAM	Alpha agonist
Hyperosmolality (in diabetic patients)	Lead
	Converting enzyme inhibitor
	Captopril, lisinopril
	Aldosterone synthetic defect
	Generalized adrenal failure
	Specific synthetic defect
	Idiopathic
	Drugs: heparin, spironolactone
	Enzyme deficiencies
	Renal aldosterone resistance
	Oliguria, low urinary Na$^+$
	Interstitial nephritis (sickle cell, systemic lupus erythematosus)
	Drugs: spironolactone
	Hydronephrosis
	Amyloidosis
	Gordon syndrome

Interpretation of Urinary Electrolytes[a]

Diagnostic Problem	Urinary Value	Primary Diagnostic Possibilities
Volume depletion	Na^+, 0 to 10 mEq/L	Extrarenal sodium loss
	Na^+, >10 mEq/L	''Renal salt wasting'' or adrenal insufficiency
Acute oliguria	Na^+, 0 to 10 mEq/L	Prerenal azotemia
	Na^+, >30 mEq/L	Acute tubular necrosis
Hyponatremia	Na^+, 0 to 10 mEq/L	Severe volume depletion; edematous states
	Na^+, ≥dietary intake	Inappropriate antidiuretic hormone ADH secretion; adrenal insufficiency
Hypokalemia	K^+, 0 to 10 mEq/L	Extrarenal potassium loss
	K^+, >20 mEq/L	Renal potassium loss
Metabolic alkalosis	Cl^-, 0 to 10 mEq/L	Chloride-responsive alkalosis
	Cl^-, ≥ dietary intake	Chloride-resistant alkalosis

[a] For purposes of this table, it is assumed that the patient is not receiving diuretics.

BIBLIOGRAPHY

Anderson RJ, Chung HM, Kluge R, et al. Hyponatremia: A prospective analysis of its epidemiology and the pathogenetic role of vasopressin. Ann Intern Med 1985;102:164–168.

Arieff AI, Llach F, Massry SG. Neurological manifestations and morbidity of hyponatremia: Correlation with brain water and electrolytes. Medicine 1976;55:121–129.

Ashraf N, Locksley R, Arieff AI. Thiazide-induced hyponatremia associated with death or neurologic damage in outpatients. Am J Med 1981;70:1163–1168.

Bartter F, Schwartz WB. The syndrome of inappropriate secretion of antidiuretic hormone. Am J Med 1967;42:790.

Berl T. Treating hyponatremia — Damned if we do and damned if we don't. Kidney Int 1990;37:1006– 1018.

Berl T, Anderson RJ, McDonald KM, et al. Clinical disorders of water metabolism Kidney Int 1976;10:117–132.

Carrilho F, Bosoh J, Arroyo V, et al. Renal failure associated with demeclocyline in cirrhosis. Ann Intern Med 1977;87: 195–197.

DeFronzo RA, Thier SO. Pathophysiologic approach to hyponatremia. Arch Intern Med 1980;140:897.

Fichman MT, Vorherr H, Kleeman CP, et al. Diuretic-induced hyponatremia. Ann Intern Med 1971;75:853.

Forrest JN Jr, Cox M, Hong C, et al. Superiority of demeclocycline over lithium in the treatment of chronic syndrome of inappropriate secretion of antidiuretic hormone. N Engl J Med 1978;298:173–177.

Gullans SR, Verbalis JG. Control of brain volume during hy-

perosmolar and hypoosmolar conditions. Annu Rev Med 1993;44:289–301.

Hantman O, Rossier B, Zohlman R, et al. Rapid correction of hyponatremia in the syndrome of inappropriate secretion of antidiuretic hormone. Ann Intern Med 1973;78:870–875.

Harrington JT, Cohen JJ. Clinical disorders of urine concentration and dilution. Arch Intern Med 1973;131:810.

Leaf A, Cotran R. Renal pathophysiology. New York: Oxford University Press, 1976.

Leaf A. The clinical and physiologic significance of the serum sodium concentration (Part 1). N Engl J Med 1962;267:24–30.

Leaf A. The clinical and physiologic significance of the serum sodium concentration (Part 2). N Engl J Med 1962;267:77–83.

Lee WH, Packer M. Prognostic importance of serum sodium concentration and its modification by converting-enzyme inhibition in patients with severe chronic heart failure. Circulation 1986;73:257–267.

Narins RG, Jones ER, Stom MC, et al. Diagnostic strategies in disorders of fluid, electrolyte and acid-base homeostasis. Am J Med 1982;72:496–519.

Potassium in Clinical Medicine. Searle and Co. Monograph, Medcom, Inc., 1973.

Renal and Electrolyte Disorders. 4th ed. Schrier RW, ed. Philadelphia: Lippincott-Raven, 1997.

Robertson GL, Aycinena P. Neurogenic disorders of osmoregulation. Am J Med 1982;72:339–353.

Rose BD. Clinical physiology of acid-base and electrolyte disorders. 4th ed. New York: McGraw-Hill, 1994.

Schrier RW, Ed. Renal and electrolyte disorders. 4th ed. Philadelphia: Lippincott-Raven, 1997.

Schrier RW. Pathogenesis of sodium and water retention, high-output and low-output cardiac failure, nephrotic syndrome, cirrhosis, and pregnancy. N Engl J Med 1988;319: 1065–1072, 1127–1134.

Sterns RH. Severe symptomatic hyponatremia: Treatment and outcome. A study of 64 cases. Ann Intern Med 1987;107: 656–664.

The Sea within Us. Searle & Co. Monograph. New York: Science and Medicine Publishing Co., Inc, 1975.

Valtin H, Schafer JA. Renal function: mechansims preserving fluid and solute balance in health. 3rd ed. Boston: Little, Brown & Co., 1995.

C·H·A·P·T·E·R

52

Acid-Base Disorders

Julie A. Breyer

The acidity of body fluids is expressed in terms of the hydrogen ion concentration ($[H^+]$). The $[H^+]$ is normally 40 nanoequivalents per liter (nEq/L) and is usually expressed in terms of pH, which is the negative log of the $[H^+]$. Figure 52.1 shows the relationship between the pH measured in a patient's blood and the $[H^+]$—the two most commonly employed units for specifying the level of acidity. Figure 52.1 shows several important points:

- pH and the $[H^+]$ are inversely related. As the $[H^+]$ increases, pH decreases.
- A normal pH of 7.4 corresponds to a normal $[H^+]$ of 40 nEq/L.
- A reasonably accurate estimate of proton concentration can be made from pH by exploiting the nearly linear relationship between pH and the $[H^+]$ between pH 7.1–7.5. In this pH range, the $[H^+]$ will change by 1 nEq/L for each 0.01 unit change in pH.

To illustrate the pH:$[H^+]$ relationship, given that a normal pH of 7.4 corresponds to a proton concentration of 40 nEq/L, if a patient's pH is 7.2, the proton concentration equals 60 nEq/L:

Change in pH = 0.2 units

Change in $[H^+]$ = (0.2 ÷ 0.01) nEq/L = 20 nEq/L

Therefore,

$[H^+]$ at 7.2 = (40 + 20) nEq/L = 60 nEq/L

Estimating the $[H^+]$ is important for doing calculations with acid-base data. Another method that relates pH to $[H^+]$ compensates for the true curvilinear relationship between pH and $[H^+]$. Although slightly more complex than the preceding technique for estimating $[H^+]$, this method is more accurate

and works over a broader pH range. This method begins at the point at which pH = 7.40 and $[H^+]$ = 40 nEq/L and proceeds as follows:

- To calculate the $[H^+]$ for each 0.1 pH decrement, sequentially multiply 40 nEq/L by 1.25.
- To calculate the $[H^+]$ for each 0.1 pH increment, sequentially multiply 40 nEq/L by 0.8.

This relationship appears in Table 52.1.

As serum pH falls below 7.36, a patient is said to be acidemic. Conversely, as the pH rises above 7.44, a patient is said to be alkalemic. Acidemia and alkalemia are descriptions of the patient's actual blood pH. Acidosis and alkalosis are descriptions of pathophysiologic processes that, if unopposed, may lead to acidemia and alkalemia. In acidosis, the plasma bicarbonate concentration may be below normal, while in alkalosis the plasma bicarbonate concentration may be above normal. For example, if a patient is vomiting, he or she will have a high bicarbonate (32 mEq/L) and thus an alkalosis, but if at the same time the patient has respiratory failure and a high P_{CO_2} (e.g., 75 mm Hg), arterial pH may actually be in the acidemic range (e.g., pH = 7.25).

ACID-BASE TERMINOLOGY

The principal terms in acid-base disorders are defined as follows:

- Acidemia–An increase in $[H^+]$ and a decrease in arterial pH
- Alkalemia–A decrease in $[H^+]$ and an increase in arterial pH
- Acidosis–A process that acidifies body fluids (i.e., lowers plasma bicarbonate) and if unopposed will lead to a fall in pH and acidemia

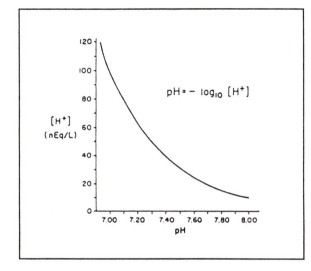

Figure 52.1. Relationship between pH and hydrogen ion concentration, the two most commonly employed units for specifying the level of acidity. (With permission from Cohen JJ, Kassirer JP. Acid-base chemistry and buffering. In: Acid/Base. Boston: Little Brown & Co, 1980:5.)

Table 52.1. Relationship Between pH and $[H^+]$	
pH	**$[H^+]$ (nEq/L)**
7.80	16
7.75	18
7.70	20
7.65	22
7.60	25
7.55	28
7.50	32
7.45	35
7.40	40
7.35	45
7.30	50
7.25	56
7.20	63
7.15	71
7.10	79
7.05	89
7.00	100
6.95	112
6.90	126
6.85	141
6.80	159

From Cohen JJ, Kassirer JP Acid-base chemistry and buffering. In: Acid/Base. Boston, Mass: Little Brown & Co, 1980:5

- Alkalosis—A process that alkalinizes body fluids (i.e., raises plasma bicarbonate) and if unopposed will lead to an increase in pH and an alkalemia

THE BODY'S BUFFERS

Despite continuous acid production, the body maintains arterial pH within the narrow range of 7.35–7.45. Approximately 15 mol or 15,000 mEq of CO_2 are generated each day by tissue metabolism and are carried by hemoglobin (Hgb)-generated HCO_3 or Hgb-bound carbamino groups to the lung for excretion as CO_2. Also, approximately 70 mEq per day or 1 mEq/kg per day of a patient's body weight is generated as nonvolatile acids (mostly phosphoric and sulfuric acids) and excreted by the kidneys.

Daily acid production can be summarized as follows:

- 12,000–15,000 mEq/day of volatile acids are produced and excreted by the lungs as CO_2
- 1 mEq/kg/day of nonvolatile acids are produced and excreted by the kidneys
- The pH of body fluids is determined by: the acid produced, the buffering capacity, and the ability of the lungs and kidneys to excrete the load.

The latter is a clinically relevant fact. If a patient has renal failure and can no longer excrete the acid normally produced, the amount of HCO_3 needed to buffer the daily acid produced is 1 mEq/kg. If the patient requires more bicarbonate therapy than 1 mEq/kg to maintain the serum bicarbonate at any given level, another process, in addition to renal failure, is likely to be contributing to the acidosis.

If an extra base or acid load is introduced, the body reacts with a complex system, which is composed of buffering and activation of compensatory mechanisms. As shown in Figure 52.2, if an acid or base load is added, the first defense is extracellular buffering, followed by the intracellular and, very importantly, skeletal buffering. (The skeleton represents an enormous reservoir of alkaline salts.) As compensation develops, the respiratory system modulates the CO_2 tension and, lastly, the kidneys modulate the plasma HCO_3 concentration.

Clinical acid-base chemistry is really the chemistry of the buffers in the body. Simply stated, a buffer is a substance that can either absorb or donate protons to a solution. The most important buffer components in the extracellular fluid at physiologically relevant pH are Hgb, plasma proteins, and bicarbonate. The principal buffering system for noncarbonic acid in the extracellular fluid is the bicarbonate buffering system. Because all buffers behave as if they are in functional contact with a common pool of $[H^+]$, the determination of one buffer pair reflects the states of all other buffer pairs and also of the arterial pH. This relationship, termed the isohydric principle, shows that any alteration of the $[H^+]$ results in parallel changes in the ratio of each buffer pair within any fluid compartment:

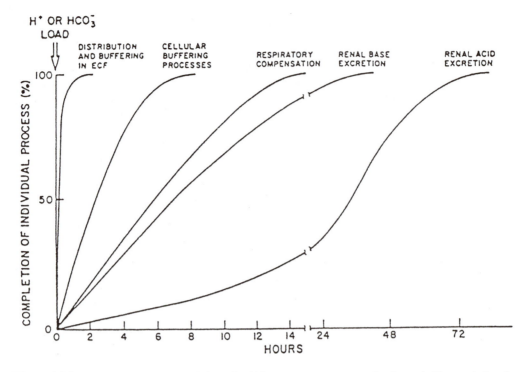

Figure 52.2. Time course for completion of acid-base compensatory mechanisms. (with permission from Cogan MG, Rector FC, Seldin DW. Acid-base disorders in the kidney. In: Brenner BM, Rector FC, eds. The Kidney. Philadelphia: W.B. Saunders, 1981:841-907.)

$$HA = H^+ + A^-$$

$$Ka = \frac{[H^+][A^-]}{[HA]}$$

$$[H^+] = \frac{K_1 H_2 CO_3}{HCO_3} = \frac{K_2 H_2 PO_4^-}{HPO_4} = \frac{KHgbH^+}{Hgb}$$

Clinically, when we assess a patient's acid-base status, we evaluate the carbonic acid bicarbonate system since it is easily measured. The most abundant extracellular buffer is HCO_3. Metabolically produced CO_2 is buffered in the red blood cells and provides the substrate for acid secretion in the kidney.

The P_{CO_2}-HCO_3 buffer system is reflected in the following formulas:

$$CO_2\ gas \rightarrow CO_2\ (dissolved) + H_2O \leftrightarrow H_2CO_3 + HCO_3^-$$

$$H^+ = \frac{KH_2CO_3}{HCO_3}$$

$$pH = pKa + \frac{(\log[HCO_3])}{H_2CO_3}$$

$$[N_2CO_3] \approx 0.03\ (P_{CO_2})\ (solubility\ coefficient)$$

The chemical species comprising this buffer system are interrelated as follows: Dissolved CO_2 is reversibly hydrated to H_2CO_3 in a slow reaction. Carbonic acid is, therefore, a volatile acid since it is in equilibrium with the gaseous CO_2. Carbonic acid dissociates spontaneously into $[H^+]$ and HCO_3.

This equilibrium reaction can be expressed in terms of the Henderson-Hasselbalch equation as the pH equals the pKa plus the log of the HCO_3 concentration over the carbonic acid concentration. Carbonic acid is present in blood in such small quantities that cannot be measured, but because carbonic acid is in equilibrium with the CO_2 in solution and the dissolved CO_2 depends on the P_{CO_2} in the arterial blood, the carbonic acid term of the equation can be replaced by the term P_{CO_2} times the solubility coefficient (0.03). The Henderson-Hasselbalch equation follows:

$$pH = pKa + \frac{\log [HCO_3]}{(0.03)P_{CO_2}} = \frac{kidney}{lung} = \frac{metabolic}{respiratory}$$

$$7.4 = 6.1 + \frac{\log [24]}{(0.03)(40)}$$

(pH is determined by the ratio of HCO_3/P_{CO_2} to P_{CO_2}.)

Thus the pH—that is, the $[H^+]$ of the blood—is determined by the ratio of the serum bicarbonate concentration to the partial pressure of CO_2 in the arterial blood. The bicarbonate concentration is regulated by the kidney. Metabolic processes, such as metabolic acidosis and metabolic alkalosis, primarily affect the bicarbonate concentration of the blood. The P_{CO_2} is regulated by the lung, and respiratory acidosis and alkalosis are reflected in primary changes in the P_{CO_2}.

The Henderson-Hasselbalch equation can be rearranged and simplified to form the following equation:

$$[H^+] = \frac{24 \times P_{CO_2}}{[HCO_3]}$$

As noted previously, the $[H^+]$ is calculated from the pH, given that a pH of 7.4 equals an $[H^+]$ of 40 nEq/L and that there is a linear relationship between pH and $[H^+]$ between a pH of 7.1–7.5. Also noted, for every 0.01 change in pH, there is a 1 nEq/L change in the $[H^+]$ concentration. The advantage of using this simplified equation is that it facilitates the calculation of one unknown parameter from two known parameters. For example, if the plasma bicarbonate concentration and the pH are known, the P_{CO_2} can be calculated. Also, this equation allows one to check the validity of simultaneous laboratory measurements of pH, bicarbonate concentration, and P_{CO_2}. When the reported HCO_3 concentration and P_{CO_2} are entered into the right side of the equation, the equation should solve to equal the $[H^+]$ predicted by the arterial pH. If it does not, then one of the reported values is wrong. (Many an intern has racked his or her brain trying to analyze a patient's acid-base problem without checking to see if the numbers are consistent using this equation.)

SIMPLE ACID-BASE DISORDERS

Clinical disorders of acid-base equilibrium are classified according to which of the two variables, P_{CO_2} or bicarbonate concentration, is directly affected by the primary pathologic process:

- Clinical disorders initiated by a primary change in the bicarbonate are referred to as metabolic disorders.
- Clinical disorders initiated by a change in the P_{CO_2} are referred to as respiratory disorders.
- Decreases in the plasma bicarbonate result in metabolic acidosis, whereas increases in the plasma bicarbonate result in metabolic alkalosis. Hypercapnia, an increase in the P_{CO_2}, results in a respiratory acidosis; hypocapnia results in a respiratory alkalosis.

In each of the four primary disturbances shown in Table 52.2, the initiating process not only alters the acid-base equilibrium directly, but also sets in motion secondary compensatory responses that change the other member of the P_{CO_2}-bicarbonate pair:

- In metabolic acidosis, the primary disturbance is a fall in the bicarbonate. The body, in an attempt to return the pH or $[H^+]$ back toward normal, induces a fall in P_{CO_2} (via hyperventilation) so that the ratio approaches normal.
- In metabolic alkalosis, the primary increase in bicarbonate is compensated for by a decrease in ventilation and an increase in P_{CO_2}.
- In respiratory acidosis, the compensatory response is a rise in the serum bicarbonate due to decreased renal excretion of bicarbonate and increased renal net acid excretion.
- In respiratory alkalosis, the primary fall in P_{CO_2} is compensated by increased renal excretion of bicarbonate and a resultant fall in serum bicarbonate.

If one remembers the basic principles relating P_{CO_2} and bicarbonate to pH or $[H^+]$ and that the body's goal is to maintain a nearly normal pH, then all these clinical compensatory responses can be simply predicted.

If only one of these primary processes is present, then the patient has a simple acid-base disturbance with an appropriate compensatory response. On the other hand, if two or more primary abnormalities are present, the patient is said to have a mixed acid-base disorder. For example, a patient may have a heart attack, become hypotensive, underperfuse his or her organs, and develop a metabolic acidosis due to the accumulation of lactic acid, but also have pneumonia, respiratory failure, and a respiratory acidosis. This patient is said to have a mixed acid-base disorder with two primary processes.

COMPENSATORY RESPONSES

The role of compensatory processes can be summarized as follows:

- These processes may return the ratio of HCO_3 to P_{CO_2} back toward normal and thus help normalize the arterial pH.
- Compensation, with one exception (primary respiratory alkalosis), never returns the pH fully back to normal.
- Compensatory responses require normally functioning lungs and kidneys and take time to occur.

Table 52.2. The Four Primary Acid-Base Disturbances

Type of Disturbance	Primary Alteration	Compensatory Response	Mechanism of Compensatory Response
Metabolic acidosis	Decrease in plasma $[HCO_3]$	Decrease in Pa_{CO_2}	Hyperventilation
Metabolic alkalosis	Increase in plasma $[HCO_3]$	Increase in Pa_{CO_2}	Hypoventilation
Respiratory acidosis	Increase in Pa_{CO_2}	Increase in plasma $[HCO_3]$	Increased $[HCO_3]$ reabsorption by the kidney
Respiratory alkalosis	Decrease in Pa_{CO_2}	Decrease in plasma $[HCO_3]$	Decreased $[HCO_3]$ reabsorption by the kidney

- The lack of compensation in an appropriate interval defines the presence of a second primary disorder.
- The compensatory response creates a second laboratory abnormality.
- The appropriate degree of compensation can be predicted.

Compensatory processes may return the ratio of the bicarbonate and the P_{CO_2} back toward normal and thus help normalize the arterial pH, but the compensatory response will never return the pH completely to normal. For example, if a patient has a metabolic acidosis and, thus, a low serum bicarbonate, the compensatory response of a fall in the P_{CO_2} will raise the arterial pH. However, the patient will still be acidemic; that is the arterial pH will still be below 7.38. The primary process can be determined by looking at the arterial blood gas levels and deciding whether the bicarbonate or the P_{CO_2} have moved in the right direction to lead to that change in pH. In our example of simple metabolic acidosis, the patient will be acidemic since the fall in the bicarbonate (the primary process) produces the fall in pH. Although the compensatory fall in P_{CO_2} increases the pH, it does not return it to normal and is clearly a secondary event. One exception to this rule is chronic respiratory alkalosis for more than 2 weeks: the compensatory fall in bicarbonate may return the pH to normal. The primary disorder in this setting has to be determined by history.

Compensatory responses require normally functioning kidneys and lungs. A patient with significant renal failure cannot develop full metabolic compensation to a primary respiratory disorder. Similarly, a patient on a ventilator whose respiratory rate is mechanically controlled cannot develop a compensatory respiratory response. Compensatory responses take up to 12–24 hours to develop fully. Thus, one cannot say that a patient has failed to compensate if he or she has not yet had time to do so. If an appropriate amount of time has passed and an adequate compensatory response has not developed, then this failure defines the presence of a second primary disorder. A clinical example of this could be the patient with diabetic ketoacidosis and severe metabolic acidosis who is obtunded. If the arterial blood gas shows a pH of 7.10, P_{CO_2} of 30, and bicarbonate concentration of 9 mEq/L, one can conclude that the respiratory compensation, although present, is incomplete. Thus, the patient has a mixed acid-base disorder consisting of metabolic and respiratory acidosis.

Finally, the limits of appropriate metabolic compensation (change in HCO_3) for any given degree of primary respiratory acidosis or alkalosis and the limits of respiratory compensation (change in P_{CO_2}) for a given degree of primary metabolic acidosis or alkalosis have been defined. A P_{CO_2} that lies outside these limits in a patient with a primary metabolic disorder defines a coexistent respiratory disorder. Similarly, an HCO_3 that lies outside the expected limits of compensation in a patient with a primary respiratory disorder defines a coexistent metabolic disorder. Nomograms such as Figure 52.3 (which shows 95% confidence limits of compensations for primary "simple" acid-base disturbances) plot the HCO_3, pH, and P_{CO_2} values expected in primary acid-base disorders. Points within the star-like figure are consistent with, but not diagnostic of, a simple acid-base disorder with a single primary disor-

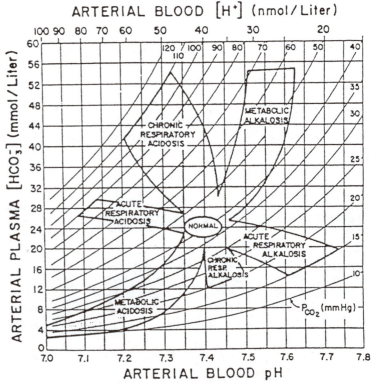

Figure 52.3. Acid-base nomogram. To predict the pH change with changes in $[HCO_3^-]$ or in P_{CO_2}, trace along the diagonal lines for changes in $[HCO_3^-]$ with constant P_{CO_2}; trace along the horizontal lines for changes in P_{CO_2} with constant $[HCO_3^-]$. (With permission from Cogan MG, et al. Acid-base disorders. In: Breenner BM, Rector FC, eds. The Kidney. Philadelphia: W.B. Saunders, 1981:860.)

Table 52.3.   Expected Compensatory Changes in Simple Acid-Base Disorders

Primary Disorder	Compensatory Change*	
	Acute (24 hours)	*Chronic (2–3 days)*
Metabolic acidosis	$P_{CO_2} = 1.5\,[HCO_3^-] + 8 \pm 2$	Same
	$P_{CO_2} =$ last 2 digits of the pH	
Metabolic alkalosis	$P_{CO_2} = 40 + 0.6\,(\Delta[HCO_3^-])$	Same
Respiratory acidosis	$\uparrow \Delta[HCO_3^-] = \Delta[HCO_3^-]/10$	$\uparrow \Delta[HCO_3^-] = 3.5 \times \Delta P_{CO_2}/10$
Respiratory alkalosis	$\downarrow \Delta[HCO_3^-] = 2 \times \Delta P_{CO_2}/10$	$\downarrow \Delta[HCO_3^-] = 5 \times \Delta P_{CO_2}/10$

* Note that some equations give the answers in terms of the change in the plasma measurement (*e.g.* $\Delta[HCO^-_3]$, ΔP_{CO_2}), whereas other equations give the absolute value of the measurement (*e.g.*, P_{CO_2}). Adapted from Narins RG, Emmett M. Simple and mixed acid-based disorders: A practical approach. Medicine 1980;59:161–187.

der and appropriate compensation. Mixed acid-base disorders that include more than one primary acid-base abnormality have values that fall within the star-like figure between two or three contributing acid-base disorders. It should be noted that values falling outside the star-like figure generally predict a mixed disorder, but values that fall within the star-like figure, although usually representing simple disorders, can result from coincidental mixed disturbances. The mild alkalemia shown in the area of pure chronic respiratory acidosis and the nearly consistent hypercapnia with metabolic alkalosis are still somewhat controversial.

One need not rely exclusively on nomograms. Rather, the degree of compensation and its appropriateness can be calculated with equations that predict the expected degree of compensation (Table 52.3). The most useful and most often used equation is the expected respiratory compensation in metabolic acidosis. Note that the degree of compensation in respiratory acidosis and alkalosis varies depending on whether the primary process is acute or chronic.

PRIMARY ACID-BASE DISORDERS

METABOLIC ACIDOSIS

Key information:

- Definition: Begins with fall in serum HCO_3 due to accumulation of nonvolatile acids.
- Primary Defect: Fall in HCO_3. Accumulation of metabolic acids is caused by:
  - Excess acid production that overwhelms renal capacity for excretion (e.g., diabetic ketoacidosis)
  - Loss of alkali, Leaving unneutralized acid behind (e.g., diarrhea)
  - Renal excretory failure: Normal total acid production in face of poor renal function (e.g., chronic renal failure of any cause)
- Compensatory Change:
  - Tissues and red blood cells act to increase serum HCO_3 by exchanging intracellular Na and K for extracellular H^+, raising serum HCO_3 and K.

- Pulmonary ventilation increases. A fall in P_{CO_2} brings pH back toward normal.

Before causes of metabolic acidosis can be further discussed, the anion gap must be reviewed. Total serum anions include chloride and bicarbonate, routinely measured on the SMA-6, as well as the unmeasured anions. Total anions equal the total cations in blood, which include sodium and unmeasured cations. The unmeasured anions in healthy persons exceed the unmeasured cations, a difference called the anion gap. The anion gap can be estimated by subtracting the sum of the chloride and bicarbonate concentrations from the sodium concentration, as shown in the following equations:

$$UA + Cl + HCO_3 = UC + Na$$

$$UA - UC = \text{Anion Gap} = Na - (Cl + HCO_3) = 12$$

In a healthy state, the value is approximately 12. The anion gap can be increased because of a decrease in unmeasured cations, an increase in unmeasured anions, or laboratory error in the measurement of Na, Cl, or HCO_3 (Table 52.4).

Metabolic acidosis is frequently associated with an increased anion gap. In fact, metabolic acidoses are categorized clinically by the presence or absence of an abnormally elevated anion gap. In a high-anion-gap acidosis, the proton that titrates bicarbonate is accompanied by an unmeasured anion, resulting in the accumulation of that anion in the blood and a high-anion-gap acidosis (Figure 52.4). If the anion accompanying the proton is chloride, then the patient has a metabolic acidosis with a normal anion gap, since the fall in HCO_3 is matched by an increase in chloride. This is, by definition, a hyperchloremic acidosis. For example, a patient can have a loss of HCO_3 in the stool with an increase in chloride secondary to volume depletion. The result is a normal anion gap acidosis or hyperchloremic acidosis. Clinically, the anion gap should be calculated for every patient each time one draws a set of electrolytes (Figure 52.5).

The causes of high-anion-gap metabolic acidosis include:

- Ketoacidosis
- Lactic acidosis
- Uremia

Table 52.4. Causes of Anion Gap Changes	
Causes of Decreased Anion Gap	*Causes of Increased Anion Gap*

• Increased unmeasured cation
  – Increased concentration of normally present cation: hyperkalemia, hypercalcemia, hypermagnesemia
  – Retention of abnormal cation: 1 G-globulin, tromethamine (TRIS) buffer, lithium
  – Decreased unmeasured anion hypoalbuminemia
• Laboratory error
  – Systemic error: hyponatremia due to viscous serum, hyperchloremia in bromide intoxication
  – Random error: falsely decreased serum sodium, or falsely increased serum chloride or bicarbonate.
	• Decreased unmeasured cation
	  – Hypokalemia, hypocalcemia, hypomagnesemia
	• Increased unmeasured anion
	  – Organic anions: lactate, ketone acids
	  – Inorganic anions: phosphate, sulfate
	  – Proteins: hyperalbuminemia (transient)
	  – Exogenous anions: salicylate, formate, nitrate, penicillin, carbenicillin, etc.
	  – Incompletely identified: anion accumulation in paraldehyde, ethylene glycol, methanol and salicylate poisoning, ureinia, hyperosmolar hyperglycemic nonketotic coma
	• Laboratory error
	  – Falsely increased serum sodium
	  – Falsely increased serum chloride or bicarbonate

Basic Acid-Base Terminology (Breyer)

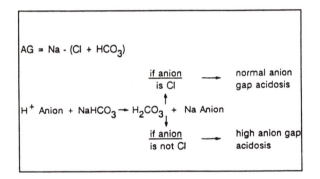

Figure 52.4.   Anion gap in metabolic acidosis.

• Salicylate toxicity
• Ethylene glycol toxicity
• Methanol toxicity
• Paraldehyde toxicity
• Massive rhabdomyolysis

If a patient has an elevated anion gap, lactic acidosis and ketoacidosis are the most common causes. One can measure the serum levels of these organic anions. Intoxications with aspirin, antifreeze, methanol, or paraldehyde can also cause an anion-gap acidosis and should be considered (Figure 52.6), especially in an unconscious patient. (As noted above, the "normal" anion gap is approximately 12.) When a patient has an increased anion gap, most anions that will account for this are associated with a single proton. In an uncomplicated high-anion-gap acidosis, for every 1 mmol/L rise in the anion gap, there should be a concomitant fall of 1 mmol/L in the bicarbonate (HCO_3) concentration. The difference between the patient's anion gap and a "normal" anion gap is called

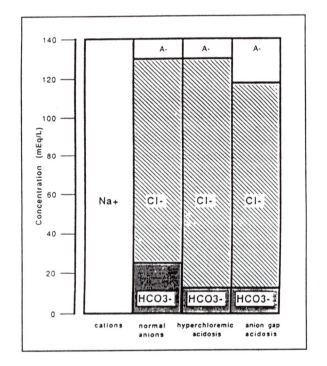

Figure 52.5.   The anion gap. (With permission from Breyer MD, Jacobson HR. Approach to the patient with metabolic acidosis or metabolic alkalosis. In: Kelley, ed. Textbook of Internal Medicine. Philadelphia: W.B. Saunders, 1989:923.)

the delta anion gap (ΔAG). The ΔAG and ΔHCO_3 are calculated by the following formulas:

$$\Delta AG = \text{observed AG} - \text{upper normal AG}$$

$$\Delta HCO_3 = \text{lower normal } HCO_3 - \text{observed } HCO_3$$

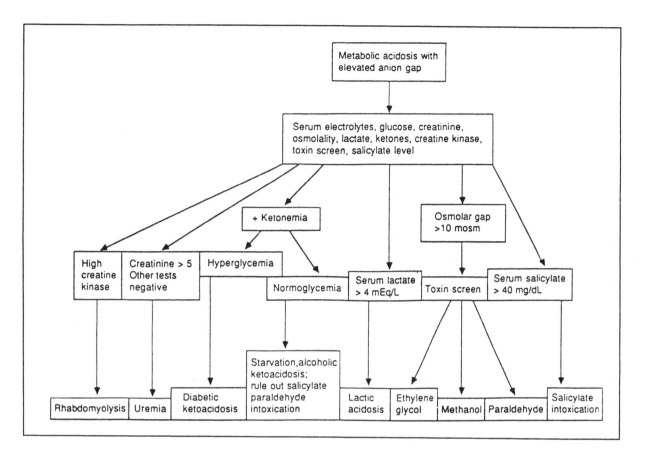

Figure 52.6. Diagnostic algorithm for metabolic acidosis with elevated anion gap. (With permission from Breyer MD, Jacobson HR. Approach to the patient with metabolic acidosis or metabolic alkalosis. In: Kelley, ed. Textbook of Internal Medicine. Philadelphia: W.B. Saunders, 1989:926.)

For example, a patient with an anion gap of 20 has a $\Delta AG = 20 - 12 = 8$. The eight unmeasured anions would account for a decrease in the serum bicarbonate concentration of 8 mmol/L. Any significant deviation from this rule implies the existence of a mixed acid-base disorder. When the fall in bicarbonate (ΔHCO_3) is greater than the rise in AG (ΔAG) ($\Delta HCO_3 >> \Delta AG$), two possible situations exist if laboratory error is excluded. Most commonly, there is either a mixed-high-anion-gap and normal-anion-gap acidosis, or a mixed-high-anion-gap acidosis and "chronic" respiratory alkalosis with a compensating hyperchloremic acidosis. Conversely, when the anion gap is greater than the ΔHCO_3 ($\Delta AG >> \Delta HCO_3$), there is almost always a mixed high anion gap acidosis and primary metabolic alkalosis.

The presence of a hyperchloremic or normal anion gap acidosis suggests a completely different set of diagnoses, including renal tubular acidosis (RTA) diarrhea, ileal conduits, and HCl ingestions (Table 52.5). The diagnostic algorithm appears in Figure 52.7.

In patients with a hyperchloremic metabolic acidosis, the urine anion gap can be used to distinguish whether the cause of the acidosis is caused by a renal tubular defect or by other causes, such as diarrhea. The urine anion gap is calculated as follows:

Table 52.5.   Causes of Hyperchloremic Metabolic Acidosis

Hypokalemic
  Proximal renal tubular acidosis drug induced: acetazolamide, coumarin, sulfamyalon
  Distal renal tubular acidosis
  Posthypocapnea
  Diarrhea
  Ureterosigmoidostomy/ileal loop
  Pancreatic fistula/biliary drainage
  Correction phase of diabetic ketoacidosis
Hyperkalemic/Normokalemic
  Type IV renal tubular acidosis: interstitial nephritis, hypoaldosteronism, hydronephrosis
  HCI ingestions/infusions: hyperalimentation, cholestyramine, $CaCl_2$, NH_4Cl
  Dilutional acidosis

$$AG = (urine\ Na^+ + urine\ K^+) - (urine\ Cl^-)$$

Since ammonium is excreted in the urine with chloride, this index can be used to estimate the concentration of ammonium in the urine in a patient with hyperchloremic metabolic

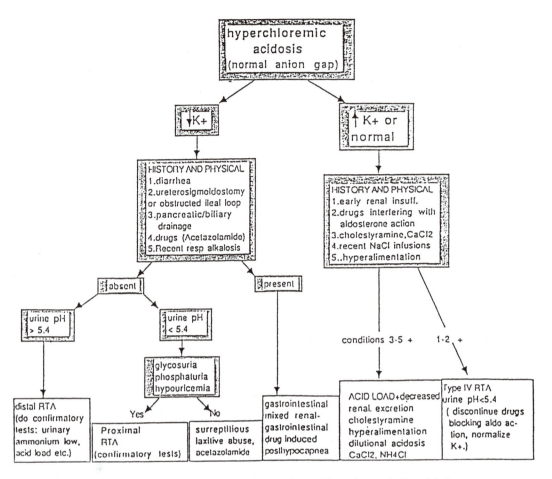

Figure 52.7. Diagnostic algorithm for hyperchloremic metabolic acidosis.

acidosis. A negative urine anion gap ($Cl^- >> Na^+ + K^+$) suggests the appropriate excretion of ammonium in the urine with Cl^- and the presence of gastrointestinal loss of HCO_3. A positive urine anion gap ($Cl^- < Na^+ + K^+$) suggests the presence of an RTA with a distal acidification defect and inadequate ammonium excretion in the urine.

METABOLIC ALKALOSIS

Key information:

- Definition: A rise in the concentration of serum HCO_3
- Primary Defect: Rise in serum HCO_3, with two requirements:
  - New HCO_3 must be added to the blood from renal or extrarenal sources (the process of generation).
  - Kidney must increase its net reabsorptive capacity to maintain the higher level of serum [HCO_3]. (The stimuli that increase renal HCO_3 reabsorption are high PCO_2, extracellular fluid contraction, CI depletion, steroid excess, and K^+ depletion.)
- Compensatory Change:
  - Tissues and red blood cells act to lower serum HCO_3 by exchanging intracellular H^+ for

extracellular K and Na, lowering both serum HCO_3 and K.
- Alkalosis tends to cause hypoventilation and elevation of PCO_2. Compensation for alkalosis is more erratic than for acidosis. Generally PCO_2 rarely is > 55 mg Hg.

The causes of metabolic alkalosis can be divided: those associated with a high urinary excretion of chloride and those associated with a low excretion of chloride and, therefore, responsive to saline administration (Table 52.6 and Figure 52.8).

RESPIRATORY ACIDOSIS

Key information:

- Definition: Decreases pulmonary clearance of CO_2
- Primary Defect: Increases PCO_2
- Compensatory Change: In acute syndromes, tissues and red blood cells generate HCO_3 by taking up H^+ in exchange for NA and K^+. Acts to increase serum HCO_3 and K. In chronic syndromes, renal HCO_3 synthesis further augments serum HCO_3.

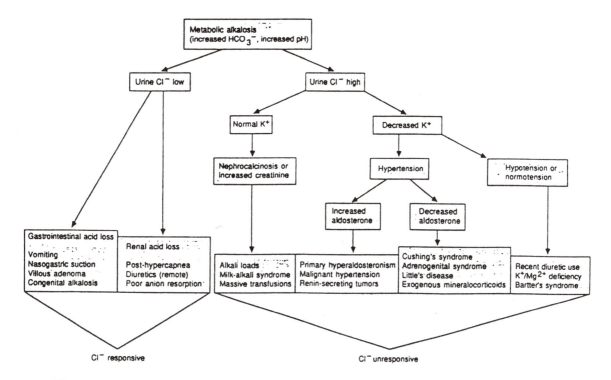

Figure 52.8. Diagnostic algorithm for metabolic alkalosis. (With permission from Breyer MD, Jacobson HR. Approach to the patient with metabolic acidosis or metabolic alkalosis. In: Kelley, ed. Textbook of Internal Medicine. Philadelphia: W.B. Saunders, 1989:932.)

Table 52.6. Urinary Chloride Concentration in Metabolic Alkalosis

Less than 20 mEq/L	*Greater than 30 mEq/L*
Vomiting	Primary hyperaldosteronism
Nasogastric suction	Cushing's syndrome: adrenal, ectopic ACTH, pituitary
Chloride wasting diarrhea	Exogenous steroid: licorice glucocorticoid,
Colonic cillous adenoma	carbenoxalone
Diuretic therapy (remote ingestion)	Adrenal 11 or 17 Hydroxylase defects
Post-hypercapnea	Liddle's syndrome
Poorly reabsorbed anions	Bartter's syndrome
Glucose refeeding	K^+ and Mg^{2+} deficiency
	Milk-alkali syndrome
	Hypercalcemia with secondary hypoparathyroidism

- Acute respiratory acidosis: Duration of less than 24 hours. No time for renal compensation. Tissue and red blood cells elevate serum HCO_3 above 4 mEq/L even with very high Pco_2. Rare to see serum HCO_3 above 31 mEq/L in acute respiratory acidosis.
- Chronic respiratory acidosis: Duration of more than 24 hours. Serum HCO_3 rises further due to compensatory HCO_3 synthesis. Elevated Pco_2 stimulates renal tubular H^+ secretion and ammonia production. More acid excreted; more HCO_3 synthesized and returned to the blood. The high Pco_2 also allows kidney to reclaim new HCO_3 when filtered at glomerulus. Chloride excreted with NH_4^+ acts to lower serum chloride.

Table 52.7.   Causes of Respiratory Acidosis

Acute
- Airway obstruction: aspiration of foreign body or vomitus, laryngospasm, generalized bronchospasm, obstructive sleep apnea
- Respiratory center depression: general anesthesia, sedative overdosage, cerebral trauma or infarction, central sleep apnea
- Circulatory catastrophes: cardiac arrest, severe pulmonary edema
- Neuromuscular defects: high cervical corodotomy, botulism, tetanus, Guillain-Barre syndrome, crisis in myasthenia gravis, familial hypokalemic periodic paralysis, hypokalemic myopathy, drugs of toxic agents (*e.g.*, curare, succinylcholine, aminoglycosides, organophosphorus)
- Restrictive defects: pneumothorax, hemothorax, flail chest, severe pneumonitis, infant respiratory distress syndrome (hyaline membrane disease), adult respiratory distress syndrome
- Mechanical ventilators

Chronic
- Airway obstruction: chronic obstructive lung disease (bronchitis, emphysema)
- Respiratory center depression: chronic sedative depression, primary alveolar hypoventilation (Ondine's curse), obesity-hypoventilation syndrome (Pickwickian syndrome), brain tumor, bulbar poliomyelitis
- Neuromuscular defects: poliomyelitis, multiple sclerosis, muscular dystrophy, amyotrophic lateral sclerosis, diaphragmatic paralysis, myxedema, myopathic disease (*e.g.*, polymyositis, acid maltase deficiency)
- Restrictive defects: kyphoscoliosis, spinal arthritis, fibrothorax, hydrothoras, interstitial fibrosis, decreased diaphragmatic movement (*e.g.*, ascites), prolonged pneumonitis, obesity

From Cohen JJ, Kassirer JP. Acid-base chemistry and buffering. In Acid/Base, Boston, Mass, Little Brown & Co, 1980:325.
Basic Acid-Base Terminology (Breyer)

Causes of respiratory acidosis are summarized in Table 52.7.

RESPIRATORY ALKALOSIS

Key information:

- Definition: Increased pulmonary clearance of CO_2
- Primary Defect: Fall in P_{CO_2}
- Compensatory Change:
  - Acute respiratory alkalosis: Duration of less than 24 hours. No renal compensation acutely. By exchanging intracellular H^+ for extracellular NA and K, tissue and red blood cells act to lower HCO_3, which rarely falls below 15 mEq/L, and K. Metabolic acid production (lactate) increases slightly.
  - Chronic respiratory alkalosis: Chronic alkalosis impairs the kidney's ability to excrete acid. Retained acid further lowers serum HCO_3. More complete compensation. Duration longer than 2 weeks is associated with alkalemia. Greater duration may elicit normal pH. Only acid-base disturbance compensation in which pH may return to normal.

The causes of respiratory alkalosis are listed in Table 52.8. Table 52.9 contains common clinical situations in which more than one primary acid-base problem presents, that is, a mixed disorder.

A few clues may be helpful in assessing the presence of a mixed acid-base disturbance:

- Normal pH (with exception of respiratory alkalosis). With the sole exception of chronic respiratory alkalosis, a normal pH value in the setting of an abnormal P_{CO_2}, or bicarbonate concentration signifies a mixed disturbance; compensation rarely corrects the pH to normal. The more severe the primary disorder, the less effective the compensatory mechanism at returning the pH to normal.

Table 52.8.   Causes of Respiratory Alkalosis

Hypoxia
- Decreased inspired oxygen tension
- Ventilation-perfusion inequality
- Hypotension
- Severe anemia

CNS-mediated
- Voluntary hyperventilation
- Neurologic disease: cerebrovascular accident (infarction, hemorrhage), infection (encephalitis, meningitis), trauma, tumor
- Pharmacologic and hormonal stimulation: salicylates, dinitrophenol, nicotine, xanthines, pressor hormones, pregnancy
- Hepatic failure
- Gram-negative septicemia
- Postmetabolic acidosis
- Anxiety-hyperventilation syndrome
- Heat exposure

Pulmonary disease
- Interstitial lung disease
- Pneumonia
- Pulmonary embolism
- Pulmonary edema

Mechanical overventilation

From Cohen JJ, Kassirer JP. Acid-base chemistry and buffering. In Acid/Base. Boston, Mass, Little Brown & Co, 1980:361.

Table 52.9.   Syndromes Commonly Associated With Mixed Acid-Base Disorders

Clinical Syndrome	Metabolic Alkalosis	Metabolic Acidosis	Respiratory Alkalosis	Respiratory Acidosis
Cardiopulmonary arrest	t	+	t	+
Severe pulmonary edema		+		+
Ethylene glycol + pulmonary edema		+		+
Methanol + hypoventilation		+		+
Severe hypophosphatemia		+		+
Recent alcohol binge	V	+	+	
Sepsis		+	+	
Severe liver failure	V/d	+	+	
Salicylate intoxication		+	+	
Pregnancy	V		+	
Renal failure	V	+		
Diabetic ketoacidosis	V	+		
COPD	d			+
Severe hypokalemia	+			+
Critically ill patients	V/d	+	+	+

V = vomiting
d = diuretics
t = treatment-induced.

Above are presented some clinical syndromes in which mixed acid-base disturbances are commonly seen. If metabolic alkalosis from vomiting or diuretics is frequently seen in these disorders, this is denoted by ''V'' or ''d.''
Adapted from Cohen JJ, Kassirer JP. Clinical evaluation of acid-base disorders. In: Cohen JJ, Kassirer JP, eds. Acid-Base, Boston, Mass: Little Brown & Co, 1982:405.

Table 52.10.   Disorders of Serum Chloride Concentration

Hyperchloremia
- Proportionate increase in chloride and sodium
  - Dehydration
- Disproportionate increase in chloride compared with sodium
  - Hyperchloremic metabolic acidosis
  - Renal compensation for primary respiratory alkalosis

Hypochloremia
- Proportionate decrease in chloride and sodium
  - Overhydration
- Disproportionate decrease in chloride as compared to sodium
  - Metabolic alkalosis
  - Renal compensation for primary respiratory acidosis

- P_{CO_2} + HCO_3 deviating in opposite directions–The P_{CO_2} and serum HCO_3^- concentration always deviate in the same direction in simple acid-base disorders. If they deviate in opposite directions, a mixed abnormality is present.
- pH change in the opposite direction for a known primary disorder–A pH change in the opposite direction to that predicted for a known primary disorder signifies a mixed disturbance.

The chloride and potassium concentrations can also provide clues to the underlying acid-base disorder. If the chloride concentration changes in proportion to sodium, it reflects a change in hydration (Table 52.10). However, if chloride changes in excess of serum sodium, the cause is an acid-base disorder, with hyperchloremia suggesting an acidosis and hypochloremia suggesting an alkalosis. Similarly, in a very general sense, hyperkalemia is associated with acidosis and hypokalemia is associated with alkalosis.

The approach to the patient with acid-base disorder is summarized as follows:

- Take a careful history: vomiting, diabetes, diarrhea, ingestion of toxin, sepsis.
- Perform a thorough physical examination: fever, signs of volume depletion, respiratory rate and pattern, blood pressure.
- Determine electrolytes: Na, K, CI, HCO_3.
- Calculate anion gap.
- Note that $\Delta AG = \Delta HCO_3$ in a simple disorder.
- Check internal consistencies of arterial blood gases.
- Look for clues of mixed disorder (Table 52.11).
- Check nonelectrolyte laboratory results: creatinine (renal failure), glucose (diabetes), hematocrit (volume depletion), and ketones, lactate.

Table 52.11. Representative Examples of Mixed Acid-Base Disorders

Type of Mixed Disorder	Example #	Illustrative		Laboratory			Profile		Clinical Circumstance
		pH	PaCO₂ mm Hg	HCO₃⁻	Na⁺	mEq/L K⁺	Cl⁻	Anion Gap	
Metabolic acidosis and respiratory acidosis	1.	7.10	50	15	140	5.0	102	23	Renal failure and hypercapnic respiratory failure
	2.	6.99	34	8	141	6.0	105	28	Cardiopulmonary arrest
Metabolic alkalosis and respiratory alkalosis	3.	7.69	30	35	134	4.0	84	15	Hepatic failure and nasogastric suction
	4.	7.60	40	38	131	3.6	77	16	CHF and diuretics
Metabolic alkalosis and respiratory acidosis	5.	7.44	55	36	135	3.8	84	15	COPD and diuretics
	6.	7.45	48	32	133	4.2	85	16	ARDS and acetate-rich TPN
Metabolic acidosis and respiratory alkalosis	7.	7.44	12	8	136	5.5	106	22	Renal failure and gram-negative septicemia
	8.	7.40	15	9	138	4.1	110	19	Salicylate intoxication
Metabolic acidosis and metabolic alkalosis	9.	7.43	39	25	132	3.7	84	23	Alcoholic liver disease and diuretics
	10.	7.37	35	20	138	4.0	93	25	DKA following NaHCO₃ therapy
Respiratory acidosis and respiratory alkalosis	11.	7.54	41	34	140	3.8	93	13	COPD under mechanical ventilation
	12.	7.68	28	32	137	3.5	91	14	COPD under mechanical hyperventilation
Respiratory acidosis, metabolic acidosis, and metabolic alkalosis	13.	7.38	57	33	134	4.7	77	24	COPD, diuretics, and shock
Respiratory alkalosis, metabolic acidosis, and metabolic alkalosis	14.	7.43	25	16	135	3.2	97	22	CHF, diuretics, and shock
Hyperchloremic and high anion gap metabolic acidosis	15.	7.12	16	5	137	3.6	114	18	DKA with adequate salt and water balance
Acute on chronic respiratory acidosis	16.	7.22	80	32	141	4.3	99	10	COPD and therapy with O₂-rich mixtures
Acute on chronic respiratory alkalosis	17.	7.54	12	10	132	3.2	107	15	Alcoholic liver disease and cerebral bleeding
Acute on chronic respiratory acidosis and metabolic acidosis	18.	7.09	65	19	136	3.3	105	12	COPD and diarrhea
Mixed high anion gap metabolic acidosis and respiratory acidosis	19.	7.18	44	16	133	5.7	100	17	Hepatic, renal, and pulmonary failure
Mixed high anion gap metabolic acidosis and metabolic alkalosis	20.	7.36	31	17	132	4.0	89	26	Alcoholic liver disease, vomiting, and lactic acidosis
	21.	7.40	40	24	143	5.5	95	24	DKA and lactic acidosis following bicarbonate therapy

Anion gap is calculated as $[Na^+] - ([Cl^-] + [HCO_3^-])$.

CHF = congestive heart failure; COPD = chronic obstructive pulmonary disease; ARDS = adult respiratory distress syndrome; TPN = total parenteral nutrition; DKA = diabetic ketoacidosis.

SUGGESTED READINGS

1. Emmett M, Seldin DW: Clinical syndromes of metabolic acidosis and metabolic alkalosis. In: Seldin DW, Giebisch G, eds. The Kidney: Physiology and Pathophysiology. New York, NY: Raven Press; 1985:1567–1639.
   Comprehensive, but easily readible, review of metabolic acidosis and alkalosis.

2. Narins RG, Emmett M: Simple and mixed acid-base disorders: a practical approach. Medicine 1980;59(3):161–186.
   Classic review of all acid-base disorders. This is old, but excellent.

3. Cooper DJ, Walley KR, Wiggs BR, et al: Bicarbonate does not improve hemodynamics in critically ill patients who have lactic acidosis. Ann Intern Med 1990;112:492–498.
   Prospective, randomized trial concluding that correction of acidemia does not improve hemodynamics in the ICU.

4. Narins RG, Cohen JJ: Bicarbonate therapy for organic acidosis: the case for its continued use. Ann Intern Med 1987;106:615–618.
   Good editorial reviewing the pros and cons of bicarbonate therapy.

5. Fulop M: Serum potassium in lactic acidosis and ketoacidosis. N Engl J Med 1979;300(19):1087–1089.
   Excellent review of the association between hyperkalemia and acidemia.

6. Gabow PA, Kaehny WD, Fennessey PV, et al: Diagnostic importance of an increased serum anion gap. N Engl J Med 1980;303:854–858.
   The cause of a high anion gap acidosis was studied in 57 patients hospitalized

7. Hood VL, Tannen RL: Lactic acidosis. Kidney 1989;22(1):1–6.
   Good review of the pathogenesis clinical causes and potential therapies for lactic acidosis.

8. Adrogue HJ, Wilson H, Boyd AE, et al: Plasma acid-base patterns in diabetic ketoacidosis. N Engl J Med 1982;307:1603–1610.
   In this paper 196 admissions for diabetic ketoacidosis are analyzed. The transition from a high anion gap to a hyperchloremic acidosis is well-described.

9. Jacobson HR, Seldin DW: On the generation, maintenance, and correction of metabolic alkalosis. Am J Physiol 1983;245:F425–432.
   An excellent review of the basic pathophysiology of metabolic alkalosis.

10. Wilson RF, Binkley LE, Sabo FM, et al: Electrolyte and acid-base changes with massive blood transfusions. Am Surg 1992;58:535–545.
    The impact of massive blood transfusions on acid-base status in 471 patients is analyzed.

11. Adams SL: Alcoholic ketoacidosis. Emerg Med Clin North Am 1990;(4):749–760.
    An excellent review of this unfortunate commonly seen entity.

12. Mecher C, Rackow EC, Astiz ME, et al: Unaccounted for anion in metabolic acidosis during severe sepsis in humans. Crit Care Med 1991;19:705–711.
    In this study of 30 ICU patients with the presence of an unidentified anion accounting for a portion of the anion gap is documented.

13. Rodriguez-Soriano J, Vallo A: Renal tubular acidosis. Pediatr Nephrol 1990;4:268–275.
    An excellent discussion of the use of the urinary anion gap.

14. Rothstein M, Obialo C, Hruska KA: Renal tubular acidosis. Endocrinol Metab Clin North Am 1990;19(4):869–887.
    A review of the pathogenesis and clinical approach to patients with renal tubular acidosis.

15. McLaughlin ML, Kassirer JP: Rational treatment of acid-base disorders. Drugs 1990;39(6):841–855.
    An overview of the different causes and potential therapies of common acid-base disorders.

16. Wrenn K: The delta (D) gap: An approach to mixed acid-base disorders. Ann Emerg Med 1990;19:1310–1313.
    A review of the concept of delta (D) anion gap with sample problems.

17. Brimioulle S, Kahn RJ: Effects of metabolic alkalosis on pulmonary gas exchange. Am Rev Respir Dis 1990;141:1185–1189.
    A detailed analysis of the impact of metabolic alkalosis on pulmonary /gas exchange in 8 critically ill patients.

Board Simulation: Nephrology and Hypertension

Martin J. Schreiber, Jr.

QUESTIONS

1. A 26-year-old black man presents with edema of the lower extremity, blood pressure of 170/98 mm Hg, microscopic hematuria (5–10 red blood cells [RBCs] per high-powered field [HPF]), 10.8 g of urinary protein in 24 hours, serum creatinine level of 2.9 mg/dL, and a history of heroin abuse. Potential differential diagnoses in this patient include all of the following except:

   a. Human immunodeficiency virus (HIV) nephropathy.
   b. Focal segmental glomerulosclerosis.
   c. Heroin nephropathy.
   d. Minimal change glomerulonephritis.

2. Match (in order) the most appropriate clinical entities with the following serologic markers:

   ### Serologic Markers

   1. Anti-DNase B
   2. Hepatitis B e-antigen
   3. *Escherichia coli* (verotoxin) serotype 0157:H7
   4. Antiglomerular basement membrane (anti-GBM)
   5. Cytoplasmic antineutrophil cytoplasmic antibody (C-ANCA)

   ### Clinical Entities

   A. Goodpasture's syndrome
   B. Hemolytic uremic syndrome
   C. Poststreptococcal glomerulonephritis
   D. Membranous glomerulonephritis
   E. Wegener's granulomatosis

Which of the following is the correct sequence?
   a. A, B, E, D, C.
   b. C, D, B, A, E.
   c. B, A, C, D, E.
   d. E, D, C, B, A.

3. A 24-year-old black man presents with hematuria (i.e., tea-colored urine), arthralgias, and a heart murmur. The patient was recently discharged from military service, and he developed an upper respiratory infection 10 days ago. Results of the physical examination are a swollen and tender right wrist and left elbow, prominent cervical/submandibular nodes, 2/6 systolic ejection murmur, and 2 + edema. Laboratory results are as follows:

   Urinalysis: specific gravity, 1.013; glucose, 0; pH, 6.0; protein, 3 + ; 20 RBC/HPF; 3–5 RBC casts; 5–10 white blood cells/HPF.
   Serologies: Low plasma C3 level; creatinine, 2.2 mg/dL, glucose, 51 mg/dL; increased rheumatoid factor level; FeNa, 71%; positive cryoglobulins.
   The most likely cause for this clinical scenario is:

   a. Membranous glomerulonephritis.
   b. Wegener's granulomatosis.
   c. Poststreptococcal glomerulonephritis.
   d. Acute tubular necrosis.
   e. Fanconi's syndrome.

4. A 26-year-old male executive presents to the outpatient department with increasing muscle weakness over the past 6 days. He received a living-related transplant from his mother 3 months ago. Neurologic examination reveals a decrease in muscle strength of 4.2/5 in the lower extremities, and his blood pressure

is 108/70 mm Hg. Laboratory results are as follows: serum creatinine, 1.1 mg/dL; phosphorous, 2.1 mg/dL; hemoglobin, 9.1 g/dL; hematocrit, 26.8% (with fragmented RBCs noted on peripheral smear); LDH, 342 mg/dL.

All of the following are causes for hypophosphatemia except:

a. Hyperparathyroidism.
b. Renal tubular defect.
c. Postrenal transplant.
d. Alcohol withdrawal.
e. Metabolic acidosis.

5. In patients with end-stage renal disease, bone radiography may reveal subperiosteal erosions of the phalanges, erosions of the proximal end of the tibia, and a mottled and granular (i.e., salt-and-pepper) appearance of the skull. These radiographic changes are consistent with all of the following abnormalities except:

a. Skeletal resistance to PTH.
b. Increased degradation of PTH.
c. Hypocalcemia, hyperphosphatemia.
d. Malabsorption of calcium.
e. Decreased 1,25-(OH_2)-D_3.

6. Risk factors for calcium nephrolithiasis include all of the following except:

a. High-protein diet.
b. Hyperoxaluria.
c. Hypocitraturia.
d. Hyperuricosuria.
e. High urine volume.

7. Specific diseases associated with hypercalciuria (i.e., > 300 mg per 24 hours) include all of the following except:

a. Vitamin A toxicity.
b. Hyperparathyroidism.
c. Sarcoidosis.
d. Vitamin D toxicity.
e. Hyperphosphatemia.

8. Match (in order) the description of the crystal with its appropriate composition:

Crystal

1. ''Coffin lid''
2. Envelope-shaped
3. ''Hexagonal'' benzene rings
4. Needles

Composition

A. Calcium oxalate
B. Triple phosphate
C. Cystine crystals
D. Sulfa drugs
E. Calcium carbonate

Which of the following sequences best matches the crystal descriptions?

a. B, A, C, D.
b. D, B, A, C.
c. A, B, C, D.
d. D, C, B, A.

9. A 50-year-old man who has been on hemodialysis for 12 years secondary to adult-onset diabetes presents to the emergency room with diffuse bone pain, upper leg muscle weakness, and anemia despite erythropoietin. Laboratory results are normal alkaline phosphatase level, serum calcium level of 10.9 mg/dL, and normal PTH level. The patient's past medical history is significant for parathyroidectomy 2 years ago.

Which of the following diagnoses is most consistent with this clinical scenario?

a. Sepsis.
b. Secondary hyperparathyroidism.
c. Sickle-cell disease.
d. Aluminum bone disease.
e. Erythropoietin intoxication syndrome.

10. All of the following clinical conditions are associated with papillary necrosis except:

a. Diabetes mellitus.
b. Analgesic nephropathy.
c. Sickle cell disease.
d. Pyelonephritis.
e. Penicillin allergy.

11. Which of the following statements regarding autosomal dominant polycystic kidney disease (PCKD) is false?

a. Gene linkage permits in utero PCKD diagnosis.
b. Before 30 years of age, 11 to 17% of patients have a normal renal ultrasound.
c. Before 60 years of age, 50% of patients develop end-stage renal disease.
d. Five to ten percent of patients have intracranial aneurysms.
e. High cyst penetration occurs with all antibiotics.

12. Indices of oliguric acute renal failure include all of the following except:

a. Urinary H_2O, <350 mOsm/kg.
b. Urinary Na, >40 mEq/L.
c. Urine/plasma creatinine, <20

d. FeNa, >1

e. Negative urinary anion gap.

13. Uric acid nephropathy occurs in patients with all of the following conditions except:

   a. Myelolymphoproliferative malignancies with tumor lysis.
   b. Lesch-Nyhan syndrome.
   c. Rhabdomyolysis, crush injury.
   d. Sarcoidosis.
   e. Metastatic breast cancer with tumor necrosis.

14. The differential diagnosis of pulmonary hemorrhage and glomerulonephritis includes all of the following except:

   a. Goodpasture's syndrome.
   b. Wegener's granulomatosis.
   c. Poststreptococcal glomerulonephropathy.
   d. Anaphylactoid Henoch-Schönlein purpura.
   e. Cryoglobulinemia.

15. Renal manifestations of HIV infection include:

   a. Hyponatremia.
   b. Tubuloreticular inclusions.
   c. Focal segmental glomerular sclerosis.
   d. Acute tubular necrosis.
   e. All of the above.

16. Which of the following statements regarding pregnancy, renal disease, and urinary tract infection are false?

   a. Of patients with asymptomatic bacteriuria, 30% develop pyelonephritis.
   b. Pyelonephritis is associated with intrauterine fetal death.
   c. Asymptomatic bacteriuria should be treated with single-dose antibiotics.
   d. Patients with symptomatic pyelonephritis should be hospitalized.
   e. Long-term suppressive treatment should be used after recovery.

17. Epidemiologic aspects of hemolytic uremic syndrome include all of the following except:

   a. Temperate climate.
   b. Age.
   c. Antibiotic class.
   d. Bovine fecal contamination.
   e. Unpasteurized milk.

18. Drugs reported to cause hypertension include all of the following except:

   a. Birth control pills.
   b. Erythropoietin.
   c. Cocaine.

d. Inhaled fluorinated steroids.

e. Penicillamine.

19. All of the following laboratory test results support the diagnosis of pheochromocytoma except:

   a. Serum epinephrine and norepinephrine, ≥2000 pg/mL.
   b. 24-hour urinary metanephrine, >2 mg.
   c. Serum potassium, >3.0 mEq/L.
   d. 24-hour urinary vanillylmandelic acid, >7 mg.
   e. Suppression of plasma catecholamine, 500 pg/mL (55%).

Answers and Discussion

1. d (minimal change glomerulonephritis).

   This type of glomerulonephritis usually is not progressive, and it is uncommonly associated with hematuria. Patients typically present with periorbital and peripheral edema related to the proteinuria. Some patients can have mild-to-moderate azotemia, which can be related to intravascular volume depletion.

   The other answers are more consistent with this patient's presentation. In focal segmental glomerulonephritis, nephrotic-range proteinuria usually is detectable at presentation. Twenty to thirty percent of patients have hypertension, and 25 to 75% have microscopic hematuria. One-third of patients demonstrate a decreased glomerular filtration rate at presentation. Common clinical features in HIV nephropathy include heavy proteinuria, renal insufficiency, large and echogenic kidneys at ultrasonography, rapid progression to end stage, and strong predilection for blacks. Heroin nephropathy usually results in focal segmental glomerulosclerosis, which occurs in intravenous drug users.

2. b (C, D, B, A, E).

   Antibodies against extracellular products of streptococci, antistreptolysin, antistreptokinase (ASKase), antihyaluronidase (AHase), antideoxyribonuclease B (ADNase B), and antininicotyladenine dinucleotidase (ANADase) can be seen in patients with poststreptococcal glomerulonephritis. Hepatitis B surface and e-antigen have been identified in the immune complexes of patients with a history of hepatitis and membranous glomerulonephritis. Epidemic hemolytic uremic syndrome occurs in patients with hemorrhagic diarrhea caused by infection with specific serotypes of *E. coli,* and injury to the kidneys and lungs can be mediated by anti-GBM. ANCA are autoantibodies against proteins within the granules of neutrophils and the lysosomes of monocytes. Approximately 90% of patients with active, untreated Wegener's granulomatosis have C-ANCA.

3. c (poststreptococcal glomerulonephritis).

   The diagnosis of poststreptococcal glomerulonephritis should be entertained on the basis of patient history, urinary findings, and hypocomplementemia (i.e., low plasma C3 level). The antistreptolysin titer is elevated in approximately

75% of patients with pharyngitis. The low plasma C3 level occurs during the first week, and elevated rheumatoid factor titers and circulating cryoglobulins can be found in most patients. Membranous glomerulonephritis, Wegener's granulomatosis, acute tubular necrosis, and Fanconi's syndrome are not associated with low plasma C3 levels. Other entities associated with low C3 level, with or without a low C4 level, include membranoproliferative glomerulonephritis, cryoglobulinemia, systemic lupus erythematosus, subacute bacterial endocarditis, acute poststreptococcal glomerulonephritis, hemolytic uremic syndrome, thrombotic thrombocytopenic purpura, severe malnutrition, and hepatic failure.

4. e (metabolic acidosis).

Both respiratory and metabolic alkalosis may induce hypophosphatemia, and extracellular alkalosis results in intracellular alkalosis, which causes phosphorous to shift into the intracellular space (with subsequent hypophosphatemia). Persistent elevation in parathyroid hormone (PTH) levels and an intrinsic renal tubular defect in phosphorus reabsorption result in post-transplant hypophosphatemia. Renal tubular acidosis and hypokalemia are associated with increased urinary excretion of phosphorus, and the poor oral intake associated with alcohol withdrawal can lead to hypophosphatemia.

5. b (increased degradation of PTH).

Radiographic changes seen in patients with chronic renal failure are accompanied by serologic alterations, which include hypocalcemia, hyperphosphatemia, low 1,25-vitamin D_3 levels, and decreased absorption of calcium from the gastrointestinal tract. Renal synthesis of calcitriol worsens with advancing renal failure, and calcitriol deficiency may lead to impaired gastrointestinal absorption of calcium and negative calcium imbalance. Degradation of PTH is not increased in patients with chronic renal failure.

6. e (high urine volume).

Risk factors for calcium nephrolithiasis include hypercalcemia, decreased tubular calcium reabsorption (i.e., renal tubular acidosis), low urine volume, loop diuretics, protein loading, phosphate depletion, hyperuricosuria, hypocitraturia, and hyperoxaluria.

7. e (hyperphosphatemia).

Hypercalciuria usually is idiopathic, but it can be seen in patients with primary hyperparathyroidism, renal tubular acidosis, sarcoidosis, or familial hypercalciuric syndromes. The mechanism of hypercalcemia in sarcoidosis is an increase in both intestinal calcium absorption and bone reabsorption. Hypercalcemia can occur in patients with hypervitaminosis A because of enhanced bone reduction.

8. a (B, A, C, D).

Those crystals found in alkaline urine include triple phosphate (i.e., ammonium, magnesium, phosphate), amorphous phosphates, calcium carbonate, calcium phosphate, and ammonium barrettes. Struvite crystals (i.e., triple phosphate) are prismatic or "coffin lid" in appearance. Those crystals fre-

quently found in acidic urine are uric acid, calcium oxalate, and amorphous urates. Cystine crystals are colorless, refractile, hexagonal plates with equal or unequal sides. Most sulfonamide drugs precipitate as sheaves of either clear or brown crystals, which are soluble in acetone.

9. d (aluminum bone disease).

Aluminum-containing antacids and calcium citrate increase the risk of aluminum accumulation and toxicity. Citrate augments the intestinal absorption of aluminum. The combination of an intact PTH level of less than 200 pg/mL (normal, <65 pg/mL) and an increment in serum aluminum of greater than 150 mg/L have excellent predictive value for aluminum bone disease. Features of aluminum-related bone disease include proximal muscle weakness, recurrent fractures, severe pain on any motion against gravity, serum calcium levels in the upper range of normal, PTH levels usually lower than expected for patients receiving dialysis (10–20% of patients consistent with osteitis fibrosa), and normal levels of 1,25-(OH)-D_3. Patients also demonstrate hypochromic microcytic anemia, with suboptimal response to erythropoietin.

10. e (penicillin allergy).

Renal papillary necrosis results from abnormalities of tubular interstitial nephropathy that are accompanied by compromised medullary blood flow, which produces ischemic necrosis in a portion of the renal medulla. Conditions commonly associated with renal papillary necrosis include diabetes mellitus, urinary tract obstruction, pyelonephritis, analgesic abuse, sickle-cell hemoglobinopathy, and infants with hypoxia and jaundice. Penicillin allergy has not been associated with renal papillary necrosis.

11. e (high cyst penetration occurs with all antibiotics).

In 90 to 95% of patients, PCKD results from a mutation on the short arm of chromosome 16. Genetic linkage studies may be performed to diagnose the PCKD in patients with a greater than 50% risk for this disorder (i.e., a sibling, child, or parent with the gene).

The sensitivity of ultrasonography in detecting this disorder is 22% for children younger than 10 years, and it increases to 86% in those from 20 to 30 years of age. Approximately 10 to 20% of patients with PCKD have intracranial aneurysms, and ruptured aneurysms occur more frequently in patients with a family history of hemorrhage.

Cyst infections should be treated with antibiotics that penetrate the cyst, such as trimethoprim-sulfamethoxazole, chloramphenicol, metronidazole, vancomycin, erythromycin, and clindamycin. Treatment should consist of a 6-week course. It is important to remember, however, that not all antibiotics have a high cyst penetration characteristic.

12. e (negative urinary anion gap).

A negative urinary anion gap (i.e., $Na^+ + K^+ - Cl^-$) indicates normal acidification and can be seen in patients with diarrhea. A positive value indicates impaired ammonium excretion, thus suggesting renal tubular acidosis. The most common indices depicting oliguric renal failure include answers a through d.

Urinary net charge equals $[Na^+ + K^+]_u$ minus $[Cl^-]$. Thus, if urinary NH_4^+ is increased, urinary Cl^- exceeds the $[Na^+ + K^+]$. This suggests an extrarenal cause for the acidosis (i.e., diarrhea, parenteral hyperalimentation with acidic amino acid). If the $[Na^+ + K^+]_u$ is greater than the $[Cl^-]_u$, the urinary NH_4^+ conservation is low, thus suggesting renal tubular acidosis.

The urinary anion gap is not used as an index of oliguric acute renal failure.

13. d (sarcoidosis).

Several hematologic malignancies are associated with excessive degradation of nucleic acids, which increases urate production. This can be prevented by alkalizing the urine and maintaining a low urinary acid concentration. Uric acid nephropathy is not seen with sarcoidosis. The main categories associated with uric acid nephropathy are myelolymphoproliferative malignancies with lysis; metastatic cancer of the breast, lungs, or stomach; rhabdomyolysis; seizures; thyrotoxicosis; and Lesch-Nyhan syndrome. Hypercalcemic nephropathy is seen with sarcoidosis and other granulomatous diseases.

14. c (poststreptococcal glomerulonephropathy).

The clinical picture of Goodpasture's syndrome can be seen in patients with other types of vasculitis, such as periarteritis nodosa or cryoglobulinemia (i.e., Meltzer's syndrome, Raynaud's phenomenon, thrombocytopenia, positive rheumatoid factor, circulating cryoglobulins). Anaphylactoid purpura may have pulmonary hemorrhage on occasion.

15. e (all of the above).

Of patients infected with HIV, 60% have low serum sodium levels because of volume depletion and dilute fluid replacement. The syndrome of inappropriate antidiuretic hormone can be seen in patients with pulmonary and intracranial diseases, including pneumocystosis, toxoplasmosis, and tuberculosis. Endothelial tubuloreticular inclusion bodies are a marker of HIV infection, and histologically, HIV may demonstrate findings similar to those of focal segmental glomerular sclerosis (FSG) (i.e., diffuse epithelial cell changes and prominent collapse of the glomerular tuft). Acute tubular necrosis in HIV infection can occur in patients with hypovolemia, shock, sepsis, and in those who are receiving nephrotoxic drugs. Drug-induced acute interstitial nephritis can be seen along with interstitial edema from malnutrition, proteinuria, and hypoalbuminemia. Hemolytic uremic syndrome also may be seen in patients with HIV.

16. c (asymptomatic bacteriuria should be treated with single-dose antibiotics).

Asymptomatic bacteriuria has been associated with babies who are small for gestational age. Of women with asymptomatic bacteria, 30% develop pyelonephritis, which is associated with intrauterine fetal death and with premature labor. All pregnant patients with symptomatic pyelonephritis should receive intravenous antibiotics and hydration. Single large-dose antibiotic therapy should not be used during pregnancy. Long-term suppressive therapy should be used after recovery from an acute event.

17. c (antibiotic class).

Several chemotherapeutic and other medications (e.g., cyclosporine, penicillin, metronidazole, penicillamine, sulfonamides, oral contraceptives) have been associated with hemolytic uremic syndrome. No specific antibiotic class has been consistently responsible for hemolytic uremic syndrome, however. Epidemics among younger populations have occurred in more temperate climates and resulted from fecal-contaminated meat and cider as well as from unpasteurized milk.

18. e (penicillamine).

Many drugs have been associated with hypertension, but penicillamine has not been associated with secondary hypertension. Hypertension due to erythropoietin results from a rise in systemic vascular resistance. Cocaine can cause tachycardia, chest pain, dilated pupils, combativeness, and an acute increase in blood pressure, but cocaine is less apt to cause chronic hypertension. Oral contraceptive medications can produce a rise in both systolic and diastolic blood pressure; oral contraceptives do not suppress renin release effectively. Estrogen administration results in enhanced synthesis and release of angiotensinogen from the liver. Anabolic steroids, inhaled fluorinated steroids, bromocriptine, cadmium, and lead induce hypertension.

19. e. (suppression of plasma catecholamine, 500 pg/ml [55%]).

Individuals experiencing a decrease in the plasma catecholamine level to 500 pg/mL or a suppression of greater than 50% most likely do not have a pheochromocytoma as the cause of their resistant hypertension. Increases in the serum catecholamine level to greater than 2000 pg/mL, urinary metanephrine values of more than 2 mg in 24 hours, serum potassium level of greater than 3 mEq/L, and urinary catecholamines (norepinephrine and epinephrine) of more than 100 mg per 24 hours support the diagnosis of pheochromocytoma. Scintigraphy with ^{131}I-labeled meta-iodobenzylguanidine (MIBG) can be used to localize a pheochromocytoma; computed tomography is a reliable method for preoperative localization.

SUGGESTED READINGS

QUESTION 1

Artero M, Biava C, Amend W, Tomlanovich S, Vincenti F. Recurrent focal glomerulosclerosis: natural history and response to treatment. Am J Med 1992;92:375–383.

Bourgoignie JJ. Renal complications of human immunodeficiency virus type I. Kidney Int 1990;37:1571–1584.

Cameron JS, Turner, DR, Ogg CS, et al. The nephrotic syndrome in adults with 'minimal change' glomerular lesion. Q J Med 1974;43:461–468.

Cunningham EE, Brentjens JR, Zielezny MA, et al. Heroin nephropathy: a clinical, pathologic, and epidemiologic study. Am J Med 1980;68:47–53.

Cantor ES, Kimmel PL, Bosch JP. Effect of race on the expression of age-associated nephropathy. Arch Intern Med 1991;151:125–128.

Kilcoyne MM, Gocke DJ, Meltzer JI, et al. Nephrotic syndrome in heroin addicts. Lancet 1972;1:17–20.

QUESTION 2

Glassock RJ. Secondary membranous glomerulonephritis. Nephrol Dial Transplant 1992;7:64–71.

Hellmark T, Johansson C, Weislander J. Characterization of anti-GBM antibodies involved in Goodpasture's syndrome. Kidney Int 1994;46:823–829.

Hoffman GS, Kerr GS, Leavitt RY, et al. Wegener glomerulomatosis: an analysis of 158 patients. Ann Intern Med 1992;116:488–498.

Howard AD, Moore J Jr, Gouge SF, et al. Routine serologic tests in the differential diagnosis of the adult nephrotic syndrome. Am J Kidney Dis 1990;15:24–30.

Johnson RJ, Couser WG. Hepatitis B infection and renal disease. Clinical, immunopathologic and therapeutic consideration. Kidney Int 1990;57:663–676.

Kallenberg CG, Brouwer E, Weening JJ, Cohen Tervaert JW. Anti-neutrophil cytoplasmic antibodies: current diagnostic and pathophysiological potential. Kidney Int 1994;46:1–15.

Kaplan BS, Thomson PD, DeChadarevian JP. The hemolytic uremic syndrome. Pediatr Clin North Am 1976;23:761–777.

Rodriquez-Iturbe B. Epidemic poststreptococcal glomerulonephritis. Kidney Int 1984;25:129–136.

QUESTION 3

Baldwin DS, Gluck MC, Schact RG, Gallo G. The long-term course of poststreptococcal glomerulonephritis. Ann Intern Med 1974;80:342–358.

Hebert LA, Cosio FG, Neff JC. Diagnostic significance of hypocomplementemia. Kidney Int 1991;39:811–821.

Madaio MP, Harrington JT. Current concepts. The diagnosis of acute glomerulonephritis. N Engl J Med 1983;309;1299–1302.

Roth KS, Foreman JW, Segal S. The Fanconi syndrome and mechanisms of tubular transport dysfunction. Kidney Int 1981;20:705–716.

QUESTION 4

Kreisberg RA. Phosphorus deficiency in hypophosphatemia. Hosp Pract 1977;12:121–128.

Larsson K, Rebel K, Sorbo B. Severe hypophosphatemia: a hospital survey. Acta Med Scand 1983;214:221–223.

Lentz RD, Brown DM, Kjellstrand CM. Treatment of severe hypophosphatemia. Ann Intern Med 1978;89:941–944.

QUESTION 5

Hruska KA, Teitelbaum SL. Mechanisms of disease: renal osteodystrophy. N Engl J Med 1995;333:166–174.

QUESTION 6

Coe FL, Parks JH, Asplin JR. Pathogenesis and treatment of kidney stones. N Engl J Med 1992;327:1141–1152.

Preminger GM. Renal calculi: pathogenesis, diagnosis and medical therapy. Semin Nephrol 1992;12:200–216.

QUESTION 7

Lemann J Jr, Worcester EM, Gray FW. Hypercalciuria and stones. Am J Kidney Dis 1991;17:386–391.

Levy FL, Adams-Huet B, Pak CYC. Ambulatory evaluation of nephrolithiasis: an update of a 1980 protocol. Am J Med 1995;98:50–59.

QUESTION 8

Greenberg AM. Urinanalysis. In: Primary kidney diseases: National Kidney Foundation. San Diego: Academics Press, 1994:23–33.

Schumann GB, Schweitzer SC. Examination of the urine. In: Henry JB, ed. Clinical diagnosis and management by laboratory methods. 18th ed. Philadelphia: WB Saunders, 1991:387–444.

QUESTION 9

Andress DL, Maloney NA, Endres DB, et al. Aluminum-associated bone disease in chronic renal failure: high prevalence in long-term dialysis population. J Bone Miner Res 1986;1: 391–398.

Sherrard DJ, Hercz G, Pei EY, et al. The spectrum of bone disease in end-stage renal failure: an evolving disorder. Kidney Int 1993;43:436–442.

QUESTION 10

Eknoyan G, Qunibi WY, Grissom RT, et al. Renal papillary necrosis: an update. Medicine 1982;61:55–73.

Hare WSC, Poynter JD. The radiology of renal papillary necrosis as seen in algae nephropathy. Clin Radiol 1974;25: 423–443.

QUESTION 11

Davies F, Coles GA, Harper PS, et al. Polycystic kidney disease re-evaluated: a population-based study. Q J Med 1991; 79:459–460.

Fick GN, Johnson AM, Strain JD, et al. Characteristics of very early onset autosomal dominant polycystic kidney disease. J Am Soc Nephrol 1993;3:1863–1870.

Gabow PA. Autosomal dominant polycystic kidney disease. N Engl J Med 1993;329:332–342.

Gabow PA, Bennett WM. Renal manifestations: complication management and long-term outcome of autosomal dominant polycystic kidney disease. Semin Nephrol 1991;11:643–652.

Mochizuki T, Wu G, Hayashi T, et al. PKD-2: a gene for polycystic kidney disease that encodes an integral membrane protein. Science 1996;272:1339–1342.

Parfrey PS, Bear JC, Morgan J, et al. The diagnosis and prognosis of autosomal dominant polycystic kidney disease. N Engl J Med 1990;323:1085–1090.

Sklar AH, Caruana RJ, Lammers JE, et al. Renal infections in autosomal dominant polycystic kidney disease. Am J Kidney Dis 1987;10:81–88.

QUESTION 12

Dickson BS, Anderson RJ. Non-oliguric acute renal failure. Am J Kidney Dis 1985;6:71–80.

Espinel CH, Gregory AW. Differential diagnosis of acute renal failure. Clin Nephrol 1980;13:73–77.

Goldstein MB, Bear R, Richardson RM, et al. The urine anion gap: a clinically useful index of ammonium excretion. Am J Med Sci 1986;292:198–202.

Kamel KS, Ethier JH, Richardson RM. Urine electrolytes and osmolality. When and how to use them. Am J Nephrol 1990; 10:89–102.

Miller TR, Anderson RJ, Linas SL, et al. Urinary diagnostic indices in acute renal failure: a prospective study. Ann Intern Med 1978;889:47–50.

QUESTION 13

Frei E, et al. Renal complications of neoplastic disease. J Chronic Dis 1963;16:757–776.

Kelton J, Kelley WN, Holmes EW. A rapid method for the detection of uric acid nephropathy. Arch Intern Med 1978; 138:612–615.

Kjelstrand CM, Cambell DC II, von Hartitzsch B, et al. Hyperuricemic acute renal failure. Arch Intern Med 1974;133: 349–359.

QUESTION 14

Boyce NW, Holdsworth SR. Pulmonary manifestations of the clinical syndrome of acute glomerulonephritis and lung hemorrhage. Am J Kidney Dis 1986;8:31–36.

Salant DJ. Immunopathogenesis of crescentic glomerulonephritis and lung purpura. Kidney Int 1987;32:408–425.

QUESTION 15

Berns JS, Cohen RM, Stumacher RJ, Rudnick MR. Renal aspects of therapy for human immunodeficiency virus and associated opportunistic infection. J Am Soc Nephrol 1991; 1:1061–1081.

Seney FD Jr, Burns DK, Silva FG. Acquired immunodeficiency syndrome and the kidney. Am J Kidney Dis 1990;16: 1–13.

Humphreys MH. Human immunodeficiency virus associated nephritis. Kidney Int 1995;48:311–320.

Masharani U, Schambelan M. The endocrine complications of acquired immunodeficiency syndrome. Adv Intern Med 1993;38:323–336.

Rao TK. Clinical features of human immunodeficiency virus associated nephropathy. Kidney Int 1991;35(Suppl): S13–S18.

QUESTION 16

Bint AJ, Hill D. Bacteriuria of pregnancy: an update on significance, diagnosis and management. J Antimicrob Chemother 1994;33(Suppl A):93–97.

Cunningham FG, Lucas MJ. Urinary tract infections complicating pregnancy. Clin Obstet Gynecol 1994;8:353–373.

QUESTION 17

Cleary TG, Lopez EL. The shiga-like toxin-producing *Escherichia coli* in hemolytic uremic syndrome. Pediatr Infect Dis J 1989;8:720–724.

Goldstein MH, Churg J, Strauss L, et al. Hemolytic uremic syndrome. Nephron 1979;23:263–272.

Kahn SI, Tolkan SR, Kothari O, et al. Spontaneous recovery of the hemolytic uremic syndrome with prolonged renal and neurologic manifestations. Nephron 1982;32:188–191.

Remuzzi G, Ruggenenti P, Berhani T. Thrombotic microangiopathies. In: Tisher CC, Brenner BM, eds. Renal pathology. 2nd ed. Philadelphia: JB Lippincott, 1994:1154–1184.

Schieppati A, Ruggenenti P, Cornejo RP, et al., for the Italian Registry of Hemolytic Uremic Syndrome. Renal function at hospital admission as a prognostic factor in adult hemolytic uremic syndrome. J Am Soc Nephrol 1992;2:1640–1644.

QUESTION 18

Abraham PA, Opsahl JA, Keshaviah PR, et al. Body fluid spaces and blood pressure in hemodialysis patients during amelioration of anemia with erthyropoietin. Am J Kidney Dis 1990;16:438–446.

Buckner FS, Eschbach JW, Haley NR, et al. Hypertension following erthyropoietin therapy in anemic hemodialysis patients. Am J Hypertens 1990;3:947–955.

Grossman E, Messerli FH. High blood pressure: a side effect of drugs, poisons and food. Arch Intern Med 1995;155:450–460.

Harris PWR. Malignant hypertension associated with oral contraceptives. Lancet 1969;2:466–467.

Hollander JE. Management of cocaine-associated myocardial ischemia. N Engl J Med 1995;333:1267–1272.

Saruta T, Saade GA, Kaplan NM. A possible mechanism for hypertension induced by oral contraceptives. Arch Intern Med 1970;126:621–626.

QUESTION 19

Bravo EL. Evolving concepts in the pathophysiology, diagnosis and treatment of pheochromocytoma. Endocrine Reviews 1994;15:356–368.

Bravo EL. Pheochromocytoma: New concepts and future trends. Kidney Int 1991;40:544–546.

Grossman E, Goldstein DS, Hoffman A, Keiser HR. Glucagon and clonidine testing in the diagnosis of pheochromocytoma. Hypertension 1991;17:733–741.

Gastroenterology

C • H • A • P • T • E • R

54A

Liver Disease: Hepatology

Kevin D. Mullen

This chapter reviews viral hepatitis, drug-induced hepatic injury, and selected inherited metabolic liver diseases. It is not exhaustive, focusing rather only on essentials. Readers are assumed to have some basic knowledge of these topics already. Sherlock and Dooley's *Diseases of the Liver and Biliary System* is recommended as the best text for additional information.

VIRAL HEPATITIS

ACUTE VIRAL HEPATITIS

Hepatitis A, B, C, delta (or D), and E all can present with acute viral hepatitis syndromes. Most often, these involve a prodrome of malaise, anorexia, mild fever, nausea, and some vomiting that usually is not distinguishable from other viral syndromes. If jaundice appears, it quickly becomes obvious that acute viral hepatitis is a likely diagnosis. Great caution should be taken to ensure the problem is not caused by drug-induced liver injury or bacterial cholangitis. In patients with acute viral hepatitis, transaminase levels typically are at least 10 to 20 times normal during the symptomatic phase of the illness. Current serologic testing has made the diagnosis relatively easy:

- *Acute Hepatitis A:* Hepatitis A immunoglobulin (Ig) M antibody must be positive.
- *Acute Hepatitis B:* Hepatitis B IgM antibody to core and hepatitis B surface antigen must be positive.
- *Acute Hepatitis C:* Hepatitis C antibody only becomes positive at 4 to 6 weeks.
- *Acute Delta Hepatitis:* Delta antibody and Hepatitis B surface antigen positive.
- *Acute Hepatitis E:* Usually in patients from high-risk areas (e.g., Pakistan/Bangladesh) in whom other tests

are negative. (The Centers for Disease Control and Prevention offer a kit for diagnosis.)

Some other atypical possibilities also should be considered. First, in severe/fulminant acute hepatitis B, patients can be surface antigen negative and e antigen negative (e antigen implies that whole virus is present). This happens because of a grossly overaggressive immune response. Hepatitis B virus will be cleared, but the liver is destroyed. IgM antibody to core may be the only positive test. In patients with gross acute hepatitis, acute hepatitis B should be considered even if the surface antigen test is negative.

Another scenario is acute hepatitis C. Though fairly rare, the appearance of antibodies to hepatitis C may be delayed for 4 to 6 weeks after the onset of high transaminase levels. Serum hepatitis C RNA or retesting for hepatitis C antibody are the best options for further tests in patients with seronegative acute hepatitis.

Sequelae to acute viral hepatitis include:

1. Protracted jaundice. Most often, viral hepatitis is self-limiting, but jaundice can persist for months in approximately 10% of patients even though transaminase levels normalize. This is seen especially in patients with hepatitis A.
2. Recurrent attack of acute hepatitis. In 10 to 20% of patients, hepatitis A can be notable for a relapse occurring with high transaminase levels. Stool is once again positive for the virus (by electron microscopy). This resolves without sequelae.
3. Evolution to chronic hepatitis. This never happens in patients with hepatitis A or E. It does, however, occur in 5 to 10% of those with hepatitis B, 70 to 85% of those with hepatitis C, and perhaps, 30 to 50% of those with delta hepatitis.
4. Fulminant viral hepatitis occurs in 0.1% of patients

573

with hepatitis A, 1% of those with hepatitis B, less than 1% of those with hepatitis C, 3% of those with delta hepatitis, and less than 1% of those with hepatitis E (except during pregnancy, in which there may be a 20% mortality rate).

CHRONIC VIRAL HEPATITIS

Chronic Hepatitis B

All patients with chronic hepatitis B have hepatitis B surface antigen. Active liver injury, as evidenced by raised transaminase levels, is attributable to hepatitis B if intact hepatitis B virus is present in the blood. Three tests are available for this: serum hepatitis B DNA, DNA polymerase activity in blood, and hepatitis B e antigen. The last test is used most frequently. Remember that liver injury during hepatitis B infection predominantly results from immune attack on viral-infected cells.

If there is no intact virus, there should be no hepatitis. When a patient has hepatitis B surface antigen–positive results and raised transaminase levels but no evidence of intact virus in the blood (e.g., no hepatitis B e antigen, no hepatitis B DNA), then other causes for the liver injury should be sought. In patients with a history of intravenous drug use, delta hepatitis should be high on the list of considerations; other possibilities are hepatitis A and C or conditions such as drug-induced hepatic injury.

In patients with hepatitis B, always check whether hepatitis B e antigen is present. One rare scenario in the United States is mutant-strain hepatitis B. This strain, which is more common in Asia, simply consists of hepatitis B virus replication but no presence of e antigen. Serum hepatitis B DNA levels are high in these patients as well. This is one of the few instances during chronic hepatitis B infection in which active liver damage occurs without detectable e antigen. (The other circumstance in which this occurs is at the point of seroconversion from e antigen to e antibody positive.)

Often, a brisk bout of hepatitis occurs as the immune system clears the virus. This is seen either spontaneously or during interferon therapy. At present, interferon therapy is recommended only in hepatitis B surface antigen–E antigen–positive patients with raised transaminase levels, and it is used only if the liver disease is well compensated (i.e., near-normal albumin and prothrombin time).

Chronic Hepatitis C

Chronic hepatitis C is extraordinarily common in the United States. It has a *prevalence of approximately* 4 million cases, compared with a maximum of 1 million cases of hepatitis B.

Serum Hepatitis C Testing The best initial test is simple enzyme-linked immunosorbent assay (ELISA) antibody to hepatitis C virus. False-negative results occur in patients with immunodeficiency (e.g., acquired immunodeficiency syndrome, transplantation drugs) and, possibly, in those with ure-

mia. False-positive results tend to occur in patients with autoimmune disease, with or without hypergammaglobulinemia. In patients with raised transaminase levels (even if mild), a risk factor for parenteral hepatitis (e.g., intravenous drug use, transfusions, and so on), and a positive test for hepatitis C antibody, a diagnosis of chronic hepatitis C (if enzymes are documented to be elevated for 6 months) is certain.

Wells of ELISA plates are coated with synthetic fragments of hepatitis C virus. If antibodies to one or more hepatitis C antigen are present in the patient's blood, they will adhere to the reaction well.

The recombinant immunoblot assay (RIBA) test is a bit different. It uses the same bits of virus protein but layers them in strips separately. The test is positive if two or more bands become visible. A single band constitutes an indeterminate test, but it usually indicates that viral antibodies are real and that virus remains present.

Serum hepatitis C RNA testing now is widely available. There are two main assays: the signal amplification assay, and the polymerase chain reaction (PCR) assay. Both are quantitative tests. Signal amplification is easy to perform but lacks sensitivity, detecting hepatitis C virus only when 200,000 to 350,000 (or more) virions are present per milliliter. The new PCR assay detects virus at numbers as low as 100 per milliliter. Serum hepatitis C RNA levels are used for the following:

- To determine if hepatitis C is present in patients with normal liver enzymes.
- To decide if patient response to interferon is likely (e.g., patients with less than 2 million virions per milliliter respond better).
- To measure the impact of interferon therapy. For example, if the PCR is negative at 3 months, there is a good chance of sustained response. If the PCR is positive at 3 months, there is no chance of response, and the utility of continued interferon therapy is uncertain.

Natural History The natural history of hepatitis C has been delineated best in cases acquired through blood transfusions. This natural history is as follows:

- *10 years:* Active hepatitis (chronic hepatitis develops in 70 to 85% of patients).
- *10–20 years:* Cirrhosis (in approximately 30% of patients).
- *20–30 years:* Cirrhosis decompensation and hepatoma.

Treatment According to the recent National Institutes of Health Consensus Development Conference, definite candidates for interferon therapy are those patients with active hepatitis on liver biopsy but without frank cirrhosis (a hotly debated topic). Much uncertainty remains about treatment recommendations.

In the United States, 30% of liver transplantations now are performed in patients with hepatitis C, with or without alcohol use. Alcohol intake is an important cofactor in many patients.

Chronic hepatitis C is associated with a variety of extrahepatic problems, including vasculitis in lower limbs, glomerulonephritis, lichen planus, neuropathy, eye ulcers, and if there is additional iron overload, a condition called porphyria cutanea tarda. This condition leads to crusty, scaling lesions on the back of the hands.

The key points about chronic hepatitis C can be summarized as follows:

1. Normal transaminase levels do not mean that hepatitis C is cured (check serum hepatitis C RNA).
2. Approximately 30% of patients will get cirrhosis (this percentage is rising every few years).
3. Liver biopsy still is recommended before interferon therapy.
4. There is some evidence that iron overload and regular alcohol intake worsens hepatitis C.
5. There is recent, good evidence that alcohol abuse accelerates hepatitis C injury.
6. Interferon cures 25% of patients at most.

DRUG-INDUCED LIVER INJURY

As mentioned, always consider drug-induced liver injury. Specifically, be alert for drug use in the patient history. If a patient develops abnormal liver tests, jaundice, and so on while taking a drug, consider the possibility of drug-induced liver injury. Usually, the drug should be discontinued (or substituted) until the cause of the changes in the liver tests are determined (e.g., viral hepatitis, biliary stone obstruction, and so on). This is not as critical in patients with asymptomatic, modest elevations in transaminase levels (e.g., from one to two times normal); in these patients, a monitoring approach can be used. If the patient has jaundice or very high transaminase levels, it is vital to stop the drug as soon as possible, and in the case of acetaminophen, specific measures need to be employed.

Acetaminophen liver toxicity is of great concern at present. Unlike most hepatotoxic drug reactions, which are unpredictable and rare, acetaminophen used in moderate to high doses (10–15 g) is toxic to the liver. A one-time ingestion of 10 to 15 g can be lethal unless the antidote N-acetylcysteine is given before severe liver injury occurs. An algorithm based on blood levels since ingestion of the overdose is useful for predicting who will have liver injury. Administration of N-acetylcysteine in those at risk works well to prevent severe liver injury. Patients seen late, when their liver tests are already high, still derive benefit from this treatment, but its efficacy is greatly reduced. An arterial pH of less than 7.3 at presentation is a good predictor of who will have total liver failure.

Standard therapeutic doses of acetaminophen do not cause liver injury, because *hepatic glucuronidation* efficiently clears the drug. When higher doses are taken (e.g., ≥ 2 g), more of the drug is metabolized by the P450 2E1 enzyme, which gives rise to a metabolite called N-acetyl-p-benzoquinonenemine (NAPQI). This metabolite damages the liver in cases of acute overdose, and it also is responsible for liver injury when individuals exceed the normal doses. Induction of the P450 2E1 enzyme by alcohol abuse makes this even more likely to occur. In the normal liver, a secondary protective mechanism is present to bind/detoxify NAPQI:glutathione. N-acetylcysteine is a precursor for this compound, which is why it is given as treatment. In cases of overdose or an alcoholic liver, glutathione is depleted, thus allowing the toxic metabolite NAPQI to cause damage by covalent binding to cell proteins.

Acetaminophen hepatotoxicity and other types of drug-induced hepatotoxicity are important in clinical practice. Lee as well as Sherlock and Dooley have written excellent reviews of these topics.

INHERITED METABOLIC LIVER DISEASE
HEREDITARY HEMOCHROMATOSIS

The carrier frequency for hereditary hemochromatosis (HHC) is estimated to be between 1 in 8 to 1 in 12 among people of Northern European descent (i.e., heterozygotes). Individuals who are homozygous for this disorder have an inappropriate increase in intestinal iron absorption, thus resulting in progressive iron accumulation in the liver and other organs (e.g., heart, pancreas). If the condition is diagnosed before organ damage (e.g., cirrhosis, cardiomyopathy, diabetes), iron depletion with phlebotomy can prevent virtually all sequelae of this disorder. The recent major discovery in this field has been the finding of a hemochromatosis gene on the short arm of chromosome 6 within the HLA region in 85% of patients with HHC. How a major histocompatibility complex class I–like protein, which is the gene product, controls iron absorption, however, is not yet known.

The diagnosis of HHC is made on the basis of iron overload, and this will remain so until new technology for genetic testing is available. The percentage transferrin saturation now is the classic and best screening test for this disorder. This measurement is calculated by dividing the serum iron level by the total iron-binding capacity and then multiplying by 100. All patients with extensive liver disease will have saturations of greater than 70%; earlier in the course of this disease, approximately 55% is the cut-off point for adults with evolving iron overload. If the ferritin level is greater than 1000 ng/mL and the saturation is greater than 55%, the condition is likely to be hemochromatosis.

The only way to be certain about the diagnosis of hemochromatosis is to perform a liver biopsy and use part of the specimen for quantitative iron measurements. Because iron accumulation occurs over time, use of the hepatic iron index is recommended. This is liver iron (in μmol/g) divided by age. The hepatic iron index is greater than 1.9 in patients with genetic hemochromatosis. Each unit of blood contains 250 mg of iron. Phlebotomy is performed weekly until the hematocrit drops to 35; thereafter 1 U of blood is drawn off every 2 to 3 months to keep the patient's iron stores low.

If started early enough, phlebotomy prevents all clinical manifestations. If started before cirrhosis is present, it can reverse cardiomyopathy, glucose intolerance, hepatomegaly, and pigmentation of the skin. If started after cirrhosis is present, it cannot reverse cirrhosis or the risk of hepatoma, but it still should be done to prevent liver function from getting worse. Testicular atrophy is irreversible.

WILSON'S DISEASE

Multiple gene abnormalities seem to cause Wilson's disease. The basic defect is a decreased hepatic excretion of copper. Copper accumulates in the liver, thus leading to fatty liver, a hepatitis-like clinical picture, and ultimately, cirrhosis. Once the liver is copper-loaded, copper spills into the circulation and deposits in the brain (i.e., basal ganglia), eyes (i.e., Kayser-Fleischer rings), renal tubules (renal tubular defect leads to loss of amino acids, uricuria), and rarely, causes cardiomyopathy. An acute liver syndrome with hemolysis also is rarely seen, and osteopenia can be a feature.

The usual features of Wilson's disease are:

- Ceruloplasmin, <20 mg/dL (a marker for the disease but not a primary cause of copper accumulation).
- Urine copper, >100 μg/day.
- Kayser-Fleischer rings visible to the naked eye or on slit-lamp examination.
- Hepatic histology abnormal
- Hepatic copper, >250 μg/g dry weight.

Indications for testing are:

- Unexplained liver disease in children or young adults.
- Hemolysis with liver disease.
- Neurologic disease in young patients (e.g., Parkinsonism, gait disturbance, psychosis).
- Fanconi syndrome.
- Hypouricemia.
- Kayser-Fleischer rings in eyes.
- Sunflower cataracts.
- Siblings of affected patients.

Diagnostic tests include ceruloplasmin, slit-lamp examination, urine copper levels, and liver biopsy with quantitative copper levels. Treatment is penicillamine, 250 to 500 mg four times a day before meals, plus pyridoxine; oral zinc is used if penicillamine is not tolerated. Many patients improve or at least stabilize. Liver transplant is curative.

α_1-ANTITRYPSIN DEFICIENCY

α_1-Antitrypsin deficiency is a relatively common disorder in people of northern European and Scandinavian ancestry. In the United States, approximately 1 in 2000 people are homozygous for the abnormal Z_1 alleles. Only 10 to 15% of (i.e., Homozygotes) individuals are affected with liver disease. The gene defect is on the long arm of chromosome 14, and it seems to be a production of defective α_1-antitrypsin, which accumulates in the endoplasmic reticulum of the hepatocyte.

P_1 ZZ individuals may not have symptoms (for unknown reasons), or they may have one of following three problems:

- Premature emphysema, especially in smokers.
- Neonatal hepatitis (10%).
- Active hepatitis in adolescents or cirrhosis in adults.

It is not common for adults to have a history of neonatal jaundice, but adults rarely will have both lung and liver problems.

The diagnosis is established by measuring the serum α_1-antitrypsin level. In P_1 ZZ individuals, levels of α_1-antitrypsin are only 10% of normal. There are a confusing array of different phenotypes in this disorder as well. The classic ZZ type has very low levels of α_1-antitrypsin. The "α_1-peak" in a routine serum protein electrophoresis mainly results from α_1-antitrypsin; consequently, the α_1-peak is reduced in patients with α_1-antitrypsin deficiency.

Treatment includes management of the complications from liver disease, surveillance for development of hepatoma, transplantation, and family screening.

SUGGESTED READINGS

HEPATITIS

Sherlock S, Dooley J, ed. Diseases of the liver and biliary system. 10th ed. Oxford: Blackwell Science, 1997:265–336.

Management of hepatitis C. Hepatology 1997;26(Suppl 1).

This entire issue (155 pages) is devoted to all aspects of Hepatitis C. It represents the report of The National Institutes of Health Consensus Development Conference held on March 24–26, 1997.

DRUG-INDUCED LIVER INJURY

Lee WM. Drug induced hepatotoxicity. N Engl J Med 1997, 333:1118–1127.

Sherlock S, Dooley J, eds. Diseases of the liver and biliary system. 10th Ed. Oxford: Blackwell Science, 1997:337–369.

INHERITED METABOLIC LIVER DISEASE

Sherlock S, Dooley J, eds. Diseases of the liver and biliary system. 10th ed. Oxford: Blackwell Science, 1997:405–412, 417–423,445–447.

54B

Liver Disease: Complications of Cirrhosis

Arthur J. McCullough

In 1995, cirrhosis was the tenth-leading cause of death in the United States for all age groups, and it was the seventh-leading cause of death for those between 45 and 64 years of age (1). The average 5- and 10-year survival rates for patients with cirrhosis are 44 and 25%, respectively (Table 54B.1). These survival rates are similar regardless of the cause, except for alcoholic cirrhosis, which has 5- and 10-year survival rates of 23 and 7%, respectively; these survival rates are significantly lower than those for patients with cirrhosis of other causes (2). The survival rate is not uniform across all cirrhotic groups, however. It depends on disease severity, which is best predicted by the Child's-Pugh classification.

The major complications and causes of death and their relative frequency in patients with cirrhosis are:

- Variceal bleeding, 20%
- Bacterial peritonitis, 24%
- Hepatic encephalopathy/liver failure, 20%
- Hepatocellular carcinoma, 11%
- Renal insufficiency, 9%

Sixteen percent of patients will die from nonhepatic causes.

VARICEAL BLEEDING

Esophageal varices are a common occurrence in patients with cirrhosis and an important cause of morbidity and mortality. Patients with cirrhosis and varices have a 20% higher 2-year mortality and a 30% higher 5-year mortality rate than those without varices. The mean 2-year incidence of variceal bleeding is 30%, and the mortality rate of a bleeding episode approaches 50%. Therefore, preventing the first episode of variceal bleeding has received widespread interest (3).

The risk of bleeding in all patients with cirrhosis, regardless of cause, depends on three parameters:

1. Severity of liver disease (i.e., Child's class),
2. Size of varices, and
3. Presence of red signs on varices (4).

The mortality of a bleeding episode depends mainly on the Child's class (5). Table 54B.2 shows the various therapies that have been used as prophylaxis against the initial bleed as well as against secondary esophageal variceal bleeding.

PREVENTION

It now is recognized that patients with grade II (i.e., medium) or larger varices benefit from prophylaxis with nonselective β-blockers. Many analyses have found that the rate of first-time hemorrhages is reduced statistically significantly with such therapy, which also is cost-effective (3). β-Blockers must be taken on a regular basis; compliance is extremely important. The goal of therapy is to decrease the basal pulse rate by 25%. This decrease in pulse rate does not correlate extremely well, however, with the decrease in portal pressure, but it is the best way to monitor patients.

The average dose of the nonselective β-blocker propranolol is 20 mg three times a day. Propranolol cannot be tolerated, however, in 10 to 15% of patients with cirrhosis. Nadolol is better tolerated, with a discontinuance rate of 4 to 5%, but it is more expensive. The combination of β-blockers with isosorbide may be better than monotherapy alone for preventing bleeding.

Two other prophylactic therapies are sclerotherapy and surgical decompression. Both, however, are less cost-effective than β-blockers and should not be used currently. The utility of screening endoscopy is debated, but it sometimes is used at 1-year intervals for patients with grade I varices or at 2-year intervals for those with no varices.

Table 54B.1.   Survival Rates in Patients with Cirrhosis

Cause	Patients (n)	Survival (%)	
		5 Years	10 Years
Alcohol	82	23	7
Cryptogenic	13	33	20
Hepatitis C virus	62	38	24
Hepatitis B virus	42	48	20
Hemochromatosis	20	41	22
Autoimmune	16	46	23
PBC*	36	56	39

Data from Propst A, Propst T, Sangerl G, Ofner D, Judmaier G, Vogel W. Prognosis and life expectancy in chronic liver disease. Dig Dis Sci 1995;40: 1805–1815.

* PBC = primary sclerosing cholangitis

Table 54B.2.   Therapy for Varices

	Primary	Secondary
Pharmacologic		
β-Blockers	X	X
Somatostatin		X
Vasopressin + NTG*		X
Glypressin		X
Endoscopic		
Sclerotherapy	X	X
Band Ligation		X
Radiologic-TIPS		X
Surgery	X	X

* NTG = nitroglycerin

TREATMENT

Initial treatment for any patient with variceal hemorrhage is resuscitation. As many as 50% of patients with cirrhosis and upper gastrointestinal hemorrhage are bleeding from nonvariceal sources. However all patients with cirrhosis and upper gastrointestinal hemorrhage should be assumed to have varices as the source of their bleeding. They also should be treated as such until the bleeding site is identified definitively. Clotting abnormalities should be corrected and fluid resuscitation (with limited saline load) initiated while attempts are made to control the bleeding. Ample evidence suggests that intravenous somatostatin or octreotide should be given immediately as a bolus and then hourly at least for the next 24 to 48 hours. Studies also indicate that during the early treatment of acute variceal bleeding, somatostatin is approximately as effective as sclerotherapy (75–90% versus 80–95%, respectively) or ligation of varices, and it is safer than intravenous vasopressin

used alone. If used, vasopressin should be combined with nitroglycerin to limit ischemic side effects.

Initial pharmacologic therapy also has the added advantage of clearing the field for subsequent endoscopy, and diagnostic endoscopy should then be performed to confirm the cause of the bleeding. It also may be accompanied by therapeutic endoscopy (i.e., injection sclerotherapy or endoscopic variceal band ligation). When it can be performed, band ligation is superior to sclerotherapy.

Once the acute esophageal bleeding is controlled, the standard approach is to repeat ligation or sclerotherapy sessions until the varices are obliterated. This usually is combined with β-blocker therapy. Use of both the endoscopic and the pharmacologic approaches after controlling the initial bleeding, however, is controversial. A recent Veterans Administration study indicates that sclerotherapy helps to prevent rebleeding, but that it does not affect the survival rate. In addition, β-blockers are not as effective for preventing secondary bleeding as they are when used prophylactically against an initial bleed. Nonetheless, the current standard approach is repeated endoscopy to obliterate the varices combined with drug therapy to decrease the portal pressure.

In approximately 5–10% of patients, bleeding esophageal varices cannot be controlled despite use of pharmacologic and endoscopic therapies. In such patients, balloon tamponade (85–90% effective) should be performed only by those experienced with this technique because of the recognized, associated life-threatening complications. Esophageal balloon tamponade should be performed only in an intensive care unit, and if the patient has any degree of obtundation (as often is the case), endotracheal intubation should be performed before the balloon is placed. If the patient continues to bleed or rebleeds and is a candidate for liver transplantation, placement of a transjugular intrahepatic portosystemic shunt (TIPS) is appropriate. If the patient is not a candidate for liver transplantation, a surgical shunt or esophageal devascularization usually is performed. The surgical mortality rate, however, is so high in Child's Class C patients with cirrhosis that TIPS may

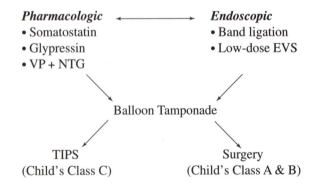

Figure 54B.1.   Treatment of variceal bleeding (to control acute episode). EVS = endoscopic variceal sclerotherapy; VP = vasopressin; NTG = nitroglycerine.

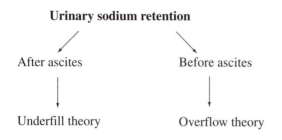

Urinary sodium retention

After ascites   Before ascites

Underfill theory   Overflow theory

Figure 54B.2.   Pathophysiology of ascites.

be considered even if liver transplantation is not an option (Fig. 54B.1).

ASCITES

Ascites is the most common complication of cirrhosis, occurring in approximately 50% of patients who have had the disease for 10 years. Its development is a poor prognostic sign, because once ascites occurs, the 2-year survival rate is only 50% (6). The ascites is caused by increased sodium reabsorption by the kidney (predominantly in the distal tubule). The prominent mechanism involved in renal sodium reabsorption is an increase in the renin-aldosterone-angiotensin (RAAS) system. In addition, the sympathetic nervous system and, perhaps, hyperinsulinemia are responsible for sodium absorption in the more proximal renal tubule. Whether sodium reabsorption by the kidney appears before or after development of ascites has led to the overfill and underfill hypotheses of ascites development (Fig. 54B.2). Most recently, however, the peripheral arterial vasodilatation theory, which combines the overfill and the underfill theories, has been proposed. According to this theory, the large capacitance of the splanchnic venous system becomes dilated because of sinusoidal-induced portal hypertension. This increase in splanchnic venous blood pooling decreases the effective plasma volume at a time when no ascites has developed, which then triggers the RAAS system and causes sodium to be reabsorbed before ascites develops but after the effective plasma volume decreases. This increased sodium and fluid reabsorption by the kidney, combined with an increased hepatic sinusoidal pressure, then causes fluid to accumulate in the abdominal cavity.

TREATMENT

Treatment of ascites is necessary to avoid certain complications. Early satiety and a 10% increase in energy expenditure frequently exacerbates muscle wasting and cachexia in patients with this disease. In addition, treatment increases cardiac output and decreases the risks of hernia, umbilical rupture, and spontaneous bacterial peritonitis.

The diagnosis is suspected on the basis of the patient history and physical examination. It usually is confirmed by the results of ultrasonography, abdominal paracentesis, or

both. There is general consensus that new onset ascites or ascites suspected of having a complication such as an infection or a malignancy should be tapped. There also is an emerging opinion that all hospitalized patients should undergo diagnostic paracentesis. Abdominal paracentesis with appropriate fluid analysis is the most rapid and cost-effective method for diagnosing the cause of ascites. In view of the fact that 10 to 27% of patients with cirrhosis and ascites have an ascitic fluid infection, a surveillance tap at this time may detect unexpected infection, especially when there is clinical concern. Complications of diagnostic paracentesis have been reported in approximately 1% of patients, even though more than 70% of patients have an abnormal prothrombin time. There are few contraindications to paracentesis, and coagulopathy should preclude paracentesis only when there is clinically evident fibrinolysis or disseminated intravascular coagulation. Bleeding is sufficiently uncommon to preclude the need for prophylactic fresh-frozen plasma or platelets.

Table 54B.3 details the laboratory analysis of ascitic fluid. If uncomplicated cirrhotic ascites is suspected, only screening tests (i.e., cell count and differential, albumin concentration, bacterial culture in blood culture bottles) are performed with the initial specimen. Additional testing is performed on the basis of the screening tests and clinical judgment; further testing usually necessitates another paracentesis. The serum ascites-albumin gradient (SAAG) categorizes ascites better than total protein measured on the basis of the exudate/transudate concept and better than the modified peripheral fluid exudate/transudate criteria (7). The SAAG is calculated by subtracting the ascitic fluid albumin concentration from the serum albumin concentration. If the SAAG ascites is greater than 1.1 g/dL, the patient has portal hypertension ascites; if the SAAG is less than 1.1 g/dL, the patient does not have portal hypertension. This test is approximately 95% accurate for distinguishing between ascites caused by portal hypertension and that from other causes (Table 54B.4). Bedside inoculation of blood culture bottles with ascitic fluid is the best way to demonstrate bacterial growth.

Table 54B.5 outlines the basic treatment of ascites. The mainstay of therapy for patients with cirrhosis and ascites is education regarding sodium restriction and oral diuretics. Restricting sodium to less than 2 g/day (≈ 88 mmol) theoreti-

Table 54B.3.   Laboratory Analysis of Ascites Fluid

Routine	*Optional/Unusual*
Cell count with differential	Gram stain
Albumin (first specimen)[a]	Amylase[a]
Culture (bedside inoculation)	Triglyceride[a]
Total protein	Cytology
Glucose	TB smear/culture
Lactate dehydrogenase	

[a] Requires simultaneous blood sample.

Table 54B.4. Classification of Ascites (Albumin Gradient)

High (≥ 1.1 g/dL)	*Low (< 1.1 g/dL)*
Cirrhosis	Peritoneal carcinomatosis
Alcoholic hepatitis	Peritoneal TB
Heart failure	Pancreatic ascites
Hepatic metastases	Biliary ascites
FHF*	Nephrotic syndrome
Budd-Chiari	Serositis
Venous occlusive disease	Bowel obstruction
Portal-vein thrombosis	
Myxedema	
Fatty liver of pregnancy	
''Mixed''	

Data from Runyon BA, McMutchison JG, Antillon MR, et al. Short course us. long course antibiotic treatment of spontaneous bacterial peritonitis: a randomized controlled trial of 100 patients. Gastroenterology 1991;100: 1737–1742.
* FHF = fulminant hepatic failure.

Table 54B.5. Management of Ascites

Tolerable salt restriction
Diuresis with spironolactone ± loop diuretic
Paracentesis is a safe and effective adjunct therapy
    Volume expansion is controversial
    Dextran 70 vs. albumin
Poorly responsive ascites
    TIPS
    Peritoneovenous shunt
    Extracorporeal ultrafiltrational reinfusion

cally speeds weight loss, but it is such a stringent restriction that compliance is less likely. Sodium rather than fluid restriction results in weight loss. Fluid restriction is necessary only if the patient has spontaneous or diuretic-induced hyponatremia.

Even though 10 to 15% of patients respond to bed rest alone, this is impractical, and there have been no controlled trials to *support this approach*. The usual diuretic regime consists of oral spironolactone combined with the loop diuretic furosemide, beginning with 100 mg of aldactone and *40 mg of furosemide*. The doses of both agents can be increased simultaneously to a maximal dose of 400 mg/day for spironolactone and 160 mg/day for furosemide. The presence of hyperkalemia or hyponatremia may require a downward adjustment in the doses of spironolactone and of furosemide, respectively. Single morning doses maximize compliance. The combined approach of dietary sodium restriction and dual-diuretic therapy has been effective in 90% of patients (8). The rate of weight loss, however, depends on whether edema is present. If edema is present, there is no limit to the daily weight loss that can be obtained; once the edema has resolved, 0.5 kg/day is probably the maximum daily weight loss that should be sought (9). If encephalopathy, hyponatremia (<120 mmol/dL), or a serum creatinine level greater than 2 mg/dL develops, the clinical situation must be reassessed and second-line options considered. The patient also should be questioned about use of any drugs that inhibit renal prostaglandins and have an anti-diuretic effect (e.g., aspirin). In hospitalized patients with tense ascites, a single, large-volume paracentesis should be performed. This large-volume paracentesis does nothing to correct the underlying problem that led to ascites formation, however, and the recommendations described here for sodium restriction and diuretic therapy should be initiated. Diuretic-sensitive patients optimally should be treated with a sodium-restricted diet and oral diuretics rather than with serial paracentesis. Liver transplantation should be considered for all patients with cirrhosis and ascites.

REFRACTORY ASCITES

Refractory ascites is defined as fluid overload that is unresponsive to a two week treatment regimen of a sodium-restricted diet and high-dose diuretic therapy (400 mg/day of spironolactone and 160 mg/day of furosemide) in the absence of prostaglandin inhibitors such as nonsteroidal anti-inflammatory drugs. Refractory ascites develops in less than 10% of patients with cirrhosis and ascites.

Several treatment options are available for these patients:

1. Serial therapeutic paracentesis should be performed as needed, usually approximately every 2 to 3 weeks. Postparacentesis volume expansion is optional because of its expense; however, one recent study (10) indicated that volume expansion with albumin is more effective than dextran 70 or polygeline in preventing postparacentesis circulatory dysfunction.
2. For acceptable candidates, liver transplantation should be considered.
3. For patients who are not transplant candidates, a peritoneovenous shunt may be considered, as might be a TIPS procedure (11–13).

SPONTANEOUS BACTERIAL PERITONITIS

The diagnosis of spontaneous bacterial peritonitis (SBP) is established on the basis of a positive ascitic fluid bacterial culture and an elevated ascitic fluid polymorphonuclear (PMN) count (>250 cells/mL) without an intra-abdominal source of infection. If SBP is clinically suspected, paracentesis should be performed. The ascitic fluid PMN count is readily available, and it is accurate in determining the need for empiric antibiotic coverage. Broad-spectrum antibiotic therapy is warranted until the culture susceptibility is available. Cefotaxime or a similar third-generation cephalosporin usually is consid-

Study	Dose	SBP Resolution (%)	Hospital Survival (%)
Felizart, 1985	2 g per 4 hours	86	73
Ariza, 1991	1 g per 3 hours	81	42
Runyon et al. (15)	2 g per 8 hours		
5 Days		93	67
10 Days		91	42
Spanish	2 g per 6 hours	75	69
Multicenter	2 g per 12 hours	79	79

Table 54B.6.   Cefotaxime for Spontaneous Bacterial Peritonitis

Table 54B.7.   Treatment of Spontaneous Bacterial Peritonitis

High index of suspicion
 Improved culture technique
Early aggressive therapy
 Cefotaxime for 5 days
Exclude second-degree bacterial peritonitis
Prevent recurrence
 Prophylactic antibiotics
 Consider early transplant

ered to be the treatment of choice (Tables 54B.6 and 54B.7). This drug is given at a dose of 2 g intravenously every 8 hours until specific bacterial sensitivities are known (14). A recent randomized, controlled trial (15) showed that 5 days of treatment is as efficacious as 10 days. Occasionally, secondary bacterial peritonitis, which is an ascitic fluid infection caused by a surgically treatable, intra-abdominal source, can complicate ascites. Such infections usually result from free perforation of a viscus or a loculated abscess. The characteristic ascitic fluid analysis in patients with free perforation is an elevated PMN count, multiple organisms, and two or three of the following:

1. Total protein level > 1 g/dL.
2. Glucose level < 50 mg/dL, and
3. *Lactate dehydrogenase level* greater than the upper limit of the normal serum values.

The source of free perforation should be sought in these patients, and a 48-hour follow-up PMN count should be obtained. Most patients with the typical presentation of SBP do not need a repeat paracentesis to document sterility.

A previous episode of SBP, ascitic fluid protein concentration less than 1 g/dL, and acute variceal hemorrhage have been identified as predictors for the development of SBP. Nor-

floxacin, 400 mg/day, has been reported to prevent SBP in patients with low protein ascites and in patients with previous SBP (16). Norfloxacin, 400 mg twice daily, also has been beneficial in patients with variceal hemorrhage. Because superimposed fungal infections have been reported to result from prolonged therapy with ciprofloxacin in patients with a liver transplant, intermittent dosing with regimes such as 750 mg of ciprofloxacin once per week or 5 doses of trimethoprim-sulfamethoxazole per week may be appropriate to prevent infections without selecting resistant flora. Therefore, long-term outpatient therapy should be reserved for those who have survived a previous episode of SBP.

HEPATIC ENCEPHALOPATHY

Hepatic encephalopathy is a clinical syndrome that is characterized by a wide spectrum of neuropsychiatric abnormalities. It is associated with significant liver disease but is potentially fully reversible. It generally is considered to be caused by toxins present in the splanchnic circulation that bypass the liver during portosystemic shunting and gain entrance to the central nervous system. The exact cause of hepatic encephalopathy remains elusive (17), but the following hypotheses have been proposed:

- Ammonia neurotoxicity
- Synergistic neurotoxins (e.g., ammonia, mercaptans, fatty acids)
- False neurotransmitters
- Imbalance of true neurotransmitters (γ-aminobutyric acid [GABA])
- Endogenous benzodiazepines

CLINICAL PRESENTATION

The different forms of hepatic encephalopathy are listed in Table 54B.8. Subclinical encephalopathy and both single and recurrent overt hepatic encephalopathy in patients with cirrhosis are most common. Subclinical encephalopathy appears to be the single most common form. If psychometric testing is performed (18), most patients with cirrhosis are found to have subclinical hepatic encephalopathy. Similarly, most will have an abnormal electroencephalographic tracing as well. Whether subclinical encephalopathy has the same cause as clinically overt hepatic encephalopathy, however, remains unknown.

Table 54B.8.   Hepatic Encephalopathy in Cirrhosis

Subclinical encephalopathy	Very common
Single/recurrent overt hepatic encephalopathy	Common
Chronic cerebral degeneration	Very rare
Spastic paraparesis	Very rare

Table 54B.9.   Factors Precipitating Hepatic Encephalopathy

Diuretics/renal failure	29%
Sedatives/analgesics	24%
Gastrointestinal bleeding	18%
Metabolic alkalosis	11%
Excess dietary intake	9%
Infection	3%
Constipation	3%
Hepatic injury	3%

Clinical features associated with hepatic encephalopathy are:

- Asterixis
  - The most consistent finding
  - 1–3 beats per second, bilateral, asynchronous
  - A nonspecific finding
- Fetor hepaticus
  - Sweetish, musty odor
  - Mercaptans (i.e., dimethylsulfide)
- Decerebrate rigidity
  - Prognosis poor but still reversible

Laboratory abnormalities associated with hepatic encephalopathy are:

- Nonspecific abnormalities
  - Liver function tests
  - Renal function/hypoglycemia
  - Respiratory alkylosis
- More specific abnormalities
  - Blood ammonia (predictive value, 85–90%)
  - Cerebrospinal fluid glutamine more helpful than ammonia
  - Electroencephalography: bilateral, synchronous slow (delta) waves (3–4 per second, frontal lobe)

For the most part, these clinical and laboratory features are nonspecific. The clinician must rule out other causes of decreased mentation in patients with cirrhosis.

Very few patients with cirrhosis develop encephalopathy without a precipitating factor that provokes development of an acute-on-chronic encephalopathy. These risk factors are listed in Table 54B.9. The clinician must carefully evaluate each patient for these complications. A recent analysis at my hospital found the three most common causes to be diuretic-induced abnormalities; sedatives, analgesics, or both; and gastrointestinal bleeding. Gastrointestinal bleeding appears to precipitate encephalopathy because hemoglobin lacks isoleucine, which makes it a low-quality form of protein. Often, the first sign of sepsis in a patient with cirrhosis is mild encephalopathy.

TREATMENT

Potential precipitating factors should be recognized and treated immediately. If the patient remains alert, oral lactulose therapy is appropriate (19), but diarrhea should be prevented to avoid fluid and electrolyte abnormalities. If the patient is comatose, lactulose should not be given through a nasogastric tube because of a decrease in gastrointestinal motility (20); regular enemas should be instituted in these patients.

Chronic hepatic encephalopathy has become a problem for patients with liver disease who are not candidates for transplantation. Long-term treatment commonly is necessary. A vegetarian diet is preferred to meat, but such a diet enhances bloating of the abdomen and often is not logistically feasible. Long-term use of neomycin has decreased because of the ototoxicity and renal toxicity associated with this therapy. Other therapies such as metronidazole, sodium benzoate, and L-dopa have been examined in small studies, but their use remains experimental. They should not be used clinically at present.

Many studies have examined the use of branch-chained amino acids in treatment of chronic hepatic encephalopathy. The early success of such treatment in pilot studies has not been confirmed with larger, randomized control trials. The general approach to the treatment of patients with hepatic encephalopathy is:

- Exclude other causes of encephalopathy
- Identify and correct precipitating factors
- Commence empiric treatment
  - Stop GI bleeding
  - Restrict protein
  - Stop drugs
  - Clean out gut
  - Start lactulose

Most patients can be controlled by treating the precipitating factors and initiating lactulose. The effects of lactulose are:

- Suppresses colonic absorption of NH_3 and GABA
- Suppresses NH_3 generation (i.e., bacterial and intestinal)
- Stimulates nitrogen excretion (i.e., NH_3 incorporated into stool)
- Increases intestinal transit time.
- Decreases short-chain (i.e., 3–6 carbon) fatty acids (i.e., acetate increases)

If the encephalopathy persists, long-term therapy with lactulose, with or without increasing the proportion of vegetable protein in the diet, can treat most patients successfully. Only in a minority of patients are these and other potential but unproven therapies necessary.

HEPATOCELLULAR CARCINOMA

Hepatocellular carcinoma is among the 10 most common malignancies worldwide. Unfortunately, symptomatic patients have only a 6-month life expectancy. Epidemiologic data suggest that infection with hepatitis B or C virus and cirrhosis are risk factors for development of hepatocellular carcinoma (21). Approximately 80% of patients with hepatoma worldwide have evidence of hepatitis B infection. Hepatitis C also now is recognized as a major risk factor in the development of carcinoma. Of the many causes of cirrhosis, only Wilson's disease and autoimmune chronic active hepatitis do not appear to be associated with an increased risk of hepatocellular carcinoma. On the basis of a recent cost-effectiveness model, it now is recommended that high-risk patients should have an α-fetoprotein and ultrasound performed at 6-month intervals (22). In these high-risk patients, standard liver tests have little benefit when a hepatoma is suspected clinically. α-Fetoprotein levels greater than 500 ng/mL are diagnostic of this malignancy in the absence of certain other rare diseases (i.e., ataxia telangectasia). Ultrasonography is the most sensitive radiographic technique, but magnetic resonance imaging may be helpful considering its specificity (23).

In patients with cirrhosis, small cancers can grow slowly and, therefore, remain undetected. In one recent study (24), 20 to 40% of patients who died of cirrhosis had unsuspected hepatocellular cancer, and unsuspected tumors often are identified within the explanted liver of patients with cirrhosis undergoing liver transplantation. Natural history studies indicate that 13% of patients with untreated tumors may survive 3 years, but most die within 4 months after the onset of symptoms (25). At the time of death, 50% of patients with hepatocellular carcinoma have regional or distant metastases. The most frequent cause of death is hepatic failure resulting from local spread or preexisting cirrhosis, followed by hemorrhage from tumor rupture or variceal bleeding. Accurate disease staging is crucial for selecting the most appropriate treatment.

SURGICAL TREATMENT

Surgical resection remains the mainstay for treatment of hepatocellular carcinoma, and it is the only chance for long-term, tumor-free survival. Surgical resection, however, should be restricted to patients with well-preserved liver function and negligible expected risks for morbidity or mortality caused by the surgery. Therefore, evaluation of the hepatic function and the hepatic reserve is key to the treatment of these patients.

A number of single tests and composite indexes have been proposed to evaluate the hepatic reserve, but the Child's-Pugh classification remains the most widely used. Elevated portal pressure also may have prognostic value in addition to the Child's-Pugh modified classification in this setting (26). Perioperative mortality rates following hepatic resections for hepatocellular carcinoma range from 2 to 10%. The decision to resect a tumor is made on the basis of excluding extrahepatic spread and the segmental anatomy of the liver. Resection can be facilitated by using intraoperative ultrasonography to improve identification of the site, the number of lesions, and the relationship between the lesions and the adjacent vessels.

The morbidity rate associated with even small resections of cirrhotic liver should not be underestimated. Most authors report a 1-year survival rate of between 55 and 80%—and a 5-year survival rate of 1%—after hepatic resection. Survival rates are improved in patients with encapsulated tumors of less than 3 cm, with negative resection margins, and without capsular invasion of tumor cells. Multifocal tumors have a significant influence on survival rates, and the recurrence rate is higher in these patients. Unfortunately, the pathologic stage cannot be determined with ease preoperatively, and the long-term results of resection have been disappointing, mainly because of the high rate of intrahepatic recurrence. Hepatic resection leaves patients with cirrhosis exposed to development of metachronous or synchronous tumor deposits and death from underlying liver dysfunction.

LIVER TRANSPLANTATION

Because of the limited benefit from hepatic resection, liver transplantation, which initially was considered to be a poor treatment option, has been used more frequently and is associated with recently improved results (27, 28). Overall, the survival rate after transplantation (47% at 3 years) appears to be similar to that for resection (50% at 3 years). Survival without recurrence, however, may be better than for resection (46% versus 27%, respectively). There is a survival advantage from transplantation for small uninodular or binodular tumors, but patients with diffuse tumors or those with more than two nodules (i.e., >3 cm), or patients with tumor thrombus in the portal vein, have done poorly with either operative approach. Therefore, if liver transplantation does carry an advantage in the treatment of this disease, it should be restricted to those patients who have small, encapsulated tumors restricted to one lobe and without vascular or capsule invasion.

NONSURGICAL TREATMENT

Few patients have resectable hepatocellular carcinomas at presentation; therefore, several nonsurgical treatment modalities have been tried. Systemic chemotherapy using both individual and combination therapies has been uniformly unsuccessful. Very poor results and the high incidence of severe side effects dictate that systemic chemotherapy has only a minor, if any, role in treatment and palliation of hepatocellular carcinoma. Therefore, several other tumor-targeting therapies have been employed.

Arterial Embolization or Ligation

Arterial embolization or ligation is based on the fact that the hepatic artery supplies almost all blood to the tumor, especially if the tumor has a capsule and is small. Compared with an untreated group of patients, however, those undergoing hepatic arterial ligation had a higher 7-day mortality rate (33% versus 6%,respectively) and a lower median survival time (34 versus 58 days, respectively) (29).

Hepatic arterial infusion therapy has been used to achieve higher local levels of chemotherapy in the liver and to reduce systemic toxicity. It appears to be more effective than intravenous chemotherapy, but such treatment has not uniformly demonstrated a definite survival advantage. Its efficacy depends on whether the patient has portal vein thrombosis.

Recently, chemotherapeutic agents also have been combined with lipiodol, which is an iodized oil taken up selectively by the tumor and which remains within the tumor for significant periods of time. Greater tumor necrosis has been demonstrated with this approach, and the combination of 5-fluorouracil and cisplatinum with lipiodol, given as a continuous hepatic arterial infusion, achieved a 1-year survival rate of 61% among 21 patients in an uncontrolled study (30).

Transcatheter Arterial Chemotherapeutic Embolization

The technique of transcatheter arterial chemotherapeutic embolization (TACE) involves use of interventional angiography to embolize the tumor's arterial supply with gelatin-sponge particles or chemotherapeutic agents and lipiodol. Initial results show only modest success, and though TACE is a useful treatment for some patients with unresectable hepatocellular carcinoma, no prospective, randomized studies have compared this treatment with liver resection or transplantation. The respective merits of embolization with chemotherapy or chemotherapy alone in treatment of advanced hepatic malignancy have not been established.

Percutaneous Ethanol Injection Therapy

Percutaneous ethanol injection therapy is effective in tumors smaller than 5 cm. In one recent study (31), patients with Child's Class A and B cirrhosis who had a single, small (i.e., <5 cm) hepatocellular carcinoma were treated with resection, ethanol injection, or no treatment. In Child's Class A patients, the cumulative 3-year survival rates were 79% for surgery, 71% for ethanol injection, and 26% for no treatment. In Child's Class B patients, the 3-year survival rates were 40% for surgery, 41% for ethanol injection, and 13% for no treatment. Ethanol injection does not appear to benefit patients with larger tumors.

Cryoablation

Cryoablation, which is the destruction of tissue by a freeze/thaw process, has been suggested as a useful tool in the treatment of hepatic cancer. One poorly controlled study suggested that the 1-, 3-, and 5-year survival rates for all groups were 52, 21, and 11%, respectively, but these results are difficult to interpret.

OTHER TREATMENTS

Radiation therapy has limited value in treatment of hepatocellular carcinoma. Immunotherapy recently has been attempted as treatment, but early results are not encouraging. Because of these poor results, various combinations of multiple modalities have been attempted. The results of these proposed therapies are too preliminary, however, and they do not provide sufficient information on which to base a sound clinical approach.

At present, patients who are surgical candidates with potentially resectable lesions should be considered for hepatic resection or liver transplantation. In those patients who are not surgical candidates, experimental protocols employing local or systemic therapy such as alcohol injection and cryotherapy should be offered.

REFERENCES

1. Rosenberg HM, Ventura SJ, Maurer JD. Births and deaths: United States, 1995. Monthly Vital Statistics Rep 1995;45(Suppl 2):31–36.
2. Propst A, Propst T, Sangerl G, Ofner D, Judmaier G, Vogel W. Prognosis and life expectancy in chronic liver disease. Dig Dis Sci 1995;40:1805–1815.
3. Teran JC, Imperiale TF, Mullen KD, Tavill AS, McCullough AJ. Primary prophylaxis of variceal bleeding in cirrhosis: a cost-effectiveness analysis. Gastroenterology 1997;112:473–482.
4. The North Italian Endoscopic Club for the Study and Treatment of Esophageal Varices. Prediction of the first variceal hemorrhage in patients with cirrhosis of the liver and esophageal varices. N Engl J Med 1988;319:983–989.
5. Graham DY, Smith JL. The course of patients after variceal hemorrhage. Gastroenterology 1981;80:8090–809.
6. Runyon BA. Care of patients with ascites. N Engl J Med 1994;330:337–342.
7. Runyon BA, Montano AA, Akriviadis EA, Antillon MR, Irving MA. McHutchison JG. The serum-ascites gradient is superior to the exudate-transudate concept in the differential diagnosis of ascites. Ann Intern Med 1992;117:215–220.
8. Stanley MM, Ochi S, Lee KK: Peritoneovenous shunting as compared with medical treatment in patients with alcoholic cirrhosis and massive ascites. N Engl J Med 1989;321:1632–1638.
9. Pockros PJ, Reynolds TB. Rapid diuresis in patients with ascites from chronic liver disease. The importance of peripheral edema. Gastroenterology 1986;90:1827–1833.
10. Gines A, Fernandez-Esparrach G, Monescillo A, et al. Randomized trial comparing albumin, Dextran 70, and polygeline in cirrhotic patients with ascites treated by paracentesis. Gastroenterology 1996;111:1002–1010.
11. Lebrec D, Giuily N, Hadengue A, et al. Transjugular intrahepatic portosystemic shunts: comparison with para-

centesis inpatients with cirrhosis and refractory ascites: a randomized trial. J Hepatol 1996;25:135–144.

12. Wong F, Sniderman K, Liu P, Allidina Y, Sherman M, Blendis L. Transjugular intrahepatic portosystemic stent shunt: Effects on hemodynamics and sodium hemostasis in cirrhosis and refractory ascites. Ann Intern Med 1995; 122:816–822.

13. Gines P, Arroyo V, Vargas V, et al. Paracentesis with intravenous infusion of albumin as compared with peritoneovenous shunting in cirrhosis with refractory ascites. N Engl J Med 1991;325:829–835

14. Felisart J, Rimola A, Arroyo V, et al. Randomized comparative study of efficacy and nephrotoxicity of ampicillin plus tobramycin versus cefotaxime in cirrhotics with severe infections. Hepatology 1985;5:457–462.

15. Runyon BA, McHutchison JG, Antillon MR, et al. Short course vs. long course antibiotic treatment of spontaneous bacterial peritonitis: a randomized controlled trial of 100 patients. Gastroenterology 1991;100:1737–1742.

16. Gines P, Rimola A, Planas R, et al. Norfloxacin prevents spontaneous bacterial peritonitis recurrence in cirrhosis: results of a double blind, placebo controlled trial. Hepatology 1990;12:716–724.

17. Ferenci P, Puspok A, Steindl P. Current concepts in the pathophysiology of hepatic encephalopathy. Eur J Clin Invest 1992;22:573–581.

18. Gitlin N, Lewis DC, Hinkley L. The diagnosis and prevalence of subclinical encephalopathy in apparently health, ambulatory, non-shunted patients with cirrhosis. J Hepatol 1986;3:75–82.

19. Conn HO, Leevy CM, Vlahcevic ZR, et al. Comparison of lactulose and neomycin in the treatment of chronic portal-systemic encephalopathy. Gastroenterology 1977; 72:573–583.

20. Van Thiel DH, Gafuiolo S, Wright HI, Chien MC, Gavaler JS. Gastrointestinal transit in cirrhotic patients: effect of hepatic encephalopathy and its treatment. Hepatology 1994;19:67–71.

21. Johnson PJ. The epidemiology of hepatocellular carcinoma. Eur J Gastroenterol Hepatol 1996,8:845–849.

22. McMahon BJ, London T. Workshop on screening for hepatocellular carcinoma. J Natl Cancer Inst 1991;83: 916–919.

23. Huang GT, Sheu JC, Yang PM, Lee HS, Wang TH, Chen DS. Ultrasound-guided cutting biopsy for the diagnosis of hepatocellular carcinoma—a study based on 420 patients. J Hepatol 1996;25:334–338.

24. DiBisceglie AM, Rustgi VK, Hoofnagle JH, Dusheiko GM, Lotze ML. Hepatocellular carcinoma. Ann Intern Med 1988;108:390–401.

25. Rasmussen I, Garden OJ. The management of liver cell cancer. Eur J Gastroenterol Hepatol 1996;8:861–867.

26. Bruix J, Castells A, Bosch J, et al. Surgical resection of hepatocellular carcinoma in cirrhotic patients: prognostic value of pre-operative portal pressure. Gastroenterology 1996;111:1018–1022.

27. Iwatsuki S, Starzl TE, Sheahan DG, et al. Hepatic resection versus transplantation for hepatocellular carcinoma. Ann Surg 1991;214:221–229.

28. Bismuth H, Chiche L, Adam R, Castaing D, Diamond T, Dennison A. Liver resection versus transplantation in cirrhotic patients. Ann Surg 1993;218:145–151.

29. Lai E, Choi T, Tong S, Ong GB, Wong J. Treatment of unresectable hepatocellular carcinoma: results of a randomized controlled trial. World J Surg 1986;10:501–509.

30. Toyoda H, Nakano S, Kumada T, et al. The efficacy of continuous local arterial infusion of 5-fluorouracil and cisplatin through an implanted reservoir for severe advanced hepatocellular carcinoma. Oncology 1995;52: 295–299.

31. Livraghi T, Bolondi L, Buscarini L, et al. No treatment resection and ethanol injection in hepatocellular carcinoma. J Hepatol 1995;22:522–526.

Pancreatic Diseases

Darwin L. Conwell

This chapter addresses the following conditions:

- Acute pancreatitis
- Chronic pancreatitis
- Pancreatic adenocarcinoma
- Endocrine neoplasms of the pancreas
  - Gastrinomas
  - VIPomas
  - Glucagonomas
  - Somatostatinomas

ACUTE PANCREATITIS

Each year, more than 100,000 patients are hospitalized for pancreatitis in the United States, and approximately 2000 of these patients die from severe pancreatitis. Pancreatitis has numerous causes, obscure pathogenesis, and few effective treatments. Most cases are mild (75%), but as many as 25% can be severe, with sequelae of systemic organ dysfunction.

ANATOMY AND PHYSIOLOGY

The pancreas is a retroperitoneal organ approximately 12 to 20 cm in length and 70 to 120 g in weight. The organ head is apposed to the curvature of the duodenum, and the organ tail extends obliquely, posterior to the stomach, toward the hilum of the spleen.

The pancreas has a very rich blood supply, which is supplied by branches of the celiac, superior mesenteric, and splenic arteries. Venous drainage of the pancreas enters the hepatic portal system. Both sympathetic and parasympathetic efferent fibers supplied by the vagus and splanchnic nerves innervate the pancreas via the celiac plexuses.

The functional unit of the pancreas is the pancreatic acinus, which is composed of acinar and ductal cells. The acinar cells have a very rich and highly specialized intracellular matrix for synthesis, storage, and secretion of large amounts of proteins, mainly as digestive enzymes. The ductal cells primarily secrete water and electrolytes.

There are three primary phases to postprandial pancreatic secretion:

1. Cephalic
2. Gastric
3. Intestinal

The cephalic phase is stimulated by the thought, sight, taste, or smell of food via vagal cholinergic innervation. The gastric phase occurs in response to gastric distension, which also is mediated by vagal cholinergic reflexes. The intestinal phase, which is the major phase of postprandial pancreatic secretion, is regulated primarily by release of secretin and cholecystokinin (CCK). Secretin released into the blood from the duodenum is responsible for bicarbonate and water secretion from pancreatic ductal cells. CCK released into the circulation is primarily responsible for protease enzyme secretion from the acinar cells; it also mediates secretin-stimulated electrolyte secretion.

There is experimental evidence in rats for feedback inhibition of pancreatic enzyme secretion by intraduodenal pancreatic proteases such as trypsin, chymotrypsin, and elastase. These pancreatic proteases inhibit release of CCK and, thus, decrease pancreatic secretion.

PATHOPHYSIOLOGY

The pathophysiology of acute pancreatitis has been studied extensively in experimental models, which reveal a disruption

Table 55.1. Causes of Acute Pancreatitis

Gallstones	45%
Alcohol	35%
Idiopathic	10%
Other	10%

Drugs
    Azathioprine
    Thiazide
    Valproic acid
    2′,3′-Dideoxyinosine
    Sulfasalazine
    Trimethoprim-sulfamethoxazole
    Pentamide
    Tetracycline
Trauma
Postoperative
Hyperlipidemia
Hypercalcemia
Infectious agents
    Mumps
    Coxsackie B virus
    Cytomegalovirus
    Candida sp.
    Human immunodeficiency virus
    Salmonella sp.
    Shigella sp.
    Escherichia coli
    Legionella sp.
    Leptospirosis
Ductal obstruction

in the normal separation of lysosomal and pancreatic enzymes with formation of condensing vacuoles. This exposure of pancreatic proenzymes to lysosomal enzymes such as cathepsin B activates trypsinogen and leads to premature activation of other pancreatic enzymes. In turn, this results in pancreatic autodigestion and the potential for profound systemic complications once the activated enzymes leak into the bloodstream.

ETIOLOGY

Numerous patients with pancreatitis have been described. As Table 55.1 shows, acute pancreatitis is caused by gallstones in approximately 45% of patients, by alcohol consumption in approximately 35%, is idiopathic in approximately 10%, and results from other causes in approximately 10%.

CLINICAL PRESENTATION

Typical symptoms of acute pancreatitis include acute abdominal pain, nausea, and vomiting. Patients also may have re-

duced bowel sounds secondary to ileus. Jaundice may be evident with gallstones or compression of the common bile duct by an edematous pancreatic gland. Patients may show evidence of subcutaneous necrosis on skin examination as well.

Laboratory features may include a transient, mild hypoglycemia; hypocalcemia; hyperbilirubinemia; and mild elevations in the serum alanine aminotransferase (ALT) and alkaline phosphatase levels. Patients with a bilirubin level greater than 2.5 times the normal value and a serum ALT of twice the normal value are very likely to have gallstone pancreatitis.

DIAGNOSIS

Acute pancreatitis usually is diagnosed on the basis of clinical findings (described earlier) and elevated serum amylase and lipase levels. It also is important to consider other causes of hyperamylasemia, such as small-bowel obstruction, perforation, infarction, or perforated duodenal ulcers, in the differential diagnosis.

When a patient presents with acute pancreatitis, ultrasonography of the right upper quadrant is the imaging modality of choice. This will help to delineate the presence or absence of gallstones and give some idea of the pancreatic morphology. Computed tomography (CT) is only recommended for those patients with severe pancreatitis who show no improvement clinically after 72 hours of supportive therapy.

PROGNOSIS

The degree of elevation in the serum amylase and lipase levels does not provide any prognostic value when determining the severity of pancreatitis. The most accurate method of determining severity within the first 48 hours after hospital admission is well described in the Ranson criteria (Table 55.2).

Table 55.2. Ranson Prognostic Criteria for Severity of Acute Pancreatitis

At Admission
Age >55 years
Leukocyte count $> 16,000$ μ/L
Plasma glucose > 200 mg/dL
Serum lactate dehydrogenase > 350 μ/L
Serum aspartate aminotransferase > 250 μ/L
During the Initial 48 Hours
Hematocrit decrease of $> 10\%$
Serum urea nitrogen increase of > 5 mg/dL
Serum $Ca^{++} < 8$ mg/dL
$Pao_2 < 60$ mm Hg
Base deficit > 4 meq/L
Fluid sequestration > 6 L

The mortality rate increases considerably in patients with an increasing number of Ranson criteria. Those patients with three or more criteria have severe pancreatitis.

The Ranson criteria are not valid 48 hours after admission. The APACHE II score is more reliable after this time period. Patients with a score of eight or greater have severe pancreatitis.

A dynamic CT scan, which is indicated in patients with severe pancreatitis, will help to determine whether a patient has necrotizing pancreatitis. Uniform enhancement on the CT scan implies an intact microcirculation and is suggestive of interstitial pancreatitis. Areas of nonenhancement indicate disruption of pancreatic microcirculation, which is strongly suggestive of pancreatic necrosis. The infection rate in patients with interstitial pancreatitis is approximately 1%, whereas that in patients with necrotizing pancreatitis is as high as 50%.

TREATMENT

Treatment of acute interstitial pancreatitis usually is supportive, with intravenous fluids and analgesia. Patients with severe pancreatitis (i.e., Ranson score, ≥3; APACHE score, ≥8; or organ dysfunction) require fine-needle aspiration of necrotic areas in the pancreas to rule out infection. These patients also require monitoring in an intensive care unit. Antibiotics do not decrease mortality, but they are strongly recommended. Antibacterial agents with good pancreatic tissue penetration are preferred (e.g., imipenem, ciprofloxacin). If the Gram stain of aspirated pancreatic tissue shows evidence of bacterial colonization, surgical debridement is recommended.

Patients with severe pancreatitis can have other systemic complications, such as renal failure, acute respiratory distress syndrome, gastrointestinal bleeding, or hypotension. Local pancreatic complications can include pancreatic abscess or pseudocyst formation. Pancreatic abscesses primarily are infected with *Escherichia coli* and require both antibiotic therapy and early surgical intervention. Pancreatic pseudocysts occur in approximately 20% of patients with acute pancreatitis and they should be drained only if they are causing symptoms.

Patients with gallstone pancreatitis who are deteriorating clinically or have evidence of biliary sepsis should undergo emergent endoscopic retrograde cholangiopancreatography (ERCP) for removal of impacted gallstones. This should be followed by a cholecystectomy.

CHRONIC PANCREATITIS

ETIOLOGY

The most common cause of chronic pancreatitis, alcohol consumption, accounts for 70% of cases, and approximately 20% of cases are idiopathic. Remaining miscellaneous causes include trauma and prolonged metabolic disturbances (i.e., hy-

percalcemia, hypertriglyceridemia). Chronic pancreatitis also can be inherited as an autosomal dominant disorder (i.e., hereditary pancreatitis).

The underlying physiology involves basal hypersecretion of pancreatic proteins, with a concomitant decrease of protease inhibitors. This changes the biochemical composition of the pancreatic juice, and it predisposes the patient to the formation of protein plugs and pancreatic stones. Blockage of small ducts results in premature activation of pancreatic enzymes, with resultant development of acute pancreatitis that, over time, causes permanent structural damage to the gland.

CLINICAL PRESENTATION

The two most common clinical presentations of patients with chronic pancreatitis are abdominal pain and weight loss. The mechanism for abdominal pain is controversial, but it may involve inflammation of the pancreas, increased intrapancreatic pressure, neuroinflammation, or extrapancreatic causes such as stenosis of the common bile duct and duodenum. The weight loss initially results from a decreased caloric intake because of fear of precipitating abdominal pain. Later, as the pancreatitis advances, patients will develop pancreatic insufficiency manifested as malabsorption or diabetes mellitus.

DIAGNOSIS

The diagnosis of chronic pancreatitis is strongly suggested by the patient history and is confirmed through laboratory tests and imaging studies. The secretin or CCK-stimulation test, which directly measures pancreatic bicarbonate secretion, has a sensitivity and specificity of approximately 90%. An indirect test of pancreatic function that measures urinary chymotrypsin output, the bentiromide test, has a sensitivity of approximately 85% and specificity of 90%.

The presence of diffuse calcifications throughout the pancreas on radiographs, ultrasounds, or CT scans is diagnostic of chronic pancreatitis. Plain-film radiography of the abdomen should be the first diagnostic test, because it is both simple and inexpensive. Ultrasonography has a sensitivity of 70% and specificity of 90%. CT increases the sensitivity and specificity by 10 to 30% over that of ultrasonography alone.

ERCP is the most sensitive and specific diagnostic test for chronic pancreatitis, but it is an expensive procedure with a low but significant rate of complications, notably ERCP-induced pancreatitis. ERCP should be reserved for those patients in whom the diagnosis cannot be established clearly or for evaluation of complications from chronic pancreatitis.

TREATMENT

Treatment of chronic pancreatitis usually is supportive and involves control of pain, avoidance of alcohol, and use of adequate analgesics. At present, the mainstay of treatment involves use of pancreatic enzymes to cause feedback inhibition of pancreatic secretion and, thus, decreased pancreatic ductal pressure.

Nonenteric, coated-enzyme supplementation provides pancreatic protease (i.e., trypsin) to the duodenum in patients with pancreatic insufficiency. Enzyme supplementation decreases the pain of chronic pancreatitis, and enteric-coated preparations that protect lipase from gastric acid destruction help in treatment of steatorrhea. H_2-receptor antagonist or proton-pump inhibitors to decrease gastric acidity may be needed if enteric-coated preparations are not effective in decreasing steatorrhea. It also is important to rule out other causes of steatorrhea, such as celiac sprue, Crohn's disease, or bacterial overgrowth, in patients who are refractory.

Surgery is effective in decreasing abdominal pain, producing relief in 60 to 80% of patients. (The mortality associated with surgery is 5% or less.) A pancreaticojejunostomy is the procedure of choice in most patients.

COMPLICATIONS

The most common complications in patients with chronic pancreatitis include development of pancreatic pseudocysts, ascites, and splenic-vein thrombosis:

- Pancreatic pseudocysts occur in approximately 25% of patients. Asymptomatic pseudocysts can be followed with serial ultrasonograms or CT scans. Most pseudocysts will resolve in time. Large pseudocysts (usually $\geq$ 6 cm) causing symptoms should be drained, either surgically or radiologically.
- Patients with pancreatic ascites require ERCP to document the area of duct disruption, and medical treatment with total parenteral nutrition and octreotide supplementation has been shown to be effective. Those patients who do not respond to medical treatment will require surgical intervention.
- Splenic-vein thrombosis occurs in approximately 4% of patients. Patients are predisposed to gastrointestinal bleeding from gastric varices. The diagnosis is confirmed by celiac angiography, and splenectomy is curative.

PANCREATIC ADENOCARCINOMA

ETIOLOGY: RISK FACTORS

Risk factors for developing pancreatic carcinoma include cigarette smoking, high-fat diet, chronic pancreatitis, hereditary pancreatitis, and industrial exposure to coal-tar derivatives. Patients with chronic pancreatitis have a relative risk for development of pancreatic cancer that increases over time. In addition, hereditary pancreatitis increases the risk of developing pancreatic cancer fivefold.

CLINICAL PRESENTATION

The clinical presentation of pancreatic adenocarcinoma is pain, jaundice, weight loss, or new-onset diabetes. The patient also may have superficial thrombophlebitis, gastrointestinal bleeding, or psychiatric disturbances.

DIAGNOSIS

The diagnosis usually is established through fine-needle aspiration of a mass seen on an ultrasonogram or CT scan of the abdomen. ERCP has a sensitivity of approximately 90% in those patients with negative imaging studies.

TREATMENT AND PROGNOSIS

Surgery offers the only chance for cure; however, only 10% of patients have resectable tumors. The surgery of choice, a Whipple procedure in those patients with carcinoma at the head of the pancreas, carries a mortality rate of approximately 2%. Palliative procedures such as gastrojejunostomy and endoscopic stenting procedures are undertaken in those patients with metastatic disease. Numerous attempts at radiation therapy and chemotherapy have met with poor results and produced no statistically significant beneficial effect on patient survival. Pancreatic ductal carcinoma has a 5-year survival rate of only 1%.

ENDOCRINE NEOPLASMS OF THE PANCREAS

Pancreatic endocrine tumors originate from the neurendocrine cell system. The histologic classification fails to describe the growth pattern of the tumor or to determine whether it is malignant. Malignancy can be determined only if the patient has evidence of metastatic disease. The malignant potential of these tumors varies on the basis of histologic type. Pancreatic endocrine tumors also may be part of the multiple endocrine neoplasia (MEN) type I syndrome.

GASTRINOMAS

Gastrinomas are found in the pancreas or peripancreatic area in 90% of patients. In 15%, they are located in the duodenal wall.

CLINICAL PRESENTATION

Zollinger-Ellison syndrome is characterized by gastric acid hypersecretion, peptic ulceration, and diarrhea. Approximately 25 to 30% of patients with gastrinomas have MEN-type I syndrome. A serum gastrin concentration greater than

1000 pg/mL in patients who produce gastric acid is diagnostic of gastrinoma.

DIAGNOSIS

The diagnosis can be confirmed by the secretin test. An absolute increase in serum gastrin level to greater than 100 pg/mL above baseline confirms the diagnosis. CT or octreotide scanning can localize the tumor.

TREATMENT AND PROGNOSIS

Patients with Zollinger-Ellison syndrome should be explored surgically for isolated tumors. Patients with multifocal tumors and metastatic disease are not candidates for resection. Omeprazole minimizes symptoms, and total gastrectomy can be performed in patients who do not respond to medical treatment. Chemotherapy with streptozocin and 5-fluorouracil is effective. Approximately 50% of patients with gastrinoma die within 10 years because of metastatic disease.

VIPOMAS

Patients with VIPomas usually present with watery secretory diarrhea and profound hypokalemia. VIPomas tend to be large and may be detected on CT scans or ultrasonograms. The diagnosis is established by an elevated serum vasoactive intestinal polypeptide concentration of greater than 200 pg/mL and by a pancreatic endocrine tumor on imaging studies. The definitive therapy is surgical resection; in many patients, octreotide controls diarrheal symptoms.

GLUCAGONOMAS

Glucagonomas are extremely rare tumors of the pancreatic alpha cells. The clinical presentation includes diabetes; a migratory, necrolytic, erythematous rash; stomatitis; glossitis; and weight loss. The diagnosis is confirmed by an elevated fasting plasma-glucagon level of greater than 400 pg/mL with a characteristic skin rash. Surgical resection is the definitive therapy; symptoms can be controlled with octreotide.

SOMATOSTATINOMAS

Somatostatinomas are pancreatic tumor cells that arise from D cells. The characteristic triad of symptoms includes diabetes, cholelithiasis, and diarrhea with steatorrhea. The diagnosis is established by a somatostatin level of greater than 200 pg/ml. There is no known effective treatment, but chemotherapy with streptozotocin and 5-fluorouracil may have some value.

REVIEW EXERCISES

QUESTIONS

1. A 76-year-old woman with ERCP-induced pancreatitis continues to have fevers (39°C) with a rising white-blood-cell count on the fourth hospital day. A dynamic CT scan reveals an area of nonenhancement in the pancreas. What is the next appropriate step in treatment of this patient?
   a. Fine-needle aspiration of the pancreas.
   b. Angiography.
   c. Magnetic resonance imaging.
   d. Start total parenteral nutrition.

2. A 21-year-old woman has had recurrent abdominal pain since 3 years of age. She gives a history of similar symptoms in an uncle, who died of pancreatic cancer at age 45. A KUB shows extensive calcification in the upper abdomen. This patient most likely has what diagnosis?
   a. Celiac sprue.
   b. Zollinger-Ellison syndrome.
   c. Hereditary pancreatitis.
   d. Gastric carcinoma.

3. A 50-year-old man with diabetes and a history of intermittent diarrhea is noted to have a small pancreatic mass during laparoscopic cholecystectomy for gallstones. What serologic test would you perform?
   a. Vasoactive intestinal polypeptide.
   b. Calcitonin.
   c. Somatostatin.
   d. Urinary 5-hydroxyindoleacetic acid.

Answers

1. a

2. c

3. c

SUGGESTED READINGS

Nortan JA, et al. Endocrine tumors of the pancreas. World J Surg 1993;17:425–519.

Information from a symposium on endocrine tumors of the pancreas.

Steer ML, et al. Chronic pancreatitis. N Engl J Med 1995; 332:1482–1490.

A comprehensive update from one of the leaders in pancreatic diseases.

Steinberg W, et al. Acute pancreatitis. N Engl J Med 1994; 330:1198–1210.

A comprehensive update of our present knowledge of acute pancreatitis.

Warshaw AL, et al. Pancreatic carcinoma. N Engl J Med 1992; 326:455–465.

A review assessing the diagnosis and staging of pancreatic carcinoma, with an overview of treatment.

56

Esophageal Diseases

Joel E. Richter

The esophagus is a relatively simple, tubular organ connecting the oropharynx with the stomach. The pleasures of eating and maintaining adequate nutrition require a normal, healthy esophagus, which has three major functions:

1. To transport ingested material from the oropharynx to the stomach,
2. To prevent regurgitation of food and gastric contents from the stomach into the esophagus, and
3. To vent ingested air to reduce abdominal bloating.

ANATOMY AND PHYSIOLOGY

The esophagus can be divided into three functional regions:

1. The upper esophageal sphincter (UES),
2. The esophageal body, and
3. The lower esophageal sphincter (LES).

UPPER ESOPHAGEAL SPHINCTER

The UES consists of striated muscle, which is formed primarily by the horizontal fibers of the cricopharyngeus muscle at the level of the C5-6 vertebrae. Similar to the striated muscles of the oropharynx and upper portion of the esophagus, the UES is innervated like skeletal muscle, and it receives motor input directly from the brainstem (i.e., nucleus ambiguous) to the motor end plates in the muscle. The UES is tonically closed, and it opens momentarily in response to a swallow (i.e., the first function). The UES also forms a secondary barrier that prevents aspiration of gastroesophageal contents (i.e., the second function).

ESOPHAGEAL BODY

The esophageal body consists of an empty tube lined by squamous mucosa, which is comprised of a submucosal layer and two layers of muscles (i.e., the inner circular and outer-longitudinal muscles). There is no serosa overlying the muscle layers. The upper portion of the esophagus is primarily striated muscle, whereas the lower two-thirds are predominately smooth muscle.

The nerve network for the esophageal body lies between the muscle layers. Meissner's (submucosa) plexus is between the muscularis mucosa and the circular muscle layer; Auerbach's (myenteric) plexus is between the circular and longitudinal muscles. Similar to the LES, innervation of the smooth muscle portion of the esophageal body occurs primarily via the vagus nerve, from neurons arising in the dorsal motor nucleus of the brainstem, and nerve endings in the myenteric plexus.

At rest, the esophageal body is quiet, without motor activity. Normal esophageal motor activity is characterized by orderly progression (i.e., peristalsis) of a contraction along the esophagus, in coordination with relaxation and contraction of the UES and LES. Figure 56.1 represents the pressure sequence of a normal, primary peristaltic wave as measured with esophageal manometry. Note the single pressure complex that begins in the pharynx and progressively opens the UES, then moves sequentially down the esophageal body through an opened LES. The food bolus literally is pushed ahead by this peristaltic wave, through the opened LES and into the stomach.

These activities are initiated by the voluntary act of swallowing. Perpetuation through the distal esophagus, however, is controlled by the enteric nervous system.

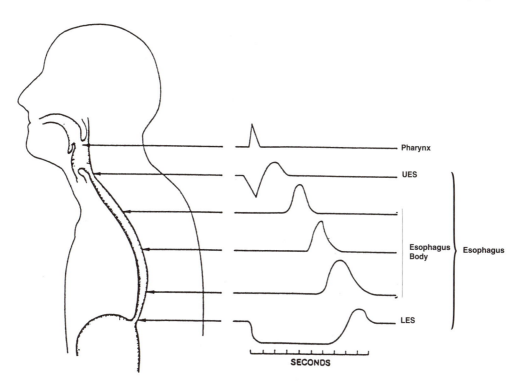

Figure 56.1. Pressure sequences in swallowing.

LOWER ESOPHAGEAL SPHINCTER

The LES is a high-pressure zone of smooth muscle straddling the diaphragm, it is composed of the smooth muscle of the distal esophagus and striated muscle of the crural diaphragm, and it is the major component of the antireflux barrier. At rest, the sphincter is tonically contracted, thus preventing reflux of gastric contents. On swallowing, the LES relaxes, and it stays relaxed until the peristaltic wave reaches the end of the esophagus and produces sphincter closure. LES relaxation is vagally mediated via preganglionic cholinergic nerves and postganglionic, noncholinergic, nonadrenergic nerves. Candidates for inhibitory neurotransmitters include vasoactive intestinal peptide (VIP) and nitric oxide.

Tonic contractions of the LES predominately result from intrinsic muscle activity. LES pressure fluctuates greatly over time, even from minute to minute. Much of this results from various extraesophageal factors that modulate LES pressure, including:

- Food ingested during meals (proteins increase and fats decrease LES pressure)
- Cigarette smoking (decreases LES pressure)
- Gastric distension (decreases LES pressure)

Gastric distension is a critical trigger for transient LES relaxation, which is important in venting ingested gases. In response to transient increases in intra-abdominal pressure, LES pressure increases to a greater degree than the increases occurring in the abdomen below, thus preventing gastroesophageal reflux (GER). In addition, many hormones and peptides affect LES pressure. Those that increase LES pressure include:

- Gastrin
- Motilin
- Substance P
- Pancreatic polypeptide

Those that decrease LES pressure include:

- Secretin
- Cholecystokinin
- Glucagon
- VIP

DIAGNOSTIC PROCEDURES

A thorough patient history and physical examination, which are critical in evaluating patients with esophageal disorders, often will identify the appropriate diagnosis and direct further testing (Fig. 56.2).

IMAGING TECHNIQUES

The barium esophagram is the single most important test for the diagnosis of structural and motor abnormalities in the esophagus. A proper examination should include videotaping the oropharyngeal and esophageal portions of swallowing, as well as full-column and air-contrast views of the distended esophagus, to identify mucosal irregularities, masses, and re-

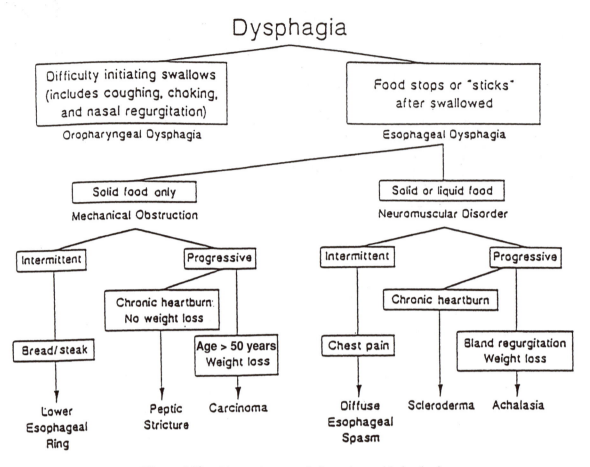

Figure 56.2.   Diagnostic approach for patients with dysphagia.

gions of luminal narrowing. A solid bolus, such as a marsh-mallow or tablet, should be administered to any patient with solid-food dysphagia in whom a liquid study has been nondiagnostic. Esophageal peristalsis can be assessed in the prone position, with the patient taking five to 10 single swallows of barium; this technique approximates esophageal manometry. To identify GER, the ease and extent of barium reflux should be evaluated by rolling the patient from side to side, coughing, the Valsalva maneuver, and the water-siphon test.

Solid-food scintigraphy with the patient upright best approximates normal food ingestion and bolus transport. This is an excellent technique for measuring the completeness of LES relaxation and esophageal emptying, and it is especially helpful in patients with achalasia.

A new imaging technique, endoscopic ultrasonography is useful in diagnosing and staging both benign and malignant esophageal neoplasms. This modality is superior to computed tomography in evaluating depth of tumor infiltration and assessing regional lymph node metastases.

ESOPHAGEAL MOTILITY STUDIES

Manometry is the definitive test for diagnosing esophageal motility disorders, because it allows accurate measurements of sphincter pressures and esophageal pressure waves and more completely evaluates abnormalities of esophageal peristalsis. The test is performed by placing a small catheter into the esophagus and simultaneously measuring, at multiple sites, changes in intraluminal pressure. Normal values over a broad range of ages have been developed using commercially available equipment.

Esophageal manometry does have limitations, however. It accurately records esophageal pressures, but it does not reliably evaluate other important aspects of esophageal function, including completeness of sphincter relaxation, bolus movement, and esophageal emptying. These can be evaluated best with video-imaging techniques.

ENDOSCOPY AND MUCOSAL BIOPSY

Fiberoptic endoscopy with biopsies and brush cytologies is the best method for identifying mucosal abnormalities of the esophagus. The procedure usually is performed on outpatients, with local and, sometimes, intravenous anesthesia. A small, flexible endoscope, which is passed orally, permits a thorough evaluation of the esophagus, stomach, and duodenum. Endoscopy is the preferred method for identifying reflux esophagitis, infectious esophagitis, and neoplasms. Mucosal biopsies are most helpful in identifying Barrett's esophagus, mild esophagitis, neoplasms, and infectious causes of esophagitis.

AMBULATORY ESOPHAGEAL pH MONITORING

Prolonged ambulatory monitoring of the esophagus for as long as 24 hours is the most reliable means of diagnosing GER. The pH probe is placed transnasally, 5 cm above the LES, and GER is defined as a drop in esophageal pH to less than 4. Data are collected in a light-weight box worn on a waist belt, and the information is analyzed by computer. This test usually is performed on outpatients, which allows physiologic activities to be monitored in the supine and upright positions, both while awake and asleep and while fasting and after eating. Recording units have an event marker that can be triggered when symptoms occur. This technique allows accurate quantitation of acid reflux, and it permits correlation between subjective symptoms such as chest pain, cough, heartburn, wheezing, and acid reflux.

TESTS FOR ASSESSING ESOPHAGEAL SENSORY MECHANISMS

Tests that assess esophageal sensory mechanisms are used when the esophagus is suspected of causing atypical symptoms of chest pain. The most commonly used tests include the acid-perfusion Bernstein test for identifying an acid-sensitive esophagus and the edrophonium (Tensilon) test for identifying the esophagus as the source of chest pain. Other provocative tests include:

- Injection of bethanechol, pentagastrin, and ergonovine
- Infusion of hypertonic solutions
- Esophageal balloon distension

GASTROESOPHAGEAL REFLUX DISEASE

Gastroesophageal reflux disease (GERD)—with heartburn its major symptom—is the most common disorder of the esophagus, the major indication for antacid consumption, and probably the most prevalent condition originating from the gastrointestinal tract. According to a recent Gallup survey, 44% of U.S. adults experience heartburn at least once every month, and 10% complain of weekly symptoms. More than 40% take antacids for their heartburn, but only 25% discuss this complaint with a physician. Pregnant women have the highest prevalence of heartburn, with at least 25% having daily symptoms, usually in the third trimester.

GERD is defined as the sequelae, both clinical and histopathologic, of the chronic movement of gastroduodenal contents into the esophagus. GERD, however, is a spectrum of disease; for example, it occurs without adverse consequences in many healthy individuals. Episodes of ''physiologic reflux'' typically are postprandial, short lived, asymptomatic, and almost never occur at night. Pathologic reflux leads to inflammatory changes and mucosal injury (i.e., reflux esophagitis) and, usually, symptoms.

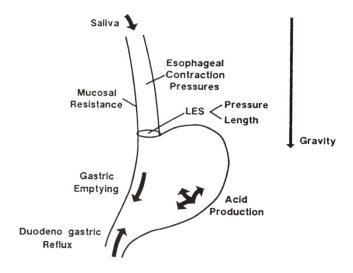

Figure 56.3.   Pathogenesis of GER.

PATHOPHYSIOLOGY

The pathophysiology of GERD results from the complex interplay of multiple factors (Fig. 56.3). The common denominator for acid reflux is creation of a common cavity, representing equilibration of intragastric and intraesophageal pressures. The LES is the major barrier against GER, with a secondary barrier formed by the crural diaphragm during inspiration, but measurement of a single LES pressure is not very discriminatory. In fact, recent studies determined that transient LES relaxation, occurring with either normal or low LES pressures, is the major mechanism promoting free reflux of gastric contents. Transient relaxation accounts for nearly all episodes of reflux in normal subjects and 65% of episodes in patients with GERD. Other patients experience reflux because of very low baseline LES pressures, with either transient increases in intra-abdominal pressure (i.e., stress reflux) or spontaneous reflux across an atonic sphincter.

Esophageal acid clearance normally occurs as a two-step process:

1. Swallow-induced, peristaltic esophageal contractions rapidly clear fluid volume from the esophagus, and
2. The small amount of residual acid is neutralized by saliva, which has a pH of 6.4 to 7.8.

Dysfunction of esophageal clearance mechanisms contributes to esophagitis, particularly in patients with severe motility disorders (e.g., scleroderma) or sicca complex.

Both the nature and volume of gastric contents are important. The primary role of acid is indisputable, but its mechanism of mucosal damage involves the action of coexisting pepsin more than direct damage from acid alone. In animal models, bile salts and pancreatic enzymes can produce esophagitis, but their importance in human disease is unknown. Acid hypersecretory states (e.g., Zollinger-Ellison syndrome) may be associated with a high prevalence of esophagitis. Delayed gastric emptying promotes GER but is an important factor in only 10 to 15% of patients with GERD.

The same degree of acid exposure may lead to variable degrees of mucosal damage, which probably relates to individual variations in esophageal mucosal resistance. Factors contributing to mucosal resistance include:

- Mucus
- Bicarbonate ions secreted by submucosal glands
- Stratified squamous cells and their tight junctions
- Mucosal blood flow

The relationship between a sliding hiatal hernia and development of GERD remains controversial. Most patients with esophagitis have a sliding hiatal hernia, but many patients with hiatal hernias do not have GERD. Recent evidence suggests that a large, nonreducible hernia may interfere with normal esophageal clearance by acting as a fluid trap, thus promoting acid reflux during swallow-induced LES relaxations, particularly in the supine position.

CLINICAL PRESENTATION

Symptoms of GERD include:

- Heartburn
- Associated symptoms
  - Dysphagia
  - Odynophagia
  - Regurgitation
  - Water brash
  - Belching

Patients describe their heartburn as a retrosternal burning pain, which also may be noted in the epigastrium, neck, throat, and, occasionally, the back. Frequently, it occurs postprandially, and it is exacerbated by recumbency or bending over. In patients with heartburn, dysphagia is suggestive of a peptic stricture. Other alternative diagnoses include severe inflammation without stricture, peristaltic dysfunction, and an esophageal cancer arising in Barrett's esophagus. Odynophagia usually represents ulcerative esophagitis. The effortless regurgitation of acidic fluid, especially postprandially and at night, is highly suggestive of GERD. Water brash is the sudden appearance in the mouth of a slightly sour or salty fluid from the salivary glands in response to intraesophageal acid exposure.

GERD may present with extraesophageal symptoms, including:

- Chest pain
- Respiratory complaints
- Ear, nose, and throat problems

In these patients, the clinical symptoms of heartburn or regurgitation may be mild or even absent. Recent studies indicate that GERD may be the major cause of noncardiac chest pain in as many as 50% of patients. Chronic cough, recurrent aspiration pneumonia, and pulmonary fibrosis may relate to GERD, and some studies suggest a close association between asthma and GERD, with up to 80% of patients with asthma having evidence of excessive acid reflux on pH testing. Hoarseness, sore throat, halitosis, dental erosions, vocal-cord granuloma, and even laryngeal cancer may be caused by intermittent aspiration of gastric contents.

DIAGNOSIS

In most patients with classic symptoms of heartburn or regurgitation, the history is sufficiently typical to permit a trial of therapy without diagnostic tests. The following situations should lead to early investigation:

- Esophageal symptoms not responding to medical therapy
- Dysphagia and atypical presentations of suspected GERD
- Possible complications of reflux disease
- Before considering patients for antireflux surgery

Tests for GERD evaluate different variables in the disease spectrum, including:

- Potential for reflux
  - Hiatal hernia
  - Manometry
- Esophageal damage
  - Barium esophagram
  - Endoscopy
  - Mucosal biopsy
- Acid sensitivity
  - Acid-perfusion Bernstein test
  - 24-hour pH test with symptom correlation
- Presence of abnormal reflux
  - Barium esophagram
  - 24-hour pH test

There is no single best selection of tests. These tests must be applied selectively and on the basis of the information desired.

All patients with persistent symptoms of reflux or with frequent relapses after H_2-antagonist therapy should have endoscopy to identify possible esophagitis or other complications of GERD. Patients with esophagitis and complications should undergo biopsy to exclude associated malignancies and Barrett's esophagus. One must remember, however, that most patients with GERD have no evidence of esophagitis at endoscopy.

The barium esophagram should be the first diagnostic procedure in most patients with dysphagia. An optimally administered, double-contrast barium esophagram detects erosive and ulcerative esophagitis in approximately 90% of patients. Radiologic detection of mild (i.e., nonerosive) esophagitis, however, is unreliable. The barium esophagram also is the preferred method for identifying hiatal hernia, and it is good for identifying GER fluoroscopically, particularly when provocative maneuvers are done.

Prolonged esophageal pH monitoring is helpful in patients with atypical presentations or difficult treatment problems, and it has essentially replaced the acid-perfusion Bernstein test. The most common indications include:

- Noncardiac chest pain
- Suspected pulmonary or ear, nose, and throat presentations of GERD
- Intractable reflux symptoms associated with a negative workup

Prolonged pH monitoring also should be conducted before antireflux surgery if there is any question about the diagnosis. It is the single best test for diagnosing GERD, with a sensitivity of 85% and specificity of greater than 95%.

Manometry of LES pressure is not considered to be a sensitive diagnostic test, because fewer than 25 to 50% patients with GERD have a low resting LES pressure (<10 mm Hg). Manometry is reserved for patients in whom another diagnosis (e.g., achalasia) is suspected, and it is mandatory before antireflux surgery to ensure adequate esophageal pump function.

TREATMENT

The rationale for GERD therapy depends on a careful definition of specific aims (Table 56.1). In patients without esophagitis, the goal is simply to relieve the acid-related symptoms; in patients with esophagitis, the ultimate goal also is to heal esophagitis while preventing further complications, such as strictures and Barrett's metaplasia. These goals are set against a complex background, however. GERD is a chronic condition, and patients with esophagitis generally relapse when medical therapy is stopped.

Lifestyle Modifications

Lifestyle changes—the cornerstone of effective reflux treatment in all patients—are summarized in Table 56.2.

Antacids and Alginic Acid

Antacids and alginic acid are useful for treating mild, infrequent reflux symptoms, especially those brought about by lifestyle indiscretions. They are not effective in healing esophagitis, however. Antacids work primarily by neutralizing acid, albeit for relatively short periods. Therefore, patients need to take these agents frequently, usually 20 to 30 minutes after meals and at bedtime. Aluminum hydroxide antacids containing alginic acid form a highly viscous solution, which floats on the surface of the gastric pool and acts as a mechanical barrier. Recent studies confirm that alginic acid tablets (Gaviscon) effectively prevent upright acid reflux.

Prokinetic Drugs

Bethanechol and metoclopramide are prokinetic drugs that effectively relieve symptoms of heartburn, but their efficacy in treating esophagitis is equivocal. Bethanechol (25 mg) and metoclopramide (10 mg) are given 30 minutes before meals and at bedtime. Side effects are common in both young and elderly patients. The new prokinetic drug, cisapride, is more effective than placebo and equal to H_2 antagonists in controlling symptoms of reflux and healing mild esophagitis. Cisapride acts by promoting release of acetylcholine at the myenteric plexus, thereby increasing LES pressure, improving peristalsis amplitude, and accelerating gastric emptying. At a dose of 10 mg taken 30 minutes before meals and at bedtime, cisapride has minimal side effects, with abdominal cramps, borborygmi, and diarrhea being the most common. Cisapride also may be useful in maintenance therapy for patients with reflux symptoms and mild esophagitis.

H_2 Antagonists

Use of H_2 antagonists achieved the first real breakthrough in treatment of GERD, and it continues to be the backbone of therapy for mild reflux esophagitis. Despite advertising to the contrary, all H_2 antagonists (i.e., cimetidine, ranitidine, famotidine, nizatidine), when properly dosed, are equally effective at improving symptoms of reflux and healing mild to moderate

Table 56.1. General Approach to the Treatment of GERD

	Symptoms Without Esophagitis	Mild Esophagitis	Severe Esophagitis or Intractable Symptoms
Acute	Lifestyle changes PRN medication H_2 antagonists Antacids Alginic acid Prokinetics	Lifestyle changes Daily medications H_2 antagonists Cisapride	Lifestyle changes Daily medications Proton-pump inhibitor
Maintenance	PRN medications as above	H_2 antagonists Cisapride	Proton pump inhibitor Antireflux surgery

Table 56.2.   Lifestyle Modifications for Patients with GERD

Decrease LES Pressure	Improve Acid Clearance	Direct Esophageal Irritants	Decrease Gastric Distension

Avoid certain foods
    Fats
    Chocolate
    Coffee
    Carminatives
Avoid certain medications
    Theophylline
    Progesterone
    Antidepressants
    Nitrates
    Calcium channel blockers
	Elevate head of bed
	Upright position after meals
		Avoid citrus, spicy, or
		    tomato-based products
		Avoid medications causing
		    pill-induced esophagitis
			Avoid large meals
			Take evening meals several
			    hours before retiring
			Lose weight

GERD. H_2 antagonists usually are given once, or preferably twice, a day. Recent data on patterns of acid exposure show that most acid reflux occurs during the early evening hours after dinner, and that it decreases markedly during the sleeping hours. Therefore, it may be preferable to take an H_2 antagonist 30 minutes after the evening meal rather than at bedtime. Heartburn can be significantly decreased by H_2 antagonists and esophagitis healed in approximately 60% of patients after up to 12 weeks of treatment. Healing rates differ in individual trials, however, depending primarily on the degree of esophagitis before therapy. Mild esophagitis heals in 75 to 90% of patients, whereas moderate to severe esophagitis heals in only 40 to 50% of patients. Studies also suggest that H_2 antagonists are effective at preventing relapse of GERD in patients with reflux symptoms and mild esophagitis. Recently, the H_2 antagonists are now available over-the-counter at lower doses. Their efficacy is similar to antacids, although the duration of symptom relief may be longer.

Proton-Pump Inhibitors

Omeprazole and lansoprazole are potent, long-acting inhibitors of both basal and stimulated acid secretion. They act by selective, noncompetitive inhibition of the H^+/K^+-ATPase pump on the parietal cell. Proton-pump inhibitors completely abolish reflux symptoms in most patients with severe GERD, usually within 1 to 2 weeks; complete healing of esophagitis occurs after 8 weeks in 80% of patients. Omeprazole and lansoprazole are superior to H_2 blockers at relieving symptoms and healing esophagitis, particularly in patients with severe esophagitis.

Side effects are minimal with short-term use, but the long-term safety of these drugs is not established. Proton-pump inhibitors cause profound hypoacidity, which stimulates gastrin release, which in turn promotes proliferation of enterochromaffin-like cells in the gastric fundus. In the rat model, prolonged use of omeprazole causes gastric carcinoids; however, such carcinoids have not been reported to date in humans treated for uncomplicated reflux or ulcer disease. This class

of drugs is most effective in patients with severe reflux symptoms and severe esophagitis, as well as in maintenance therapy to prevent relapse of esophagitis for up to 1 year.

Antireflux Surgery

Antireflux surgery, done either openly or by laparoscopic techniques, attempts to maintain a segment of the tubular esophagus below the diaphragm and usually includes wrapping the stomach around the distal esophagus to produce increased LES pressure. Long-term relief of symptoms occurs in approximately 80% of patients followed for up to 20 years. Preservation of esophageal function, as confirmed with esophageal testing before surgery, is critical for successful antireflux surgery. So is a skillful surgeon. Indications for antireflux surgery include:

* Younger patients with severe GERD who otherwise would require lifelong medical therapy
* Recurrent, difficult-to-dilate strictures
* Nonhealing ulcers
* Severe bleeding from esophagitis
* Aspiration symptoms from related reflux disease

COMPLICATIONS

PEPTIC STRICTURES

Peptic strictures represent the end-stage of ongoing reflux, mucosal damage, healing, and secondary fibrosis. Strictures present with slowly progressive dysphagia for solids, usually without much weight loss. Radiographically, peptic strictures commonly are found in the lower esophagus, and they are characterized by smooth-walled, tapered, circumferential narrowings. In all patients, the benign nature of the stricture must be confirmed with endoscopy and biopsy. Therapy for peptic strictures consists of a careful review of dietary and medication habits, aggressive antireflux therapy, and bougienage. Patients should chew their food well, take fluids liberally, and avoid potentially damaging pills (e.g., aspirin, nonsteroidal anti-inflammatory drugs [NSAIDs], potassium chloride). Aggressive acid suppression, particularly with proton-pump inhibitors, may reduce the need for subsequent dilations. Dilating (i.e., stretching) the narrowed distal esophagus with blunt bougies, either passed freely or over a guidewire, can markedly relieve symptoms of dysphagia.

BARRETT'S ESOPHAGUS

Barrett's esophagus, secondary to severe esophagitis, produces a unique reparative process in which the original squamous epithelial lining is replaced by metaplastic columnar epithelium. The prevalence of Barrett's esophagus varies depending on the population being studied. Patients with symptomatic GERD have a prevalence rate of 5 to 12%, whereas those with esophagitis, scleroderma, or peptic strictures can have higher rates (11–44%). The diagnosis is best made with endoscopy and confirmed with biopsy. Barrett's epithelium may comprise three types of mucosa, but only the specialized columnar epithelium has malignant potential. Therapy is no different than that for any other form of esophagitis. The major concerns are the increased prevalence and incidence of esophageal adenocarcinoma. The prevalence rate is estimated at 10%, which is a 30- to 40-fold increase over that of the general population. The incidence rates are quite variable, however, ranging from one in 46 to one in 441 patient-years of follow-up. As with colonic adenomas, the columnar lining of the esophagus may evolve through increasing degrees of dysplasia to cancer over time. For this reason, endoscopic surveillance is recommended in patients with Barrett's esophagus to detect high-grade dysplasia or early cancer, thereby permitting curative surgical resection.

OTHER INFLAMMATORY DISORDERS OF THE ESOPHAGUS

Other disorders of the esophagus usually are acute in onset and characterized clinically by odynophagia and dysphagia. An algorithm for evaluating patients with odynophagia is shown in Figure 56.4.

INFECTIOUS ESOPHAGITIS

Infections of the esophagus are rare in the general population. When present, however, they should prompt a search for an underlying abnormality of immunity. Esophageal infection is seen primarily in three groups of immunocompromised patients:

1. Patients infected with the human immunodeficiency virus (HIV),
2. Patients with cancer and granulocytopenia after chemotherapy, and
3. Organ-transplant patients receiving immunosuppressive therapy.

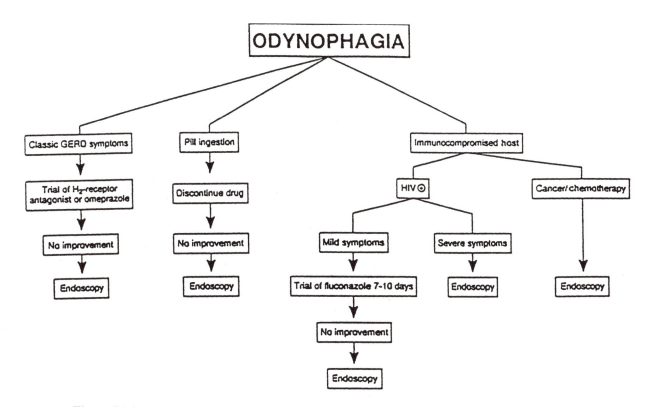

Figure 56.4. Diagnostic approach for patients with odynophagia. (With permission from Wilcox CM, Karowe NW. Esophageal infection: etiology, diagnosis, and Management. Gastroenterologist 1994;2:188–206.)

Other predisposing conditions include:

- Malignancy
- Alcoholism
- Diabetes mellitus
- Therapy with corticosteroids or other immunosuppressive agents

The most common causes of infectious esophagitis are:

- *Candida* sp.
- Herpes simplex virus
- Cytomegalovirus

Candida esophagitis most commonly is seen in patients infected with HIV or who have granulocytopenic cancer. Viral esophagitis predominates in patients with bone marrow transplants. Both candida and viral esophagitis are encountered after solid-organ transplantation. Other less common causes of infectious esophagitis include:

- Histoplasmosis
- *Mycobacterium tuberculosis*
- *Mycobacterium avium-intracellulare* complex
- *Cryptosporidium* sp.
- *Pneumocystis carinii*
- Epstein-Barr virus
- HIV
- Gram-negative and gram-positive bacteria

Mixed infections are present in approximately 30% of patients, and esophageal infections should be suspected in immunocompromised patients presenting with odynophagia, dysphagia, or chest pain. Oral thrush commonly is sought, but its presence does not preclude infections with organisms besides *Candida* sp. Its absence, in addition, does not preclude *Candida* sp. Double-contrast barium esophagram has neither high sensitivity nor specificity for infectious esophagitis. Endoscopy with brush cytology, biopsy, and culture is the best initial diagnostic test.

Candidiasis is recognized by discrete, 3- to 5-mm, raised, yellowish plaques or confluent cheesy exudates. The diagnosis is established most easily by brushing the plaques, smearing the material on a clear glass slide, allowing it to dry, and then applying 10% potassium hydroxide. It is examined for the typical branched hyphae and budding yeast. Fungal cultures and histologic examination of biopsy specimens also are helpful. Treatment of candida esophagitis is determined by the severity of the infection and the nature of the underlying immune defect (Table 56.3).

Herpetic esophagitis is characterized by clear vesicles early in its course. Because these vesicles are short lived, however, the usual finding is discrete, small, superficial ulcers with a punched-out appearance and raised yellow edges. The intervening mucosa often appears normal. Brushings and biopsy specimens show cytologic changes that may be suggestive of herpetic infection (i.e., Cowdry type A inclusions).

Cytomegalovirus esophagitis appears as an extensive area of mucosal injury with inflammatory exudate and ulcerations. The ulcers are very deep, progress in size, and, occasionally,

Table 56.3.   Treatment for Common Esophageal Infections

Infection	Treatment
Candida	
Minimal compromise (i.e. diabetes, steroids)	Nystatin, 1–3 million u QID or Clotrimazole, 100 mg TID
Acquired immunodeficiency syndrome	Ketoconazole, 200–400 mg/day or Fluconazole, 100 mg/day Failure of above: Amphotericin B, 0.3 56.4mg/kg per day
Herpes simplex virus	
Immunocompetent patient	Supportive care Analgesics Topical anesthetics
Immunocompromised patients	
Mild cases	Acyclovir, 200–400 mg 5 times per day orally
More severe cases	Acyclovir, 15 mg/kg per day IV
Cytomegalovirus	Ganciclovir, 5 mg/kg IV q 12 hours or Foscarnet, 60 mg/kg per day IV q 8 hours
HIV	Prednisone, 40 mg daily

Modified with permission from Wilcox CM, Karowe NW. Esophageal infection: etiology, diagnosis, and Management. Gastroenterologist 1994;2: 188–206.

perforate. Biopsy specimens, brush cytologies, or viral cultures may show evidence of this virus. More recently, esophageal ulcerations have been described in patients who seroconvert to HIV. These patients present with a syndrome characterized by fever, myalgia, maculopapular rash, and odynophagia. Endoscopy shows multiple, discrete esophageal ulcerations, and electron microscopy of tissue shows retroviral organisms, thus indicating HIV as the direct cause.

Table 56.3 summarizes treatment of these common esophageal infections.

PILL-INDUCED ESOPHAGITIS

More than half of cases of pill-induced esophagitis result from tetracycline or tetracycline derivatives (particularly doxycycline). Other commonly prescribed medications causing esophageal injury include:

- Slow-release potassium chloride
- Iron sulfate
- Quinidine

Chapter 56 Esophageal Diseases **601**

- Corticosteroids
- NSAIDs

A common factor among these patients is a history of improper ingestion. Nearly half the reported patients have taken little or no fluids while swallowing their pills, or they took their pills just before bedtime. Patients with pill-induced esophageal injury generally complain of odynophagia and retrosternal burning; only a minority report that pills get stuck in their chest. Endoscopy, which is the first investigative study, usually reveals discrete ulcers at aortic arch or distal esophagus.

Patients with pill-induced esophagitis improve after withdrawal of the offending medication. Symptomatic resolution and endoscopic healing usually are evident after 3 days to 6 weeks. In addition to drug discontinuation, other therapies include palliation of odynophagia with viscous lidocaine, prevention of acid reflux, and assurance of adequate nutrition. Rarely, patients will develop strictures requiring dilation. To prevent further pill-induced esophageal injuries, patients should be encouraged to ingest all pills with 8 ounces of water while standing or sitting upright, and they should be discouraged from taking pills just before bedtime.

ESOPHAGEAL MOTILITY DISORDERS

Functional disturbances of the esophagus, resulting from either neurologic or muscular disorders, may involve the striated, smooth, or both muscle segments. The most common motility abnormalities involve the distal smooth muscle.

ACHALASIA

Achalasia is characterized by a double defect in esophageal function. The LES does not relax appropriately, thus offering resistance to the flow of liquids and solids from the esophagus into the stomach. In addition, there is loss of peristaltic muscle movement in the lower two-thirds (i.e., smooth muscle portion) of the esophagus. Achalasia usually presents between 25 and 60 years of age, and men and women are affected equally. The cause is unknown, but the two most popular theories suggest achalasia is secondary to an infection or a degenerative disease of the neurons. In South America, infection with the protozoan *Trypanosoma cruzi* produces ganglion damage and an achalasia-like syndrome with megaesophagus, but this rarely is seen in the United States.

Pathophysiology

Abnormalities in both muscle and nerves can be detected in patients with achalasia, but a neural lesion is thought to be of primary importance. Three major neuroanatomic anatomic changes are described:

1. Loss of ganglion cells within the Auerbach's plexus.
2. Degeneration of the vagus nerve.

3. Qualitative and quantitative changes in the dorsal motor nucleus of the vagus.

There is selective damage to inhibitory neurons, with marked reduction in the levels of VIP and nitric oxide receptors, which can account for the observed motility disturbances. Further evidence of denervation is the exaggerated contractions in the LES and esophageal body that are observed when these patients are given methacholine; this response indicates denervation hypersensitivity.

Clinical Presentation

Nearly all patients with achalasia have dysphagia for solids, and most also have dysphagia for liquids. The onset is gradual, and most have symptoms for an average of 2 years before the diagnosis is made. Postural changes, such as throwing the shoulders back, lifting the neck, and performing a rapid Valsalva maneuver, help to improve esophageal emptying. Fullness in the chest and regurgitation of undigested, nonacidic food are seen in many patients as well. Undigested food may be regurgitated postprandially or at night, thereby causing choking, cough, and aspiration pneumonia. Chest pain occurs in some patients and is more common in younger patients with earlier disease. Surprisingly, heartburn sometimes is described, presumably because of the fermentation of intraesophageal contents. Weight loss is very common and usually increases with the duration of the disease.

Diagnosis

In a patient with suspected achalasia, the first diagnostic test is a barium esophagram. Early in the course of disease, the esophagus may appear normal in diameter but has a loss of normal peristalsis. As the disease progresses, the esophagus becomes more dilated and tortuous, with retained food and air-fluid levels. The distal esophagus is characterized by a smooth, symmetric, tapering, "bird-beak" appearance. Clues to the diagnosis also may be found on chest radiographs, including:

- Widened mediastinum
- Thoracic air-fluid level
- Absence of the gastric air bubble

As Table 56.4 shows, the diagnosis of achalasia is confirmed by esophageal manometry that reveals such characteristic features as:

- Absence of peristalsis in the distal smooth muscle esophagus
- Incomplete or abnormal LES relaxation
- Elevated LES pressure
- Elevated intraesophageal pressures relative to gastric pressures

All patients with achalasia should undergo upper gastrointestinal endoscopy to differentiate primary achalasia from

Table 56.4.   Manometric Characteristics of Esophageal Motility Disorders

| | Achalasia | Spastic Motor Disorder | | | Scleroderma |
		DES	Nutcracker	Hypertensive LES	
Striated muscle/UES	Normal	Normal	Normal	Normal	Normal
Smooth muscle	Aperistalsis	Intermittent peristalsis Simultaneous, repetitive High amplitude Long duration Spontaneous	Normal peristalsis High amplitude	Normal peristalsis	Low-amplitude peristalsis or aperistalsis
LES	Abnormal relaxation High pressure	Occasional LES dysfunction	Normal	High pressure Normal relaxation	Low or no pressure

DES, diffuse esophageal spasm.

pseudoachalasia, which usually is secondary to an adenocarcinoma.

Treatment

The goal of therapy in patients with achalasia is to diminish the high residual LES pressure after swallowing. If esophageal emptying is improved, esophageal stasis and its consequences are reduced. Peristalsis rarely returns, but patients feel as if swallowing is nearly normal. Three treatments are available:

1. Pharmacologic therapy
2. Pneumatic dilation
3. Surgical myotomy

Pharmacologic Therapy   Smooth muscle relaxants, including sublingual isosorbide dinitrate or calcium antagonists such as nifedipine, can be used prophylactically with meals or as necessary for pain or dysphagia. These medications provide variable relief of symptoms, but their effectiveness tends to decrease with time. Recently, botulinum toxin injection into the LES during the time of endoscopy has been shown to improve symptoms for 3 months to 1 year.

Pneumatic Dilation   Pneumatic dilation involves placement of a balloon across the LES, which then is inflated to a pressure adequate to tear the muscle fibers of the sphincter. Good to excellent results occur in 50 to 90% of patients. The procedure can be performed on an outpatient basis, recovery is rapid, and discomfort is short lived. Approximately 30% of patients may require subsequent dilations, however, and perforation is a major complication, being reported in approximately 5% of patients and usually requiring surgical repair.

Surgical Myotomy   Heller myotomy involves incising the circular muscle of the LES and the more distal esophagus down to the mucosa and allowing the muscle to protrude through the incision. Myotomy produces good to excellent results in 60 to 90% of patients, and the operative mortality rate is low. Disadvantages of myotomy include:

- Morbidity associated with the operation
- Long hospital stay
- Increased costs compared with those of pneumatic dilation
- Increased risk of postoperative GER

To prevent postoperative GER, many surgeons now add a loose, antireflux operation to the myotomy. Laparoscopic and thoracoscopic techniques for esophageal myotomy currently are under investigation.

SPASTIC MOTILITY DISORDERS

Spastic manometric patterns differ from those of achalasia by the following characteristics:

- Normal peristalsis intermittently interrupted by simultaneous contractions
- High-amplitude or long-duration waves
- Dysfunction of the LES

Confusion has arisen, however, concerning whether these manometric abnormalities represent separate, distinct entities or variations of diffuse esophageal spasm (Table 56.4). The similarities among these disorders in presentation, natural history, and treatment suggest these syndromes frequently overlap, and that they should be designated as spastic motility disorders of the esophagus.

Pathophysiology

The cause and pathogenesis of these disorders are unknown, and no specific, characteristic pathologic lesion is present. Spastic motility abnormalities commonly are associated with other medical conditions, particularly GER. Central nervous system processing could produce some of these manometric abnormalities. Psychologically stressful interviews, loud noises, or difficult mental tasks can produce simultaneous waves and increase contraction amplitudes in the distal esophagus of both normal persons and patients with spastic motility disorders. These patients also appear to have both a motor and a sensory component to their spastic disorder. Acid instillation may stimulate sensitive neural receptors, thus producing discomfort independent of motility changes. Esophageal balloon distension can reproduce esophageal pain at low distending volumes without noticeable motor changes.

Clinical Presentations

Spastic disorders of the esophagus, which generally present during middle age, occur more commonly in women. Dysphagia and chest pain are the cardinal symptoms; most patients present with both. Dysphagia for liquids and solids is present in 30 to 60% of patients. The symptom is intermittent, however, and it varies daily from mild to very severe, though usually is not progressive or severe enough to interfere with eating or to cause weight loss. Intermittent anterior chest pain, sometimes mimicking that of angina pectoris, is reported by most patients. Episodes of pain last from minutes to hours and may require narcotics or nitroglycerin, thereby further confusing the distinction between esophageal and cardiac pain. Many patients also have symptoms compatible with those of irritable bowel syndrome, as well as urinary and sexual dysfunction in women.

Diagnosis

Spastic motility disorders are best defined with esophageal manometry. The patient's chief symptom is an important factor in the prevalence and type of motility disorder identified. In patients with diffuse esophageal spasm, the barium esophagram may reveal severe, lumen-obliterating, tertiary contractions that trap barium and delay transit, thereby producing to-and-fro movement of the bolus. Other spastic motility disorders frequently have a normal barium esophagram. Endoscopy may be done, but its major role is to identify possible structural lesions or to rule out reflux esophagitis. Provocative tests, such as Tensilon and balloon distension, may be able to provoke chest pain. Ambulatory 24-hour pH monitoring is useful to identify associated GERD, which is present in 20 to 50% of these patients.

Treatment

Many patients respond favorably to confident reassurance that their chest pain is not coming from their heart and has an esophageal origin. GER should be identified and aggressively treated; otherwise, no single drug has a proved efficacy in treatment of spastic esophageal motility disorders. Smooth muscle relaxants such as long-acting nitrates, calcium channel blockers, and anticholinergics may decrease high-amplitude contractions, but they do not consistently relieve chest pain.

Antidepressant medications may reduce the amount of discomfort experienced (as well as the patient's reaction to pain), but the esophageal motility abnormality does not change. Passive dilation of the esophagus has no value; however, pneumatic dilation helps some patients with diffuse esophageal spasm or hypertensive LES who complain of severe dysphagia and have documented delays in esophageal emptying. Rarely, a long, surgical myotomy may help some patients. Aggressive interventions must be used cautiously, however, because symptoms may not be relieved.

SCLERODERMA

Esophageal involvement is seen in 70 to 80% of patients with scleroderma, and more than 90% will have associated Raynaud's phenomena. Esophageal involvement is seen in patients with either progressive systemic sclerosis or in those with CREST (calcinosis, Raynaud's, esophageal involvement, sclerodactyly, and telangiectasias) syndrome. The pathophysiology involves an abnormality in muscle excitation and responsiveness resulting from muscle atrophy and decreased cholinergic excitation.

The classic manometric features of advanced scleroderma include:

- Low LES pressure
- Peristaltic dysfunction of the smooth muscle portion of the esophagus, which is characterized by low-amplitude contractions or aperistalsis
- Preserved function of the striated esophagus and oropharynx (Table 56.4)

Because of these manometric abnormalities, patients may have dysphagia and severe GERD. Surprisingly, dysphagia for solids and liquids is reported by fewer than half of patents with scleroderma. More severe dysphagia is suggestive of esophagitis, often with an associated stricture. Esophagitis is present in most patients.

Treatment of scleroderma centers around GER and its complications. Patients should chew their food well and drink plenty of fluids. GERD should be identified and aggressively treated using H_2 antagonists or proton-pump inhibitors. Strictures respond to frequent dilations. In severe cases, antireflux surgery may be warranted.

ESOPHAGEAL TUMORS

More than 90% of esophageal tumors are malignant. Squamous cell carcinoma, which primarily is a disease of black males, remains the most common malignant tumor of the esophagus. On the other hand, adenocarcinoma, which is seen mainly in white males, is a recognized complication of Barrett's esophagus. Recently, there has been a striking, five- to sixfold increase in the incidence of adenocarcinoma of the esophagus, thus changing the squamous cell:adenocarcinoma ratio from 90:10 to 60:40.

Other types of malignant tumors of the esophagus, which

are rare conditions, include lymphoma and melanoma. Common benign tumors of the esophagus include:

- Leiomyomas
- Lipomas
- Granular cell tumors
- Squamous cell papillomas
- Esophageal cysts

MISCELLANEOUS ESOPHAGEAL DISORDERS

ESOPHAGEAL DIVERTICULA

An esophageal diverticulum is an outpouching of one or more layers of the esophageal wall. It occurs in three main areas:

- Immediately above the UES (i.e., Zenker's diverticulum)
- Near the midpoint of the esophagus (i.e., traction diverticulum)
- Immediately above the LES (i.e., epiphrenic diverticulum)

Zenker's diverticulum presents in older patients, who complain of cervical dysphagia, gurgling in the throat, halitosis, regurgitation of foul food, and, sometimes, a neck mass. Originally believed to relate to discoordination of UES relaxation, recent studies have shown the sphincter opens incompletely because of reduced muscle compliance. To compensate for this decreased cross-sectional area, the hypopharyngeal bolus pressure increases, thus leading to dysphagia and diverticulum formation.

Traction diverticula usually are asymptomatic. They are believed to occur either secondary to external inflammatory processes (e.g., tuberculosis) or to a localized segmental motility disorder.

Epiphrenic diverticula are invariably associated with esophageal motility disorders, especially achalasia.

Diverticula are best diagnosed with a barium esophagram; endoscopy rarely is required. Treatment of symptomatic diverticula requires surgery.

ESOPHAGEAL TEARS AND PERFORATIONS

Esophageal tears and perforations can result from:

- Prolonged and violent vomiting after a meal or alcoholic binge
- Instrumentation of the esophagus
- Ingestion of foods containing bones or sharp foreign objects

A mucosal tear at the gastroesophageal junction is known as a Mallory-Weiss tear. It can be asymptomatic or associated with significant upper gastrointestinal bleeding.

On the other hand, spontaneous esophageal rupture (i.e., Boerhaave's syndrome) is a rare, life-threatening condition that is characterized by a full-thickness tear of the esophageal wall. Patients with Boerhaave's syndrome present with:

- Severe, substernal epigastric pain
- Dysphagia
- Odynophagia
- Dyspepsia

Findings include hypotension, fever, tachycardia, and subcutaneous emphysema. Radiographs frequently reveal:

- Pleural effusions
- Parenchymal infiltrates
- Pneumothorax
- Pneumomediastinum
- Mediastinal widening

The diagnosis is confirmed with a barium esophagram using a water-soluble contrast agent (Gastrografin). On confirmation, a nasogastric tube to provide continuous suction should be placed and the patient given broad-spectrum antibiotics. Small, self-contained leaks can be treated successfully with conservative management, but larger tears require immediate surgery.

RINGS AND WEBS

The lower esophageal (i.e., Schatzki's) ring, which is located at the squamocolumnar junction, is the most common source of intermittent dysphagia for solids. Rings usually are found in patients older than 50 years of age; they rarely are found in those younger than 30 years. The origin of the lower esophageal ring is unknown, but recent studies suggest it is a complication of GERD. The diagnosis is made with:

- Barium swallow using the prone position
- Valsalva maneuver
- Having the patient swallow a marshmallow or tablet to bring out the ring

Treatment includes:

- Simple reassurance, with guidance for adjustment of eating habits
- Dilation of the ring with a blunt bougie
- Therapy for associated GERD

Webs are membranous narrowings covered entirely by squamous mucosa. They can occur anywhere along the esophagus but are found primarily in the upper 2 to 4 cm. Some webs are congenital; others are associated with iron deficiency anemia (i.e., Patterson-Kelly or Plummer-Vinson syndrome). Most webs are asymptomatic and are discovered as incidental radiologic findings. Symptomatic patients usually are women reporting dysphagia for solids rather than for liquids. The diagnosis is made with the lateral view of the barium esophagram. Treatment with bougienage often is successful.

REVIEW EXERCISES

QUESTIONS

1. Which of the following are the components of the LES?
   a. Distal esophageal smooth muscle.
   b. Distal esophageal striated muscle.
   c. Crural portion of the diaphragm.
   d. a and c.

2. A patient presents with intermittent dysphagia for solids only, and especially for bread and meat. What is the cause?
   a. Lower esophageal (i.e., Schatzki's ring).
   b. Esophageal cancer.
   c. Zenker's diverticulum.
   d. Achalasia.

3. The most effective medication for relieving heartburn symptoms and healing esophagitis is:
   a. Antacids.
   b. Cisapride.
   c. H_2 blockers.
   d. Proton-pump inhibitors.

4. Achalasia usually is not characterized by which of the following symptoms?
   a. Dysphagia for solids and liquids.
   b. Dysphagia for solids only.
   c. Bland regurgitation.
   d. Heartburn.

5. The most common pill associated with esophagitis is:
   a. NSAIDs.
   b. Quinidine.
   c. Doxycycline.
   d. Slow-release potassium.

6. Which one of these diseases has *not* been associated with GERD?
   a. Noncardiac chest pain.
   b. Asthma.
   c. Dental erosion.
   d. Laryngeal cancer.
   e. All of the above.

Answers

1. d

The LES has two components. Basal pressure is generated by the distal esophageal smooth muscle. The increased sphincter pressure that occurs during inspiration is generated by the crural diaphragm. This augmentation prevents GER with deep inspiration efforts.

2. a

The lower esophageal ring presents classically with dysphagia for solids and no weight loss. Esophageal cancer has progressive dysphagia and weight loss. Achalasia presents with dysphagia for solids and liquids and regurgitation of non-acidic, undigested food and saliva. Zenker's diverticulum present with cervical dysphagia, bland regurgitation, and halitosis.

3. d

Proton-pump inhibitors decrease acid secretion by at least 80%, thus inhibiting both nocturnal and meal-stimulated acid secretion; they are the most effective medications for relieving symptoms of reflux and healing esophagitis. Antacids, which only neutralize acid in the stomach, are best for intermittent relief of mild heartburn. Cisapride, which improves LES pressure, esophageal clearance, and gastric emptying, is most effective for relieving mild to moderate reflux symptoms, usually without esophagitis. H_2 blockers inhibit acid secretion best at night, and they are best for mild to moderate heartburn associated with mild esophagitis.

4. b

Dysphagia for solids suggests an anatomic (i.e., structural) rather than a functional (i.e., motility) disorder.

5. c

All these medications are associated with pill-induced esophagitis. The most frequent culprit, however, is doxycycline, because it is a widely used antibiotic. Classically, young adults taking doxycycline for acne will present with dysphagia and odynophagia, because they take their medication either with a minimal amount of water or immediately before bedtime.

6. e

More than 50% of patients with noncardiac chest pain have acid reflux. Extraesophageal presentations of GERD include damage to the lungs (i.e., asthma) and oropharynx (e.g., hoarseness, vocal-cord granulomas, dental erosions, laryngeal cancer) secondary to high reflux.

SUGGESTED READINGS

Baehr PH, McDonald GB. Esophageal infections: risks factors, presentation, diagnosis and treatment. Gastroenterology 1994;106:509–532.

Baron TH, Richter JE. The use of esophageal function tests. Adv Intern Med 1993;38:3661–3686.

Biot WJ, Devesa SS, Kneller RW, Fraumeni JF Jr. Rising incidence of adenocarcinoma of the esophagus and gastric cardia. JAMA 1991;265:1287–1289.

Champion GL, Richter JE. Atypical presentations of gastroesophageal reflux disease: chest pain, pulmonary, and ear, nose, throat manifestations. Gastroenterologist 1993;1:18–33.

Kim-Deobold J, Kozarek RA. Esophageal perforation: an 8-year review of a multispeciality clinic's experience. Am J Gastroenterol 1992;87:1112–1119.

Parkman HP, Reynolds JC, Ouyang A, Rosato EF, Eisenberg JM, Cohen S. Pneumatic dilatation or esophagomyotomy treatment for idiopathic achalasia: clinical outcome and cost analysis. Dig Dis Sci 1993;38:75–85.

Sloan S, Rademaker AW, Kahrilas PJ. Determinants of gastroesophageal junction incompetence: hiatal hernia, liver esophageal sphincter, or both? Ann Intern Med 1992;117:977–982.

Sontag SJ. The medical management of reflux esophagitis. Gastroenterol Clin North Am 1990;19:683–712.

Spechler SJ. Department of Veterans Affairs Gastroesophageal Reflux Disease Study Group. Comparison of medical and surgical therapy for complicated gastroesophageal reflux disease. N Engl J Med 1992;326:786–792.

Peptic Ulcer Disease

Gary W. Falk

Peptic ulcer disease (i.e., gastric and duodenal ulcers) is a common clinical problem. Approximately 500,000 new cases and 4 million recurrences are seen in the United States each year. The mortality rate from peptic ulcer disease is low (i.e., <10,000 deaths annually), but the cost of the disorder is staggering, with estimates for its diagnosis and treatment at $3 to $4 billion each year.

Peptic ulcer disease once was thought of simply as a problem of acid hypersecretion. Today, however, it is clear that an ulcer is the end result of an imbalance between aggressive and defensive factors in the gastroduodenal mucosa. Much of this imbalance clearly relates to infection with *Helicobacter pylori*.

EPIDEMIOLOGY

The lifetime prevalence of peptic ulcer disease is approximately 5 to 10%. A variety of risk factors predispose patients to peptic ulcer disease, including a family history of ulcers, smoking, ingestion of nonsteroidal anti-inflammatory drugs [NSAIDs], and infection with *H. pylori*. Certain diseases are associated with peptic ulcer disease as well. The unopposed hypergastrinemia of Zollinger-Ellison syndrome (i.e., sporadic and multiple endocrine neoplasia, type 1 [MEN-1]) causes gastric acid hypersecretion, as do the elevated histamine levels in systemic mastocytosis and basophilic leukemia. The mechanisms whereby other disorders, including cirrhosis, chronic obstructive pulmonary disease, chronic renal failure, renal transplantation, and α_1-antitrypsin deficiency, are associated with peptic ulcer disease are unknown.

A number of "myth" factors clearly are not associated with development of ulcers. Stress, personality, occupation, alcohol consumption, and diet have no relationship to the pathogenesis of peptic ulcer disease.

GASTRODUODENAL MUCOSAL OFFENSIVE AND PROTECTIVE FACTORS

Formation of ulcers requires acid and peptic activity in gastric secretions. Acid secretion occurs in the parietal cells, which are located in the oxyntic glands of the fundus and body of the stomach (Fig. 57.1). These cells may be stimulated to secrete acid by three different pathways. The neurocrine pathway involves vagal release of acetylcholine. The paracrine pathway is mediated by release of histamine from both mast and enterochromaffin-like cells in the stomach. The endocrine pathway is mediated by release of gastrin from antral G cells. Each of these transmitters has a specific receptor located on the basolateral surface of the parietal cell, and stimulation of these receptors activates the intracellular second-messenger systems. In these second-messenger systems, gastrin and acetylcholine promote accumulation of intracellular calcium, and histamine causes a stimulatory G protein to activate adenylate cyclase, which in turn generates cyclic adenosine monophosphate. These intracellular messengers then activate protein kinases that activate the proton pump (i.e., the H^+,K^+-ATPase enzyme), which is located at the apical surface of the parietal cell, to secrete hydrogen ions in exchange for potassium ions. Prostaglandins and somatostatin inhibit parietal cell function through binding to receptors that act through inhibitory G proteins to inhibit adenylate cyclase. Acid is necessary to convert pepsinogen, which is secreted from gastric chief cells, into pepsin, which is a proteolytic enzyme that is inactive at a pH greater than 4.

Under normal circumstances, gastroduodenal surface epithelial cells resist injury through several protective mechanisms. First, these cells secrete mucus and bicarbonate, which creates a pH gradient in the mucus layer between the acidic gastric lumen and the cell surface. Second, the surface cells resist back-diffusion of acid by intrinsic mechanisms. Finally, prostaglandins enhance mucosal protection by:

Figure 57.1. Acid secretion by the parietal cell. Each transmitter has a specific receptor located on the basolateral surface of the parietal cell. Stimulation of these receptors leads to activation of intracellular second-messenger systems: gastrin and acetylcholine promote accumulation of intracellular calcium, and histamine causes a stimulatory G protein (G_s) to activate adenylate cyclase, which in turn generates cyclic adenosine monophosphate (cAMP). These intracellular messengers then activate protein kinases that activate the proton pump (i.e., the H^+,K^+-ATPase enzyme), which is located at the apical surface of the parietal cell, to secrete hydrogen ions in exchange for potassium ions. Prostaglandins and somatostatin inhibit parietal cell function through binding to receptors that act through inhibitory G proteins (G_i) to inhibit adenylate cyclase. Dotted arrows indicate sites of action of various drugs that inhibit acid secretion. *ATP,* adenosine triphosphate; *ECL,* enterochromaffin-like cells.

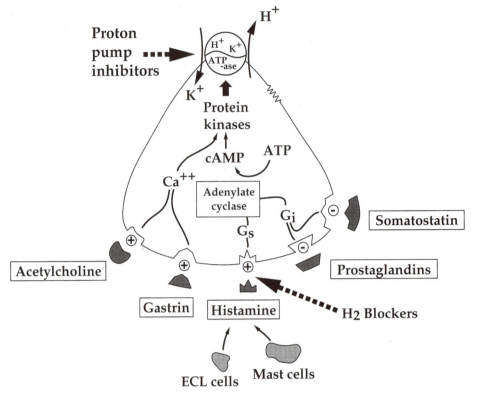

1. Increasing mucus secretion,
2. Increasing bicarbonate production, and
3. Maintaining mucosal blood flow.

PATHOPHYSIOLOGY

Peptic ulcers develop when the equilibrium between acid peptic activity and mucosal defenses is disrupted. *H. pylori,* NSAIDs, and acid-secretory abnormalities are the major factors that disrupt this equilibrium. Acid peptic injury is necessary for ulcers to form, but acid secretion is normal in almost all patients with gastric ulcers. In addition, acid secretion is increased in approximately one-third of patients with duodenal ulcers. Zollinger-Ellison syndrome accounts for 0.1% of patients who present with peptic ulcer disease. A defect in bicarbonate production and, hence, acid neutralization in the duodenal bulb, also is seen in patients with duodenal ulcer disease. This abnormality resolves with eradication of *H. pylori,* however, if it is present.

HELICOBACTER PYLORI

Helicobacter pylori is a Gram-negative, curved, flagellated rod that is found only in the gastric epithelium or in gastric metaplastic epithelium in the duodenum and esophagus. The organism has a characteristic urease activity, resides in the mucus layer between the junction of gastric epithelial cells, and rarely penetrates the cells. *H. pylori* clearly causes histo-

logic gastritis, and it is responsible for most cases of gastritis that are not associated with a known, primary cause such as eosinophilic gastritis or autoimmune gastritis. *H. pylori* antral gastritis occurs in 80 to 95% of patients with duodenal ulcers and in 70 to 90% of patients with gastric ulcers.

Clearly, *H. pylori* causes histologic gastritis, but only a minority of patients with *H. pylori* gastritis develop peptic ulcer disease or gastric cancer. There is a clear, age-related prevalence of infection with *H. pylori* in healthy subjects, increasing from 10% in those younger than 30 years of age to 60% in those older than 60 years. *H. pylori* colonization rates also are higher in blacks, lower socioeconomic classes, and inhabitants of custodial institutions. Unless treated, infection with *H. pylori* typically is lifelong.

PATHOGENESIS OF *HELICOBACTER PYLORI*–INDUCED INJURY

Helicobacter pylori is a noninvasive organism. It usually resides in the mucus layer overlying the gastric epithelium, but some organisms actually adhere to cells. How the organism escapes the bactericidal effects of gastric acid, colonizes the gastric mucosa, and damages the epithelial cells is not well understood. Important factors in the organism's ability to colonize the stomach include its flagella, which facilitate locomotion, its ability to adhere to the mucus layer, and its production of urease. Urease increases the juxtamucosal pH, thus creating a microclimate more hospitable than that of the acidic stomach. Colonization then results in a response of both acute and chronic inflammatory cells and, hence, gastritis. *H. pylori* also induces gastric epithelial cells to produce inflammatory cytokines.

Subsequent clinical outcomes depend on a complex interplay between virulence factors of the organism, host response, environmental factors, and age at the time of infection. There clearly are different strains of *H. pylori,* with different virulence factors. The *vacA* gene encodes a vacuolating cytotoxin that damages epithelial cells and is more common in patients with peptic ulcer disease. This often is seen together with the *cagA* gene, which also more commonly is seen in patients with peptic ulcer disease. The most common end point of infection with *H. pylori* is chronic superficial gastritis, which may persist for years. Duodenal and gastric ulcers develop in a minority of patients. Atrophic gastritis is another end result of infection, and this may increase the risk of gastric cancer. Finally, the mucosal lymphocytic response to infection may produce a monoclonal B-cell proliferation in mucosa-associated lymphoid tissue (MALT), thus resulting in MALT lymphoma as well as more aggressive lymphomas.

The inflammatory response to *H. pylori* is heterogeneous, as is peptic ulcer disease. Acute infection results in short-lived gastric acid hyposecretion, which resolves despite persistence of the organism. Chronic infection increases the basal gastrin, gastrin response to a meal, basal unstimulated acid output, and gastrin-stimulated acid output. All of these abnormalities resolve after eradication of the organism. Regulation of antral G cells may be altered by abnormalities in the ability of adjacent somatostatin-producing D cells to shut down gastrin release. Eradication of *H. pylori* causes an increase in production of D-cell mRNA and in the number of D cells themselves. Increased gastric acid secretion results in exposure of the duodenal bulb to an increased acid load and, hence, development of gastric metaplasia, which typically is colonized with *H. pylori.*

USE OF NSAIDS

Ingestion of NSAIDs is associated with an increased risk of developing gastric and duodenal ulcers, with the risk for gastric ulcers approximately six times greater than that for duodenal ulcers. NSAID-induced ulceration occurs with all drugs in this class, regardless of enteric coating or delivery as a prodrug formulation. Certain compounds such as salsalate, nabumetone (Relafen), and etodolac (Lodine), however, may be associated with a decreased risk of ulceration. New NSAIDs that selectively inhibit inducible cyclo-oxygenase enzymes and release nitric oxide may have less gastrointestinal toxicity.

Two types of mucosal injury are caused by NSAIDs. The first develops after acute ingestion and relates to direct topical injury of mucosal cells. Acute aspirin ingestion causes a decrease in mucosal potential difference, enhanced back-diffusion of hydrogen ions, and local inflammation. Hyperemia,

subepithelial hemorrhage, and superficial erosions are seen endoscopically. In the second, which occurs with longer-term NSAID use, these types of lesions disappear and frank peptic ulceration may develop. Chronic NSAID ingestion results in inhibition of mucosal prostaglandin synthesis and, hence, a decrease in mucus and bicarbonate production and mucosal blood flow.

The risk of NSAID-induced ulceration is dose related, and it increases with age, female sex, smoking, concurrent use of corticosteroids, increasing duration of therapy, and history of ulcer disease. Serious complications such as bleeding, perforation, and gastric outlet obstruction develop in 2 to 4% of patients receiving NSAIDs and typically occur without antecedent symptoms. Risk factors for these serious complications are age older than 75 years, previous peptic ulcer disease, previous peptic ulcer bleed, and underlying cardiovascular disease.

The frequencies of *H. pylori* infection and NSAID ingestion increase with age. It remains to be seen, however, if eradication of *H. pylori* results in decreased frequency of NSAID-induced peptic ulcers.

CLINICAL PRESENTATION

Epigastric, burning abdominal pain that is relieved by antacids and often awakens the patient at night classically has been associated with peptic ulcer disease. Unfortunately, epigastric pain as a marker for ulcer disease has a low sensitivity and specificity, and epigastric pain more commonly does not result from an ulcer. Dyspepsia, which is the classic symptom of peptic ulcer disease, is defined as a pain centered in the upper abdomen or as discomfort characterized by fullness, bloating, distention, or nausea. Symptoms may be chronic, recurrent, or of new onset. Dyspepsia is a common clinical problem, and it may be seen in 13 to 40% of adults. The differential diagnosis of dyspepsia is extensive and includes:

- Peptic ulcer disease
- Gastroesophageal reflux disease
- Gastric cancer
- Gastroparesis
- Functional dyspepsia

Ulcers also may be asymptomatic, especially in patients ingesting NSAIDs. Patients also may present with complications of ulcer disease; hemorrhage may develop in 20%, perforation in 5%, and gastric outlet obstruction in 2%.

DIAGNOSIS

There are four possible diagnostic approaches to a patient with dyspepsia:

1. A short trial of empiric antisecretory therapy.
2. Immediate endoscopy.

3. Empiric antibiotic therapy for *H. pylori,* without testing for *H. pylori* infection.
4. Noninvasive testing for *H. pylori* infection, followed by treatment with antibiotics or endoscopy in positive patients.

No randomized, controlled, clinical trials have produced results that would allow physicians to make evidence-based decisions about the approach to dyspepsia in the *H. pylori* era.

The approach of empiric antisecretory therapy was endorsed by the American College of Physicians in 1985, and there have been no updated guidelines since then. Empiric therapy for 6 to 8 weeks using standard doses of an H_2-receptor antagonist, combined with withdrawal of offending agents such as NSAIDs and cigarettes, was recommended for patients with intermittent dyspepsia but no clinically obvious disease. A diagnostic evaluation without initial empiric therapy, however, was indicated for patients with obvious systemic symptoms, such as weight loss, bleeding, nausea, and vomiting. Immediate investigation also was deemed to be appropriate in patients older than 45 to 50 years of age with new-onset dyspepsia in whom gastric neoplasia was a consideration. In addition, diagnostic studies were indicated for the following patients:

- Those failing to respond to 7–10 days of therapy
- Those with persistent symptoms after 6–8 weeks of therapy.
- Those with symptom recurrence.

Immediate endoscopy was advocated by Bytzer et al., who found that prompt endoscopy in patients with dyspepsia resulted in fewer physician visits, less use of antisecretory drugs, decreased number of sick days, and greater patient satisfaction than in patients who were treated empirically with H_2-receptor antagonists. This study did not deal with *H. pylori* infection, however. Silverstein et al., using a decision-analysis model, found the decision between empiric antisecretory therapy and initial endoscopy to be essentially a "toss-up."

Also using decision-analysis models, Fendrick et al. and Ofman et al. found a strategy of initial noninvasive testing for *H. pylori* in patients with uncomplicated dyspepsia, followed by antimicrobial therapy in positive patients, to be the most cost-effective approach to this population. This is the so-called "test and treat" approach.

To date, empiric treatment of patients with dyspepsia using antibiotics for presumed *H. pylori* infection without proof of infection is not supported by results with any model. Indiscriminate, widespread use of antimicrobial therapy also may be associated with illnesses related to the alteration of normal human flora, increased resistance of *H. pylori* and other bacteria that are not a target of therapy, and a host of adverse effects (e.g., *Clostridium difficile* colitis).

Given the limitations of the available data, what is the

Table 57.1. Diagnostic Approaches for Patients with Dyspepsia

1. Immediate endoscopy mandatory for alarm signs of:
   Weight loss
   Anorexia
   Nausea or vomiting
   Evidence of bleeding (anemia, melena)
   Age > 50 years with new-onset dyspepsia
   Gastric ulcer or lesion suspicious for cancer on barium radiographs
2. Immediate endoscopy optional for:
   Young patients
   Short duration of symptoms
   Absence of alarm signs
   NSAID use
3. Noninvasive *H. pylori* testing in patients without alarm signs (serology preferred):
   Positive patients → antimicrobial treatment
   Negative patients → antisecretory treatment
4. Endoscopy in patients with persistent symptoms after antisecretory or antimicrobial therapy:
   Assess response after 2 weeks

most rational strategy? Perhaps the most thoughtful approach is that of Graham and Rabeneck (Table 57.1).

Upper endoscopy and double-contrast radiography are comparable in diagnostic accuracy for ulcers. Radiology still has a cost advantage, but far too many obsolete and inaccurate single-contrast studies are still performed. Upper endoscopy has the advantages of direct mucosal visualization, biopsy capabilities for gastric ulcers and *H. pylori,* and therapeutic options for bleeding ulcers and gastric outlet obstruction.

DIAGNOSTIC TESTS FOR *H. PYLORI*

Testing for *H. pylori* is essential in patients with peptic ulcer disease. A negative test will focus the subsequent diagnostic evaluation on other causes of peptic ulcer disease, such as NSAID consumption or gastrinoma. Furthermore, a negative test precludes antimicrobial therapy to eradicate *H. pylori.* Prior administration of proton-pump inhibitors, bismuth, antibiotics, or sucralfate may suppress *H. pylori* temporarily, thus resulting in false-negative test results.

Several diagnostic tests are available for detecting infection with *H. pylori.* These are best subdivided into invasive and noninvasive techniques:

- Invasive (endoscopic biopsy required)
  - Culture
  - Histology
  - Rapid urease test

- Noninvasive
  - Serology
  - ^{13}C urea breath test

Demonstration of *H. pylori* by either culture or histology of the organism is the gold standard. Culture is tedious, however, and it is less sensitive than histologic review of a biopsy specimen, which classically shows chronic superficial gastritis. The organism is best seen with special stains, such as Warthin-Starry, Giemsa, or Genta. Classically, biopsy specimens have been taken from the antrum. The organism may have a patchy distribution, however, and the yield of biopsy specimens is increased by sampling the fundus as well as the antrum. Because they require endoscopy, both biopsy and culture are invasive and expensive. The passage of several days also is necessary to obtain the diagnosis. Mucosal biopsies may be directly inoculated into a urea-containing medium with a pH-sensitive indicator that turns red when ammonia is metabolized from urea by the urease of the organism (i.e., the rapid urease test). The first of the rapid urease tests, the CLO test (*C*ampylobacter-*L*ike *O*rganism), has a sensitivity of approximately 90%, but the specificity approaches 100%. Rapid urease tests are easy to perform and inexpensive, thus making them the endoscopic method of choice to detect *H. pylori.*

The urease activity of *H. pylori* also may be detected noninvasively by ingestion of ^{13}C-labeled urea. The urease splits off labeled carbon dioxide, which may be detected in the patient's breath. The urea breath test is accurate, with a sensitivity and specificity of approximately 95% each. The ^{13}C-urea breath test is the ideal noninvasive test to document *H. pylori* eradication, because it does not involve exposure to radiation and reflects current infection only. The other noninvasive test is serologic testing for antibodies to *H. pylori.* The enzyme-linked immunoabsorbent assay (ELISA) is simple, inexpensive, and commercially available, and detection of immunoglobulin (Ig) G antibody has a sensitivity of up to 99% and specificity of up to 100% for diagnosis of the organism. The antibody level falls after eradication, but the time course of this fall is uncertain. It may remain positive for up to 3 years after bacterial eradication, thereby limiting its role in documentation of eradication. Furthermore, to document a decreased antibody titer, both pretreatment and posttreatment samples must be run in parallel, thus making such testing impractical. Rapid, inexpensive, office-based serologic tests with good operating characteristic are available, but their accuracy is somewhat less than that of laboratory-based assays.

On the basis of cost, accuracy, and simplicity, the rapid urease test is the endoscopic method of choice for diagnosis of infection with *H. pylori.* Recent treatment with antibiotics or proton-pump inhibitors, however, decreases the yield of the test. Histology should be performed only if the rapid urease test is negative and the bacteria still suspected. Serology of IgG antibodies to *H. pylori* by ELISA is the noninvasive method of choice to detect *H. pylori* infection, because it is inexpensive, widely available, and accurate. The urea breath test is the test of choice to document eradication of infection

in selected patients, such as those with complicated peptic ulcer disease (i.e., bleeding, perforation, or obstruction) and recurrent symptoms after a course of antibiotic therapy.

Because treatment suppresses the organism even if it is not eradicated, confirmation of cure should be done no sooner than 4 weeks after treatment. Routine monitoring for relapse, reinfection, or treatment failure is not recommended except in those who have suffered from complications of an ulcer such as bleeding.

TREATMENT

INITIAL TREATMENT

Several excellent treatment options are available—and hard to beat—for healing peptic ulcers. H_2-receptor antagonists heal 90 to 95% of duodenal ulcers and 88% of gastric ulcers at 8 weeks. Proton-pump inhibitors heal 80 to 95% of duodenal ulcers at 4 weeks and 95% of gastric ulcers at 8 weeks. Peptic ulcer disease is a chronic disorder, however, and carries a relapse rate at 1 year of 50 to 90% after successful antisecretory therapy for both duodenal and gastric ulcers. This relapse rate was once reduced to between 10 and 30% at 1 year using chronic, low-dose (i.e., half-strength), maintenance therapy with any H_2-blocker. Treatment of *H. pylori* infection has revolutionized treatment of peptic ulcer disease.

TREATMENT OF *H. PYLORI* INFECTION

Eradication of *H. pylori* accelerates the rate of healing for duodenal and gastric ulcer healing to approximate that with use of omeprazole at 4 weeks. Eradication markedly changes the natural history of both duodenal and gastric ulcers. In patients with healed gastric and duodenal ulcers, the relapse rate at 1 year is 13% and 12%, respectively, in those treated with ranitidine and triple therapy, compared with 74% and 95%, respectively, in those treated with ranitidine alone. The annual reinfection, rate is approximately 1%. Eradication of *H. pylori* should be attempted in all patients with current or past peptic ulcer disease and evidence of infection.

Treatment of *H. pylori* infection is not simple, however, and several obstacles await both the physician and the patient:

- None of the antimicrobial regimens used for *H. pylori* infection are 100% effective. Despite in vitro sensitivity to a variety of antibiotics, the in vivo activity of these same drugs against H. pylori is disappointing. As such, eradication of the organism is difficult. Factors such as compliance and antibiotic resistance, especially to clarithromycin and metronidazole, influence treatment efficacy as well.
- There is no agreement on a single best regimen.
- There is no agreement on dosage, frequency, and duration of therapy.
- Many studies involve small sample sizes.

Table 57.2.   Efficacy and Cost of 14 Days of Therapy for *H. pylori* Infection

Regimen	Wholesale Cost ($)	Efficacy (%)
"BMT"	30	90
Bismuth, 2 tablets q.i.d.		
Metronidazole, 250 mg q.i.d.		
Tetracycline, 500 mg q.i.d.		
Helidac	75	90
BMT + omeprazole, 20 mg b.i.d.	132	95
Helidac + omeprazole, 20 mg b.i.d.	177	95
Ranitidine bismuth, 400 mg b.i.d. Clarithromycin, 500 mg t.i.d.	186	80
Omeprazole, 40 mg q.i.d. Clarithromycin, 500 mg t.i.d.	239	80
Lansoprazole, 30 mg b.i.d. Amoxicillin, 1 g b.i.d. Clarithromycin, 500 mg b.i.d.	198	90
Metronidazole, 500 mg b.i.d. Omeprazole, 20 mg b.i.d. Clarithromycin, 250 mg b.i.d.	201	90

Eradication of *H pylori* is defined as absence of the organism at 4 weeks (or later) after completion of therapy. Treatment options, efficacy, and costs are shown in Table 57.2.

Triple therapy with bismuth subsalicylate, two tablets four times a day, combined with tetracycline, 500 mg four times a day, and metronidazole, 250 mg four times a day, for 14 days yields consistently high eradication rates (i.e., close to 90%). This regimen has now been approved by the U.S. Food and Drug Administration (FDA) and is marketed as Helidac (Protor & Gamble). Side effects are common, however, and dosing is both complex and inconvenient. Compliance is a key factor in predicting the efficacy of triple therapy. Subjects taking less than 60% of trial medication had an eradication rate of 69%, compared with 96% in those taking more than 60% of trial medication. Multidrug therapy also is complicated by adverse effects, especially diarrhea, nausea, and vomiting, which may occur in 19% of patients. Addition of omeprazole, 20 mg two times a day, to triple therapy increases the eradication rate to more than 95%, and it may decrease the occurrence of side effects as well. As such, triple therapy remains the gold standard for compliant patients.

The combination of omeprazole, 40 mg daily, with clarithromycin, 500 mg three times a day, for 14 days received FDA approval as the first sanctioned therapy for infection with *H. pylori*. This combination has an efficacy of approximately 80%, and dosing is far easier than that of conventional triple therapy. The cost of this regimen, however, is in excess of $200.

Another FDA-approved, dual-therapy option is ranitidine bismuth (Tritec, Glaxo Wellcome), 400 mg two times a day, plus clarithromycin, 500 mg three times a day, which also has an eradication rate of approximately 80% and is slightly less expensive than omeprazole plus clarithromycin. Both of these regimens, however, are simpler for patients to take and are well tolerated, but this is achieved at the price of decreased efficacy.

Another well-tolerated regimen is omeprazole, 20 mg two times a day, combined with metronidazole, 500 mg two times a day, and clarithromycin, 250 mg two times a day, for 14 days, which has an eradication rate of approximately 88%. This regimen is simple to take and highly efficacious, but treatment failure may result in resistance to both metronidazole and clarithromycin.

Dual therapy with amoxicillin and omeprazole is no longer appropriate because of its poor efficacy. Unfortunately, it is unclear how best to treat patients who fail a course of anti–*H. pylori* therapy. In the future, therapeutic immunization after infection may offer the best treatment, especially in the developing world. Additional combinations of agents and shorter courses of therapy are under investigation as well.

Antacids

Antacids are highly effective agents for healing ulcers and controlling symptoms. From a practical perspective, however, inconvenient dosing frequency and adverse effects limit their use to control of symptoms only.

H₂-Receptor Antagonists

H_2-receptor antagonists remain a mainstay of therapy for ulcers. Acid secretion is decreased by competitively and selectively inhibiting the histamine H_2-receptor of the parietal cell.

This class of drugs is uniformly safe and well-tolerated. The risk of adverse effects is slightly increased with cimetidine, however, because of binding to cytochrome P-450 and, hence, increased drug interactions. Given as a single, full dose at bedtime, each of the available compounds (i.e., cimetidine, 800 mg; ranitidine, 300 mg; famotidine, 40 mg; nizatidine, 300 mg) has a comparable efficacy for healing ulcers. Typical healing rates at 8 weeks are 90 to 95% for duodenal ulcers and 88% for gastric ulcers. Cimetidine now is available in a generic formulation, thus making it the least expensive H_2-receptor antagonist.

Proton-Pump Inhibitors

Omeprazole and lansoprazole belong to a class of gastric antisecretory drugs called proton-pump inhibitors. These drugs irreversibly inhibit the H^+,K^+-ATPase enzyme of the parietal cell, thus resulting in potent, long-lasting suppression of acid secretion.

Proton-pump inhibitors are safe and well tolerated. Life-long administration of high doses to rats results in development of carcinoid tumors of the stomach. This finding relates to the elevated gastrin level that occurs with use of omeprazole and lansoprazole because of the loss of normal feedback inhibition on gastrin release caused by intragastric acid. There have been no reports of gastric carcinoid tumors in humans with the short-term therapy for peptic ulcer disease.

More importantly, we now know that long-term therapy with proton-pump inhibitors in patients infected with *H. pylori* increases the severity of gastritis and leads to gastric atrophy in 31% of patients after 5 years of treatment. Gastric atrophy is a precursor lesion of gastric cancer; therefore, an attempt at *H. pylori* eradication may be indicated in infected patients committed to long-term therapy with proton-pump inhibitors.

Proton-pump inhibitors result in more-rapid healing of duodenal ulcers than occurs with H_2-receptor antagonists. Healing rates of 80 to 95% have been reported at 4 weeks. At a dose of 40 mg daily for 8 weeks, omeprazole heals up to 95% of gastric ulcers and is superior to conventional doses of histamine H_2-receptor antagonists. Comparable results for gastric ulcer healing are found with lansoprazole at a dose of 30 mg daily for 8 weeks. Omeprazole and lansoprazole are both FDA approved for treatment of duodenal ulcers, and omeprazole is FDA approved for treatment of gastric ulcers.

The cost of a 4-week course of therapy with these drugs is similar to an 8-week course with H_2-receptor antagonists. The correct doses for healing duodenal ulcers are omeprazole, 20 mg daily, and lansoprazole, 15 mg daily, for 4 weeks. Omeprazole, 40 mg daily for 8 weeks, is the approved dose for gastric ulcers.

Sucralfate

Sucralfate is a complex salt of sucrose sulfate and aluminum hydroxide, and it is as effective as H_2-receptor antagonists in treatment of duodenal ulcer disease. The drug is well tolerated and has few adverse effects. Evidence for efficacy in gastric ulcer disease is less compelling, and sucralfate is not FDA approved for this indication. The mechanism of action for sucralfate is unclear, but it appears to enhance mucosal defenses. The correct dose is 1 g four times a day.

Treatment and Prophylaxis of NSAID-Induced Ulceration

There are two clinical problems in patients treated with NSAIDs: treatment of ulcers that develop during therapy, and prophylaxis of ulceration. For patients who develop ulcers while ingesting NSAIDs, therapy should be stopped and the patient placed on conventional doses of H_2-receptor antagonists or proton-pump inhibitors. The *H. pylori* status of these patients should be assessed and the organism eradicated if present. For patients who need to continue NSAID therapy, the dosage should be reduced as much as possible. Small ulcers (i.e., ≤5 mm) in the stomach or duodenum will heal with coadministration of H_2-receptor antagonists; larger gastric ulcers will heal with coadministration of double-dose proton-pump inhibitors.

Before considering prophylaxis of NSAID-induced mucosal damage, one should remember that the number of patients taking NSAIDs is large. In addition, the risk of developing a complication is low for any given individual.

Misoprostol is a prostaglandin E_1 analogue that is effective for prophylaxis of NSAID-induced gastric and duodenal ulcers. It acts by prostaglandin-dependent pathways to decrease gastric acid secretion and to enhance mucosal defenses. Misoprostol can prevent acute damage to the gastroduodenal mucosa and decrease the frequency of developing both gastric and duodenal ulcers in patients requiring long-term therapy with NSAIDs. Lower doses of misoprostol, 200 μg two or three times a day, are just as effective as administration four times a day for prevention of duodenal and gastric ulcers. Adverse effects are no more common than with placebo at these lower doses, in contrast to the common reports of diarrhea and abdominal cramps in patients treated with full doses (i.e., 200 μg four times a day).

Until recently, there was no proof that administration of misoprostol decreased serious gastrointestinal complications. A recent study by Silverstein et al., however, has demonstrated a reduction in serious gastrointestinal complications, such as bleeding, perforation, and gastric outlet obstruction, when misoprostol, 200 μg four times a day, was administered for 6 months to patients with rheumatoid arthritis.

Histamine H_2-receptor antagonists may be used in selected patients for prophylaxis of NSAID-induced ulceration, but other agents, such as misoprostol and proton-pump inhibitors, may be more effective. High-dose famotidine, 40 mg two times a day, is more effective than placebo at preventing both duodenal and gastric ulcers in patients receiving long-term NSAID therapy. Conventional doses of famotidine and other histamine H_2-receptor antagonists are effective for prophylaxis of duodenal ulcers.

Nevertheless, the high cost of routine administration of prophylactic medications and the fact that NSAID use is so common do not justify routine NSAID prophylaxis. Rather, such prophylaxis should be used only in high-risk individuals, such as those older than 75 years of age or with underlying cardiovascular disease, previous peptic ulcer disease, or previous ulcer bleeding. A possible approach to treatment of NSAID-induced ulceration and NSAID prophylaxis is seen in Table 57.3.

NONHEALING ULCERS

Approximately 10% of ulcers fail to heal after standard acid-suppression therapy (i.e., 8 weeks of histamine H_2-receptor antagonists or 4 weeks of proton-pump inhibitors for duodenal ulcers, 12 weeks of H_2-receptor antagonists or 8 weeks of proton-pump inhibitors for gastric ulcers). Persistence of symptoms and macroscopic ulceration do not necessarily correlate.

Considerations for nonhealing ulcers are:

- Noncompliance
- Cigarette smoking

Table 57.3.   Treatment of NSAID-induced Ulceration and NSAID Prophylaxis

1. Discontinue NSAIDs
2. If NSAIDs are necessary, use the lowest dose possible
3. Consider prophylactic therapy for at-risk populations, which include those with:

    Age > 75 years
    History of peptic ulcer disease
    History of bleeding peptic ulcer
    Cardiovascular disease

4. For gastric ulcer prophylaxis, use:

    Misoprostol, 200 μg two or three times a day
    Famotidine, 40 mg two times a day

5. For duodenal ulcer prophylaxis, use:

    Misoprostol, 200 μg two times a day
    Famotidine, 20 mg two times a day
    Ranitidine, 150 mg two times a day

- NSAID ingestion
- Acid hypersecretion
  - Zollinger-Ellison syndrome
  - Idiopathic
- Cancer (gastric ulcers)
- *H. pylori*

Each of these issues should be addressed before the institution of additional therapy. Infection with *H. pylori* and surreptitious use of NSAIDs have emerged as the two leading causes of refractory peptic ulcers. Determination of salicylate levels and platelet aggregation studies may be useful in these patients.

There is no advantage to switching from one H_2-blocker to another. Omeprazole at a dose of 40 mg will heal almost all peptic ulcer disease refractory to conventional doses of therapy. Eradication of *H. pylori,* if present, should be attempted in these patients.

MAINTENANCE THERAPY

Maintenance therapy with a long-term, low dose (i.e., half strength) of any H_2-blocker now is an obsolete concept. Before the role of *H. pylori* in peptic ulcer disease was determined, the ulcer relapse rate was reduced to between 10 to 30% at 1 year using this strategy. Today, maintenance therapy is indicated only for a small subset of patients with chronic peptic ulcer disease. Patients with *H. pylori*–positive peptic ulcer disease should be placed on maintenance therapy if eradication is unsuccessful. Patients with *H. pylori*–negative peptic ulcer disease should be placed on maintenance therapy if they have three or more relapses each year or a history of ulcer complications, such as bleeding or perforation, and multiple other medical problems.

BLEEDING PEPTIC ULCERS

Peptic ulcer disease is the most common cause of upper gastrointestinal bleeding. Whereas bleeding ceases spontaneously in 80% of patients, the mortality rate from bleeding ulcers remains unchanged, at 6 to 7% over the last 30 years. The major risk factor for bleeding ulcers is consumption of NSAIDs.

Several predictors of adverse outcome in patients with bleeding ulcers will help in clinical decision making. These include:

- Hemodynamic instability at presentation
- Bright red blood per rectum and via the nasogastric tube
- Age > 60 years
- An increasing number of underlying medical illnesses

All patients with upper GI bleeding should undergo early upper endoscopy, which allows for both therapeutic intervention and determination of other predictors for rebleeding. Rebleeding rates are approximately 5% for patients with clean-based ulcers, 10% for patients with ulcers having flat spots, 22% for patients with adherent clots, 43% for patients with nonbleeding visible vessels, and 55% for patients with active oozing or spurting from an ulcer. Patients with large ulcers (i.e., >1 cm in size) also have higher rebleeding and mortality rates.

Endoscopic therapy with bipolar or thermal coagulation and injection of epinephrine clearly improves the outcome in patients with bleeding ulcers. This improvement occurs by decreasing the length of hospital stay, number of blood transfusions, and need for emergency surgery. Results of a recent meta-analysis also indicate that endoscopic therapy improves the mortality rate in these patients. Because most bleeding recurs within 3 days of initial presentation, patients with active bleeding or stigmata of hemorrhage, such as pigmented spots in an ulcer crater or clot, can be discharged within 3 days if stable. Given the excellent prognosis for patients with clean-based ulcers, discharge within 24 hours of presentation also is reasonable. Patients failing endoscopic therapy are candidates for surgical intervention, or, if deemed to represent too high a surgical risk, they can be treated angiographically with either intra-arterial vasopressin or embolization techniques.

Patients with bleeding peptic ulcers who are infected with *H. pylori* have a marked decrease in rebleeding after *H. pylori* eradication, whereas failure to cure the infection results in a rebleeding rate of approximately 33% at 1 year. Therefore, all patients with bleeding peptic ulcers should have their *H. pylori* status determined. Antibiotic therapy should be given to patients who are infected; these patients should have cure of their infection confirmed with the urea breath test. Failure to cure *H. pylori* infection mandates long-term, even indefinite, maintenance therapy with half-dose histamine H_2-receptor antagonists.

H. PYLORI AND FUNCTIONAL DYSPEPSIA: TREATMENT IMPLICATIONS

The literature on *H. pylori* and functional dyspepsia is confusing. Approximately 50% of patients with functional dyspepsia are infected with the organism; however, the prevalence of *H. pylori* probably is not higher among patients with functional dyspepsia than among asymptomatic controls. Trials assessing treatment of *H. pylori* in patients with functional dyspepsia have had serious methodologic flaws. As such, treatment of *H. pylori* in patients with functional dyspepsia should be avoided at present. This disorder more likely relates to an abnormal perception of events in the gut resulting from abnormal visceral afferent hypersensitivity.

H. PYLORI AND GASTRIC NEOPLASIA

Infection with *H. pylori* is an important risk factor for development of gastric cancer, which is the second-leading cause of death from cancer worldwide. Approximately 40 to 60% of tumors of the gastric body or antrum are associated with *H. pylori* infection. The incidence of gastric cancer in the United States is decreasing, however, and it is estimated that only 1% of infected Americans will ever develop cancer.

Possible mechanisms of carcinogenesis include:

1. Injurious effects of metabolic products of the organism;
2. Rapid turnover of cells because of chronic inflammation, which may increase the risk of mutation and cellular transformation; and
3. Toxic effects of inflammatory products causing cellular injury, mutation, and transformation.

Because most infected patients never develop cancer, other factors such as diet, strain diversity, and age at infection probably play a role. Recent work by Hannson et al. demonstrated that the risk of developing gastric cancer increases in patients with gastric ulcer disease, but that it decreases in patients with duodenal ulcer disease. More importantly, chronic therapy with proton-pump inhibitors in *H. pylori*–infected patients increases the severity of gastritis and leads to gastric atrophy in 31% of patients after 5 years of treatment. Gastric atrophy is a precursor lesion of gastric cancer; therefore, an attempt at *H. pylori* eradication may be indicated in infected patients who are committed to long-term therapy with proton-pump inhibitors. Mass screening for *H. pylori* in middle-aged U.S. adults, however, is not indicated at present. Parsonnet et al. estimated that the cost to screen all Americans between 50 and 54 years of age and to treat the infected patients would be $996 million.

H. pylori infection also is associated with gastric non-Hodgkin's lymphoma and with MALT lymphoma, which is a low-grade, B-cell subtype of non-Hodgkin's lymphoma of the stomach. Eradication of *H. pylori* may cure approximately 70% of individuals with MALT-type lymphoma.

ZOLLINGER-ELLISON SYNDROME

Patients with Zollinger-Ellison syndrome are characterized by marked hypersecretion of acid resulting from high circulating levels of gastrin because of a gastrin-secreting tumor. Approximately 25% of gastrinomas are associated with MEN-I; the remainder are sporadic. These patients often are discovered fortuitously by an elevated gastrin level as part of an evaluation of nonhealing or chronic peptic ulcers. Gastrinomas are a relatively uncommon cause of hypergastrinemia, however. Patients with hypochlorhydria related to decreased intraluminal acid in the setting of atrophic gastritis or antisecretory therapy are the most common causes, and *H. pylori* infection also causes hypergastrinemia. As such, the presence of acid hypersecretion, as documented by gastric acid analysis, is necessary for the diagnosis of Zollinger-Ellison syndrome to be made. A secretin stimulation test should be considered only if acid hypersecretion is documented. The single best imaging test for gastrinomas is somatostatin-receptor scintigraphy, which is superior to ultrasonography, computed tomography, magnetic resonance imaging, and angiography for tumor localization.

Surgical therapy is the preferred treatment of sporadic Zollinger-Ellison syndrome. The tumors often are found in the duodenum as well as in the pancreas. Multiple pancreatic tumors are the classic finding in gastrinomas as part of the MEN-I syndrome, and as such, the role of surgery in these patients is less clear. These patients, as well as those in whom a tumor cannot be localized, should be managed with acid-suppression therapy. Because of their potency in decreasing acid secretion, proton-pump inhibitors are the clear choice in these patients.

STRESS-RELATED MUCOSAL DAMAGE

Stress-related mucosal damage develops in most critically ill patients, and overt upper gastrointestinal bleeding may occur in as many as 15% of untreated patients. Critical illnesses associated with a risk for stress-related mucosal injury include burns, trauma, central nervous system injury, prolonged hypotension, sepsis, respiratory failure, hepatic failure, and multiorgan failure. The mortality rate of these patients who go on to bleed is increased; however, the incidence of major bleeding in critically ill patients recently has decreased. The reason for this is uncertain and cannot necessarily be attributed to the widespread use of prophylactic therapy.

Stress-related mucosal injury is caused by mucosal ischemia, which impairs mucosal resistance to acid back-diffusion and the presence of acid. Hyperemia of the mucosa evolves into erosions and, then, frank ulceration in the stomach and duodenum.

Several prophylactic treatment strategies are effective in

preventing upper gastrointestinal bleeding in critically ill patients. There is no proof that one strategy is more effective than another, however, and none influences the mortality rate, length of hospital stay, or transfusion requirements. Antacids administered every 2 hours neutralize gastric acid but have the disadvantages of inconvenience, increased nursing time, and diarrhea. Sucralfate requires placement of a nasogastric tube, but a dose of 1 g every 4 hours may decrease the risk of late-onset nosocomial pneumonia. H_2-receptor antagonists, given either as a continuous infusion or by bolus injection every 12 hours (in the case of more potent agents such as famotidine), are safe, convenient, and should be titrated to an intragastric pH of greater than 4 to minimize the activity of pepsin. Fewer side effects are encountered with ranitidine and famotidine than with cimetidine.

Should all patients in the intensive care unit (ICU) receive prophylaxis, especially in this era of cost constraints? The answer is no. A recent large, multicenter, Canadian study of 2252 medical and surgical ICU patients identified coagulopathy and respiratory failure requiring mechanical ventilation for 48 hours or longer as the only risk factors for clinically significant bleeding in the ICU. Only 1.5% of all patients had clinically significant bleeding in this large study. Therefore, patients with coagulopathy or mechanical ventilation should continue to receive prophylaxis. Other patients who should receive "targeted" prophylaxis include those with CNS trauma, burns, organ transplantation, or a history of peptic ulcer disease with or without bleeding. Admission to the ICU does not automatically warrant prophylaxis for stress gastropathy anymore.

SUGGESTED READINGS

Bytzer P. Diagnosing dyspepsia: any controversies left? Gastroenterology 1996;110:302–306.

Bytzer P, Hansen JM, Schaffalitzky de Muckadell OB. Empirical H_2-blocker therapy or prompt endoscopy in management of dyspepsia. Lancet 1994;343:811–816.

Cook DJ, Fuller HD, Guyatt GH, et al. Risk factors for gastrointestinal bleeding in critically ill patients. N Engl J Med 1994; 330:377–381.

Cutler AF, Havstad S, Ma CK, Blaser MJ, Perez-Perez GI, Schubert TT. Accuracy of invasive and noninvasive tests to diagnose *Helicobacter pylori* infection. Gastroenterology 1995;109:136–141.

Dooley CP, Cohen H, Fitzgibbons PL, et al. Prevalence of *Helicobacter pylori* infection and histologic gastritis in asymptomatic persons. N Engl J Med 1989;321:1562–1566.

Falk GW. *H. pylori* 1997: testing and treatment options. Cleve Clin J Med 1997;64:187–192.

Falk GW. Omeprazole: a new drug for the treatment of acid-peptic diseases. Cleve Clin J Med 1991;58:418–427.

Feldman M, Burton ME. Histamine₂-receptor antagonists. Standard therapy for acid-peptic disease. N Engl J Med 1990; 323:1672–1680,1749–1755.

Fendrick AM, Chernew ME, Hirth RA, Bloom BS. Alternative management strategies for patients with suspected peptic ulcer disease. Ann Intern Med 1995;123:260–268.

Gibril F, Reynolds JC, Doppman JL, et al. Somatostatin receptor scintigraphy: its sensitivity compared with that of other imaging methods in detecting primary and metastatic gastrinomas. Ann Intern Med 1996;125:26–34.

Graham DY, Lew GM, Klein PD, et al. Effect of treatment of *Helicobacter pylori* infection on the long-term recurrence of gastric or duodenal ulcer. Ann Intern Med 1992;116: 705–708.

Graham DY, Rabeneck L. Patients, payers and paradigm shifts: what to do about *Helicobacter pylori*? Am J Gastroenterol 1996;91:188–191.

Hansson LE, Engstrand L, Nyren O, et al. *Helicobacter pylori* infection: independent risk indicator of gastric adenocarcinoma. Gastroenterology 1993;105:1098–1103.

Hansson LE, Nyren O, Hsing AW, et al. The risk of stomach cancer in patients with gastric or duodenal ulcer disease. N Engl J Med 1996;335:242–249.

Health and Public Policy Committee, American College of Physicians. Endoscopy in the evaluation of dyspepsia. Ann Intern Med 1985;102:266–269.

Jensen DM, Cheng S, Kovacs TOG, et al. A controlled trial of ranitidine for the prevention of recurrent hemmorhage from duodenal ulcer. N Engl J Med 1994;330:382–386.

Kuipers EJ, Lundell L, Klinkenberg-Knol EC, et al. Atrophic gastritis and *Helicobacter pylori* infection in patients with reflux esophagitis treated with omeprazole or fundoplication. N Engl J Med 1996;334:1018–1022.

Laine L. The long term management of patients with bleeding ulcers: *Helicobacter pylori* eradication instead of maintenance antisecretory therapy (editorial). Gastrointest Endosc 1995; 41:77–79.

Laine L, Peterson WL. Bleeding peptic ulcer. N Engl J Med 1994;331:717–727.

Lanas AI, Remacha B, Esteva F, Sainz R. Risk factors associated with refractory peptic ulcers. Gastroenterology 1995;109: 1124–1133.

Levine JS. Misoprostol and nonsteroidal anti-inflammatory drugs: a tale of effects, outcomes and costs (editorial). Ann Intern Med 1995;123:309–310.

Logan RP, Bardhan KD, Clestin LR, et al. Eradication of *Helicobacter pylori* and prevention of recurrence of duodenal ulcer: a randomized, double-blind, multicenter trial of omeprazole with or without clarithromycin. Aliment Pharmacol Ther 1995;9:417–423.

McCarthy DM. Sucralfate. N Engl J Med 1991;325:1017–1025.

McGowan CC, Cover TL, Blaser MJ. *Helicobacter pylori* and gastric acid: biological and therapeutic implications. Gastroenterology 1996;110:926–938.

National Institutes of Health Consensus Development Conference Statement. *Helicobacter pylori* in peptic ulcer disease. JAMA 1994;272:65–69.

Ofman JJ, Etchason J, Fullerton S, Kahn KL, Soll AH. Management strategies for *Helicobacter pylori*-seropositive patients with dyspepsia: clinical and economic consequences. Ann Intern Med 1997;280–291.

Parsonnet J, Friedman GD, Vandersteen DP, et al. *Helicobacter pylori* infection and the risk of gastric carcinoma. N Engl J Med 1991;325:1127–1131.

Parsonnet J, Hansen S, Rodriguez L, et al. *Helicobacter pylori* infection and gastric lymphoma. N Engl J Med 1994;330:1267–1271.

Parsonnet J, Harris RA, Hack H, Owens DK. Modeling cost-effectiveness of *Helicobacter pylori* screening to prevent gastric cancer: a mandate for clinical trials. Lancet 1996;348:150–154.

Peek RM, Blaser MJ. Pathophysiology of *Helicobacter pylori*–induced gastritis and peptic ulcer disease. Am J Med 1997;102:200–207.

Peura DA. *Helicobacter pylori:* a diagnostic dilemma and a dilemma of diagnosis (editorial). Gastroenterology 1995;109:313–315.

Piper JM, Ray WA, Daugherty JR, Griffin MR. Corticosteroid use and peptic ulcer disease: role of nonsteroidal anti-inflammatory drugs. Ann Intern Med 1991;114:735–740.

Prod'hom G, Leuenberger P, Koerfer J, et al. Nosocomial pneumonia in mechanically ventilated patients receiving antacid, ranitidine, or sucralfate as prophylaxis for stress ulcer. Ann Intern Med 1994;120:653–662.

Raskin JB, White RH, Jackson JE, et al. Misoprostol dosage in the prevention of nonsteroidal anti-inflammatory drug-induced gastric and duodenal ulcers: a comparison of three regimens. Ann Intern Med 1995;123:344–350.

Roggero E, Zucca E, Pinotti G et al. Eradication of *Helicobacter pylori* infection in primary low-grade gastric lymphoma of mucosa-associated lymphoid tissue. Ann Intern Med 1995;122:767–769.

Silverstein FE, Graham DY, Senior JR, et al. Misoprostol reduces serious gastrointestinal complications in patients with rheumatoid arthritis receiving nonsteroidal anti-inflammatory drugs. Ann Intern Med 1995;123:241–249.

Silverstein MD, Petterson T, Talley NJ. Initial endoscopy or empirical therapy with and without testing for *Helicobacter pylori* for dyspepsia: a decision analysis. Gastroenterology 1996;110:72–83.

Soll AH. Medical treatment of peptic ulcer disease. Practice guidelines. JAMA 1996;275:622–629.

Soll AH. Pathogenesis of peptic ulcer disease. N Engl J Med 1990;322:909–916.

Soll AH, Weinstein WM, Kurata J, McCarthy D. Nonsteroidal anti-inflammatory drugs and peptic ulcer disease. Ann Intern Med 1991;114:307–319.

Taha AS, Hudson N, Hawkey CJ et al. Famotidine for the prevention of gastric and duodenal ulcers caused by nonsteroidal antiiflammatory drugs. N Engl J Med 1996;334:1435–1439.

Walsh JH, Peterson WL. The treatment of *Helicobacter pylori* infection in the management of peptic ulcer disease. N Engl J Med 1995;333:984–991.

Walt RP. Misoprostol for the treatment of peptic ulcer and antiinflammatory-drug-induced gastroduodenal ulceration. N Engl J Med 1992;327:1575–1580.

Wolf MM, Soll AH. The physiology of gastric acid secretion. N Engl J Med 1988;319;1707–1715.

Yousfi MM, el-Zimaity HM, al-Assi MT, Cole RA, Genta RM, Graham DY. Metronidazole, omeprazole and clarithromycin: an effective combination therapy for *Helicobacter pylori* infection. Aliment Pharmacol Ther 1995;9:209–212.

58

Colorectal Carcinoma

Carol A. Burke

Colorectal carcinoma—the second-most common cancer (and cause of cancer deaths) in the United States—is of major public health importance. As shown in Table 58.1, both men and women face a lifetime risk for developing invasive colorectal cancer of 1 in 17.

It is estimated that more than 130,000 new cases of colorectal cancer will be diagnosed in 1997, and that 54,000 deaths from colorectal cancer will occur (1). Both screening and postpolypectomy surveillance studies report a reduced colorectal cancer mortality rate through early detection of disease and polyp removal. Unfortunately, however, more than 45% of patients present with stage III or IV disease, which carry a 5-year survival rate of 50% and 7%, respectively.

ETIOLOGY

Most colorectal carcinomas are believed to arise from a precursor lesion known as an adenoma, which is a benign, neoplastic polyp with malignant potential. It is not precisely known how long an adenoma takes to develop into an invasive cancer, but data from multiple observational studies suggest 10 years. Support for the adenoma–carcinoma sequence stems from indirect evidence (2), including:

- Anatomic distribution and patient demographics are similar for both adenomas and colorectal cancers.
- Risk of dysplasia/cancer increases with increasing polyp size and villous architecture, and most cancers are associated with adenomatous polyps.
- Progressive genetic alterations have been found as adenomas progress to cancer.
- Colonoscopic polypectomy has been associated with a diminished incidence of cancer.

RISK FACTORS

Colorectal carcinogenesis results from complex interactions between genetic susceptibility and environmental as well as dietary factors. Genetic predisposition is an essential factor in tumorigenesis for many patients, but epidemiologic studies have implicated dietary variables (e.g., high fat, low fiber) as cofactors in development of colorectal cancer and polyps. The risk for adenomatous polyps and cancer is low before age 40, but it increases with age, to a peak in the seventh and eighth decades of life. There does not appear to be a sex or a race predilection, except in blacks, who have a slightly higher incidence of stage IV disease. Approximately 70% of newly diagnosed colorectal cancers arise in patients without known risk factors. In approximately 30% of patients with colorectal cancer, risk factors have been identified, including:

- Personal history of adenomatous polyps or colorectal cancer
- Inherited adenomatous polyposis syndromes

Familial adenomatous polyposis (FAP) is an autosomal dominant disease with nearly 90% penetrance. The gene (*APC*) has been identified on the long arm of chromosome 5. Patients with FAP develop hundreds to thousands of colonic adenomas in the second decade of life, and all of these patients will develop colon cancer by age 40 if prophylactic colectomy is not performed. Upper gastrointestinal adenomas are common in this population, and periampullary cancer is the second-leading cause of death from cancer in this population.

Gardner's syndrome is thought to be a phenotypic variant of FAP. In addition to the colonic adenomatous polyposis, benign soft-tissue tumors, osteomas, dental abnormalities, desmoid tumors, and congenital hypertrophy of the retinal pigment epithelium are found.

Turcot's syndrome is an autosomal recessive disorder in

Table 58.1. Percentage of U.S. Population Developing Invasive Colorectal Cancer				
	Birth–39 y	*40–59 y*	*60–79 y*	*Lifetime Risk*
Male	0.06 (1 in 667)	0.92 (1 in 109)	4.27 (1 in 23)	6.02 (1 in 17)
Female	0.05 (1 in 2000)	0.70 (1 in 143)	3.24 (1 in 31)	5.77 (1 in 17)

* 1991–1993 data from NCI Surveillance, Epidemiology, and End Results Program, 1996. Parker SL, Tong T, Bolden S, et al. Cancer statistics, 1997. CA Cancer J Clin 1997;47:5–27.

which brain tumors are associated with the colonic adenomatous polyposis.

- Hereditary nonpolyposis colon cancer (HNPCC)

Hereditary nonpolyposis colon cancer is an autosomal dominant disease with nearly complete penetrance. This type of cancer occurs at a young age and often is right-sided. At least four genes have been identified in the germline of 30% of patients with HNPCC; alterations in these genes produce abnormalities in repair of DNA. Diagnosis of HNPCC includes:

1. Three or more relatives with colorectal cancer, with one being a first-degree relative of the other two,
2. One cancer diagnosed before age 50, and
3. At least two successive generations affected.

There is a subset of HNPCC families with gastric, ovarian, and endometrial carcinomas in addition to colon cancer.

- Ulcerative or Crohn's colitis

The extent and duration of ulcerative colitis is indicative of the risk for colorectal cancer. Risk is highest in patients with pancolitis and is negligible in patients with proctosigmoiditis. After a decade of disease, the cancer risk increases yearly by from 1 to 2%.

- First-degree relative with colon cancer or adenomatous polyp diagnosed before age 60

First-degree relatives of patients with colorectal cancer have a two- to threefold increased risk of colorectal cancer and adenomatous polyps (3, 4). First-degree family members of patients with adenomatous polyps also have an increased risk of colorectal cancer, particularly when the adenoma is diagnosed before age 60 (5).

- Individuals with a personal history of breast, ovarian, or uterine cancer (6)

PATHOGENESIS

Colorectal tumorigenesis results from multiple, acquired genetic alterations within tumor tissue, which in turn result in promotion of malignant transformation (i.e., oncogenes) or loss in the inhibition of cellular proliferation (i.e., tumor-sup-

Table 58.2. Genetic Alterations in Colorectal Tumorigenesis		
Oncogenes	*Tumor-Suppressor Genes*	*Mismatch Repair Genes*
kras	5q (*APC*)	2p (*MSH2*)
	17p (*p53*)	3p (*MLH1*)
	18q (Deleted in colon cancer)	2 (*PMS1*)
		7 (*PMS2*)

pressor genes) (7). Recently, a new class of genes resulting in defective DNA repair (i.e., mismatch repair genes) have been identified and implicated in carcinogenesis in HNPCC (Table 58.2).

CLINICAL PRESENTATION

Colon polyps rarely are symptomatic, but the most common presentation is occult gastrointestinal bleeding. Anemia and hematochezia are less common presentations. Adenocarcinomas produce symptoms when the tumors are advanced, whereupon bleeding (i.e., occult, anemia, hematochezia), change in bowel habits, obstruction, or symptoms of local invasion occur.

DIAGNOSIS

The diagnosis of colorectal cancer most often is made during a colonic evaluation performed for gastrointestinal symptoms or evidence of blood loss. Adenomatous polyps usually are detected on screening or surveillance examinations.

PATHOLOGY

"Polyp" is an inexact term that indicates a protuberance of tissue into the colonic lumen. Histologic analysis of polyps, however, has allowed for a meaningful classification scheme based on their malignant potential (Table 58.3). Neoplastic polyps are premalignant, and nonneoplastic polyps have no malignant potential.

Table 58.3.   Classification of Colorectal Polyps

Neoplastic	Nonneoplastic
Adenoma	Hyperplastic
Tubular	Hamartoma
Tubulovillous	Lymphoid aggregate
Villous	Inflammatory

Table 58.4.   Adenoma Size, Histology, and Cancer Risk

	Percentage with Invasive Cancer		
Histology	<1 cm	1–2 cm	>2 cm
Tubular adenoma	1	10	35
Tubulovillous adenoma	4	7	46
Villous adenoma	10	10	53

Adapted from Muto T, Bussey HJR, Marson BC. The Evolution of cancer of the colon and rectum. Cancer 1975;36:2251.

Adenomas account for approximately two out of every three colonic polyps. Both the size of the polyp and the degree of villous features are predictive for the risk of malignancy within the polyp (Table 58.4).

Hyperplastic polyps are the second-most common type of polyp, and they account for approximately 10 to 30% of colonic polyps. Hyperplastic polyps most often are found in the rectosigmoid and have no clinical significance. Unfortunately, however, hyperplastic polyps and adenomas are indistinguishable at endoscopy. Therefore, all polyps detected in the colon and rectum should be removed and sent for histologic analysis.

SCREENING

The purpose of screening is to apply an accurate, low-cost, low-risk test to a population with an average risk of a common disease that is associated with high morbidity and mortality rates and is known to have an effective treatment. Various methods are available for colorectal cancer screening, and the cost-effectiveness of these modalities is under study (Table 58.5) (8,9).

Fecal Occult Blood Testing

Fecal occult blood testing (FOBT) is the most widely studied screening method. Because large polyps and cancers intermittently bleed FOBT can be an effective screening tool. The peroxidase activity of hemoglobin can be detected by a color change when it catalyzes the oxidation of guaiac by a peroxide reagent. Compliance rates are low, however, possibly because of both the need for a special diet (i.e., meat-free, high-residue, and without vegetables having peroxidase activity, such as turnips and horseradish) for at least 24 hours before specimen collection and the requirement of three separate stool specimens collected at least 1 day apart. Any positive FOBT warrants colonoscopy.

A randomized trial of screening FOBT involving 46,551 volunteers found a 33% decrease in the mortality rate from colorectal cancer in a group that underwent annual screening (10). This reduced mortality rate also was accompanied by improved survival and a shift to earlier-stage cancer being detected. Overall compliance was low, however, with only 46% of volunteers completing all the screening. Slide rehydration increased the sensitivity from 81 to 90%, but it decreased the specificity from 98 to 90% and the positive predictive value from 5.6 to 2.2%. In addition, 38% of the annual-screening group underwent colonoscopy, which may have affected the reduction in mortality.

Sigmoidoscopy

Sigmoidoscopic screening allows a portion of the colorectal mucosa to be visualized directly and diagnostic biopsy to be performed at the time of examination. Both the sensitivity and specificity for detection of polyps and cancers in the segment of the bowel examined is high. Unfortunately, however, nearly 40% of polyps and cancers are beyond the limits of detection for the longest (i.e., 60 cm) flexible sigmoidoscope.

Opinions regarding the need to perform colonoscopy for patients with a single tubular adenoma smaller than 0.5 cm found on flexible sigmoidoscopy vary, but the prevalence of proximal neoplasms in such patients may be substantial enough to warrant screening colonoscopy. In one recent study, one-third of patients with distal adenomas smaller than 0.5 cm harbored more proximal adenomas, and 6% had advanced lesions (11).

Results of several case-control studies show a reduction in deaths from colorectal cancer in patients who undergo predominantly rigid sigmoidoscopic examinations. The reported reduction in mortality varies from between 59 and 80%. The most well-known study (12) reviewed the use of sigmoidoscopic screening in 261 patients who died from cancer of the

Table 58.5.   Cost, Sensitivity, and Specificity of Screening Tests for Colorectal Cancer

	Cost per test ($)	Sensitivity (%)	Specificity (%)
FOBT	10–20	26–92	90–98
Flexible sigmoidoscopy	150–500	90	98
Air-contrast barium enema	300–500	60–80	98
Colonoscopy	1000–1500	75–95	100

distal colon or rectum and compared these patients to 868 controls. Screening reduced the rectosigmoid cancer mortality rate by 60%, and the protective effect of sigmoidoscopy was noted to last for up to 10 years. This reduction in mortality may have resulted from earlier detection of cancers and removal of premalignant polyps.

Fecal Occult Blood Testing and Sigmoidoscopy

In one controlled trial (13), 12,479 people underwent annual screening with rigid sigmoidoscopy or rigid sigmoidoscopy combined with FOBT. A reduction in the colorectal cancer mortality rate, detection of earlier-stage cancer, and longer survival were seen in patients undergoing both FOBT and rigid sigmoidoscopy.

Barium Enema

Barium enema has the advantage of imaging the entire colon. It can be performed in two ways: single-contrast, using barium alone to identify filling defects; or air-contrast, in which air is instilled after most of the barium has been evacuated to outline the colonic mucosa. Air-contrast barium enema has replaced the single-contrast enema for detection of polyps and cancers, but one recent study found no statistically significant difference in sensitivity and specificity between these two modalities for the detection of large cancers (14). Single-contrast barium enema is inaccurate for the detection of polyps, however, and should not be used for polyp screening (15). Because the rectosigmoid is not always well visualized by air-contrast barium enema, flexible sigmoidoscopy should be performed as well for a complete examination. As of this writing, no trials have addressed use of barium enema in screening for colorectal cancer.

Colonoscopy

Colonoscopy is the only technique with both diagnostic and therapeutic applications. It has been considered to be the ''gold standard'' for detection of colonic neoplasms, and it can be completed in more than 95% of examinations. As of this writing, no published studies have examined the effectiveness of colonoscopic screening in prevention of colorectal cancer, but one large, multicenter trial will soon begin in the United States. In one cohort study of 1418 patients who underwent colonoscopy and polypectomy (16), a lower-than-expected incidence of colorectal cancer was observed.

Recommendations

The American Cancer Society guidelines for colorectal cancer screening were updated in 1997. Recommendations for average-risk patients, who begin screening at age 50, include:

- Annual FOBT plus flexible sigmoidoscopy every 5 years, or
- Colonoscopy every 10 years, or
- Double-contrast barium enema every 5 to 10 years

The above recommendations are supported by other organizations as well (17). Patients with a greater-than-average risk for colorectal cancer should undergo total colonic surveillance individualized according to the risk of cancer, which involves the following factors:

- History of adenomatous polyps

  Once polyps are removed, the next surveillance examination should occur in 3 years. A study of 1418 patients randomized to surveillance colonoscopy at 1 and 3 years after polypectomy (versus those randomized to 3 years alone) found no difference in the percentage of patients with polyps of advanced pathologic features (i.e., >1 cm, high-grade dysplasia, invasive cancer) (18). After one negative result at a 3-year examination, the interval can be increased to 5 years (19). The surveillance interval for large (i.e., >2 cm) and sessile polyps, multiple polyps, polyps removed piecemeal, or polyps with malignancy and favorable prognostic features is individualized and may be as short as 3 to 6 months.

- History of colorectal cancer

  In patients undergoing curative surgical intervention for a colorectal cancer and who have a normal preoperative colonoscopy, the subsequent surveillance examination should occur at 3 years and, if negative, every 5 years thereafter.

- Inherited adenomatous polyposis syndromes

  Patients with FAP should receive genetic counseling and be offered genetic testing. Beginning at puberty, gene carriers or those with indeterminate status should undergo yearly flexible sigmoidoscopy.

- Inherited nonpolyposis colon cancer

  Patients with HNPCC should receive genetic counseling and be offered genetic testing. Colonoscopy should be performed every 1 to 2 years beginning at age 25 (or at an age 10 years younger than that of the youngest relative with colon cancer). After age 40, surveillance examinations should be conducted yearly.

- Ulcerative or Crohn's colitis

  Colonoscopy generally is performed every 1 to 2 years after 8 years of pancolitic disease. Patients with disease involving the left colon should begin surveillance after 12 to 15 years of disease.

- Two first-degree relatives with colon cancer at any age or adenomatous polyps or colorectal cancer in a first-degree relative relative diagnosed before age 60

  A full colonic evaluation every 5 years beginning at age 40 (or at an age 10 years younger than that of the relative with cancer) is appropriate.

- Personal history of breast, ovarian, or uterine cancer

Surveillance of patients with a personal history of breast, ovarian, and uterine cancer should be individualized. A full colonic evaluation at an interval recommended for average-risk patients is advisable.

TREATMENT

The curability, recurrence, and survival of colorectal cancer is determined on the basis of the disease stage. For most early stage cancers (i.e., Duke's A and B), surgery alone is curative (Table 58.6). For more advanced disease, surgery and adjuvant chemotherapy are recommended to prevent recurrence and prolong survival.

ADJUVANT TREATMENT

Treatment of metastatic colorectal cancer is aimed at reducing recurrence and improving survival. Chemotherapy with 5-fluorouracil (5-FU) has been a mainstay for treatment despite a convincing lack of survival benefit. In 1989, 5-FU plus levamisole was shown to reduce the risk of colon cancer recurrence by 41%, and the death rate by 33%, in 929 patients with Duke's stage C disease versus those receiving surgery alone (20); results in 318 patients with Duke's stage B2 colon cancer were equivocal. In another study of 218 patients with stage B2 disease, a 31% reduction in recurrence was found among patients receiving 5-FU and levamisole, but no demonstrable

Table 58.6.   Comparison of Duke's and TNM Staging

Dukes	Stage	TNM			5-Year Survival (%)
A	I	T1 or T2	N0	M0	90
B1	II	T3	N0	M0	75
B2		T4	N0	M0	
C	III	Any T	N1–N3	M0	35–60
D	IV	Any T	Any N	M1	<10

Primary Tumor (T)
TIS   Carcinoma in situ
T1   Tumor invades submucosa
T2   Tumor invades muscularis propria
T3   Tumor invades through muscularis propria
T4   Tumor invades serosa, nodes and adjacent organs
Metastases (M)
M0   No distant metastases
M1   Distant metastases
Regional Nodes (N)
N0   negative nodes
N1   1–3 positive (+) nodes
N2   >3 (+) nodes
N3   (+) nodes on vascular trunk

effect on survival was noted (21). Patients with Duke's stage C colon cancer should receive adjuvant therapy with 5-FU and levamisole; those with Duke's stage B2 disease should be encouraged to participate in on-going trials.

The combination of postoperative radiation and 5-FU significantly reduces the rates of recurrence, cancer-related deaths, and overall mortality in patients with stage II and III rectal cancer compared with radiation therapy alone (22).

HEPATIC METASTASES

The prognosis of patients with hepatic metastases is poor, with virtually no survivors at 3 years. A multi-institutional study reviewing hepatic resection as treatment of colorectal cancer metastases found a 5-year survival rate of 33% and disease-free survival rate of 21% (23). Favorable prognostic factors included a resection margin of greater than 1 cm and two or fewer metastases smaller than 8 cm.

PREVENTION

Chemoprevention is one of the most exciting potential preventive measures against colorectal cancer. High consumption of fruits and vegetables is consistently associated with a lower risk of colorectal cancer. The mechanism by which fiber may prevent cancer is unknown, but a small, randomized, double-blind and placebo-controlled study identified a statistically significant reduction in fecal bile acid concentrations among patients receiving a wheat-bran fiber and calcium supplement (24). Results of epidemiologic studies show that diets high in carotenoid vegetables, cruciferous vegetables, garlic, and tofu (or soybeans) are associated with decreased prevalence of adenoma (25). Nonsteroidal anti-inflammatory drugs, particularly aspirin, substantially reduce the risk of colorectal cancer, anywhere from 4 to 60%. In two large, prospective cohort studies, regular aspirin use in doses similar to those taken for cardioprotection was associated with decreased risk of colorectal cancer (26, 27). Long-term randomized, controlled trials examining use of aspirin for the prevention of colorectal cancer are currently underway.

CONCLUSIONS

Colorectal cancer is one of the leading causes of cancer and death from carcinoma in the United States. Increasing awareness regarding the preventable nature of this disease along with widespread use of screening should favorably affect the incidence of colorectal cancer. Colorectal cancer screening and polyp removal can save lives, and the most exciting area of future research will be primary prevention of adenomas and colorectal cancer through chemoprevention.

REVIEW EXERCISES

QUESTIONS

For the scenarios in questions 1 through 4, choose the appropriate recommendation from the following (may be used more than once):

   a. Colonoscopy and polypectomy.
   b. Yearly FOBT and flexible sigmoidoscopy every 5 years.
   c. Colonoscopy at age 40.
   d. Colonoscopy in 3 years.
   e. Colonoscopy in 1 year.

1. A single, 3-mm, rectal adenoma found on flexible sigmoidoscopy in a 32-year-old woman.

2. A 62-year-old man who just underwent colonoscopy for an 18-year history of pancolitis.

3. A 54-year-old woman with a lifelong history of irritable bowel syndrome.

4. A 68-year-old black man with recent removal of a 1-cm, villous, pedunculated polyp.

For questions 5 through 9, which statements about colorectal cancer and polyps are true, and which are false?

5. A 70-year-old man undergoing curative resection of Duke's stage A colon cancer found on a surveillance colonosocopy can wait 3 years until the next examination.

6. A 53-year-old woman with one tubular adenoma and one tubulovillous adenoma removed at colonoscopy is at increased risk of subsequent cancer and should undergo repeat colonoscopy in 1 and 3 years.

7. A 34-year-old man who has a 52-year-old brother with colon cancer, a sister with ovarian cancer, and a father who died of colon cancer at age 58 should undergo colonoscopy at age 50.

8. All patients with colon cancer should be offered adjuvant therapy with levamisole and 5-FU.

9. A patient with FAP has a 50% chance of transmitting the disease to his or her children.

10. A 62-year-old woman arrives in your office with recent-onset abdominal pain and a change in bowel habit. She has no family history of cancer and otherwise is in good health. Physical examination reveals some tenderness in the suprapubic area but otherwise is normal. FOBT reveals one of six smears to be positive. Which of the following options is most appropriate?
   a. Repeat FOBT.
   b. Schedule a colonoscopy.
   c. Order a flexible sigmoidoscopy and, if negative, no further evaluation.
   d. Reassure the patient she has symptoms of irritable bowel syndrome and treat with fiber.

Answers

1. a
2. e
3. b
4. d
5. True
6. False
7. False
8. False
9. True
10. b

REFERENCES

1. Parker SL, Tong T, Bolden S, Wingo PA. Cancer statistics, 1997. CA Cancer J Clin 1997;47:5–27.
2. Morson BC. The evolution of colorectal carcinomas. Clin Radiol 1984;35:425–431.
3. St. John DJ, McDermott F, Hopper J, et al. Cancer risk in relatives of patients with common colorectal cancer. Ann Intern Med 1993;118:785–790.
4. Bazzoli F, Fossi S, Sottili S, et al. The risk of adenomatous polyps in asymptomatic first-degree relatives of persons with colon cancer. Gastroenterology 1995;109:783–788.
5. Winawer S, Zauber A, Gerdes H, et al. Risk of colorectal cancer in the families of patients with adenomaotus polyps. N Engl J Med 1996;334:82–97.
6. Schoen R, Weissfeld J, Kuller L. Are women with breast, endometrial or ovarian cancer at increased risk for colorectal cancer? Am J Gastroenterol 1994;89:835–842.
7. Vogelstein B, Fearon E, Hamilton S, et al. Genetic alterations during colorectal-tumor development. N Engl J Med 1988;319:525–532.
8. Day DW, Morson BC. Pathology of adenomas in the pathogenesis of colorectal cancer. In: Morson BC, ed. Major problems in pathology. Philadelphia: WB Saunders; 1978:43–57.
9. Lieberman DA. Cost-effectiveness model for colon cancer screening. Gastroenterology 1995;109:1781–1790.
10. Mandel JS, Bond JH, Church TR, et al. Reducing mortality from colorectal cancer by screening for fecal occult blood. Minnesota Colon Cancer Control Study. N Engl J Med 1993;328:1365–1371.
11. Read TE, Read JD, Butterly LF. Importance of adenomas 5 mm or less in diameter that are detected by sigmoidoscopy. N Engl J Med 1997;336:8–12.
12. Selby JV, Friedman GD, Quesenberry CO, Weiss NS. A case-control study of screening sigmoidoscopy and mortality from colorectal cancer. N Engl J Med 1992;326:653–657.
13. Winawer SJ, Flehinger BJ, Schottenfeld D, Miller DG. Screening for colorectal cancer with fecal occult blood testing and sigmoidoscopy. J Natl Cancer Inst 1993;85:1311–1318.
14. Rex D, Rahmani E, Haseman J, et al. Relative sensitivity of colonoscopy and barium enema for detection of colorectal cancer in clinical practice. Gastroenterology 1997;112:17–23.
15. Gilbertsen VA, Williams SE, Schuman L, McHugh R. Colonoscopy in the detection of carcinoma of the intestine. Surg Gynecol Obstet 1979;149:877–878.
16. Winawer SJ, Zauber AG, Ho MN, et al. Prevention of colorectal cancer by colonoscopic polypectomy. N Engl J Med 1993;329:1977–1981.
17. Winawer SJ, Fletcher R, Miller L, et al. Colorectal cancer screening: clinical guidelines and rationale. Gastroenterology 1997;112:594–642.
18. Winawer S, Zauber A, O'Brien M, et al. Randomized comparison of surveillance intervals after colonoscopic removal of newly diagnosed adenomatous polyps. N Engl J Med 1993;328:901–906.
19. Bond JH. Polyp guideline: diagnosis, treatment and surveillance for patients with nonfamilial colorectal polyps. Ann Intern Med 1993;119:836–842.
20. Moertel C, Fleming T, MacDonald J, et al. Levamisole and fluorouracil for adjuvant therapy of resected colon carcinoma. N Engl J Med 1990;322:352–358.
21. Moertel CG, Fleming TR, Macdonald JS. Intergroup study of fluorouracil plus levamisole as adjuvant therapy for stage II/Duke's stage B2 colon cancer. J Clin Oncol 1995;13:2935–2943.
22. Krook J, Moertel C, Gunderson L, et al. Effective surgical adjuvant therapy for high-risk rectal carcinoma. N Engl J Med 1991;324:709–715.
23. Hughes KS, Simon R, Songhorabodi S, et al. Resection of the liver for colorectal carcinoma metastasis: a multi-institutional study of indications for resection. Surgery 1990;103:278–288.
24. Alberts DS, Ritenbaugh C, Story JA, et al. Randomized, double-blinded, placebo-controlled study of effect of wheat bran fiber and calcium on fecal bile acids in patients with resected adenomatous colon polyps. J Natl Cancer Inst 1996;88:81–92.
25. Witte JS, Longnecker MP, Bird C, et al. Relations of vegetable, fruit, and grain consumption to colorectal adenomatous polyps. Am J Epidemiol 1996;144:1015–1025.
26. Giovannucci E, Egan KM, Hunter DJ, et al. Aspirin and the risk of colorectal cancer in women. N Engl J Med 1995;333:6009–6014.
27. Giovannucci E, Rimm E, Stampfer M, et al. Aspirin use and the risk for colorectal cancer and adenoma in male health professionals. Ann Intern Med 1994;121:241–246.

SUGGESTED READINGS

Krook J, Moertel C, Gunderson L, et al. Effective surgical adjuvant therapy for high-risk rectal carcinoma. N Engl J Med 1991;324:709–715.

Study showing improved mortality rate and reduction in recurrence of advanced rectal cancer by adjuvant radiation and chemotherapy.

Mandel JS, Bond JH, Church TR, et al. Reducing mortality from colorectal cancer by screening for fecal occult blood. Minnesota Colon Cancer Control Study. N Engl J Med 1993; 328:1365–1371.

Landmark study showing a colorectal cancer mortality benefit from FOBT screening.

Moertel C, Fleming T, MacDonald J, et al. Levamisole and fluorouracil for adjuvant therapy of resected colon carcinoma. N Engl J Med 1990;322:352–358.

Study setting the standard of care for Duke's C colon cancer, in which a decrease in colon cancer deaths and recurrence was noted with adjuvant therapy with levamisole and 5-FU.

Selby JV, Friedman GD, Quesenberry CO, Weiss NS. A case-control study of screening sigmoidoscopy and mortality from colorectal cancer. N Engl J Med 1992;326:653–657.

Lower-than-expected death rate from colorectal cancer in patients screened with sigmoidoscopy.

Vogelstein B, Fearon E, Hamilton S, et al. Genetic alterations during colorectal-tumor development. N Engl J Med 1988; 319:525–532.

Landmark study of the spectrum of genetic alterations as adenomas progress to colon cancer.

Winawer SJ, Fletcher R, Miller L, et al. Colorectal cancer screening: clinical guidelines and rationale. Gastroenterology 1997;112:594–642.

Current expert opinion and clinical practice guidelines regarding the complex topic of screening for colorectal cancer.

Winawer S, Zauber A, O'Brien M, et al. Randomized comparison of surveillance intervals after colonoscopic removal of newly diagnosed adenomatous polyps. N Engl J Med 1993; 328:901–906.

Randomized study showing no difference in the percentage of patients with polyps of advanced pathologic features at surveillance colonoscopy 1 and 3 years after polypectomy versus at 3 years alone.

Winawer SJ, Zauber AG, Ho MN, et al. Prevention of colorectal cancer by colonoscopic polypectomy. N Engl J Med 1993;329:1977–1981.

First study showing patients who undergo colonoscopy and polypectomy have a lower-than-expected incidence of colorectal cancer.

59

Inflammatory Bowel Disease

Aaron Brzezinski

Ulcerative colitis and Crohn's disease are inflammatory conditions of the gastrointestinal system; their origin is unknown. Other conditions that are considered to be idiopathic inflammatory bowel diseases (IBDs) include lymphocytic colitis and collagenous colitis. The hallmark of these diseases is uncontrolled inflammation. Ulcerative colitis and Crohn's disease have a bimodal distribution and mostly affect young individuals, but collagenous and lymphocytic colitis mostly affect middle-aged women. Because Crohn's disease and ulcerative colitis are more prevalent, this chapter emphasizes these entities.

ETIOLOGY

EPIDEMIOLOGY

The incidence of ulcerative colitis has remained stable, at from 2 to 10 per 100,000 individuals, whereas the incidence of Crohn's disease is increasing, with current estimates as high as from 1 to 6 per 100,000. There is great geographic variation in the incidence of these diseases, with an inverse relationship between levels of sanitation and incidence of IBD. IBD is more prevalent in Northern Europe and the northern parts of North America (i.e., the northern United States and Canada) compared with the southern regions. In Third World countries, where infectious gastroenteritis is common, IBD is uncommon.

There is a slight female preponderance, and the age at presentation is bimodal, with the greatest peak occurring between 15 and 25 years of age and a second, lesser peak after the sixth decade of life. Both diseases can occur in children, but ulcerative colitis is more common among this population.

RISK FACTORS

All populations are at risk, but whites more commonly are affected. Ashkenazi Jews in Europe and in the United States have a two- to fourfold increased risk of ulcerative colitis and a six- to eightfold increased risk of Crohn's disease compared with the general population in those same areas. Ashkenazi Jews in Israel, however, have a lower risk of IBD compared with those in Europe or the United States.

An interesting association also exists between cigarette smoking and IBD. A greater-than-expected number of patients with Crohn's disease are cigarette smokers, whereas a less-than-expected number of patients with ulcerative colitis smoke.

PATHOGENESIS

The cause of IBD remains unknown. There is a genetic predisposition to the disease, however, and there are as-yet-unknown environmental or infectious agents that trigger the disease. IBD does not follow a mendelian pattern of inheritance, but 10 to 25% of patients have a first-degree relative with IBD, and the lifetime risk of IBD among first-degree relatives of patients is 9% for offspring and siblings and 3.5% for parents. A strong disease concordance exists as well. Relatives of patients with ulcerative colitis usually have ulcerative colitis, and relatives of patients with Crohn's disease usually develop Crohn's disease. The concordance rates for monozygotic twins is 100%.

The gastrointestinal system is in a constant state of controlled inflammation. It is continuously exposed to lumenal antigens; therefore, it is logical that these can trigger an abnormal inflammatory response. These antigens may be dietary, infectious, or environmental. To date, however, no specific antigens have been identified, though many have been proposed, including *Mycobacterium paratuberculosis* and proteins from bacterial cell-wall membranes. Whatever the trigger may be, mucosal activation of macrophages leads to increased release of proinflammatory cytokines (i.e., interleukin [IL]-1, tumor necrosis factor, IL-6, IL-8), which in turn leads to cell destruction by different mechanisms (including clonal expansion of natural killer cells and cytotoxic T cells), B-cell proliferation (with increased production of mucosal immunoglobulin G), and increased production of thromboxane A_2, leukotriene B, and platelet activating factor (PAF) (i.e., proinflammatory mediators that amplify the inflammatory response by recruiting and activating neutrophils).

SPECIFIC CONDITIONS

Specific IBDs include ulcerative colitis and Crohn's disease.

ULCERATIVE COLITIS

Clinical Features

The presenting symptoms of ulcerative colitis depend both on the extent and severity of the disease. Patients with ulcerative colitis usually present with nonbloody diarrhea that rapidly progresses to bloody diarrhea. At presentation, the disease is limited to the rectum and sigmoid colon in more than 50% of patients. In most, the initial presentation is mild to moderate, and at least 90% achieve remission with medical treatment. Fewer than 10% present with a severe or fulminant attack. The mortality rate from the initial attack is less than 0.5%.

Diagnosis

The diagnosis of ulcerative colitis relies on the clinical picture, stool testing, endoscopic appearance, and histologic findings. To provide optimal medical treatment and establish the prognosis, it is important to determine the extent of disease. In patients with untreated ulcerative colitis, there is always rectal involvement. Histology is the most sensitive way of establishing disease extent, and colonoscopy with biopsy is indicated for patients in whom ulcerative colitis is suspected. Biopsies also are useful in screening patients for dysplasia, because those with extensive and longstanding disease have an increased risk of colorectal cancer. Colonoscopy is not necessary to assess patient response to medical treatment or for routine follow-up of patients with ulcerative colitis. When determining extent of the disease, colonoscopy without biopsy is less sensitive, and radiology is the least sensitive. In fact, both of these modalities underestimate the true extent of disease.

Stool Samples Stool studies are useful in excluding infectious causes that can mimic ulcerative colitis. These include *Salmonella* sp., *Shigella* sp., *Campylobacter* sp., *Clostridium difficile, Yersinia* sp., and *Escherichia coli* 0157:H7. In endemic areas, stool examination for *Entamoeba histolytica* is indicated, because amebic colitis may mimic ulcerative colitis and use of corticosteroids in these patients has disastrous results. In patients who are immunosuppressed (by chemotherapy, transplantation, or acquired immunodeficiency syndrome), other infectious agents, such as cytomegalovirus, *Mycobacterium avium* complex, *Neisseria gonorrhoeae,* or chlamydia, should be excluded.

Endoscopy Patients with untreated ulcerative colitis always have rectal involvement. The earliest endoscopic findings in patients with ulcerative colitis are blurring of the blood vessels and hyperemia. In patients with more severe inflammation, the mucosa becomes granular, friable, and finally, with severe ulcerative colitis, ulcerated. In patients with severe ulcerative colitis, blood, mucus, and pus are present in the lumen as well. Overall, the mucosa is diffusely involved in a continuous pattern. In chronic disease, the colon becomes tubular in appearance, and pseudopolyps may be present. A sharp demarcation between diseased and healthy mucosa also may be seen.

Radiology In patients with severe or fulminant colitis, intestinal perforation or pneumatosis coli should be excluded before endoscopy by plain-film radiography. Double-contrast barium enema is safe in patients with mild or moderately severe ulcerative colitis, but this modality underestimates the extent of disease and does not allow concurrent histologic sampling. In patients with longstanding ulcerative colitis, the haustral folds are lost, and the colon is shortened and narrow (i.e., "stem-pipe colon"). Pseudopolyps can be visualized easily at double-contrast barium enema. In addition, strictures can be diagnosed by contrast barium enema and patients should undergo colonoscopy with biopsy and brush cytology to rule out dysplasia or cancer when strictures are present.

Histology Inflammatory changes in ulcerative colitis primarily are confined to the mucosa, with infiltration by neutrophils, lymphocytes, plasma cells, and macrophages; cryptitis with crypt abscesses; and goblet-cell depletion. In patients with chronic disease, there is architectural distortion, with crypt atrophy and shortened glands that lose their normal "test-tube array."

Severity Truelove and Witts proposed a classification of severity based on symptoms and laboratory tests (Table 59.1). Such a classification is useful to determine prognosis and treatment. Since its initial description, few modifications have been made.

Differential Features See "Differential Features of Ulcerative Colitis and Crohn's Disease."

Table 59.1.   Severity Criteria for Ulcerative Colitis, Modified

	Mild	*# Severe*	*Fulminant*
Stool frequency	<4/day	>6/day	>10/day or, at times, no bowel movements
Blood in stool	Small amounts	Macroscopic with all bowel movements	Continuous
Temperature	No fever	>37.8°C on 2 of 4 days	>37.8°C
Heart rate	Normal	>90	>90
Hemoglobin	Normal	<75% of normal (12 g/dL)	Transfusion-requiring
Erythrocyte sedimentation rate	<30 mm/h	>30 mm/h	>30 mm/h
Radiography	Normal	Thumbprinting	Edematous, dilated
Clinical signs	Normal or mild tenderness	Abdominal tenderness	Abdominal distension, absent bowel sounds, tenderness

Moderate: Between mild and severe.
Modified from Truelove SC, Witts LJ. Cortisone in ulcerative colitis. Br Med J 1955;1:1041–1048.

Treatment

Patients with mild or moderate disease do not require hospitalization and are treated with 5-aminosalicylic compounds. Patients with severe disease are best treated with corticosteroids. Patients with fulminant or toxic megacolon require hospitalization and, frequently, emergency surgery. (See "Treatment.")

Prognosis

Most patients with ulcerative colitis have intermittent attacks, with remissions lasting from a few weeks to many years. Approximately 10 to 15% have a chronic, continuous course, and 5 to 10% present with a severe attack that requires urgent colectomy. The course and prognosis largely are determined by the extent of disease. In 70% of patients presenting with proctitis, the disease remains confined to the rectum; in the other 30%, the disease will extend proximally when patients are followed for up to 30 years. The risk of eventual colectomy is proportional to the extent of disease, and it is significantly greater in those patients with pancolitis. The rate of colectomy is as high as 30% during the first year of disease in those patients with pancolitis at presentation. After the first year, however, the colectomy rate for all patients with ulcerative colitis, regardless of extent, is 1% per year.

Patients with ulcerative colitis have an increased risk of colorectal cancer. This risk depends on the duration and extent of disease; more recently, increased risk has been associated with cholestatic liver disease, such as primary sclerosing cholangitis. The risk of colorectal cancer increases after 7 years in patients with pancolitis, and it has been estimated to increase by 1% per year after 15 or 20 years. In patients with left-sided ulcerative colitis, risk of colorectal cancer also is increased, but there is no agreement on how high this risk actually is. Patients with proctitis have no increased risk and do not require different screening than the general population.

Colorectal cancer in patients with ulcerative colitis usually, but not always, is preceded by dysplasia. For this reason, patients with pancolitis for more than 7 years are advised to undergo surveillance colonoscopies with biopsies. The optimal timing between colonoscopies is uncertain, however. Generally, patients are advised to undergo their first screening colonoscopy with multiple biopsies 7 years after the onset of symptoms. Four quadrant biopsy samples are obtained at 10-cm intervals, and extra biopsy samples are taken from suspicious areas, such as strictures or masses. Dysplastic changes can be found in areas remote from where a cancer might be; therefore, the entire colon should be screened. If no dysplasia is found, colonoscopy is repeated at 1- to 3-year intervals. If high-grade dysplasia is found and confirmed by another experienced pathologist, colectomy is recommended. For low-grade dysplasia, debate continues regarding the best recommendation. Some pathologists and gastroenterologists treat dysplasia—whether low- or high-grade—as premalignant and advise colectomy. Others recommend repeat colonoscopies and biopsies every 6 months in patients with low-grade dysplasia either until there is no dysplasia (in which case patients return to yearly screening) or colectomy (if high-grade dysplasia is found). Because of sampling error, however, dysplasia may be missed with this approach. I view dysplasia—whether low- or high-grade—as premalignant and advise colectomy.

CROHN'S DISEASE

Crohn's disease is heterogeneous and has different clinical presentations. It can affect any segment of the gastrointestinal system, but the most common involvement is ileocolonic disease (≈45% of patients), small-bowel involvement alone

(≈33%), and colonic involvement alone (≈20%). Esophageal and gastroduodenal involvement occurs in 0.5 to 4.0% of patients. Most patients with gastroduodenal involvement also have evidence of Crohn's disease elsewhere in the gastrointestinal system. Clinically, Crohn's disease can be inflammatory, stenotic, fistulizing, or mixed. The signs, symptoms, and treatment depend on the site of involvement and disease behavior.

Clinical Presentation

Patients with ileocolic disease usually present with nonbloody diarrhea, crampy abdominal pain (usually worse after meals), weight loss, and low-grade fever. The onset usually is subacute, but it can be acute and confused with acute appendicitis. On examination, patients are pale, can have decreased bowel sounds, and experience tenderness on palpation in the right lower quadrants, where a palpable mass may be present. More than 90% of patients with ileocecal disease eventually require surgery, the most common indications for which are internal fistulae, abscess, or obstruction.

Small-bowel disease most commonly is localized in the terminal ileum, but it can be diffuse, involving the jejunum and the ileum. Such patients present with diarrhea, abdominal pain consistent with intermittent and incomplete small-bowel obstruction, and weight loss. Patients tend to be older at presentation, and the most common indication for surgery is obstruction. Patients with jejunal involvement have malabsorption and steatorrhea.

Patients with Crohn's disease usually have inflammatory disease and present with diarrhea and hematochezia. Obstruction may occur because of strictures, and fistulae both to and from the colon generally are found. In patients who require surgery, differentiating Crohn's colitis from ulcerative colitis is of primary importance. In 10% of patients, however, a specific diagnosis cannot be established; such patients are labeled as having "indeterminate colitis." Approximately 50% of patients with Crohn's colitis require surgery and the most common indications in this group are perianal disease and obstruction. Approximately 30% of patients with Crohn's disease have perianal disease, and approximately 10% of female patients with Crohn's colitis develop rectovaginal fistulae.

Gastroduodenal Crohn's disease may be difficult to distinguish from peptic ulcer disease and erosions caused by nonsteroidal anti-inflammatory drugs (NSAIDs). Patients usually present with nausea, vomiting, and abdominal pain that improve with antacids. When patients develop gastrocolic fistulae, these usually originate from the colon rather than the stomach. Patients with gastrocolic fistulae present with diarrhea and malabsorption or with feculent emesis. Gastric outlet obstruction occurs in approximately 30% of patients and is the most common indication for surgery in this group.

Rectal and perianal involvement occurs in 10 to 30% of patients, and it usually manifests by perianal abscess or fistulae. Rectal and perianal disease can occur without colonic involvement and, at times, before there is evidence of Crohn's disease elsewhere in the gastrointestinal tract.

Diagnosis

Diagnosis of Crohn's disease is based on clinical, laboratory, radiologic, endoscopic, and histologic criteria. The clinical presentation (described earlier) depends on the site of involvement and disease behavior.

Laboratory Testing Most often, laboratory testing confirms the clinical suspicion and helps to rule out conditions that mimic Crohn's disease, such as infectious or parasitic enteritis or colitis. More often, the abnormalities found at laboratory testing reflect the inflammatory and chronic nature of Crohn's disease. Patients frequently are anemic and have leukocytosis, thrombocytosis, and elevated erythrocyte sedimentation rate and orosomucoid acid level. Perinuclear antinuclear cytoplasmic antibodies are found in only 10% of patients with Crohn's disease, compared with more than 70% of patients with ulcerative colitis.

Radiology Radiology plays a major role in diagnosis of Crohn's disease. The small intestine is well visualized with a small-bowel series, and dedicated small-bowel series provide better mucosal detail than upper gastrointestinal series with small-bowel follow-through. Small-bowel enema is indicated only in a small group of patients. The findings on radiographs include mucosal ulceration, loop separation, strictures, fistulae, and cobblestoning. For those patients in whom an abscess is suspected, computed tomography is useful, because it not only confirms presence of an abscess but also provides guidance for percutaneous drainage.

Endoscopy Colonoscopy and esophagogastroduodenoscopy allow direct visualization of the mucosa as well as mucosal sampling for histology. Because Crohn's disease is discontinuous, areas of abnormal mucosa with normal intervening mucosa, which are referred to as "skip lesions," are visualized at endoscopy. Patients with Crohn's disease may have rectal sparing as well. When discrete ulcers are seen, "aphthoid" ulcers are considered to be "pathognomonic" of Crohn's disease; aphthoid ulcers are 3 to 5 mm in size and have a surrounding red halo. Cobblestoning frequently is seen. Fistulae are a feature of Crohn's disease but not ulcerative colitis.

Differential Features of Ulcerative Colitis and Crohn's Disease Distinguishing ulcerative colitis from Crohn's disease can be difficult, especially in patients with fulminant colitis (Table 59.2). Histopathologic examination can be very useful in making this distinction. The histologic findings seen in Crohn's disease but not in ulcerative colitis are aphthous ulcers, noncaseating granulomas, microscopic skip lesions, and transmural involvement.

The principal possibilities in the differential diagnosis of IBD are infectious enteritis or colitis, ischemia, radiation enteritis, lymphoma, Behcet's disease, endometriosis, diverticulitis, and NSAID-induced enteropathy or colopathy. A

Table 59.2.   Differential Features of Ulcerative Colitis and Crohn's Disease

	Ulcerative Colitis	Crohn's Disease
Clinical features		
Rectal bleeding	Usual	Sometimes
Abdominal mass	Absent	Often
Perianal disease	Extremely rare	≤30%
Upper gastrointestinal symptoms	Unrelated	Frequent
Malnutrition	Rare, mild	Frequent, moderate to severe
Endoscopic and radiologic features		
Rectal involvement	Present	Variable
Continuous disease	Always	Rare
Discrete linear ulcers	Rare	Frequent
Aphthoid ulcers	Absent	Common
Cobblestoning	Absent	Common
Skip areas	Absent	Common
Small-bowel disease	Absent[a]	Common
Fistulae	Absent	Common
Pathologic features		
Aphthous ulcers	Absent	Common
Noncaseating granulomas	Absent	10–30%
Crypt abscess	Common	Frequent
Transmural involvement	Absent	Present
Microscopic skip lesions	Absent	Frequent

[a] Except backwash ileitis.

careful patient history, physical examination, and laboratory tests are critical to exclude conditions that mimic IBD.

EXTRAINTESTINAL MANIFESTATIONS

To date, more than 100 extraintestinal manifestations of IBD have been described. Some parallel the disease activity; others follow an independent course. Patients with colonic disease have more frequent extraintestinal manifestations. Complications that parallel disease activity include:

- Peripheral arthritis
- Erythema nodosum
- Pyoderma gangrenosum
- Keratoconjunctivitis
- Episcleritis
- Hypercoagulability

Extraintestinal manifestations that run an independent course include:

- Ankylosing spondylitis, which more commonly occurs in patients with ulcerative colitis who are positive for HLA-B27
- Sacroiliitis
- Anterior uveitis

ARTHRITIS

Arthritis of IBD usually is nonerosive, mono- or pauciarticular, asymmetric, and migratory. There is no synovial destruction, and large joints more commonly are affected. Peripheral arthritis is more common in female patients and correlates with disease activity. Axial arthritis relates to HLA-B27 and does not correlate with disease activity.

SKIN AND EYES

Erythema nodosum occurs in approximately 3% of patients with IBD. Characterized by tender, subcutaneous nodules, it generally occurs along the shins. The area affected is erythematous and exquisitely sensitive to touch.

Pyoderma gangrenosum is characterized by an ulcerating lesion that becomes purulent, necrotic, and when it heals, leaves a scar. Commonly found at sites of minimal trauma, these lesions occur in both ulcerative colitis and Crohn's disease. Treatment frequently involves immunosuppressant therapy.

Ocular manifestations of IBD include iritis, keratoconjunctivitis, episcleritis, and uveitis. Patients with uveitis generally are positive for HLA-B27. Frequent symptoms include blurred vision, photophobia, and a painful eye. Ocular manifestations are emergencies, because if they are not treated properly, they can lead to blindness. Such patients should be treated in consultation with an ophthalmologist.

LIVER DISEASE

Cholestatic liver disease is the most common manifestation of hepatic involvement in patients with IBD. It occurs in 5% of patients, and it does not parallel disease activity. Primary sclerosing cholangitis (PSC) occurs in from 1 to 5% of patients with ulcerative colitis and rarely in patients with Crohn's colitis. PSC runs a course independent from disease activity, and it can either precede the diagnosis of ulcerative colitis or present years after colectomy for ulcerative colitis. In most patients, early diagnosis depends on detection of biochemical abnormalities, such as an elevated alkaline phosphatase (ALP) level. Levels of ALP can fluctuate, however, and even return to normal in patients with established PSC. During the late stages of disease, PSC can be complicated by cholangiocarcinoma.

TREATMENT

Because the etiology of IBD remains unknown, other than surgery, which arguably ''cures'' patients with ulcerative colitis, the treatment of IBD remains palliative. The goals of medical treatment are to improve symptoms, decrease complications, decrease the need for surgical intervention, and improve the patient's quality of life. Treatment can be divided in two phases: therapy of the acute attack, and maintenance of remission.

PHARMACOLOGIC TREATMENT

Medications used to treat patients with IBD include:

- 5-aminosalicylic acid (5-ASA)
- Antibiotics
- Corticosteroids
- Immunosuppressive medications

5-Aminosalicylic Acid

The 5-ASA mediators are anti-inflammatory agents that act at the mucosal level and decrease inflammation, possibly by inhibiting formation of both prostaglandin and leukotriene metabolites (Table 59.3). The 5-ASA medications also are effective at maintaining remission in patients with ulcerative colitis. As mentioned, ulcerative colitis is characterized by periods of activity and periods of quiescence. With continuous use of 5-ASA, remission can be prolonged in a significant number of patients with ulcerative colitis.

Keep in mind that the therapeutic effect of 5-ASA is local, at the mucosal level, and not systemic. For the medication to be therapeutic, it must be delivered to the site of the disease. If a preparation that releases 5-ASA in the colon is given to patients with small-bowel disease only, no therapeutic effect will be observed. Given orally, 5-ASA is rapidly absorbed in the proximal small bowel, acetylated by the liver, and excreted in the urine. To prevent proximal absorption and allow the 5-ASA to exert its anti-inflammatory effect at the disease site, different delivery systems are available, including:

- Creating a larger molecule by binding it to a carrier or another 5-ASA via an azo-bond
- Coating 5-ASA with a pH-sensitive resin
- Using delayed-release preparations

Other 5-ASA preparations currently used are in the form of suppositories and enemas. Suppositories effectively induce remission in patients with ulcerative proctitis; the recommended dose is 500 mg twice a day for 4 to 6 weeks. Enemas effectively induce remission in patients with proctosigmoiditis; the recommended dose is 4 g per 60 mL at bedtime for 4 to 6 weeks. Both suppositories and enemas can maintain remission in patients with ulcerative proctitis or proctosigmoiditis.

Table 59.3. Aminosalicylic Acid Formulations

	FDA Indication	*Common Use*	*Dose*
Azo compounds, (Sulfasalazine [Sulfapyridine–5-ASA])	Mild to moderate ulcerative colitis Adjuvant in severe maintenance of remission in ulcerative colitis	Same Crohn's colitis, mild	Acute disease, 4–8 g/day Maintenance, 2–4 g/day
Olsalazine (5-ASA–5-ASA) (Dipentum)	Maintenance of remission of ulcerative colitis in patients intolerant of Sulfasalazine	Same Induce remission in mild to moderate ulcerative colitis in patients allergic to intolerant of Sulfasalazine	250 mg/day orally b.i.d. with meals
pH-Sensitive preparations (Mesalamine, polymer-coated Asacol)	Mildly to moderately active ulcerative colitis Maintenance of remission in ulcerative colitis	Same Active mild to moderate Crohn's colitis Maintenance of remission in Crohn's colitis (debatable)	FDA approved: 1.2–2.4 g/day Common use: 2.4–4-8 g/day, higher dose for active Crohn's 2.4–4.8 g/day for maintenance of remission
Delayed-release preparations (Mesalamine, ethylcellulose-coated Pentasa)	Induction of remission in patients with mild to moderate active ulcerative colitis	Mild to moderate Crohn's ileitis or ileocolitis Maintenance of remission in Crohn's disease (debatable)	Active disease, 4 g/day Maintenance of remission, 2 g/day

FDA, U.S. Food and Drug Administration.

Azo-Bond Compounds Sulfasalazine, which is a 5-ASA molecule bound to sulfapyridine by an azo-bond, was the first 5-ASA preparation found to be effective in treatment of IBD. Sulfapyridine serves as a carrier and has no therapeutic effect. The azo-bond is split by an azo-reductase that is produced by colonic bacteria. Therefore, the main therapeutic use of sulfasalazine is in patients with colonic involvement, whether it is ulcerative colitis or Crohn's colitis. Sulfasalazine effectively induces remission in patients with mild or moderate disease, but patients with severe disease should be treated with corticosteroids.

A therapeutic effect from sulfasalazine is seen in 60 to 80% of patients with mild or moderate ulcerative colitis. The therapeutic dose is 4 to 6 g daily, divided into four doses. To improve tolerance, start at a low dose (e.g., 500 mg three or four times a day), and then increase the dose gradually. Thirty percent of patients are either allergic or intolerant to sulfapyridine, and they require discontinuation of sulfasalazine. The most common side effects include headache, nausea, anorexia, oligospermia, and dyspepsia; less common side effects include skin rash, pruritus, urticaria, and hemolytic anemia. Rarely, patients can develop life-threatening reactions, such as aplastic anemia or anaphylactic reactions. Because sulfapyridine decreases folic acid absorption by competitive inhibition, patients receiving sulfasalazine should take supplemental folic acid (0.4–1.0 mg/day).

Intolerance and allergy to sulfasalazine more commonly result from sulfapyridine rather than 5-ASA. A 5-ASA compound that does not contain sulfapyridine can be used in patients who are intolerant to sulfasalazine or allergic to sulfa. Olsalazine (Dipentum) is 5-ASA that is bound by an azo-bond to another molecule of 5-ASA. It is safe in patients who are allergic to sulfa. The azo-bond in olsalazine also is split by azo-reductase from colonic bacteria, so the site of action is colonic as well. Unfortunately, however, as many as 17% of patients on olsalazine develop secretory diarrhea; this side effect can be minimized by giving the olsalazine with meals.

pH-Sensitive Preparations The only pH-sensitive preparation available in the United States is Asacol, which is 5-ASA coated with a methacrylic acid copolymer B (called Eudragit-S) that dissolves at pH 7.0 (i.e., the pH in the colon). The main indication, therefore, is colonic disease. The recommended dose in patients with active mild or moderate ulcerative colitis or Crohn's colitis is 2.4 g per 24 hours in three or four divided doses. Tolerance is good, and larger doses (i.e., 4.8–6.0 g per 24 hours) produce better results. Asacol is well tolerated, and very few patients develop diarrhea.

Delayed-Release Preparations The only delayed-release preparation currently available is Pentasa, which is an ethyl-cellulose-coated mesalamine preparation that releases 5-ASA throughout the small and large intestine. Pentasa is approved for use in patients with ulcerative colitis. In clinical trials, it has effectively induced remission in patients with mild or moderate symptoms of inflammatory Crohn's disease of the small intestine, with or without colonic involvement. Like all 5-ASA medications, the higher the dose, the more effective it is. The recommended dose is 4 g per 24 hours in four divided doses.

Antibiotics

Primary treatment with antibiotics is indicated only in patients with Crohn's disease, and controlled data are available only for metronidazole and ciprofloxacin. Metronidazole is particularly effective in patients with Crohn's colitis or perianal disease. The most common side effects leading to discontinuation of metronidazole are gastrointestinal intolerance and peripheral neuropathy. Metronidazole is contraindicated during pregnancy because of the risk of cleft palate; in addition, all patients should be warned of its potential Antabuse effect. For those patients that do not tolerate metronidazole, ciprofloxacin is used with simular results.

Corticosteroids

Corticosteroids play a major role in medical treatment of IBD. They are indicated in patients with moderate or severe ulcerative colitis or Crohn's disease and in those who fail to respond to 5-ASA. Corticosteroids effectively induce remission, but they are not indicated for maintaining remission. In patients with ulcerative colitis, 40 to 60 mg of oral prednisolone or prednisone per day is recommended; for patients with Crohn's disease, a starting dose of 1 mg/kg per day is recommended. Oral corticosteroids are tapered slowly (i.e., 5 mg every 5 to 7 days) once remission is achieved. If remission is not achieved quickly with oral corticosteroids, however, patients should be admitted to the hospital and treated with intravenous steroids.

Patients with more severe ulcerative colitis are best treated in a hospital with intravenous corticosteroids. Hydrocortisone and methylprednisolone are equally effective. Hydrocortisone usually is prescribed at a dose of 300 mg per 24 hours. Controlled data are not available, but intravenous hydrocortisone may be more effective when given by continuous infusion rather than by an intravenous bolus every 8 hours. If the patient fails to respond in 5 to 7 days, surgery or other medical treatments should be considered. Adrenocorticotropic hormone rarely is used and is only marginally more effective—and only then in those patients who have never been treated with corticosteroids.

Corticosteroid enemas are useful in patients with ulcerative proctosigmoiditis, and newer steroids are under investigation. Budesonide has potent anti-inflammatory effects. Because of high first-pass liver metabolism, however, it has less systemic effects and less adrenal suppression than prednisone. Budesonide is not yet available for clinical use in the United States.

The many side effects of corticosteroids, which are the major factors limiting their use in patients with IBD, include moon facies, buffalo hump, striae, posterior subcapsular cataracts, aseptic necrosis of bone, glaucoma, osteoporosis, immunosuppression, hyperglycemia, acne, mood swings, insomnia, weight gain, and adrenal insufficiency. Arrest of growth occurs in children, but this can be lessened by administering corticosteroids on alternate days rather than daily. Patients should be informed about the potential risks of corticosteroids and the need for glucocorticoid supplementation in case of surgery for up to 1 year after corticosteroid cessation. Patients also should be warned about the severe risks of sudden discontinuation of corticosteroids.

Immunosuppressive Drugs

The main indications for immunosuppressive drugs in patients with IBD are refractory disease and steroid-dependent disease. Immunosuppressive drugs also are used to promote fistula healing and in patients with steroid-resistant pyoderma gangrenosum. Substantial patient experience exists with 6-mercaptopurine (6-MP) and Azathioprine (i.e., an S-substituted form of 6-MP); experience with cyclosporine and with methotrexate is more limited. The exact mechanism by which immunosuppressive drugs improve symptoms in patients with IBD is unclear, but it may result from blocking lymphocyte proliferation and activation as well as by affecting humoral responsiveness.

The therapeutic benefit of 6-MP and azathioprine is slow in onset. It usually is delayed by at least 3 months, and therapeutic benefits have been observed even as late as 12 months after initiation of treatment. Historically, these medications allow steroid reduction or discontinuation in approximately 75% of the patients who are steroid dependent, improve symptoms in approximately 70% of patients with refractory disease, and promote fistula healing in approximately 60% of patients. In those with ulcerative colitis, benefit is observed in 50 to 75% of patients. The role of these medications is less clear in these patients, however, because surgery is seen as "curative" for ulcerative colitis. The main side effects of 6-MP and azathioprine are pancreatitis (3%), allergic-type reactions (2%), bone-marrow suppression (2%), and with long-term use, cervical cancer and lymphoma. Patients receiving these drugs also are more susceptible to infections, and it is important for them to understand the need for routine blood tests while on these medications.

Cyclosporine is a potent immunosuppressant that frequently is used to prevent rejection in patients undergoing organ transplantation. Cyclosporine does not maintain remission in patients with IBD, and its use may be restricted to those with severe ulcerative colitis who do not respond to intravenous corticosteroids and would like to avoid surgery. Because of significant side effects, this medication should be used only by experienced physicians, and preferably in tertiary-care centers. The most common side effects include nephrotoxicity, seizures, paresthesia, hypertrichosis, hypertension, and infections.

Information on methotrexate is limited, but an intramuscular dose of 25 mg once a week is useful at inducing remission in patients with Crohn's disease. Patients receiving methotrexate also should receive folic acid, 1 mg/day, for the duration of treatment, which usually is 16 weeks. The most serious toxicities are hypersensitivity pneumonitis, teratogenicity, hepatotoxicity, and bone-marrow suppression. Patients should be strongly advised against drinking alcohol, and women with childbearing potential should practice adequate contraception. The risk of hepatotoxicity is greater in patients who are obese and in those who consume alcohol.

SURGICAL TREATMENT

Between one-third and one-half of patients with IBD will require surgery. Patients with ulcerative colitis and extensive Crohn's colitis require surgery because of failure to respond to medical treatment, hemorrhage, toxic dilatation, perforation, strictures causing obstruction, and dysplasia or cancer. The type of surgery performed is different for patients with Crohn's disease than for those with ulcerative colitis. Depending on the indication, patients with Crohn's disease may have segmental resection or stricturoplasty. Patients with ulcerative colitis should undergo subtotal colectomy regardless of disease extent. A pelvic pouch formed from the terminal ileum and anal anastomosis avoids permanent ileostomy, but it is complicated by pouchitis in 5 to 10% of patients.

Recurrence is frequent in patients with Crohn's disease. Approximately 50% will require surgery within 5 years, and 80% within 10 years, of the previous surgery. The endoscopic and histologic recurrence rate is almost 100% at 1 year, but the symptomatic recurrence rate is lower. Symptomatic recurrence can be delayed in some patients by using 5-ASA , 6-MP, or azathioprine postoperatively, but use of these medications cannot be recommended in all patients and should be individualized.

SYSTEMIC COMPLICATIONS

Systemic complications are more common in patients with Crohn's disease. The most common systemic complications are weight loss, malabsorption, urinary stones, gallstones, thrombotic and embolic events, sepsis, and amyloidosis. Many of the systemic complications in patients with Crohn's disease relate to involvement of the small intestine and depend on the extent of disease. Weight loss is common as well, the main reason for which is decreased oral intake either because of anorexia or postprandial symptoms. Malabsorption, which also is frequent, results from extensive mucosal involvement, thus leading to decreased absorptive surface area or protein-losing enteropathy, or from fistulous tracts that bypass the small bowel.

Gallstones and kidney stones are complications that relate primarily to alterations of small-bowel pathophysiology, thus leading to excess absorption of oxalate and abnormal recirculation of bile salts. Vitamin B_{12} is selectively absorbed in the distal 100 cm of the terminal ileum; if this segment is diseased or removed surgically, patients will develop vitamin B_{12} malabsorption, with subsequent vitamin B_{12} deficiency. In such patients, the optimal route for supplementation is parenteral. Likewise, hydroxy bile acids are absorbed in the distal 100 cm of the terminal ileum. Thus, when less than 100 cm are diseased or surgically removed, the malabsorbed hydroxy bile acids enter the colon and cause secretory diarrhea; these patients respond to oral cholestyramine, which binds bile salts. Conversely, when more than 100 cm of terminal ileum are surgically removed, patients deplete their pool of bile acid and develop malabsorption and steatorrhea. Such patients respond to a low-fat diet that is supplemented by medium-chain triglycerides, which do not require bile salts for absorption.

Patients with Crohn's disease also can develop malab-sorption because of small-bowel bacterial overgrowth. This bacterial overgrowth can result from strictures or fistulae, or it can occur after surgery because of a resected ileocecal valve and ileocolic anastomosis.

Hypercoagulability, which leads to thrombotic and embolic phenomena in patients with IBD, currently is the third-leading cause of disease-related mortality in patients with IBD. The leading causes are colorectal cancer and sepsis. Amyloidosis was a frequent complication in the past, but it is rarely seen now. Amyloidosis occurs more frequently in patients with unremitting fistulous disease or septic complications. Other rare, extraintestinal complications of IBD include pancreatitis, immune-mediated neutropenia, and immune-mediated thrombocytopenia.

REVIEW EXERCISES

QUESTIONS

1. A 26-year-old white woman presents to your office because of diarrhea. Her history reveals:

- An episode of self-limited diarrhea 3 years ago that lasted 3 weeks and was diagnosed as irritable bowel syndrome.
- Four weeks before consultation, she developed three to four loose bowel movements per day.
- She has cramps with urgency before defecation, which are followed by a small, loose bowel movement.
- On two occasions, she has had nocturnal bowel movements.
- She denies blood with the stool.
- She has no systemic symptoms.
- Two months ago, she discontinued cigarette smoking after an episode of shortness of breath.
- Her past medical history is unremarkable.
- She takes Ibuprofen for menstrual cramps.

Examination reveals the following:

- In no distress, a heart rate of 84, a respiratory rate of 16, and a temperature of 37.6°C.
- Abdomen reveals normal bowels sounds, is soft, and is tender to palpation in the left lower quadrant.
- Rectal examination reveals soft stool, which is trace positive for occult blood.

1a. Your initial impression is:
   a. Irritable bowel syndrome.
   b. Infectious diarrhea.
   c. Ulcerative colitis.
   d. Crohn's colitis.
   e. Collagenous colitis.

1b. The best diagnostic test is:
   a. Complete blood count/differential.
   b. Stool for *C. difficile.*
   c. Flexible sigmoidoscopy with biopsies.
   d. Air-contrast barium enema.
   e. Small-bowel series.

1c. Your recommendation is:
   a. Admit to hospital..
   b. Flagyl, 500 mg orally three times a day for 1 week
   c. Fiber and an anticholinergic agent.
   d. Prednisone, 40 mg orally once a day.
   e. 5-ASA enemas HS.

2. A 34-year-old patient with ulcerative colitis for the previous 12 years comes to see you. She is pregnant and would like to discuss subsequent medical treatment during pregnancy and lactation. Her history reveals:

- She presented at 22 years of age with bloody diarrhea and initially was treated with prednisone. Since then, she has received sulfasalazine.
- She has mild flare-ups in the spring every year, which are controlled by increasing the dose of sulfasalazine from a maintenance dose of 2 to 4 g/day.
- She otherwise is healthy.
- She does not take any other medications.

Your recommendation is:
   a. Discontinue sulfasalazine because of the risk of kernicterus and start Asacol.
   b. Discontinue sulfasalazine, and do not treat unless she has an exacerbation.
   c. Continue sulfasalazine at the present dose.
   d. Add folic acid, 1 mg orally once a day.
   e. Discontinue sulfasalazine postpartum to decrease the risk of kernicterus.

Answers

1. c, c, e

This patient has new-onset ulcerative colitis, which is mild. Her symptoms are those of distal ulcerative colitis; therefore, the best initial treatment is a topical 5-ASA product.

2. d

All 5-ASA compounds are safe during pregnancy and lactation, and they should be continued to decrease the risk of a flare up with potentially disastrous consequences. Though Sulfasalazine has sulfapyridine and all sulfas have the potential for inducing kernicterus, this is a theoretical concern; kernicterus has yet to be reported in association with Azulfidine. Folic acid should be added because Azulfidine interferes with folic acid absorption and to decrease the risk of spina bifida.

SUGGESTED READINGS

Brzezinski A, Rankin GB, Seidner DL, Lashner BA. Use of old and new oral 5-aminosalicylic acid formulations in inflammatory bowel disease. Cleve Clin J Med 1995;62:317–323.

D'Haens GR, Lashner BA, Hanauer SB. Pericholangitis and sclerosing cholangitis are risk factors for dysplasia and cancer in ulcerative colitis. Am J Gastroenterol 1993;88:1174–1178.

Ekbom A, Helmick C, Zack M, Adami HO. Increased risk of large bowel cancer in Crohn's disease with colonic involvement. Lancet 1990;336:357–359.

Ekbom A, Helmick CG, Zack M, Holmberg L, Adami HO. Survival and causes of death in patients with inflammatory bowel disease. A population-based study. Gastroenterology 1992;103:954–960.

Farmer RG, Easley KA, Rankin GB. Clinical patterns, natural history, and progression of ulcerative colitis: a long-term follow up of 1,116 patients. Dig Dis Sci 1993;38:1137–1146.

Farmer RG, Whelan G, Fazio VW: Long-term follow-up of patients with Crohn's disease: relationship between clinical pattern and prognosis. Gastroenterology 1985;88:1818–1825.

Feagan BG, Rochon J, Fedorak RN, et al. Methrotexate for the treatment of Crohn's disease. N Engl J Med 1995;332:292–297.

Fockens P, Tytgat GNJ. Role of endoscopy in follow-up of inflammatory bowel disease. Endoscopy 1992;24:582–584.

Gendre JP, May JY, Florent C, et al. Oral mesalamine (Pentasa) as maintenance treatment in Crohn's disease: a multicenter placebo-controlled study. Gastroenterology 1993;104:435–439.

Gillen CD, Walmsley RS, Prior P, Andrews HA, Allan RN. Ulcerative colitis and Crohn's disease: a comparison of the colorectal cancer risk in extensive colitis. Gut 1994;35:1590–1592.

Greenberg GR, Feagan BG, Martin F, et al. Oral budesonide for active Crohn's disease. N Engl J Med 1994;331:836–841.

Greenstein AJ, Lachman P, Sachar DB, et al. Perforating and non-perforating indications for repeated operations in Crohn's disease: evidence for two clinical forms. Gut 1988;29:588–592.

Gumaste V, Sachar DB, Greenstein AJ. Benign and malignant colorectal strictures in ulcerative colitis. Gut 1992;33:938–941.

Kirsner JB. Problems in the differentiation of ulcerative colitis and Crohn's disease of the colon: the need for repeated diagnostic evaluation. Gastroenterology 1975;68:187–191.

Lashner BA. Recommendations for colorectal cancer surveillance in ulcerative colitis: a review of research from a single university-based surveillance program. Am J Gastroenterol 1992;87:168–175.

Lashner BA. Risk factors for small bowel cancer in Crohn's disease. Dig Dis Sci 1992;37:1179–1184.

Lashner BA, Provencher KS, Seidner DL, Knesebeck D, Brzezinski A. The effect of folic acid supplementation on the risk for cancer or dysplasia in ulcerative colitis. Gastroenterology 1997;112:29–32.

Lashner BA, Shaheen NJ, Hanauer SB, Kirschner BS. Passive smoking is associated with an increased risk of developing inflammatory bowel disease in children. Am J Gastroenterol 1993;88:356–359.

Lashner BA, Turner BC, Bostwick DG, et al. Dysplasia and cancer complicating strictures in ulcerative colitis. Dig Dis Sci 1990;35:349–352.

Lock MR, Farmer RG, Fazio VW, Jagelman DG, Lavery IC, Weakley FL. Recurrence and reoperation for Crohn's disease: the role of disease location in prognosis. N Eng J Med 1981;304:1586–1588.

Malchow H, Ewe K, Brandes JW, et al. European Cooperative Crohn's Disease Study: results of drug treatment. Gastroenterology 1984;86:249–266.

Michener WM, Caulfield M, Wyllie R, Farmer RG. Management of inflammatory bowel disease: 30 years of observation. Cleve Clin J Med 1990;37:685–691.

Pennington L, Hamilton SR, Bayless TM, Cameron JL. Surgical management of Crohn's disease: influence of disease at margin of resection. Ann Surg 1980;192:311–318.

Persson PG, Ahlbom A. Hellers G. Inflammatory bowel disease and tobacco smoke: a case-control study. Gut 1990;31:1377–1381.

Petras RE, Mir-Madjlessi SH, Farmer RG. Crohn's disease and intestinal carcinoma: a report of 11 cases with emphasis on associated epithelial dysplasia. Gastroenterology 1987;93:1307–1314.

Prantera C, Pallone F, Brunetti G, et al. The Italian IBD Study Group. Oral 5-aminosalicylic acid (Asacol) in the maintenance treatment of Crohn's disease. Gastroenterology 1992;103:363–368.

Present DH, Korelitz BI, Wisch N, et al. Treatment of Crohn's disease with 6-mercaptopurine. A long-term, randomized, double-blind study. N Engl J Med 1980;302:981–987.

Reiser JR, Waye JD, Janowitz HD, Harpaz N. Adenocarcinoma in strictures of ulcerative colitis without antecedent dysplasia by colonoscopy. Am J Gastroenterol 1994;89:119–122.

Riddell RH, Goldman H, Ransofhoff DF, et al. Dysplasia in

inflammatory bowel disease: standardized classification with provisional clinical implications. Hum Pathol 1983;14:931–968.

Sachar DB, Andrews H, Farmer RG, et al. Proposed classification of patient subgroups in Crohn's disease. Working Team Report 4. Gastroenterol Int 1992;3:141–154.

Silverstein MD, Lashner BA, Hanauer SB, Evans AA, Kirsner JB. Cigarette smoking in Crohn's disease. Am J Gastroenterol 1989;84:31–33.

Steinhart AH, Hemphill DJ, Greenberg GR. Sulfasalazine and mesalazine for the maintenance therapy of Crohn's disease: a meta-analysis. Gastroenterology 1994;106:A778.

Sutherland LR, Ramcharan S, Bryant H, Fick G. Effect of cigarette smoking on recurrence of Crohn's disease. Gastroenterology 1990;98:1123–1128.

Truelove SC, Witts LJ. Cortisone in ulcerative colitis. Br Med J 1955;1:1041–1048.

Woolrich AJ, DaSilva MD, Korelitz BI. Surveillance in the routine management of ulcerative colitis: the predictive value of low-grade dysplasia. Gastroenterology 1992;103:431–438.

C·H·A·P·T·E·R

60

Diarrhea and Malabsorption

Edy E. Soffer

Diarrhea is best defined by increased stool weight, which essentially results from increased water content. For most individuals on a typical Western diet, diarrhea implies 24-hour stool output in excess of 250 g. A more practical definition is abnormal looseness of the stool, which usually is associated with increased stool weight and frequency of bowel movements.

Assimilation of food occurs in two phases: digestion, and absorption. Maldigestion occurs when there is a defect in the luminal phase of assimilation. Malabsorption occurs when there is a defect in the mucosal absorption of food elements.

The small intestine absorbs water, electrolytes, and nutrients. The latter require bile and pancreatic enzymes so that the products of digestion—monosaccharides, amino acids, small peptides, and fatty acids—can cross the cell membranes. The colon absorbs mostly water. Sites of intestinal absorption are:

Duodenum
  Iron
Jejunum
  Carbohydrates, iron, folate, calcium, proteins, lipids, vitamins, electrolytes ← water
Ileum
  Bile salts, vitamin B$_{12}$
Cecum
  Electrolytes ← water

Of the approximately 10 L of fluids that enter the duodenum daily, 2 L enter the colon, and only 100 mL are excreted in the stool. Colonic absorptive capacity is 5.5 to 6.0 L/day. Therefore, diarrhea may not be present even with moderate small-bowel disease, but it will be observed with even mild colonic dysfunction.

MECHANISM OF DIARRHEA

Water is absorbed passively in the gut, and this absorption depends on osmotic gradients. As such, diarrhea results from an excess of osmotically active substances in the stool, which in turn result from either decreased absorption of nutrients and electrolytes, excess secretion of electrolytes, or both. There are four mechanisms of diarrhea, with the two major ones being secretory and osmotic.

OSMOTIC DIARRHEA

Osmotic diarrhea results from an unabsorbable, or a poorly absorbable, solute that causes excessive water output. Poorly absorbable solute exerts an osmotic pressure effect across the intestinal mucosa. Because the diarrhea results from the solute, it tends to stop during fasting. In addition, there is a stool ''osmotic gap.'' Normally, most stool osmolality can be accounted for by adding sodium and potassium and then multiplying by two for the associated anions. If a nonabsorbable solute is in the fecal fluid, the concentration of electrolytes is lower. Therefore, adding sodium and potassium and then multiplying by two will result in a number that is lower than the total osmolality. Because of some technical problems associated with measuring total fecal osmolality, one can assume the total should be 290 mOsm, which is close to serum osmolality.

In a study of normal volunteers in whom diarrhea was induced using different agents, the osmotic gap in secretory diarrhea always was less than 50 mOsm. In all forms of osmotic diarrhea, however, the gap always was greater than 50 mOsm. A fecal fluid pH below 5.6 helps to distinguish diarrhea resulting from malabsorption of a sugar, such as lactulose.

638

Causes of osmotic diarrhea are:

- Disaccharidase deficiency
- Malabsorption
- Poorly absorbed sugars:
  - Lactulose
  - Sorbitol
  - Mannitol
- Laxatives
  - Magnesium
  - Sodium citrate
  - Sodium phosphate
- Antacids
  - Magnesium

SECRETORY DIARRHEA

In secretory diarrhea, there is abnormal ion transport across the intestinal epithelial cells, which results from the active secretion of ions. In these patients, there is no osmotic gap, and because the diarrhea does not relate to the intestinal content, it typically will not cease with fasting.

The most striking example of secretory diarrhea is that associated with a bacterial toxin, such as that of cholera. Causes of secretory diarrhea are

- Infections (cholera)
- Celiac sprue
- Collagenous colitis
- Stimulant laxatives
  - Phenolphthalein
  - Senna
  - Docusate sodium
- VIP producing tumors
- Carcinoid tumor
- Hyperthyroidism

DIARRHEA CAUSED BY ALTERED MOTILITY

Motility disturbances of the gastrointestinal tract can result in decreased absorption, and any anatomic disruption, such as gastrectomy or vagotomy, can produce diarrhea. Proving altered motility as the sole cause of diarrhea, however, is very difficult. Dysmotility-induced diarrhea often is a diagnosis of exclusion. One consequence of reduced intestinal motility may be bacterial overgrowth, which aggravates the diarrhea and causes malabsorption of fat.

Causes of diarrhea resulting from altered motility are:

- Irritable bowel syndrome (possibly)
- Postsurgical
  - Vagotomy
  - Cholecystectomy
  - Gastrectomy
- Hyperthyroidism

EXUDATIVE DIARRHEA

Extensive injury of the small bowel or colonic mucosa may result in loss of fluid and protein into the intestinal lumen and ensuing diarrhea. Exudation rarely is the only mechanism accounting for the diarrhea, however. Causes of exudative diarrhea also include inflammatory bowel disease and invasive bacterial infections (e.g., *Shigella* sp., *Salmonella* sp., and so on).

More than one mechanism may exist. For example, in infectious and inflammatory conditions, both malabsorption, leading to osmotic diarrhea, and active secretion can coexist.

MALABSORPTION

MECHANISMS

Malabsorption can result from abnormal digestion or absorption. Digestion involves the breakdown of nutrients into smaller molecules, which then can be absorbed by transport across the intestinal epithelium. The digestive process starts in the stomach with acid and pepsin, and it continues in the upper small bowel with bile and pancreatic enzymes such as lipase, amylase, and trypsin. As a result, fats are broken down into fatty acids and monoglycerides, proteins into amino acids and peptides, and carbohydrates into monosaccharides and disaccharides. Further breakdown of these nutrients occurs at the brush border of the intestinal mucosal cells by disaccharidases and oligopeptidases, with final absorption across the large surface area of the small intestine.

Of all the nutrients ingested, lipids require the most complex digestive process before they are absorbed. Lipolysis starts in the stomach and is completed in the jejunum by pancreatic lipase, thus resulting in formation of free fatty acids and glycerol. Bile salts manufactured in the liver are necessary to facilitate absorption through micellar formation. The bile salts then are reabsorbed themselves in the terminal ileum to be used over and over again (i.e., enterohepatic circulation). Therefore, fat malabsorption can occur because of gastrectomy, pancreatic insufficiency, advanced liver disease or biliary obstruction, and absent or markedly diseased ileum. In addition, the action of bile salts can be impaired by deconjugation, which occurs with bacterial overgrowth.

Causes of malabsorption are:

- Mucosal defect
  - Disaccharidase deficiency
  - Sprue
  - Whipple's disease
  - Crohn's disease
  - Abetalipoproteinemia
- Infection
  - Giardiasis
  - Tropical sprue
- Lymphatic obstruction
  - Intestinal lymphangiectasia

- • Lymphoma
- • Multiple mechanisms
  - • Gastrectomy
  - • Crohn's disease
  - • Ileal resection
- • Drugs
  - • Neomycin
  - • Laxatives
  - • Cholestyramine
- • Miscellaneous
  - • Defect in intraluminal phase
  - • Pancreatic insufficiency
  - • Bile-salt deficiency
  - • Bacterial overgrowth

CLINICAL PRESENTATION

Symptoms of malabsorption are multiple. Diarrhea almost universally is present, and stools often are described as bulky and sticky. Floating stools do not necessarily indicate malabsorption.

Unless there is an inflammatory etiology (i.e., inflammatory bowel disease) or pancreatic disease, abdominal pain is mild. Weight loss can be either mild or advanced, depending on severity of the malabsorption.

Malabsorption may lead to multiple manifestations from various nutritional deficiencies. These include anemia because of iron, vitamin B_{12}, or folic acid deficiency; hypocalcemia; and tendency to bleed because of vitamin K deficiency.

The patient history can provide important clues. A surgical history should be taken, with particular attention paid to the exact site and extent of any resected organ. Alcohol abuse or previous attacks of abdominal pain may lead to the diagnosis of chronic pancreatitis. A drug history should be taken as well, along with a history of travel and sexual practices.

DIAGNOSIS OF DIARRHEA AND MALABSORPTION

PATIENT HISTORY

An appropriate diagnostic workup for diarrhea starts with a thorough interview. The first step is to establish that diarrhea actually is present. Patients are unable to report the exact amount and weight of stool passed over a period of time, but through proper questioning, one at least can establish if the diarrhea is of the "small volume" or "large volume" type. In small-volume diarrhea, the patient has frequent, urgent defecation of small amounts of stool. In large-volume diarrhea, large amounts of frequent stools are passed. Small-volume diarrhea usually is associated with diseases of the left colon and rectum, and indicates an irritability of the rectosigmoid, which leads to frequent passage of small amounts of stools. Large-volume diarrhea more likely is associated with diseases of the small bowel or right colon.

Before proceeding to the next step in the workup, it is important to detect the occasional patient who does not actually have diarrhea but is consulting because of fecal incontinence. This information may not be submitted voluntarily. Often, it must be identified by careful questioning of the patient.

There are many ways to classify diarrhea on a clinical basis. A good start, however, is to establish if the diarrhea is acute or chronic. Acute diarrhea is defined as that having a duration of less than 1 month. Chronic diarrhea is defined as that having a duration of more than 1 month. Most frequently, acute diarrhea results from infection.

The patient history also should identify other symptoms accompanying the diarrhea. In chronic diarrhea, abdominal pain may indicate pancreatic disease. Blood in the stool indicates an inflammatory or infectious cause, but mucus in the stool rarely indicates a serious disorder. Frothy, mushy stools may indicate malabsorption; however, these descriptions usually are not reliable. Nocturnal diarrhea is suggestive of an organic cause, though it is not incompatible with irritable bowel syndrome. Other important factors to inquire about include fever, weight loss, travel history, sexual habits, relation of diarrhea to diet (particularly milk), and any medications being used.

TESTS FOR CHRONIC DIARRHEA

Blood Tests

A complete blood count and set of routine biochemistry tests can be helpful. Anemia, hypocalcemia, hypokalemia, and a low serum albumin level are good indicators of partial or total malabsorption.

Hydrogen Breath Test

A lactose hydrogen breath test is a simple way to detect carbohydrate malabsorption. Fifty grams of lactose solution are given, and hydrogen is measured in the breath at intervals of up to 2 hours. A rise of more than 20 parts per million over the basal level is suggestive of lactose malabsorption. This test is based on the fact that malabsorbed lactose is fermented by colonic bacteria, and that hydrogen diffuses through the mucosa and is exhaled in the breath. In clinical practice, abstention from milk and dairy products that leads to symptomatic improvement may be sufficient to make the diagnosis of lactase deficiency.

D-Xylose Test

D-Xylose is a pentose that is easily absorbed by the intestinal mucosa. Because its absorption requires little intraluminal action, the D-xylose test is meant to be specific for a mucosal absorptive defect. A dose of 25 mg of D-xylose is given by mouth, and 4 to 5 mg should be collected in the urine over the following 5 hours. If there is malabsorption, the urine content will be lower. Unfortunately, this test is affected by poor fluid intake, renal dysfunction, ascites, patient age, diabetes, and certain drugs, such as NSAIDs. Because of these problems, the test is not used as widely today as it has been in the past.

Glucose Hydrogen Breath Test

The glucose hydrogen breath test is similar to the lactose breath test, except that glucose is substituted for lactose. In patients with malabsorption, a high amount of hydrogen is found in the breath. An abnormal test usually is considered to be a sign of bacterial overgrowth, with high amounts of H_2 resulting from the action of bacteria on glucose. Rapid transit without bacterial overgrowth, however, may cause glucose malabsorption and produce an abnormal test.

Tests of Pancreatic Function

Collection of pancreatic secretions after stimulation with secretin is a good indicator of pancreatic function. This test demands close attention, however, and it may be affected by technical factors. The bentiromide test is a tubeless test that involves ingestion of *p*-aminobenzoic acid. The compound is broken down by pancreatic enzymes, and the byproduct is excreted in the urine. Measurement of the urine byproducts gives an indication of pancreatic function.

Various imaging methods of the pancreas are used to establish a pancreatic abnormality. Depending on the pathology that is suspected, ultrasonography, computed tomography, or endoscopic retrograde cholangiopancreatography may be indicated.

Schilling Test

Malabsorption of vitamin B_{12} can result from intrinsic factor deficiency (i.e., pernicious anemia). Malabsorption of vitamin B_{12} also can result from pancreatic insufficiency impairing the transfer of vitamin B_{12} from R-protein to intrinsic factor, bacterial overgrowth causing binding of vitamin B_{12} by bacteria in the small bowel, and lack of ileal receptors for absorption of vitamin B_{12}–intrinsic factor complex, such as occurs following ileal resection or in advanced ileal disease.

The Schilling test, as traditionally performed, distinguishes cobalamin deficiency from malabsorption. If the first phase of the test is abnormal, there is vitamin B_{12} malabsorption. If the addition of intrinsic factor corrects the test result, malabsorption is secondary to intrinsic factor deficiency. The test may be repeated after administration of tetracycline (i.e., third phase), and if the result is corrected, this is a sign of bacterial overgrowth. The Schilling test is quite cumbersome for detection of bacterial overgrowth, however. A more simple approach is to treat the patient empirically with antibiotics for a short period of time and see if the diarrhea decreases significantly.

Qualitative Stool Fat Test

The qualitative stool fat test is quick, cheap, simple, and infrequently used. In this test, a small amount of stool is examined under the microscope after staining with Sudan III. Fat droplets indicate an increased amount of triglycerides in the stool and a defect in the intraluminal phase of lipid absorption (i.e., pancreatic insufficiency). After heating and acidification, fatty acids take up the Sudan III stain, thus indicating preserved breakdown of triglycerides but poor absorption of fatty acids (i.e., mucosal disease).

In many studies, the qualitative stool fat test has been both reproducible and a reliable indicator of malabsorption. It needs special attention by an interested technician, however, and most laboratories do not perform the test often enough to provide this.

Quantitative Fecal Fat Test

In the quantitative fecal fat test, stools are collected for 2 days while the patient is on a 100 g–fat diet for the 2 days preceding the test as well as during the period of the test itself. Medications that interfere with absorption or motility should be discontinued. The test can be accomplished very well on an outpatient basis.

Normal fecal fat excretion is 7 g or less over 24 hours. Mild steatorrhea occurs in patients with conditions such as gastrectomy and bacterial overgrowth. More severe steatorrhea occurs in patients with sprue and pancreatic insufficiency. Overall, the highest values often are seen in patients with pancreatic insufficiency; however, there is considerable overlap in the magnitude of the steatorrhea as produced by different conditions.

The 72-hour stool collection is the best test to establish the presence of steatorrhea with certainty. It also is a good way to determine if the patient is suffering from diarrhea or simply the frequent passage of small stools. The total weight of the stool should be provided by the laboratory.

Structural Studies

Small-bowel radiography or an endoscopic examination when indicated can provide useful clues for the diagnosis. In the past, small-bowel biopsy specimens were obtained by using different capsules. The test was tedious, uncomfortable, and sometimes, unsuccessful. It is almost universally accepted today, however, that adequate specimens can be obtained by endoscopic means. The findings at small-bowel biopsy rarely are specific, but the procedure is invaluable in the diagnosis of sprue and Whipple's disease.

DIAGNOSTIC APPROACH TO ACUTE DIARRHEA

Acute diarrhea typically results from infection. A patient history should be obtained regarding recent travel, food and water ingestion, antibiotic use, and sexual habits. Fever, leukocyto-

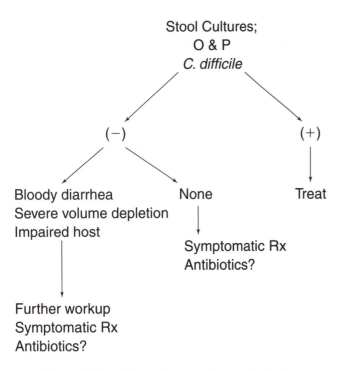

Figure 60.1.   Diagnostic approach to acute diarrhea.

sis, and blood in the stool are suggestive of invasive organisms such as *Salmonella* sp., *Shigella* sp., *Yersinia* sp., *Entamoeba histolytica,* and hemorrhagic *Escherichia coli.* Organisms that cause little or no inflammation include viruses, *Giardia lamblia,* and toxin-producing bacteria such as *E. coli* and *Staphylococcus aureus;* diarrhea caused by this group of agents usually is milder and of shorter duration than that caused by invasive organisms. Acute diarrhea that begins during hospitalization usually is iatrogenic, and infection with *Clostridium difficile* is a common cause. Figure 60.1 outlines the diagnostic approach to acute diarrhea.

DIAGNOSTIC APPROACH TO CHRONIC DIARRHEA

Chronic diarrhea is defined as that which lasts for more than 1 month. Major causes include malabsorption (particularly lactose intolerance), inflammatory bowel disease, microscopic/collagenous colitis, and irritable bowel syndrome. With the exception of *Giardia lamblia,* infections are rare.

Findings at the initial evaluation can help to determine the cause as either malabsorption (i.e., weight loss, anemia, biochemical deficiencies), inflammatory bowel disease (i.e., evidence of inflammation such as fever, leukocytosis, elevated sedimentation rate, bloody diarrhea) or irritable bowel syndrome (i.e., none of the listed abnormalities). In patients with documented diarrhea and a negative diagnostic investigation, an attempt should be made to exclude factitious drug ingestion. If all tests are negative, bile salt–binding drugs or opiates can be tried. In most patients with chronic idiopathic diarrhea,

the disorder is self-limited and resolves within 6 to 24 months. Figure 60.2 outlines the diagnostic approach to chronic diarrhea.

TREATMENT

MALABSORPTION

Treatment of malabsorption depends on the specific cause. Examples of treatment include antibiotics for bacterial overgrowth, a gluten-free diet for celiac sprue, and a low-fat diet for bile-salt deficiency. Care should be taken to address more than one factor, however, because there often are multiple mechanisms operating in these disorders. Vitamin and mineral supplementation may be required regardless of the cause.

CELIAC SPRUE

Celiac sprue is a malabsorptive disorder. It results from injury to the small bowel caused by gluten and similar proteins in certain foods (e.g., wheat, barley, oats, rye). There is a high prevalence among first-degree relatives, and manifestations vary from asymptomatic iron-deficiency anemia to severe malabsorption. Conditions that may be associated with sprue include insulin-dependent diabetes mellitus, microscopic/collagenous colitis, dermatitis herpetiformis, thyroid disease, and selective immunoglobulin A deficiency. Small-bowel biopsy is diagnostic, but antigliadin and antiendomysial antibody tests have a high sensitivity and specificity and are helpful in screening. Celiac sprue is associated with an increased risk of malignancy, specifically that of gastrointestinal origin; therefore, a gluten-free diet is recommended in asymptomatic individuals.

MICROSCOPIC/COLLAGENOUS COLITIS

Microscopic/collagenous colitis is a spectrum of disease that is characterized by diarrhea and mucosal histologic abnormalities but normal endoscopic and radiographic features. The mean age at presentation is in the sixth decade of life, with a predominance of female patients. Microscopic/collagenous colitis can be associated with autoimmune disorders and celiac sprue. Typically, there are no biochemical deficiencies, and random biopsies of the colon are required for diagnosis.

DIARRHEA IN ACQUIRED IMMUNODEFICIENCY SYNDROME

As many as two-thirds of patients with acquired immunodeficiency syndrome (AIDS) develop diarrhea during the course of their disease, and there is an increasing array of infectious and noninfectious causes of diarrhea in this population. These include pathogens found in immunocompetent hosts, those related to sexually transmitted organisms, organisms associ-

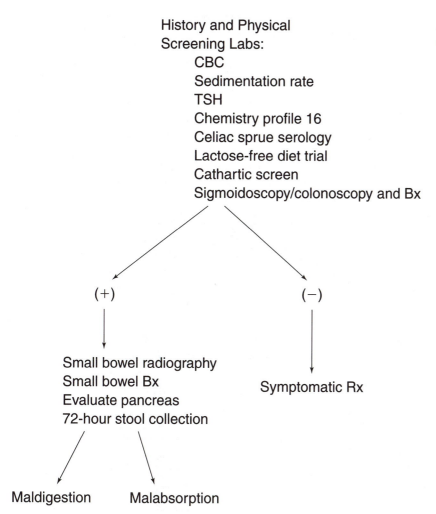

History and Physical
Screening Labs:
    CBC
    Sedimentation rate
    TSH
    Chemistry profile 16
    Celiac sprue serology
    Lactose-free diet trial
    Cathartic screen
    Sigmoidoscopy/colonoscopy and Bx

(+)   (−)

Small bowel radiography
Small bowel Bx
Evaluate pancreas
72-hour stool collection

Symptomatic Rx

Maldigestion   Malabsorption

Figure 60.2. Diagnostic approach to chronic diarrhea.

ated with an immuncompromised host, and noninfectious causes. Stool analysis is the most productive investigation, followed by flexible sigmoidoscopy. Upper endoscopy may be performed if the workup to identify small-bowel pathogens is negative.

Causes of diarrhea in patients with AIDS are:

- Infections
  - Organisms affecting immunocompetent hosts
    - *Salmonella* sp.
    - Shigella sp.
    - *C. difficile*
    - *G. lamblia*
    - *Entamoeba histolytica*
  - Sexually transmitted pathogens
    - *Neisseria gonorrhoeae*
    - Chlamydia
    - *Treponema pallidum*
  - Organisms affecting the immunocompromised host
    - *Mycobacterium avium intracellulare*
    - Cytomegalovirus
    - *Cryptosporidium* sp.
    - Microsporidia
- Malignancy
  - Kaposi's sarcoma
  - Non-Hodgkin's lymphoma
- ''AIDS enteropathy''

REVIEW EXERCISES

QUESTIONS

1. A 68-year-old woman complains of diarrhea and occasional fecal incontinence but otherwise is healthy. Her appetite is good, and her weight is stable. What helps you to decide if her diarrhea is significant?
   a. Passage of liquid stools.
   b. Frequent passage of stools.
   c. Large bowel movements.
   d. A 24-hour stool weight of more than 250 grams.
   e. A 24-hour stool weight of more than 125 grams.

2. Secretory diarrhea may be distinguished from osmotic diarrhea because:
   a. Secretory diarrhea decreases or disappears with fasting.
   b. There usually is no osmotic gap in secretory diarrhea.
   c. Osmotic diarrhea often is accompanied by bleeding.
   d. Larger volumes of stool are produced in secretory diarrhea.

3. A 52-year-old man presents with a 2-year history of diarrhea and weight loss. There is no bleeding. He admits to heavy alcohol intake in the past but has been ''dry'' for several years. His diabetes is well-controlled with insulin, and he underwent cholecystectomy 6 years ago. Results of laboratory tests are normal except for mild anemia, and radiographs of the small bowel and colon are reported as normal. The next test should be:
   a. Endoscopic retrograde cholangiopancreatography.
   b. Small-bowel biopsy.
   c. A 72-hour stool collection for volume and fat.
   d. Glucose hydrogen breath test.
   e. Colonoscopy with biopsy.

4. A 59-year-old black woman presents with a 6-year history of diarrhea and occasional abdominal pain. Results of laboratory and stool tests are normal. For this patient, you would proceed with:
   a. Upper gastrointestinal endoscopy and biopsy.
   b. Treatment with anticholinergics.
   c. Colonoscopy and random biopsies.
   d. Hydrogen breath test for lactose intolerance.

5. A 55-year-old woman with diarrhea is found to have lymphocytic colitis. She has iron-deficiency anemia and diarrhea that is hard to control. For this patient, you would proceed with:
   a. Iron supplementation.
   b. Antigliadin antibody.
   c. Small-bowel radiography.
   d. A 72-hour stool collection for fat.
   e. Small-bowel biopsy.

Answers

1. d
2. b
3. c
4. d
5. e

SUGGESTED READING

Achkar E, Carey WD, Petras R, et al. Comparison of suction capsule and endoscopic biopsy of small bowel mucosa. Gastrointest Endosc 1986;32:278–281.

Afzalpurkar RG, Schiller LR, Little KH, et al. The self-limited nature of chronic idiopathic diarrhea. N Engl J Med 1992; 327:1849–1852.

Bai JC, Andrush A, Matelo G, et al. Fecal fat concentration in the differential diagnosis of steatorrhea. Am J Gastroenterol 1989;84:27–30.

Bertomeu A, Ros E, Barragágan V, et al. Chronic diarrhea with normal stool and colonic examinations: organic or functional? J Clin Gastroenterol 1991;13:531–536.

Corazza GR, Menozzi MG, Strocchi A, et al. The diagnosis of small bowel bacterial overgrowth. Reliability of jejunal culture and inadequacy of breath hydrogen testing. Gastroenterology 1990;98:302–309.

Craig RM, Atkinson AJ. D-Xylose testing: a review. Gastroenterology 1988;95:223–231.

Cummings JH, Sladen GE, James OFW, et al. Laxative-induced diarrhoea: a continuing clinical problem. Br Med J 1974;1:537–541.

Dandalides SM, Carey WD, Petras R, et al. Endoscopic small bowel mucosal biopsy: a controlled trial evaluating forceps size and biopsy location in the diagnosis of normal and abnormal mucosal architecture. Gastrointest Endosc 1989;35: 197–200.

Danielsson Å, Nyhlin H, Persson H, et al. Chronic diarrhoea after radiotherapy for gynaecological cancer: occurrence and aetiology. Gut 1991;32:1180–1187.

DiMagno EP, Go VLW, Summerskill WHJ. Relations between pancreatic enzyme outputs and malabsorption in severe pancreatic insufficiency. N Engl J Med 1973;288:813–815.

Drummey GD, Benson JA, Jones CM. Microscopical examination of stool for steatorrhoea. N Engl J Med 1961;264: 85–87.

Eherer AJ, Fortran JS. Fecal osmotic gap and pH in experimental diarrhea of various causes. Gastroenterology 1992; 103:545–551.

Fordtran JS, Santa Ana CA, Morawski SG, et al. Pathophysiology of chronic diarrhoea: insights derived from intestinal perfusion studies in 3l patients. Clin Gastroenterol 1986;15: 477–490.

French JM, Gaddie R, Smith N. Diarrhoea due to phenolphthalein. Lancet 1956;i:55l.

Goggins M, Kelleher D. Celiac disease and other nutrient related injuries to the gastrointestinal tract. Am J Gastroenterol 1994;89:S2–S17.

Grohmann GS, Glass RI, Pereira HG, et al. Enteric viruses and diarrhea in HIV-infected patients. N Engl J Med 1993; 329:14–20.

Haeney MR, Culank LS, Montgomery RD, et al. Evaluation of xylose as measured in blood and urine. A one-hour blood xylose screening test for malabsorption. Gastroenterology 1978;75:393–400.

Hofman AF. Bile acid malabsorption caused by ileal resection. Arch Intern Med 1972;130:597–605.

Jesserun J, Yardley JH, Lee EL, et al. Microscopic and collagenous colitis: different names for the same condition? Gastroenterology 1986;9l:1583–1584.

Khouri MR, Huang G, Shiau YF. Sudan stain of fecal fat: new insights into an old test. Gastroenterology 1989;96:421–427.

King CE, Toskes PP. Intestinal bacterial overgrowth. Gastroenterology 1979;76:1035–1055.

Kotler DP, Orenstein JM. Chronic diarrhea and malabsorption associated with enteropathogenic bacterial infection in a patient with AIDS. Ann Intern Med 1993;119:127–128.

Manabe YC, Vinetz JM, Moore RD, et al. *Clostridium difficile* colitis: an efficient clinical approach to diagnosis. Ann Intern Med 1995;123:835–840.

McGill DB, Miller LJ, Carney JA, et al. Hormonal diarrhea due to pancreatic tumor. Gastroenterology 1980;79:571–582.

Newcomer AD, McGill DB, Thomas PJ, et al. Prospective comparison of indirect methods for detecting lactase deficiency. N Engl J Med 1975;293:1232–1236.

Phillips S, Donaldson L, Geisler K, et al. Stool composition in factitial diarrhea: a 6-year experience with stool analysis. Ann Intern Med 1995;123:97–100.

Saslow SB, Camilleri M. Diabetic diarrhea. Semin Gastrointest Dis 1995;6:187–193.

Sellin JH, Hart R. Glucose malabsorption associated with rapid intestinal transit. Am J Gastroenterol 1992;87:585–589.

Simon D, Brandt LJ. Diarrhea in patients with the aqcuired immunodeficiency syndrome. Gastroenterol 1993;105: 1236–1242.

Smith P, et al. Intestinal infections in AIDS. Ann Intern Med 1988;108:328–333.

Valdimarsson T, Lennart F, Grodzinsky E, et al. Is small bowel biopsy necessary in adults with suspected celiac disease and IgA anti-endomysium antibodies? Dig Dis Sci 1996;41: 83–87.

Vogelsang H, Genser D, Wyatt J, et al. Screening for celiac disease: a prospective study on the value of noninvasive tests. Am J Gastroenterol 1995;90:394–398.

Wilcox CM, Schwartz DA, Cotsonis G, Thompson SE. Chronic unexplained diarrhea in human immunodeficiency virus infection: determination of the best diagnostic approach. Gastroenterology 1996;110:30–37.

C•H•A•P•T•E•R

61

Board Simulation: Gastroenterology

John J. Vargo

QUESTIONS

1. A 64-year-old woman with significant dysphagia to solids and liquids should undergo which diagnostic test?

   a. Esophageal manometry.
   b. Barium swallow.
   c. 24-Hour pH probe.
   d. Upper endoscopy.
   e. Bernstein test.

2. A 36-year-old man with a history of intermittent retrosternal chest pain and a previous evaluation with a normal cardiac stress test and normal endoscopy should receive which diagnostic test?

   a. Esophageal manometry.
   b. Barium swallow.
   c. 24-Hour pH probe.
   d. Upper endoscopy.
   e. Bernstein test.

3. An 86-year-old man recently suffered a stroke and now is noted to cough or choke when eating. A chest radiograph reveals a right middle lobe infiltrate. Which diagnostic test should he receive?

   a. Esophageal manometry.
   b. Barium swallow.
   c. 24-Hour pH probe.
   d. Upper endoscopy.
   e. Bernstein test.

4. A 52-year-old woman is positive for human immunodeficiency virus (HIV) and presents with severe odynophagia refractory to oral fluconazole for presumed esophageal candidiasis. The patient's CD4 count is less than 50 μL. Which diagnostic test should she receive?

   a. Esophageal manometry.
   b. Barium swallow.
   c. 24-hour pH probe.
   d. Upper endoscopy.
   e. Bernstein test.

5. A 74-year-old woman with chronic renal insufficiency and aortic valvular disease presents with guaiac-positive stool on numerous occasions and an iron deficiency anemia that requires transfusion. Which diagnosis is appropriate?

   a. Mallory-Weiss tear.
   b. Dieulafoy's lesion.
   c. Cecal arteriovenous malformations.
   d. Esophageal varices.
   e. Diverticular bleeding.

6. A 34-year-old man who uses nonsteroidal anti-inflammatory agents presents with a third episode of hematemesis. Results of two previous upper endoscopies have been normal. Which diagnosis is appropriate?

   a. Mallory-Weiss tear.
   b. Dieulafoy's lesion.
   c. Cecal arteriovenous malformations.
   d. Esophageal varices.
   e. Diverticular bleeding.

7. A 45-year-old woman is noted to have hematemesis

after a protracted bout of nausea and vomiting. Which diagnosis is appropriate?

a. Mallory-Weiss tear.
b. Dieulafoy's lesion.
c. Cecal arteriovenous malformations.
d. Esophageal varices.
e. Diverticular bleeding.

8. A 74-year-old man with a significant history of ethanol abuse presents with painless hematochezia. A nasogastric tube aspirate is unremarkable. Which diagnosis is appropriate?

a. Mallory-Weiss tear.
b. Dieulafoy's lesion.
c. Cecal arteriovenous malformations.
d. Esophageal varices.
e. Diverticular bleeding.

9. A 34-year-old man with known, chronic hepatitis B and a history of intravenous drug abuse presents with lethargy, jaundice, and new-onset ascites. Which diagnosis is most likely?

a. Hepatitis A.
b. Hepatitis B.
c. Hepatitis C.
d. Hepatitis D.
e. Cytomegalovirus.

10. A 23-year-old woman presents with fatigue, lethargy, and jaundice. The physical examination reveals mild, tender hepatomegaly. The patient also spent her spring break volunteering in the flooded Ohio Valley region with the Red Cross. Which diagnosis is most likely?

a. Hepatitis A.
b. Hepatitis B.
c. Hepatitis C.
d. Hepatitis D.
e. Cytomegalovirus.

11. A 45-year-old woman who recently underwent orthotopic liver transplantation for primary biliary cirrhosis presents with lethargy and fatigue. Her medications include cyclosporine, prednisone, and azathioprine. Which diagnosis is most likely?

a. Hepatitis A.
b. Hepatitis B.
c. Hepatitis C.
d. Hepatitis D.
e. Cytomegalovirus.

12. A 56-year-old health care worker presents with a history of fluctuating, asymptomatic elevation in transaminase levels. Which diagnosis is most likely?

a. Hepatitis A.
b. Hepatitis B.

c. Hepatitis C.
d. Hepatitis D.
e. Cytomegalovirus.

13. A 24-year-old man is evaluated in the emergency room for midepigastric pain, nausea, and melena. The patient is a nonsmoker who occasionally uses ibuprofen for headaches. There is no history of hepatitis or ethanol use.

The physical examination reveals a blood pressure of 126/68 mm Hg, a pulse of 76 bpm, and no evidence of orthostasis. There are no cutaneous stigmata of chronic liver disease. There is mild, midepigastric tenderness without hepatosplenomegaly. Laboratory analyses reveals a hematocrit of 38%, platelet count of 225,000 μL, and a normal prothrombin time. Upper endoscopy reveals a clean-based, bulbar duodenal ulcer.

Which of the following actions is most appropriate?

a. Admit for observation and administer an intravenous H_2 blocker.
b. Discharge, then treat for 8 weeks with an H_2 blocker.
c. Admit for observation, transfuse to a hematocrit of 40%, and obtain *Helicobacter pylori* serology.
d. Discharge, then treat with an 8-week course of an H_2 blocker and repeat endoscopy in 8 weeks for biopsies and to document healing.
e. Discharge, treat with an 8-week course of an H_2 blocker, and obtain *H. pylori* serologies.

14. A 34-year-old woman is evaluated for a 9-month history of fatigue and a 1-week history of dark urine. The physical examination is notable for jaundice, spider angiomata on the chest, a liver edge palpated 5 cm below the right costal margin, and a spleen palpable 4 cm below the left costal margin. Results of the laboratory tests are:

Complete blood count	Normal
Alanine aminotransferase	550 U/L
Aspartate aminotransferase	680 U/L
Serum bilirubin	16.8 mg/dL
Direct bilirubin	9.6 mg/dL
Alkaline phosphatase	135 U/L
Serum albumin	2.5 g/dL
Serum globulin	9.0 g/dL

The best way to confirm the diagnosis is with:

a. Ultrasonography with a portal-vein Doppler study.
b. Endoscopic retrograde cholangiopancreatography.
c. HIDA scintigraphy.
d. Percutaneous liver biopsy.
e. Serum ceruloplasmin and slit-lamp examination.

15. Continuing with the patient from question 14, the appropriate treatment of the most likely diagnosis is:

a. Interferon-α, 3 million U subcutaneously three times a week.
b. Ursodeoxycholic acid, 300 mg three times a day.
c. Methotrexate, 15 mg/wk.
d. D-penicillamine, 750 mg/day.
e. Prednisone, 30 mg/day.

16. A 42-year-old man with a history of Crohn's disease presents with an 18-hour history of severe abdominal pain, which began in the right flank but now is noted in the right lower quadrant and groin. Current medications include prednisone, 20 mg/day, and sulfasalazine, 1 gm three times a day. The physical examination is notable for a patient who is clearly uncomfortable and writhing on the examination table. The resting pulse is 110 bpm, without orthostatic changes or fever. There are hypoactive bowel sounds with right costovertebral angle tenderness and mild, right lower quadrant tenderness. There is no rebound tenderness. An acute abdominal series shows a nonspecific, small-bowel gas pattern and no evidence of free air. Results of the laboratory studies are:

Hematocrit	46%
Leukocyte count	14,600/uL, with 60% polymorphonuclear leukocytes
Serum amylase	105 U/L
Serum lipase	65 U/L
Alanine aminotransferase	25 U/L
Aspartate aminotransferase	30 U/L
Urinalysis	Red blood cells: many/hpf White blood cells: 3–5/hpf Amorphous protein and mucus noted

The best test to confirm the diagnosis is with:

a. HIDA scan.
b. Intravenous urography.
c. Computed axial tomography.
d. Laparoscopic appendectomy.
e. Gastrografin enema.

17. Continuing with the patient from question 16, the cause of the most likely diagnosis is:

a. Enteric hyperoxaluria.
b. Decreased enterohepatic circulation of bile salts.
c. Inflammatory occlusion of the appendiceal orifice.
d. Interval development of an enterovesical fistula.
e. "Silent perforation" of the terminal ileum, which is masked because of steroid therapy.

18. A 32-year-old man presents with a 2-month history of abdominal distention and jaundice. The patient had immigrated from the Far East to the Unites States at the age of 7 years. There is no history of intravenous drug use, transfusions, or ethanol use.

The physical examination is notable for spider angiomata, jaundice, a liver edge palpable 3 cm below the right costal margin, and a spleen tip palpable 4 cm below the left costal margin. There is a fluid wave and shifting dullness. Serologic studies show:

Hepatitis B surface antigen	Positive
Hepatitis B core antibody	Positive
Hepatitis B e antigen	Positive
Antibody to surface antigen	Negative
Antibody to e antigen	Negative

Which statement best describes the patient's current serologic status?

a. He was previously infected with hepatitis B virus, has recovered, and is immune to hepatitis B.
b. He is a chronic carrier of hepatitis B virus and minimally infectious.
c. He is a chronic carrier of hepatitis B virus and highly infectious.
d. He is in the incubation period, is minimally infectious, and is likely to develop acute hepatitis B.
e. He is in the incubation period, is highly infectious, and is likely to develop acute hepatitis B.

19. Continuing with the patient from question 18, the patient undergoes a diagnostic paracentesis, which reveals the following:

Leukocyte count	190/uL, with 90% lymphocytes
Albumin	2.3 g/dL
Amylase	0 U/L
Serum albumin	2.6 g/dL

Which of the following statements concerning the most likely cause for the patient's ascites are false?

a. Ultrasonography of the liver reveals a hyperechoic mass in the right lobe, with an otherwise shrunken, irregular liver.
b. The serum alpha-fetoprotein level is elevated.
c. The ascites will rapidly respond to dietary sodium restriction and spironolactone, 200 mg/day.
d. Surgical treatment such as limited resection or orthotopic liver transplantation can be considered.
e. Vertical transmission of the hepatitis B virus at birth is the most likely route of infection.

20. Squamous cell cancer is three to four times more common in women than in men. True or false?

21. *H. pylori*–associated dysplastic changes in the squamous mucosa are a precursor lesion. True or false?

22. Combined radiation therapy and chemotherapy results in a higher survival rate than that with radiotherapy alone. True or false?

23. Development of Barrett's esophagus increases the risk of squamous cell cancer. True or false?

24. Endoscopic ultrasonography is more sensitive than computed tomography (CT) in detecting local spread through the esophageal wall and into adjacent structures. True or false?

Questions 25–28
For questions 25 to 28, state whether the condition is associated with development of chronic pancreatitis (true or false).

25. Coxsackie B virus. True or false?

26. Gallstones. True or false?

27. Trauma. True or false?

28. Type IV hyperlipidemia. True or false?

29. A 36-year-old man with a history of Crohn's ileitis was recently treated for a psoas abscess with CT-guided drainage and broad-spectrum antibiotics. He now presents with worsening diarrhea despite increasing the oral prednisone dose. Flexible sigmoidoscopy reveals foci of adherent, yellowish-white plaques in the rectum and sigmoid colon. What is the therapy for this patient's diarrhea?

    a. Tetracycline, 250 mg orally three times a day.
    b. Cholestyramine.
    c. Low-fat diet.
    d. Fiber supplementation.
    e. Metronidazole, 250 mg three times a day for 14 days.

30. A 20-year-old man has diarrhea after resection of a 30-cm segment of strictured terminal ileum. What is the therapy for this patient's diarrhea?

    a. Tetracycline, 250 mg orally three times a day.
    b. Cholestyramine.
    c. Low-fat diet.
    d. Fiber supplementation.
    e. Metronidazole, 250 mg three times a day for 14 days.

31. A 65-year-old woman who underwent a Bilroth II anastomosis for peptic ulcer disease has experienced chronic diarrhea. The glucose breath test is positive. What is the therapy for this patient's diarrhea?

    a. Tetracycline, 250 mg orally three times a day.
    b. Cholestyramine.
    c. Low-fat diet.
    d. Fiber supplementation.
    e. Metronidazole, 250 mg three times a day for 14 days.

32. A 30-year-old man has experienced intermittent diarrhea and associated left lower quadrant abdominal pain that is relieved with defecation. There is no history of fever, weight loss, or hematochezia. A recent barium enema, small-bowel series, and stool samples for ova, parasites, and bacterial cultures have been unremarkable. What is the therapy for this patient's diarrhea?

    a. Tetracycline, 250 mg orally three times a day.
    b. Cholestyramine.
    c. Low-fat diet.
    d. Fiber supplementation.
    e. Metronidazole, 250 mg three times a day for 14 days.

Answers and Discussion

1. a
   The patient has dysphagia to *both* solid and liquids, which is an important indicator that a motility disorder (e.g., achalasia) is present. Esophageal manometry therefore is the diagnostic test of choice.

2. c
   In this patient, cardiac ischemia and structural esophageal abnormalities have been effectively excluded. Atypical gastroesophageal reflux can manifest as intermittent retrosternal chest pain and can be addressed with a 24-hour pH probe.

3. b
   The patient's symptoms suggest oropharyngeal dysphagia secondary to a recent stroke and further complicated by an aspiration pneumonia. A videoesophagram (i.e., a videotaped version of a barium swallow) can be used to assess suspected cases of pharyngeal dysphagia. Typically, laryngeal penetration and, sometimes, frank aspiration can be observed.

4. d
   This patient who is HIV positive and has a low CD4 count has *failed* traditional therapy for presumed esophageal candidiasis. Endoscopy with biopsy and viral cultures can be used to clarify the cause of the odynophagia (e.g., cytomegalovirus, herpes virus, or HIV-associated esophageal ulceration).

5. c
   There is no history of melena or hematochezia, thus suggesting a slow, intermittent blood loss, which is classic for cecal arteriovenous malformations. The patient has two risk factors for such malformations: renal failure, and aortic valvular disease.

6. b
   Dieulafoy's lesions are essentially "visible vessels" without an associated, surrounding ulceration, and they are notoriously difficult to identify except during active bleeding. Dieulafoy's lesions can occur in the esophagus, duodenum, or colon but are most common in the stomach. These lesions usually respond to endoscopic therapy.

7. a
   This is the classic presentation of a Mallory-Weiss tear:

hematemesis or coffee ground emesis *following a bout of retching or nausea/vomiting.*

8. e

Though the patient has a history of ethanol abuse, the negative nasogastric tube aspirate effectively rules out esophageal varices or a Mallory-Weiss tear. Diverticular bleeding frequently presents as painless hematochezia, and it can be diagnosed endoscopically. In some patients, however, when a view of the lumen can not be obtained, angiography can be useful in making the diagnosis.

9. d

In patients with established chronic hepatitis B who suddenly present with a decompensated clinical picture, hepatitis D should be considered. Suprainfection with hepatitis D often leads to a fulminant picture.

10. a

The key is the history of potential exposure. The patient was exposed to hepatitis A (fecal-oral transmission) because of the potentially unsanitary conditions that are common after a flood.

11. e

This scenario is unlikely to represent a sudden recurrence of primary biliary cirrhosis, and the systemic symptoms would not be seen with rejection. The patient is being treated with a triple-drug immunosuppressive regimen, which places the patient at risk for reactivation of cytomegalovirus.

12. c

This is a common presentation for hepatitis C. Approximately 50% of patients who are exposed to hepatitis C develop chronic hepatitis, and approximately 50% of patients with chronic hepatitis C develop cirrhosis.

13. e

This patient has a clean-based ulcer with no evidence of hemodynamic instability or comorbid illness. A clean-based ulcer has a less than 5% chance of rebleeding. Duodenal ulcers also are associated with *H. pylori* in more than 90% of patients. Almost all duodenal ulcers are benign, and repeat endoscopy usually is not indicated unless a malignant process is suspected.

14. d

The patient primarily has a hepatocellular pattern of liver injury with pronounced hypergammaglobulinemia. The latter usually is seen in patients with autoimmune, chronic, active hepatitis. There is no abdominal pain to suggest cholelithiasis or choledocholithiasis.

15. e

After confirming the diagnosis through a liver biopsy, treatment with corticosteroids usually leads to prompt biochemical and clinical improvement. Wilson's disease can present similarly but without the striking hypergammaglobulinemia.

16. b

The hematuria and pattern of abdominal pain are critical for clarifying the diagnosis in this patient.

17. a

Patients with Crohn's disease of the small bowel are at risk for enteric hyperoxaluria. Exposure of the colonic mucosa to bile salts and fatty acids alters colonocyte permeability and leads to enhanced oxalate absorption.

18. c

This patient is a chronic carrier of hepatitis B, as denoted by the positive HbsAg. Presence of the e antigen correlates with a high level of infectivity.

19. c

The *low* serum-ascites albumin gradient is consistent with a possible malignant ascites. This patient was exposed to hepatitis B during birth (i.e., vertical transmission), developed cirrhosis, and then hepatocellular carcinoma. Malignant ascites traditionally is difficult to treat with diuretic therapy.

20. False

Squamous cell cancer is three to four times more common in men.

21. False

H. pylori is not associated with squamous cell cancer of the esophagus.

22. True

Combined radiation therapy and chemotherapy is associated with increased morbidity, but this regimen is superior to radiation therapy alone in improving survival rates among patients with squamous cell esophageal cancer.

23. False

The specialized columnar type of Barrett's mucosa is a risk factor for *adenocarcinoma* of the esophagus.

24. True

Endoscopic ultrasonography is superior to CT for the locoregional staging of esophageal cancer.

25. False

26. False

27. True

28. True

Chronic pancreatitis most commonly is caused by ethanol. Trauma and prolonged metabolic disturbances also may precipitate chronic pancreatitis. Gallstones and the Coxsackie B virus can lead to acute pancreatitis.

29. e

This patient exhibits the classic endoscopic finding of pseudomembranous colitis, which in this case most likely was precipitated by the recent course of broad-spectrum antibiotics. Treatment with metronidazole is associated with a 20% relapse rate.

30. b

Resection of less than 100 cm of terminal ileum is associated with a bile-salt diarrhea, which results from the irritant effects of the bile salts on the colonic mucosa. Treatment with bile salt–binding agents (e.g., cholestyramine) can lead to improvement.

31. a

The positive glucose breath test is suggestive of bacterial overgrowth, which can be seen following gastrointestinal surgery during which a "blind" limb is created. Other causes include achlorhydria, motility disorders, and structural abnormalities such as small-bowel diverticulosis, strictures, adhesions, and fistulas.

32. d

The patient's symptoms and normal evaluation are characteristic of irritable bowel syndrome. In many patients, treatment with fiber can normalize stool consistency and improve symptoms.

Cardiology

Evaluation of Patients with Coronary Artery Disease

Thomas H. Marwick

WHAT IS "SIGNIFICANT" CORONARY ARTERY DISEASE?

In patients with coronary stenoses, flow of blood is preserved at rest until the lumen diameter is reduced by 90 to 95%, at which time rest pain occurs. Patients with milder lesions develop ischemia during stress, when, despite dilation of the distal coronary vasculature, coronary flow becomes restricted by the stenosis. This usually occurs with stenoses of greater than 50%, and almost always with lesions of greater than 70%, of the artery diameter. In the 50% range, flow reduction is modulated by collateral flow, location and length of stenoses, relation to bends and bifurcations, and other variables. Thus, the "gold standard" of coronary artery disease (CAD) is stenoses of greater than 50% diameter (some centers use > 70%) at coronary angiography.

There certainly are a number of problems with this criterion, including poor correlation between severity of stenosis and reduction of flow and interobserver variability in subjective interpretation. Nonetheless, a reference standard is needed, and this is the best that is currently available.

STATISTICAL APPROACH TO ASSESSING STRESS TESTS

No noninvasive test used for the diagnosis of CAD is perfect. The aim of testing is to inform the ordering physician about the likelihood of disease being present as well as its severity and prognosis. Not every patient with a positive test proceeds to coronary angiography; therefore, separation of "diagnostic" and "prognostic" testing is artificial. The functional data permit a judgement to be made regarding whether the cost, risk, and discomfort of coronary angiography will be worthwhile.

Several values are used to measure the ability of noninvasive tests to predict the presence of significant coronary stenoses. These include sensitivity, specificity, accuracy, and both positive and negative predictive value (PV). Sensitivity and specificity are the most widely used, because they depend less on disease prevalence than the other variables. Definitions of statistical terms relating to accuracy are:

Sensitivity = True positives/All patients with CAD

Specificity = True negatives/All patients without CAD

PV of positive test = True positives/All positive tests

PV of negative test = True negatives/All negative tests

Accuracy = All correct results/All patients

CLINICAL EVALUATION

Regardless of a patient's clinical status, stress testing is not appropriate for the diagnosis or exclusion of CAD. Applying Bayes' theorem, the posttest probability of disease depends not only on the accuracy of the test but also on the pretest probability of CAD, which may be defined on the basis of age, gender, and symptom status (Table 62.1). The relationship between accuracy, pretest probability, and posttest probability is summarized in Figure 62.1, which shows that patients with a very low (<20%) or very high (>80%) pretest probability of disease will remain in these categories regardless of test results and accuracy. Thus, in patients with high or low probability of disease, the usefulness of noninvasive testing for diagnostic purposes is limited. These tests may, however, provide useful prognostic data (e.g., exercise capacity, site and extent of ischemia, severity of left ventricular dysfunction), which may influence treatment. (The following sections assume that appropriate decisions about investigation are

Figure 62.1. Relation of pretest and posttest probability with tests of (**A**) low accuracy and (**B**) high accuracy.

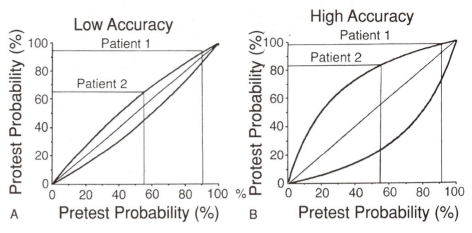

Table 62.1. Diagnosis of Myocardial Ischemia: Pretest Probability in Men				
Age (yr)	**Asymptomatic**	**Nonanginal**	**Atypical**	**Typical**
30–39	2	5	22	70%
40–49	6	14	46	87%
50–59	10	22	59	92%
60–69	12	28	67	94%

made on clinical grounds, even though in clinical practice, these ''rules'' are constantly broken.)

DIAGNOSTIC TESTS

There are a bewildering number of combinations stress-testing methodologies and electrocardiography (ECG) or imaging techniques for the detection of ischemia (Table 62.2). No single test is optimal for the diagnosis of CAD in the population as a whole, but the two major determinants of appropriate testing are interpretability of the stress ECG and ability of the patient to exercise maximally. Patients who can exercise maximally should do so, because exercise testing provides useful functional and prognostic information independent of whether ischemia is detected. If the ECG is nondiagnostic (discussed later), an imaging test should be performed, and this should be planned for all patients who undergo pharmacologic stress because of an inability to exercise. The latter groups (nondiagnostic ECGs) now constitute the majority of tests performed in most tertiary centers (Fig. 62.2).

EXERCISE ELECTROCARDIOGRAPHY

Who Should Undergo Exercise Electrocardiography?

Patients should undergo exercise ECG if they can exercise maximally and have an interpretable ST segment. In contrast

Table 62.2. Noninvasive Diagnosis of Ischemia	
Stress Techniques	**Diagnostic Tests**
Exercise	ECG only
Bicycle	
Treadmill	
Pharmacologic	Perfusion
Adenosine	^{201}Tl
Dipyridamole	Tc-MIBI
Dobutamine	Other ^{99m}TC
Pacing + other (e.g.,	Function
cold pressor)	2D echocardiography
	Nuclear left ventriculography
	New approaches
	PET
	MRI
	Fast CT

CT, computed tomography; *MRI*, magnetic resonance imaging; *2D*, two-dimensional.

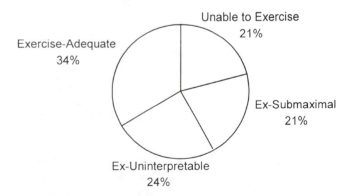

Figure 62.2. Distribution of patients able to exercise and with interpretable ECG among patients attending a hospital exercise laboratory. Ex-Submaximal = patients who are able to exercise but are unable to increase their heart rate to 85% of the age predicted maximum. Ex-Uninterpretable = uninterpretable ECG due to resting ECG changes.

Table 62.3.   Costs, Reimbursements, and Charges for Common Diagnostic Methodologies as a Multiple of the Cost for an Exercise Stress ECG

	Charges	*Reimbursement (Medicare)*	*Cost*
Exercise ECG	2.5	0.4	1.0
Exercise ^{201}Tl	13.3	3.2	5.1
Exercise echocardiography	7.7	1.6	1.4
Coronary angiography	31.8	9.1	13.4

to the expense of imaging tests (which can exceed $1000), exercise ECG is "low-tech" and relatively inexpensive. It is difficult to obtain current, specific cost and charge data at most institutions, but the multiples between different tests change little. Table 62.3 lists these multiples for costs, reimbursements, and charges involved with the common diagnostic methodologies.

Despite the potential cost savings of a given methodology, we must consider its effectiveness as well. Exclusive use of standard exercise ECG would have clear disadvantages in relation to accuracy. Only about one-third of patients exercise maximally and have an interpretable stress ECG, and among these patients, equivocal results (e.g., borderline ST-segment changes without angina) may necessitate performance of a stress-imaging test anyway.

Indications for exercise ECG tests in addition to those used for the diagnosis of CAD are:

- Diagnostic evaluation of chest pain
- Physiologic significance of known CAD
- Prognosis of CAD (especially after myocardial infarction)
- Evaluation of therapy (e.g., drug, percutaneous transluminal coronary angioplasty, coronary artery bypass graft)
- Screening for CAD in "at-risk" individuals
- Evaluation of arrhythmias, pacing
- Heart failure (especially evaluation of treatment)
- Estimation of functional capacity
- Follow-up of patients with congenital and valvular diseases

Provided that the contraindications are observed, exercise ECG testing is quite safe, with a recorded serious-event rate of 1:1000 or lower. Contraindications are:

- Acutely unstable coronary syndromes[1]
- Symptomatic, severe aortic stenosis[1]
- Uncontrolled heart failure

- Uncontrolled serious cardiac dysrhythmias[1]
- Severe hypertension
- Recent pulmonary embolism
- Serious acute noncardiac disorder
- Inability to cooperate

Performing Exercise Electrocardiography

Exercise ECG testing simply involves performance of a standardized exercise protocol while the patient undergoes ECG monitoring for evidence of ischemia. The end points of testing are:

- Patient request/exhaustion
- Severe angina, marked ST-segment depression (>3 mm) or elevation (>2 mm)
- Fall of systolic blood pressure below resting despite more work
- Poor perfusion, central nervous system symptoms
- Serious arrhythmias
- Hypertension (>280/115 mm Hg)

Note attaining the "maximum" pulse rate is not an indication to stop in most instances.

A test is identified as being "positive" by a horizontal or downsloping ST-segment depression of greater than 0.1 mV (Fig. 62.3). Upsloping depression is accepted if it occurs 0.06 or 0.08 seconds after the J point, but this is less specific than the other changes. Unless it occurs in leads with Q waves, ST-segment elevation is a reliable sign of transmural ischemia. The presence of angina, exercise capacity, hemodynamic response, and rhythm during testing are useful adjunctive results. These data have been combined into various global exercise scores, but these have not been widely accepted.

Accuracy of Exercise Electrocardiography

Results of studies having minimal referral bias have shown that both the sensitivity and specificity of standard exercise ECG is in the mid-70% range (Table 62.4). The accuracy is somewhat lower in female subjects, but the reasons for this are not well understood.

Selection of exercise ECG testing must be made with the knowledge that this technique is less accurate than stress-imaging approaches. Equivocal results such as a negative test response in a high-probability patient may occur, thus causing a stress-imaging test or angiography to be performed to clarify the matter.

In patients who are unable to exercise, the ECG component of either dipyridamole or dobutamine stress is insensitive for the identification of myocardial ischemia. Consequently, if either dipyridamole or dobutamine is selected as a stressor in these patients, a stress-imaging technique should be performed as well.

[1] Lesser degrees of these problems, especially after treatment, may benefit from exercise testing.

Figure 62.3. Exercise-induced ST-segment depression consistent with myocardial ischemia.

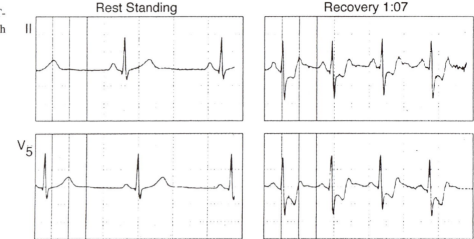

Rest Standing

Recovery 1:07

II

V₅

Table 62.4. **Exercise Electrocardiography: Sensitivity and Specificity**		
	Sensitivity (n [%])	*Specificity (n [%])*
Sketch (JAMA '80)	40/59 (68)	39/48 (81)
Melin (Circ '81)	73/99 (74)	43/61 (70)
Patterson (AJC '82)	27/50 (54)	35/46 (76)
Weintraub (AJC '84)	73/101 (72)	37/46 (80)
Hung (AHJ '85)	99/117 (85)	34/54 (63)
Combined male patients	312/426 (73)	188/255 (74)
Hung (JACC '86)	20/28 (71)	38/64 (59)
Melin (Circ '85)	27/44 (61)	72/91 (79)
Combined female patients	47/72 (65)	110/155 (71)

STRESS-IMAGING TECHNIQUES

Who Should Undergo Stress Imaging?

Stress imaging typically is used in patients with nondiagnostic ST segments. This includes patients with the following conditions:

- Left bundle-branch block
- Left ventricular hypertrophy with strain
- Digitalis therapy
- Resting ST-segment changes, Wolff-Parkinson-White syndrome

Stress imaging also is used in patients who require pharmacologic stress because of their inability to exercise maximally, such as those with the following conditions:

- Peripheral vascular disease
- Orthopedic problems (e.g., back, legs)
- Chronic respiratory disease
- Cerebrovascular disease

- Medications, poor motivation
- Poor physical capacity

To these, one also might add patients with normal resting ST segments in whom exercise ECG may be unreliable, such as women and patients with left ventricular hypertrophy.

Performing Stress Imaging

Standard nuclear methodologies comprise stress ventriculography and myocardial perfusion imaging. Ventriculography has a poor specificity and is intrinsically insensitive for identification of segmental ischemic dysfunction. It may have some value in combination with ^{99m}Tc-methoxyisobutylisonitrile (MIBI) perfusion imaging for exclusion of false-positive perfusion defects resulting from soft-tissue attenuation. Otherwise, however, it has been superseded by other methodologies for the diagnosis of CAD.

Widespread application of single-photon emission computed tomography (SPECT) to myocardial perfusion imaging has enhanced our ability to localize CAD and to appreciate its extent. Thallium is innately unfavorable for imaging because of its low-energy photon emission, which leads to tissue attenuation and scatter; unfavorable radiation dosimetry, which also contributes to low photon counts; and long half-life, which precludes a true resting scan and leads to ambiguity regarding the presence of infarction and ischemia. These constraints are not shared by ^{99m}Tc, however, which has been attached to various isonitriles, the most widespread of which is MIBI. The benefits of MIBI include:

1. Better image quality.
2. A small increment of accuracy, particularly in the posterior territories of the heart, which are the most poorly visualized areas at ^{201}Tl imaging).
3. Ability to perform ventriculography simultaneously with perfusion measurements.
4. Absence of redistribution, thus allowing injection of this tracer at one time and imaging at a later time,

which is useful in the emergency room or during acute intervention.

Recent work has combined the benefits of ^{201}Tl (i.e., assessment of viability, lesser expense) with those of MIBI (i.e., absence of washout, high-quality images), thus producing a dual-isotope approach that enhances the performance speed of nuclear scintigraphic studies. The benefits of using MIBI in this approach, however, are obtained at a significant increase in cost.

Positron-emission tomography (PET) is a sophisticated imaging technique that may be used to examine myocardial perfusion using the tracers ^{13}N-ammonia, ^{15}O-water, or ^{82}Rb. This technology provides accurate measurements of myocardial perfusion, but further development of PET for diagnostic purposes has been inhibited by its cost. Whether the expense of PET is justified on the basis of better prognostic assessment or prevention of a substantial number of unnecessary catheterizations remains unresolved.

Stress echocardiography involves comparison of regional function at rest as well as both during and after stress to identify myocardial ischemia. Usually, this process is facilitated by a side-by-side display of digitized images in a cineloop format. Its accuracy, however, depends on the ability of the observer to identify often subtle changes in regional function. The clinical interpretation of all stress-imaging approaches involves some degree of subjectivity, but a trained observer is especially important during stress echocardiography.

Accuracy of Stress Imaging

Tomographic myocardial perfusion imaging (i.e., SPECT) offers a greater sensitivity for CAD than planar approaches, but this may occur at the cost of lower specificity (Table 62.5). To an extent, this may reflect referral bias. Perfusion scintigraphy has a particularly low specificity in subgroups of patients with left ventricular hypertrophy and left bundle-branch block. Thus, whereas perfusion scintigraphy has the benefit of much experience with its use, recent concerns have focused on its cost as well as on its false-positive rate. It remains an

excellent choice, however, in patients with previous infarction and at centers without a major commitment to high-quality stress echocardiography.

The accuracy of PET for the diagnosis of CAD is greater than 90%, though many of the studies have been small and included an unacceptable number of patients with previous myocardial infarction (Table 62.6). Comparisons of cardiac PET with SPECT have shown a benefit to PET in terms of accuracy, which mirrors the underlying benefits of PET regarding accurate localization of tracer, ability to obtain high counts (and, therefore, excellent image quality), and capacity to perform attenuation correction. Clinically, these benefits include a better ability to resolve moderate (i.e., 50–70% diameter) coronary stenosis, reduction of false-positive results because of soft-tissue attenuation artifacts, and ability to accurately diagnose CAD involving the posterior parts of the heart (reflecting the benefits of attenuation correction, reduction of scatter, and higher counts). Both the cost and availability of PET, however, mandate a selective and sparing use of this technology. For diagnostic purposes, its high specificity is attractive in patients with a lower probability of CAD, and its high diagnostic accuracy is attractive in patients for whom angiography is inappropriate. It also may be useful for studying patients who otherwise are difficult to image (e.g., obese patients). Nonetheless, the major value of PET relates to evaluating the physiologic significance of known coronary lesions as well as investigating issues of myocardial viability.

The sensitivity and specificity of exercise echocardiography for identification of CAD are approximately 85% each (Table 62.7). As with other noninvasive tests, however, these values vary among studies relative to the mix of patients, and particularly relative to the prevalence of multivessel disease and previous infarction, which augment the recorded sensitivity of all stress-imaging tests. Two particular problems for stress echocardiography are identification of multivessel disease in patients without previous infarction and detection of ischemia in the setting of resting wall-motion abnormalities. Currently, stress echocardiography has the disadvantage of involving subjective interpretation. It has advantages, how-

Table 62.5. Exercise Tl-SPECT Diagnosis of Coronary Artery Disease: Sensitivity and Specificity

	Sensitivity (%)		Specificity (%)	MI (in CAD) (%)
	Overall	No MI		
Tamaki ($n = 104$)	96	96	91	39
DePasquale ($n = 210$)	95	92	74	26
Iskandrian ($n = 461$)	82	78	60	18
Maddahi ($n = 183$)	95	90	56	47
Mahmarian and Verani (1991) ($n = 360$)	87	79	87	33
Van Train ($n = 262$)	94	90	43	40
Total	90	85	70	31

MI, myocardial infarction.

Table 62.6.   Accuracy of PET for Detection of Coronary Artery Disease

	Tracer	MI (%)	Sensitivity (n [%])	Specificity (n [%])
Schelbert (1982)	^{13}N	?	31/32 (97)	13/13 (100)[a]
Yonekura (1987)	^{13}N	43	37/38 (97)	13/14 (93)[a]
Tamaki*(1988)	^{13}N	74	47/48 (98)	3/3 (100)[a]
Go (1990)	^{82}Rb	47	142/152 (93)	39/50 (78)
Stewart (1991)	^{82}Rb	42	50/60 (83)	19/21 (90)

MI, myocardial infarction.
[a] Including normal volunteers.

Table 62.7.   Digital Exercise Echocardiography: Sensitivity and Specificity

	Sensitivity (n [%])	Specificity (n [%])
Armstrong (JACC '87)	40/51 (78)	19/22 (86)
Ryan (JACC '88)	31/40 (78)	24/24 (100)
Crouse (AJC '91)	170/175 (97)	34/53 (64)
Marwick (JACC '92)	96/114 (84)	31/36 (86)
Quinones (Circ '92)	64/86 (74)	21/26 (81)
Hecht (JACC '93)	127/137 (93)	37/46 (80)
Ryan (JASE '93)	192/211 (91)	76/98 (78)
Combined	720/814 (88)	242/305 (79)

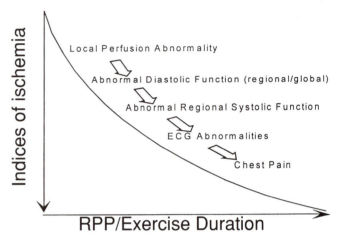

Figure 62.4.   The "ischemic cascade," during which less-sensitive tests become positive at higher workloads. RPP = rate-pressure product.

ever, in relation to cost, safety, and patient convenience. In addition, it may be the test of choice for patients with left ventricular hypertrophy and, possibly, those with left bundle-branch block.

COMPARATIVE STUDIES

The sensitivity of stress imaging exceeds that of exercise ECG. This result can be readily anticipated from the "ischemic cascade" (Fig. 62.4).

The overall accuracy of stress echocardiography is comparable to that of nuclear scintigraphy. Scintigraphy has a slightly higher sensitivity, however, and echocardiography has a higher specificity. The strengths of stress echocardiography are its speed, cost, accuracy in patients with left ventricular hypertrophy or left bundle-branch block, and acquisition of data about resting left ventricular function, valves, and pericardium. Scintigraphy is more sensitive for single-vessel disease, is better for recognizing multivessel disease, and may be better for distinguishing ischemia and infarction. It also is more quantitative, though both techniques require both technical and interpretive expertise.

The decision between echocardiography and nuclear testing is made predominantly on the basis of local expertise and availability. This is particularly true for stress echocardiography, which undoubtedly is the most demanding of the techniques.

EVALUATION OF PATIENTS UNABLE TO EXERCISE

As discussed, pharmacologic stress ECG (without imaging) is not a good option in patients who are unable to exercise. Because myocardial perfusion scintigraphy essentially depends on the evaluation of differences in regional hyperemia, coronary vasodilators (e.g., dipyridamole, adenosine) are the optimal pharmacologic stressors for this test. For echocardiography, dobutamine is a better stressor than coronary vasodilators, which rarely cause ischemia in a functional sense.

Exercise and pharmacologic stress-imaging tests have comparable accuracy. The additional data provided by exercise, however, including correlation of stress with daily life, exercise capacity, ST-segment and rhythm evaluation, all favor use of exercise whenever a patient can exercise maximally.

PROGNOSIS

In clinical practice, diagnosis rarely is separate from prognostic assessment. In addition, further investigations rarely are determined by the prediction of CAD alone but on the basis of an assessment of the severity and, hence, the implications of the diagnosis in each individual.

The outcome of patients with CAD is determined by their left ventricular function, amount of jeopardized myocardium, exercise capacity, and noncardiac factors such as age and diabetes. As functional testing provides most of these data, it is not surprising that its predictive power exceeds that of coronary angiography, which supplies anatomic data. At exercise testing, exercise capacity, hypotension, and dysrhythmias predict outcome at exercise testing more so than ST-segment changes. At imaging, the extent of ischemic or all abnormal myocardium is the strongest predictor of outcome.

CONCLUSIONS

Recent advances in stress testing have enhanced our ability to identify CAD by noninvasive means. Over the last decade, SPECT, stress echocardiography, and PET have become accepted clinical tools, and some initial data point toward their specific utility in individual situations. Nonetheless, the standard exercise ECG stress test remains the backbone of functional testing for CAD. Indeed, the challenge of the next few years will be to incorporate these new techniques into the cost-effective treatment of patients with suspected CAD.

REVIEW EXERCISES

QUESTIONS

1. A 56-year-old woman with arthritis has atypical pain but a normal ECG. The best diagnostic option is:
   a. Stress (exercise or dobutamine) ECG.
   b. Coronary angiography.
   c. Exercise echocardiography.
   d. Dipyridamole-thallium imaging.
   e. None of the above.

2. A 28-year-old woman presents with left-sided pain at rest and exercise. The best diagnostic option is:
   a. Exercise ECG.
   b. Coronary angiography.
   c. Exercise echocardiography.
   d. Exercise thallium imaging.
   e. None of the above.

3. A 68-year-old man presents with central retrosternal pain at exercise. The best diagnostic option is:
   a. Exercise ECG.
   b. Coronary angiography.
   c. Exercise echocardiography.
   d. Exercise thallium imaging.
   e. None of the above.

4. A 48-year-old man with hypertensive left ventricular hypertrophy complains of atypical chest pain. The best diagnostic option is:
   a. Exercise ECG.
   b. Coronary angiography.
   c. Exercise echocardiography.
   d. Dipyridamole-thallium imaging.
   e. None of the above.

5. Problems may occur with exercise thallium imaging except in patients with:
   a. Left bundle-branch block.
   b. Left ventricular hypertrophy.
   c. Female sex.
   d. Obesity, posterior circulation disease.
   e. Left Anterior Descending (LAD) Coronary Artery disease.

6. A 52-year-old woman has an uninterpretable ECG and atypical pain. The least expensive option is:
   a. Exercise thallium imaging.
   b. Coronary angiography.
   c. Exercise echocardiography.
   d. Dipyridamole PET imaging.
   e. None of the above.

7. A 52-year-old man needs a femoropopliteal bypass. What would you recommend first for risk stratification?

a. Exercise ECG.
b. Coronary angiography.
c. Dobutamine echocardiography.
d. Dipyridamole-thallium imaging.
e. Clinical evaluation.

8. The following probably constitute significant CAD except:
   a. Proximal LAD stenosis of 80%.
   b. LAD stenosis of 60% with angina.
   c. Right Coronary Artery stenosis of 50%.
   d. Left Circumflex Coronary Artery stenosis of 50% with positive exercise ECG.

9. Which of the following patients has the greatest probability of CAD?
   a. A 48-year-old woman with atypical chest pain.
   b. A 25-year-old man with typical angina.
   c. A 45-year-old man with atypical chest pain.
   d. A 70-year-old man with atypical chest pain.

10. In what proportion of patients is an exercise ECG adequate for the diagnosis of CAD?
    a. Most (approximately 80%).
    b. Majority (approximately 60%).
    c. Minority (approximately 40%).
    d. Few (approximately 10%).

11. What is the accuracy of exercise ECG for diagnosis of CAD?
    a. Sensitivity 85%, specificity 85%
    b. Sensitivity 85%, specificity 65%
    c. Sensitivity 75%, specificity 75%
    d. Sensitivity 75%, specificity 95%

12. In a patient with intermediate pretest CAD probability, which of the following tests is least sensitive?
    a. Stress echocardiography.
    b. Exercise thallium-SPECT.
    c. Exercise ECG.
    d. Exercise nuclear ventriculography.

13. In a middle-aged woman with atypical pain, which of the following tests is most accurate?
    a. Exercise ECG.
    b. Exercise thallium-SPECT.
    c. PET.
    d. Exercise nuclear ventriculography.

14. In a patient with hypertensive LVH and atypical pain, which of the following tests is most accurate?
    a. Exercise ECG.
    b. Exercise thallium-SPECT.
    c. PET.
    d. Exercise echocardiography.

Answers

1. d	8. c
2. e	9. d
3. b	10. c
4. c	11. c
5. e	12. c
6. c	13. c
7. e	14. d

SUGGESTED READINGS

Berman DS, Kiat HS, van Train KF, et al. Myocardial perfusion imaging with technetium-99m-sestamibi: comparative analysis of available imaging protocols. J Nucl Med 1994;35: 681–688.

Detrano R, Froelicher VF. Exercise testing: uses and limitations considering recent studies. Prog Cardiovasc Dis 1988; 31:173–204.

Diamond GA, Forrester JS. Analysis of probability as an aid in the clinical diagnosis of coronary artery disease. N Engl J Med 1979;300:1350–1358.

Fletcher GF, Balady G, Froelicher VF, et al. AHA Medical/ Scientific Statement. Exercise standards. A statement for healthcare professionals from the AHA. Circulation 1995;91: 580–615.

Gibbons RJ, Balady GJ, Beasley JW et al. Guidelines for exercise testing. A report of the ACC/AHA task force on assessment of cardiovascular procedures. Circulation 1997;96: 345–354.

Kahn JK, McGhie I, Akers MS, et al. Quantitative rotational tomography with ^{201}Tl and ^{99m}Tc-methoxyisobutylisonitrile. A direct comparison in normal individuals and patients with coronary artery disease. Circulation 1989;79:1282–1290.

Mahmarian JJ, Verani MS. Exercise thallium-201 perfusion scintigraphy in the assessment of coronary artery disease. Am J Cardiol 1991;67:2D–11D.

Marwick T, Willemart B, D'Hondt AM, et al. Selection of the optimal nonexercise stress for the evaluation of ischemic regional myocardial dysfunction and malperfusion: comparison of dobutamine and adenosine using echocardiography and Tc-99m MIBI single photon emission computed tomography. Circulation 1993;87:345–354.

Picano E, Lattanzi F, Orlandini A, Marini C, L'Abbate A. Stress echocardiography and the human factor: the importance of being expert. J Am Coll Cardiol 1991;17:666–669.

Pryor DB, Shaw L, McCants CB, et al. Value of the history and physical in identifying patients at increased risk for CAD. Ann Intern Med 1993;118:81–90.

C•H•A•P•T•E•R

63

Clinical Electrocardiography: A Visual Board Review

Donald A. Underwood and Richard Grimm

The electrocardiogram (ECG) is an important clinical tool in both the acute and chronic evaluation and treatment of patients. It is often the first information gathered, after the history, for patients who present with chest pain syndromes, syncope, and abrupt changes in respiratory status. It has also emerged as the pivotal piece of information in the modern treatment of acute myocardial infarction, frequently representing the gate through which patients must pass to be considered for thrombolytic therapy. As isolated information, the electrocardiogram has value, but it is important to remember that it is just one clinical tool and has its greatest meaning when related to the individual patient who may present with any of a number of symptoms and histories. Mastery of electrocardiography evolves over many years of clinical experience. In fact, it is never truly mastered. Skills with observation and integration merely continue to be refined, and even the most

senior electrocardiographer can find new variations and clinical relationships related to electrocardiograms.

A review like this cannot "teach" electrocardiography. As mentioned, that requires time, repeated clinical correlation, and the help of one of the many excellent available texts on electrocardiography. Instead, this review intends to remind you of clinical situations that you have experienced in which the electrocardiogram was of importance and to cement that memory into your basic fund of clinical knowledge. These are not examples of rare conditions, nor are the electrocardiograms at all unusual or unique. They are common tracings you have encountered in patients, which, it is hoped, will reinforce important ECG concepts, reassure you in your experience, and perhaps give some guidance in suggesting additional reading.

ELECTROCARDIOGRAMS FOR INTERPRETATION

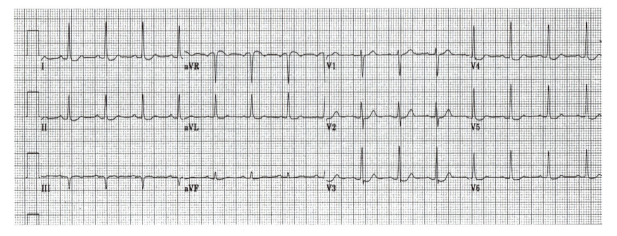

ECG 1. This patient has a sinus rhythm. The main abnormality is ST segment depression that is scooping in quality. The QT interval is also relatively short. This is most compatible with digitalis effect. It is an example of ST depression that has an appearance specific enough for a definite diagnosis.

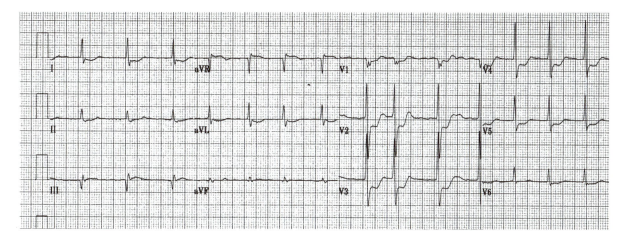

ECG 2.   This patient shows atrial fibrillation (an irregularly irregular ventricular response and no definite atrial activity). There is also ST segment depression in lead I, not inconsistent with digitalis effect. In the midprecordial leads, however, the ST segment depression is deeper, horizontal, and downsloping. This could be digitalis effect, but subendocardial ischemia or infarction should also be considered.

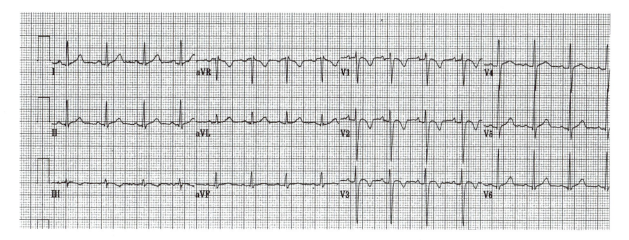

ECG 3.   This electrocardiogram shows a sinus rhythm. Midprecordial T-wave changes are present; these could be abnormal. The patient, however, is a young girl, age 7, and in this case the T-wave changes are normal and represent a juvenile pattern.

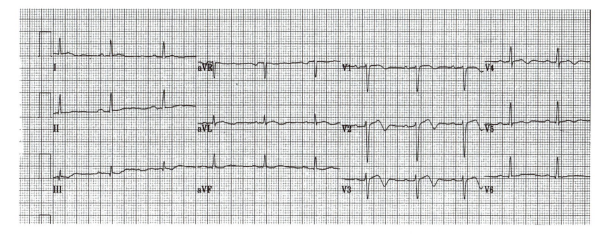

ECG 4.   This electrocardiogram also shows T-wave changes. They extend as inversions to lead V_5. The T-wave in lead V_6 is low. This is a nonspecific T-wave abnormality. The electrocardiogram is not normal, but the specific disease process would need to be determined clinically.

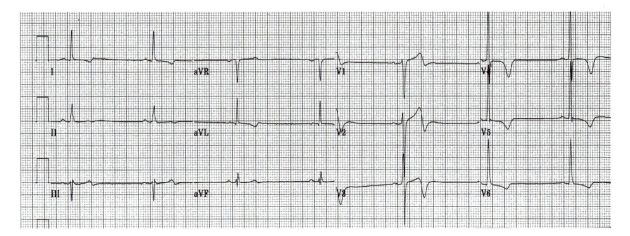

ECG 5.   This electrocardiogram shows a sinus bradycardia. There are T-wave changes that in the midprecordium are biphasic and terminally symmetric. This also is a nonspecific T-wave abnormality. T-waves like this, however, are commonly seen in patients with coronary artery disease. Sometimes this appearance can be seen with ventricular hypertrophy, especially hypertrophic cardiomyopathy. Again, clinical correlation is necessary.

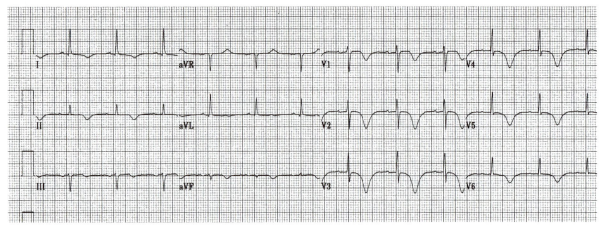

ECG 6.   This electrocardiogram shows T-wave abnormalities. They are generalized and are found throughout the electrocardiogram. The T-waves are deeply inverted and symmetric. The QT interval is prolonged. This can be seen in coronary disease. Also in the differential diagnosis is significant central nervous system (CNS) injury, which was the case in this patient.

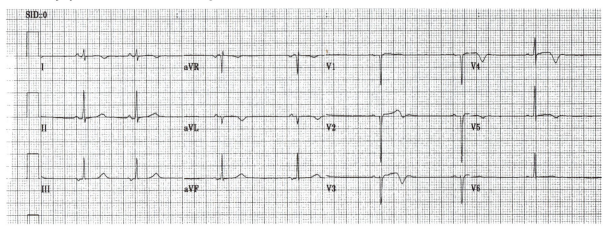

ECG 7.   This electrocardiogram shows T-wave changes with terminal symmetry in the midprecordium. It also shows poor R-wave progression. This is suggestive of myocardial injury, and although definite Q-waves are not present, the combination of T-waves of this type with minimal R-waves is often seen following myocardial injury with wall motion abnormalities found in wall motion studies. This electrocardiogram is from a young woman with Ehlers-Danlos syndrome of the vascular type, who suffered an anterior descending dissection and rupture with infarction.

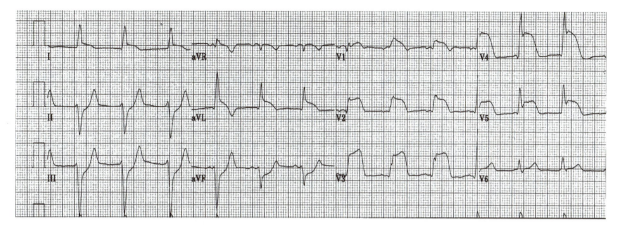

ECG 8.   ST segment elevation is the hallmark of acute myocardial infarction, which is the case on this electrocardiogram. ST elevations of significance are seen in the anterior and lateral leads. A sinus rhythm is in the middle portion of the electrocardiogram. To the left and right, however, the complexes are broader and P-waves are absent. This is an accelerated idioventricular rhythm seen in the face of the acute infarct. Accelerated idioventricular rhythm is not uncommonly seen as a reperfusion arrhythmia after thrombolytic therapy for myocardial infarction.

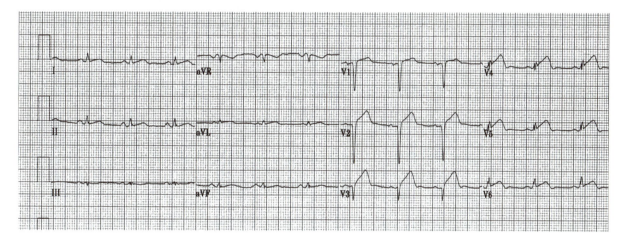

ECG 9.   This is an acute anterior infarct. The ST segment is elevated, the QT interval is relatively prolonged, and there is straightening in the upslope of the ST segment into the T-wave. There are no reciprocal changes, which is not an uncommon finding in acute anterior infarction, unlike that in acute inferior or lateral infarcts.

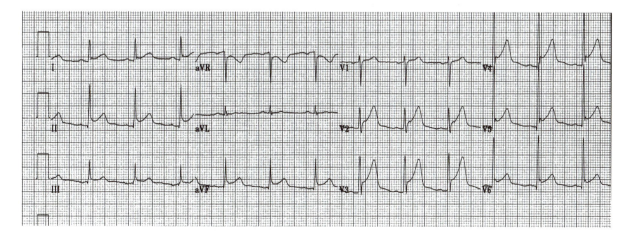

ECG 10.   ST segment elevation does not always represent an acute myocardial infarction. In this case, there is definite ST segment elevation. This is seen in all leads except aVR. This is an example of acute pericarditis. Occasionally PR segment deviation can be seen, as in this case in which there is a PR segment elevation in lead aVR.

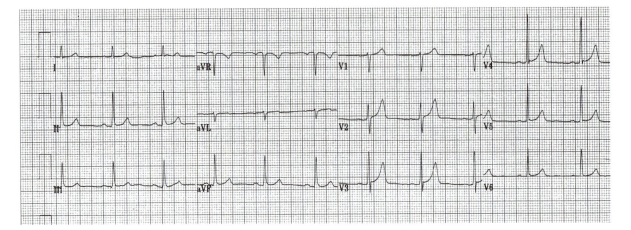

ECG 11.   ST segment elevation, which is regional, often is due to myocardial infarction, but it is always important to remember early repolarization, a normal variant. The J point is distinct with elevation in lead V_2 and especially lead V_3. The QT interval is not prolonged. The upslope of the T-wave is not straightened. This is a normal ECG with early repolarization.

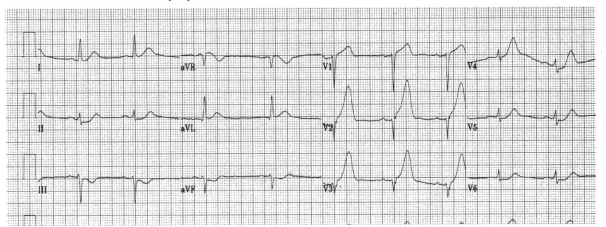

ECG 12.   In this electrocardiogram, the broad, somewhat symmetric T-waves are the dominant finding. The QT interval is also prolonged. There is minimal ST elevation in the midprecordial leads. This represents the acute T-wave phase of an acute myocardial infarction, which often is not seen on electrocardiography because it occurs when the patient is in process of reaching the hospital, and the electrocardiogram is still evolving through this picture.

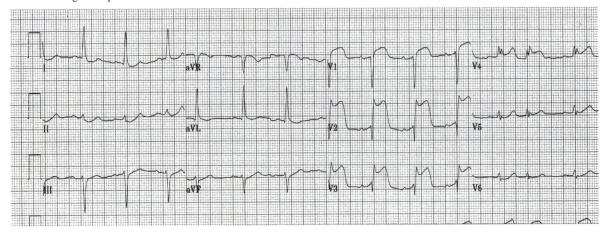

ECG 13.   This is the same patient as in ECG no. 12, 40 minutes later. Very clear ST segment elevation is seen in the midprecordial leads, and the diagnosis of acute anteroseptal myocardial infarction is clear. In addition, there are premature atrial contractions. Once again, definite reciprocal changes are not seen.

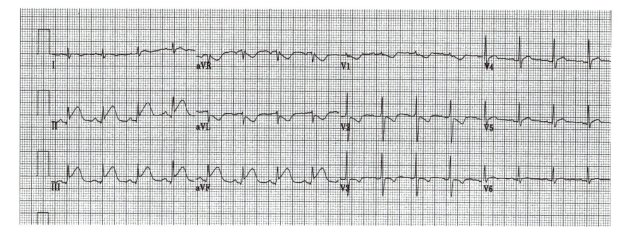

ECG 14.   This electrocardiogram shows ST segment elevation, this time in the inferior leads II, III, and aVF. There is ST depression in aVL that is probably reciprocal. This is an example of an acute inferior infarct.

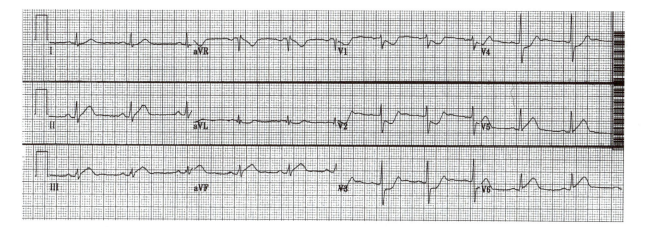

ECG 15.   This also is an acute inferior infarction. There is some slight ST elevation in leads III and aVF. There are reciprocal depressions in leads V_1, V_2, and V_3. The T-waves are broad. The upslope of the T-wave is straightened. These changes are also seen in leads V_5 and V_6. The differential diagnosis of the ST segment depression in the right precordium, which is seen with an acute inferior infarct, is simple reciprocal change "ischemia at a distance," and posterior infarction. Posterior infarction is more likely to be the case here in view of the acute ST-T wave changes that are seen in V_5 and V_6 in addition to the acute inferior abnormalities.

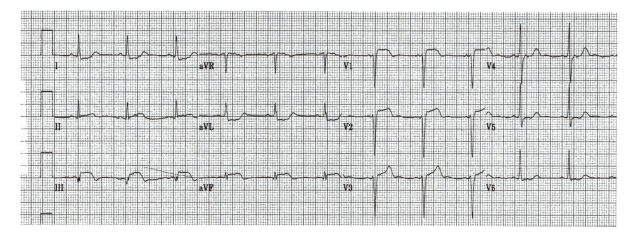

ECG 16.   The ST segment elevation in leads III and aVF associated with depressions in leads I and aVL suggests acute inferior infarction. In addition, there is ST segment elevation in leads V_1 and V_2. Elevations in the right precordial leads, in the face of an inferior infarct, should strongly suggest right ventricular infarct, which can be confirmed with right-sided chest leads, although in this case that would not be necessary as this is a fairly characteristic RV infarct.

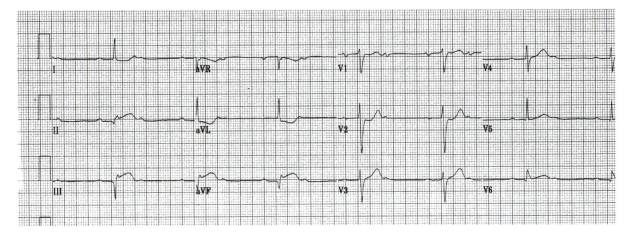

ECG 17.   Acute inferior infarctions can be associated with a variety of sinus and AV node conduction abnormalities. This is an example of one of those. This ECG shows an acute inferior infarct pattern with elevation in the inferior leads and reciprocal depressions in lead I and especially aVL. In addition, a 2:1 block can be seen.

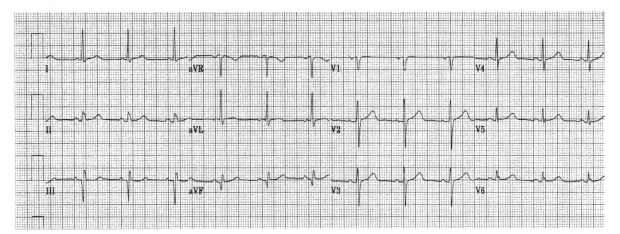

ECG 18.   This is an old inferior infarction. Well-established Q-waves are seen in leads III and aVF; aVF is the key lead. Here, the Q-wave is broad, being 0.04 seconds in duration. The ST segment abnormalities have resolved. T-waves are back to normal. This is a well-established (old or remote) infarct.

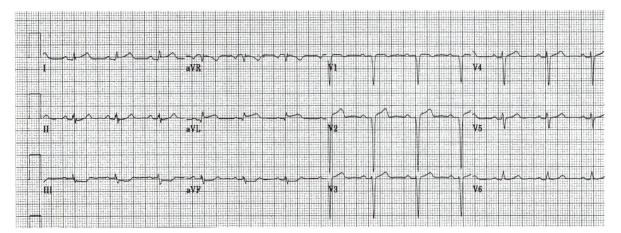

ECG 19.   ST segment elevation, which is slight but definite, is seen in lead aVL. This is supported by some elevation in lead I and reciprocal changes in the inferior leads, especially leads III and aVF. This is an example of an acute high lateral infarction. The precordium is fairly unremarkable, and this is a type of infarct that can sometimes evolve as a surprise, resulting in high enzyme elevations in what seems to be an electrocardiographically limited event. The high lateral wall is relatively electrically silent, and changes in those leads need to be respected.

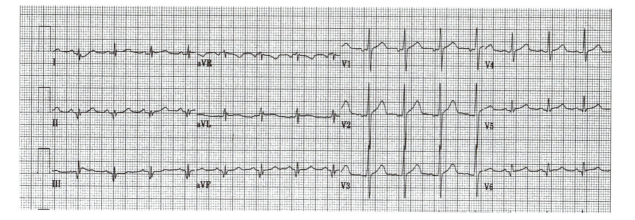

ECG 20. In this electrocardiogram, the inferiorly directed Q-waves are obvious. They are broad and deep relative to the R-waves and without question represent an inferior infarct. Lead V_6 has similar Q-wave duration and QR ratio. Importantly, the R-wave in lead V_1 is prominent, greater or at least equal to the S-wave in that lead with T-waves upright. This is an example of an inferoposterior infarction. (See also ECG no. 15.)

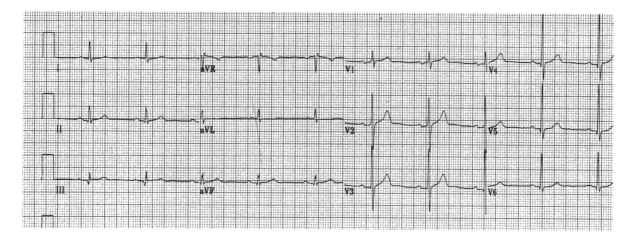

ECG 21. This electrocardiogram shows small inferior Q-waves. Those in lead III are prominent, but those in leads II and aVF are below the diagnostic level. V_1, however, shows prominence of the R-wave with an R>S and an upright T-wave. This is an example of posterior infarction.

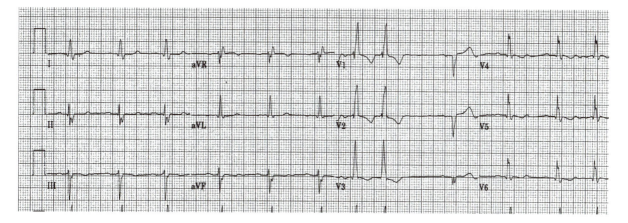

ECG 22. Electrocardiograms sometimes reveal their secrets in only a few beats. This ECG shows a right bundle branch block with left-axis deviation. In the middle panel, a premature atrial contraction can be seen, and following the compensatory reset, normal intraventricular connection is permitted to occur. The "normal beat" after the pause shows Q-waves that extend from V_1 to V_3. This is an old anteroseptal infarct uncovered by the PAC, also an example of a rate-dependent right bundle branch block.

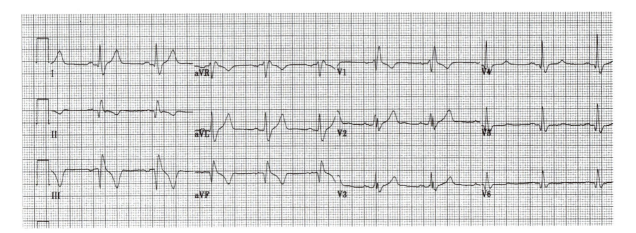

ECG 23. Right bundle branch block does not obscure the diagnosis of myocardial infarction. Right bundle branch block is defined by a terminal vector that results in the large R′ in V_1 and broad terminal S in V_6 and often in lead I. Infarcts are defined in the initial portion of the QRS, so these diagnoses are not mutually exclusive on the electrocardiogram. This is an example of a right bundle branch block with broad Q-waves in the inferior leads of an old inferior infarct. Probably there also is some lateral involvement with the Q-waves in leads V_5 and V_6.

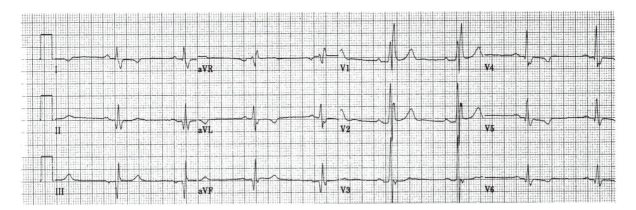

ECG 24. This electrocardiogram, which is similar to the previous tracing, has some important differences. It is a right bundle branch block and an old inferior infarction. Usually with a right bundle branch block there are T-wave inversions in the right precordial leads. In this case, the T-wave is upright, suggesting a primary T-wave abnormality and supporting the diagnosis of inferior and posterior infarction in the face of a right bundle branch block. Ordinarily, right bundle branch block prevents the diagnosis of posterior infarction, but in this case, the initial vector is prominent and the T-wave is upright in V_1, representing inferoposterior infarct.

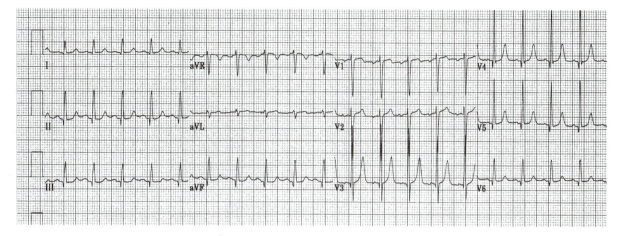

ECG 25. T-waves in this electrocardiogram are prominent. The QT interval actually is relatively prolonged, although with tachycardia that is sometimes hard to assess. There is some slight ST segment elevation, especially in lead V_3, which represents early repolarization. Although the ST segment elevation and prominent T-waves are seen with myocardial infarction, in this case the narrow symmetry of the T-waves should suggest hyperkalemia.

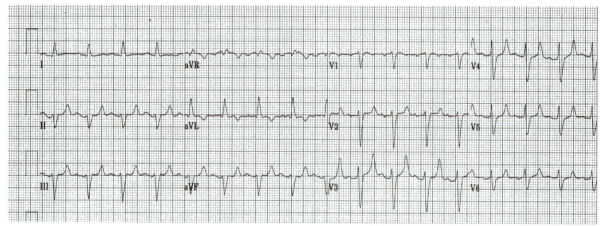

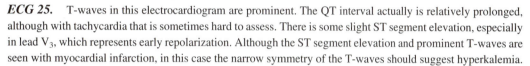

ECG 26. This electrocardiogram also shows prominent symmetric T-waves. It is associated with broadening of the QRS, which is generalized. This is an example of hyperkalemia, but it is hyperkalemia at a level at which the resting membrane potential has become less negative, activation of the action potential in phase 0 is prolonged, and the intraventricular conduction is prolonged. As hyperkalemia evolves, broadening of the QRS producing an intraventricular delay is commonly seen.

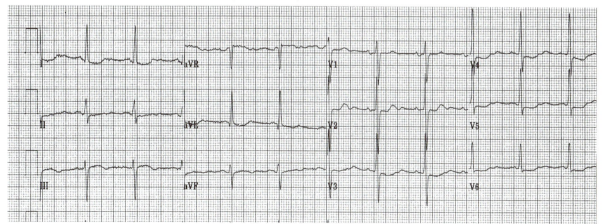

ECG 27. This is an example of hypokalemia that shows ST segment depression in the midprecordium. The T-waves are low and broad, and the U-waves have become prominent with T-U fusion and U-waves that are more prominent than the T-waves with which they are associated.

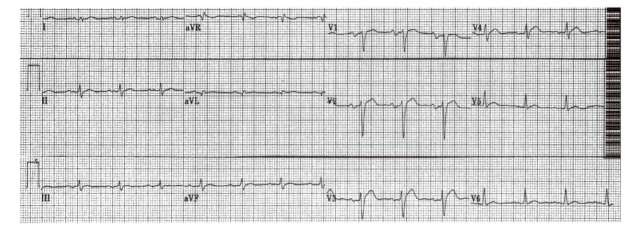

ECG 28. In this electrocardiogram, the T-waves are normal in appearance, but the QT interval is relatively short. This might be passed as a normal electrocardiogram, but it is in fact an example of hypercalcemia.

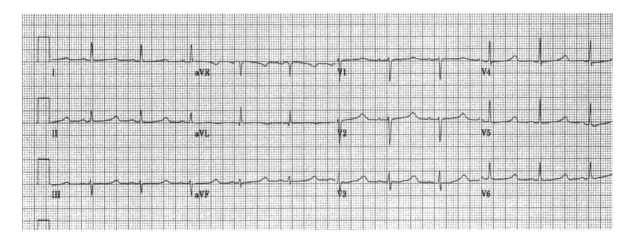

ECG 29. This ECG is the opposite of the last tracing. It shows prolongation of the QT interval. The T-wave, however, has a fairly normal appearance, as is seen with hypocalcemia.

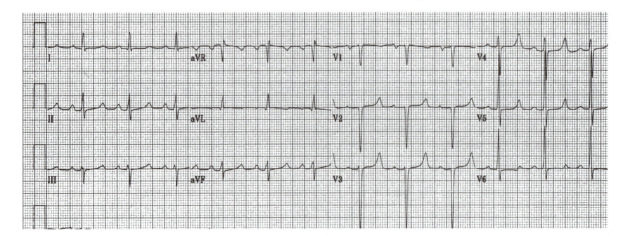

ECG 30. This is a mixed electrolyte abnormality. The QT interval is prolonged, suggesting hypocalcemia. T-waves are symmetric, especially in the midprecordial leads, compatible with hyperkalemia. This was a patient with renal insufficiency in need of dialysis.

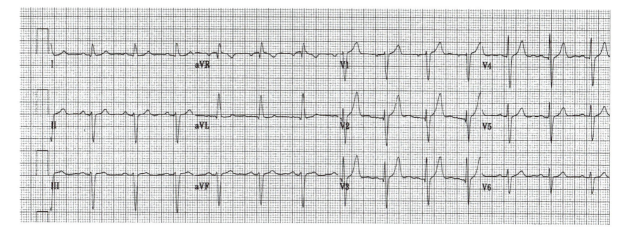

ECG 31. In this electrocardiogram, the dominant finding is marked left-axis deviation. It is associated with small Q-waves in leads I and aVL. The total complex is not wide. This is an example of an anterior hemiblock. The presence of small Q-waves in the right precordial leads is part of the anterior hemiblock pattern and not a sign of myocardial infarction.

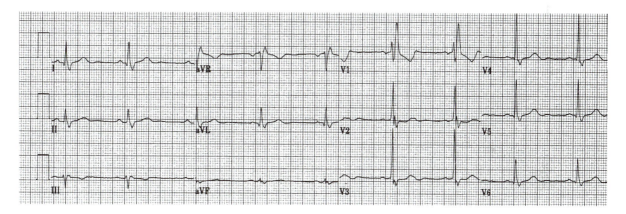

ECG 32. This is a right bundle branch block. This is defined by the broadening of the complex, the terminal wide vector in V_1, and the terminal negative vector in V_6. These are produced by the right ventricular depolarization, unopposed by left ventricular vectors.

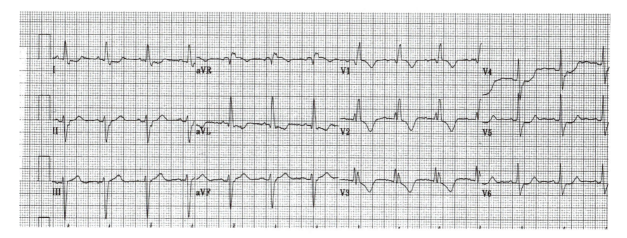

ECG 33. This patient's ECG shows a sinus rhythm with normal PR interval. There is a right bundle branch block with broad R' in lead V_1 and a terminal S in V_6. There also is marked left-axis deviation and small Q-waves in leads I and aVL. This is an example of a bifascicular block: right bundle branch block and anterior fascicular block.

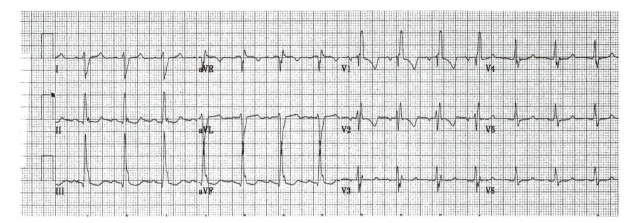

ECG 34. This electrocardiogram shows a sinus rhythm with normal PR interval. There is a right bundle branch block and right-axis deviation. This could be a bifascicular block with right bundle branch block and posterior fascicular block, but posterior fascicular block is a clinical diagnosis. The patient should be examined and right ventricular enlargement excluded before making that diagnosis.

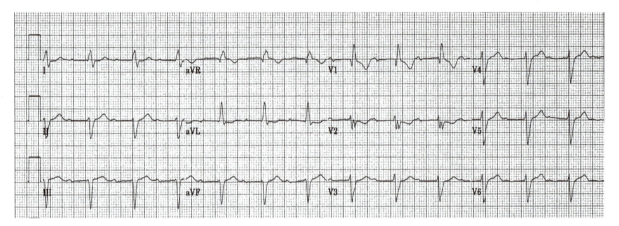

ECG 35. In this electrocardiogram, there is a right bundle branch block with broad R′ in V_1, broad terminal S in V_6, an anterior hemiblock, and first-degree AV block. This is at least a bifascicular block and certainly could be trifascicular, although that cannot be stated with certainty based on the electrocardiogram alone.

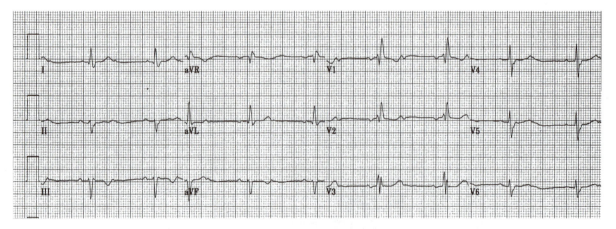

ECG 36. In this electrocardiogram, there are a right bundle branch block and an anterior fascicular block. In addition, most of the electrocardiogram shows a 2:1 AV block. Usually with conducting system defects and a 2:1 block, the AV conduction abnormality is Mobitz type II. In this ECG, however, a Wenckebach sequence is seen at the second and third QRS complexes. The PR interval has a sequential increase followed by a dropped beat with a 3:2 block. If Wenckebach AV block is in one location, it is likely to be the basis of pauses elsewhere. This is not a trifascicular block.

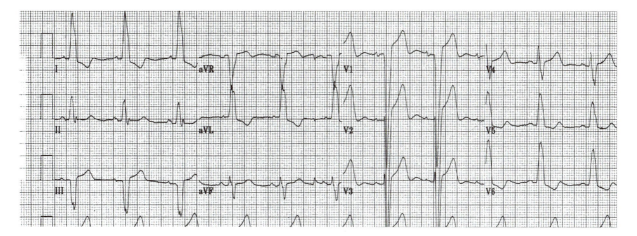

ECG 37.   This is a left bundle branch block. The complexes are > 120 msec; there are no Q-waves in I or V₆ (which would represent normal septal depolarization); and there are secondary repolarization changes in the lateral leads. Based on the QRS, other diagnoses should not be made in the face of a left bundle branch block.

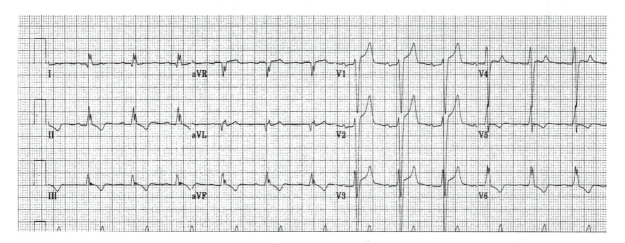

ECG 38.   This electrocardiogram has a wide complex that in V₆ has an appearance suggesting left bundle branch block. There are, however, Q-waves in lead I. Left bundle branch block is defined by the absence of septal Q-waves, and this ECG is more properly interpreted as an intraventricular conduction defect. There is a possibility of a lateral infarct also.

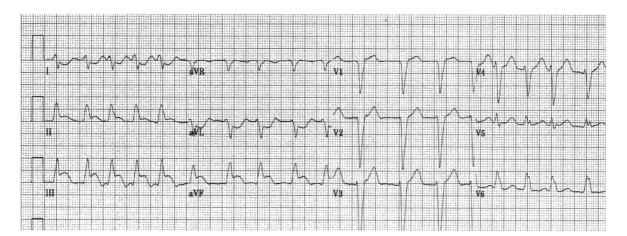

ECG 39.   This is a left bundle branch block with ST segment elevation in the inferior leads and depressions in aVL and lead I, which probably are reciprocal. This is an example of acute inferior infarct in the face of left bundle branch block. The infarct is defined by the ST segment elevation, which is a primary repolarization defect not appropriate for the bundle branch block.

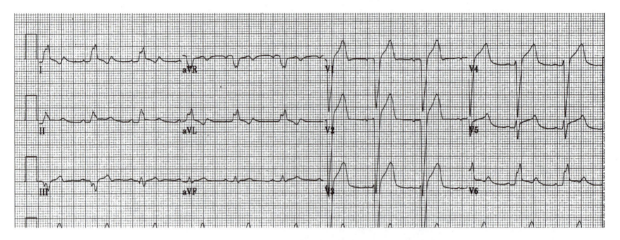

ECG 40. This electrocardiogram also has a bundle branch block. There is generalized ST elevation. This is a primary repolarization finding. The diffuse nature suggests pericarditis. This tracing and the previous one are examples of electrocardiographic diagnoses made with left bundle branch block, based on repolarization changes and not on the basic QRS complexes.

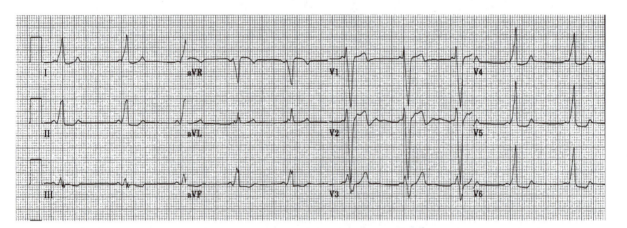

ECG 41. An appearance on this ECG suggests left bundle branch block. It is, however, preexcitation with a short PR interval and a delta wave giving a pseudo bundle branch block appearance. Wolff-Parkinson-White syndrome can mimic almost everything, so always be aware of short PR intervals and delta waves.

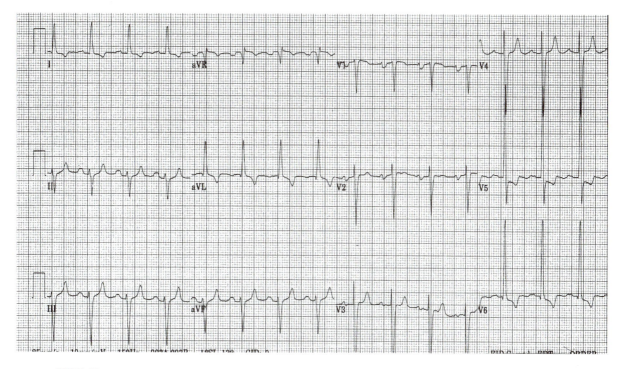

ECG 42. This is a classic example of left ventricular hypertrophy. The voltage is prominent with secondary ST and T-wave changes laterally ("strain"), left-axis deviation, prolongation of the QRS, and left atrial enlargement. The left atrial enlargement is diagnosed by the width of the P-wave, with notching as seen in lead II and the broad terminal negative portion of the P-wave in V_1.

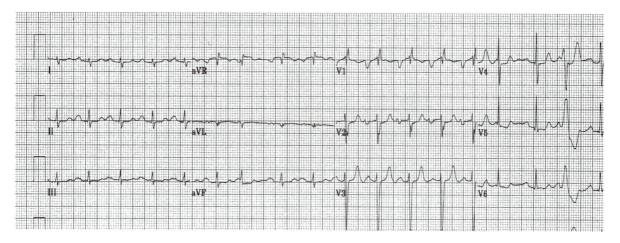

ECG 43. This patient also has left atrial enlargement with a broad P-wave in lead II and a broadly negative terminal component of the P-wave in V_1. This is right ventricular hypertrophy rather than left. It is suggested by the prominent R′ in lead V_1 with T-wave inversion and right-axis deviation. This is a patient with mitral stenosis. There also is one premature ventricular beat.

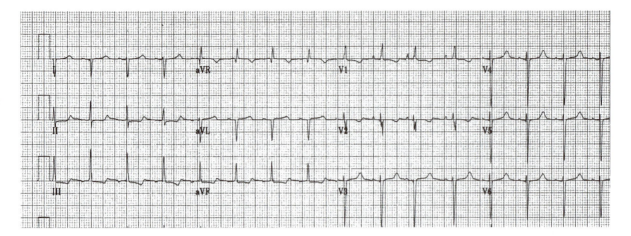

ECG 44. This is another example of right ventricular hypertrophy. In this case it is a dominant R-wave with no S-wave and with T-wave inversion in V_1. This was a young woman with primary pulmonary hypertension. In addition to the prominent R-wave in V_1 with T-wave inversion, there is right-axis deviation, and the S-waves are deep relative to R in the lateral leads.

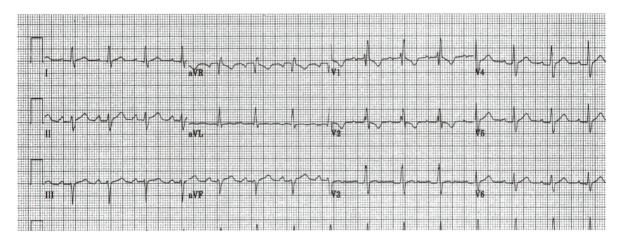

ECG 45. Here is an incomplete right bundle branch block with rSR′ and R′>S with T-wave inversion, suggesting right ventricular hypertrophy. This pattern of right ventricular hypertrophy can be seen with mitral stenosis and also with atrial septal defects. The usual atrial septal defect will have right-axis deviation. An atrial septal defect in which left-axis deviation is seen is usually an ostium primum defect. Notching of the P-wave raises the possibility of left atrial enlargement. This was a young man with ostium primum atrial septal defect, cleft mitral valve, and significant mitral insufficiency.

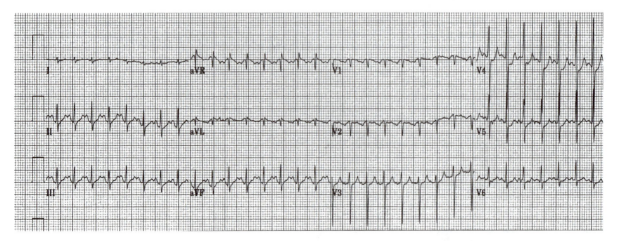

ECG 46. This electrocardiogram shows a significant tachycardia. The differential diagnosis for narrow complex tachycardia is extensive. In this case, the patient's condition is a sinus tachycardia.

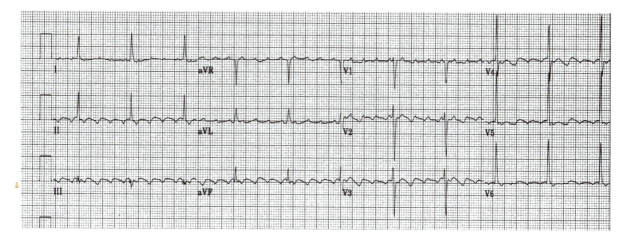

ECG 47.   This is another patient with tachycardia. The ventricular rate is controlled. The atrial rate is very rapid at around 300. It has a negative ''sawtooth'' appearance in the inferior leads and demonstrates classic atrial flutter. The patient either is taking a medication that is slowing AV conduction or he or she also has associated AV conduction disease.

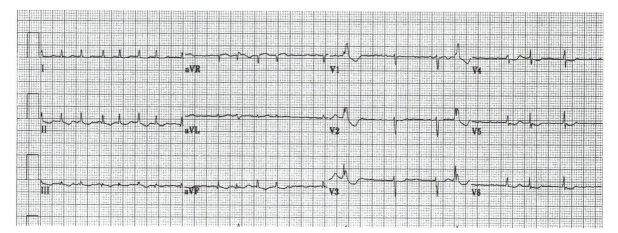

ECG 48.   This is an irregularly irregular rhythm: atrial fibrillation. There are occasional wider beats that have a right bundle branch block configuration. These are examples of Ashman's phenomenon.

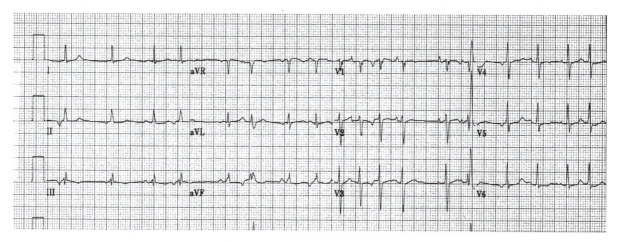

ECG 49.   This also is an irregularly irregular narrow complex tachycardia. There are fairly distinct atrial waves, however. They are chaotic, and there is a wide variety of wave forms. This is an example of multifocal atrial tachycardia. The 6th and 14th beats have right bundle branch block aberrancy and also are examples of Ashman's phenomenon. Multifocal atrial tachycardia is usually related to decompensated lung disease. Its treatment is best accomplished through treating the pulmonary problem.

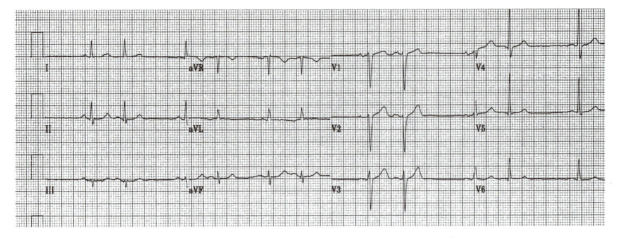

ECG 50.　In this ECG, the rhythm is sinus. It has a bigeminal pattern. Each of the premature beats is preceded by a P-wave—but a P-wave that has a configuration different from the basic sinus rhythm. This is atrial bigeminy.

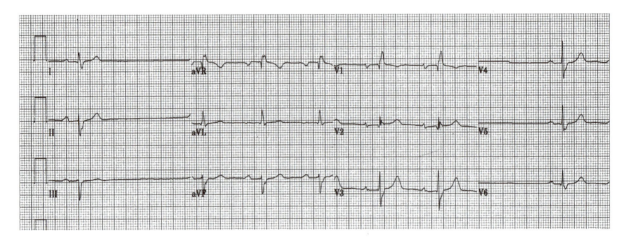

ECG 51.　In this electrocardiogram, the obvious problem is the pauses that are seen. There is no obvious premature activity that has resulted in the pause, so this is either a sinus arrest or sinus exit block.

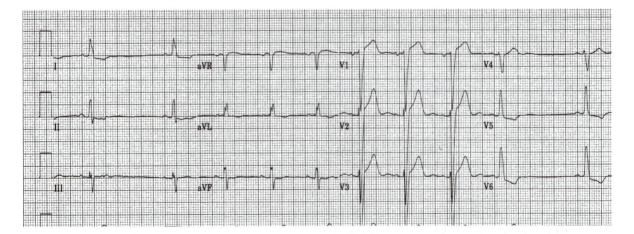

ECG 52.　In this electrocardiogram, which shows an incomplete left bundle branch block, there are also pauses. Here, however, the T-wave preceding the pause can be seen to have a distorted shoulder and a modified downslope that represents an atrial depolarization. This is an example of blocked premature atrial beats.

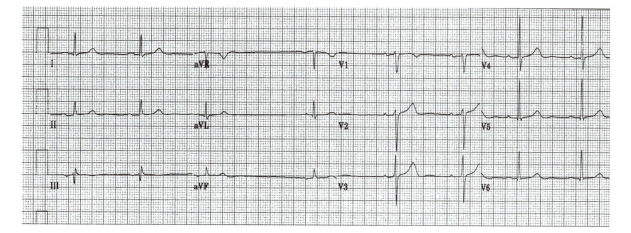

ECG 53. This electrocardiogram shows a pause. It also is a blocked PAC. It is a subtle finding with slight peaking of the T-wave preceding the pause compared to other T waves in the same lead.

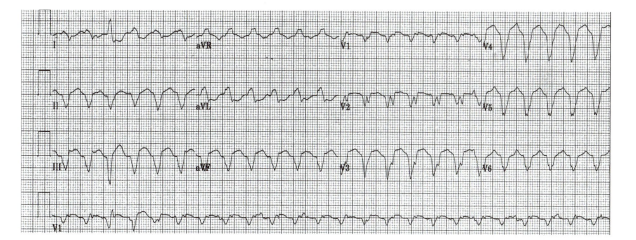

ECG 54. This is an example of a wide complex tachycardia, ventricular tachycardia. The key things to look for are AV dissociation, which is evident here as P-waves that pass through the regular ventricular activity (especially seen in the V_1 rhythm strip). Additionally, the third beat is a hybrid or a fusion beat. AV dissociation has good specificity for ventricular tachycardia, but fusion beats are especially specific. This ECG does show morphologic changes that go along with ventricular tachycardia in that there is anterior negative concordance of voltage.

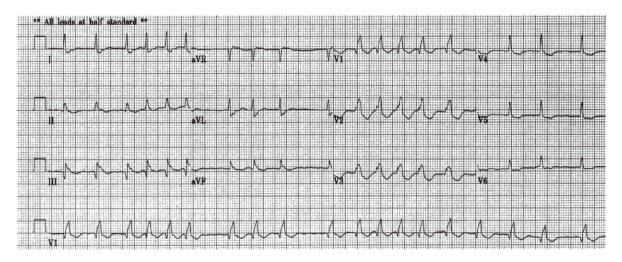

ECG 55.   This is a wide complex tachycardia. It has a right bundle branch-like pattern. It is grossly irregular. Although ventricular tachycardia can be subtly irregular, it never is irregular to this degree. This is atrial fibrillation with an intraventricular conduction defect—in this case, a right bundle branch block.

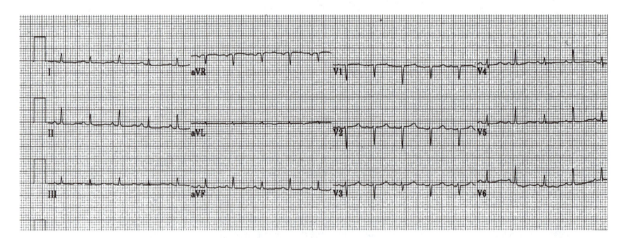

ECG 56.   The rhythm is sinus tachycardia. The voltage is low and alternates. This is an example of electrical alternans in a patient with cardiac tamponade, a potential cardiac emergency.

Valvular Heart Disease

Brian P. Griffin

Valvular heart disease remains an important cause of cardiac morbidity, despite a decline in the incidence of rheumatic valvular disease in the developed world. Congenital valvular anomalies (e.g., bicuspid aortic valve, which is seen in approximately 2% of the population) and myxomatous degeneration of valvular tissue (e.g., mitral valve prolapse) are the most common conditions encountered today.

Valvular heart disease may cause problems when the valve becomes stenotic, is regurgitant, or as frequently occurs, there is a combined stenotic and regurgitant lesion. Multiple valves often are either affected by the primary disease process (e.g., rheumatic fever) or secondarily affected by the pressure or volume effects of another valve lesion. For instance, tricuspid regurgitation commonly is associated with mitral disease because mitral disease increases pulmonary pressures, thus causing the right ventricle to dilate. Right ventricular dilatation causes the tricuspid valve ring or annulus to dilate and, thus, causes the valve to leak.

Stenotic lesions produce problems by reducing cardiac output, particularly during stress, and by increasing the pressure in the chambers proximal to the valve. The heart chambers respond to increased pressure first by hypertrophying and then by dilating. Conversely, regurgitant lesions cause problems by increasing the volume load on the ventricles. For instance, in mitral and aortic regurgitation, the left ventricle dilates to maintain a normal cardiac output. Eventually, with more severe degrees of regurgitation, ventricular dilatation fails to compensate for the regurgitation, and cardiac output falls.

CLINICAL PRESENTATION

Many patients with valvular heart disease are asymptomatic for years. The onset of symptoms often is insidious, and pa-

tients often unwittingly decrease their activities to reduce their symptoms. An acute onset of symptoms may signal valvular disruption (e.g., acute myocardial infarction with papillary muscle rupture or following endocarditis), an acute volume load (e.g., as in pregnancy), or the onset of a tachyarrhythmia (e.g., atrial fibrillation). Symptoms include the following:

- Dyspnea is the most common symptom in valvular heart disease. It usually results from high pulmonary venous pressures, which increase the transudation of fluid into the alveoli and result in diminished gas exchange. It is seen relatively early in mitral stenosis and later in the course of aortic and mitral regurgitation and of aortic stenosis. It is important to determine how limiting the dyspnea is, because therapeutic interventions usually are based on the severity of symptoms rather than on the severity of the disease process itself.
- Chest discomfort may be anginal because of oxygen supply/demand mismatch (e.g., aortic or mitral stenosis) or nonanginal (e.g., mitral valve prolapse).
- Syncope usually results from an inability to increase cardiac output during peripheral vasodilatation (e.g., with exercise). It is seen in conditions that severely limit cardiac output (e.g., aortic stenosis, mitral stenosis with pulmonary hypertension).
- Palpitations result from an arrhythmia (e.g., atrial fibrillation in mitral disease).
- Embolic events may occur when material on abnormal valves (e.g., calcium) embolizes. An important cause of embolization is endocarditis, and another important cause of embolization is thrombus formation in the left atrium during mitral valve disease.
- Fatigue is common in all forms of valvular heart disease, particularly those associated with low cardiac output (e.g., mitral or aortic stenosis).

DIAGNOSIS

PHYSICAL EXAMINATION

The physical examination is critical to the evaluation of patients with valvular heart disease. It is important to examine thoroughly all aspects of the cardiovascular system. These aspects include:

- *Pulse:* Best palpated at the carotid artery. Assess the rhythm, rate, character (e.g., slow upstroke in aortic stenosis, collapsing in aortic regurgitation).
- *Venous pressure:* Height, wave pattern: large "A" waves in pulmonary hypertension, pulmonary stenosis; large "V" waves in tricuspid regurgitation.
- *Blood pressure:* Narrow pulse pressure (i.e., difference between systolic and diastolic blood pressure) in aortic stenosis, wide pulse pressure with low diastolic pressure in aortic regurgitation.
- *Facies:* Cyanosis, often marked peripherally in low output. "Mitral facies" in mitral stenosis (i.e., purplish red cheeks).

HEART EXAMINATION

Palpation

Palpate for cardiomegaly and the position of the apex beat. In addition, palpate for the following:

- *Thrills:* Thrills occur with significant valvular lesions and result from turbulent blood flow at the site of the valve lesion. They can be systolic or diastolic in timing, and they are most common with aortic stenosis, ventricular septal defect, and pulmonic stenosis. Diastolic thrills are less common, but they occur with mitral stenosis and aortic regurgitation.
- *Character of apex beat:* Tapping is less sustained than normal in mitral stenosis and is more sustained than normal or heaving in left ventricular hypertrophy.
- *Right ventricular heave:* Right ventricular heave is felt along left sternal border in right ventricular hypertrophy.
- *Other sounds:* The second heart sound often is palpable in pulmonary hypertension, and S_3 and S_4 may be palpable as well.

Auscultation

Auscultate for the following:

- *First heart sound:* The first heart sound is loud in mitral/tricuspid stenosis and soft in mitral regurgitation.
- *Second heart sound:* The second heart sound has a loud pulmonary component in pulmonary hypertension and a soft aortic component in severe aortic stenosis.
- *Third heart sound:* The third heart sound is a low-pitched, filling sound best heard with the bell of a stethoscope. It is common during severe mitral regurgitation and left ventricular dilatation and may be physiological in young people.
- *Fourth sound:* The fourth heart sound is the atrial filling sound. It is heard during conditions with left ventricular hypertrophy (e.g., aortic stenosis).
- *Opening snap:* The opening snap is heard at the lower left sternal border during mitral stenosis. The opening snap follows S_2. The shorter the time interval between S_2 and the opening snap, the more severe the mitral stenosis.
- *Ejection sounds:* Early systolic sounds at the base of the heart are heard in congenitally abnormal but mobile valves (e.g., bicuspid aortic valve).
- *Midsystolic clicks:* Systolic sounds heard with myxomatous mitral valve prolapse because of tensing of the redundant leaflets.

Assess murmurs in terms of timing, location, intensity, and provocative maneuvers. Timing involves the following:

- Systolic
    - Ejection (peaking in midsystole): Aortic stenosis, pulmonic stenosis, hypertrophic cardiomyopathy.
    - Pansystolic (heard throughout systole, may encompass S_1 and S_2): Mitral regurgitation, tricuspid regurgitation.
    - Late systolic: Mitral valve prolapse, ischemic mitral regurgitation because of papillary muscle dysfunction.
- Diastolic
    - Early, decrescendo: Aortic regurgitation, pulmonary regurgitation.
    - Mid: Mitral stenosis, tricuspid stenosis.
    - Presystolic (late diastole): Mitral stenosis in normal sinus rhythm.

Location involves the following:

- *Apical:* Mitral murmurs; aortic murmur may radiate to the apex.
- *Base:* Aortic, pulmonary murmurs.
- *Sternal border:* Tricuspid murmurs, aortic and pulmonary regurgitation.
- *Radiation:* To axilla with mitral, to neck and apex with aortic.

Regarding intensity, severity of the lesion often relates to the loudness of the murmur in systolic murmurs (e.g., aortic stenosis, mitral regurgitation). The severity of diastolic murmurs relates more to the duration of the murmur than to intensity.

Provocative maneuvers include:

- *Respiration:* Right-sided lesions are louder with inspiration (i.e., increased flow through the right heart). Left-sided are louder with expiration.
- *Valsalva:* The Valsalva maneuver decreases intracardiac

volume and reduces the intensity of most murmurs. Exceptions are the murmurs of hypertrophic cardiomyopathy, which becomes louder, and of mitral valve prolapse, which becomes longer and louder. A reduction in intracardiac volume accentuates outflow obstruction in hypertrophic cardiomyopathy and prolapse in mitral valve prolapse syndrome.

- *Position:* With standing, intracardiac volume decreases; therefore, most murmurs decrease in intensity (except those of hypertrophic cardiomyopathy and mitral valve prolapse). Squatting accentuates intracardiac volume. Therefore, most murmurs become louder, but those of mitral valve prolapse and hypertrophic cardiomyopathy usually decrease.

STUDIES

Electrocardiography

During electrocardiography, look for atrial fibrillation, left or right atrial enlargement, and signs of left ventricular or right ventricular hypertrophy.

Chest Radiography

A chest radiograph is useful in detecting cardiac chamber enlargement, pulmonary venous hypertension, and more overt signs of pulmonary congestion.

Doppler Echocardiography

Echocardiography is the most important test currently used for the diagnosis of valvular heart disease. It can define the specific valves that are affected, the type of lesion (i.e., stenosis or regurgitation), and the severity of the lesion. Transesophageal echocardiography is especially useful when chest-wall images are poor, a prosthesis has been implanted, and while looking at the left atrium for thrombus.

Severity of Stenosis Planimetry using 2-dimensional echocardiography can directly measure the area of the valve opening in mitral stenosis. This is the most reliable measurement in mitral stenosis, but it often is technically difficult.

Velocity across the valve as measured by Doppler can be converted to a pressure gradient using the Bernoulli equation:

$$Pressure\ gradient = 4 \times Velocity^2$$

Thus, for example, if a peak velocity measured across the aortic valve is 4 m/s, then the peak pressure gradient across the valve is 64 mm Hg.

The pressure gradient depends on the flow across the valve. The higher the flow for any given area, the higher the

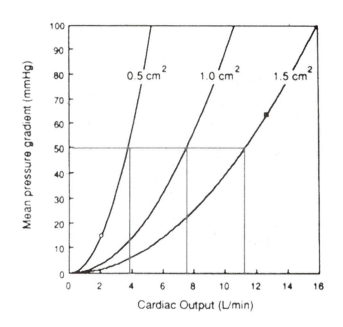

Figure 64.1. Relationship of flow to pressure gradient and valve area. A mean pressure gradient of 50 mm Hg across the aortic valve is possible with valve area of 0.5 to 1.5 cm^2 depending on the flow (i.e., cardiac output) through the valve.

pressure gradient will be (Fig. 64.1). Therefore, pressure gradients should be interpreted with knowledge of the cardiac output and function.

Estimation of Valve Area The continuity equation usually is applied to the aortic valve. Because of the law of conservation of mass–energy, the flow into the valve is equivalent to that leaving the valve. Flow (F) is the product of the cross-sectional area (A) at a given point and the velocity (v) at that point, or

$$F = Av$$

The velocity (v_p) and cross-sectional area (A_p) below the aortic valve in the left ventricular outflow tract can be measured readily, as can the velocity at the site of maximal narrowing at the aortic valve (v_d), which is highest velocity recorded (Fig. 64.2). The cross-sectional area at the valve itself (A_d) can be derived as:

$$A_d = A_p v_p / v_d$$

Pressure Half-Time In mitral stenosis, severity of stenosis inversely relates to the time it takes for the initial pressure to fall to half its original value. The valve area has been empirically derived as 220/Pressure Half-Time. The shorter the pressure half-time, the less severe the stenosis.

Assessment of Regurgitant Lesions Qualitative assessment of lesion severity is done by using the flow disturbance associated with the regurgitation on color-flow mapping. Quantitative assessment uses the determination of flow across the

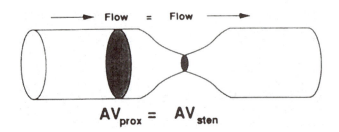

Figure 64.2.   Flow is the product of area and velocity at a given point, and the continuity equation uses this to calculate the aortic valve area. Flow in the left ventricular outflow tract below the valve can be calculated from the known velocity (v) and area (A) at this level (A_{prox} v_{prox}). The stenotic valve area can be derived from the velocity at this point (v_{sten}) as $\frac{A_{prox}\ v_{prox}}{v_{sten}}$.

regurgitant valve and across a normal valve. Regurgitant flow is the total flow through the regurgitant valve minus that through the normal valve. The regurgitant fraction equals the regurgitant volume divided by the total volume flow (i.e., forward plus backward).

Newer methods are becoming available to measure regurgitant flow directly and the size of the regurgitant orifice. These use the flow field that is proximal to the regurgitant orifice (proximal convergence or pisa).

ASSESSMENT OF EFFECTS OF VALVULAR DISEASE ON VENTRICULAR FUNCTION

Increasing ventricular size over time in the absence of symptoms is an indication for surgical intervention in patients with mitral and aortic regurgitation. The response of the left ventricle, both in size and function, to exercise stress is increasingly used to assess the effect of valvular regurgitation on contractile function and to help determine optimal timing for surgery.

CARDIAC CATHETERIZATION

Cardiac catheterization is less critical today because of reliable, noninvasive measures. It still is used, however, when there is a discrepancy between clinical findings and noninvasive techniques or to confirm noninvasive findings in selected patients. It also is necessary when coronary disease is suspected or must be excluded (e.g., in patients who need surgery).

With cardiac catheterization, the pressure gradients across the valves can be measured directly rather than simply being derived, as they are with Doppler. The effects of maneuvers such as exercise also can be used to determine the severity of a lesion. Valve area is derived empirically using the Gorlin equation from the flow (thermodilution or Fick technique) and the pressure gradient across the valve.

Regurgitation usually is assessed semiquantitatively, by direct injection of dye into the left ventricle to assess mitral regurgitation or into the aorta to assess aortic regurgitation. The opacification of the chamber receiving the regurgitant flow is then determined.

TREATMENT

General principles for treating patients with valvular heart disease include:

1. Assess severity of symptoms.
2. Determine the nature of the valvular lesion and its severity.
3. Assess the effects of the lesion on ventricular function.
4. Assess for other cardiac (or other) pathologies.

Intervention is indicated in the following situations:

- Limiting symptoms with significant stenosis
- Limiting symptoms with significant regurgitation
- Significant left ventricular dysfunction or progressive left ventricular dilatation with severe mitral or aortic regurgitation

Prophylaxis for endocarditis is indicated whenever blood flow at a structurally abnormal valve is turbulent. The benefits of prophylaxis have never been fully established, but it is usual to err on the side of administration. Patients with mild leaks in otherwise normal valves (e.g., physiologic leaks at the mitral, tricuspid, or most commonly, pulmonic valve) have a relatively low risk for endocarditis and probably do not require prophylaxis.

SPECIFIC VALVE LESIONS

MITRAL STENOSIS

Mitral stenosis is twice as common in women as in men. It usually is rheumatic in origin, though congenital mitral stenosis also occurs. The valve becomes fibrosed and tends to calcify with time. Reduction in the size of the mitral valve orifice lowers the cardiac output, and it tends to raise left atrial and pulmonary venous and arterial pressures. In patients with severe mitral stenosis, pulmonary hypertension as high as that of the systemic vasculature may occur. Flow across the mitral valve occurs in diastole and is critically dependent on the heart rate; therefore, reduction in the time for diastolic filling by increased heart rate worsens the symptoms and can cause acute pulmonary edema. Symptomatic deterioration often results from the onset of atrial fibrillation.

Complications of mitral stenosis may include atrial arrhythmia, atrial fibrillation, and thromboembolism. Left atrial enlargement and atrial fibrillation predispose patients to atrial thrombus and thromboembolism. This may occur in as many as 25% of those who are not anticoagulated, and it often occurs silently.

Diagnosis

The symptoms of mitral stenosis are:

*   Dyspnea
*   Fatigue
*   Hemoptysis (from pulmonary venous hypertension)
*   Angina, even syncope, if there is pulmonary hypertension
*   Edema secondary to right heart failure

   The signs of mitral stenosis are:

*   Tapping apex beat from a loud first heart sound if the valve is pliable.
*   Diastolic thrill in severe stenosis (classically described as being like a purring cat).
*   Palpable P_2 if there is pulmonary hypertension.
*   Loud S_1 because the valve remains open at the end of diastole and shuts abruptly with the onset of systole. As the valve calcifies, the S_1 gets softer.
*   Opening snap indicates a pliable valve and disappears as the valve calcifies. The opening snap often is heard at the left sternal border rather than at the apex, and with the diaphragm rather than with the bell of the stethoscope.
*   Diastolic murmur with presystolic accentuation in sinus rhythm.
*   Best heard at apex with the bell of the stethoscope and the patient on his or her left side.
*   Associated pulmonary hypertension leads to a loud P_2, right ventricular heave, tricuspid regurgitation. and pulmonary insufficiency (i.e., Graham-Steel murmur).
*   Occasionally, no murmur is heard if flow through the valve is very low (e.g., as with severe pulmonary hypertension).

Signs indicating severe stenosis include a long diastolic murmur; short duration of the interval between S_2 and the opening snap, thus indicating high atrial pressure even at the end of systole; and a loud P_2.

Differential Diagnosis The differential diagnosis of diastolic murmur includes tricuspid stenosis, Austin-Flint murmur of aortic regurgitation (i.e., aortic regurgitant jet hits the mitral valve and prevents full diastolic opening), left atrial myxoma, and cor triatriatum. Silent mitral stenosis with pulmonary hypertension simulates primary pulmonary hypertension.

Studies Electrocardiography shows left atrial enlargement, right atrial enlargement, right axis, and right ventricular hypertrophy. Chest radiography may show left atrial enlargement, prominence of main pulmonary artery Kerley B lines with edema, and pulmonary hemosiderosis. Doppler echocardiography shows the following:

*   Doming of the mitral valve, which has restricted opening. The opening may be measured directly by

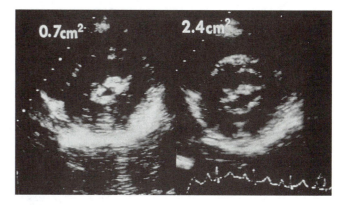

Figure 64.3. Planimetry of the mitral valve by echocardiography. The mitral valve area increases after balloon valvuloplasty (**right panel**) compared with baseline (**left panel**).

planimetry in the short-axis (Fig. 64.3), which usually is the most reliable method for assessing severity of the narrowing.
*   Pressure gradient across the valve (normal, < 5 mm Hg) may be as high as 20 mm Hg in those with severe mitral stenosis. The valve area also is derived empirically from the pressure half-time (discussed earlier).
*   Decrease in valve area (normal, 4–6 cm^2), to less than 1 cm^2 in patients with critical mitral stenosis.
*   Mitral valve score based on thickness, calcification, mobility, and involvement of subvalvular apparatus on transthoracic echocardiography is used to determine the likelihood of success for percutaneous mitral valvuloplasty. The score may vary from 0 to 16. If score is greater than 8, valvuloplasty will have less chance of success.
*   Presence of associated lesions such as mitral, aortic, or tricuspid regurgitation is sought.
*   Stress echocardiography is increasingly used to assess functional capacity and the effects of exercise on valve pressure gradients and pulmonary pressures (as derived from the velocity of tricuspid regurgitation). This is especially useful when patients have severe stenosis but deny symptoms or when the degree of stenosis apparently is mild but the symptoms are more severe than would be anticipated.

   Cardiac catheterization is used to determine the presence of accompanying coronary disease, and it also is useful in confirming the severity of mitral disease. Knowledge regarding the effect of exercise on the mitral pressure gradient may be useful when severity of the lesion is in doubt. Cardiac catheterization is necessary for percutaneous mitral valvuloplasty (Fig. 64.4).

Treatment

Survival rates are lower among patients with mitral stenosis in whom symptoms have appeared. Patients increasingly are

Figure 64.4. The mitral valve gradient is shaded area between left atrial (LA) and left ventricular (LV) pressure in diastole. **Left,** The gradient before percutaneous valvuloplasty. **Right,** The reduced gradient after successful balloon valvuloplasty.

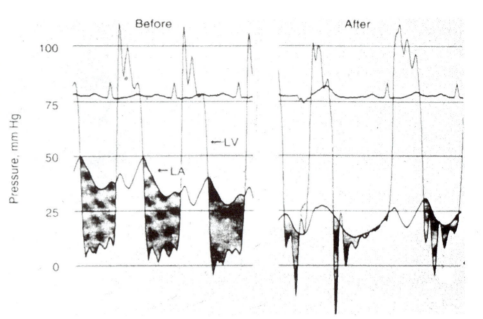

treated with balloon valvuloplasty, which has results similar to those of open mitral commissurotomy regarding symptoms and valve area at 2 years. Balloon valvuloplasty is feasible if the valve is pliable and relatively uncalcified (as assessed by the echocardiographic splitability score), if no more than mild mitral regurgitation is present (i.e., mitral regurgitation usually increases one grade with the balloon procedure), if no thrombus is present in the left atrium (i.e., a thrombus could be dislodged by wires during valvuloplasty), and if severe tricuspid regurgitation is absent (i.e., severe tricuspid regurgitation often persists following a balloon procedure).

Asymptomatic patients usually can be treated conservatively. Indications for intervention in patients without symptoms include significant pulmonary hypertension, prophylaxis in those undergoing major surgery during which a large volume shift might be encountered, or women of childbearing age with severe stenosis who wish to start a family.

With symptomatic patients, consider intervention with balloon valvuloplasty or surgery. Valve replacement is indicated in patients with calcified valves or severe mitral regurgitation.

Patients with mitral stenosis must be monitored closely during pregnancy, because the volume load and tachycardia may cause severe, symptomatic deterioration even in those with mild mitral stenosis. The risk of heart failure is greatest during the first trimester and at delivery. Careful monitoring and slowing of the heart rate will allow most patients with mitral stenosis to carry their pregnancy to term without intervention. In those with severe, symptomatic deterioration, commissurotomy (preferably with a balloon) is indicated.

With medical treatment, control of heart rate in patients with atrial fibrillation is important. In older patients who are not considered to be good surgical candidates, rate control and diuretics may effectively reduce symptoms. In younger patients, prophylaxis against rheumatic fever usually is required. Patients with chronic atrial fibrillation and mitral stenosis have a high risk for thromboembolism and should receive anticoagulation.

Surgical treatment consists of open commissurotomy in which the fused mitral valve leaflets are opened under direct vision by the surgeon or prosthetic valve insertion.

MITRAL REGURGITATION

Etiology

Primary mitral regurgitation is an abnormality of the valve or apparatus. The causes of primary mitral regurgitation are:

- *Rheumatic:* More often men than women
- *Myxomatous:* Mitral valve prolapse
- *Congenital:* Endocardial cushion defect with primum atrial septal defect.
- *Endocarditis:* Bacterial, marantic, Libman-Sacks disease
- *Ischemic:* Papillary muscle dysfunction or rupture.
- *Young people (<35 years):* Mitral regurgitation most often results from myxomatous disease

Secondary mitral regurgitation results from dilatation of the left ventricle from any cause. This can include ischemia, cardiomyopathy, or aortic valve disease.

Pathophysiology

When there is volume load on the left atrium and left ventricle, the left ventricle initially responds by pumping more vigorously and emptying more completely. Subsequently, there is progressive dilatation, with eventual impairment of left ventricular function. This may be permanent despite valve surgery.

Diagnosis

Mitral regurgitation often is asymptomatic for many years. Dyspnea and heart failure are the most common symptoms, and right heart failure with hepatic congestion and cachexia also are seen.

Signs include no specific pulse findings. The jugular venous pressure often is elevated because of right heart failure.

The murmur generally is holosystolic, louder in expiration, best heard at the apex, and radiates to the axilla. A murmur that radiates to the back indicates a posterior-directed jet (e.g., anterior prolapse of the mitral valve). It often is associated with an S_3 gallop, which is consistent with severe mitral regurgitation and a dilated left ventricle. S_1 usually is soft, and S_2 may be loud in patients with pulmonary hypertension.

Studies Electrocardiography shows a volume overload pattern and left atrial enlargement. Echocardiography allows the anatomy of the valve and cause of the leak to be delineated precisely. It also is useful in determining the severity of the leak, either semiquantitatively by the size and extent of the regurgitant jet on color Doppler or quantitatively as the regurgitant volume. The leak can be quantified by a new color Doppler technique proximal to the hole through which the leaks occurs (i.e., regurgitant orifice). Size of the regurgitant orifice also can be estimated; in patients with severe mitral regurgitation, it usually is greater than 0.3 cm^2.

Change in size of the chambers, particularly the left ventricle, over time is useful for monitoring progress of the lesion and determining need for surgery. The contractile function of the left ventricle is difficult to assess accurately through noninvasive means, because the ventricle is volume loaded and ejects much of its blood back into the lower-pressure left atrium. Left ventricular function always appears to be better than it really is when using ejection indices such as ejection fraction. An ejection fraction of less than 60% should suggest possible contractile dysfunction in this condition.

Increasingly, left ventricular volume measurements are made to determine the appropriate timing of surgery. We have used response of the left ventricle to exercise stress as a means of determining contractile reserve in this condition.

Chest radiography shows left atrial and left ventricular enlargement as well as congestive changes (Fig. 64.5), and cardiac catheterization can determine the severity of mitral regurgitation (using ventriculography) or the presence of coronary disease. Large "V" waves in pulmonary-wedge tracings also suggest severe mitral regurgitation. A succession of pressure–volume loops, as defined using high-fidelity catheters and by changing the loading conditions, allows myocardial elastance to be measured. This is the best load-independent measure of true contractile function in this condition. It remains a research tool, however, because it is difficult to mea-

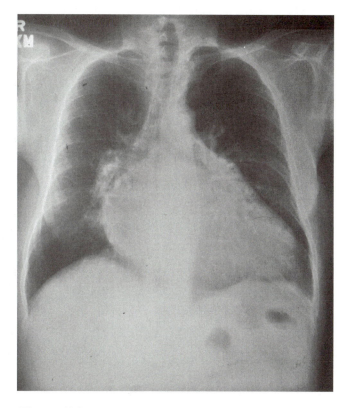

Figure 64.5. Chest radiograph of a patient with chronic mitral regurgitation, showing left atrial and left ventricular enlargement.

sure and requires catheterization as well as intravenous pressors and vasodilators for its measurement.

Treatment

Medical Treatment No treatment is needed for mild regurgitation, but these patients should undergo serial echocardiography. Afterload reduction usually is not indicated in those with primary mitral regurgitation, because this has not been shown to postpone surgical intervention. Antibiotic prophylaxis generally is necessary. If congestive heart failure is present, treatment includes diuretics, digoxin, and afterload reduction. In patients with secondary mitral regurgitation, the primary disease should be treated. Use vasodilators or afterload reduction in patients with cardiomyopathy.

Surgical Treatment Patients with mitral regurgitation eventually develop heart failure. The onset of heart failure is associated with reduced survival rates, as is significant ventricular dysfunction. Mitral regurgitation should be corrected before signs of left ventricular dysfunction or failure become overt. Indications for surgery, therefore, are severe mitral regurgitation with symptoms of heart failure, dyspnea, evidence of deteriorated left ventricular function, or progressive left ventricular enlargement. In asymptomatic patients, an end-systolic dimension of 2.6 cm/m^2 is considered to be an indication for surgery. Because patients with mitral regurgitation should

Figure 64.6.   Effects of exercise on left ventricular ejection fraction (LVEF) and end-systolic volume (ESV) in patients A (**top 3 panels**) and B (**bottom 3 panels**), both of whom have severe mitral regurgitation. In patient A, LVEF increases at peak exercise and ESV falls, thus indicating preserved left ventricular systolic function. The LVEF remains normal following mitral valve repair. In patient B, LVEF declines and ESV increases at peak exercise, thus indicating latent left ventricular dysfunction, which becomes overt once the volume loading effects that mask it are removed following mitral valve repair.

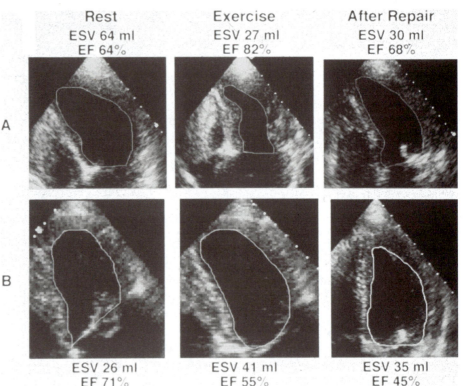

have hyperdynamic function, even a low-normal left ventricular ejection fraction (i.e., <60%) should be considered to be a sign of incipient left ventricular dysfunction, and surgery should be recommended accordingly. Patients in whom the left ventricular ejection fraction fails to increase, or the end-systolic volume fails to decrease, on exercise likely have contractile dysfunction and should be considered for early surgery (Fig. 64.6).

Types of surgical therapy include mitral valve repair and mitral valve replacement.

Mitral valve repair is the surgical intervention of choice. It is very successful in selected patients, especially those with myxomatous valves (i.e., prolapse) or mitral regurgitation from ischemia. It is less likely to be feasible, however, in patients with endocarditis or rheumatic disease. Mitral valve repair has lower mortality rate than replacement (i.e., 1–2%) and allows better preservation of left ventricular systolic function through conservation of valve-supporting structures. Long-term success rates are not known, but initial and intermediate-term results are encouraging.

Mitral valve replacement is indicated when repair is not feasible, especially in rheumatic or elderly patients with calcified valves. Replacement has both a higher mortality rate (i.e., ≥5%) and morbidity rate with thromboembolic complications, especially involving mechanical valves.

MITRAL VALVE PROLAPSE

Mitral valve prolapse is a relatively common condition and is associated with myxomatous degeneration of the mitral valve.

There is an increased amount of acid mucopolysaccharides in the valve tissue. Mitral valve prolapse is associated with Marfan's syndrome, but it usually occurs as an isolated entity involving the mitral valve. Occasionally, however, the tricuspid and the aortic valves also are involved. In prolapse, the annulus may be dilated, and there is elongation of the chordae. The valve leaflets often are redundant, with excess tissue that causes them to prolapse. The degree of abnormality tends to increase with age.

Mitral valve prolapse is associated with a spectrum of abnormality, varying from asymptomatic to severe heart failure resulting from mitral regurgitation. It is most common in young women, and an autosomal-dominant inheritance with incomplete penetrance has been suggested on the basis of familial clustering. Mitral valve prolapse usually is a relatively benign condition, especially in women. In many women, prolapse becomes less prominent with age, which may reflect a relative disproportion between the size of the valve leaflets and the ventricle, which is lessened as the ventricle dilates with increasing age.

Diagnosis

Mitral valve prolapse often is asymptomatic at presentation and detected by a midsystolic click on auscultation. Another presentation is with congestive heart failure from severe mitral regurgitation that results from acute chordal rupture. Patients with prolapse and regurgitation are prone to endocarditis, and they may present as such.

In young women especially, a syndrome of chest pain

of nonanginal quality, paresthesia, and arrhythmia (especially ventricular ectopy) is seen. These symptoms have been attributed to autonomic imbalance, but they are as common in matched populations without prolapse as in those with prolapse.

Complications of mitral valve prolapse (i.e., severe mitral regurgitation, endocarditis, a need for surgery) are more common in older men, though mitral valve prolapse itself is more prevalent in women. Other, more rare presentations include transient ischemic attack, syncope, or sudden death.

Signs are a midsystolic click, with or without a systolic apical murmur. The murmur typically occurs after the click in late systole, but in those with more severe prolapse, the murmur may be holosystolic. Clicks may be present even without echocardiographic prolapse. Maneuvers that decrease intracardiac volume accentuate the click and murmur, causing them to begin earlier in systole.

Studies Electrocardiography commonly shows inferior T-wave inversion. Mitral valve prolapse is a cause of false-positive stress electrocardiograms.

Echocardiography reveals late systolic prolapse of the posterior leaflet on M-mode, as well as thickening and redundancy of the leaflets and chordae. Prolapse of either leaflet (posterior is much commoner) or both can be seen on a two-dimensional echocardiogram. It is important to make the diagnosis with the parasternal or apical long-axis views rather than with the apical views. In apical views, apparent prolapse of the mitral leaflets occurs even in normal patients, because the mitral annulus is not a flat plane but is saddle-shaped. Thus, in this view, the mitral leaflets often appear to be displaced superior to the annular plane. Mitral regurgitation of varying severity may be present as well.

Treatment

If severe mitral regurgitation is present, surgery is indicated. Reassuring patients of the relatively benign nature of this condition often is beneficial. Autonomic symptoms and ventricular ectopy often respond to treatment with β-blockade (in small doses).

According to the American Heart Association guidelines, antibiotic prophylaxis is indicated for dental work and selected procedures if both a click and a murmur are present, but such prophylaxis usually is not required for a click alone.

AORTIC STENOSIS

Aortic stenosis is increasingly common. Approximately 2% of the population have a bicuspid aortic valve, and 80% of cases occur in males. Aortic stenosis may occur at, above, or below the valve.

Etiology

The causes of aortic (valvular) stenosis are:

- Congenital (bicuspid, occasionally unicuspid)
- Rheumatic
- Degenerative (valvular calcification)

Subaortic (nonvalvular) stenosis occurs because of a congenital membrane that is seen below the aortic valve in the left ventricular outflow tract. Hypertrophic cardiomyopathy is a dynamic obstruction of the left ventricular outflow tract as the left ventricle contracts. Supravalvular aortic stenosis is associated with hypercalcemia.

Pathophysiology

Obstruction of the aortic valve initially leads to increased left ventricular hypertrophy and then to left ventricular dilatation and failure. The normal aortic valve opens from 3 to 4 cm^2. The valve area is greater than 1.5 cm^2 in patients with mild aortic stenosis, 1.0 to 1.5 cm^2 in those with moderate stenosis, and less than 1 cm^2 in those with severe stenosis. Critical aortic stenosis is present when the valve area is less than 0.75 cm^2. Normalization of the valve area, as based on the body surface area, often is useful. A valve area of less than 0.5 cm^2/m^2 is considered to be critical stenosis.

The pressure gradient across the valve also is used to indicate the severity of aortic stenosis, but this depends on the flow. In patients with normal heart function and without significant aortic regurgitation, a mean gradient of 50 mm Hg by Doppler or a peak-to-peak gradient of 50 mm Hg at cardiac catheterization is consistent with severe aortic stenosis. In patients with heart failure, flow may be reduced, thus giving a small gradient across the aortic valve and underestimating the degree of stenosis. Aortic regurgitation increases the flow across the valve and, in turn, the gradient for any degree of stenosis. It generally is best to measure the valve area rather than relying on the pressure gradient alone.

Diagnosis

The symptoms of aortic stenosis are:

- Angina in patients without coronary disease because of mismatch between the blood supply and demand, especially of the subendocardium of the hypertrophied heart.
- Dyspnea because of increased pulmonary capillary pressure.
- Syncope caused by inability of the heart to increase output with systemic vasodilatation, thus leading to decreased cerebral perfusion. Arrhythmia also can cause syncope or sudden death in these patients.

The signs of aortic stenosis are:

- Pulse is anacrotic (i.e., pulsus parvus et tardus), with slow delayed upstroke. This is the most reliable physical sign of significant aortic stenosis.
- Pulse usually is best examined at the carotid artery.
- Systolic thrill often is felt in patients with critical aortic stenosis.

- In young people with mobile valves, an ejection click may be heard.
- A harsh ejection systolic murmur over aortic area radiating to neck, usually with a soft S_2 and S_4, is heard. The murmur often radiates to the apex as well.

Studies Electrocardiography reveals left atrial enlargement and left ventricular hypertrophy. Doppler echocardiography reveals a thickened, abnormal valve, and this study can define severity of the lesion with the pressure gradient and valve area. Cardiac catheterization is used to assess the valve area and pressure gradient, but it usually is not indicated if Doppler gradients appear to be reliable, the patient is younger than 40 years, and does not have angina (Fig. 64.7).

Treatment

Survival rates are lower among patients in whom symptoms have appeared. Once left ventricular dysfunction or congestive heart failure occurs, the 2-year survival rate is very low. Asymptomatic patients with severe aortic stenosis, except for young patients with severe congenital aortic stenosis, have a relatively low risk of death. In studies, patients who died suddenly with aortic stenosis usually had the onset of symptoms before death. In older patients, especially those with calcific aortic stenosis, the asymptomatic interval in severe aortic stenosis usually is relatively short (typically 2–3 years).

Therefore, patients with symptoms of syncope, angina, or dyspnea and severe aortic stenosis should be considered for surgery. No treatment usually is indicated in patients without symptoms, except in those with severe stenosis and resultant left ventricular dysfunction or in those with severe aortic stenosis and pressure gradients of greater than 100 mm Hg who may have an increased risk of sudden death. Asymptomatic, severe aortic stenosis patients must be monitored closely with serial echocardiography at 6-month intervals (at least) and must be alerted to report their symptoms. In older patients with calcific aortic stenosis, elective surgery may be considered, even among those who are asymptomatic, given the high likelihood of its being necessary anyway. Asymptomatic patients with severe aortic stenosis should avoid heavy exertion, and young patients with aortic stenosis should refrain from competitive sports.

In young patients with fused commissures, aortic valvotomy provides good palliation for years. Often, this treatment results in significant aortic regurgitation, but it also obviates a prosthesis while growth is still occurring. Prosthetic valve replacement may be either mechanical or bioprosthetic. Biologic valves should be avoided in young patients, because early degeneration is common. The mortality rate typically is from 2 to 3%, though it is less in young patients.

Homograft implantation using cadaveric human valves has good intermediate-term results, but the long-term results are not known. This procedure does not require long-term anticoagulation. Aortic valve repair is possible at some centers in selected patients with congenitally bicuspid valves.

The Ross procedure involves autotransplantation of the native pulmonic valve to the aortic position and a pulmonary homograft to the pulmonary position. This is indicated in adolescent patients, because the autograft grows with the patient. The procedure, however, is technically complex.

Balloon valvuloplasty accomplished with percutaneous dilatation of the aortic valve is feasible in patients with congenital stenosis and even calcific stenosis. Results are better in younger patients. In older patients, it is used as a palliative procedure in those who cannot withstand surgery, and most often as a bridge to surgery. Short-term hemodynamic results are reasonable, and early restenosis (≤6 months) is the rule. Survival rates are not affected in those patients who cannot undergo valve replacement. Morbidity and mortality rates,

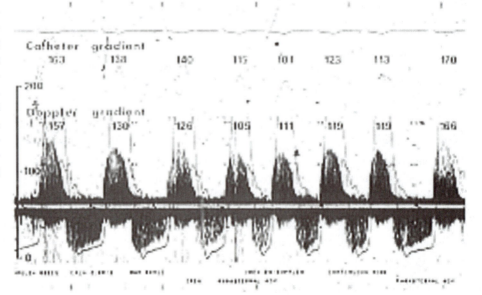

Figure 64.7. Simultaneous left ventricular (LV) and left aortic (LA) pressure gradients and Doppler tracings indicating excellent agreement between Doppler and catheter aortic transvalvular gradient despite atrial fibrillation. (Reprinted with permission from Currie PJ, Seward JB, Reeder GS, et al. Continuous-wave Doppler echocardiographic assessment of severity of calcific aortic stenosis. Circulation 1995; 71:1162–1169.)

however, are substantial (i.e., 5%). This procedure is not an alternative to surgery in older patients.

AORTIC REGURGITATION

Etiology

The causes of aortic regurgitation are:

- Congenital anomaly (e.g., bicuspid valve, aortic valve prolapse).
- Rheumatic disease.
- Diseases of the aorta such as aortic root aneurysm because of Marfan's syndrome or aortic dissection involving the ascending aorta. The mechanism of aortic regurgitation usually involves dilatation of the aortic root with poor coaptation of leaflets.
- Aortitis cause by connective tissue disease or syphilis.
- Endocarditis.
- Degenerative (an area of leaflet coaptation becomes friable with aging).
- Aortic regurgitation (rarely, if ever, caused by ischemic heart disease).

Pathophysiology

Aortic regurgitation causes volume overload of the left ventricle, which dilates to compensate for the volume load. Left ventricular dilatation is well tolerated for a long time, but eventually, it leads to impaired systolic function and heart failure. The pressure gradient between the aorta and left ventricle is greatest at aortic valve closure and falls progressively throughout diastole, thus giving rise to the decrescendo nature of the aortic regurgitation murmur.

Diagnosis

Aortic regurgitation often is asymptomatic for years. If it is acute, such as in dissection or endocarditis, it may give rise to congestive symptoms that are poorly tolerated. Chest pain of an anginal nature also may be reported.

The signs of aortic regurgitation are:

- High-volume pulse with rapid fall-off as blood leaks back into the left ventricle (i.e., collapsing or Corrigan's water-hammer pulse). Increased capillary pulsation also is seen (i.e., Quincke's pulse) at the nail bed, where alternate flushing and pallor of the skin is seen when light pressure is applied to the nail tip. Other signs of severe aortic regurgitation are pistol-shot femoral artery pulses and Duroziez's sign (i.e., a to-and-fro murmur over the femoral artery when it is lightly compressed with a stethoscope).
- The pulse pressure is widened, with a high systolic and a low diastolic pressure.
- Prominent pulsation of the carotid arteries are seen.

- The apex beat is hyperdynamic, and a diastolic thrill may be felt on occasion.
- The murmur of valvular aortic regurgitation is decrescendo and is heard over the aortic area and along the left sternal border. The murmur is best heard during expiration, with the patient leaning forward. When aortic regurgitation results from aortic root dilatation, the murmur frequently is heard at the right rather than the left sternal border.
- Aortic regurgitation usually is associated with an ejection systolic murmur, even in patients without clinically significant stenosis. The ejection murmur reflects increased flow across the aortic valve.
- S_3 and S_4 may be heard.
- During severe aortic regurgitation, the jet may impinge on the opening of the anterior mitral valve leaflet and cause a mid-diastolic murmur (i.e., Austin-Flint murmur).

Studies Electrocardiography reveals diastolic volume overload and left ventricular hypertrophy. Doppler echocardiography can quantify and determine the mechanism of the aortic regurgitation. Serial echocardiography is used to follow left ventricular size and function over time. The chest radiography shows cardiomegaly and a prominent aorta.

Cardiac catheterization aortography is used to determine semiquantitatively the severity of aortic regurgitation. It currently is the gold standard for assessing such severity.

Treatment

Acute, severe aortic regurgitation needs urgent surgical treatment. Afterload reduction with sodium nitroprusside can stabilize the patient while he or she is waiting for surgery. Intraaortic balloon counterpulsation increases the severity of aortic regurgitation by increasing the diastolic pressure in the aorta, and it should not be used for treatment of this condition.

Chronic aortic regurgitation is well tolerated for many years. Valve surgery is indicated once symptoms occur or left ventricular dysfunction manifests. After left ventricular dysfunction is present for more than 1 year, it may not normalize—even after aortic valve replacement. Sudden death is more likely once left ventricular size is greatly increased; therefore, careful follow-up of patients with significant regurgitation is required.

Echocardiography is used to follow both the size and function of the left ventricle. Even in asymptomatic patients, surgery should be considered if the left ventricle end-systolic dimension is greater than 5 cm, because surgical intervention in patients with large ventricles is associated with poor outcome. Surgery may be considered at smaller end-diastolic and end-systolic dimensions if the left ventricular enlargement is rapidly progressive or left ventricular function is declining. In asymptomatic patients with left ventricular dilatation, afterload reduction with nifedipine delays the need for surgery. Valve surgical options are similar to those for aortic stenosis, except that aortic valve repair is more likely to be possible in patients with aortic regurgitation as compared to those with aortic stenosis.

TRICUSPID STENOSIS

Tricuspid stenosis is less common than mitral stenosis. Tricuspid stenosis occurs in 5 to 10% of patients with severe mitral stenosis. Carcinoid is an additional rare cause.

Tricuspid stenosis leads to elevated right atrial pressure. In turn, this leads to peripheral edema, ascites, and low cardiac output.

Diagnosis

Isolated tricuspid stenosis is rare, but it may lead to low cardiac output and peripheral edema. The signs include a jugular pressure with a large ''A'' wave if the patient is in normal sinus rhythm. Elevated jugular venous pressure is present as well. Auscultation reveals a diastolic murmur similar to that of mitral stenosis, except that it is best heard during inspiration and over the left sternal margin and xiphoid.

Studies   Electrocardiography shows right atrial enlargement. Doppler echocardiography is used to measure the gradient across the tricuspid valve.

Treatment

Right-sided symptoms should be treated with diuretics first. Balloon valvuloplasty is feasible in suitable candidates, and surgical treatment should be considered in patients undergoing mitral surgery if the mean tricuspid gradient is greater than 4 or 5 mm Hg. If surgical repair is unsuccessful, prosthetic replacement usually is performed with a tissue valve (because of the increased risk of thrombosis with mechanical prostheses at this position).

TRICUSPID REGURGITATION

Tricuspid regurgitation may be either primary or secondary. Primary tricuspid regurgitation usually results from rheumatic disease. Other causes include carcinoid, congenital abnormalities (e.g., Ebstein's anomaly), right ventricular ischemia or infarction, tricuspid valve prolapse, trauma, or endocarditis.

Secondary tricuspid regurgitation results from conditions that cause pulmonary hypertension with resultant right ventricle dilatation and dilatation of the tricuspid annulus. Tricuspid regurgitation leads to reduced cardiac output with peripheral edema as well as hepatic and gastrointestinal congestion.

Diagnosis

Tricuspid regurgitation causes symptoms of low cardiac output (e.g., fatigue) or right-sided failure (e.g., anorexia) from passive congestion of the liver and gastrointestinal tract. The signs include large ''V'' waves in the jugular venous pulse. Auscultation reveals a pansystolic murmur, which is heard best during inspiration at the left sternal border and subxiphoid area.

Studies   Electrocardiography reveals right atrial enlargement and right ventricular hypertrophy. Doppler echocardiography can be used to determine both the severity of the regurgitation and its cause.

Treatment

Isolated, severe tricuspid regurgitation may not require any treatment apart from diuretics. Surgical repair or replacement might be considered in patients with congestive symptoms that are refractory to medical treatment. In patients with secondary tricuspid regurgitation, the primary condition should be treated. In those with tricuspid regurgitation secondary to mitral or aortic valve disease, however, tricuspid annuloplasty should be considered at the time of surgery for the primary condition.

REVIEW EXERCISES

QUESTIONS

1. Mitral stenosis usually is rheumatic.

   a. True.
   b. False.

2. Mitral stenosis is more common in men.

   a. True.
   b. False.

3. Mitral stenosis presents early with dyspnea.

   a. True.
   b. False.

4. Mitral stenosis is best treated with surgery before symptoms appear.

   a. True.
   b. False.

5. Consider the following hemodynamic data: left atrial pressure, 25 mm Hg; left ventricular pressure, 120/10 mm Hg; aortic pressure, 120/80 mm Hg; and cardiac index, 1.9 L/min per m^2. These are most consistent with which valvular lesion?

   a. Mitral stenosis.
   b. Mitral regurgitation.
   c. Aortic stenosis.
   d. Aortic regurgitation.

6. In patients with mitral regurgitation, left ventricular function often appears to be normal until late in the disease.

   a. True.
   b. False.

7. In patients with mitral regurgitation, no treatment is indicated until symptoms appear.

   a. True.
   b. False.

8. In patients with mitral regurgitation, left ventricular function often improves following surgical treatment.

   a. True.
   b. False.

9. In patients with mitral regurgitation, prosthetic replacement is generally superior to valve repair.

   a. True.
   b. False.

10. Surgical treatment is indicated in patients with aortic stenosis if they are asymptomatic but the valve area is 0.9 cm^2.

    a. True.
    b. False.

11. Surgical treatment is indicated in patients with aortic stenosis if they have dyspnea on exertion and the valve area is 0.9 cm^2.

    a. True.
    b. False.

12. Surgical treatment is indicated in patients with aortic stenosis if they are 15 years of age and have a pressure gradient of 100 mm Hg across the valve.

    a. True.
    b. False.

13. Consider the following hemodynamic data: left atrial pressure, 15 mm Hg; left ventricular pressure, 220/15 mm Hg; aorta pressure, 100/60 mm Hg; and cardiac index, 1.9 L/min per m^2. These are most consistent with which valvular lesion?

    a. Mitral stenosis.
    b. Mitral regurgitation.
    c. Aortic stenosis.
    d. Aortic regurgitation.

14. Surgical treatment is indicated in asymptomatic patients with aortic regurgitation if the regurgitation is severe and both left ventricle size and function are normal.

    a. True.
    b. False.

15. Surgical treatment is indicated in asymptomatic patients with aortic regurgitation if regurgitation is severe but the left ventricle is 5 cm in size at the end of systole.

    a. True.
    b. False.

16. Surgical treatment is indicated in patients with aortic regurgitation if regurgitation is severe and left ventricular dysfunction is present.

    a. True.
    b. False.

17. A 27-year-old woman has recent onset of shortness of breath going up stairs and a history of palpitations. The physical examination reveals a regular pulse, loud S_1, and an apical diastolic murmur. The most likely diagnosis is:

a. Aortic stenosis.
b. Mitral stenosis.
c. Aortic regurgitation.
d. Tricuspid stenosis.

18. What is the appropriate treatment for a patient with mitral stenosis who had moderate symptoms and a pliable valve but now has severe mitral stenosis without significant mitral regurgitation?

a. Medical treatment.
b. Open commissurotomy.
c. Mitral valve replacement.
d. Balloon valvuloplasty.

19. A 59-year-old man with severe myomatous mitral regurgitation is asymptomatic, with a left ventricular ejection fraction of 55% and an end systolic diameter index (ESDI) of 2.9 cm/in^2. The most appropriate treatment is:

a. Mitral valve replacement.
b. No treatment.
c. Angiotensin-converting enzyme inhibitor.
d. Mitral valve repair.
e. Digoxin and diuretics.

Answers

1. a (true)
Mitral stenosis is nearly always rheumatic. Occasionally, congenital mitral stenosis may occur.

2. b (false)
Women are affected more commonly.

3. b (false)
Mitral stenosis usually presents late, and it is asymptomatic for many years.

4. b (false)
Normally, it is best to wait for symptoms to appear. Mitral valvuloplasty is the best initial intervention.

5. a
There is a diastolic pressure gradient of 15 mm Hg across the mitral valve and reduced cardiac output.

6. a (true)
Latent left ventricular dysfunction is masked by volume loading.

7. b (false)
Symptoms often are late, and increasing left ventricle size and decreasing function may occur before symptoms.

8. b (false)
Left ventricular function usually is worse than it appears. Before surgery it appears to decline after surgery.

9. b (false)
Valve repair usually is preferable, because the surgical risk is lower and the ventricular function better conserved with repair than with replacement.

10. b (false)
Symptoms usually are the main indication for surgery in patients with moderately severe (noncritical) aortic stenosis.

11. a (true)
See explanation for question 10.

12. a (true)
There is an increased risk of sudden death with a high pressure gradient in this age group.

13. c
There is a systolic pressure gradient across the aortic valve, and the cardiac index is reduced.

14. b (false)
Asymptomatic patients with severe aortic regurgitation and normal left ventricle size and function are followed closely for signs of left ventricle enlargement and dysfunction.

15. a (true)
Increased left ventricle size (of >5 cm) is an indication for surgery in patients with aortic regurgitation despite lack of symptoms.

16. a (true)
See explanation for question 14.

17. b
Mitral stenosis is the lesion most likely to be responsible for all these findings.

18. d
A pliable valve in symptomatic mitral stenosis without mitral regurgitation might make valvuloplasty feasible.

19. d
Mitral valve repair is the best option, if feasible, because of lower mortality and morbidity rates. Surgery is indicated given increased left ventricle size and decreased left ventricular function. (LV dysfunction is usually present once LVEF is <60% in patients with severe mitral regurgitation).

SUGGESTED READINGS

Braunwald E. Valvular heart disease. In: Harrrison's principles of internal medicine. 12th ed. New York: McGraw-Hill, 1991:938–952.

Durack DT, Lukas AS, Bright DK. New criteria for diagnosis of infective endocarditis: utilization of specific echocardiographic findings. Am J Med 1994;96:200–209.

Griffin BP. Valvular heart disease. Sci Am Med 1998;11:1–12.

Griffin BP, ed. Valvular heart disease. Curr Opin Cardiol 1995;Vol 10(2):99–154.

Griffin BP, ed. Valvular heart disease. Curr Opin Cardiol 1996;11(2):93–154.

Reyes, Raju BS, Wynne J, et al. Percutaneous balloon valvuloplasty compared with open surgical commissurotomy for mitral stenosis. N Engl J Med 1994;331:961–967.

Scognamiglio R, Rehuintoole SH, et al. Nifedipine in asymptomatic patients with severe aortic regurgitation and normal left ventricular function. N Engl J Med 1994;331:689–694.

Arrhythmias

Mina K. Chung

Cardiac arrhythmias can be categorized on the basis of mechanisms, rates, and associated risk. When considering rate, tachycardias generally consist of arrhythmias with rates of more than 100 beats per minute (bpm). Significant bradycardias generally consist of arrhythmias with rates of less than 60 bpm. The appropriate diagnosis and assessment of the risk associated with arrhythmias are important to their treatment.

Tachyarrhythmias

MECHANISMS

The mechanisms underlying cardiac arrhythmias usually are categorized into disorders of impulse formation, impulse conduction, or a combination of both.

DISORDERS OF IMPULSE FORMATION

Automaticity

Automaticity is the property of a cell or fiber to initiate a spontaneous impulse without previous stimulation. Spontaneously discharging cardiac cells that initiate spontaneous action potentials during phase 4 diastolic depolarization result in automaticity. The rate at which the sinus node discharges usually is faster than, and suppresses, the discharge rate of other potential latent or subsidiary automatic pacemaker sites. Normal or abnormal automaticity at the sinus node or other ectopic sites, however, can lead to rates that are faster and can gain control of the cardiac rhythm for one or more cycles. This may manifest if the discharge rate of the sinus node slows or that of the latent pacemaker increases.

Normal Automaticity Cells that can exhibit spontaneous phase 4 diastolic depolarization are located in the sinus node, atria, atrioventricular (AV) junction, and the His-Purkinje system. Normal automaticity generally occurs in normal cells with normal membrane resting potentials. It can be suppressed by overdrive pacing, but generally resumes after termination of pacing. Subsidiary pacemakers can become dominant in the settings of acidosis, ischemia, sympathetic stimulation, and use of certain drugs. Examples of arrhythmias in this category include sinus tachycardia that is inappropriate to the clinical situation and, possibly, ventricular parasystole.

Abnormal Automaticity Normal myocardial cells maintain membrane resting potentials in the range of -90 mV, and they depolarize only when stimulated. Abnormal automaticity, however, can occur in cells with reduced maximum diastolic potentials, often at membrane potentials positive to -50 to -60 mV. The partial depolarization and failure to reach or maintain the normal maximum diastolic potential may induce automatic discharge. Examples of tachycardias that likely result from abnormal automaticity include accelerated junctional rhythm (i.e., nonparoxysmal junctional tachycardia), accelerated idioventricular rhythms, certain atrial tachycardias, some ventricular tachycardias (VTs) in patients without structural heart disease, exercise-induced VT, VT during the first several hours of myocardial infarction (MI), and some VTs in patients with marked electrolyte imbalance.

Triggered Activity

Unlike automaticity, which does not require previous stimulation to occur, triggered activity is initiated by oscillations in the membrane potential (i.e., afterdepolarizations) that are induced by preceding action potentials. Afterdepolarizations that occur before full repolarization is completed are called early afterdepolarizations (EADs); those that occur after completion of repolarization, during phase 4, are called delayed afterdepolarizations (DADs). If afterdepolarizations reach threshold potential, an action potential can be generated, which potentially can trigger another or repetitive afterdepolarizations.

Early Afterdepolarizations   Occurring during phase 2 or 3 of the action potential, EADs are thought to be responsible for VTs associated with prolonged repolarization, such as long QT syndromes (acquired or congenital) and torsades de pointes. Rapid rates and magnesium both suppress EADs as well as these arrhythmias. Experimentally, EADs can be produced by hypoxia, cesium, as well as class IA (e.g., quinidine) and III (e.g., sotalol) antiarrhythmic agents.

Delayed Afterdepolarizations   Occurring after repolarization during phase 4, DADs have been demonstrated in Purkinje fibers as well as in atrial and ventricular fibers exposed to digitalis. Faster rates may augment DADs and are associated with an increase in intracellular calcium overload. Clinically, DADs have been classically implicated in digitalis toxicity as well as in tachyarrhythmias associated with catecholamine excess, acidosis, MI, and possibly, certain VTs (e.g., verapamil-responsive VT).

DISORDERS OF IMPULSE CONDUCTION

Conduction delay or block can produce bradyarrhythmias or tachyarrhythmias. The most common mechanism of tachyarrhythmias is reentry. Classically, reentry requires:

1. Alternate or separate pathways of conduction as defined by anatomic barriers (e.g., myocardial scar, AV node and accessory pathway [AP]) or functional properties (e.g., no anatomic boundaries but contiguous fibers with different electrophysiologic properties, such as local differences in refractoriness, excitability, or anisotropic intercellular resistances),
2. An area of unidirectional block in one pathway, and
3. An area of conduction in the alternate pathway that is slow enough for the propagating and returning impulse to meet and excite tissue proximal to the block that has recovered (Fig. 65.1).

Reentry is thought to be the mechanism underlying most recurrent paroxysmal tachycardias. These include atrial flutter, atrial fibrillation, AV nodal reentry, AV reentry involving APs (including Wolff-Parkinson-White syndrome), and most VTs associated with ischemic heart disease and previous MI.

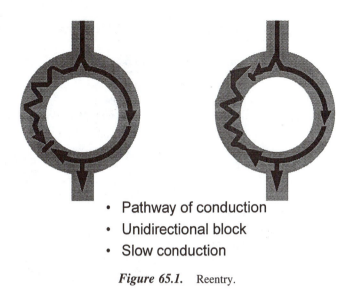

- Pathway of conduction
- Unidirectional block
- Slow conduction

Figure 65.1.   Reentry.

DIAGNOSIS

PATIENT HISTORY AND PHYSICAL EXAMINATION

The key to diagnosing and appropriately treating patients with arrhythmias is determination of the underlying, predisposing cardiac substrate. Known structural heart disease, particularly in patients with known coronary artery disease or ischemic or nonischemic cardiomyopathies, can greatly influence both treatment and diagnosis. Patients presenting with wide QRS-complex tachycardias and previous MI almost always have VT. Triggering agents (e.g., inotropic or QT-prolonging drugs) or events may be important to longer-term treatment and subsequent prevention of arrhythmias. In addition to hemodynamic status and evidence of underlying valvular or ventricular dysfunction, helpful physical findings include evidence of AV dissociation (i.e., cannon A waves in the jugular venous pulse) and termination or slowing with vagal maneuvers (e.g., carotid sinus massage, Valsalva, cough, cold-water immersion) or adenosine.

DIFFERENTIAL DIAGNOSIS

Tachyarrhythmias can be classified into wide versus narrow QRS complex and regular versus irregular tachycardia (Table 65.1). Electrocardiographic (ECG) evaluation of tachycardias should begin by assessing the rate, regularity, and QRS width. Narrow QRS tachycardias, which are defined as tachycardias with a QRS width of less than 120 milliseconds, implies ventricular activation over the rapidly conducting His-Purkinje system, which in turn suggests a supraventricular tachycardia (SVT; a tachycardia requiring atrial or AV junctional tissue for initiation or maintenance). Irregularity of the ventricular rate during an SVT suggests atrial fibrillation, atrial flutter with variable block, or multifocal atrial tachycardia. A wide

Table 65.1.	**Differential Diagnosis of Tachycardias**	
	Regular Rhythm	*Irregular Rhythm*
Narrow QRS Complex	Sinus tachycardia Sinus node reentry Atrial tachycardia Atrial flutter AV nodal reentry Orthodromic AV reentry	Atrial fibrillation Atrial flutter with variable AV block Multifocal atrial tachycardia
Wide QRS Complex	Ventricular tachycardia Supraventricular tachycardia Preexisting BBB Functional BBB Preexcitation Antidromic AV reentry Bystander AP	Ventricular tachycardia Atrial fibrillation with Preexisting BBB Functional BBB Preexcitation Torsades de Pointes

Adapted with permission from McKiernan TL and Prater S, Critical Care Board Review Syllabus 1996

QRS tachycardia may result from VT or SVT and is discussed later.

NARROW QRS TACHYCARDIAS

Electrocardiographic evaluation of narrow QRS tachycardias should include assessment of:

- Rate
- Regularity
- QRS width
- Atrial activation pattern and relationship to the QRS (RP/PR relationship, morphology of the P wave)
- QRS morphology
- Effect of bundle-branch block (BBB) aberration (if present)
- Mode of initiation
- Effect of vagal maneuvers and drugs

SVTs may be classified as:

- Sinus node tachycardias
  - Inappropriate sinus tachycardia
  - Sinus node reentry
- Atrial tachycardias
  - Automatic
  - Reentrant
- Atrial flutter
- Atrial fibrillation
- Multifocal atrial tachycardia
- Junctional tachycardias
  - Nonparoxysmal
  - Automatic
- AV nodal reentry
  - Typical
  - Atypical
- AV reciprocating tachycardia and other SVTs associated with APs

In narrow QRS-complex tachycardias, the relationship of the QRS and P waves can be important in establishing the diagnosis. The QRS and P-wave relationships and configurations commonly seen in patients with various SVTs are shown in Figure 65.2, and they are discussed further in later sections on specific arrhythmias. In typical AV nodal reentrant tachycardia (AVNRT), which is characterized by near-simultaneous atrial and ventricular activation, the P wave is buried in the QRS, and it either is not visible or is detected at the end of the QRS (within 80 ms) in 94% of cases. In 2% of cases, the P wave barely precedes the QRS and can be diagnostic. Atypical AVNRT occurs in 4% and is characterized by a long RP interval and a short PR interval, with inverted P waves in the inferior (i.e., II, III, aVF) leads. In orthodromic AV reentrant tachycardia (AVRT) mediated by a retrograde-conducting AP, the retrograde P wave often can be detected early in the ST segment. Slowly conducting retrograde APs can have long RP intervals. Atrial tachycardias, sinus tachycardia, and sinus node reentrant tachycardia (SANRT) will have long RP and short PR intervals, with the P-wave morphology differing from that of sinus rhythm in ectopic atrial tachycardias but similar in SANRT or sinus tachycardia.

Thus, close examination of the PR and RP intervals can be helpful. The differential diagnosis of short RP (i.e., RP interval shorter than the PR interval) and long RP (i.e., RP interval longer than the PR interval) SVTs is shown in Figure 65.3. Short RP narrow-complex tachycardias most likely result from AVNRT or orthodromic AVRT mediated by a retrograde-conducting AP; atrial tachycardia is a much less likely cause. Long RP narrow-complex tachycardias result from atrial (or sinus) tachycardias, atypical AVNRT, or orthodromic AVRT mediated by a slow-conducting AP.

WIDE QRS-COMPLEX TACHYCARDIA

Wide-complex tachycardia (WCT) has a QRS duration of 120 milliseconds or longer, with a ventricular rate of 100 bpm or more.

Differential Diagnosis

The differential diagnosis of WCT includes:

- VT
- SVT
  - SVT with preexisting BBB or intraventricular conduction defect

Normal Sinus Rhythm

Sinus Tachycardia
Sinus Node Reentrant Tachycardia

100%

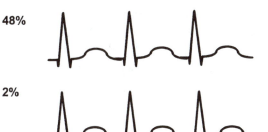

Ectopic Atrial Tachycardia

100%

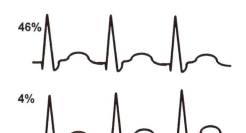

AV Node Reentrant Tachycardia (AVNRT)

48%

2%

46%

4%

Orthodromic AV Reentrant Tachycardia (AVRT) mediated by a retrogradely conducting accessory pathway

91%

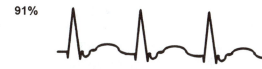

9%

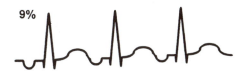

Figure 65.2.   Relationships and configurations of QRS and P waves in SVT. (Adapted with permission from Josephson ME. Clinical cardiac electrophysiology: techniques and interpretation. 2nd ed. Malvern, PA: Lea & Febiger, 1993:269.)

- SVT with aberrant His-Purkinje system conduction (i.e., functional BBB)
- Ashman's phenomenon after long-short RR interval
- Rate-related, acceleration-dependent BBB
- Maintenance of functional BBB by transseptal concealed conduction (i.e., linking)
- SVT with antegrade conduction via an AP
  - Antidromic SVT with antegrade conduction via an AP
  - Atrial fibrillation/flutter/tachycardia with antegrade conduction via an AP
  - AVNRT with antegrade conduction down a bystander AP
- SVT with slowed conduction because of electrolyte/metabolic imbalance or an antiarrhythmic drug

The diagnosis of WCT often can be established on the basis of clinical presentation, physical examination, ECG findings, and provocative maneuvers. As a general rule, however, treat as a VT when in doubt, particularly in patients with structural heart disease.

Clinical Presentation

In multiple studies, VT was the correct diagnosis in more than 80% of patients presenting with WCT. VT is more likely to occur in older patients, but age alone is not a useful marker. In very young patients (<20 years), SVT is a more frequent cause of WCT. VT can occur in younger patients with structurally normal hearts, but this is uncommon. Hemodynamic instability is a poor discriminating factor, because hemodynamic stability depends on rate, ventricular function, cardiac disease, and concomitant pharmacologic therapy. A history of structural heart disease, particularly of coronary artery disease with previous MI, is important. In patients with a history of MI, 98% of WCTs result from VT; a history of MI and symptoms of tachycardia starting only after the MI strongly favor VT.

Physical Examination

Rate and blood pressure are not useful in determining the cause of WCTs. The finding of AV dissociation, however,

Normal Sinus Rhythm

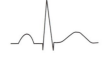

Short R-P Tachycardias

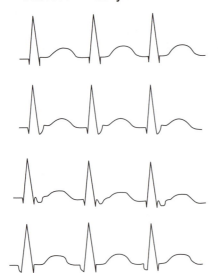

AVNRT*
Other junctional tachycardias
Orthodromic AVRT mediated by a
retrogradely conducting AP

AVNRT*
Other junctional tachycardias
Orthodromic AVRT mediated by a
retrogradely conducting AP

Orthodromic AVRT mediated by a
retrogradely conducting AP*
AVNRT

AVNRT

Long R-P Tachycardias

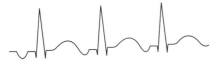

Atypical AVNRT (anterograde fast,
retrograde slow conduction pathway)
Orthodromic AVRT mediated by a slow,
decrementally conducting retrograde AP
Atrial tachycardia

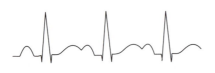

Atrial tachycardia
Sinus node reentrant tachycardia
Sinus tachycardia

* = most common

Figure 65.3. Differential diagnosis of SVTs by RP/PR relationships and P-wave configurations. *, most common. (Adapted with permission from Josephson ME. Clinical cardiac electrophysiology: techniques and interpretation. 2nd ed. Malvern, PA: Lea and Febiger, 1993:270.)

strongly favors VT. This is because approximately two-thirds of patients with VT will have AV dissociation at electrophysiology study, and AV dissociation is rare in SVT. Asynchronous contraction of the atria and ventricles can cause cannon A waves in the jugular venous pulsation, wide split heart sounds, variable S_1, and variability in blood pressure resulting from changes in stroke volume with AV dissociation.

Provocative Maneuvers

Vagal maneuvers can depress sinus node automaticity and slow AV nodal conduction. Gradual slowing of the rate of the

WCT suggests sinus tachycardia. Termination of the rhythm suggests reentry involving the AV node or sinus node (e.g., SANRT, AVNRT, AVRT). Transient block with reinitiation suggests atrial tachycardia, atrial fibrillation, or atrial flutter. VT rarely is affected by vagal maneuvers.

It is important that intravenous verapamil *not* be used to treat WCT, because hemodynamic collapse and death have been reported, regardless of the cause of the WCT. Adenosine has a much shorter duration of action (i.e., seconds) and is delivered intravenously as a 6- to 12-mg rapid bolus. Like vagal maneuvers, adenosine can terminate supraventricular arrhythmias resulting from reentry involving the AV or sinus node, or it can allow demonstration of atrial flutter waves, atrial tachycardia, or atrial fibrillation. Some uncommon forms of VT in structurally normal hearts can be terminated by vagal maneuvers or adenosine.

Electrocardiographic Findings

In patients with preexisting complete BBB, the QRS complex will be wide, and comparison with previous ECGs can be helpful. The QRS may be wide in any supraventricular rhythm, however, if functional aberrancy occurs. Patients receiving antiarrhythmic drugs, particularly class IC agents, may develop rate-related aberrancy. Preexcitation via an anterograde-conducting AP (i.e., Wolff-Parkinson-White syndrome) also causes a wide QRS. The ECG should be analyzed with specific attention to the AV relationship, presence of capture or fusion beats, and QRS duration, axis, and morphology.

Fusion beats occur when conducted supraventricular impulses depolarize the ventricle coincident with ventricular depolarization from the VT circuit. A narrower, usually intermediate-width QRS results. Narrow beats during WCT strongly favor the diagnosis of VT, but they are not pathognomonic (e.g., premature ventricular contraction [PVC] during SVT with BBB could also result in a narrower QRS complex).

Capture beats represent conduction of a supraventricular impulse to the ventricle and depolarization before it is depolarized by the VT circuit. It appears as a narrow-complex beat with a shorter coupling interval than the tachycardia interval, which indicates that the WCT is VT. Capture beats virtually exclude SVT with aberrancy, because they occur after a

shorter interval with a narrow QRS and aberrancy with wider QRS complexes is more likely to occur after shorter rather than longer intervals.

Atrioventricular dissociation strongly favors the diagnosis of VT, but this feature is not always identifiable on surface ECGs. One-third of VTs may have 1 : 1 VA conduction. Even so, variable retrograde VA conduction, or VA Wenckebach conduction, strongly suggests VT. Rare SVTs may exhibit VA dissociation (e.g., automatic junctional tachycardia with retrograde block). Recording of an atrial electrogram by a right atrial or an esophageal electrode may facilitate assessment.

QRS morphology can help to distinguish SVT with aberrancy from VT. QRS concordance in leads V_1 through V_6 is predictive of VT but also can be seen in patients with Wolff-Parkinson-White syndrome. Delayed or slowed initial QRS deflection suggests VT. The QRS morphology can be classified into a left BBB (LBBB) or a right BBB (RBBB) pattern on the basis of QRS polarity in V_1. RBBB morphology has a predominantly positive QRS deflection, and LBBB morphology a predominantly negative QRS deflection, in V_1. In RBBB morphology, WCT (Fig. 65.4), a monophasic R, qR, RS, or R greater than r' pattern in V_1 favors VT. In V_6 a QS, QR, or monophasic R pattern also favors VT. In contrast, triphasic complexes in V_1 or V_6 favor SVT. In LBBB morphology, WCT (Fig. 65.5), an R in V_1 or V_2 of 40 milliseconds or greater, notched downstroke on the S wave in V_1 or V_2, any Q in V_6, or more than 60 milliseconds from the QRS onset to the S nadir in V_1 or V_2 favors VT.

A commonly used, four-level algorithm for distinguishing VT from SVT (i.e., the Brugada criteria) is shown in Fig-

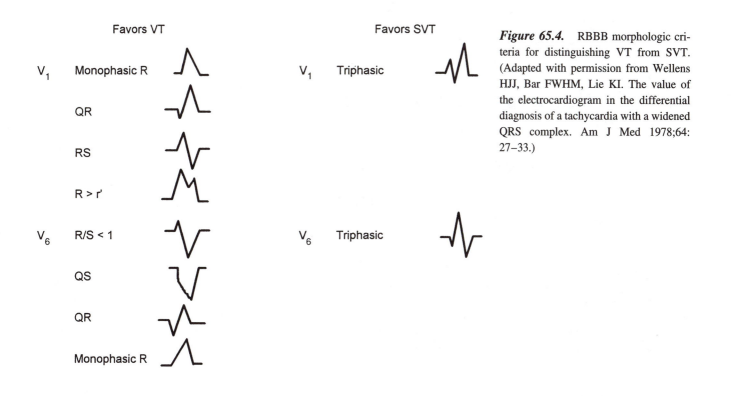

Figure 65.4. RBBB morphologic criteria for distinguishing VT from SVT. (Adapted with permission from Wellens HJJ, Bar FWHM, Lie KI. The value of the electrocardiogram in the differential diagnosis of a tachycardia with a widened QRS complex. Am J Med 1978;64: 27–33.)

Figure 65.5. LBBB morphologic criteria for VT in leads V_1 and V_6. (Adapted with permission from Kindwall KE, Brown J, Josephson ME. Electrocardiographic criteria for ventricular tachycardia in wide complex left bundle branch block morphology tachycardias. Am J Cardiol 1988;61:1279–1283.)

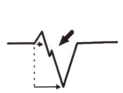
V_1 or V_2

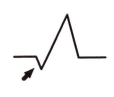
V_6

1   R in V_1 or V_2 ≥ 40 ms sec.

2   >60 msec from QRS onset to S nadir in V_1 or V_2.

3   Notched downstroke S wave in V_1 or V_2.

4   Any Q in V_6.

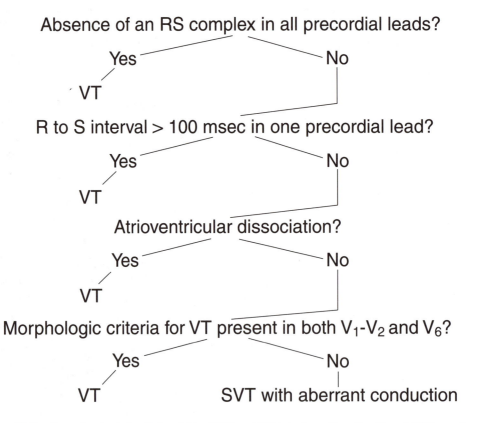

Absence of an RS complex in all precordial leads?

Yes — No

VT

R to S interval > 100 msec in one precordial lead?

Yes — No

VT

Atrioventricular dissociation?

Yes — No

VT

Morphologic criteria for VT present in both V_1-V_2 and V_6?

Yes — No

VT — SVT with aberrant conduction

Figure 65.6. Brugada criteria for distinguishing VT from SVT in tachycardia with widened QRS complexes. (Reprinted with permission from Brugada P, Brugada J, Mont L, Smeets J, Andries EW. A new approach to the differential diagnosis of a regular tachycardia with a wide QRS complex. Circulation 1991;83:1649–1659.)

ure 65.6. This algorithm was prospectively validated for more than 500 WCTs with electrophysiologic diagnoses. It had a high sensitivity (0.987) and specificity (0.965). Using these criteria, if no RS can be identified in any precordial lead, VT is diagnosed. If an RS complex is present and the RS interval is longer than 100 milliseconds, VT is diagnosed. If the RS interval is shorter than 100 ms, evidence of AV dissociation indicates VT. If none of the first three criteria are met, then morphologic criteria for VT are analyzed in leads V_1-V_2, and V_6. If both leads fulfill the criteria for VT, then VT is diagnosed; otherwise, the diagnosis of SVT with aberrancy is made by exclusion of VT.

Other ECG clues include consistent initiation of WCT by premature atrial contractions, which favors a supraventricular rhythm. Initiation of WCT preceded by constant PP intervals but a short PR interval (with the QRS fused to the P wave) in patients without preexcitation suggests VT. Grossly irregular RR intervals suggest atrial fibrillation. If a rapid, irregular WCT has beat-to-beat variation in the QRS duration, Wolff-Parkinson-White syndrome should be suspected. Comparison with previous sinus rhythm ECGs is helpful to determine preexisting preexcitation or baseline BBB/intraventricular conduction defect.

A QRS duration of longer than 140 milliseconds with WCT of RBBB morphology or of longer than 160 milliseconds with LBBB morphology favors the diagnosis of VT. Most SVTs with aberrancy have QRS durations of 140 milliseconds or less, but wide QRS durations can be seen with preexcitation and marked baseline intraventricular conduction defects. In addition, from 15 to 35% of patients with VT also may have QRS durations of 140 milliseconds or less.

QRS-axis deviation with a right superior axis (i.e., negative in I, aVF) suggests VT. Left superior axis (i.e., left-axis deviation; negative in aVF, II; positive in I) in WCT with RBBB morphology suggests VT, but it is not helpful in WCT with LBBB morphology.

Treatment

For hemodynamically unstable WCT, including pulmonary edema or severe angina, cardioversion should be performed (including 200 J to between 300 and 360 J if initially unsuccessful). Sedation should be given before cardioversion if the patient is awake. For hemodynamically stable WCT, a clinical history (including cardiac disease, previous arrhythmias, previous MI, drug use) should be elicited and physical examination performed (including inspection for cannon A waves). A 12-lead ECG and laboratory studies to exclude electrolyte/metabolic abnormalities, ischemia, hypoxia, or drug toxicity should be obtained. If the diagnosis is in doubt, placement of an esophageal lead can be considered. Adenosine, 6 to 12 mg delivered intravenously as a rapid bolus, can be given. Lidocaine or procainamide can be attempted as well, and if the WCT persists, bretylium or intravenous amiodarone can be considered. Cardioversion under anesthesia or overdrive pace termination can be attempted for persistent WCT. If WCT is incessant, consider the possibility of electrolyte abnormalities, digitalis toxicity, acute severe ischemia, reperfusion arrhythmias, proarrhythmia, or torsades de pointes. Consideration also should be given to empiric $MgSO_4$, treatment for acute ischemia or MI, and intravenous amiodarone.

Evaluation after termination of WCT should include consideration of electrophysiologic testing to determine the WCT etiology. Subsequent therapy depends on the diagnosis, but it can include pharmacologic, ablation, or device therapies.

SPECIFIC SUPRAVENTRICULAR ARRHYTHMIAS

ATRIAL PREMATURE DEPOLARIZATIONS

Atrial premature depolarizations can be frequent and occasionally, symptomatic. Though not associated with significant risk, they can be associated with underlying cardiovascular or pulmonary disease. Treatment generally includes reassurance, avoidance of precipitating factors (e.g., caffeine, sympathomimetic agents), and occasionally, β-blockers or calcium channel blockers.

SINUS TACHYCARDIA

Sinus tachycardia is defined in an adult as having a sinus rate of greater than 100 bpm. The sinus node is located in the high right atrium and is sensitive to catecholamines and autonomic tone. Therefore, sinus tachycardia may be secondary to many physiologic and pathologic states. It is a normal response to exertion, anxiety, and a variety of stresses, including fever, hypotension, hypovolemia, hyperthyroidism, congestive heart failure, pulmonary embolism, myocardial ischemia or infarction, inflammation, and drugs, such as catecholamines, caffeine, alcohol, or nicotine. Because of the location and automatic properties associated with the sinus node, physiologic sinus tachycardia has normal P-wave morphology (i.e., upright in II, III, and aVF) and exhibits gradual rate acceleration and deceleration that varies with changes in the autonomic tone and volume. Treatment should focus on the cause of sinus tachycardia, avoidance of stimulants, fluid replacement in patients with hypovolemia, fever reduction, and possibly, β-blockers or calcium channel blockers.

Inappropriate Sinus Tachycardia

Inappropriate sinus tachycardia, in which otherwise healthy patients have chronic, nonparoxysmal sinus tachycardia without apparent cause or at an inappropriate rate, may result from increased automaticity, increased sympathetic tone, increased sensitivity to catecholamines, decreased vagal tone, or an automatic atrial focus located near the sinus node. Treatment may require β-blockers, calcium channel blockers, digitalis, or sinus node radiofrequency modification or surgical ablation.

Sinus Node Reentry

Sinus node reentry, which only rarely occurs, may be difficult to distinguish from sinus tachycardia. The onset typically is sudden and paroxysmal, and it often is precipitated by a premature atrial beat, which is important in establishing the diagnosis. The heart rate can vary from 80 to 200 bpm but generally is slower than other SVTs, with an average rate of 130 to 140 bpm. The rate also can fluctuate with the autonomic tone. P-wave morphology demonstrates a high-to-low atrial activation sequence (i.e., upright in II, III, aVF) that is identical to sinus rhythm in morphology. The PR interval relates to the SVT rate, with a long RP interval and a shorter PR interval. AV block can occur (e.g., Wenckebach) without affecting the tachycardia. Vagal maneuvers (e.g., carotid sinus massage, Valsalva maneuver) or adenosine can slow and terminate the tachycardia. Drugs such as β-blockers or calcium channel blockers, as well as class I or III antiarrhythmic agents, also have been used successfully. Surgical or radiofrequency catheter ablation occasionally may be indicated.

ATRIAL TACHYCARDIAS

Tachycardias originating in the atria at sites other than the sinus or AV node are called atrial, or ectopic atrial, tachycardias. Heart rates generally are regular, ranging from 100 to 250 (generally 150–200) bpm, with a P-wave morphology differing from that in sinus rhythm and isoelectric periods between P waves, thus distinguishing it from atrial flutter or atrial fibrillation. There usually is a long RP interval (with a shorter PR interval) that is variable in duration. AV conduction block (i.e., spontaneous Wenckebach second-degree AV block or AV block induced by carotid sinus massage, other vagal maneuvers, or adenosine) typically does not terminate the tachycardia. A positive or biphasic P wave in aVL suggests a right atrial origin. A positive P wave in V$_1$ suggests a left atrial focus. At physical examination, rapid "A" waves in the jugular venous pulse may be evident.

Atrial tachycardia can occur paroxysmally in short, nonsustained or in longer, sustained runs, and they occasionally may be incessant, potentially leading to a tachycardia-mediated cardiomyopathy. It often is associated with significant structural heart disease, pulmonary disease, hyperthyroidism, or digitalis intoxication. Three mechanisms of atrial tachycardias have been described: abnormal automaticity, reentry, and triggered activity. In general, and depending on the clinical situation, treatment in patients not receiving digitalis may include AV node–blocking agents (e.g., calcium channel blockers, β-blockers, digitalis); class IA, IC, or III antiarrhythmic agents; or surgical or radiofrequency catheter ablation.

Atrial Tachycardia with Block Resulting from Digitalis Toxicity

In digitalis toxicity, concomitant impairment of AV conduction can cause atrial tachycardia with block, and triggered activity (i.e., DAD) is believed to be the mechanism responsible for the atrial tachycardia. This may occur in patients with atrial fibrillation/flutter, but it can be distinguished by isoelectric periods between P waves. Treatment includes cessation of digitalis, administration of potassium (if the potassium level is not already elevated), and depending on the ventricular rate and presence of other digitalis-toxic arrhythmias, potentially a β-blocker, lidocaine, or phenytoin.

Automatic Atrial Tachycardia

Automatic atrial tachycardia generally is characterized by a "warm-up" phenomenon, in which the heart rate gradually accelerates after initiation. Usually, it can be overdrive suppressed, but not terminated, by pacing. Automatic atrial tachycardia can occur in all age groups and be seen in association with MI, lung disease, alcohol ingestion, and metabolic abnormalities.

Reentrant Atrial Tachycardia

Reentrant atrial tachycardia can result from anatomic abnormalities, including surgical scars or atriotomy incisions. It can be initiated by premature atrial stimuli that induce conduction delay or block, usually can be terminated by atrial pacing, and not uncommonly is associated with atrial flutter.

Multifocal Atrial Tachycardia

Multifocal atrial tachycardia (MAT) is characterized by a heart rate of greater than 100 bpm, multiple (>3) P-wave morphologies, and variable PP, PR, and RR intervals. The multiple P-wave morphologies result from multiple depolarizing foci in the atria. The irregularly irregular ventricular rate can mimic atrial fibrillation, and differentiation from "coarse" atrial fibrillation can be made by isoelectric periods between P waves. MAT predominantly occurs in patients who are elderly or critically ill with advanced chronic pulmonary disease. Other commonly associated conditions include pneumonia, infection or sepsis, postoperative states, lung cancer, pulmonary embolism, cor pulmonale, congestive heart failure, hypertensive heart disease, and other acute cardiac or pulmonary processes. Rarely, digoxin toxicity, hypokalemia, and hypomagnesemia may be associated. MAT also may progress to atrial fibrillation. In critically ill patients, it is associated with a high hospital mortality rate. Treatment is directed toward the underlying disease, which often is pulmonary. Antiarrhythmic agents often are ineffective, and β-blockers can be effective but often are contraindicated in patients with severe bronchospastic disease. Verapamil, amiodarone, and potassium as well as magnesium replacement have been helpful. The mechanism underlying MAT may be enhanced automaticity or triggered activity.

ATRIAL FLUTTER

The incidence of atrial flutter is lower than that of atrial fibrillation, and two general categories of atrial flutter have been described. The typical (i.e., type I) form is caused by macroreentry in the right atrium. Atrial depolarization in this reentrant circuit typically propagates in the counterclockwise direction craniocaudally down the free wall, through a corridor of functionally slow-conducting tissue in the posterolateral to posteromedial right atrium, and caudalcranially up the atrial septum. This pattern of atrial activation inscribes the typical "sawtooth" flutter waves on the surface ECG that typically are negative in the inferior leads (i.e., II, III, aVF). The atrial rate usually is 250 to 350 bpm, but this may be slowed by class IA, IC, and III antiarrhythmic drugs. Type I atrial flutter often can be terminated by atrial pacing. It also can be cured, with a success rate of 75 to 90%, by radiofrequency catheter ablation, with application of radiofrequency energy to produce a line of conduction block across the posterior corridor.

The atypical (i.e., type II) atrial flutter has an atrial rate that usually is greater than 350 to 400 bpm and generally cannot be influenced or terminated by atrial pacing. In some patients, it may result from clockwise propagation along the posterior corridor reentrant circuit, as described in type I atrial flutter (and can be classified as type I clockwise atrial flutter), or other pathways of conduction.

In untreated patients with type I atrial flutter, the atrial rate usually is 300 bpm, with 2:1 AV conduction and a ventricular rate of 150 bpm. Slower rates may occur with treatment (e.g., AV node–blocking agents) or AV nodal disease. The ventricular response often occurs with 2:1, 4:1, alternating 2:1/4:1, or variable conduction patterns. Thus, the ventricular rate may be constant or variable and irregular. Occasionally, 1:1 AV conduction can be seen in patients with preexcitation syndromes (e.g., Wolff-Parkinson-White syndrome), with hyperthyroidism, or in children, and this can be a medical emergency. Slowing of the atrial rate, such as by antiarrhythmic agents, also may result in 1:1 AV conduction. Vagal maneuvers or adenosine can help to establish the diagnosis by blocking the ventricular response and enhancing appreciation of the flutter waves. Esophageal or intracardiac atrial electrogram recordings can help in patients for whom the diagnosis remains unclear.

Paroxysmal atrial flutter can occur in patients without structural heart disease, but chronic, persistent atrial flutter usually occurs in patients with underlying heart disease. Conditions associated with atrial flutter include coronary artery disease, rheumatic heart disease, cardiomyopathy, hypertensive heart disease, pulmonary disease with or without cor pulmonale, hyperthyroidism, alcohol ingestion, pericarditis, acute MI, pulmonary embolism, septal defects, congenital heart disease, after surgical repair of congenital defects, and other causes of atrial dilatation.

Treatment of atrial flutter commonly involves controlling the ventricular response with agents such as verapamil, diltiazem, β-blockers, or digoxin. Synchronized direct current (DC) cardioversion is effective and may require only low energies (i.e., 50–100 J). Rapid atrial overdrive pacing may terminate type I atrial flutter. Antiarrhythmic agents (i.e., class IA, IC, III) have been used successfully, but because facilitation of AV conduction may occur during use of class IA agents with vagolytic activity or class I or III agents that slow the atrial rate enough to allow 1:1 conduction, concomitant negative dromotropic (i.e., AV nodal slowing) agents may be required. Long-term prevention of atrial flutter has been difficult with medical treatment. As noted, however, type I atrial flutter can

be cured, with a success rate of 75 to-90%, by radiofrequency catheter ablation, with application of radiofrequency energy to produce a line of conduction block across the posterior corridor.

ATRIAL FIBRILLATION

Atrial fibrillation is the most common sustained tachyarrhythmia. During atrial fibrillation, electrical activation of the atria occurs in rapid, multiple waves of depolarization, with continuously changing, wandering pathways. Intra-atrial activation can be recorded as irregular, rapid depolarizations, often at rates exceeding 300 to 400 bpm. Mechanically, this pattern of rapid, disordered atrial activation results in loss of coordinated atrial contraction. Irregular electrical inputs to the AV node lead to irregular ventricular rates.

On the surface ECG, atrial fibrillation is characterized by absence of discrete P waves, presence of irregular fibrillatory waves, or both, and an irregularly irregular ventricular response. Complete BBB or aberrancy (i.e., Ashman's phenomenon) can mimic VT. At physical examination, the pulse is irregularly irregular, variable stroke volumes may produce pulse deficits, and the jugular venous waveform will lack A waves.

The incidence of atrial fibrillation increases with age. The most common underlying cardiovascular diseases associated with atrial fibrillation are hypertension and ischemic heart disease. Age, valvular disease, congestive heart failure, hypertension, and diabetes mellitus are independent risk factors for atrial fibrillation. Other associated conditions include rheumatic heart disease (especially mitral valve disease), nonrheumatic valvular disease, cardiomyopathies, congenital heart disease, pulmonary embolism, thyrotoxicosis, chronic lung disease, sick sinus syndrome/degenerative conduction system disease, Wolff-Parkinson-White syndrome, pericarditis, neoplastic disease, postoperative states, and normal hearts affected by high adrenergic states, alcohol, stress, drugs (especially sympathomimetics), excessive caffeine, hypoxia, hypokalemia, hypoglycemia, or systemic infection.

One of the most important clinical consequences of atrial fibrillation is its association with thromboembolic events and stroke. Recommended guidelines for antithrombotic therapy are listed in Table 65.2.

Short-Term Treatment

Short-term treatment of atrial fibrillation that is symptomatic with an increased heart rate should include consideration of urgent cardioversion if the patient is hemodynamically unstable (e.g., hypotensive) or has evidence of ischemia or pulmonary edema. For moderate-to-severe symptoms, acute control of the ventricular rate usually can be achieved with intravenous β-blockers, verapamil, diltiazem, or digoxin (Table 65.3). Digoxin can be used safely in patients with heart failure, but it has a delayed peak onset of heart rate–lowering effect, a narrow therapeutic window, and is less effective in

Table 65.2.   Guidelines for Antithrombotic Therapy for Atrial Fibrillation

American College of Chest Physicians Guidelines
Strongly consider long-term oral warfarin therapy (INR, 2.0–3.0) for:
   All patients > 65 years with atrial fibrillation
   Patients < 65 years with any of the following risk factors:
      Previous transient ischemic attack or stroke
      Hypertension
      Heart failure
      Diabetes
      Clinical coronary artery disease
      Mitral stenosis
      Prosthetic heart valves
      Thyrotoxicosis
   Oral anticoagulation is recommended for these patients instead of aspirin because of the greater reduction in stroke
      provided by anticoagulation
   Patients with atrial fibrillation who are poor candidates for anticoagulation therapy or who refuse anticoagulation
      Aspirin, 325 mg/day
Patients < 65 years with no risk factors for stroke:
   Either aspirin or no antithrombotic therapy
Patients 65–75 years without the above risk factors:
   Patient and physician should balance the low risk of stroke with the possible side effects of antithrombotic therapy in
      selecting either aspirin or oral anticoagulants
Patients > 75 years:
   Oral anticoagulant therapy is recommended
   This must be balanced against the age-related risks of bleeding
   Anticoagulation at the lower end of the therapeutic range (INR, 2.0–3.0) may be appropriate
For electrical cardioversion of patients in atrial fibrillation, it is strongly recommended that:
   Warfarin therapy (INR, 2.0–3.0) should be given for 3 weeks before elective cardioversion of patients who have been in
      atrial fibrillation for > 2 days, and it should be continued until normal sinus rhythm has been maintained for 4 weeks
   Consideration should be given to treating patients in atrial flutter in the same manner as patients in atrial fibrillation
   Long-term anticoagulation beyond the 4 weeks after cardioversion should be considered if there also is cardiomyopathy,
      history of previous embolism, or mitral valve disease
   Heparin anticoagulation followed by oral anticoagulation may be indicated for patients requiring emergency cardioversion
      for hemodynamic instability, in the presence of mitral valve disease, or following cardioversion if spontaneous echo
      contrast in the left atrium or left atrial appendage is detected
Contraindications to Anticoagulation:
   Hemorrhagic tendencies
   Recent intracranial hemorrhage or neurosurgery
   Recent major hemorrhage or trauma
   Uncontrolled diastolic hypertension with blood pressure > 105 mm Hg
Other critical considerations include:
   Patients at risk of falling
   Alcohol abuse
   Drug interactions
   Poor compliance or follow-up
   Concomitant use of nonsteroidal anti-inflammatory drugs
It should be noted that many of these patients were excluded from the multicenter trials on atrial fibrillation.
There is an increased risk of bleeding that correlates with the level of anticoagulation (ie, INR > 4).
A marked decrease in efficacy is noted at INR < 2.0

Adapted with permission from Laupacis A, Albers G, Dalen J, et al. Antithrombotic therapy in atrial fibrillation. Chest 1995;108:352S–359S.
INR, international normalized ratio.

Table 65.3.   Medical Treatment for Ventricular Rate Control in Supraventricular Arrhythmias, including Atrial Fibrillation

Agent	Loading Dose	Maintenance Dose	Side Effects/Toxicity	Comments
Digoxin	0.25–0.50 mg IV, then 0.25 mg IV q 4–6 h to 1 mg in the first 24 h	0.125–0.250 mg PO or IV q.d.	Anorexia, nausea, AV block, ventricular arrhythmias; accumulates in renal failure	Used in congestive heart failure vagotonic effects on the AV node, delayed onset of action, narrow therapeutic window, less effective in paroxysmal atrial fibrillation or high adrenergic states
Class II (β-blockers)			Bronchospasm, congestive heart failure, ↓ blood pressure	Effective in heart rate control even with exercise, rapid onsets of action
Propranolol	1 mg IV q 2–5′ to 0.1–0.2 mg/kg	10–80 mg PO t.i.d.–q.i.d.		
Metoprolol	5 mg IV q 5′ to 15 mg	25–100 mg PO b.i.d.		
Esmolol	500 μg/kg IV over 1′	50 μg/kg IV for 4′; repeat load PRN and ↑ maintenance 20–50 μg/kg/min q 5–10′ PRN		Esmolol short-acting
Class IV (calcium channel blockers)			↓ blood pressure, congestive heart failure	Rapid onset, can be used safely in chronic obstructive pulmonary disease and diabetes mellitus
Verapamil	2.5–10.0 mg IV over 2′	5–10 mg IV q 30–60′ or 40–160 mg PO t.i.d.	↑ Digoxin level	
Diltiazem	0.25 mg/kg over 2′, repeat prn q 15′ at 0.35 mg/kg	5–15 mg/h IV or 30–90 mg PO q.i.d.		
Class III				
Sotalol		80–240 mg PO b.i.d.	Bradycardia, congestive heart failure, bronchospasm, ↓ blood pressure, ↑ QT, Torsade de Pointes, proarrhythmia	
Amiodarone	600–1600 mg/day, divided	100–400 mg PO q.d.	Bradycardia, pulmonary, thyroid, liver, skin, gastrointestinal, ophthalmologic	Drug interactions
Adenosine	6–18 mg IV rapid bolus		Transient sinus bradycardia, sinus arrest, AV block, flushing, chest discomfort, bronchospasm; may precipitate atrial fibrillation by shortening of atrial refractoriness	Not effective in controlling ventricular rate in atrial fibrillation flutter, but may be useful diagnostically; can terminate reentrant paroxysmal SVTs utilizing the AV node

rate control of paroxysmal atrial fibrillation or rapid rates during hyperadrenergic states when the vagal tone is low, such as in the intensive care unit, because of increased sympathetic tone. Pharmacologic or electrical cardioversion, use of antiarrhythmic agents, and anticoagulation should be considered. If the duration of atrial fibrillation is more than 48 hours, anticoagulation with warfarin for 3 weeks versus transesophageal echocardiographically guided cardioversion with anticoagulation should be considered. For shorter durations of atrial fibrillation (i.e., <48 hours), anticoagulation should be considered if the patient has underlying heart disease or risk factors for thromboembolism.

Long-Term Treatment

Long-term treatment of atrial fibrillation should include evaluation for underlying structural heart disease, risk factors, and potentially, other precipitating arrhythmias. Anticoagulation with warfarin or aspirin should be considered as well. Control of the ventricular rate with β-blockers, calcium channel blockers, or digoxin also may be required (Table 65.3). In addition, restoring and maintaining sinus rhythm with cardioversion, maintenance antiarrhythmic therapy, or both can be considered. Available primary antiarrhythmic agents that may effectively maintain sinus rhythm include class IA (i.e., quinidine, procainamide, disopyramide), class IC (i.e., flecainide, propafenone), class IA/B/C (i.e., moricizine), and class III (i.e., sotalol, amiodarone) antiarrhythmic drugs (Table 65.4). Nonpharmacologic approaches for refractory patients could include permanent pacemaker implantation for symptomatic bradyarrhythmias, including mode-switching, dual-chamber devices for paroxysmal atrial fibrillation; complete AV junction ablation with implantation of a rate-responsive, permanent pacemaker; AV junction modification; or the maze operation. The maze procedure was designed to cure atrial fibrillation by dividing the atria into ''maze-like'' corridors and blind alleys, which limit development of reentry by limiting the available path length. Newer investigational approaches to atrial fibrillation include an implantable atrial defibrillator, a catheter-based mazed procedure, and novel pacing approaches.

JUNCTIONAL TACHYCARDIAS

Abnormal junctional tachycardias can be divided into nonreentrant and reentrant tachycardias.

Nonparoxysmal Junctional Tachycardia

Nonparoxysmal AV junctional tachycardia is characterized by gradual onset and termination, and it likely results from accelerated automatic discharge in or near the bundle of His. In this form of accelerated junctional rhythm, AV junctional tissue may exhibit faster discharge rates or usurp the dominant pacemaker status during sinus slowing. Heart rate generally ranges from 70 to 130 bpm, but it can be faster. Nonparoxysmal AV junctional tachycardia occasionally occurs in patients with underlying heart disease, such as acute MI, myocarditis, after open-heart surgery (particularly valve procedures), or with digitalis intoxication. It also can occur in otherwise healthy, asymptomatic individuals. In infants or children, it is associated with a high mortality rate. Incessant tachycardia may lead to a tachycardia-mediated cardiomyopathy. Treatment generally is supportive and directed toward the underlying disease. Standard treatment for digitalis toxicity may be required. β-Blockers and class IA, IC, and III antiarrhythmic agents have been used, as has radiofrequency catheter ablation.

Atrioventricular Nodal Reentrant Tachycardia

The most common form of paroxysmal reentrant SVT is AVNRT, which accounts for between 60 to 70% of patients with paroxysmal supraventricular tachycardia. Reentry occurs within the AV node and perinodal tissue, and at least two functional pathways of conduction can be demonstrated within the AV node in patients with AVNRT (Fig. 65.7). Typically, one (fast) pathway conducts rapidly, with a relatively long refractory period. A second (slow) pathway conducts more slowly, and usually with a shorter refractory period. During sinus rhythm, conduction generally occurs over the fast pathway. A premature atrial depolarization that blocks conduction in the fast pathway because of the longer refractory period, however, still may conduct over the slow pathway. If conduction through this pathway is slow enough that the fast-pathway refractory period ends and the impulse can travel retrogradely back to the atrium, then AV node reentry can occur. In common, or typical, AVNRT, anterograde conduction occurs via the slow pathway and retrograde conduction via the fast pathway. Rapid retrograde activation of the atrium via the fast pathway occurs nearly simultaneously with the ventricular activation, and it usually causes the P wave to be simultaneous with, or buried within, the QRS. In between 5 and 10% of patients with AVNRT, atypical or uncommon AVNRT occurs, in which anterograde conduction takes place via the fast pathway and retrograde conduction via the slow pathway. This causes retrograde P waves that usually are negative in the inferior leads (i.e., II, III, aVF) and are separated from the QRS, with an RP interval that is longer than the PR interval (i.e., a mechanism of long RP tachycardia).

Clinically, AVNRT commonly occurs in patients with no structural heart disease, and 70% of patients are women. It may occur at any age, but most patients present during the fourth or fifth decade of life. Symptoms may include palpitations, lightheadedness, near-syncope, weakness, dyspnea, chest pain, rarely syncope, and frequently neck pounding with prominent A waves that can be seen on the jugular pulse, representing atrial contraction against a closed tricuspid valve.

Electrocardiographically, the rate of AVNRT usually is 150 to 200 bpm, though rates as high as 250 bpm can occur. Initiation of typical AVNRT usually occurs with a premature

Table 65.4. Class I and III Antiarrhythmic Agents

Antiarrhythmic Drug	Dose	Side Effects/Comments
Class IA		↑ QT, proarrhythmia/TdP, potential ↑ AV node conduction can be seen with all three
Quinidine	200–400 mg PO t.i.d.–b.i.d.	Diarrhea, nausea, ↑ digoxin levels
Procainamide	10–15 mg/kg IV at ≤50 mg/min or 500–1000 mg PO q 6 h (sustained release)	↓ Blood pressure, congestive heart failure, drug-induced lupus; metabolite NAPA (class III) can accumulate in renal failure
Disopyramide	100–300 mg PO t.i.d.	Anticholinergic effects (e.g., urinary retention, dry eyes/mouth), congestive heart failure
Class IB		
Lidocaine	50–100 mg IV (0.5–1.5 mg/kg) bolus, infusion of 1–4 mg/min, and rebolus in 5–15 mins	Reduce dosage in congestive heart failure, elderly, hepatic dysfunction; bradycardia, hypotension, central nervous system (tremors, seizures, altered mental status) side effects
Mexiletine	150–300 mg PO q 8 h	Gastrointestinal side effects (nausea, vomiting) common, may be minimized by dosing with meals; central nervous system effects (tremor, dizziness, nervousness)
Tocainide	400–600 mg PO q 8 h	Gastrointestinal side effects (nausea, vomiting), central nervous system less common (dizziness, vertigo, nervousness); rare but potentially life-threatening agranulocytosis and pulmonary fibrosis
Phenytoin	100 mg PO q 8 h; loading up to 1 g in divided doses; or 20–50 mg/min IV to maximum 1 g	Rarely used as an antiarrhythmic agent outside of digitalis toxicity; central nervous system side effects common; dermatologic reactions
Class IC		Proarrhythmia
Flecainide	50–200 mg PO b.i.d.	Visual disturbance, dizziness, congestive heart failure, avoid in coronary artery disease or left ventricular dysfunction
Propafenone	150–300 mg PO t.i.d.	Congestive heart failure, ? avoid in coronary artery disease/left ventricular dysfunction
Class IA/B/C		
Moricizine	200–300 mg PO t.i.d.	Proarrhythmia, dizziness, gastrointestinal/nausea, headache, caution in coronary artery disease/left ventricular dysfunction
Class III		
Sotalol	80–240 mg PO b.i.d.	Congestive heart failure, bronchospasm, bradycardia, ↑ QT, proarrhythmia/TdP; renally excreted
Bretylium	5–10 mg/kg IV bolus; 1–2 mg/min IV infusion	Hypotension; transient increased arrhythmias possible due to initial norepinephrine release; reduce dose in renal failure
Amiodarone	600–1600 mg/d loading in divided doses PO, 100–400 mg PO q.d. maintenance; IV available	Pulmonary toxicity, bradycardia, hyper- or hypothyroidism, hepatic toxicity, gastrointestinal (nausea, constipation), neurologic, dermatologic, and ophthalmologic side effects, drug interactions

NAPA, N-acetylprocalnamide; TdP, torsade de pointes.

Figure 65.7. AVNRT.

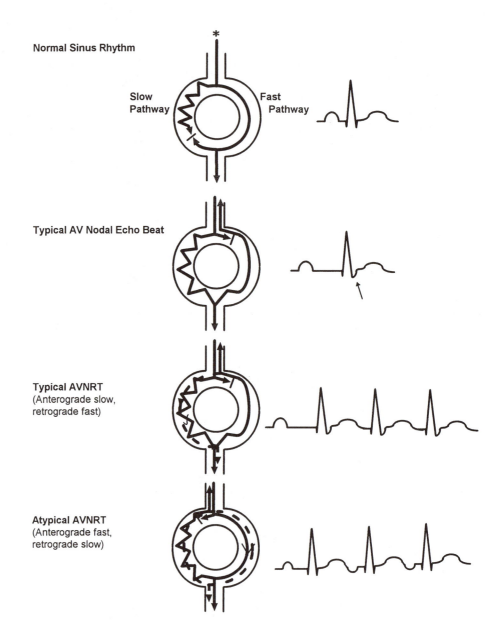

atrial contraction that is followed by a long PR interval, thus indicating blocked conduction in the fast pathway and conduction down the slow pathway. Because atrial and ventricular activation occur simultaneously during the tachycardia, P waves generally are buried in the QRS. A pseudo r′ in V$_1$ may be seen during typical AVNRT. A longer RP interval indicates retrograde conduction via a slower retrograde pathway.

Treatment

Vagal maneuvers (e.g., carotid sinus massage, Valsalva maneuver) may slow or terminate the tachycardia. Adenosine, 6 to 12 mg administered as a rapid intravenous bolus, is the initial drug of choice. Termination of a narrow-complex tachycardia by vagal maneuvers or adenosine can be helpful

diagnostically by suggesting the AV node may be a component of the circuit (in contrast to atrial tachycardias, in which AV block can be produced with continued tachycardia). β-Blockers, verapamil, or diltiazem also can be successful. Long-term use of these agents or of class IA, IC, or III antiarrhythmic drugs can be successful, but radiofrequency catheter ablation, particularly of the slow AV nodal pathway, has become the standard therapy for cure of AVNRT, with success rates that can exceed 95% and less than a 1% risk of inducing complete AV block or need for a permanent pacemaker.

SUPRAVENTRICULAR TACHYCARDIA MEDIATED BY ACCESSORY PATHWAYS

Accessory pathways are bands of excitable conducting tissue that connect the atrium and the ventricle, thus bypassing either all or part of the normal AV conduction system. Preexcitation syndromes are disorders in which anterograde ventricular or retrograde atrial activation occurs, either in part or totally, through anomalous pathways distinct from the normal conduction system. Anterograde conduction (i.e., from atrium to ventricle) via an AP during sinus rhythm causes manifest ventricular preexcitation (i.e., Wolff-Parkinson-White syndrome). This results in wide QRS complexes, because the AP inserts into the ventricular myocardium with activation occurring from myocyte to myocyte rather than via the faster-conducting His-Purkinje system. On ECG, a short PR interval and a delta wave (i.e, initial slurring of the QRS) usually are seen. Approximately 1 to 3 per 1000 ECGs show ventricular preexcitation. APs that conduct only in the retrograde direction are called concealed (i.e., no ventricular preexcitation or delta wave seen on surface ECG), yet these still may participate in SVT. Typical APs conduct rapidly and nondecrementally. Variant APs include those with slow, decremental conduction and connections from the atrium to the distal AV node, the atrium to the His bundle, and the atrium to the right bundle, distal Purkinje network, or apex via a duplicate AV node–His bundle-like connection (i.e., Mahaim fiber). Congenital abnormalities associated with APs include Ebstein's anomaly, coarctation of the aorta, hypertrophic cardiomyopathy, ventricular septal defects, and D-transposition of the great arteries.

Atrioventricular Reentrant Tachycardia

During AVRT, the AP as well as the atria and ventricles are essential parts of the circuit (Fig. 65.8). In orthodromic AVRT, anterograde conduction occurs via the AV node and retrograde conduction via the AP. In antidromic AVRT, anterograde conduction occurs via an AP and retrograde conduction via the AV node or a second AP. Other AP-associated tachycardias include atrial fibrillation, atrial flutter, atrial tachycardia, or AVNRT with conduction via a ''bystander'' AP, in which the AP is not integral to the tachycardia but conducts to the ventricle. Slowly conducting, concealed APs, which usually are located in the posteroseptum, can mediate near-incessant orthodromic SVT with retrograde, slow conduction via the AP (i.e., permanent form of junctional reciprocating tachycardia); these can present as a tachycardia-mediated cardiomyopathy. The most common tachycardias

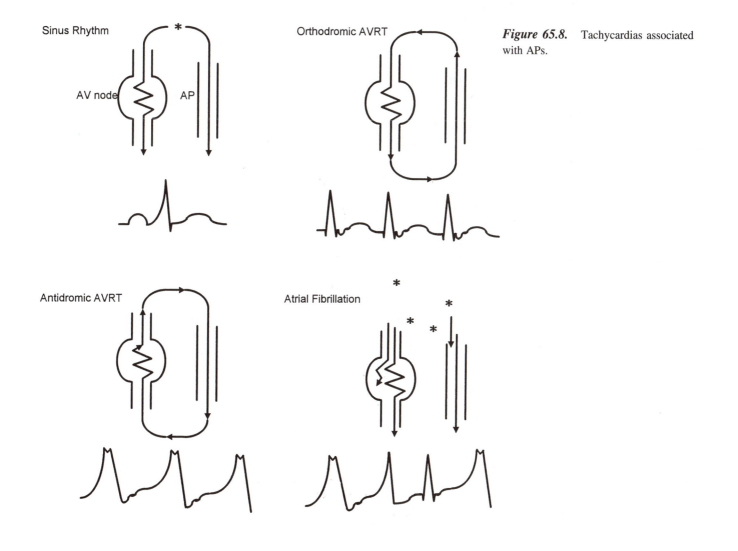

Figure 65.8. Tachycardias associated with APs.

associated with APs are discussed in the following sections; their treatment is summarized in Table 65.5.

Orthodromic Atrioventricular Reentrant Tachycardia

Orthodromic AVRT is the most common SVT in patients with APs, occurring in 90% of those who are symptomatic. Antero-grade conduction occurs via the AV node and His-Purkinje system, inscribing a narrow QRS (with no preexcitation) on the surface ECG unless BBB aberrancy occurs. Because retro-grade conduction is via the AP, patients with either manifest or concealed APs can experience orthodromic AVRT. The heart rate of the tachycardia usually is 150 to 250 bpm, and the tachycardia usually initiates with an atrial or ventricular premature depolarization. Because the atria and ventricles are requisite parts of the circuit, a 1:1 relationship must be present. Demonstration of AV dissociation or intermittent AV block during SVT excludes AVRT as a diagnosis. The P wave commonly is visualized in the early part of the ST segment, with a constant RP interval despite the tachycardia rate. Spon-taneous or induced BBB during orthodromic AVRT that slows the tachycardia rate indicates participation of an AP ipsilateral to the side of the BBB (Fig. 65.9). For example, during ortho-dromic AVRT utilizing a left free-wall AP as the retrograde limb, production of block in the left bundle forces ventricular activation to occur via the right bundle, thus requiring conduc-tion through a longer, ventricular myocardial path back up to the AP and slowing the tachycardia cycle length.

Short-term treatment of the two common, regular, nar-row-complex tachycardias (i.e., orthodromic AVRT and AVNRT) is similar, because the AV node is an integral part of the circuit in the anterograde direction. To terminate the tachycardia, vagal maneuvers or adenosine are the first op-tions of choice, followed by intravenous β-blockers, vera-pamil, or diltiazem. Adenosine can shorten atrial refractory periods and, occasionally, precipitate atrial fibrillation with a rapid ventricular response. In patients with very rapid SVT and hemodynamic impairment, DC cardioversion is the initial treatment of choice. Longer-term treatment may include β-blockers, verapamil, diltiazem, digoxin, or class IA, IC, or III antiarrhythmic drugs. Radiofrequency catheter ablation, however, can be curative, with high success rates; in many patients, it can be considered as a first-line or early therapeutic option.

Antidromic Atrioventricular Reentrant Tachycardia

Antidromic AVRT is uncommon, occurring in less than 5 to 10% of patients with Wolff-Parkinson-White syndrome. The anterograde limb of the circuit is via an AP. In 33 to 60% of patients with antidromic AVRT, however, multiple APs are present, and the retrograde limb may be via either the AV node or another AP. Because ventricular activation occurs via an AP, the QRS is wide, bizarre, and preexcited. Mahaim

---

Table 65.5.   Management of Preexcitation Syndromes

Initial evaluation:
Determine presence or absence of symptoms
Characterize symptoms, including frequency and severity
Determine previous treatment regimens and effectiveness
Document specific arrhythmias present during symptoms
Determine presence of concomitant heart disease
Acute treatment of arrhythmias associated with
    preexcitation syndromes:
Orthodromic SVT
    Vagal maneuvers (e.g., Valsalva, carotid sinus massage)
    Adenosine IV (6–12 mg rapid IV bolus)
    Verapamil IV (5–10 mg IV)
    Procainamide IV (1 g over 20–30 min)
    Cardioversion
Antidromic SVT (retrograde conduction may occur via a
    second AP or the AV node)
    Procainamide IV
    Cardioversion
Atrial fibrillation (digoxin and verapamil may accelerate
    ventricular rate and should not be used)
    Procainamide IV
    Cardioversion
Long-term treatment of patients with preexcitation
    syndromes:
Pharmacologic management
    Concealed AP
        Digoxin/verapamil/β-blocker
        Class IC; flecainide/propafenone
        Class IA; disopyramide/quinidine/procainamide
        Class III; sotalol/amiodarone
    Manifest AP
        Class IC; flecainide/propafenone
        Class IA; disopyramide/quinidine/procainamide
        Class III; sotalol/amiodarone
Indications for nonpharmacologic management
    Life-threatening ventricular rate during atrial
        fibrillation/flutter
    SVT refractory to medical therapy
    Intolerance to medical therapy
    Alternate first-line therapy in patients with symptomatic
        arrhythmias or high-risk occupations
Nonpharmacologic approaches
    Radiofrequency catheter ablation
    Surgical ablation (rarely required)
    Antitachycardic devices (rarely required)
Indications for electrophysiology studies
    Delineation of the mechanism of arrhythmias
    Localization/mapping of pathways for ablation
    Assess efficacy of antiarrhythmic agents
    Assessment of the refractory periods of the AP as an
        indicator of the risk of sudden death

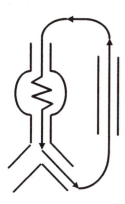

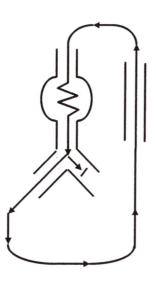

Figure 65.9. Orthodromic AVRT with BBB ipsilateral to the AP.

Orthodromic AVRT   Orthodromic AVRT with Ipsilateral BBB

fibers, which are APs with decremental conduction properties that connect the atrium to the distal right bundle branch or apex via a duplicate AV node–His bundle-like connection, also can mediate a form of antidromic AVRT with LBBB morphology. In antidromic AVRT, if the AV node comprises the retrograde limb, then vagal maneuvers or adenosine may terminate the tachycardia, but these measures will not be effective if both limbs are via APs. In the short term, treatment may require DC cardioversion or procainamide.

Atrial Fibrillation and Wolff-Parkinson-White Syndrome

In patients with manifest APs having a short refractory period, rapid conduction to the ventricles during atrial fibrillation via the AP can provoke ventricular fibrillation. The shortest pre-excited RR interval during atrial fibrillation gives an indication as to the refractory period of the AP. Short refractory periods (<250 ms) are associated with increased risk of sudden death. Verapamil can increase the ventricular rate during atrial fibrillation; intravenous verapamil may precipitate ventricular fibrillation and should *not* be given. The treatment of choice is procainamide or DC cardioversion.

SPECIFIC VENTRICULAR ARRHYTHMIAS

Ventricular tachycardia is defined as three or more consecutive ventricular beats at a rate of 100 bpm or more. Nonsustained VT is defined as VT lasting three or more beats under 30 seconds in duration and that does not require intervention for termination. Sustained VT is VT lasting 30 seconds or more or requiring intervention for termination. QRS morphology may be either monomorphic (i.e., uniform) or polymorphic (i.e., variable). The usual heart rate of VT ranges from 100 to 280 bpm. VT is wide because of the slower rate of conduction through ventricular tissue compared with that through Purkinje fibers. Hemodynamic stability depends on

the rate, underlying cardiac disease, ventricular function, and concomitant pharmacologic treatment. VA dissociation occurs in 60 to 70% of these patients, but it may be evident on surface ECGs only in one-third of patients.

PREMATURE VENTRICULAR DEPOLARIZATIONS

Isolated premature ventricular depolarizations are not associated with significant risk in patients without structural heart disease, but frequent or complex premature ventricular complexes can be markers for potential increased risk in those with structural heart disease. Treatment of isolated, symptomatic premature complexes generally includes assessment of risk if there is structural heart disease or risk factors, avoidance of precipitating factors (e.g., caffeine, sympathomimetic agents), and reassurance, with occasional β-blockers or, rarely, other antiarrhythmic agents for persistently symptomatic patients.

VENTRICULAR TACHYARRHYTHMIAS AFTER MYOCARDIAL INFARCTION

Premature ventricular complexes, nonsustained or sustained VT, ventricular fibrillation, and polymorphic VT can occur during the acute phases of ischemia/infarction. Coronary reperfusion has been associated with accelerated idioventricular rhythms and ventricular tachyarrhythmias. Nonsustained or sustained VT, which often results from reentry, can occur late after MI.

Use of lidocaine as prophylaxis for ventricular fibrillation in patients with suspected acute MI has been controversial. Prophylactic lidocaine may produce a small decrease in the incidence of ventricular fibrillation. It has not been shown to improve the mortality rate, however, and significant side effects can occur. Potential adverse effects include asystole, bradyarrhythmias, neurologic symptoms, seizures, respiratory arrest, nausea, and vomiting. Current data suggest that routine use of prophylactic lidocaine in patients with suspected acute MI should be avoided when facilities and personnel for prompt resuscitation are available, but when defibrillation is unavailable, prophylactic lidocaine might be beneficial. In other words, during situations in which facilities or personnel are unavailable, the benefits of lidocaine prophylaxis may outweigh its risks.

Short-term treatment of ventricular arrhythmias following MI depends on the hemodynamic status of the patient and presence of on-going or recurrent ischemia (as well as other precipitating factors). The long-term prognosis depends on the timing of these arrhythmias in relation to the acute infarction as well as to the degree of ventricular dysfunction. Asymptomatic premature ventricular complexes or nonsustained VT generally do not require short-term therapy, but they may be associated with an increased mortality rate when they are frequent or complex, detected late in the course of MI, or associated with left ventricular dysfunction. Accelerated idioventricular rhythms have been associated with coronary reperfusion, but they have not been specific or highly sensitive as predictors of reperfusion and generally do not require specific short-term therapy. Early VT/fibrillation that is sustained is associated with an increased in-hospital mortality rate. Among hospital survivors, however, it does not signify a worsened long-term prognosis. Short-term therapy may require DC countershock, antiarrhythmic therapy, correction of electrolyte and metabolic imbalances, or assessment and treatment of associated recurrent or on-going ischemia.

Long-term treatment requires assessment of prognostic significance. Frequent or complex ventricular arrhythmias occurring after the acute phase of MI (i.e., the first 48–72 hours) are more frequent in patients with significant myocardial dysfunction. They also are an independent prognostic factor. Empiric suppression of PVCs or nonsustained VT using antiarrhythmic agents, however, with the possible exception of amiodarone, is associated with the potential for an increased mortality rate. Patients with nonsustained VT and LVEF ≤35% after MI should be considered for electrophysiology study with implantation of a cardioverter-defibrillator if the study induces sustained VT or reproducible ventricular fibrillation that is not suppressed by an antiarrhythmic drug. Sustained ventricular arrhythmias after the acute phase of MI are associated with a high rate of recurrence, and further electrophysiologic assessment as well as treatment with pharmacologic agents or an implantable cardioverter-defibrillator may be indicated. β-blockers and angiotensin-converting enzyme inhibitors have also been associated with improved survival rates in many studies.

VENTRICULAR ARRHYTHMIAS ASSOCIATED WITH NONISCHEMIC CARDIOMYOPATHY

Ventricular tachycardia or fibrillation associated with nonischemic cardiomyopathy may result from reentry, triggered activity, or increased automaticity. A form of macroreentry caused by bundle-branch reentry is more common in patients with nonischemic dilated cardiomyopathy and preexisting His-Purkinje system disease, as can be manifested by an intraventricular conduction delay in sinus rhythm, most commonly of the left BBB–type. Bundle-branch reentrant VT most commonly presents as a rapid VT of left BBB morphology, though rare right BBB morphologies have been described. This arrhythmia potentially can be cured by selective radiofrequency ablation of one of the bundle branches (most commonly the right).

ARRHYTHMOGENIC RIGHT VENTRICULAR DYSPLASIA

Arrhythmogenic right ventricular dysplasia results from a cardiomyopathy, possibly familial in some patients (i.e., chromosome 14), that predominantly involves the right ventricle with hypokinetic and thinned areas that often have fatty infiltration. It can cause ventricular arrhythmias in patients with an apparently normal left ventricle. VTs associated with arrhythmogenic right ventricular dysplasia generally have a LBBB morphology and may result from reentry. Pharmacologic therapies with antiarrhythmic drugs, surgery, implantable cardioverter-defibrillator therapy, and radiofrequency ablation have been used as treatments of ventricular arrhythmias in patients with arrhythmogenic right ventricular dysplasia.

VENTRICULAR TACHYCARDIAS IN PATIENTS WITH STRUCTURALLY NORMAL HEARTS

Syndromes of repetitive, monomorphic, nonsustained or sustained VT and paroxysmal VTs can present in patients with structurally normal hearts. Right ventricular outflow tract VT can present with symptomatic, minimally symptomatic, or asymptomatic frequent, repetitive, or paroxysmal nonsustained or sustained VT, or with frequent symptomatic PVCs. It may be precipitated by stress, exercise, or high catecholamine states. Vagal maneuvers or adenosine may terminate the tachycardia. The PVCs or VT is monomorphic and characterized by left BBB morphology with an inferior axis (i.e., positive QRS in aVF, II, III). The VT often is associated with a gradual onset (i.e., ''warm-up'') and offset, may not be inducible with programmed ventricular extrastimulation (i.e., at electrophysiology study), but may occur during rapid pacing or infusion of isoproterenol. The mechanism may result from triggered activity or increased automaticity. Radiofrequency catheter ablation has been effective in abolishing the right ventricular outflow tract focus, and treatment also may include β-blockers, calcium channel blockers, and type I or III antiarrhythmic agents. Idiopathic left VT or fascicular tachycardia may present as a paroxysmal VT and usually can be induced by programmed ventricular extrastimulation, rapid pacing, isoproterenol, or exercise. It is characterized by right BBB morphology, usually with left superior axis (i.e., left-axis deviation; negative in II, aVF), and it usually arises in the left inferoposterior septum through a mechanism believed to result from fascicular reentry or triggered activity. It may be terminated or suppressed by verapamil or diltiazem, and it has been successfully treated using radiofrequency catheter ablation at sites where the VT is preceded by a fascicular potential.

TORSADE DE POINTES

A form of polymorphic VT, torsade de pointes (TdP) is a potentially life-threatening condition that can occur as a complication of several medications or in association with congenital long QT syndromes. The heart rate ranges from 150 to 250 bpm with twisting of the QRS complexes around the baseline. QT prolongation and QTU abnormalities are characteristic but may be present only in beats preceding TdP. TdP typically is rate dependent, and sinus bradycardia, bradycardia resulting from AV block, or abrupt prolongation of the RR interval (e.g., with a pause after a premature complex) can trigger its onset. It usually initiates with "long-short" coupled intervals, which may occur because of a PVC on the previous, long QT–associated T wave. A pause followed by a subsequent sinus or supraventricular beat and another PVC with a short coupling interval then may initiate TdP.

Acquired and congenital forms of long QT syndromes also can predispose to TdP. Congenital syndromes include the Romano-Ward syndrome (i.e., autosomal dominant) and Jervell-Lange-Nielson syndrome (i.e., double dominant, associated with deafness). Linkage studies have revealed multiple separate loci (including on chromosomes 3, 4, 7, 11, and 21) that cause abnormalities in K^+ or Na^+ channels. The acquired long QT syndromes, many of which are associated with drugs that can prolong repolarization, are more common.

Congenital conditions associated with TdP include:

- Romano Ward syndrome
- Jervell-Lange-Nielson syndrome

Acquired conditions associated with TdP include:

- Antiarrhythmic drugs that prolong QT interval
  - Quinidine
  - Procainamide (including its metabolite *N*-acetylprocainamide)
  - Disopyramide
  - Sotalol
  - Amiodarone
  - Bepridil
- Tricyclic antidepressants
- Phenothiazines
- Antibiotics
  - Erythromycin
  - Pentamidine
  - Trimethoprim-sulfamethoxazole
  - Ampicillin
  - Ketoconazole
  - Itraconazole
  - Spiramycin
- Nonsedating antihistamines
  - Terfenadine
  - Astemizole

- Other QT-prolonging drugs
  - Probucol
  - Ketanserin
  - Cisapride
- Organophosphates
- Electrolyte abnormalities
  - Hypokalemia
  - Hypomagnesemia
  - Hypocalcemia (uncommon)
- Bradyarrhythmias
- Hypothyroidism
- Liquid protein and other diets, anorexia
- Central nervous system abnormalities, particularly affecting sympathetic outflow
  - Subarachnoid hemorrhage
  - Brainstem, cervical cord lesions

Treatment includes avoidance of offending agents and may require acceleration of the heart rate, which can be accomplished with either pharmacologic agents (e.g., isoproterenol) or pacing, and intravenous magnesium. Lidocaine, mexiletine, or phenytoin can be tried as well.

PHARMACOLOGIC THERAPY

The most commonly accepted classification of antiarrhythmic drugs is the Vaughan-Williams classification (Harrison's modification). All drug classifications possess shortcomings, and specific agents may block more than one ion channel with effects that are characteristic of multiple classes. This scheme, however, has proved useful. Class I antiarrhythmic drugs block Na^+ channels, thereby decreasing action-potential upstroke velocity (i.e., phase 0) and slowing conduction. Class I drugs are further divided into three subdivisions. Class IA agents, which prolong repolarization or action-potential duration, have a moderate effect on conduction slowing and depression of phase 0. Class IB drugs have little effect on conduction and phase 0 in normal tissue, but they exhibit moderate effects in abnormal tissue. In addition, they show either no effect or a shortening of repolarization/action-potential duration. Class IC agents have a marked effect on conduction slowing and phase 0, with mild or no effects on repolarization or action potential duration. Class II contains the β-adrenergic blocking agents, and class III agents prolong repolarization/action potential duration. Class IV contains calcium channel blockers. Tables 65.3 and 65.4 list commonly used antiarrhythmic agents and their suggested dosages.

Another strategy for classifying drugs has been the Sicilian Gambit approach, in which an attempt is made to identify the mechanism of a specific arrhythmia, the vulnerable electrophysiologic parameter of the arrhythmia (e.g., refractory period, conduction, excitability, phase 4 depolarization, action-potential duration), and the ionic target that most likely will modulate the vulnerable parameter. The Sicilian Gambit encourages consideration of drug actions irrespective of the Vaughan-Williams classification.

Bradyarrhythmias

SINUS NODE DYSFUNCTION

Sinus node dysfunction includes a range of abnormalities, including sinus bradyarrhythmias (e.g., sinus pauses, sinus bradycardias, chronotropic incompetence, sinus pauses or sinus arrest, sinoatrial exit block), sick sinus syndrome, and tachycardia-bradycardia syndrome (e.g., paroxysmal or persistent atrial tachyarrhythmias with periods of bradyarrhythmia). Other forms of sinus node dysfunction that cause tachycardias (e.g., sinus tachycardia, inappropriate sinus tachycardia, sinus node reentry) were discussed previously.

SINUS BRADYCARDIA

Sinus bradycardia, which generally is defined as heart rates of less than 60 bpm, is common in young, healthy adults (especially in athletes), with normal rates during sleep falling to as low as 35 to 50 bpm. It usually is benign, but it can be associated with diseases such as hypothyroidism, vagal stimulation, increased intracranial pressure, MI, and drugs such as β-blockers (including those used for glaucoma), calcium channel blockers, amiodarone, clonidine, lithium, and parasympathomimetic drugs. Treatment often is unnecessary if the patient is asymptomatic. Patients with chronic bradycardia or chronotropic incompetence and symptoms of congestive heart failure or low cardiac output, however, may benefit from permanent pacing.

SINUS PAUSES OR SINUS ARREST

Sinus pauses or arrest may result from degenerative changes of the sinus node, acute MI, excessive vagal tone or stimuli, digitalis toxicity, sleep apnea, or stroke. Symptomatic or very long pauses may require permanent pacing.

SINOATRIAL EXIT BLOCK

Sinoatrial exit block results from a block in conduction from the sinus node to the atria. It usually appears as absence of a P wave, with the sinus pause duration being a multiple of the basic PP interval (i.e., type II). In Type I (Wenckebach pattern) sinoatrial exit block, the PP interval shortens before the pause, and the pause is less than two PP intervals. Sinoatrial exit block usually is transient but may be caused by drugs, vagal stimulation, or degenerative disease of the sinus node and atrium. Therapy for symptomatic sinoatrial exit block involves avoidance of precipitating factors and, potentially, pacing for persistent symptoms.

SICK SINUS SYNDROME

Sick sinus syndrome includes a variety of sinus nodal disorders, such as inappropriate sinus bradycardia, sinus pauses/ arrest/sinoatrial exit block, combinations of sinoatrial and AV conduction abnormalities, and tachycardia-bradycardia syndrome, in which periods of rapid atrial tachyarrhythmias as well as periods of slow atrial and ventricular rates occur. Treatment depends on the basic rhythm disturbance. Drug therapy for rapid atrial arrhythmias may aggravate the bradyarrhythmias, and permanent pacing may be required.

HYPERSENSITIVE CAROTID SINUS SYNDROME

Carotid sinus hypersensitivity can produce sinus arrest or AV block leading to syncope, and it may be demonstrable with carotid sinus massage. Two types of responses are noted. A cardioinhibitory component with pauses of longer than 3 seconds and/or a vasodepressor component with a decrease in systolic blood pressure may be provoked with carotid sinus massage. Symptomatic patients may require pacemaker implantation to treat the cardioinhibitory component. Continued symptoms caused by vasodepressor reactions, even after pacemaker implantation, may require further treatment, including support stockings, high-sodium diets, or sodium-retaining drugs.

ATRIOVENTRICULAR DISSOCIATION

Atrioventricular dissociation refers to independent depolarization of the atria and ventricles. It may be caused by:

1. Physiologic interference resulting from slowing of the dominant pacemaker (e.g., sinus node) and escape of a subsidiary or latent pacemaker (e.g., junctional or ventricular escape),
2. Physiologic interference resulting from acceleration of a latent pacemaker that usurps control of the ventricle (e.g., accelerated junctional tachycardia or VT), and
3. AV block preventing propagation of the atrial impulse from reaching the ventricles, thus allowing a subsidiary pacemaker (e.g., junctional or ventricular escape) to control the ventricles.

Note that patients with complete AV block have AV dissociation and, generally, a ventricular rate that is slower than the atrial rate. Patients with AV dissociation, however, may have complete AV block or dissociation resulting from physiologic interference, with the latter typically having an atrial rate that is slower than the ventricular rate.

ATRIOVENTRICULAR BLOCK

AV block occurs when the atrial impulse either is not conducted to the ventricle or is conducted with delay at a time when the AV junction is not refractory. It is classified on the basis of severity into three types.

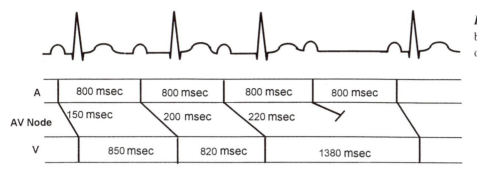

Figure 65.10. Second-degree AV block Mobitz type I (Wenckebach) periodicity.

In first-degree AV block, conduction is prolonged (PR interval > 200 ms), but all impulses are conducted. The conduction delay may occur in the AV node, the His-Purkinje system, or both. If the QRS complex is narrow and normal, the AV delay usually occurs in the AV node.

In second-degree AV block, an intermittent block in conduction occurs. In Mobitz type I (i.e., Wenckebach) second-degree AV block, progressive prolongation of the PR interval occurs before the block in conduction. In the usual Wenckebach periodicity (Fig. 65.10), the PR interval gradually increases, but with a decreasing increment, thus leading to a gradual shortening of the RR intervals. The longest PR interval usually precedes the block, and the shortest PR interval usually occurs after the block, thereby resulting in the long RR interval of the blocked impulse being shorter than twice the basic PP interval. Variants of this pattern are not uncommon. In Mobitz type II second-degree AV block, PR intervals before the block are constant, and there are sudden blocks in P-wave conduction. Advanced or high-degree AV block refers to a block of two or more consecutive impulses. In Mobitz type I block, the level of the block is almost always at the AV node. Rarely, type I Wenckebach periodicity in the His-Purkinje system may be seen in patients with BBB. In contrast, Mobitz type II block is almost always at the level of the His-Purkinje system and has a higher risk of progressing to complete AV block.

In third-degree (i.e., complete) AV block, no impulses are conducted from the atria to the ventricles. The level of the block can occur at the AV node (usually congenital), His bundle, or in the His-Purkinje system (usually acquired). Escape beats that are junctional at rates of 40 to 60 bpm generally occur with congenital complete AV block. Escape beats that are ventricular in origin often are slow, ranging from 30 to 40 bpm.

INDICATIONS FOR PERMANENT PACING

Conditions for which permanent pacing is or is not indicated are outlined in Table 65.6, based upon a three-part classification as follows:

- *Class I:* Conditions for which there is general agreement that permanent pacemakers should be implanted.
- *Class II:* Conditions for which pacemakers frequently are used but for which there is disagreement regarding their necessity.
- *Class III:* Conditions for which there is general agreement that pacemakers are unnecessary.

INDICATIONS FOR TEMPORARY PACING

In general, temporary pacing is indicated for patients with medically refractory, symptomatic bradyarrhythmias without contraindications to pacing. In the absence of acute MI, particularly while awaiting implantation of a permanent pacemaker (if indicated), temporary pacing can be warranted for patients with medically refractory, symptomatic or hemodynamically compromising sinus node bradyarrhythmias, second- or third-degree AV block, or third-degree AV block with a wide QRS escape rhythm or a ventricular rate of less than 50 bpm. In the presence of acute MI, temporary pacing is indicated for the following:

- Third-degree AV block
- Second-degree AV block
  - Mobitz II with anterior MI
  - Mobitz II with inferior MI and wide QRS complex or recurrent block with narrow QRS
  - Mobitz I with marked bradycardia and symptoms
- AV block associated with marked bradycardia and symptoms (e.g., hypotension, heart failure, low cardiac output)
- BBB
  - New bifascicular block
  - Alternating BBB
  - New BBB with anterior MI
  - Bilateral BBB of indeterminate age with anterior or indeterminate MI
  - Bilateral BBB with first-degree AV block

Table 65.6. Indications for Permanent Pacemakers and Recommended Pacing Modes

Disorder	Class of Indication	Recommended Pacing Mode
Sinus node dysfunction	I. Sinus node dysfunction with documented symptomatic bradycardia, possibly a consequence of necessary long-term drug therapy II. Sinus node dysfunction with heart rates < 40 bpm; no clear associations between symptoms and bradycardia III. No symptoms	AAI if no AV node or other conduction tissue disease DDD if concomitant AV node or conduction disease present DDDR if chronotropic incompetence DDIR or AMS if episodes of supraventricular arrhythmias present
AV block	I. Symptomatic 2° or 3° AV block, asymptomatic 3° AVB with heart rate ≤ 40 bpm or periods of asystole ≥ 3.0 seconds, or consequence of His bundle ablation II. Asymptomatic 2° type II or 3° AV block with heart rates <40 bpm; asymptomatic 2° type I at intraHis or infraHis levels III. 1° AV block or asymptomatic 2° AV block type I at the AV node level	DDD if chronotropically competent VVI(R) if no organized atrial activity DDDR or VVIR if chronotropically incompetent
AV block associated with myocardial infarction	I. Persistent advanced 2° AV block or 3° AV block with block in the HPS (bilateral BBB); transient advanced AV block and associated BBB II. Persistent advanced AV block at the AV node III. Transient AV block in the absence of IVCDs or in the presence of isolated LAFB; acquired LAFB without AV block; persistent 1° AV block with BBB not demonstrated previously	DDD if chronotropically competent VVI(R) if no organized atrial activity DDDR or VVIR if chronotropically incompetent
Bifascicular or trifascicular block	I. Fascicular block with intermittent 3° AV block associated with symptoms, or 2° type II AV block with or without symptoms II. HV > 100 msec or fascicular block associated with syncope that cannot be ascribed to other causes; pacing-induced infra-His block III. Asymptomatic fascicular block or fascicular block with associated 1° AV node block	DDD if chronotropically competent VVI(R) if no organized atrial activity DDDR or VVIR if chronotropically incompetent
Neurocardiogenic syncope or carotid sinus hypersensitivity	I. Recurrent syncope provoked by carotid sinus stimulation; pauses of >3 seconds induced by minimal carotid sinus pressure II. Syncope associated with bradycardia reproduced by head upright tilt; recurrent syncope without clear provocative events and with a hypersensitive cardioinhibitory response III. Recurrent syncope in the absence of a cardioinhibitory response	DDD or DDI
Cardiomyopathy	I. None II. Severely symptomatic patients with HOCM refractory to drug therapy (controversial) III. Severely symptomatic pts with dilated cardiomyopathy (may become class II in future)	DDD if chronotropically competent DDDR if chronotropically incompetent

Adapted with permission from Kusumoto FM, Goldschlager N. Cardiac pacing. N Engl J Med 1996;334:89–98; and Dreifus LS, Fisch C, Griffin JC, Gillette PC, Mason JW, Parsonnet V. Guidelines for implantation of cardiac pacemakers and antiarrhythmia devices: a report of the American College of Cardiology/American Heart Association Task Force on Assessment of Diagnostic and Therapeutic Cardiovascular Procedures (Committee on Pacemaker Implantation). Circulation 1991;84:455–467.

HOCM, hypertrophic obstructive cardiomyopathy; HPS, His Purkinje System; IVCDs, intraventricular conduction defect; LAFB, left anterior fascicular block.

SUGGESTED READINGS

Akhtar M, Shenasa M, Jazayeri M, Caceres J, Tchou PJ. Wide QRS complex tachycardia: reappraisal of a common clinical problem. Ann Intern Med 1988;109:905–912.

Brugada P, Brugada J, Mont L, Smeets J, Andries EW. A new approach to the differential diagnosis of a regular tachycardia with a wide QRS complex. Circulation 1991;83:1649–1659.

Dreifus LS, Fisch C, Griffin JC, Gillette PC, Mason JW, Parsonnet V. Guidelines for implantation of cardiac pacemakers and antiarrhythmia devices: a report of the American College of Cardiology/American Heart Association Task Force on Assessment of Diagnostic and Therapeutic Cardiovascular Procedures (Committee on Pacemaker Implantation). Circulation 1991;84:455–467.

Ganz LI, Friedman PL. Supraventricular tachycardia. N Engl J Med 1995;332:162–173.

Kindwall KE, Brown J, Josephson ME. Electrocardiographic criteria for ventricular tachycardia in wide complex left bundle branch block morphology tachycardias. Am J Cardiol 1988;61:1279–1283.

Kusumoto FM, Goldschlager N. Cardiac Pacing. N Engl J Med 1996;334:89–98.

Laupacis A, Albers G, Dalen J, Dunn M, Feinberg W, Jacobson A. Antithrombotic therapy in atrial fibrillation. Chest 1995;108:352S–359S.

Task Force of the Working Group on Arrhythmias of the European Society of Cardiology. The Sicilian Gambit. Circulation 1991;84:1831–1851.

Wellens HJJ, Bar FWHM, Lie KI. The value of the electrocardiogram in the differential diagnosis of a tachycardia with a widened QRS complex. Am J Med 1978;64:27–33.

Zipes DP. Genesis of cardiac arrhythmias: electrophysiological considerations. In: Braunwald E, ed. Heart disease: a textbook of cardiovascular medicine. 5th ed. Philadelphia: WB Saunders, 1997:565–577.

Zipes DP. Specific arrhythmias: diagnosis and treatment. In: Braunwald E., ed. Heart disease: a textbook of cardiovascular medicine. 5th ed. Philadelphia: WB Saunders, 1997:640–704.

66

Adult Congenital Heart Disease

Douglas S. Moodie

Adult congenital heart disease will become increasingly important over the next 20 years. Children who have undergone corrective or palliative operations during infancy and childhood are surviving well into adulthood, and cardiologists who care for these children now are faced with young or middle-aged adults who require a lifetime of follow-up. In addition, many patients first present with their congenital heart lesion as adults. These patients are an increasingly important area in adult cardiovascular disease, as evidenced by numerous publications on this topic (1–9).

Treating adults with congenital heart disease is difficult, because physicians involved in such care have not been trained to deal with the issues involved. Many pediatric cardiologists stop following their patients after 20 years of age, turning them over to adult cardiologists. Adult cardiology programs generally have not concentrated on the problems of adults with congenital heart disease, focusing mainly on acquired heart disease. Thus, adult patients with congenital heart disease who had surgery as children or initially present as adults encounter physicians who are somewhat ill-equipped to deal with their problems.

Where these patients should receive care can be problematic as well. It is difficult for adults to obtain care in the setting where most pediatric cardiologists practice (i.e., children's hospitals). The special needs of adults with congenital heart disease also are not always evident in adult institutions, which primarily are equipped to deal with acquired coronary or valvular heart disease. Thus, it is increasingly important for pediatric and adult cardiologists to work closely together, and for a "new breed" of congenital cardiologists to appear. These cardiologists most likely will come from pediatric cardiology settings, but they also must feel comfortable dealing with adult congenital heart disease. At my institution (Cleveland Clinic), all patients with congenital cardiac disease are followed by the pediatric cardiologist from infancy to late adulthood. Board-certified internists who are advanced fellows in cardiology rotate on the congenital cardiology service. These fellows manage the complications and problems seen in adult medicine that are unfamiliar to pediatric cardiologists. The major cardiac problems, however, are managed by a cardiologist who is trained in specific congenital lesions.

It is important that cardiologists caring for adults with congenital cardiac disease know how individuals present as adults. Current studies (10, 11) have dealt primarily with infants and children followed into adulthood. This chapter concentrates on experience at my institution in adults who presented with their defects as adults. The congenital lesions we have encountered most commonly in adults are atrial septal defect, ventricular septal defect, patent ductus arteriosus, coarctation of the aorta, tetralogy of Fallot, pulmonary stenosis, corrected transposition of the great arteries, and Ebstein anomaly.

Atrial Septal Defect

If congenitally bicuspid aortic valve and mitral valve prolapse are excluded, atrial septal defect (ASD) is the most common form of congenital heart disease in adults, constituting approximately 22 to 25% of these patients (1). Some 65 to 75% of all ASDs are of the ostium secundum type, 15 to 20% are of the ostium primum type (i.e., partial atrioventricular canal), and 5 to 10% are the sinus venosus type, which is associated with partial anomalous pulmonary venous connection of the right upper pulmonary veins. ASDs account for 7 to 11% of all cardiac defects in general. The female:male ratio is approximately 2:1.

In young adults, the dominant shunt is left to right, because the left atrial pressure exceeds the right atrial pressure during the major portion of the cardiac cycle. Immediately after atrial systole, the right atrial pressure may briefly exceed that of the left, and blood may shunt right to left. Despite the marked increase in pulmonary blood flow (i.e., as high as three to four times the systemic blood flow), pulmonary artery pressure almost always is normal until later in adult life, and though pulmonary arteries may have medial hypertrophy and intimal proliferation, pulmonary vascular changes greater than grade II are rare even in middle-aged adults.

Between 1956 and 1981, we saw 295 patients with ASD, who eventually underwent surgical closure. There were 219 women and 76 men. Patients ranged in age from 19 to 70 years, with a mean age of 40 years.

CLINICAL PRESENTATION

The most common presenting symptoms were shortness of breath (51%) and easy fatigability (43%). Forty-three percent also reported palpitations, 12% experienced atrial fibrillation, and 15% were asymptomatic. Eleven percent reported one or more episodes of heart failure, 4% had cyanosis, and 3% had suffered a stroke.

Seventy-six patients were New York Heart Association (NYHA) Functional Class I, 179 were Class II, 34 were Class III, and 6 were Class IV. Twenty-nine percent of patients were taking digoxin, and 18% were on diuretics. Six percent were taking antiarrhythmics, and 9% were on other medications. There was a positive family history for ASD in 27% of patients. A heart murmur was detected in 97%, and a fixed, split S_2 was noted in 54%.

RADIOGRAPHIC FEATURES

Chest radiography demonstrated cardiomegaly in 71% of patients. Fifty-one percent had mildly increased vascularity, 38% were normal, 11% had moderately increased vascularity, and 1% had greatly increased vascularity.

ELECTROCARDIOGRAPHIC FEATURES

Electrocardiography revealed sinus rhythm in 92% of patients. There was right ventricular hypertrophy in 52%, atrial fibrillation in 7%, and complete heart block in 1%. The mean QRS axis was 82°, with a range of 0 to 160°; the mean P axis was 72°, with a range of 30 to 150°. Right ventricular hypertrophy correlated strongly with pulmonary artery pressure but did not correlate with age. Preoperative atrial fibrillation correlated with both increasing pulmonary artery pressure and age.

CARDIAC CATHETERIZATION

Cardiac catheterization was performed on 290 patients. The systolic pulmonary artery pressures varied from 13 to 146 mmHg, with a mean pressure of 40 mm Hg. Left atrial pressures ranged from 2 to 28 mm Hg, with a mean of 8.5 mm Hg, and right atrial pressures were slightly lower, with a mean of 7 mm Hg. The mean pulmonary flow:systemic flow ratio (Qp/Qs) was 2.8:1, with a range of 1.2 to 10:1. Mean total pulmonary vascular resistance (RP) was 3.9 U, with a range of 1.4 to 8.6 U. Mean systemic resistance was 28 U.

Thirteen percent of these patients were noted to have anomalous pulmonary venous connection. Nine percent had coronary artery disease, 5% had pulmonary stenosis, and 1% had tricuspid insufficiency and aortic valve disease. Fifteen percent of the patients had pulmonary vascular disease.

Left ventricular function, as assessed by ventriculography, was normal in 96%, mildly impaired in 2%, moderately impaired in 2%, and severely impaired in none. Mitral insufficiency was noted in 7% of the patients, being mild in 5%, moderate in 1%, and severe in 1%. Eighty-six percent of the defects were of the ostium secundum type, and ostium primum and sinus venosus defects were each found in 6% of the patients.

Ventricular Septal Defect

In 1879, Henri Roget wrote, "The congenital defect of the heart compatible with life and perhaps a long one, one of the most frequent which I have encountered . . . is the communication between the two ventricles because of failure of occlusion of the interventricular septum and its upper portion" (12). Ventricular septal defect (VSD) is a common anomaly, occurring in approximately 10% of adult patients with congenital heart disease (1). Campbell (13) has described the natural history of adults with VSD in his practice: 27% of his patients died by age 20, 53% by age 40, and 69% before age 60.

Our experience with 79 patients over 18 years of age having isolated VSD seen between 1951 and 1981 involved 42 men and 37 women. These patients ranged in age from 18 to 59 years, with a mean age of 34 years. Twelve patients had surgical closure soon after presentation, whereas 67 were treated medically.

CLINICAL PRESENTATION

The medical group consisted of 67 patients—33 men and 34 women—who ranged in age from 18 to 59 years at presentation, with a mean age of 33 years. At the time of diagnosis, 42 of these patients were in NYHA Functional Class I, 15 in Class II, 8 in Class III, and 2 in Class IV. Only 29% were taking medication, with digitalis and diuretics being most common. The most common symptoms among these patients are listed in Table 66.l.

Almost all patients had a holosystolic murmur of VSD audible along the left sternal border. Seventy-four percent were grade 2–4/6, and 51% had a palpable thrill. The physical findings among these patients are summarized in Table 66.2.

Table 66.1.   Adult Ventricular Septal Defect (Medical Group): Symptoms in 87 Patients

Symptom	Patients (n [%])
Dyspnea	19 (28)
Exercise intolerance	16 (24)
Shortness of breath	15 (22)
Edema	13 (19)
Hypertension	3 (4)
Fever	2 (3)
None	23 (34)

Table 66.2.   Adult Ventricular Septal Defect (Medical Group): Physical Findings in 67 Patients

Finding	Patients (n [%])
Systolic murmur	66 (99)
Split S_2	57 (85)
Normal pulmonary component	38 (57)
Increased pulmonary component	22 (33)
Systolic thrill	34 (51)
Cyanosis	11 (16)
Clubbing	6 (9)
S_3	10 (15)
Right ventricular lift	7 (10)
Hepatomegaly	5 (7)
Systolic click	2 (3)
S_4	1 (1)

Chest radiography showed cardiomegaly in 32% of the patients. The pulmonary vascularity was increased in 28%.

The initial electrocardiogram revealed a variety of rhythm patterns. Normal sinus rhythm was the most common, occurring in 58 of the 67 patients (Table 66.3).

CARDIAC CATHETERIZATION

Forty-six patients had cardiac catheterization; however, only 38% of these patients had sufficient data available to calculate the pulmonary artery resistance. Results of these catheterizations are listed in Table 66.4. After the initial evaluation, 8 patients were placed on medication, and 58 required no treatment.

COURSE

The medical group was followed from between 1 month and 24 years, with a mean follow-up of 9 years. Patient age at follow-up ranged from 24 to 74 years, with a mean age of 42 years. At follow-up, 51 patients were alive, and 15 had ex-

pired. Only one patient had bacterial endocarditis and succumbed. The most common causes of death among these patients are listed in Table 66.5. Of the catheterization data available for the medically followed patients who died, 73%

Table 66.3.   Adult Ventricular Septal Defect (Medical Group): Electrocardiographic Findings in 67 Patients

Finding	Patients (n [%])
Sinus rhythm	58 (87)
Sinus bradycardia	6 (9)
Sinus tachycardia	2 (3)
Supraventricular tachycardia	1 (1)
First-degree atrioventricular block	4 (6)
Premature ventricular contractions	2 (3)
Right ventricular hypertrophy	16 (24)
Left ventricular hypertrophy	2 (3)
Biventricular hypertrophy	3 (4)

Table 66.4.   Adult Ventricular Septal Defect (Medical Group): Cardiac Catheterization Findings in 46 Patients

Finding	Mean	Patients (n)
Femoral artery pressure (mm Hg)		
Systolic	127 ± 24	45
Diastolic	79 ± 14	45
Femoral artery saturation (%)	92 ± 6	31
Mixed venous saturation (%)	69 ± 16	29
Pulmonary artery saturation (%)	78 ± 8	37
Left ventricular pressure (mm Hg)		
Systolic	128 ± 24	42
Diastolic	12 ± 6	42
Right ventricular pressure (mm Hg)		
Systolic	53 ± 44	43
Diastolic	8 ± 6	43
Pulmonary artery pressure (mm Hg)		
Systolic	50 ± 42	43
Diastolic	23 ± 24	43
Cardiac index (L/min/m^2)	3.2 ± 1.2	26
Pulmonary index (L/min/m^2)	5.0 ± 5.5	25
Qp/Qs	1.6 ± 1.4	26
Pulmonary resistance (units)	10.3 ± 13.8	26
Pulmonary arteriolar resistance (units)	6.4 ± 13.7	11
Systemic resistance (units)	35.8 ± 16.2	24
Left-to-right shunt (%)	30 ± 23	20

Table 66.5.   Adult Ventricular Septal Defect (Medical Group): Cause of Death in 15 Patients

Cause	(%)
Heart failure	45
Myocardial infarct	45
Sudden death	31
Pulmonary embolus	29
Renal failure	37
Noncardiac, other	42
Heart failure and endocarditis	42
Cerebrovascular accident	43
Major hemorrhagic complications and pulmonary hypertension	43

Table 66.6.   Adult Ventricular Septal Defect (Medical Group): Pulmonary Artery Pressure in Patients Who Died

Patient No.	Pulmonary Systolic Pressure (mm Hg)	Pulmonary Diastolic Pressure (mm Hg)
1	122	58
2	96	52
3	88	50
4	98	54
5	48	4
6	38	15
7	30	12
8	173	80
9	100	55
10	115	70
11	118	72

had a systolic pulmonary artery pressure of greater than 50 mm Hg (Table 66.6).

Fifteen patients continued to have symptoms, including palpitations, atypical chest pain, dysrhythmias, shortness of breath, angina, and fatigability. Fourteen patients were maintained on medication. At follow-up, 42 patients were NYHA Functional Class I, 8 were Class II, and 2 were Class III. Only one patient was severely restricted in physical activity, and 32 patients continued to work. Excluding those patients who died, only three deteriorated, with the remainder either stable or improved.

Patients who were Class I at presentation had a better survival rate than the more symptomatic patients. Survival at 10 years was 90% for Class I patients and 58% for others. Cardiomegaly at initial presentation significantly reduced the chance for survival. Ten-year survival was 90% for patients without cardiomegaly and 50% for those with elevated pulmonary artery pressure ($P < .001$) in the medical group.

Patent Ductus Arteriosus

Between 1951 and 1984, we evaluated 117 patients with the diagnosis of isolated patent ductus arteriosus (PDA). These patients ranged in age from 18 to 81 years, with a mean age of 36 years. There were 95 women and 22 men. Follow-up was obtained for 114 of these patients.

Thirty-three patients received no therapy, and 12 received medical therapy alone. Sixty-eight patients underwent surgical closure of the PDA. All patients were classified functionally at the initial diagnosis. Fifty-seven were in NYHA Functional Class I, 51 in Class II, 7 in Class III, and 2 in Class IV. There was no significant difference between the surgical and nonsurgical groups on the basis of functional class.

CLINICAL PRESENTATION

Symptoms at diagnosis were comparable in the two groups (Table 66.7). Thirty-seven of the 117 patients presented with exercise intolerance. And 29% complained of dyspnea. Cyanosis was more frequent in the nonsurgical group. Thirty-seven patients were asymptomatic at initial presentation.

Ninety-seven percent of these patients presented with a systolic murmur, which generally was of grade 2–4/6 in intensity. It was best heard at the left upper sternal border in most patients. The intensity of the murmur was comparable in both groups. A continuous murmur was heard in 61%, and four patients presented with no heart murmur. Only 38% of the nonsurgical patients presented with a diastolic murmur, whereas 71% of the surgical patients had a diastolic murmur, which ranged in intensity from grade 2–4/6 ($P < .0001$). The pulmonary component of S_2 was heard with equal intensity in the nonsurgical and surgical groups. The frequency of a systolic thrill or S_3 was not different in the two groups.

There was no difference between the surgical and nonsur-

Table 66.7.   Adult Patent Ductus Arteriosus: Symptoms in 117 Patients

Symptom	Nonsurgically Treated (n [%])	Surgically Treated (n [%])
Patients	45 (100)	72 (100)
Asymptomatic	19 (42)	18 (25)
Symptomatic	25 (58)	54 (75)
Exercise intolerance	11 (24)	26 (38)
Dyspnea	11 (24)	23 (32)
Cyanosis	9 (20)	0 (0)
Peripheral edema	5 (11)	4 (5)
Clubbing	3 (7)	0 (0)

Reprinted with permission from Fisher RC, Moodie DS, Sterga R, Gill C. Patent ductus arteriosus in adults—long-term follow-up: nonsurgical versus surgical treatment. J Am Acad Cardiol 1986;8:281–284.

gical groups on the basis of type or amount of medications taken at initial presentation. Eighty-nine patients were taking no medication. Endocarditis was seen in three of the patients preoperatively.

RADIOGRAPHIC FEATURES

Sixteen patients demonstrated calcification of the ductus, either at chest radiography or surgery. In the surgical group, 11 patients had calcification; their ages ranged from 28 to 70 years, with a mean age of 49 years. In the nonsurgical group, five patients had calcification; their mean age of 61 years was somewhat greater.

Cardiomegaly was found in 46% of the patients. Sixteen patients demonstrated increased pulmonary vascularity.

ELECTROCARDIOGRAPHIC FEATURES

The electrocardiogram revealed normal sinus rhythm in 95% of patients. In the nonsurgical group, 13 patients demonstrated right ventricular hypertrophy, and 5 demonstrated left ventricular hypertrophy. In the surgical group, 10 patients had evidence of right ventricular hypertrophy, and 13 had evidence of left ventricular hypertrophy

Coarctation of the Aorta

Between 1952 and 1970, 69 adult patients—49 men and 20 women—underwent surgical correction for coarctation of the aorta and were evaluated preoperatively. Their ages ranged from 18 to 50 years, with a mean age of 30.5 years.

CLINICAL PRESENTATION

Fifty-eight percent (40 of 69) of these patients were asymptomatic. Twenty-three percent (16 of 69) had exercise intolerance, and 17% (12 of 69) complained of claudication. Ten percent experienced dyspnea and had angina, and one patient was cyanotic. Ninety percent (62 of 69) were hypertensive, and 44% (30 of 69) had a heart murmur. Ten percent had already experienced bacterial endocarditis, 4% had a myocardial infarction, and 1% had aortic dissection. Five patients had suffered a stroke.

As mentioned, 62 of these patients had hypertension, and 21 were on antihypertensive medication or diuretics. The mean blood pressure in this group was 152/86 mm Hg, with systolic blood pressure ranging from 100 to 260 mm Hg and diastolic from 40 to 148 mm Hg. Femoral pulses were absent in 18%, normal in 2%, and diminished in 80%.

Tetralogy of Fallot

Tetralogy of Fallot was the most common form of cyanotic congenital heart disease. It is estimated that without sur-

gical intervention, only approximately 10% of these patients survive beyond 21 years of age (14–16). Several studies have examined the adult with tetralogy of Fallot (17–21).

Between 1951 and 1981, we saw 13 patients over the age of 18 years for total intracardiac repair of tetralogy of Fallot. These 13 patients included 8 men and 5 women. Three had no previous palliation. Of the 10 who had undergone previous palliation, 6 had a Potts anastomosis and 3 a Blalock shunt. One patient had an aortopulmonary artery graft. Patient age at palliation ranged from 5 months to 19 years, and time from palliation to total repair ranged from 2 to 80 years, with a mean time of 20 years. Patient age at total intracardiac repair ranged from 18 to 42 years, with a mean age of 30 years.

CLINICAL PRESENTATION

Cyanosis and dyspnea on exertion were the most common symptoms before total repair. Other, less frequent findings were fatigue, restricted activity, hemoptysis, pneumonia, headache, syncope, and endocarditis. On the NYHA Functional Classification, one patient was Class I, one was Class II, 10 were Class III, and one was Class IV.

Cyanosis was present in 11 patients, and clubbing was present in 10. No patient had heart failure, but all had a systolic murmur. Other findings were as noted in Table 66.8.

RADIOGRAPHIC FEATURES

Cardiomegaly was present in five patients. Seven patients had evidence of right ventricular enlargement, whereas two had evidence of left ventricular enlargement. Decreased pulmonary vascularity was apparent in only one patient.

Table 66.8. Adult Tetralogy of Fallot: Physical Findings in 13 Patients

Finding	Patients (n [%])
Cyanosis	11 (85)
Clubbing	10 (77)
Right ventricular lift	9 (64)
Systolic thrill	5 (39)
Systolic click	3 (22)
Single S_2	8 (62)
Diminished pulmonary component	4 (31)
S_4	1 (7)
Systolic murmur	13 (100)
Continuous murmur	4 (29)
Diastolic murmur	0 (0)

Reprinted with permission from Kreindel M, Moodie DS, Sterba R, Gill C. Total repair of tetralogy of Fallot in the adult: the Cleveland Clinic experience, 1951–1981. Cleve Clin Q 1985; Fall:375–381.

ELECTROCARDIOGRAPHIC FEATURES

All patients had normal sinus rhythm. Eleven had evidence of right ventricular hypertrophy, and nine showed right-axis deviation. Three patients had complete right bundle branch block. One patient had first-degree atrioventricular block.

CARDIAC CATHETERIZATION

Hemodynamic data were obtained in 11 of these patients (Table 66.9). Right ventricular systolic pressure ranged from 70 to 130 mm Hg, and right ventricular outflow tract gradients were measured in 9 patients. These gradients ranged from 50 to 112 mm Hg. In addition, pulmonary artery pressures were measured in 10 patients. Systolic pressure ranged from 18 to 85 mm Hg, and diastolic pressure ranged from 15 to 65 mm Hg.

Pulmonary Stenosis

Between 1951 and 1981, we saw 68 patients older than 20 years of age with pulmonary stenosis (PS). Thirty-seven of these patients had PS with associated defects, and 31 had isolated PS. Of those patients with associated defects, 19 had a VSD, 10 an ASD, 4 aortic insufficiency, 3 mitral valve prolapse, 2 mitral insufficiency, 2 corrected transposition of the great arteries, 2 univentricular heart, 2 congenital coronary

Table 66.9.   Adult Tetralogy of Fallot: Hemodynamic Data

Patient No.	RVSP (mm Hg)	RVOG (mm Hg)	PAP (mm Hg)
1	82	57	25/15
2	—	—	—
3	130	—	—
4	130	112	18[a]
5	110	—	—
6	115	90	25/15
7	110	85	25/20
8	115	—[b]	85/65
9	120	100	20[a]
10	95	75	20[a]
11	—	—	—
12	70	50	20/15
13	125	85	40/25

Reprinted with permission from Kreindel M, Moodie DS, Sterba R, Gill C. Total repair of tetralogy of Fallot in the adult: the Cleveland Clinic experience, 1951—1981. Cleve Clin Q 1985; Fall:376.
PAP, pulmonary artery pressure; *RVOG*, right ventricular outflow tract gradient; *RVSP*, right ventricular systolic pressure; —, not obtained.
[a] Systolic.
[b] Previous Potts shunt.

anomalies, 2 isolated dextrocardia, and 1 patient each with PDA, supravalvular PS, aortic stenosis, tricuspid stenosis, bicuspid aortic valve, subvalvular PS, double-outlet right ventricle, and double-outlet left ventricle.

Of the 31 patients with isolated PS, 13 were men, and 18 were women. These patients ranged in age from 18 to 51 years. Sixty-five percent were on no medication. Only one patient had hepatomegaly.

CLINICAL PRESENTATION

Of the 31 patients with isolated PS, 13 had shortness of breath, 11 exercise intolerance, 7 dyspnea on exertion, 3 tachypnea or edema, and 1 each hypertension and cyanosis. There were 5 patients in NYHA Functional Class I, 16 in Class II, and 10 in Class III or IV.

All patients had systolic murmurs. Twelve had at least a grade 3/6 systolic murmur, and 21 had systolic murmurs ranging in severity from grade 3–5. No patient had a diastolic murmur.

Four had a right ventricular lift and 12 a systolic thrill. The S_2 could be appreciably auscultated as split in 23 patients. S_4 was heard in 5 patients and S_3 in 4 patients.

RADIOGRAPHIC FEATURES

Heart size was normal in 28 patients, and 5 patients had cardiomegaly. Vascularity was normal in 28, increased in 2, and decreased in 1.

ELECTROCARDIOGRAPHIC FEATURES

Electrocardiography showed sinus rhythm in all patients. One had sinus bradycardia, and two had first-degree atrioventricular block. Fifteen showed right ventricular hypertrophy. Sixteen demonstrated no hypertrophy of either the right or left ventricle.

Corrected Transposition of the Great Arteries

Congenitally corrected transposition of the great arteries is an unusual cardiac malformation in that normal hemodynamic pathways are not altered by the anatomic abnormalities. The entity originally was described by Von Rokitansky in 1875 (22), and in most patients, it is accompanied by associated anomalies that dictate the symptomatology and considerably affect the prognosis. We use this term to refer to patients with ventricular inversion and to those in whom the aorta is anterior and to the left of the pulmonary artery.

We reviewed patient records from 1960 to 1986, which revealed 18 patients with corrected transposition. These patients ranged in age from 10 to 67 years at initial assessment.

Fifteen patients were older than 20 years at initial assessment, and 3 patients younger than 20 years were included as their follow-up extended well into adulthood.

CLINICAL PRESENTATION

Seventeen of these patients had associated cardiac lesions. The most common were left atrioventricular valve insufficiency (11 patients), VSD (7 patients), ASD (4 patients), and PS (3 patients).

Six patients were NYHA Functional Class I, six Class II, five Class III, and one Class IV. Patients presenting with Class III or IV had hemodynamically significant, associated lesions, which may have accounted for their poor clinical status, and one of these patients had a cardiomyopathic systemic ventricle.

ELECTROCARDIOGRAPHIC FEATURES

Fifteen patients were in sinus rhythm, and three had permanent pacemakers inserted for complete heart block. In two patients, the complete heart block was congenital, and in one, it occurred following closure of a VSD.

COURSE

Our data suggest that the morphologic right ventricle can function for a long time as the systemic ventricle, even in patients with associated lesions that pose a significant hemodynamic load. Using radionuclide angiographic techniques, Benson et al. (23) provided data that suggested a normal response for the morphologic right ventricle to exercise in adolescent patients with isolated corrected transposition of the great arteries. Clearly, what may determine the long-term outlook for these patients is the associated lesions.

Ebstein Anomaly

Between 1950 and 1985, we saw 22 patients with Ebstein anomaly. These patients ranged in age from 15 to 58 years.

CLINICAL PRESENTATION

Seventeen of these patients had easy fatigability and dyspnea on exertion, and 5 had palpitations and shortness of breath. Two patients presented with heart failure, and 2 patients were asymptomatic. There was no family history of Ebstein anomaly in these patients, but there were four siblings in these families with either an ASD or a VSD.

On physical examination, six patients were cyanotic.

Eighteen had a widely split and a questionable fixed S_2. All patients had a systolic heart murmur that was grade 2–4/6 in intensity, and 2 patients had a diastolic murmur. Ebstein anomaly has been called ''the great masquerader,'' in that it may manifest with different presentations, but 19 of our 22 patients had cardiomegaly.

ELECTROCARDIOGRAPHIC FEATURES

Electrocardiography demonstrated complete or incomplete right bundle-branch block in 16 patients. There was right atrial enlargement in 4 patients and first-degree atrioventricular block in 3. One patient had Wolff-Parkinson-White syndrome.

Five patients had atrial fibrillation, with three before and two after cardiac surgery. Two patients had complete heart block after surgery and required a permanent pacemaker. Two patients had paroxysmal supraventricular tachycardia, and four had unifocal premature ventricular contractions. The single patient with Wolff-Parkinson-White syndrome eventually underwent surgical ablation.

CARDIAC CATHETERIZATION

Cardiac catheterization was performed in all 22 patients. Twelve demonstrated at least a moderate ASD, 8 severe tricuspid insufficiency, 4 mitral insufficiency and mitral valve prolapse, 2 tricuspid stenosis, and 1 each PS and VSD. In a single patient, the diagnosis was missed at cardiac catheterization but confirmed at surgery. No deaths occurred during the catheterizations in these patients. Two patients sustained ventricular tachycardia in the catheterization laboratory and required cardioversion.

COURSE

Follow-up for these patients extended for between 2 to 25 years. Eight of the 22 patients died, with two of these deaths occurring after cardiac surgery.

In those patients treated nonsurgically, one died suddenly at age 24 during competitive athletics. Another patient died of a stroke at age 57, and two patients died of heart failure, one at age 45 and one at age 48.

Fourteen of these patients are alive. Six who underwent surgery are NYHA Functional Class I, and 8 who were treated medically are currently Class II.

One patient had four miscarriages, with increasing shortness of breath during pregnancy. Another patient had three pregnancies with no difficulties. Three patients underwent one pregnancy each without difficulty, and one patient had four pregnancies with slight shortness of breath and normal deliveries.

REFERENCES

1. Fuster V, Bradenburg RO, McGoon DC, et al. Clinical approach management of congenital heart disease in the adolescent and adult. Cardiovasc Clin North Am 1980: 161–197.
2. Kusumoto M, Amemiya K. Congenital heart disease in patients over 40 years old who have not undergone cardiac surgery. Jpn Circ J 1981;45:243–248.
3. Abinader EG, Oliven M. Congenital heart disease in the middle aged and elderly. J Ir Med Assoc 1980;73: 201–205.
4. Danielson GK, McGoon DC. Surgical therapy and results. In: Roberts WC, ed. Adult congenital heart disease. Philadelphia: FA Davis, 1987:543–560.
5. Nicks R, Halliday EJ. Surgery for congenital heart disease in adults. Med J Aust 1971;5:424–428.
6. Gonzalez-Lavin L, Neirotti R, Ross JK, et al. Surgical correction of congenital malformation of the heart and great vessels in patients over 20 years of age. Mich Med 1975;74:9–12.
7. Bekoe S, Magovern GJ, Liebler GA, et al. Congenital heart disease in adults. Surgical management. Arch Surg 1975;110:960–964.
8. Fetzer JA. Congenital heart disease in the adult. J Alpha Omega Alpha 1973;72:1150–1155.
9. Shibuya M. The natural history of adult congenital heart disease. Jpn Circ J 1972;36:832.
10. Roberts WC. Congenital heart disease in adults. In: Brest A, ed. Cardiovascular Clinics. Philadelphia: FA Davis, 1987.
11. Roberts WC. Adult congenital heart disease. Philadelphia: FA Davis, 1987.
12. Perloff JK. The clinical recognition of congenital heart disease. Philadelphia: WB Saunders, 1978:396.
13. Campbell M. Natural history of ventricular septal defect. Br Heart J 1971;33:246–257.
14. Freisinger GC, Bahnson HT. Tetralogy of Fallot. Report of a case with total correction at 54 years of age. Am Heart J 1966;71:107–111.
15. Holladay WE, Witham AC. The tetralogy of Fallot. Arch Intern Med 1957;100:400–414.
16. Higgins CB, Mulder DC. Tetralogy of Fallot in the adult. Am J Cardiol 1972;29:837–846.
17. Abraham KA, Cherian G, Rao VD, et al. Tetralogy of Fallot in adults. A report on 147 patients. Am J Med 1979; 66:811–816.
18. Garson AJ, Nihill MR, McNamara DG, et al. Status of the adult and adolescent after repair of tetralogy of Fallot. Circulation 1979;59:1232–1240.
19. Garson AJ, McNamara DG, Cooley DA. Tetralogy of Fallot in adults. Cardiovasc Clin 1979;10:341–364.
20. Beach PM, Bowman FO, Kaiser GA, et al. Total correction of tetralogy of Fallot in adolescents and adults. Circulation 1971;5(Suppl I):37–44.
21. Abraham KA, Cherian G, Sukumar IP, et al. Hemodynamics in adult tetralogy of Fallot. Indian Heart J 1979; 31:88–91.
22. Von Rokintansky D. Die Defecte der Scheidewonde Meczens. Vienna: W Braumuller, 1875:81.
23. Benson LN, Burns R, Schwaiger M, et al. Radionuclide angiographic evaluation of ventricular function isolated congenitally corrected transposition of the great vessels. Am J Cardiol 1986;48:319–324.

Acute Myocardial Infarction

Curtis M. Rimmerman

Acute myocardial infarction (MI) remains the leading cause of death worldwide. Despite advances in both prevention of coronary artery disease and treatment of acute MI, significant morbidity and mortality rates remain.

EPIDEMIOLOGY

Almost 900,000 people suffer an acute MI in the United States each year. Of these, approximately 25% die, with 50% of these deaths occurring in the prehospital setting, before effective treatment can be given. Invariably, these prehospital deaths are arrhythmogenic in origin. To minimize out-of-hospital deaths from acute MI, a multipronged approach is essential, including:

- Patient education
- Rapid evaluation
- Prompt initiation of thrombolytic therapy

Successful early infarct–related coronary artery reperfusion reduces both the infarct size and the incidence of subsequent complications, including congestive heart failure, arrhythmia, and death.

CLINICAL PRESENTATION

Approximately 50% of patients will suffer prodromal chest discomfort before an acute MI. Chest discomfort can occur during periods of physical or emotional stress, but the relationship is not clearly causal. Chest symptoms often are described as discomfort, not pain, and are located in the midsubsternal region, with frequent radiation to the neck, throat, jaw, and left as well as right arms. The discomfort generally is prolonged, lasting at least 30 minutes. Occasionally, the discomfort is epigastric in origin, which may simulate symptoms arising from a gastrointestinal source and, therefore, produce a delay in seeking medical attention. In patients with prodromal chest discomfort, the discomfort of infarction is similar in quality but more intense and persistent. Other associated symptoms of myocardial infarction include profound diaphoresis, nausea and vomiting, dyspnea, and palpitations.

When a patient presents with severe chest discomfort of acute onset, important differential diagnostic considerations include pulmonary embolism and aortic dissection. Patients with pulmonary embolism frequently will demonstrate unexplained hypoxemia not supported by physical examination or chest radiographic findings. Frequently, there is an antecedent history of immobility, previous congestive heart failure, or previous pulmonary embolism. Patients with acute aortic dissection have a history of hypertension (often severe) in the setting of ''ripping'' chest, interscapular and back pain (not discomfort) in the setting of pulse deficits, and a widened mediastinum on chest radiographs.

DIAGNOSIS

PHYSICAL EXAMINATION

During an acute MI, patients often appear to be restless and unable to find a comfortable position. Diaphoresis and skin pallor often are visible, and the pulse is regular and rapid. Premature systoles are common as well. The blood pressure response varies, including:

- Hypertensive (in the setting of increased adrenergic stimulation)
- Normal
- Hypotensive (particularly in patients with larger infarctions and superimposed left ventricular failure)

The jugular venous pulse usually is normal, unless a right ventricular infarct is present. Rales may be present on pulmonary examination, reflecting a larger, left-sided infarction and a component of heart failure. Cardiac examination frequently demonstrates an S_4 gallop, and a dyskinetic cardiac apex may be palpable precordially, particularly during an anterolateral infarction. A third heart sound may be either preexisting or new, with a newly discovered third heart sound reflecting a more extensive MI. Newly audible systolic murmurs, which are reflective of transient or persistent mitral regurgitation, commonly are detected during the peri-infarction period.

The combined findings of a carefully obtained patient history and physical examination will strongly suggest the diagnosis of MI in most patients. Additional essential studies include electrocardiography and serum analysis of cardiac enzyme levels.

ELECTROCARDIOGRAPHY

Diagnostic Findings

The diagnosis of acute MI can be made on the basis of electrocardiographic criteria, including ST-segment elevation of greater than 1 mm in at least two contiguous leads. Reciprocal ST-segment depression is an associated and helpful finding that makes the possibility of acute pericarditis mimicking acute infarction less likely. Electrocardiographically, ST-segment elevation is thought to represent acute myocardial injury. In contrast, Q-wave formation is most appropriately labeled as infarction, and Q waves in the setting of ST-segment elevation are best labeled as acute infarction. In the absence of ST-segment elevation, Q waves represent an MI of indeterminate age.

An electrocardiogram (ECG) also provides an estimate of infarction size, particularly if the ECG demonstrates ST-segment elevation in leads V_{2-6}, I, and aVL, which collectively are indicative of an extensive, anterolateral MI. The ECG is an indispensable adjunct to the patient history and physical examination, but it sometimes can provide inconclusive information despite an ongoing acute MI. Less-specific electrocardiographic findings include ST-segment depression and T-wave inversion. Infarction involving the left circumflex coronary artery, which most commonly is reflected in leads V_5, V_6, I, and aVL, also frequently is "electrocardiographically silent."

Q-Wave vs. Non-Q-Wave Infarction

The electrocardiographic development of Q waves in patients with a serum analysis consistent with acute MI is termed a *Q-wave myocardial infarction.* There are several important distinctions between a Q-wave and a non-Q-wave infarction. First and foremost, it is not possible to ascertain whether a Q-wave infarction truly is transmural and a non-Q-wave in-

farction nontransmural. There is significant overlap, and it is best to limit oneself to an electrocardiographic description. Despite this, Q-wave infarctions typically demonstrate an occlusive thrombus in more than 80% of patients during an acute MI, compared with only 10 to 20% of patients with non-Q-wave infarctions. Patients with Q-wave infarcts tend to suffer larger infarctions and have less prominent coronary collaterals, lower associated ejection fractions, and higher peak cardiac enzyme levels. In-hospital mortality is greater among patients with Q-wave infarctions, which likely is secondary to their larger size. Importantly, postinfarction ischemia is more common in patients with non-Q-wave infarctions, as is reinfarction. The 3-year mortality rate is similar for both groups.

LABORATORY STUDIES

Serial testing of serum cardiac enzyme levels should be performed routinely in patients with suspected acute MI. Cardiac enzyme levels assist in documenting the presence of acute infarction. In addition, larger infarctions demonstrate a greater peak enzyme level, which serves as a quantitative marker. Also, successful reperfusion (either spontaneous, via thrombolytics, or via percutaneous transluminal coronary angioplasty [PTCA]) will result in a higher and earlier peak of enzyme levels secondary to a "wash-out phenomenon," which serves as a useful clinical indicator of successful myocardial reperfusion.

Creatine Kinase

Measurement of the creatine kinase (CK)-MB isoenzyme level continues to be the most useful laboratory test for the diagnosis of acute MI. Initial elevations can be detected 3 to 4 hours after acute injury, and mean peak levels occur at approximately 24 hours (Fig. 67.1). Levels should be obtained

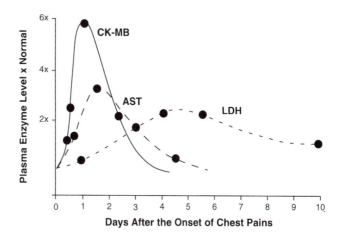

Figure 67.1. Typical plasma profiles for the MB isoenzyme of CK, AST, and LDH activities following onset of acute MI. (Reprinted with permission from J Mol Med 2:185, 1977.)

at initial presentation, 8 to 12 hours, and 16 to 24 hours after the onset of chest discomfort.

Lactate Dehydrogenase

Lactate dehydrogenase (LDH), the levels of which are helpful in documenting a recent MI, is especially useful in patients with suspected "out-of-hospital" infarction. Levels of this enzyme exceed the normal range 24 to 48 hours after the acute event, and they peak at approximately 78 to 96 hours (Fig. 67.1.) Fractionation of total LDH is important, because LDH1 is cardiac in origin. This test is best reserved for those patients in whom the suspicion for recent MI is high but the CK level has normalized.

TREATMENT

All patients with acute MI warrant hospitalization and telemetry, often in the intensive care unit.

OXYGEN

Routine administration of oxygen during the first few hours of an MI is recommended. Higher-dose mask oxygen or endotracheal intubation may be necessary as well, particularly in those with concomitant congestive heart failure.

PHARMACOLOGIC TREATMENT

Nitroglycerin

Nitroglycerin reduces both right and left ventricular preload, produces peripheral vasodilation, and reduces afterload, thereby lowering myocardial oxygen requirements and work. In addition, it has direct vasodilator effects on the coronary arteries. Intravenous administration is recommended in patients with acute MI. Long-term nitrate administration in out-of-hospital patients after an MI is not clearly beneficial, but the subgroup of patients with congestive heart failure may benefit. Intravenous nitroglycerin does remain helpful in patients with persistent ischemia or hypertension during the initial 24 to 48 hours after an acute MI; after 48 hours, continued use is appropriate in patients with recurrent ischemia or persistent heart failure.

Analgesia

Ongoing chest discomfort causes increased sympathetic output, which raises blood pressure, heart rate, and ultimately, myocardial oxygen demand. This is not desirable, and prompt administration of intravenous analgesic (e.g., morphine sulfate) is recommended.

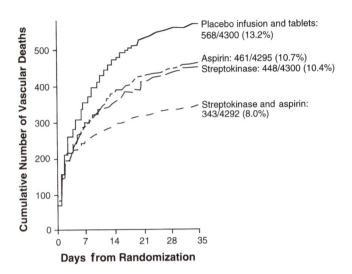

Figure 67.2. Cumulative vascular mortality for days 0 to 35 in the ISIS-II. (Reprinted with permission from ISIS-2 [Second Interventional Study of Infarct Survival] Collaborative Group. Randomized trial of intravenous streptokinase or aspirin, both or neither, among 17,187 cases of suspected acute myocardial infarction: ISIS-2. Lancet 1988;ii:349–360.)

Aspirin

Prompt administration of 160 to 325 mg of aspirin is indicated for all patients during the acute infarction phase, and daily aspirin use should continue indefinitely thereafter. The Second Interventional Study of Infarct Survival (ISIS-II) examined the efficacy of aspirin and demonstrated a reduction of 23% in the 35-day mortality rate (Fig. 67.2). Additionally, aspirin reduces the incidence of coronary reocclusion and recurrent ischemia.

Thrombolysis

Thrombolytics are indicated in patients with acute MI, ST-segment elevation in two or more contiguous leads, and chest discomfort less than 12 hours from symptom onset. Patient benefit is noted to be greater in larger (i.e., anterior) infarctions, in patients with diabetes, and in patients with previous infarctions. The benefit of thrombolytics 12 to 24 hours after symptom onset is less clear; however, patients with ongoing chest discomfort and ST-segment elevation likely will benefit.

Thrombolytics have no proven benefit in patients with ST-segment depression, and they should not be administered routinely. Patients benefiting most from thrombolytic therapy in the setting of acute MI include those with (presumably) new bundle-branch block and anterior infarction. Patients with inferior infarction also benefit, but less notably. The shorter the period between symptom onset and administration of thrombolytic therapy, the more lives are saved and the greater the benefit.

Absolute contraindications for thrombolytic administration include:

- Intracranial neoplasm
- Internal bleeding
- Previous hemorrhagic stroke or other cerebrovascular events within 1 year
- Suspected aortic dissection

Relative contraindications for thrombolytic administration include:

- Blood pressure > 180/110 mm Hg on presentation
- History of chronic, severe hypertension
- History of bleeding
- INR >2.0
- Active peptic ulcer
- Pregnancy
- Noncompressible vascular puncture
- Recent trauma
- Cardiopulmonary resuscitation (CPR)
- Recent major surgery

Heparin

It is recommended that heparin be administered routinely in patients with acute infarction who are not receiving thrombolytic therapy. In patients receiving thrombolytic therapy, indications for heparin depend on which thrombolytic agent is being used. A fibrin-specific agent (e.g., Alteplase) should have heparin coadministered at the initiation of thrombolytic infusion. Heparin administration also is recommended in patients receiving streptokinase and Anistreplase who are at high risk for systemic emboli, including those patients with a large infarction, coexisting atrial fibrillation, previous embolism, or left ventricular thrombus.

β-Blockers

β-Blockers are appropriately administered to patients within the first 12 hours of acute MI and should be continued daily thereafter. They reduce immediate, short-term, and long-term cardiac morbidity and mortality rates.

Angiotensin-Converting Enzyme Inhibitors

Early in the course of an acute MI, administration of an angiotensin-converting enzyme (ACE) inhibitor reduces mortality. The greatest benefit occurs in those patients with anterior infarctions and heart failure. Therapy with ACE inhibitors should be started promptly (i.e., within 24 hours of presentation). If left ventricular systolic function remains normal, then discontinuing ACE inhibitors 4 to 6 weeks after initiation is appropriate. If the left ventricular ejection fraction is reduced at the 35 to 40% level, ACE inhibitors should be continued indefinitely.

Calcium Channel Blockers

Calcium channel blockers are used most appropriately in the setting of acute infarction when ischemia persists and there is a contraindication to the administration of β-blockers. Calcium channel blockers have not been shown to reduce the mortality rate after acute MI, and in some patients subgroups, these agents may even increase the mortality rate.

OTHER TREATMENTS

Primary PTCA

Primary PTCA is a feasible alternative to thrombolytic therapy when prompt access to the cardiac catheterization laboratory is available. In addition, it is appropriate when there are contraindications to thrombolytic therapy and the risk:benefit ratio of thrombolysis is high. In the high-risk subpopulation of patients with acute MI in cardiogenic shock, primary PTCA, if available in a timely fashion (i.e., 60–90 minutes after symptom onset), is the preferred therapy. In these patients, PTCA also can be performed after the administration of thrombolytic therapy if the patient remains hemodynamically unstable and reperfusion is not clinically believed to have been achieved.

Hemodynamic Monitoring

Placement of a Swan-Ganz catheter and continuous measurement of right-sided cardiac pressures are indicated in select circumstances. These include:

- Severe or progressive congestive heart failure
- Cardiogenic shock
- Suspected mechanical complications of acute infarction (e.g., papillary muscle rupture, ventricular septal defect, pericardial tamponade)

Patients with severe congestive heart failure, cardiogenic shock, or both often require intravenous inotropes as well as preload- and afterload-reducing agents, which are best administered and dosed with full knowledge of the cardiac-filling pressures. This allows differentiation in critically ill patients of inadequate left ventricular volumes and an underfilled left ventricle versus a volume-replete state with extensive left ventricular systolic impairment. The routine, uncomplicated acute MI, regardless of its location, is not an indication for right-heart catheter monitoring.

Intraaortic Balloon Counter Pulsation

Intraaortic balloon counter pulsation is reserved for critically ill patients with acute MI. Particular subgroups in which this therapy is indicated include patients with:

- Persistent cardiogenic shock despite pharmacologic therapy
- Recurrent arrhythmias resulting in hemodynamic instability
- Refractory post-MI angina despite antianginal therapy

- Acute complications (e.g., ventricular septal defect, papillary muscle rupture)

COMPLICATIONS

ARRHYTHMIAS

Arrhythmias commonly are observed in patients with acute MI. Arrhythmias are more common in patients with:

- Anterior infarction
- Larger infarction
- Infarctions complicated by congestive heart failure
- Hypotension and hypoperfusion
- Older age

Arrhythmias are observed less commonly in patients receiving thrombolytic therapy.

Atrial Fibrillation

Atrial fibrillation is the most common sustained arrhythmia in this setting, occurring in approximately 10% of patients with acute MI. If hemodynamic compromise develops during an episode of atrial fibrillation, prompt electrical cardioversion is indicated. If the patient is not compromised, then cautious use of intravenous β-blockade is useful in slowing the ventricular response and attenuating superimposed ischemia. If atrial fibrillation persists, intravenous heparin should be initiated (if not already done), and antiarrhythmic therapy should be considered.

Ventricular Arrhythmias

Often fatal, ventricular arrhythmias commonly occur during acute infarction. It is important, however, to distinguish *early* ventricular fibrillation, which occurs within the first few hours of infarction, from late ventricular fibrillation, which occurs more than 48 hours after infarction (Fig. 67.3). Early ventricu-

lar fibrillation suggests a higher immediate mortality rate. The out-of-hospital mortality rate is far greater in those patients experiencing late ventricular fibrillation, however, because this often is associated with larger infarctions, greater left ventricular systolic dysfunction, and congestive heart failure.

The use of routine lidocaine administration in hospital during an acute infarction has been abandoned. Lidocaine does reduce the incidence of primary ventricular fibrillation in hospital, but it does not exert a favorable effect on mortality. Patients who receive prophylactic lidocaine are in coronary intensive care units and can be promptly resuscitated. In fact, lidocaine appears to have a negative impact on mortality, which likely is related to increased episodes of bradycardia and asystole.

In contrast, early administration of intravenous β-blockade, followed by oral doses, exerts a favorable impact on the frequency of ventricular fibrillation and should be administered routinely to patients with acute infarction but without heart block, significant hypotension, and cardiogenic shock. In addition, close monitoring of electrolyte levels, specifically of potassium and magnesium, is important in arrhythmia prevention. Treatment of ventricular fibrillation requires prompt, unsynchronized electric shock, followed by pharmaceutical therapy as outlined in the ACLS (advanced cardiac life support) protocol.

Ventricular tachycardia is classified as either nonsustained (<30 seconds) or sustained (>30 seconds). Nonsustained, nonhemodynamically compromising ventricular tachycardia does not require specific treatment other than attenuation of persistent ischemia, normalization of electrolyte levels, and β-blockade. Hemodynamically compromising sustained ventricular tachycardia requires electric shock. Sustained ventricular tachycardia, which is better tolerated, can be treated with pharmacologic agents, including intravenous lidocaine or procainamide. In addition, intravenous amiodar-

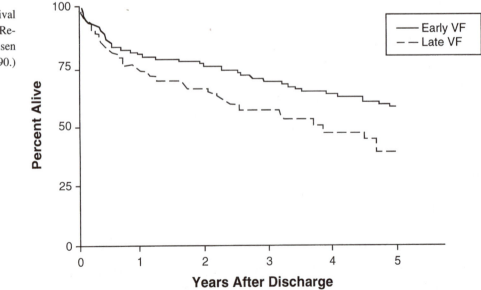

Figure 67.3. Kaplan-Meier survival curves. VF: ventricular fibrillation. (Reprinted with permission from Jeusen GVH et al. Am J Cardiol 66:10, 1990.)

one also is indicated for sustained ventricular tachycardia and is quite effective. Drug-refractory, sustained ventricular tachycardia in the setting of acute MI is best treated with β-blockade, intravenous amiodarone, balloon-pump insertion, or urgent revascularization.

BRADYARRHYTHMIAS

Sinus bradycardia is another frequent complication, especially in patients with inferior infarction and reperfusion of the right coronary artery (i.e., Bezold-Jarisch reflex). Heart block occurs in approximately 10% of patients with acute infarction, and bundle-branch block can develop as well. Patients with heart block or bundle-branch block have a greater in-hospital mortality rate, which most likely is related to the greater size of their presenting infarctions. Atropine is an effective treatment for bradycardia associated with hypotension or ischemia; it also is effective as prompt treatment for ventricular asystole or symptomatic atrioventricular (AV) block.

Temporary pacing is an effective "bridge" therapy for symptomatic bradycardia and heart block during an acute MI. It can be performed via the transcutaneous or the transvenous route. The transcutaneous mode is safer, especially in the setting of thrombolytic therapy. The transvenous mode is best used in patients with a high likelihood of proceeding to advanced heart block. Indications for temporary pacing include:

- Symptomatic bradycardia unresponsive to drug therapy
- Mobitz II AV block
- Third-degree heart block
- New bilateral bundle-branch block
- Newly acquired left bundle-branch block
- Right bundle-branch block or left bundle-branch block and first-degree AV block

Relatively few patients with acute infarction require permanent pacemakers. Rhythm disturbances that indicate a need for permanent pacing are persistent second-degree AV block in the His-Purkinje system, complete heart block, and symptomatic AV block.

MECHANICAL DEFECTS

Acute Mitral Regurgitation

Acute mitral regurgitation, which most commonly occurs 3 to 5 days after an acute infarction, more often is associated with inferior infarction. It should be suspected on physical examination when a new murmur develops, and it is best confirmed with two-dimensional echocardiography and Doppler analysis. It is an indication for prompt surgical repair, with an overall mortality rate from 40 to 90%.

Ventricular Septal Defect

Similar to acute mitral regurgitation, ventricular septal defect occurs 3 to 5 days after an acute infarction. A new murmur almost always is audible, occurring approximately two-thirds of the time in the setting of anterior infarction. This defect also can be diagnosed echocardiographically. The mortality rate in patients without surgery is greater than 90%.

Free-Wall Rupture

Free-wall rupture occurs approximately 3 to 6 days after the acute infarction and without any clear predilection for infarction location. The mortality rate approaches 100%. The incidence is thought to be reduced in patients receiving thrombolytic therapy and prompt β-blockade at the time of their initial presentation.

CONCLUSIONS

Prompt treatment of acute MI is essential. Unless contraindications exist, patients with electrocardiographic and clinical criteria for acute MI should receive intravenous thrombolytic therapy. In experienced centers, prompt, primary PTCA is an effective alternative, especially in patients with a high risk for complications from thrombolytic therapy. Pharmaceutic agents that should be administered concomitantly if no contraindications exist include:

- β-blockers
- Aspirin
- ACE inhibitors
- Intravenous nitroglycerin
- Intravenous heparin

The prognosis depends on:

- Age
- Infarction size and location
- Hemodynamic stability
- Intervening congestive heart failure
- Development of arrhythmia

All patients should be placed in coronary intensive care units, where experienced personnel can monitor them closely and attend to any complications.

REVIEW EXERCISES

QUESTIONS

1. The following items pertain to the anatomy and pathology of acute MI except:

   a. Even during an acute MI, angiography remains safe.
   b. More than 85% of infarct-related arteries are totally occluded during the acute infarction phase.
   c. The incidence of totally occluded infarct vessels is reduced after MI secondary to spontaneous thrombolysis.
   d. Most patients who die from an acute infarction have a critical obstruction in one coronary artery.

2. The following concerning risk stratification after an acute MI are true except:

   a. Women possess an improved post-MI prognosis compared with that of men.
   b. The single most important determinant of both short- and long-term survival is the residual left ventricular systolic function.
   c. Silent ischemia as detected by Holter monitoring has a similar prognosis to that of symptomatic ischemia after MI.
   d. Diabetes mellitus contributes to an increased postinfarction risk.

3. The following items are features of non-Q-wave MI except:

   a. The residual coronary artery stenosis generally is severe.
   b. Prominent collaterals serve the infarct-related artery.
   c. A greater likelihood of a previous MI exists.
   d. Recurrent infarction is less likely compared with a Q-wave infarction.

4. The following statements regarding thrombolytic therapy are true except:

   a. An improved mortality rate has been shown in patients with inferior infarction after thrombolytic administration.
   b. The earlier the thrombolytic treatment, the greater the impact on survival.
   c. Preservation of left ventricular function depends on early thrombolytic administration.
   d. CPR is an absolute contraindication for thrombolytic therapy.

5. Indications for a temporary pacemaker in patients with acute MI include the following except:

   a. New left anterior fascicular and right bundle-branch block.
   b. New second-degree Mobitz I AV block.
   c. New left bundle-branch block.
   d. Complete heart block.

Answers

1. d
   During an acute MI, angiography remains safe and, with angioplasty, often is the appropriate treatment. Importantly, most infarct-related arteries are occluded during the acute infarction phase. This is reduced after infarction secondary to spontaneous thrombolysis. Most patients who die from an acute infarction have advanced coronary atherosclerosis involving more than one coronary artery.

2. a
   Important adverse prognostic predictors after an MI include the extent of left ventricular systolic dysfunction and coexistent morbidity, including diabetes mellitus. Silent ischemia, as detected at Holter monitoring, portends a worse prognosis, as does female gender.

3. d
   Non-Q-wave infarctions are characterized by the residual, high-grade coronary stenosis, prominent collaterals, and greater likelihood of previous MI. The total creatine phosphokinase level is less, but the reinfarction rate is higher compared to patients with Q-wave infarctions.

4. d
   Thrombolytic therapy is most beneficial within the early phases of an acute MI. A reduced morbidity and mortality rate is shown for all infarcts, including inferior infarctions. Enhanced left ventricular systolic function is noted with earlier thrombolytic administration. CPR remains a relative, not an absolute, contraindication to thrombolytic therapy.

5. b
   Indications for temporary pacing during an acute MI include new-onset bifascicular block, second-degree Mobitz II AV block, and complete heart block. First-degree AV block and Mobitz I Wenckebach second-degree AV block require careful observation but not temporary pacing.

SUGGESTED READINGS

1. DeWood MA, Spona J, Notske R, et al. Prevalence of total coronary occlusion during the early hours of transmural myocardial infarction. N Engl J Med 1980;303:897–902.

   A landmark article demonstrating the high prevalence of acute coronary thrombosis in acute Q-wave MI.

2. ISIS-2 (Second Interventional Study of Infarct Survival) Collaborative Group. Randomized trial of intravenous streptokinase or aspirin, both or neither, among 17,187 cases of suspected acute myocardial infarction: ISIS-2. Lancet 1988;ii:349–360.

   The first study to demonstrate the independent benefit of aspirin in post-MI mortality. Also the first study to demonstrate the synergistic benefit of thrombolytic agents (i.e., streptokinase and aspirin).

3. Kleiman NS, White HD, Ohman EM, et al. Mortality within 24 hours of thrombolysis from myocardial infarction: the importance of early reperfusion. Circulation 1994; 90:2658–2665.

4. Ryan TJ, Anderson JL, Antman EM, et al. ACC/AHA Guidelines for the Management of Patients with Acute Myocardial Infarction: a report of the ACC/AHA Task Force on Practice Guidelines (Committee on Management of Acute Myocardial Infarction). J Am Coll Cardiol 1996; 28:1328–1428.

   An excellent review of the current guidelines for treatment of acute MI as produced by a distinguished expert panel. Also includes a rationale for treatment options.

5. TIMI 3-B Investigators. Effects of tissue plasminogen activator and a comparison of early invasive and conservative strategies in unstable angina and non Q-wave myocardial infarction: results of the TIMI-3B trial. Circulation 1994; 89:1545–1556.

Hyperlipidemia

Dennis L. Sprecher

RISK FACTORS FOR CARDIOVASCULAR DISEASE

Numerous risk factors are associated with development of cardiovascular disease. Primary risk factors include:

- Cigarette smoking
- Hyperlipidemia
- Hypertension
- Diabetes mellitus

Other risk factors include:

- Obesity
- Lack of activity
- Alcohol
- Diet
- Gender
- Age
- Family history

This chapter focuses on lipids and lipoprotein metabolism, but targeting the other risk factors, particularly cigarette use, will reduce the incidence of cardiac events. In those individuals who already have heart disease, discontinuation of cigarette use results in a 50% reduction in new events, and results of a meta-analysis on blood pressure control indicates a 17% reduction in cardiac events. Diabetes mellitus, which is present in approximately 15% of patients with coronary heart disease, remains an important risk factor to treat. Lowering the low-density lipoprotein (LDL) level in patients with diabetes mellitus profoundly reduces the risk of coronary artery disease (CAD), but the association of alcohol use, various aspects of diet, and lack of exercise with CAD remains controversial. Severe dietary restriction of fat and cholesterol as well as the transition from being sedentary to increasing functional

capacity have some ultimate benefit regarding reduction of cardiac events. However, the more common, subtle modification in these parameters among these patients may have inconsequential clinical effects.

The risk factor of gender relates not to whether disease will occur but rather to when it will occur. Women have cardiovascular disease later than men, and cardiovascular disease is the major cause of death among women in this country. The on-going Women's Health Initiative seeks to understand preventive measures and normal incidences of disease.

As noted, traditional risk factors are being supplemented with new markers thought to be relevant to CAD. Biochemical risk factors include:

- Fibrinogen
- PAI-1 (Plasminogen Activator Inhibitor-1)
- Homocysteine
- Lipoprotein A

These biochemical parameters add independent information beyond that provided by the classic risk factors.

CHOLESTEROL REDUCTION

Perhaps the most significant advance related to reduction of the cholesterol level is the association between cholesterol reduction and reduced cardiac events. In recent studies, the angiographic rate of regression following cholesterol reduction was extremely small yet statistically significant, whereas the reduction in the event rate often was much greater than 50%. Cholesterol reduction alters the organization of the plaque so that rupture and consequent myocardial infarction are less likely, and herein lies a considerable restructuring of thought. The progressive stenoses of a vessel that lead to hemodynamic compromise are not as relevant as the integrity of the plaque in predicting a future infarct, because cardiac events often result from lesions with less than 50% stenosis. Therefore, lack of hemodynamically significant stenoses may not reduce—and certainly does not exclude—the probability of a new cardiac event. Cholesterol lowering reduces the incidence of myocardial infarction, and according to large clinical trials (i.e., Scandinavian Simvastatin Survival Study [4S], West of Scotland Study [WOSCOPS], and Cholesterol and Recurrent Events [CARE]), the time to plaque stabilization, if it is to occur, will be between 6 months and 2 years of continuous treatment.

RECENT STUDIES

Results of numerous recent trials have demonstrated a reduction of cardiac events that is associated with a reduction in cholesterol serum levels. The 4S study evaluated more than patients with cardiac disease who were randomized to either Simvastatin, which is a 3-hydroxy-3-methylglutaryl coenzyme A (HMG-CoA) reductase inhibitor, or placebo. Therapy with Simvastatin was associated with a reduced incidence of death and nonfatal myocardial infarction. This was the first cholesterol-lowering study to definitely indicate a reduced mortality rate with therapy.

The WOSCOPS study involved primary prevention and demonstrated the benefit of Pravastatin compared with placebo. This benefit consisted of a 30% reduction in death and nonfatal myocardial infarction.

The CARE study tested Pravachol in patients with CAD but whose LDL cholesterol level was either low or normal (i.e., 115–175 mg/dL). Again, the results were comparable to those of other studies and suggested that even with LDL values as low as 125 mg/dL, there was a benefit to further reduction with therapy. It remains unclear, however, whether baseline LDL values less than 125 mg/dL also are worth lowering in secondary prevention.

Saphenous vein grafts are protected through lowering the LDL level as well. In the Post Coronary Artery Bypass Graft (Post-CABG) Trial using Mevacor (Lovastatin), the LDL level was lowered from a baseline mean of 155 mg/dL to either 135 mg/dL (modest treatment) or 95 mg/dL (aggressive treatment). Benefit was observed angiographically over time. Coumadin was not found to be of value.

Most of the patients in the primary and secondary studies were selected through use of very high, isolated LDL cholesterol elevations. When a patient also has a low high-density lipoprotein (HDL) level, high triglyceride levels, or other related risk factors, the benefit of LDL-lowering therapy was maintained. The CARE study demonstrated benefits in patients with LDL levels of 125 to 175 mg/dL, regardless of HDL levels. The angiographic HARP study indicated no improvement in CAD lesions with LDL levels of less than 140 mg/dL over a 2.5-year period.

SCREENING AND TREATMENT GUIDELINES

There have been two iterations of the adult treatment guidelines for cholesterol. The most recent amendments to these guidelines include recognition that older age in both men and woman constitutes a risk factor for CAD. Further, data from the Framingham study indicate that HDL levels that are particularly high represent a negative risk factor (i.e., they enhance protection from cardiovascular disease). Also, given the rather strong data from interventional studies, including the Cholesterol Lowering Angiographic Study (CLAS) as well as the meta-analyses mentioned earlier, patients with coronary heart disease or previous myocardial infarctions will have lower, more stringent goals for LDL cholesterol (i.e. <100 mg/dL). This may be amended as the results of both the CLAS study and the newly reported CARE study are more carefully evaluated.

The baseline cholesterol level may have some relevance for the reduction in risk. The authors of the CARE study recognized a progression of enhanced benefit from an LDL level of 125 to 190 mg/dL. Further, the percentage reduction in LDL level was more predictive of angiographic change than the average LDL level during the study.

Numerous controversial issues have developed recently concerning the screening process itself. Results of several large meta-analyses suggest that reduction of cholesterol levels, either by diet, treatment, or both, increases the mortality rate, specifically mortality from carcinoma. Results of two large, well-publicized interventional studies, the Lipid Research Clinics Coronary Primary Prevention Trial and the Helsinki Study, suggest increased accidental and suicidal death in the treatment group. Together with carefully done meta-analyses, these studies suggest the negative impact of cholesterol lowering, and an NHLBI-supported meta-analysis carefully evaluating various combinations of studies has determined that primary prevention and cholesterol reduction have an odds ratio of 1.0, thus suggesting neither benefit nor detriment. This was before the large WOSCOPS trial, however, the results of which clearly indicate benefits from primary prevention. Another study also indicated the carcinogenic potential of HMG-CoA reductase inhibitors in rats; in contrast, other recent, large studies did not find an increase in cancer mortality or morbidity rates with cholesterol-lowering therapy. Regarding secondary prevention, results of these meta-analyses clearly indicate that cholesterol reduction has significant benefit. This latter point is a fairly accepted consensus opinion, even considering the results of older studies that used lower-potency agents.

Data on risk factor modification in women are accumulating, but the amount remains small even after more recent studies. Currently, the data suggest that cholesterol reduction is at least as beneficial in women as in men. Few reportable cardiac events occur in young adult women between 20 and 40 years of age. It remains unclear, therefore, whether such individuals should be included in the generalized National Cholesterol Education Program (NCEP) guidelines.

The baseline cardiac event rate is substantially higher among patients with CAD compared to asymptomatic subjects, and risk reduction has a more statistically significant effect in this CAD population. Clearly, cholesterol reduction is effective for both primary and secondary prevention, but the decision to treat cholesterol elevation ultimately may be an economic one. The recent guidelines for internists published by the American College of Physicians suggest that only patients with a high risk of developing the disease (i.e., those with multiple risk factors or coronary disease) should be screened for hypercholesterolemia. This conflicts with the current NCEP guidelines. Actual knowledge of a risk factor may have significant benefit to specific individuals. On the other hand, restricting the screening process potentially reduces the overall cost of basic medical care, especially in those individual who would be healthy regardless of their cholesterol value.

DIETARY FAT

The finding related to which type of fat is relevant for cholesterol-lowering prompted the U.S. Food and Drug Administration (FDA) and U.S. Department of Agriculture to focus food-product labeling on the amount of saturated fat as well as the total fat content. This new label was enacted fully in 1994 and clearly defines serving size, total calories per serving, number of calories derived from fat, total grams of fat per serving, and total saturated fat. The quick rule of thumb is that the total fat intake per serving should be less than 3 g, and that the amount of total calories from fat should be less than 50%. Several recent reviews have considered the association of diet with coronary heart disease, and issues of both compliance and targeting of fats are relevant. Cholesterol reduction from diet is as potent as that from drug therapy in reducing coronary events. On average, a 5% reduction in the LDL level can be expected.

Various groups are evaluating the quality of fat, especially of the shorter-saturated fats, including 12:0, 14:0, 16:0. The 18-carbon saturates (i.e., 18:0) do not increase the plasma cholesterol level. Further, shorter fatty acids (i.e., those with 10 or fewer carbons) result in a variation of gastrointestinal absorption and minimal effect on lipoprotein synthesis and composition. Both mono- and polyunsaturated fats may affect coagulation, and monosaturates may reduce prostaglandin-mediated platelet aggregation. Fish oil appears to decrease VLDL hepatic packaging and secretion, thus reducing triglyceride values in patients with severe hypertriglyceridemia. Fish oil has been noted, however, to increase the concentration of apolipoprotein (Apo)B and to predispose some individuals to glucose intolerance.

PHARMACOLOGIC TREATMENT

Numerous companies are working on more potent HMG-CoA reductase inhibitors, which are called "statin" agents. The following are fairly equivalent in their convenience of use and side effect profile:

- Lovastatin
- Simvastatin
- Pravastatin
- Fluvastatin
- Atorvastatin
- Cerivastatin
- Resin/statin combination
- Nicotinic acid
- Statin agent
- Gemfibrozil

Simvastatin is approximately twice as potent on a milligram-per-milligram basis as the other drugs, including Fluvastatin, which is the least expensive choice at lower dose. Atorvastatin is one of the newest of these drugs, being approved in January 1997. It can lower the LDL level by more than 60%, and it also has a significant influence on lowering the triglyceride levels. Vascular studies with this drug are anticipated. Further, a very potent combination of bile acid absorbing resin and statin agents has lowered LDL levels by more than 50%. Specifically, a low-dose combination of both (i.e., Lovastatin, 10–20 mg/day, and resin, 4–8 g/day), provided 25–30% cholesterol lowering with minimal side effects.

These various agents are particularly appropriate for isolated LDL elevations. The major laboratory tests that require monitoring with the statin agents include liver enzymes (i.e., serum glutamic-oxaloacetic transaminase and serum glutamate-pyruvate transaminase) and creatine phosphokinase (CPK). Laboratory evidence of myositis now is found in fewer patients. CPK levels should be measured at baseline, at 3 months, and subsequently if symptoms occur. More frequent findings, however, are patients with abnormalities not only of the LDL level but also—or perhaps in distinction to–triglyceride and HDL levels. Niacin and the fibric acid derivatives (e.g., Gemfibrozil) are candidate drugs for such patients. Niacin may worsen glucose intolerance in many patients, who already often are diabetic. Fibric acid derivatives (the only one currently approved in the United States is Gemfibrozil) produce moderate reduction of the LDL level (i.e., ≈15%) but excellent lowering of triglyceride and elevation of HDL levels. Statin agents also exert beneficial effects on triglyceride and HDL levels, but only moderately so. The combination of statin and Gemfibrozil poses some enhanced risk for muscle damage and liver toxicity. The combination of niacin and statin often is used in patients with mixed hyperlipidemia, but not in those who also have diabetes.

HDL/TRIGLYCERIDE ABNORMALITIES

Patients often present with either an isolated abnormality in the LDL level or an abnormality that includes triglycerides, HDL, or both. These latter subjects can present with a low HDL level alone and normal triglyceride values, with high triglyceride values and a normal HDL level, or with high triglyceride and low HDL levels. Those with a low HDL level alone have first-degree family members with a considerable enrichment in all the various phenotypes, including low HDL level alone. This lipoprotein phenotype, which is called familial hypoalpha, is a well-described phenomenon. Those patients with a high triglyceride level alone have family members with high triglyceride levels but not an enhancement in their low HDL levels. Finally, 40 to 50% of patients who present with both high triglyceride and low HDL levels are obese, and up to 50% of their family members exhibit abnormalities of HDL and triglyceride levels. The LDL distribution among these various cohorts is random. Familial hypertriglyceridemia and familial hypoalpha are part of this schema, as well as new entities, such as familial low HDL/high triglycerides. These may be insulin- or glucose-dependent abnormalities (or both).

No doubt, these abnormalities are part of a spectrum of familial disorders that present with a cluster of risk-associated factors, specifically low HDL level, high triglyceride level, obesity, high blood pressure, glucose intolerance, insulin resistance, or some combination. The genetic bases for these phenomena are unclear, but hepatic lipase and lipoprotein lipase may play a role in producing low HDL levels. The genetic etiology of phenotype B (i.e., dense LDL) has been initially localized to a section of chromosome 19, which is not distant from the LDL receptor.

In June 1992, the first homozygous familial hypercholesterolemic patients were treated with genetic-engineering technology. These patients had a substantial decrement in LDL concentrations after hepatic cells were transduced with normal LDL-receptor DNA material and readministered to the subjects. When performed on genetically familial, hypercholesterolemically defined rabbits, this same experiment demonstrated reduced LDL levels. This has now been shown in humans, though the published report is still forthcoming. In 10 to 20 years, we might expect that even the heterozygote familial hypercholesterolemic patient will be treated with genetic-engineering methodology.

OTHER ISSUES

VASOREGULATION

Data on cholesterol reduction and improvement in vasoregulation now are emerging. These data currently suggest there are alterations in vasoregulation within 3 months of cholesterol reduction, and some data suggest improvements in a much shorter time.

GENETIC MARKERS

Genetic determinants of increased risk for CAD include the protein ApoE, which has three isotypes (i.e., E2, E3, E4). ApoE4 is associated with increased incidence of CAD.

OXIDIZED LDL

Considerable animal data suggest that oxidation of LDL is associated with development of vascular disease. Human data are still minimal, however. Results of one study found that Probucol, which is a significant antioxidant, was unsuccessful in reducing femoral artery disease but was valuable in reducing restenosis after percutaneous transluminal coronary angioplasty. Results of epidemiologic studies, however, have demonstrated that some benefit is associated with use of vitamin E, but routine use of vitamin E for cardiovascular protection is not yet recommended.

REVIEW EXERCISES

QUESTIONS

1. If a person has high cholesterol and heart disease or high cholesterol and multiple risk factors, it is important to reduce the cholesterol value:

   a. To reduce the plaque size and, therefore, increase the lumen diameter.

   b. To reduce the incidence of plaque rupture and, thereby, reduce the incidence of cardiac events.

   c. To improve the total cholesterol:HDL ratio.

   d. To achieve at least a 25% reduction in the LDL level according to the NCEP guidelines.

2. M.J. is a 48-year-old man who 3 years ago suffered a myocardial infarction and had bypass surgery to place grafts in three of his vessels. His lipid profile indicated an LDL level of 150 mg/dL, an HDL level of 45 mg/dL, and a triglycerides level of 110 mg/dL. What is the recommended treatment for this patient?

   a. Initiate diet therapy for 6 months. Then, if the LDL level has not fallen to less than 100 mg/dL for LDL cholesterol, initiate medication.

   b. Begin therapy with HMG-CoA reductase inhibitor to lower the LDL level to less than 130 mg/dL.

   c. Simultaneously initiate diet therapy and an HMG-CoA reductase inhibitor to bring the LDL level to less than 100 mg/dL.

   d. Use Gemfibrozil in combination with an HMG-CoA reductase inhibitor to decrease the LDL level to less than 100 mg/dL and increase the HDL level.

3. A new food label was introduced in 1994. This label includes:

   a. The total percentage of calories from fat in each serving.

   b. The number of grams of saturated fat in the entire package.

   c. Total calories, number of calories from fat, and total fat in grams per serving.

   d. Whether the product is, indeed, healthy for you.

4. M.J. was placed on an HMG-CoA reductase inhibitor. When he returned in 6 weeks, his physician should check which of the following?

   a. Renal function.

   b. Renal, liver, and thyroid function tests.

   c. Liver function tests.

   d. Liver function tests, CPK, and ophthalmoscopic examination.

5. A.R. is a 55-year-old man with no known CAD who is totally asymptomatic. He has a family history of heart disease before 65 years of age and smokes cigarettes. His total cholesterol level is 240 mg/dL. His triglycerides level is 96 mg/dL, and his HDL level is 39 mg/dL. What is the proper treatment regimen for cholesterol control in this patient?

   a. He should be placed on an HMG-CoA reductase inhibitor because his LDL level is greater than 190 mg/dL.

   b. He should be placed on an HMG-CoA reductase inhibitor because his LDL level is greater than 160 mg/dL and he has two risk factors.

   c. His LDL level is too low; thus, he should not be placed on cholesterol-lowering therapy.

   d. Patients without CAD should not be treated for hypercholesterolemia.

6. In patients with CAD and diabetes mellitus along with an elevated LDL level, what should be suggested to prevent aggressive CAD?

   a. LDL lowering with diet and medication.

   b. Tight diabetes control.

   c. Both.

7. LDL lowering can protect both native vessels and saphenous vein grafts.

   a. True.

   b. False.

Answers

1. b

Even though regression can be significant, it often is less than 0.2 mm beyond 2 years of therapy. Generally, this is not thought to be clinically significant. Rather, organization of the plaque through cholesterol reduction appears to stabilize its components and reduce the risk of rupture. This also should reduce development of new lesions and progression of lesions already present. Epidemiologic evidence suggests the total cholesterol:HDL ratio is a valuable parameter in predicting cardiac disease. The interaction of HDL with the effects of cholesterol modification are not clearly understood, however. The NCEP guidelines suggest reducing cholesterol values below specific cut points. These guidelines may be amended in the future to target certain percentage reductions, but at present, percentage reductions are not the stated goals. Further, the NCEP provides guidelines only; they do not absolutely define medical management. Therefore, physicians must use these guidelines with individual patient data and new scientific evidence.

2. c

Considering the presence of CAD and clear-cut evidence that at 150 mg/dL, cholesterol reduction will decrease the risk of future events, treatment is crucial, because the benefit can be observed as early as 6 months after initiation. Postponing drug treatment for 6 months while the patient is on a diet, which has a low likelihood of success, no longer is reasonable. Therefore, in patients with CAD, concurrent diet and drug therapy should be initiated. Diet therapy may not yield dramatic effects, but at least 20% of patients will experience substantial reduction in the LDL level from the diet itself. Such efforts also provide continued instruction, thus targeting population-wide efforts for fat reduction in our diet. Currently, guidelines have described 100 mg/dL as the goal in patients with CAD. Results of the CARE study suggest there is no obvious impact after 5 years of treatment in patients with initial LDL levels of less than 125 mg/dL, even if their values are brought down by more than 25%. Bringing a level of 150 mg/dL down to 100 mg/dL would be an approximate 30% reduction, which should provide at least a 30 to 40% reduction in risk over the 3 to 5 years of treatment. Again, the role of HDL is not understood, and the use of Gemfibrozil in association with statins modestly increases some risk of side effects and has an unknown benefit. A high triglycerides level, low HDL level, and elevated LDL level might prompt use of such a combination.

3. c

Even though diet containing less than 30% of total calories from fat is the recommended step I American Heart Association diet, the label does not clearly indicate this percentage. Rather, it provides the total number of calories per serving and total number of calories from fat per serving, thus allowing you to calculate a percentage. A substantial advance in the food label is that some reasonable regimentation of serving size now is required. This allows comparisons between products. The comments and food label pertain to one serving, which is defined clearly at the top of the label and does not describe what is in the entire package. The main numbers at the top of the label include the total calories per serving and the total calories from fat per serving. Total fat in grams as well as saturated fat content per serving then are listed. One entire section of the label relates to the percentage of total daily calories typically consumed, being either 2000 or 2500 cal/day. It is unclear, however, to what extent this part of the label is being used by consumers. The American Heart Association originally contemplated putting out approval markers for those products determined to be appropriate for cardiovascular health, but this was superseded by the FDA food label, which does not include such a claim.

4. c

Currently, we should be most concerned about liver function test abnormalities and muscle inflammation noted by blood levels of CPK, even though both abnormalities occur in fewer than 1% of patients placed on the statin agents. The FDA requires the liver tests but not CPK, which should be tested if symptoms (i.e., muscle cramps) are noted. Considerable interest remains in measuring them, at least over the first year, on an interval basis after initiating the medication. One of the statins, Pravachol, has received FDA approval for liver tests at both baseline and 6 weeks, but not beyond as long as the dose remains constant. This is true for Simvastatin, but only during the first 6 months. There was some initial concern about cataract formation during the testing of Mevacor, the first of the statin agents approved in the United States, but there no longer is reason for such concern with these agents. No data currently suggest that HMG-CoA reductase inhibitors affect thyroid or kidney function.

5. b

For patients with LDL levels of greater than 190 mg/dL or those with levels greater than 160 mg/dL and two risk factors, it is appropriate according to the NCEP guidelines to begin a treatment regimen with diet and, subsequently, medications if the goals are not met, even in patients without known CAD. This patient has a calculated LDL level of 182 mg/dL (240 − [96/5 + 39]). In addition, he smokes cigarettes and is older than 45 years. Even though some would argue that a family history of heart disease before age 65 is a positive risk factor, the NCEP guidelines stipulate an age younger than 55 as their cut-off point for the definition of premature. Nonetheless, it is appropriate in patients without CAD, with an LDL level of greater than 160 mg/dL, and with two risk factors to begin nutritional counseling and, subsequently, diet to bring the LDL level to less than 160 mg/dL—and, ultimately, to less than 130 mg/dL. By targeting even patients without CAD who have, in essence, three risk factors, the yearly risk for such patients of a cardiac event is greater than 2%. Data from both the WOSCOPS and CARE studies certainly argue for this type of treatment.

6. a

The 4S and CARE trials found lipid lowering to be beneficial in reducing the rate of cardiac events among patients with diabetes. Data supporting diabetes control to protect against CAD, however, are not clear. Results of the University Group Diabetes Program trial suggested no benefits from use of insulin or oral agents. Results from the Diabetes Clinical Control Trial in patients with insulin-dependent diabetes mellitus (IDDM) suggest that tight diabetes control reduces the rate of microvascular complications (i.e., neuropathy, nephrotomy). Results of a recent Finnish study also suggest benefits in patients with non-IDDM. Two large, soon-to-be-reported trials will provide some insight in non-IDDM. Thus, it is reasonable that normalized glucose values would lessen the incidence of macrovascular disease, but this has not been demonstrated by the evidence. Lipid lowering is worthwhile for patients both with and without diabetes.

7. a

This is true. Results from the Post-CABG Trial and the CLAS study indicate that lipid lowering benefits saphenous vein grafts. Results of many other trials (e.g., 4S, CARE, WOSCOPS) have determined that native vessels respond to lipid lowering.

SUGGESTED READINGS

American College of Physicians. Guidelines for using serum cholesterol, high density lipoprotein cholesterol, and triglyceride levels as screening tests for preventing coronary heart disease in adults. Ann Intern Med 1996;124:515–517.

Anderson T, Meredith I, Yeung A, et al. The effect of cholesterol-lowering and antioxidant therapy on endothelium-dependent coronary vasomotion. N Engl J Med 1995;332:488–493.

Austin MA, King MC, Vranizan KM, et al. Low-density lipoprotein subclass patterns and risk of myocardial infarction. JAMA 1990;82:495–506.

Blankenhorn DH, Nessim SA, Johnson RL, et al. Beneficial effects of combined colestipol-niacin therapy on coronary atherosclerosis and coronary venous bypass grafts. JAMA 1987;257:3233–3240.

Brown B, Zhao X-Q, Sacco D, et al. Lipid lowering and plaque regression. New insights into prevention of plaque disruption and clinical events in coronary disease. Circulation 1993;87:1781–1791

Hrovat K, Harris K, Leach A, et al. The new food label, type of fat and consumer choice. (A pilot study.) Arch Fam Med 1994;3:690–695.

Kozarsky K, McKinley D, Austin L, et al. In vivo correction of low density lipoprotein receptor deficiency in the Watanabe heritable hyperlipidemic rabbit with recombinant adenoviruses. J Biol Chem 1994;269:13695–13702.

Lipid Research Clinics Program. The Lipid Research Clinics Coronary Primary Prevention Trial Results. II. The relationship of reduction in incidence of coronary heart disease to cholesterol lowering. JAMA 1984;251:365–374.

Nawroki J, Weiss S, Davidson M, et al. Reduction of LDL cholesterol by 25% to 60% in patients with primary hypercholesterolemia by atrovastatin, a new HMG-CoA reductase inhibitor. Arteriosclerosis Thromb Vasc Biol 1995;15:678–682.

Newman T, Hulley S. Carcinogenicity of lipid-lowering drugs. JAMA 1996;275:55–60.

Nishina PM, Johnson JP, Naggert JK, Krauss RM. Linkage of atherogenic lipoprotein phenotype to the low density lipoprotein receptor locus on the short arm of chromosome 19. Proc Natl Acad Sci U S A 1992;89:708–712.

Post Coronary Artery Bypass Graft Trial Investigators. The effect of aggressive lowering of low-density lipoprotein cholesterol levels and low-dose anticoagulation on obstructive changes in saphenous vein coronary artery bypass grafts. N Engl J Med 1997;336:153–162.

Reaven GM. The role of insulin resistance and hyperinsuli-nemia in coronary heart disease. Metabolism 1992;41(Suppl 1):16–19.

Rimm E, Stampfer M, Ascheria A, et al. Vitamin E consumption and the risk of coronary disease in men. N Engl J Med 1993;328:1450–1456.

Sacks F, Gibson C, Rosner B, et al. The influence of pretreatment low density lipoprotein cholesterol concentrations on the effect of hypocholesterolemic therapy on coronary atherosclerosis in angiographic trials. Harvard Atherosclerosis Reversibility Project Research Group (review). Am J Cardiol 1995;76:78C–85C.

Sacks F, Pasternak R, Gibson C, et al. Effect on coronary atherosclerosis of decrease in plasma cholesterol concentrations in normocholesterolaemic patients. Harvard Atherosclerosis Reversibility Project (HARP) Group. Lancet 1994;344:1182–1186.

Sacks F, Pfeffer M, Moye L, et al. The effect of Pravastatin on coronary events after myocardial infarction in patients with average cholesterol levels. N Engl J Med 1996;335:1001–1009.

Scandinavian Simvastatin Survival Study Group. Randomized trial of cholesterol lowering in 4444 patients with coronary heart disease: the Scandinavian Simvastatin Survival Study (4S). Lancet 1994;344:1383–1389.

Shepherd J, Cobbe SM, Ford I, et al. Prevention coronary heart disease with pravastatin in men with hypercholesterolemia. N Engl J Med 1995;333:1301–1307.

Stampfer M, Hennekens C, Manson J, et al. Vitamin E consumption and the risk of coronary disease in women. N Engl J Med 1993;328:1440–1449.

Summary of the second report of the National Cholesterol Education Program (NCEP) Expert Panel on Detection, Evaluation, and Treatment of High Blood Cholesterol in Adults (Adult Treatment Panel-II). JAMA 1993;269:3015-3023.

Thompson G, Hollyer J, Waters D. Percentage change rather than plasma level of LDL-cholesterol determines therapeutic response in coronary heart disease. Curr Opin Lipidol 1995;6:386–388.

Treasure C, Klein J, Weintraub W, et al. Beneficial effects of cholesterol-lowering therapy on the coronary endothelium in patients with coronary artery disease. N Engl J Med 1995;332:481–487.

Walldius G, Erikson U, Olsson A, et al. The effect of probucol on femoral atherosclerosis: The Probucol Quantitative Regression Swedish Trial (PQRST). Am J Cardiol 1994;74:875–883.

C·H·A·P·T·E·R

69

Heart Failure

Robert E. Hobbs

Heart failure is characterized by a disturbance of cardiac-pump function. In this syndrome, the pumping action of the heart is inadequate to meet the body's needs, thus resulting in decreased perfusion of organs and tissues as well as fluid retention. Most cases of heart failure result from systolic dysfunction, in which the contractility of the left ventricle is impaired. A smaller number of cases involve impaired relaxation of the ventricles during diastole (i.e., diastolic failure).

ETIOLOGY

The most common cause of heart failure in the United States is end-stage coronary artery disease. Other common causes include:

- Cardiomyopathies
- Valvular heart disease
- Hypertensive heart disease
- Miscellaneous other causes (e.g., congenital, high output)

  Causes of right-sided heart failure include:

- Left-sided heart failure
- Mitral stenosis and pulmonary hypertension
- Pulmonary hypertension
- Cor pulmonale secondary to chronic obstructive pulmonary disease
- Pulmonic valve disease
- Tricuspid valve disease
- Right ventricular infarction
- Arrhythmogenic right ventricular dysplasia

  Causes of high-output heart failure include:

- Thyrotoxicosis
- Arteriovenous fistula
- Pregnancy
- Paget's disease
- Anemia
- Beriberi

EPIDEMIOLOGY

Heart failure affects from 1 to 2% of the population (approximately 3 million Americans), with 400,000 new patients diagnosed each year. Heart failure also is the only cardiovascular disease now increasing in prevalence. It is the most common DRG diagnosis in Medicare patients and the most common reason for hospitalization in elderly patients.

The prevalence of heart failure increases directly with age. Approximately 10% of those older than 75 years of age have a history of heart failure. Heart failure is more common in men than in women, until very late in life.

The overall annual mortality rate from heart failure is approximately 20%, which is worse than the overall prognosis for patients with malignant tumors. In the Framingham Heart Study, men survived for a mean interval of 1.7 years after diagnosis, and females survived for a mean interval of approximately 3.2 years. Death rates are higher in patients with severe symptoms.

Each year, approximately 280,000 deaths are attributed to heart failure. Progressive pump failure accounts for approximately half of these deaths, but sudden death occurs in 40%. Heart failure is the most common predisposing factor for sudden death.

The prognosis in patients with heart failure relates to several factors. The most important indicator is exercise capacity. Patients with symptoms that occur with minimal activities have the poorest survival rate. Left ventricular function also is an important indicator; however, a low-ejection fraction without symptoms does not necessarily lead to poor outcome. Malignant cardiac arrhythmias are a poor prognostic indicator.

PATHOPHYSIOLOGY

There are two hemodynamic derangements in congestive heart failure: low cardiac output, and high intracardiac pressures. Low cardiac output accounts for the symptoms of fatigue and exercise intolerance; high intracardiac pressures account for exertional dyspnea and peripheral edema.

As heart failure progresses, the heart undergoes remodeling to compensate for low stroke volume. Remodeling consists of hypertrophy, dilatation, thinning, and rounding of the left ventricle, and it may lead to increased wall stress, mitral regurgitation, and decreased inotropic reserve.

The major compensatory mechanisms in heart failure are neurohormonal, including:

- Sympathetic nervous system activation
- Renin-angiotensin stimulation
- Release of vasopressin

Neurohormonal activation leads to vasoconstriction as well as to sodium and water retention. The immediate compensatory effects are beneficial, but the long-term effects are deleterious.

Levels of plasma catecholamines, renin, and vasopressin are elevated in patients with heart failure. These abnormalities develop because of baroreceptor dysfunction in the failing heart, which activates the sympathetic and inhibits the parasympathetic nervous system. As such, sympathetic stimulation releases catecholamines into the circulation. Catecholamines cause resting tachycardia, enhanced myocardial contractility, and vasoconstriction. They also may predispose to cardiac arrhythmias, myocyte toxicity, β-receptor dysfunction, and renin-angiotensin stimulation. Patients with the highest activation of the sympathetic nervous system have the poorest survival rates.

Renin is released from the juxtaglomerular apparatus of the kidney by several stimuli, and it acts as a substrate for conversion of angiotensinogen to angiotensin I. As angiotensin I passes through the pulmonary circuit, it is converted to angiotensin II, which stimulates the adrenal gland to release aldosterone, which in turn promotes sodium and water retention. Angiotensin II is a potent vasoconstrictor that enhances sodium retention and stimulates thirst.

Vasopressin is the third neurohormonal system to be activated in heart failure. Released from the hypothalamus because of baroreceptor or osmotic stimuli, it causes vasoconstriction as well as sodium and water retention. The action of the sympathetic nervous system, renin-angiotensin system, and vasopressin are balanced by natriuretic peptides, which are released from the atria and ventricular myocytes. Their physiologic effects include sodium excretion, water excretion, vasodilation, and inhibition of the renin-angiotensin system.

Endothelin is a potent vasoconstrictor and is derived from various sources within the cardiovascular system. Endothelin also acts as a growth factor.

Tumor necrosis factor is released from macrophages, and levels of this factor are elevated in patients with heart failure. Tumor necrosis factor is responsible for cardiac cachexia and apoptosis in the failing heart.

CLINICAL PRESENTATION

Symptoms of congestive heart failure relate to low cardiac output or congestion. Clinical manifestations of heart failure include:

- General
  - Fatigue
  - Effort intolerance
  - Decreased stamina
  - Lightheadedness
  - Mental confusion
  - Cachexia
  - Muscle wasting
  - Edema
- Respiratory
  - Dyspnea
  - Orthopnea
  - Paroxysmal Nocturnal Dyspnea (PND)
  - Cough
  - Bronchospasm
  - Respiratory distress
- Abdominal
  - Weight gain
  - Fluid retention
  - Bloating
  - Early satiety
  - Anorexia
  - Weight loss
  - Right-upper-quadrant pain
  - Nausea, vomiting

The degree of functional impairment can be stated in terms of the New York Heart Association functional classification:

I. No limitation of physical activity
No dyspnea or fatigue with ordinary physical activities
II. Slight limitation of physical activity
Dyspnea and fatigue occur with ordinary physical activities
Patient is comfortable at rest
III. Marked limitation of activity
Less-than-ordinary physical activities cause symptoms
Patient is comfortable at rest

IV. Symptoms present at rest and with any physical exertion

DIAGNOSIS

PHYSICAL EXAMINATION

Patients with severe acute congestive heart failure and pulmonary edema exhibit:

- Respiratory distress
- Tachypnea
- Diaphoresis
- Pallor
- Cyanosis
- Cool extremities
- Jugular venous distention
- Rales, both lung fields
- Rapid heat rate
- S3 and S4 gallops

Patients with chronic heart failure usually are comfortable at rest. In those with advanced heart failure, cardiac cachexia and muscle wasting may be present. The blood pressure may be normal, low, or high. The resting pulse rate is increased, and pulsus alternans is palpable. Jugular venous distention is the most important physical finding in patients with decompensated failure, and a prominent V wave from tricuspid regurgitation often is observed in the jugular venous pulse. The lungs usually are clear in chronic heart failure. Rales may be present when heart failure is decompensated. Decreased breath sounds and dullness in the lung bases reflect an underlying pleural effusion, and wheezing because of bronchospasm (i.e., ''cardiac asthma'') occasionally is heard.

Cheyne-Stokes respirations also are observed in patients with advanced heart failure. The cardiac examination reveals a diffuse point of maximal impulse (PMI), which is displaced downward and to the left. A left ventricular heave and, occasionally, a right ventricular heave are palpable. The heart rate may be rapid, and the first heart sound is accentuated. The second heart sound may be paradoxically split because of delayed electrical activation or impaired mechanical ejection of the left ventricle. The third heart sound is characteristic of heart failure, and the fourth reflects a noncompliant left ventricle. Murmurs of both mitral and tricuspid regurgitation frequently are heard on auscultation. Abdominal examination may reveal hepatomegaly, right-upper-quadrant tenderness, and ascites; pressing on the liver may further distend the jugular veins (i.e., positive hepatojugular reflux). Peripheral examination may reveal edema, muscle wasting, or cyanosis.

DIAGNOSTIC STUDIES

Electrocardiography may reveal normal sinus rhythm or atrial fibrillation. Left ventricular hypertrophy or left bundle-branch block frequently occur, and Q waves reflect previous myocardial infarction.

Chest radiography frequently shows cardiomegaly, with a cardiothoracic ratio of greater than 0.5. Increased pulmonary vascularity, redistribution of blood flow to the upper lobes, prominent pulmonary arteries, Kerley B-lines, alveolar edema, and pleural effusions are radiographic manifestations of pulmonary vascular congestion.

Echocardiography is the most useful diagnostic test. The left ventricle is dilated, and the left ventricular ejection fraction is decreased. The right ventricle may be normal or dysfunctional. There may be Doppler evidence of mitral regurgitation and tricuspid regurgitation; pulmonary artery pressures can be estimated from the Doppler waveforms. Echocardiography excludes tamponade or pericardial diseases as causes of heart failure, and Doppler measurements provide information about diastolic dysfunction.

Radionuclide ventriculography provides objective assessment of both left and right ventricular ejection fractions, and metabolic stress testing, using a modified Naughton protocol with measurement of gas exchange, provides an accurate, objective assessment of functional capacity. In normal individuals, the peak Vo_2 usually is 25 mL/kg per minute or greater. Values of less than 14 mL/kg per minute indicate severe functional impairment.

Cardiac catheterization provides hemodynamic data, which guides therapy. Coronary angiography is the most accurate means of diagnosing coronary artery disease as a cause of heart failure. The status of the cardiac valves and left ventricle also may be assessed by catheterization.

Right ventricular endomyocardial biopsy no longer is performed routinely in patients with heart failure. Myocardial tissue diagnosis may be helpful, however, in patients with restrictive cardiomyopathy.

DIASTOLIC HEART FAILURE

Systolic dysfunction is characterized by impaired contractility, whereas diastolic dysfunction is characterized by impaired relaxation. In patients with diastolic dysfunction, the left ventricular ejection fraction frequently is normal, but the diastolic filling is impaired (i.e., stiff-heart syndrome). The left ventricle is hypertrophied, left ventricular cavity size is small, and overall heart size frequently is normal. Diastolic dysfunction occurs with hypertensive heart disease, hypertrophic cardiomyopathy, restrictive cardiomyopathy, after aortic valve replacement, and ischemic heart disease.

The most important test for assessing left ventricular ejection fraction and diastolic filling patterns is echocardiography. Hemodynamically, diastolic dysfunction is characterized by elevated left ventricular end-diastolic pressure, pulmonary capillary wedge pressure, pulmonary artery pressure, right ventricular pressure, and right atrial pressure.

Treatment is directed at the underlying cause. Therapeutic goals include relieving congestion, improving relaxation, decreasing hypertrophy, and relieving ischemia. Diuretics, calcium channel blockers, antihypertensive medications, and antianginal therapy are used.

TREATMENT

Treatment of heart failure includes:

- Identifying the underlying cause of heart failure
- Determining precipitating causes for decompensation
- Initiating specific treatment
- Providing patient education

Precipitating causes of decompensated heart failure include:

- Excessive salt or fluid intake
- Noncompliance with medications
- Excessive exertion
- Arrhythmias (e.g., atrial fibrillation, heart block)
- Infection
- Renal failure
- Ischemia/myocardial infarction
- Drugs (i.e., nonsteroidal anti-inflammatory drugs, myocardial depressants)
- Pulmonary embolism
- Anemia
- Thyrotoxicosis

Patient education is an important aspect of treatment, because noncompliance is one of the most frequent causes of rehospitalization.

Treatment has changed dramatically during the past 30 years. Initially, bed rest, fluid removal, and oxygen were used. Later, efforts were directed at increasing contractility, decreasing venous return, and lowering systemic vascular resistance. Currently, newer therapies are directed at modulating the sympathetic nervous system, the renin-angiotensin system, and other neurohormonal factors. Sympathetic nervous system activity can be modulated by digoxin, β-blockers, and, perhaps, newer calcium channel blockers. Renin-angiotensin effects may be inhibited with angiotensin-converting enzyme (ACE) inhibitors or angiotensin II–receptor blockers. Therapeutic uses for natriuretic peptides, endothelin antagonists, and vasopressin inhibitors are being investigated.

INOTROPIC AGENTS

Digoxin

Digoxin, which is the only oral inotropic agent approved for clinical use, has several direct and indirect actions on the myocardium and conducting system. Hemodynamically, it is a weak inotropic agent and a weak vasoconstrictor. On a microcellular level, its action occurs through binding and inhibiting the enzyme sodium-potassium ATPase, which ultimately increases levels of intracellular calcium to enhance contractility. Recently, digoxin was found to be a centrally acting agent that restores baroreceptor dysfunction and modulates both the sympathetic nervous system and the renin-angiotensin system.

Several recent clinical trials have reestablished the importance of digoxin in symptomatic patients with heart failure. Digoxin improves exercise capacity, ejection fraction, and hemodynamics. It decreases the frequency of hospitalizations; however, it does not alter the natural course of the disease. Digoxin has a low therapeutic-toxic range, and its dose should be decreased when combined with amiodarone, verapamil, propafenone, or quinidine.

Dopamine

Dopamine, which is an intravenous inotropic agent, is a sympathomimetic amine. It is the immediate precursor of norepinephrine, and its unique physiologic properties include vasodilation, positive inotropic effects, and peripheral vasoconstriction. When used at low doses, dopamine activates dopaminergic receptors in the mesenteric and renal arteries, which enhances renal blood flow. In moderate doses, dopamine stimulates cardiac β-receptors and increases cardiac output. At high doses, it activates peripheral α-receptors, thus causing vasoconstriction.

Dobutamine

Dobutamine, which is a direct-acting, intravenous inotrope and vasodilator, is useful for treating patients with decompensated heart failure who are receiving maximal oral medical therapy. A 2- to 3-day infusion of dobutamine often results in sustained clinical and hemodynamic benefit. Patients with severe, far-advanced heart failure may receive outpatient dobutamine as palliative therapy to improve their quality of life and reduce the need for hospitalization.

Milrinone

Milrinone, which is a phosphodiesterase III inhibitor, is an intravenous inotrope and a vasodilator. It can be used either as a primary inotropic agent or in combination with dobutamine or dopamine.

DIURETICS

Most patients with heart failure benefit from diuretics, and many agents are available with different sites of action in the kidney, different potencies, and different metabolic effects. Diuretics are effective in controlling fluid volume and are useful in systolic as well as diastolic failure. Diuretics are available at relatively low cost and are administered once daily. The disadvantage of diuretics is the potential for overdiuresis, which may lower cardiac output, cause orthostatic hypotension, and activate vasoconstrictor mechanisms. Diuretics are associated with various metabolic sequelae and drug interactions.

VASODILATORS

Recently, ACE inhibitors have been the most important drugs in patients with heart failure, including those with asymptomatic left ventricular dysfunction. In addition to prolonging survival, ACE inhibitors improve symptoms, exercise tolerance, and electrolyte balance. Side effects of ACE inhibitors include hypotension, hyperkalemia, azotemia, cough, agranulocytosis, and drug rash.

β-BLOCKERS

β-Blockers may be as important as ACE inhibitors in treating heart failure. Though β-blockers modulate catecholamine excess, which may cause β-receptor desensitization or direct myocyte toxicity, their exact mechanism of action is unknown. Results of clinical trials have shown that β-blockers improve symptoms, quality of life, ejection fraction, submaximal exercise, and survival.

CALCIUM CHANNEL BLOCKERS

Calcium channel blockers are contraindicated in patients with congestive heart failure, because they depress left ventricular function, activate neurohormones, worsen symptoms, and increase the risk of death. Newer calcium channel blockers, such as amlodipine and felodipine, have a neutral effect on cardiac function. A large-scale clinical trial currently is studying the efficacy of mibefradil, which is a calcium T-channel blocker.

INTRA-AORTIC BALLOON PUMP

Intra-aortic balloon pumping temporarily improves hemodynamics in patients with severe heart failure. A balloon pump increases cardiac output by 20%, and it restores hypotensive blood pressure. However, this device may cause limb ischemia, bleeding, thrombosis, neurologic injury, and infection. Complications occur at a rate of 10% per day, and they tend to limit the usefulness of a balloon pump to a period of 1 week.

LEFT VENTRICULAR–ASSIST DEVICES

New left ventricular–assist devices (e.g., HeartMate, Novacor) are electrically powered, pusher-plate pumps that are implanted behind the abdominal wall. The inlet cannula is connected to the the apex of the heart, and the outlet cannula is attached to the ascending aorta. These devices have been used as a bridge to transplant in hundreds of patients, thus allowing patients to become physically active and rehabilitated before transplantation. Currently, the HeartMate is being evaluated as a permanent left ventricular–assist device in the REMATCH trial.

CARDIOMYOPLASTY

Cardiomyoplasty involves wrapping the latissmus dorsi muscle around the heart and then training that muscle to become fatigue-resistant. A special pacemaker senses the QRS complex, discharges a burst of electrical impulses, and stimulates the latissimus dorsi muscle to contract during systole. A randomized clinical trial is evaluating the usefulness of this surgical approach in patients with heart failure.

VENTRICULAR REDUCTION SURGERY

Ventricular reduction surgery is an investigational technique that involves resecting a triangular portion of the left ventricular myocardium from the anterolateral left ventricular wall. It often is combined with surgical repair of mitral or tricuspid regurgitation. The reconstructed left ventricle becomes a smaller and, perhaps, more efficient pumping chamber.

This procedure has been performed in the United States since May 1996. Long-term follow-up data are unavailable, but approximately half of patients have improved clinically. The anticipated 1-year mortality rate is 15%. Patients who fail to improve clinically may be listed for cardiac transplantation. Current indications include patients with dilated cardiomyopathy, no previous open-heart surgery, functional class III–IV symptoms despite a good medical regimen, and ventricular diastolic dimensions greater than 7 cm. Postoperatively, the improvement in left ventricular ejection fraction, cardiac output, and functional capacity has been modest, and medical therapy for heart failure is continued indefinitely. Unresolved issues include candidate selection and long-term benefit.

CARDIAC TRANSPLANTATION

Approximately 2300 heart transplantations are performed each year in the United States. The criteria for listing include:

- Age (generally < 65 years)
- End-stage heart disease refractory to medical or surgical therapy
- Disabling symptoms
- Anticipated poor survival

Contraindications include:

- Pulmonary hypertension
- Hepatic or renal failure
- Other serious illnesses that limit longevity or rehabilitation
- Active infection
- Recent pulmonary infarction
- Drug or alcohol abuse
- Medical noncompliance

Following transplantation, the quality of life is good, with 85% of patients active and asymptomatic. Survival rates are as follows:

- 1 month: 91%
- 1 year: 85%
- 5 years: 75%

The limiting factor in transplantation is the lack of donor hearts.

FUTURE TREATMENTS

Treatment of congestive heart failure in the twenty-first century will consist of medications to modulate extracardiac mechanisms of decompensation and newer surgical techniques to assist or replace the failing heart.

REVIEW EXERCISES

QUESTIONS

1. Which of the following is a vasodilator?

   a. Endothelin
   b. Arginine vasopressin
   c. Angiotensin II
   d. B-type natriuretic peptide
   e. Norepinephrine

2. Which of the following statements about digoxin is true?

   a. It is a powerful inotrope.
   b. It has vasodilating properties.
   c. It has a neutral effect on survival.
   d. It stimulates NA^+-K^+ ATPase.
   e. It increases atrioventricular nodal conduction.

3. Which of the following is not a side effect of ACE inhibitors?

   a. Hypokalemia.
   b. Cough.
   c. Agranulocytosis.
   d. Azotemia.
   e. Hypotension.

4. Which of the following statements about short-acting calcium channel blockers in heart failure is false?

   a. They activate neurohormoness.
   b. They elevate blood pressure.
   c. They increase the risk of death.
   d. They depress left-ventricular function.
   e. They worsen symptoms.

5. Which of the following does not cause high-output heart failure?

   a. Anemia.
   b. Pregnancy.
   c. Hypothyroidism.
   d. Arteriovenous fistula.
   e. Paget's disease.

Answers

   1. d

   2. c

   3. a

   4. b

   5. c

SUGGESTED READING

ACC/AHA Task Force Report. Guidelines for the evaluation and management of heart failure. J Am Coll Cardiol 1995; 26:1376–1398.

Armstrong PW, Moe GW. Medical advances in the treatment of congestive heart failure. Circulation 1993;88:2941–2952.

Baker DW, Konstam MA, Bottoroff M, Pitt B. Management of heart failure. Pharmacology treatment. JAMA 1994;272: 1361–1366.

CONSENSUS Trial Study Group. Effects of enalapril on mortality in severe congestive heart failure. N Engl J Med 1987; 316:1429–1435.

Corral CH, Vaughn CC. Intra-aortic balloon counterpulsation: an eleven-year review and analysis of determinants of survival. Tex Heart Inst J 1986;13:39–44.

The Digitalis Investigation Group. The effect of digoxin on mortality and morbidity in patients with heart failure. N Engl J Med 1997;336:525–533.

Dracup K, Baker DW, Dunbar SB, Dacey RA, Brocks NH, Johnson JC, et al. Management of heart failure II. Counseling, education, and lifestyle modifications. JAMA 1994;262: 1442–1446.

Furnary AP, Jessup M, Moreira LFP. Multicenter trial of dynamic cardiomyoplasty for chronic heart failure. J Am Coll Cardiol 1996;28:1175–1180.

Goodfriend TL, Elliott ME, Catt KJ. Angiotensin receptors and their antagonists. N Engl J Med 1996;334:1649–1654.

Hosenpud JD, Novick RJ, Bennett LE, Keck BM, Fiol B, Daily OP. The Registry of the International Society for Heart and Lung Transplantation: Thirteenth Official Report—1996. J Heart Lung Transplant 1996;15:655–674.

Konstam MA, Dracup K, Baker D. Heart failure: evaluation and care of patients with left ventricular systolic dysfunction. Clinical practice guideline no 11. AHCPR 94-0612. Rockville, MD: Agency for Health Care Policy and Research, Public Health Service, US Dept. of Health and Human Services, 1994.

McCarthy PM, Savage RM, Fraser CD, et al. Hemodynamic and physiologic changes during support with an implantable left ventricular assist device. J Thorac Cardiovasc Surg 1995; 109:409–418.

O'Connell JB, Bourge RC, Costanzo-Nordin MR, et al. Cardiac transplantation: recipient selection, donor procurement, and medical followup. Circulation 1992;86:1061–1079.

Packer M. The neurohormonal hypothesis: a theory to explain the mechanism of disease progression in heart failure. J Am Coll Cardiol 1992;20:248–254.

Parmley WW. Pathophysiology and current therapy of congestive heart failure. J Am Coll Cardiol 1989;13:771–785.

Unverferth DV, Magorien RD, Lewis RP, Leier CV. Long-term benefit of dobutamine in patients with congestive cardiomyopathy. Am Heart J 1980;100:622–630.

Whelton A. A symposium: current trends in diuretic therapy. Am J Cardiol 1986;57:1A–53A.

C•H•A•P•T•E•R

70

Board Simulation: Cardiology

Killian Robinson

This simulation and discussion provides some insight into the internal medicine board examination for cardiology. It is only a guide, however, to the questions that commonly are asked and the current areas of emphasis.

Common topics in the board examination include:

- Epidemiology and prevention of coronary artery disease
- Treatment of unstable angina and myocardial infarction
- Treatment of chronic, stable angina pectoris
- Treatment of valvular heart disease
- Treatment of cardiac arrhythmias
- Treatment of myocardial disease
- Treatment of pericardial disease
- Treatment of peripheral vascular disease

In addition, cardiac evaluation of patients before noncardiac surgery, cardiac disorders in pregnancy, infective endocarditis, and rheumatic fever are common topics as well.

REVIEW OF CARDIOLOGY

EPIDEMIOLOGY AND PREVENTION OF CORONARY ARTERY DISEASE

Remember the risk factors: age, sex, smoking, hypercholesterolemia, hypertension, and diabetes. You also might hear about a high homocysteine level, which has received more attention recently as a risk factor for coronary artery disease, stroke, and peripheral vascular disease. Other risk factors include family history, physical inactivity, obesity, and possibly, type A personality traits. In the United States, some 1.5 million patients suffer a myocardial infarction each year, and millions more suffer from angina. Approximately 700,000 coronary deaths occur each year, and of these, 50% die before reaching the hospital. The in-hospital mortality rate of myocardial infarction is between 10 and 15%. The strongest predictor of mortality is left ventricular function, and extent of disease also is important. The mortality rate ranges from 2% per year in those with one-vessel disease to 11% per year in those with three-vessel disease.

Treatment of Elevated Lipid Levels

The Second Report of the National Cholesterol Education Program summarizes the current recommendations. Treatment of high cholesterol (as determined on the basis of low-density lipoprotein [LDL] values) is aimed at reducing the LDL level to less than 100 mg/dL in patients with coronary disease. Patients without coronary disease but with two or more risk factors should have LDL values of less than 130 mg/dL; in those with only one risk factor, the level should be less than 160 mg/dL. Results of several large-scale trials have shown the benefit of treatment with lipid-lowering agents.

Secondary Prevention The Scandinavian, or "4S," study was a secondary prevention trial of patients with established cardiovascular disease. More than 4000 patients were randomized to receive either lipid-lowering therapy or placebo for an average of more than 5 years. The results showed a highly significant 30% reduction in the total mortality rate and a 42% reduction in the coronary mortality rate among the treated group. There was also a 37% reduction in revascularization procedures and a 34% reduction in hospital days. In this study, the 3-hydroxy-3-methylglutaryl coenzyme A (HMG-CoA) reductase inhibitor simvastatin was the investigational drug. Subsequently, the Cholesterol and Recurrent Events (CARE) study examined the effects of LDL-lowering treatment in patients with coronary artery disease and average LDL concentrations. Results of this study also demonstrated a benefit associated with lipid-lowering therapy using pravastatin. Recently, the Post-CABG Study found a benefit in the use of treatment with HMG-CoA reductase inhibitors as well. In that study, 1351 patients who had undergone coronary artery bypass graft surgery were treated with lovastatin and followed for a mean of approximately 4 years. Aggressive lowering of the LDL cholesterol level to less than 100 mg/dL reduced the progression of graft atherosclerosis. These medications are remarkable for their efficacy from drug to drug and for the relative speed with which their clinical effects become evident.

Primary Prevention   Primary prevention studies are those involving patients in whom coronary disease or other forms of atherosclerosis have not yet manifested clinically. One such study, the West of Scotland Coronary Prevention Study (WOSCOPS) demonstrated that use of another HMG-CoA reductase inhibitor (i.e., pravastatin) was associated with a reduced incidence of coronary artery disease during the treatment period. In the light of these studies, use of lipid-lowering agents likely will become more widespread.

Treatment of Unstable Angina

General measures for the treatment of angina include bed rest, pain relief, and so on. Thrombolytic agents are not used for unstable angina, because no clinical benefit has been established for their use. Bed rest, heparin, aspirin, β-adrenergic blocking agents, and nitrates are the treatments of choice for the acute episode of unstable angina. For patients in whom aspirin is unsuitable, ticlopidine may be used.

Administration of nitrates improves oxygen delivery by improving the collateral flow, and nitrates also reduce myocardial oxygen consumption, probably by a mixture of decreased preload as well as afterload. β-Adrenergic blocking agents reduce myocardial oxygen consumption by lowering blood pressure and slowing the heart rate. Calcium channel blockers may be useful as well through mechanisms similar to those of nitrates.

Coronary angioplasty may be useful in selected patients, but the associated risks are greater in patients with unstable than in stable angina. Surgery can be performed if medical therapy fails.

MYOCARDIAL INFARCTION

No details regarding how to diagnose myocardial infarction should be needed here. Right ventricular infarction, which is a common question on the board examination, is diagnosed on the basis of pain, electrocardiographic (ECG) changes, and enzyme rise. Remember to suspect right ventricular infarction if the jugular venous pressure is elevated, to record the right precordial leads on the ECG (V_{4R}), and to bear in mind these patients may need extra fluid to keep their filling pressures high enough.

Treatment includes analgesia, oxygen, bed rest, and sedation (if necessary). The cornerstone of modern therapy for the acute phase of myocardial infarction is thrombolysis. Streptokinase, which is less effective than tissue-type plasminogen activator (t-PA), usually is administered intravenously as 1.5 million U over 30 minutes. Streptokinase still is far cheaper than t-PA, but it is immunogenic. Thrombolytic therapy should be administered to patients with ST-segment elevation of greater than 0.1 mV in two or more contiguous leads, especially if the time to therapy is 12 hours or less and the patient is younger than 75 years. Such therapy also should be given to patients with left bundle-branch block that obscures ST-segment analysis, but in whom the patient history is suggestive of acute myocardial infarction. Thrombolytic therapy is more controversial in patients older than 75 years, if time to therapy is longer than 12 hours, or if blood pressure is more than 180 mm Hg systolic or 110 mg Hg diastolic. Primary percutaneous coronary angioplasty can be recommended in patients with acute myocardial infarction if it is performed by skilled individuals (i.e., those who perform >75/year) in high-volume centers (i.e., >200 procedures/year).

Myocardial infarction without ST-segment elevation or with nondiagnostic ECG changes is more common in elderly patients and in those with a history of myocardial infarction. This syndrome may relate to disruption of atherosclerotic plaque, and total coronary occlusion is less common in patients without than in patients with ST-segment elevation. Because of nondiagnostic ECGs at presentation, it may be indistinguishable clinically from unstable angina. The mortality rate may rise among those patients given thrombolytic agents, and the available data do not support thrombolysis in patients with ischemic chest discomfort and nondiagnostic ECGs.

The benefits of thrombolysis are offset by the complications of bleeding, and questions relating to this are common on the board examination. Contraindications to streptokinase include a history of active bleeding, peptic ulcers, puncture of noncompressible vessels, severe and uncontrolled hypertension, and history of major trauma or surgery within the last 2 months. Relative contraindications include old age, prolonged cardiopulmonary resuscitation, impaired hemostasis, and remote history of peptic ulcers. Adjunctive treatment includes use of heparin, which reduces complications from venous thromboembolism and also, possibly, systemic thromboembolism, and aspirin. Following myocardial infarction, β-adrenergic receptor blockers also are of use (i.e., early use may limit infarct size, long-term therapy reduces long-term mortality), as are angiotensin-converting enzyme (ACE) inhibitors (i.e., for at least 6 weeks) and nitrates as required.

VALVULAR HEART DISEASE

Board questions in internal medicine concerning valvular heart disease often relate to physical findings or laboratory investigations. Thus, a typical scenario is a patient history with physical findings and an ECG, chest radiograph, and so on. These may be mixed in groups; for example, the task may be to match physical findings with the ECG or chest radiograph in question. The following sections summarize the essentials of the major valvular and congenital diseases.

Aortic Stenosis

Symptoms of aortic stenosis include angina, syncope, and shortness of breath. Signs are a slow-rising carotid upstroke; left ventricular hypertrophy; soft second heart sound, which also may be paradoxical, becoming single on inspiration; fourth heart sound; and a harsh ejection systolic murmur radiating to both carotid arteries.

Investigations include ECG for left ventricular hypertrophy, and chest radiography may show a dilated aortic root and prominent left ventricle. The best tests are echocardiography and cardiac catheterization, which also should be undertaken to elucidate coronary anatomy in those patients with angina and older patients undergoing valve replacement.

Aortic Regurgitation

Symptoms of aortic regurgitation include shortness of breath and palpitation. Angina and syncope are not typical. Signs include a collapsing arterial pulse, which is classic, and many others that reflect the wide pulse pressure. The apex of the heart is displaced. The second heart sound may be reduced, especially with coexisting aortic stenosis, and a third heart sound is common. A typical murmur of aortic regurgitation is early diastolic (i.e., begins with the second heart sound, is high pitched, and becomes longer with increasing severity of the disorder). Investigations include ECG for left ventricular hypertrophy, and chest radiography may show a dilated aortic root and enlargement of the left ventricle. The best test is echocardiography, which may show left ventricular enlargement; color-flow Doppler will demonstrate aortic regurgitation. Cardiac catheterization is unnecessary unless complex abnormalities or coronary artery disease are suspected.

Remember that ankylosing spondylitis is associated with aortic incompetence. Tall, thin patients with skeletal abnormalities and a high arched palate may have Marfan's syndrome (autosomal dominant) which is associated with aortic dissection and acute aortic regurgitation.

Mitral Stenosis

Symptoms of mitral stenosis include dyspnea, hemoptysis, and eventually, fatigue and edema. The arterial pulse usually is normal unless atrial fibrillation is present, and the apex of the ventricle classically has a tapping impulse. A right ventricular heave often is present in those with pulmonary hypertension.

Auscultatory findings of mitral stenosis frequently are asked on the board examination. The first sound is loud, the second may be either normal or loud (with the latter in pulmonary hypertension), and diastole is marked by an opening snap. The murmur of mitral stenosis typically is heard at the

apex, preferably with the patient in the left lateral decubitus position. Like third and fourth heart sounds, the murmur is of low pitch. Auscultation is best performed with the bell of the stethoscope. (Other causes of diastolic rumbles include tricuspid stenosis, increased flow across the atrioventricular valves, mitral and tricuspid regurgitation, and atrial septal defect in which the shunt may cause increased tricuspid flow.) If sinus rhythm is still present, the first heart sound is immediately preceded by presystolic accentuation of the diastolic murmur.

An ECG showing left atrial enlargement combined with right ventricular hypertrophy should alert you to this disorder. Atrial fibrillation also is common in patients with mitral stenosis, and especially so in elderly patients. On chest radiography, enlargement of the left atrium, a small left ventricle, and enlargement of the pulmonary artery may give rise to a "straight left heart border." Echocardiography confirms the diagnosis and accurately estimates the valve area. Cardiac catheterization is not necessary unless surgery is being considered in patients who are older or have complex lesions (e.g., multiple valve abnormalities, coexisting congenital heart disease, coronary artery disease).

Mitral Regurgitation

Symptoms of mitral regurgitation include dyspnea and palpitation. The arterial pulse usually is normal, and the left ventricle is enlarged and hyperdynamic. The first heart sound may be soft, and there usually is a third heart sound, reflecting rapid left ventricular filling. The holosystolic murmur of mitral regurgitation is best heard at the apex of the heart with the diaphragm of the stethoscope.

The ECG shows left atrial enlargement, left ventricular hypertrophy, and possibly, atrial fibrillation. Chest radiography shows a large left atrium and left ventricle. The best test is echocardiography, which will confirm and quantitate regurgitant flow into the left atrium. Cardiac catheterization is unnecessary unless complex abnormalities or coronary artery disease are suspected.

CONGENITAL HEART DISEASE

Congenital abnormalities commonly questioned in the board examination include atrial and ventricular septal defect, pulmonary stenosis, coarctation of the aorta, bicuspid aortic valve, and mitral valve prolapse.

Atrial Septal Defect

The key characteristics of atrial septal defect are presentation at a young age at diagnosis, an asymptomatic murmur found at physical examination, and occasionally shortness of breath. Fixed splitting of the second heart sound is the classic finding. The ejection systolic murmur is best heard in the pulmonary area and increases on inspiration.

The ECG shows partial right bundle-branch block with right-axis deviation. These are the typical features of a secundum atrial septal defect. The ECG of the primum atrial septal defect differs in that left-axis deviation accompanies the right bundle-branch block pattern. Chest radiography shows the features of a shunt: cardiac enlargement and increased pulmonary blood flow. The diagnosis is made on the basis of echocardiography.

Ventricular Septal Defect

The typical ventricular septal defect involves patients who are young and asymptomatic (murmurs often are detected at routine physical examination) or who may be short of breath. The classic physical finding is a harsh holosystolic murmur, which is best heard at the lower left sternal border. These ventricular septal defects usually are small, but they create quite a lot of turbulence. Therefore, the murmur usually is loud and, often, accompanied by a thrill.

Nothing particularly characteristic is revealed on the ECG. Chest radiography usually is normal in patients with a small ventricular septal defect.

Pulmonary Stenosis

Often, pulmonary stenosis has no symptoms. The condition is found at a young age as an asymptomatic physical finding. The ejection systolic murmur increases on inspiration and is best heard in the pulmonary area (i.e., upper left sternal border). This is accompanied by a click, which is unusual as it is diminished by inspiration. (Right-sided cardiac events usually increase with inspiration).

The ECG may show right ventricular hypertrophy (i.e., prominent S waves in lead I and V_6 and increased R/S ratio in lead V_1). Chest radiography shows a prominent pulmonary artery. The diagnosis can be made on the basis of echocardiography, but it may be more difficult to obtain clear pictures in these patients than in those with left-sided valvular lesions. If there is any doubt, cardiac catheterization will confirm the diagnosis.

Coarctation of the Aorta

The classic manifestations of coarctation of the aorta include a patient who is asymptomatic or short of breath. Hypertension is a common presenting abnormality as well. On the board examination, if a question mentions differential hypertension in the arms with lower blood pressure in the legs, or even mentions hypertension in a young person, think of coarctation of the aorta. Other typical physical findings are radiofemoral delay and an ejection systolic murmur that usually is accompanied by a normal second sound. Pure coarctation is not accompanied by a click; however, bicuspid aortic valves commonly are associated with coarctations and may cause an ejection click. Together with the coarctation murmur, this may mimic valvular aortic stenosis.

The ECG may show left ventricular hypertrophy. Chest radiography typically shows notching on the undersurface of the ribs because of increased collateral blood flow through the intercostal arteries that overcomes the aortic obstruction.

As with all the previous cases, the patient history and physical findings of this disorder may accompany a chest radiograph on the board examination, and you may be asked to make the appropriate matches. Also, remember that Turner's syndrome (i.e., gonadal dysgenesis [45X or 46XX/45X] characterized by short stature, webbed neck, shield chest, and short fourth metacarpal) may include coarctation of the aorta.

Bicuspid Aortic Valve

Patients with a bicuspid aortic valve, which is a common abnormality, usually are asymptomatic. It may cause a systolic ejection click and systolic ejection murmur in the aortic area. Remember the common association of this abnormality with coarctation, and that both together may suggest valvular aortic stenosis.

The ECG and chest radiography are normal. The diagnosis is made on the basis of echocardiography. The importance of this abnormality is that it may cause diagnostic confusion and may predispose a patient to more severe aortic valve disease (i.e., aortic stenosis, aortic regurgitation, or both) and endocarditis in the long term.

Remember that bicuspid aortic valves also are associated with Turner's syndrome.

Mitral Valve Prolapse

Mitral valve prolapse is more common in women and in those with connective tissue disorders (e.g., Marfan's syndrome). Many patients are asymptomatic, but some may have symptoms of mitral regurgitation. Physical examination will show one (or more) ejection clicks accompanied by a late systolic murmur.

The ECG is normal. Chest radiography is normal as well. An echocardiogram allows the diagnosis to be made and any associated mitral regurgitation to be quantitated. This is important, because both atrial and ventricular arrhythmias are common and complications include mitral regurgitation. This can be dramatic in onset when resulting from another complication: rupture of chordae. Remember the important risk of infective endocarditis, as well as the risk (albeit rare) of sudden death in those with significant mitral regurgitation and ventricular tachyarrhythmias.

Patent Ductus Arteriosus

Often, patients with patent ductus arteriosus exhibit no symptoms, and the condition is diagnosed when a murmur is discovered at routine physical examination. Severe symptoms may occur in patients with Eisenmenger's syndrome (i.e., cyanosis and reversed [right to left] shunt), which also may occur with a ventricular septal defect. There may be right ventricular hypertrophy if there is pulmonary hypertension; however, usually the only abnormality is a continuous or "machinery" murmur. This murmur is heard in both systole and diastole, as are murmurs of mixed aortic valve disease (i.e., aortic stenosis with regurgitation), coronary arteriovenous fistulas, ruptured sinus of Valsalva, and pericardial rubs.

The ECG may show left ventricular hypertrophy, or even right ventricular hypertrophy if pulmonary hypertension is present. Chest radiography shows enlargement of the heart and increased pulmonary vascular markings. The diagnosis can be made on the basis of echocardiography and cardiac catheterization.

ELECTROCARDIOGRAPHY AND ARRHYTHMIAS

Electrocardiograms frequently are included in the board examination, and they often are coupled with clinical histories that are characteristic. They may be used to test knowledge of an ECG in the overall diagnosis or treatment of a patient. You should know the patterns of acute myocardial infarction; right and left ventricular hypertrophy, right and left bundle-branch block; and first-, second-, and third-degree atrioventricular nodal block (especially type I, or Wenckebach, second-degree atrioventricular block).

Common questions have included Wolff-Parkinson-White syndrome; left ventricular hypertrophy, often coupled with a suggestive patient history (e.g., systemic hypertension, aortic valve disease, coarctation); right ventricular hypertrophy (i.e., pulmonary stenosis), which, when occurring with left atrial enlargement, should suggest mitral stenosis with pulmonary hypertension; right bundle-branch block and right-axis deviation (i.e., secundum atrial septal defect); peaked (>10 mm) T waves (i.e., hyperkalemia, hyperacute infarct, central nervous system lesions, or normal). Prolongation of the QT interval is seen in some hereditary disorders (with deafness), and also in patients with hypocalcemia and in those receiving class I antiarrhythmic drugs or amiodarone.

Another common question involves profound bradycardia, which, if symptomatic, should be treated by a pacemaker. Paroxysmal atrial tachycardia with block is characteristic of digitalis toxicity.

A common topic is differential diagnosis of regular, wide QRS complex tachycardia, which can be ventricular or supraventricular. Inappropriate treatment of wide complex tachycardia with verapamil may produce profound hypotension,

and even death, in patients with poor left ventricular function. The board question may state that the patient has ischemic heart disease, which in itself makes the diagnosis of ventricular tachycardia much more likely, and it may offer you a choice between cardioversion and verapamil. In the case of any therapeutic doubt, select cardioversion. Table 70.1 shows some of the differences between supraventricular tachycardia with aberration and ventricular tachycardia. There are many more differences, but even when everything on a particular tracing is taken into account, it still might be difficult to distinguish between these two arrhythmias. In this gray area, you may be asked to choose between a potentially dangerous treatment and a safer option.

Atrial fibrillation can result from many underlying cardiovascular disorders, with coronary artery disease, hypertension, and rheumatic heart disease being the most common. Other important underlying disorders include hyperthyroidism, alcohol and lung disease, and "lone atrial fibrillation," in which the cause is obscure. Standard treatment for atrial fibrillation remains digoxin, which controls the ventricular response. Other medications may have the disadvantage of negative inotropy (e.g., calcium channel blockers, beta blockers) or a short duration of action (e.g., adenosine).

Some patients, especially those with an increased risk of thromboembolism, require anticoagulation. These include older patients and those with rheumatic heart disease, left atrial enlargement, left ventricular dysfunction, or hypertension and a history of previous vascular episodes.

PERICARDIAL DISEASE

Pericarditis

Acute pericarditis is a common topic in the board examination, which often presents with a typical history: chest pain usually is central and often sharp, is aggravated by inspiration, and is relieved by sitting. Physical examination shows a triphasic pericardial friction rub with a scratching quality. Occasionally this may be confined to systole alone, in which case it can be mistaken for a murmur. The ECG shows generalized ST-segment elevation. Other causes of ST-segment elevation include myocardial infarction (ST-segment elevation is regional, thus suggesting a problem with localized arterial supply), ventricular aneurysm (chronically present after MI;

Table 70.1. Diagnosis of Wide (≥ 120 ms) QRS Complex Tachycardia

	Supraventricular Tachycardia	Ventricular Tachycardia
Prior cardiac history	Usually none	Often (myocardial infarction or cardiomyopathy)
QRS > 140 ms	Rare	Common
If QRS morphology in V_1 resembles right bundle-branch block	Right "rabbit ears" > left "rabbit ears"	Monophasic R wave, biphasic qR, QR

this history will probably be given on the board examination), and Prinzmetal angina (caused by coronary spasm; pain at rest, at night, or both; often occurs in women; normal coronary arteries at angiography). With pericarditis, echocardiography may show an effusion.

Cardiac Tamponade

Common questions regarding cardiac tamponade generally feature a patient in shock, with low arterial and high venous pressures. There may be a prominent x descent and an absent y descent in the venous pulse, with varying degrees of hypotension and pulsus paradoxus. The ECG may show low voltage or electrical alternans (i.e., alternatively large and small QRS complexes). The diagnosis is established on the basis of echocardiography, which shows pericardial effusion and, perhaps, collapse of the right atrium as well as diastolic collapse of the right ventricle. At catheterization, right atrial, right ventricular diastolic, pulmonary artery diastolic, and wedge pressures typically are almost the same. Emergent treatment is by pericardiocentesis, which may be performed using echocardiography or under fluoroscopy.

Constrictive Pericarditis

Constrictive pericarditis is another common topic on the board examination, and it may be combined with cardiac tamponade, such as in a question comparing the two disorders (Table 70.2). Constrictive pericarditis is a chronic condition and may be caused by a host of pathologic processes, including connective tissue disorders, neoplastic and infectious diseases (especially tuberculosis), irradiation, and surgery. Essential features

Table 70.2. Comparison of Cardiac Tamponade and Constrictive Pericarditis

	Cardiac Tamponade:	Constrictive Pericarditis:
Clinical onset:	Usually Acute?	Chronic?
Elevated jugular venous pressure	Yes	Yes
Kussmaul's sign	No	Yes
Pulsus paradoxus	Yes	No
Heart sounds	Soft	Diastolic knock
Edema	No	Yes
Cardiomegaly	Often	No
Electrical alternans	Yes	No
Echocardiographic effusion	Yes	No
Catheterization:		
Equal diastolic pressures	Yes	Yes
"Dip and plateau"	No	Yes

are an elevated jugular venous pressure, which may rise further with inspiration (Kussmaul's sign). There often are chronic symptoms suggesting right-sided heart failure, weight gain, edema, and ascites. Auscultating the heart reveals the "pericardial knock," which is a filling sound associated with sudden arrest of the expanding ventricles in diastole. The ECG may show low voltage, and chest radiography may be normal. A normal chest radiograph with right heart failure is suggestive of constrictive pericarditis. As with tamponade, right-sided pressures (i.e., right atrium and ventricular diastolic, pulmonary arterial diastolic, and wedge pressures) are equal. There is a prominent y descent that is related to sudden filling of the ventricles (in contrast to tamponade), and there is an early diastolic "dip and plateau."

MYOCARDIAL DISEASES

Dilated Cardiomyopathy

There are multiple causes of dilated cardiomyopathy, including infectious processes, systemic diseases such as connective tissue disorders, drugs, and toxins. Board questions may relate to treatment, which should include digoxin, diuretics, and ACE inhibitors. To date, vasodilators are the only drugs shown to prolong life.

Hypertrophic Cardiomyopathy

Hypertrophic cardiomyopathy is a primary myocardial disease that is characterized by left ventricular hypertrophy without identifiable cause. It often is inherited as an autosomal dominant abnormality, and the ventricle has a typically hypercontractile performance. Obstruction across the outflow tract of the left ventricle also may occur, manifested by systolic anterior motion of the anterior mitral leaflet on echocardiography. The patient history often is of a healthy young person who has had a blackout; other symptoms are shortness of breath, angina, and palpitation. A jerky arterial pulse is characteristic, as is a palpable presystolic thrust at the apex. There is an ejection systolic murmur at the left sternal border not accompanied by a click, because stenosis is subvalvular, and a loud fourth heart sound often is heard. The ECG shows left ventricular hypertrophy and repolarization changes. The diagnosis is made on the basis of echocardiography; cardiac catheterization is not necessary.

Questions on the board examination regarding treatment are likely. Treatment usually involves β-blockade to slow the heart and to allow proper diastolic filling, which is impaired in these patients. Antiarrhythmic treatment may be used in selected patients, as may surgical therapy.

Echocardiography

Echocardiography has become one of the most widely used tools in clinical cardiology. Transesophageal echocardiogra-

Table 70.3. Major Uses of Transthoracic and Transesophageal Echocardiography

Transthoracic + Doppler	Transesophageal
Measurement of chamber sizes, left ventricular function	Intraoperative monitoring of left ventricular function
Assess valve obstruction, regurgitation	Measurement of intracardiac pressures
Detect vegetations, masses, abscesses	Detection of small vegetations
Detect wall motion abnormalities	Detect left atrial thrombi
Detect pericardial fluid	Guide mitral repair valvotomy, commissurotomy
View aortic root/thoracic aorta	Detect aortic dissection

phy is increasingly routine, particularly to hunt for vegetations in patients with suspected endocarditis and to examine the left atrium for clot. In addition, it is used as an adjunctive tool in those patients undergoing repair of the mitral valve or balloon mitral valvotomy. Table 70.3 provides a rough guide to the current major uses of transthoracic and transesophageal echocardiography.

SPECIAL ISSUES

It is important to be familiar with the constellation of side effects from amiodarone: photosensitivity, hyperthyroidism, hypothyroidism, pruritus, corneal deposits, alterations of liver enzymes, pulmonary fibrosis, and skin pigmentation. In addition, there are important drug interactions with digoxin and warfarin; the requirements for both of these drugs will diminish if amiodarone is started. Side effects from other commonly used cardiac drugs also are significant, especially the liver abnormalities and rhabdomyolysis of the HMG-CoA reductase inhibitors. Rhabdomyolysis is important, especially when treatment is combined with cyclosporine, gemfibrozil, or nicotinic acid. Rhabdomyolysis may be severe and cause renal failure in patients receiving the lovastatin-gemfibrozil combination. You also should be familiar with side effects from digoxin: nausea, vomiting, xanthopsia or discolored vi-

sion, almost any arrhythmia, but classically, paroxysmal atrial tachycardia with atrioventricular block. β-Adrenergic blocking agents may cause fatigue, lethargy, impotence, vivid dreams, worsening of claudication, asthma and heart failure, hypotension, and conduction disturbances. ACE inhibitors may cause hypotension, cough, and worsening of renal function. Side effects from class I antiarrhythmic drugs (e.g., quinidine, procainamide) are proarrhythmia and depression of left ventricular function. They may cause polymorphic ventricular tachycardia (i.e., torsades de pointes), and procainamide may cause a lupus-like syndrome.

Rheumatic Fever

Rheumatic fever is a rare disorder, but the criteria for its diagnosis are a common question on the board examination. Remember the major manifestations (i.e., carditis, polyarthritis, chorea, erythema marginatum, and subcutaneous nodules) as well as the minor manifestations (i.e., arthralgia, fever, elevated erythrocyte sedimentation rate, and prolonged PR interval). When supported by evidence of a recent streptococcal infection (i.e., positive throat culture, rising streptococcal antibody titer), a diagnosis of rheumatic fever can be made in patients with two major manifestations or with one major and two minor manifestations.

Infective Endocarditis

Patients at an increased or high risk for infective endocarditis are those with valvular heart disease, including rheumatic valvular heart disease, bioprosthetic and mechanical valves or those with congenital heart disease, especially ventricular septal defect. Other important lesions include mitral valve prolapse and bicuspid aortic valves, which commonly are complicated by infective endocarditis. Patients at low risk of infective endocarditis include those with secundum atrial septal defect. The mainstay of prophylaxis remains amoxicillin for dental procedures, and either erythromycin or clindamycin if patients are allergic to penicillin. High-risk patients unable to take penicillins should be given vancomycin, which should be coupled with gentamicin for prophylaxis before gastrointestinal or genitourinary procedures. Signs of infective endocarditis are fever, clubbing, splinter hemorrhages, anemia, heart failure, changing murmurs, peripheral emboli, renal failure, and valve rupture. The diagnosis is made on the basis of blood culture, and transesophageal echocardiography has an increased role in detecting vegetations.

QUESTIONS

The following sample questions cover some, but not all, of the compressed review in this chapter. In addition, these questions introduce you to the format of some board examination questions.

1. The usual features of mitral stenosis include which of the following?

   a. Loud first heart sound.
   b. Mid-diastolic rumble.
   c. Opening snap.
   d. All of the above.

2. A 17-year-old basketball player has light-headedness and dizziness on exercise. He has a jerky carotid upstroke, a double apical impulse, and an ejection systolic murmur at the apex and along the left sternal border that diminishes on squatting and increases on standing. The most likely diagnosis is:

   a. Atrial septal defect.
   b. Wolff-Parkinson-White syndrome.
   c. Hypertrophic cardiomyopathy.
   d. Tricuspid regurgitation.

3. A 26-year-old lawyer is admitted to the hospital with chest pain, and a diagnosis of myocardial infarction is made. There are no risk factors for coronary disease. The differential diagnosis should include:

   a. Possible drug abuse.
   b. Anomalies of the coronary arteries.
   c. Coronary embolus.
   d. All of the above.

4. A 59-year-old golfer is referred for evaluation of a dizzy spell. Physical examination shows a slow-rising pulse with a narrow pulse pressure. Auscultation reveals a normal first heart sound and an absent second heart sound. There is no ejection click. The late-peaking ejection systolic murmur radiates to the carotid arteries. Given these findings, the likely diagnosis is:

   a. Lung cancer.
   b. Hypertrophic cardiomyopathy.
   c. Calcific valvar aortic stenosis.
   d. Subvalvar aortic stenosis resulting from a "membranous shelf."

5. Current goals for LDL cholesterol in patients with known coronary artery disease are:

   a. Less than 200 mg/dL.
   b. Less than 180 mg/dL.
   c. Less than 140 mg/dL.
   d. Less than 100 mg/dL.

6. A 28-year-old woman develops squeezing anterior chest pain on exercise relieved by rest. The resting ECG is normal, but a stress ECG reveals a 3-mm, flat ST-segment depression that resolves during the recovery phase. The next step is:

   a. No further investigation.
   b. Coronary angiography.
   c. Advise her to buy a dog and go jogging.
   d. Exercise thallium scan.
   e. Exercise echocardiography.

7. A 20-year-old woman is referred for evaluation of hypertension. Her history and physical examination are normal except for a soft ejection systolic murmur. In your evaluation, you should pay particular attention to which of the following?

   a. History of dizziness, sweating, and palpitation.
   b. Urinary β-HCG.
   c. Radiofemoral delay.
   d. All of the above.
   e. a and c only.

8. A 46-year-old woman with established coronary disease is referred for treatment of hypercholesterolemia. You decide to start her on an HMG-CoA reductase inhibitor. Before starting therapy, you should check which of the following?

   a. Liver function tests.
   b. Barium enema.
   c. Muscle enzymes (creatine kinase).
   d. Thyroid function tests.
   e. a and c only.

9. A 55-year-old patient with a myocardial infarction is found to have 90% stenosis in the left main coronary artery. Optimal treatment for this patient should be:

   a. β-blockade.
   b. Angioplasty.
   c. Coronary artery bypass surgery.
   d. Any of the above.

10. Which of the following drugs should never be coadministered?

   a. Aspirin and heparin.
   b. Amiodarone and digoxin.
   c. Lovastatin and gemfibrozil.
   d. Amiodarone and warfarin.
   e. None of the above.

11. Which of the following features always are seen in patients with valvular aortic stenosis?

    a. Ejection systolic murmur.
    b. Ejection click.
    c. Coexisting aortic incompetence.
    d. Syncope.
    e. None of the above.

12. None of the following commonly is seen with coarctation of the aorta except:

    a. Radiofemoral delay.
    b. Early diastolic murmur.
    c. Elevated jugular venous pressure.
    d. Hypotension.

13. A 21-year-old woman has a murmur detected on routine screening. The blood pressure and pulse are normal, and the jugular venous pulse shows no abnormalities. Auscultation reveals an ejection systolic murmur heard at the left sternal border, wide and fixed splitting of the second heart sound, and a low-pitched rumble at the lower sternal border. The likely ECG findings in this patient are:

    a. Left bundle-branch block.
    b. Complete heart block.
    c. Wolff-Parkinson-White syndrome.
    d. Right bundle-branch block with right-axis deviation.
    e. All of the above.

14. Which of the following are associated with reversed splitting of the second heart sound?

    a. Left bundle-branch block.
    b. Right bundle-branch block.
    c. Right ventricular pacemaker.
    d. a and c.
    e. None of the above.

15. A 16-year-old girl presents with central chest pain that is relieved by sitting forward and worsened on breathing. Auscultation reveals a scratchy sound in both systole and diastole. The patient had a fractured femur as a child, her brother recently underwent surgery for repair of an atrial septal defect, and her mother has hypertension. Appropriate therapy for this patient would be:

    a. Streptokinase.
    b. APSAC.
    c. Heart transplantation.
    d. Nonsteroidal anti-inflammatory agents.
    e. All of the above.

16. A 21-year-old black male has recently returned from vacation in Florida, during which he suffered a severe bout of pharyngitis. He now presents with a 1-week history of pain in the ankle and small joints of his hands. Examination reveals a temperature of 99.2°F but no evidence of arthritis. A soft murmur of mitral regurgitation is heard at the apex. The ECG shows a sinus tachycardia of 105 beats per minute.

    Which of the following statements are false?

    a. Rheumatic fever is a highly likely diagnosis.
    b. The absence of a rising streptococcal antibody titer makes rheumatic fever highly unlikely.
    c. All the signs and symptoms can be explained entirely by another illness.
    d. An increased PR interval will clinch the diagnosis of rheumatic fever.

17. A 69-year-old woman presents to the emergency room with a history of weakness and dizziness of several hours' duration. She has a long history of hypertension and hyperlipidemia, and there is a remote history of myocardial infarction many years ago. Since then, she has been well. Her blood pressure measures 90/60 mm Hg, and her ECG is shown in Figure 70.1.

    Which of the following statements are true?

    a. A history of myocardial infarction in a patient with a wide complex tachycardia increases the likelihood of a ventricular origin.
    b. Any of the following increase the likelihood of ventricular tachycardia: atrioventricular dissociation, hypotension, a QRS >120 milliseconds.
    c. Satisfactory treatment options for this patient include verapamil and quinidine, digoxin, and cardioversion.

18. A 22-year-old man is referred because of a murmur detected on routine physical examination. He is asymptomatic. Physical examination reveals a harsh holosystolic murmur that is best heard at the lower left sternal border and is accompanied by a thrill. The ECG is normal, as is the chest radiograph.

    Which of these statements are true?

    a. This patient almost certainly has a small ventricular septal defect.
    b. Cardiac catheterization should be performed, because the thrill indicates the possibility of an atrial septal defect with a large shunt.
    c. Because the long-term prognosis of these patients is good, antibiotic prophylaxis against endocarditis no is longer thought to be necessary.
    d. a and b.
    e. a and c.

19. A 60-year-old man is on vacation near your office in Florida. He attends because of a history of palpitation of recent onset. There are no other cardiac symptoms, and he otherwise is well.

    Which of the following statements are true?

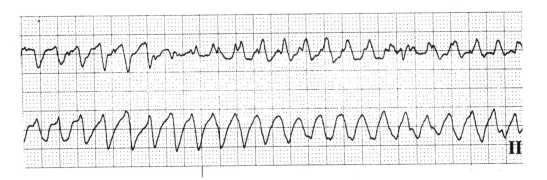

Figure 70.1.   ECG for the patient in question 17.

a. Excessive alcohol intake may be responsible.

b. The absence of weight loss, goiter, and tremor virtually excludes the diagnosis of thyrotoxicosis in this patient.

c. He should undergo electrophysiologic study, because he is at risk of sudden death.

d. Excessive tea and coffee intake rarely cause symptoms such as these.

e. These symptoms almost certainly are caused by too much sun exposure.

20. A 50-year-old businessman attends your office for a routine physical examination. He has no cardiac symptoms, takes no physical exercise, and has frequent liquid lunches. His 86-year-old mother has angina, and his father died of cancer. He is not a diabetic and has no history of hypertension. He is very overweight. The fasting lipid profile is: total cholesterol, 232 mg/dL; LDL cholesterol, 151 mg/dL; high-density lipoprotein cholesterol, 29 mg/dL; triglycerides, 258 mg/dL.

    Which of the following statements are false?

a. A history of ischemic heart disease in this patient would substantially alter your approach to his treatment.

b. Abstention from alcohol may substantially improve, and even normalize, his lipid profile.

c. The workup of this patient should include blood sugar and thyroid function tests.

d. Treatment of this patient should begin with an HMG-CoA reductase inhibitor alone, because these drugs have important side effects when combined with other treatments.

21. A 23-year-old woman has a history of intrathoracic malignancy, for which she received irradiation therapy. She now presents with swelling of the abdomen and of the ankles of several months' duration. You consider the diagnosis of constrictive pericarditis.

    Which of the following statements are true?

a. You may expect to find an elevated jugular venous pulse (with possible further rise on inspiration) together with a loud diastolic filling sound.

b. Cardiomegaly and echocardiographic investigations that pericardial fluid will be typical of this condition.

c. Pericardiocentesis can be expected to produce slow resolution of the peripheral edema.

d. All of the above.

22. An 85-year-old man who is recuperating from surgical amputation of the left lower limb has impaired kidney function, an active chest infection, and deranged electrolytes. You are consulted because of an irregular, narrow-complex tachycardia. Which ECG diagnosis is likely?

a. Sinus tachycardia.

b. Atrial flutter with 2:1 block.

c. Ventricular tachycardia.

d. Multifocal atrial tachycardia.

e. Atrial fibrillation with Wolff-Parkinson-White syndrome.

23. A 19-year-old man with a history of Ebstein's anomaly collapses on the street. At his arrival in the emergency room, an irregular, wide-complex tachycardia is seen on the monitor. Which ECG diagnosis is likely?

a. Sinus tachycardia.

b. Atrial flutter with 2:1 block.

c. Ventricular tachycardia.

d. Multifocal atrial tachycardia.

e. Atrial fibrillation with Wolff-Parkinson-White syndrome.

24. A forgetful 63-year-old woman is started on quinidine for atrial fibrillation and subsequently has a blackout. Which ECG diagnosis is likely?

a. Sinus tachycardia.

b. Atrial flutter with 2:1 block.

c. Ventricular tachycardia.

d. Multifocal atrial tachycardia.

e. Atrial fibrillation with Wolff-Parkinson-White syndrome.

Answers

1. d
2. c
3. d
4. c
5. d
6. b
7. d
8. e
9. c
10. e
11. e
12. a

13. d
14. d
15. d
16. d
17. a
18. a
19. a
20. d
21. a
22. d
23. e
24. c

SUGGESTED READINGS

Second Report of the National Cholesterol Education Program. JAMA 1993;269:3015.

Anonymous. Randomised trial of cholesterol lowering in 4444 patients with coronary heart disease: the Scandinavian Simvastatin Survival Study (4S). Lancet 1994;344(8934):1383–1389.

Sacks FM, Pfeffer MA, Moye LA, et al. The effect of pravastatin on coronary events after myocardial infarction in patients with average cholesterol levels. Cholesterol and Recurrent Events Trial investigators. N Engl J Med 1996;335(14):1001–1009.

Anonymous. The effect of aggressive lowering of low-density lipoprotein cholesterol levels and low-dose anticoagulation on obstructive changes in saphenous-vein coronary-artery bypass grafts. The Post Coronary Artery Bypass Graft Trial Investigators. N Engl J Med 1997;336(3):153–62.

Shepherd J, Cobbe SM, Ford I, et al. Prevention of coronary heart disease with pravastatin in men with hypercholesterolemia. West of Scotland Coronary Prevention Study Group. N Engl J Med 1995;333(20):1301–1307.

S•E•C•T•I•O•N

X

After the Boards

71

Medical Ethics in the 21st Century

George A. Kanoti

Medicine is changing in ways that raise serious questions about codes of medical ethics and the traditional medical-ethical-practice guidelines that flow from them. Today, the moral ground on which physicians historically have stood is shifting.

Traditionally, physicians have considered their ethical responsibilities to be rooted in and created by their professional relationship with their patients. This one-on-one relationship has created responsibilities and obligations for both physicians and patients:

- Physicians are required to be loyal to their patients and to use their knowledge and skills to achieve patient welfare: ''Always act for the good of the patient.''
- Patients are to trust their physicians and to follow their advice: ''A physician's orders must be followed.''

The physician/patient relationship is being redefined because of the professional and social changes now occurring in the practice of medicine. Two developments are directing this redefinition:

1. The impact of the consumer and individual-rights movements on the practice of medicine.
2. The intrusion of third parties into the physician/patient relationship.

Patients now seek the best value for their money and insist that physicians respect their rights to select, continue, or discontinue medical therapy. The intrusion of third parties into the patient/physician relationship pressures physicians to justify their diagnostic and therapeutic decisions both economically and managerially. Capitation and other systems of medical reimbursement require physicians to incorporate economic criteria into their diagnostic and therapeutic decisions.

An unfortunate consequence of these changes is that physicians now are seen by patients as representatives of social and economic interests rather than as protectors of patient interests. Because medical-ethical-practice guidelines historically have reflected specific circumstances of patient illnesses, social and institutional policies, and reward systems, the natural question is: Does the changing nature of the physician/patient relationship justify abandoning the traditional medical-ethical-practice guidelines built on trust and loyalty?

This chapter briefly reviews traditional training in codes of medical ethics and ethical practice guidelines, and it examines the adequacy of traditional medical ethics and institutional processes for practice in the twenty-first century. In addition, because internal medicine practitioners continue to face perennial questions in medical ethics questions—such as obligations to provide or limit life-sustaining therapy, physician-assisted suicide, euthanasia, and refusal of medical care—this chapter concludes with a brief analysis of physicians' obligations when participating in the death of their patients.

TRADITIONAL MEDICAL ETHICS TRAINING

Until recently, training in medical-ethical-practice guidelines and the process of medical ethics decision-making has been inadequate. Formal courses in medical and clinical ethics decision-making are relatively new. One unfortunate consequence of this inadequate training has been its contribution to physician stress and burnout. Sources of this stress and burnout are not limited to the pressure of time management, however. The burden of assimilating and applying vast amounts of data; the challenge of effectively communicating diagnoses, therapeutic plans, and treatment strategies; and the politics of medicine all contribute. In addition, a major player in physician stress and burnout is risk management. Lurking behind almost every clinical encounter, physicians find the shadow of real or imagined medicolegal and ethical risks of making decisions that influence a patient's life or quality of life. Too often, physician uncertainty over risk-management questions is exacerbated by minimal opportunities for education in risk management during medical school, residency, and fellowship years. Physicians find themselves ill-prepared for the complexity and uncertainty of medicolegal, and ethical choices.

Most physicians learn medical-ethical-practice guidelines (also known as medical ethical responsibilities and ethical decision-making) by observing senior physicians and then modeling their own behavior on that practice. Fortunately for patients and resident physicians, most senior physicians are responsible as well as experienced practitioners; however, their ethical advice and skills are limited by personal ethical standards and years of unique practice. Imitating the ethical practice of mentor physicians is effective if and when similar circumstances are encountered. As noted, however, physicians today face circumstances differing from those of their mentors as well as a subtle change in the ground rules for ethical medical practice. When physicians are taught ethical principles and algorithms of moral choice in academic and clinical settings, they are better equipped to apply ethical principles to these new challenges.

ROLE OF TRADITIONAL MEDICAL-ETHICAL-PRACTICE GUIDELINES

Historically, physicians have taken the position that internal rather than external constraints on their behavior are more desirable. To that end, codes of medical ethics have been developed to illustrate ethical values, that provide both justification for medical-ethical-practice guidelines and motivation for physicians to practice medicine in an ethical manner. These codes of ethics identify specific practices as either appropriate or inappropriate for clinicians; they also identify virtues that should characterize "ethical" practitioners. Physicians are expected to follow these ethical codes and guidelines and to incorporate such virtues as honesty, compassion, justice, courage, prudence, and temperance into their practice.

Despite codes of medical ethics, the complexity of medical practice creates clinical situations in which disagreement and conflict can occur between patients and physicians. These situations require some form of socially approved or institutionalized arbitration process. In the United States, the sole arbitrator outside of the medical profession, until recently, was the legislative and judicial system. The recent development of the practice of clinical bioethics however, has introduced the clinical bioethicist or the Institutional Ethics Committee as another arbitrator. These new arbitrators, though conscious of the legal precedents and tradition of medical ethics, are dedicated to teaching clinical ethics, assisting physicians to resolve medical ethics cases, and developing ethics policy.

The rejection of any role for codes of medical ethics and traditional ethical practice guidelines in addressing questions

such as those mentioned in this chapter's introduction appeals to some, who believe medicine must be more business-like, with cost-cutting, efficiency, and productivity as the major values. Others reject this argument as unprofessional, and they resist the social and professional pressures to change traditional guidelines, reasserting the importance of traditional medical ethics by mounting extensive physician and patient education programs in medical-ethical-practice guidelines as well as by political and legislative means. Both positions are in error. It is a mistake to regard the ethical wisdom acquired over centuries of medical practice as irrelevant in the new millennium, yet it also is a mistake to merely reassert traditional medical-ethical-practice guidelines without careful analysis and adaptation. The experience of those physicians who preceded today's clinicians has much to say about the practice of medicine in the twenty-first century. The traditional medical-ethical-practice guidelines evolved in different circumstances than exist today, but many of these guidelines provide insights into fundamental realities of medical practice that have not changed over time—and that very probably will not change during the next millennium. A review of the ethical values underlying traditional guidelines—respect for patients (autonomy), do no harm, and justice—may illuminate how physicians practicing internal medicine in the twenty-first century can adjust to changing circumstances without abandoning the ethical tradition that distinguishes them from entrepreneurs.

RESPECT FOR PATIENTS: POWER AND INEQUALITY

The practice of medicine involves power, and the power of physicians is obvious. They undergo rigorous education and training to acquire esoteric (almost priestly) knowledge and skills, and they use a professional language that bars lay persons from the cognoscenti. Physicians also hold the keys to accessing society's health care system. For these and other reasons, physicians possess great power.

This power creates a great imbalance, or inequality, in the physician/patient relationship. By definition, patients are not equal to physicians, and to most patients, medical language is a mystery that puts physicians in a superior position—the informed over the uninformed.

Patients have minuscule power, which is limited to avoiding medical attention, rejecting physicians' advice, nondisclosure of pertinent information, noncompliance with prescribed therapy, and institution of legal action when they perceive they have been wronged. Nonetheless, in practice, most patients' real or perceived symptoms drive them to physicians because they need an explanation of them, counsel on medical and surgical choices, guidance through the health care system, and/or compassionate care.

This imbalance of power also creates circumstances in which abuses of power are possible. Withholding information, giving obtuse and manipulative answers, spreading information to undeserving parties, and outright deception for personal gain are examples of abuses that can occur on both sides of the physician/patient relationship.

RESPECT FOR PATIENTS (AUTONOMY)

The traditional medical-ethical-practice guideline of ''respect your patients'' (also known as autonomy) was designed to respond to the imbalance of power in the physician/patient relationship by reminding physicians they are obligated to respect patients' freedom to make choices that, whether directly or indirectly, affect their health and well-being. In practical matters, physicians confront the autonomy principle whenever they communicate diagnoses and recommend therapy; that is, the obligation to behave respectfully toward patients is present every time physicians inform patients and seek their consent to proceed with therapy. Even though the concept of informed consent originated in the context of medical experimentation after World War II, and it traditionally has been linked with medical research, clinicians have the ethical responsibility to inform patients about their diagnosis, prognosis, and therapies available. The purpose of informed consent is to ensure that patients understand, both intellectually and emotionally, their diagnosis, and that they are willing to accept a therapeutic option that holds the best chance of achieving their personal goals. In turn, physicians reap important information about their patients' perceptions of their diseases and what motivations they bring to encountering their illnesses.

A physician/patient relationship begins with communicating symptoms. Physicians are taught to convey confidence and certainty in their judgments so that patients will trust them. Physicians may (and should) possess an intelligent opinion about the meaning and significance of patients' symptoms, but patients may have only a vague idea—or even no idea at all. Furthermore, patients often simultaneously desire and fear knowing a diagnosis, and in this conflicted state, they may challenge their physician's opinion and advice. When a patient questions a diagnosis or the appropriateness of a suggested therapy, physicians can feel insulted, viewing this as a naive person questioning their professional judgment. This emotional reaction by physicians to patient questioning is understandable, because one of the most tangible hallmarks of a professional is confidence in his or her professional judgment. Any challenge to that judgment can produce strong defensive (or offensive) reactions. Informed consent is the ethical and legal bulwark that protects both the physician and the patient in this situation. To communicate obtuse medical information effectively is one of the most challenging demands of practicing medicine, both today and in the twenty-first century.

Another ethical challenge in respecting patient autonomy in this era of managed care is to incorporate pertinent information about patient desires, wishes, values, end-of-life preferences, and personal goals in the written and oral communications both between and among physicians. These data are

as important as medical histories and diagnostic test results. The responsibility to properly communicate this information grows with managed care, because the structure of managed care reinforces the compartmentalization of medicine into ''efficiency units.'' In some large medical institutions, patients do not feel they have a primary physician, and in these circumstances, a great danger is that important patient-value information will not be obtained, will not be communicated, or will be lost.

Traditionally, physicians have claimed a therapeutic privilege that justifies making an exception to informed consent. This exception, it is claimed, occurs when conveying ''bad news,'' such as the diagnosis of a terminal, inoperable cancer. This exception is motivated by a desire either to avoid the emotional turmoil that can occur when ''bad news'' is conveyed or to soften the blow through ambivalent—or outright misleading—language. Probably every physician has heard during his or her training a description of a patient's suicide or suicidal ideation on being told ''bad news.'' Even if the therapeutic privilege is ethically and legally defensible as an exception to the rule of ''respect for patients,'' it is an exception that proves the rule—that patients should be given the freedom to make decisions about their care by informing them honestly about their diagnosis, treatment options, and prognosis. The traditional principle of ''respect for patients'' has a corollary that requires physicians to gain the skill of preparing patients to receive the analysis of their symptoms, especially when the diagnosis is ''bad news.'' Deception, even for compassionate reasons, is a risky practice both ethically and legally.

Finally, another area in which physicians' actions and attitudes show respect for their patients and enhance their patients' ability to exercise free choice is preparing for ''final'' illnesses. End-of-life choices are perhaps the most infrequently visited topics during physician/patient interviews. Physicians seem to avoid these discussions for a variety of reasons. This is unfortunate, however, because a discussion of patient values, goals, and expectations, as well as of the limits to their acceptance of pharmacologic and technologic medical interventions during an end-of-life illness, can increase the confidence level between physician and patient and provide the physician with valuable information. Physicians can enhance this exchange through two actions:

1. Learn what their particular state's medical advance directive laws (i.e., living wills and durable power-of-attorney for health care decisions) permit their patients.
2. Prepare their own living will or durable power-of-attorney for health care choices.

This process requires physicians to articulate their own goals, expectations, and limits of end-of-life medical care. It also requires physicians to have frank discussions about their own end-of-life wishes with their loved ones, so that their wishes are both known and understood. Patients have an uncanny ability to sense inconsistencies in physicians' language that suggest "Do as I say, not as I do." Discussing medical advance directives with patients without first preparing a personal directive will ring hollow.

DO NO HARM

"Do no harm" is a negative ethical practice guideline. It indicates in general terms what physicians should avoid in the physician/patient relationship rather than what they should achieve. To the best of their abilities, physicians are obligated to reverse disease, return patients to health, or at least reduce or make manageable the debilitating characteristics of disease and illness. This practice guideline originated with the assumption that physicians should not cause physical harm to their patients, but a strong argument exists that this guideline also should include the prevention of psychologic and social harm as well. The interaction between stress and disease is well known, and when a physician's behavior contributes to patient stress by actions such as demeaning posture, patronizing behavior, and violation of confidences, the physician violates this guideline. The complexity of modern life and the interrelationship between public and private lives, however, reduce the strength of the argument that physicians have a direct obligation to produce social and psychologic benefits to their patients. At most, physicians have an obligation to reduce or eliminate those aspects of their practice style that could cause physical, psychologic, or social harm.

This practice guideline should be interpreted more broadly than just focusing on physicians' responsibilities to their patients. It also means that physicians have a responsibility to "do no harm" to themselves. By protecting themselves, physicians contribute positively to the care of their patients. Physicians have ethical responsibilities to care for their own psychic, social, and physical health. Medical training pushes students to the limits of their psychologic, social, physical, and intellectual abilities, but when faced with such psychologic, social, physical, and intellectual overload, physicians are prone to serious errors in judgment and communication. Thus, physicians have an ethical obligation to set limits on the expenditure of their time and energy that allow them to perform at an intellectual and physical level supporting good judgment and patient communication. Practically speaking, the time to learn how to fulfill this obligation begins in the training years, when student physicians' exposure to the rigors of academic and clinical life quickly reveals their personal psychic, social, and intellectual limits. This knowledge of personal limits is important when selecting a professional environment, establishing work and recreation habits, and organizing professional schedules. For example, when seeking a position within health care organizations and negotiating terms of employment, this self-knowledge is critical, because it will set the parameters for whether to accept or reject a position.

As physicians mature in their practice, there also is an obligation to reassess the amount of time needed for physical and intellectual recreation. Physicians may find they are intellectually bored with treating patients having the inevitable seasonal diseases, such as flu and upper-respiratory-tract infections, but that they are intrigued by the patterns of disease they have seen and wish to pursue clinical research in a rigorous manner. This knowledge necessitates changes in both personal and career plans. Self-awareness and continuous reassessment are part of the ethical challenges for physician in the twenty-first century. Accompanying this reassessment is a concurrent obligation to prepare their patients for the reduced time devoted to clinical practice.

FAIRNESS TO ALL: JUSTICE

The final medical-ethical-practice guideline—"be fair to your patients"—indicates that physicians must act justly. The virtue of justice touches on a vital element of medical practice, both today and in the twenty-first century: the economic basis of medicine.

Medicine is big business today, and the future seems to hold more of the same. Traditionally, "be fair to your patients" has been interpreted to mean that physicians are required to walk the line between securing their personal economic future and being unfair or fraudulent in their billing and reimbursement practices. Medicare/Medicaid fraud is an obvious example; however, the fairness guideline extends beyond economic reimbursement. In fact, following the practice guideline of fairness in many respects is more difficult than merely not cheating patients. This guideline requires that physicians present patients with fair and objective information about their diagnoses, prognoses, and therapies. The challenge for physicians is to remove any presumptive value judgments about patients because of age, gender, race, social standing, national origin, religion, behavior patterns or other discriminating characteristics. When presenting therapeutic options for a patient's decision, for example, this value challenges physicians to identify their own presumptions concerning the moral standing of persons "of color," "of heritage," or "of economic or professional standing."

The old adage that "self-knowledge is the beginning of wisdom" is appropriate here. The moral challenge to physicians is not to change their personalities, but to act beyond and above their prejudgments about the value of persons. The hazard of acting in this manner is that it may produce a "moral schizophrenia," in which physicians act fairly to all patients but feel repugnance, anger, or hatred when treating certain patients because of racial, religious, or other prejudgments. A solution to this conflict is to understand personal prejudices and attempt to overcome them, or to create a referral base of physicians who will accept patients who precipitate emotional or moral conflicts. In the twenty-first century, these differences will not cease. In fact, our shrinking globe will actually increase the possibility that physicians will care for patients who are different culturally, morally, and religiously. The intimate nature of the physician/patient relationship places both parties in an environment where their private and personal lives, beliefs, and prejudices may surface, and the interaction between physicians and patients may produce negative or self-serving responses from both. This practice guideline reminds physicians to question whether the diagnostic choices, therapeutic options, and extended care choices are presented fairly or are skewed by a positive or negative perception of a given patient.

This practice guideline may produce ethical dilemmas for physicians practicing in managed care environments. Physicians may find themselves, or others, questioning the appropriateness of diagnostic or therapeutic decisions that will strain or exceed the economic parameters for that fiscal year, or they may find that the most appropriate therapy is not covered by patient's health care plan.

Recent economic changes have forced physicians to descend from the airy, economically sterile examining room to the stuffy, economically unsanitary board room where economic and fiscal-policy decisions are made. In many ways, this descent into the world of business and economics is good, because it requires physicians to be conscious of and responsible for the economic consequences of their decisions. Nonetheless, for many physicians, this is a ''descent into hell,'' because incorporating economic concerns into medical practice is foreign to their training and dedication. Furthermore, physicians may find themselves forced to make choices that go contrary to their best medical judgment for the patient or against institutional or social policy, thus jeopardizing their own careers and livelihood.

The new millennium brings the challenge for U.S. physicians of incorporating social rights as well as individual patient rights into their clinical algorithms. It also challenges physicians to participate in the development of local institutional economic guidelines and social policy. These physicians will bring to the negotiating table both the needs of patients and the clinical realities, which should inform fiscal policies.

PERENNIAL ETHICAL DILEMMAS

In the twenty-first century, internal medicine physicians will continue to face the classic ethical questions in their practice. These ethical dilemmas and questions concern special aspects of the physician/patient and the physician/institutional relationship, such as life and death, disclosure of information, confidentiality, and physician interventions at the beginning or end of life. Perhaps one of the most distressing questions is whether physicians should participate in their patients' deaths—and if so, to what extent.

To gain an ethical perspective on this question, a series of distinctions may be helpful. Physicians can participate in patients' deaths in a variety of ways that are ethically distinctive. Traditionally, the type and degree of physician participation have been described as:

- Withholding or withdrawing life-supporting therapies
- Physician-assisted suicide
- Euthanasia

WITHHOLDING OR WITHDRAWING LIFE-SUPPORT THERAPIES

Withholding or withdrawing life-support therapies describes situations in which physicians either do not begin or discontinue medical treatment necessary to sustain a patient's life. These treatments include ventilators, feeding tubes, cardiopulmonary resuscitation, surgery, antibiotics, blood transfusions, and any other needed therapy. When these situations occur, the ethical practice guidelines direct physicians to follow four basic steps:

1. Determine whether the life-threatening situation is temporary or part of a terminal, end-stage disease. (In some cases, this may require a second opinion.)
2. Determine patient attitudes and beliefs concerning life-sustaining therapies and end-of-life choices, either by direct conversation with the patient or family or by consulting advance directives.
3. Communicate honestly the diagnostic and prognostic information to the patient, if competent, or to the family.
4. Recommend withholding or withdrawing therapy when this is consistent with both the medical prognosis and the patient's values.

In this situation, the medical-ethical-practice guideline is to ''recommend any life-sustaining therapy only when it is consistent with medical prognosis and patient values.'' Occasionally, conflict over withholding or withdrawing therapy can occur between physicians and the patient or family. At these times, a consultation should be initiated by engaging an ethics consultant or ethics committee.

PHYSICIAN-ASSISTED SUICIDE

Physician-assisted suicide describes situations in which physicians decide to provide patients with the means or knowledge to end their own lives. This decision challenges the traditional guideline of ''do no harm,'' because death is considered by many as the ultimate harm that physicians can inflict on patients. Physicians do not directly cause the death of patients by assisting their suicide, but this distinction is not ethically significant.

Currently, there is both ethical and legal disagreement over the appropriateness of physician-assisted suicide. Ethical, legal, and public opinion are moving toward accepting physician-assisted suicide as an ethical practice under certain circumstances. Some counter that ''do no harm'' does not permit physician-assisted suicide. Use of ''do no harm'' to argue against this practice is misleading, however, mainly because ignoring a competent, terminal, end-stage patient's desire to stop the disease process can cause psychic as well as spiritual harm to the patient. Physicians have an obligation to contribute substantially to this public debate over physician-assisted suicide, because they have the necessary medical and clinical experience to craft ethically responsible guidelines.

The question of physician-assisted suicide will not fade away in the twenty-first century.

EUTHANASIA

Euthanasia describes the situation in which physicians directly kill a patient, with or without the patient's permission, for compassionate reasons. This practice is explicitly ruled out in the codes of medical ethics. It is very difficult to find circumstances justifying the direct killing of a patient without their knowledge and permission. Extreme conditions of danger to innocent third parties (e.g., war-time scenarios) or of medical futility may provide justification.

When patients are physically incapable of ending their own lives, direct killing with the patients' permission falls under the rubric of physician-assisted suicide rather than euthanasia. As in debate over physician-assisted suicide, physicians have a responsibility to contribute to the discussion and debate over euthanasia. Nonetheless, as a general practice,

physicians should indicate clearly what their personal and professional opinion is concerning participation in a patient's death.

CONCLUSIONS

Changes in reimbursement and public policy will affect the practice of physicians in the twenty-first century. Many of the traditional values that led to the establishment of ethical practice guidelines will remain the norms for assessing the ethics of individual physicians and groups of physicians. The major ethical shift in the twenty-first century will be the increasing call to incorporate social rather than individual rights into ethical assessments and decisions that clinicians and policy makers will need to make.

Medical ethics is not a static discipline. Clinical experience and outcomes research will continue to provide data for academic reassessment and clinical application of medical ethics to both group and individual decisions and policies.

Managed Care[1]

Alan E. London

The health-care industry is undergoing tremendous changes, all of which stem from the need to reduce costs. Managed care has been identified as a way to reduce costs while simultaneously improving the care that is provided to patients. As the growth of managed care plans increases, there is pressure to prove that the quality of patient care provided is equal to, or better than, that typically provided under traditional forms of health insurance. Managed care presents a challenge for all providers, but adapting to and embracing such care is necessary to survive financially in today's marketplace.

Managed care is a broad subject and includes many facets. This chapter provides a basic introduction to some of the major issues. Becoming both comfortable and knowledgeable about managed care requires a commitment on the part of physicians. On-going reading, attendance at conferences, and working closely with other physicians and professionals who deal with managed care will broaden one's base of knowledge.

EVOLUTION OF EMPLOYER-BASED HEALTH INSURANCE

The origins of managed care can be traced to the nineteenth century. What today are referred to as *health plans* were established during the early 1900s to serve specific populations, such as workers in the railroad, mining, and lumber industries (1).

During the 1920s, however, it was recognized that rising costs and the potential debt that families might incur because of a hospitalization could lead to real financial difficulties for community hospitals. These hospitals became vulnerable, and

it was recognized that the risks associated with treating a community population needed to be spread over the community as a whole. Hospital institutions needed a more reliable source of revenue. This was the need that led to development of the Blue Cross insurance program (1, 2).

In this period, the medical profession was developing the Blue Shield plan, which was intended to protect physicians and patients from "contract practice." Under contract practice, an employer selected an exclusive provider for the workforce. All other community physicians were excluded (2).

During the 1930s and 1940s, interest by the larger business community in prepaid health plans began to grow. Some precursors of the modern-day health maintenance organization (HMO) that developed at this time include the Kaiser Permanente Medical Programs, Health Insurance Plan of Greater New York, and Group Health Cooperative of Puget Sound (Seattle, WA). Broad support for this concept by employers became—and has remained—one of the major forces behind growth of managed care in the United States (1).

Since World War II, employers have been the main source of health insurance in the United States. Originally, employers wanted a way to offer employees an additional, small fringe benefit, without increasing their salaries. Health coverage was an ideal solution. Then, in 1965, the U.S. Congress passed the Medicare and Medicaid legislation to provide comprehensive health-care coverage for elderly and poor individuals (1).

During the Nixon administration in the 1970s, HMOs and the concept of managed care itself were introduced. Dr. Paul Ellwood is most noted for the rapid growth of HMOs. Ellwood concluded that the existing fee-for-service system created "perverse incentives," in which physicians and hospitals were rewarded for treating illness and discouraged from providing preventive care. Ellwood convinced the Nixon administration that a nationwide system of HMOs would link a fiscal

[1] Portions of this chapter are reprinted with permission from *Respiratory Care,* 1997 Jan;42:30–42.

strategy of prepayment with a cost-efficient system (3). Nixon's 1971 Health Message to Congress made HMOs the cornerstone of his entire national health policy, the goal of which was to make 1700 HMO programs available to 90% of the U.S. population. In 1973, Congress passed the Health Maintenance Organization Act, which provided financing and other support for the development of HMOs (3).

During the 1980s, enrollment in U.S. HMOs and preferred provider organizations (PPOs) grew from approximately 10 million at the beginning of the decade to approximately 55 million by the end (1). Employers, who were experiencing soaring health-care costs, fueled this growth by making managed care plans more economical and attractive for their employees.

Failure to pass national health-care reform legislation in the 1990s has resulted in managed care continuing to grow in popularity. Employers also now offer various benefit options to control the escalating costs of health care, and federal, state, and local governments have used various managed-care products to control health-care costs for their employees. In addition, government-sponsored programs such as Medicare, Medicaid, and worker's compensation are now some of the fastest-growing market segments in managed care today.

GROWTH IN MANAGED CARE

Managed care is defined as any system that manages delivery of health care in a way that controls its cost (4). During the 1980s and 1990s, U.S. corporations began to focus on the escalating cost of health-care benefits for their employees; as a result, managed-care insurance plans grew steadily. In 1988, approximately 50% of U.S. employees were enrolled in traditional health-care plans, and 15% were enrolled in managed-care plans, such as PPOs and point-of-service (POS) HMOs. By 1994, however, the percentage of employees enrolled in managed-care plans had increased to nearly 40% (Fig. 72.1) (5). In addition, the number of those younger than 65 years

of age receiving their care in HMOs has risen from just under 40 million U.S. patients in 1990 to approximately 60 million in 1995 (Fig.72.2) (6).

The number of Medicare recipients choosing Medicare risk HMO plans also has increased from 1 million in 1987 to approximately 4.4 million in 1996. Medicare risk enrollment has grown steadily, increasing by approximately 2% per month since 1993—or approximately 70,000 new enrollees per month. This growth will continue at an accelerated pace as the U.S. population of those 65 years of age and older grows, and also as the Health Care Financing Association (HCFA) introduces new options that will make HMOs more attractive for senior citizens (Fig. 72.3) (6).

Physicians have steadily joined managed-care networks as well. In 1992, 56% of physicians had joined such networks. In 1993, this had risen to 62%, and in 1994, 89% had joined managed-care networks (6). Some physicians have resisted the change to managed care, but many have joined these networks to maintain both their patient population and their income (Fig. 72.4). As more employers offer managed-care options (which save the employers money), traditional indemnity insurance may essentially disappear.

The growth of managed care will shift the ratio of primary-care and specialty-care physicians. A 1994 study by the Advisory Board, a membership-based research and publishing firm in Washington, D.C., projected that in a fully capitated health-care system, the required mix of physicians would shift from 34% primary-care and 66% specialty-care physicians to 60% primary-care and 40% specialty-care physicians (7). Another study by the Advisory Board (7) also showed how a fully capitated system would affect the need for specialty physicians. This study reviewed the number of U.S. physicians by specialist levels, and it compared those numbers with the needs in a fully capitated system. Table 72.1 depicts the projected surplus of physicians by specialty in such a system. It is clear from these studies that as enrollment in managed-care plans continues to grow, the need for primary-care physi-

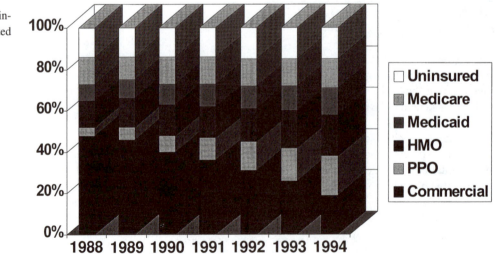

Figure 72.1. Distribution of insurance coverage in the United States, 1988–1994.

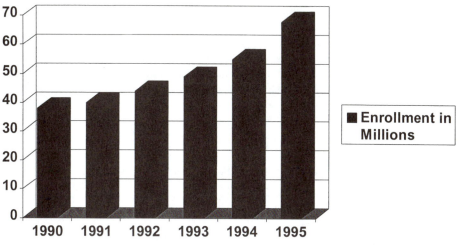

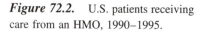

Figure 72.2. U.S. patients receiving care from an HMO, 1990–1995.

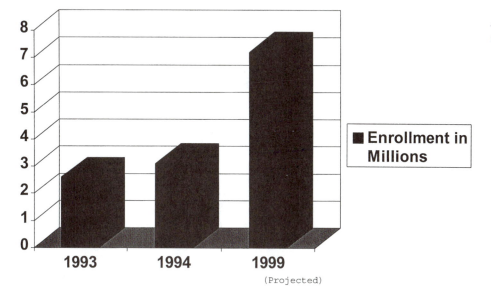

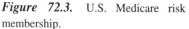

Figure 72.3. U.S. Medicare risk membership.

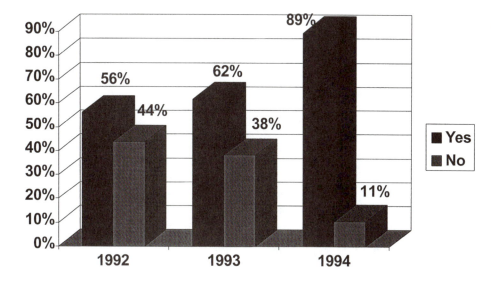

Figure 72.4. Physicians participating in managed-care networks.

Table 72.1. Effect of Capitation on Need for Specialty-Care Physicians			
Specialty	**Practicing Physicians (n)**	**Physicians Required in Capitated System (n)**	**Surplus (n [%])**
Psychiatry	36,405	9,451	29,954 (74.0)
General surgery	39,211	13,099	26,112 (66.6)
Neurology	4,501	1,658	2,843 (63.2)
Cardiology	16,478	7,074	9,404 (57.1)
Anesthesia	28,148	12,435	15,713 (55.8)
Orthopedics	20,640	12,325	8,315 (40.3)
Urology	9,452	6,356	3,096 (32.8)
Obstetrics/ gynecology	35,273	27,026	8,247 (23.4)
Emergency	15,470	12,214	3,256 (21.0)

Adapted with permission from the Grade Alliance II, the capitation strategy: the governance committee. Washington D.C., The Advisory Board Company, 1994.

cians will increase and that for specialty-care physicians will decrease.

MANAGED-CARE DELIVERY MODELS

As managed care has grown in the United States, various models of delivery have emerged, including:

- HMOs
- PPOs
- POS organizations
- Exclusive-provider organizations (EPO)
- Provider-sponsored networks (PSN)

These models have evolved from simple, staff-model HMOs to complex, risk-bearing POS organizations.

HEALTH MAINTENANCE ORGANIZATIONS

An HMO is a delivery system that provides comprehensive health care to an enrolled population, often for a prepaid, fixed (i.e., capitated) payment. The organization consists of a network of health-care providers who render a wide range of services and assume some, or all, of the financial risk in providing these services. Enrollees generally are not covered for care that is provided outside of the HMO network (8). The HMO is the most restrictive form of managed care.

PREFERRED PROVIDER ORGANIZATIONS

In the PPO organizational model, a group of selected physicians, hospitals, or both agree to provide care to members at

a negotiated fee, which often is a discount from billed charges. Members obtaining care from within the PPO network pay a predetermined level of out-of-pocket expense, such as a copayment, but have larger financial obligations if they obtain services from outside the network (often 20–30% of charges). PPOs may or may not have gatekeepers or medical, management, or referral systems (9) and is the least restrictive form of managed care.

POINT-OF-SERVICE ORGANIZATIONS

A POS organization is a health-care delivery system that groups together at least two types of plans, usually an HMO and an indemnity plan, thus allowing its members slightly more provider-selection flexibility. If members use providers outside the HMO network, they incur deductibles and copayments (8, 9).

EXCLUSIVE-PROVIDER ORGANIZATIONS

An EPO has a smaller network of providers than a PPO, with primary-care physicians serving as the care coordinators. Members who seek health care outside the network incur financial penalties (8, 9).

PROVIDER-SPONSORED NETWORKS

In a PSN, health-care providers establish a geographically diverse network and contract directly with insurers, self-funded employers, and government agencies. These networks then become the sole provider of health care for those customers who select the network (4).

A PSN is set up and controlled by the health-care providers, and it gives physicians the ability to assume and manage fully capitated risk distributed over a larger patient base. PSNs assume the responsibility for managing utilization, which is a managed-care function shifted from the insurance company to those who actually provide the patient care. PSNs have more negotiating leverage than individual providers with payors and gain some economies of scale in administering managed-care contracts (4).

INTEGRATED DELIVERY SYSTEMS

With a rapidly changing marketplace and increased pressures on all health-care providers, the desire and need for the various components of health care to come together as an integrated delivery system (IDS) has grown. An IDS is defined as "a system of health-care providers (e.g., physicians and hospitals) organized to span a large geographical area and provide a broad range of health-care services" (4).

This alignment of health-care providers, working together in a cooperative and organized system, leads to:

- Greater economies of scale
- Common information systems
- Distribution of clinical resources in a cost-effective manner
- A seamless system of patient care/avoidance of fragmented patient care
- A full continuum of care over a large geographic area
- Increased negotiating strength in managed-care contracting

There are three basic IDS models (4):

- Integration of physicians
- Integration of physicians with health-care facilities
- Integration of physicians and facilities that take on the insurer's role

An IDS can also be integrated either vertically or horizontally under one managerial hierarchy, or a contractual network (i.e., virtual integration) can be formed. Under vertical and horizontal integration, there also can be clinical integration, physician/system integration, and functional integration (10).

In an IDS, controlling medical utilization holds the most promise for controlling costs, but this requires strong medical leadership and management. Utilization management, quality-improvement activities, clinical-practice protocols, case management, network-provider profiling and reporting, and disease management all are addressed as part of medical management. Strong physician leadership in directing the care-management approach is needed to ensure both quality and cost-effective care throughout the network. Medical management information systems and processes help the organization to prove outcomes for payors and providers of care.

The benefits to a physician participating in an IDS are numerous, and they include:

- Participating in the governance of the IDS

- Retaining the ability to participate in defining the medical standards by which care is rendered
- Retaining autonomy in their own practices
- Being part of a larger system committed to downsizing and reducing the costs of practicing medicine

EFFECT ON QUALITY OF PATIENT CARE

Measuring quality in health care is complex. The managed-care enrollee's perception of quality actually may have little to do with the quality of clinical care that he or she receives, and many questions have been raised about whether the financial incentives offered to managed-care providers negatively affect the quality of care compared with that provided to patients under traditional fee-for-service insurance.

In 1995, the Advisory Board reviewed the effects of capitation on physician utilization patterns in groups of California physicians. Figure 72.5 shows the declining rates for five cardiology and gastroenterology procedures; a 77% reduction in angioplasty procedures within this group of physicians is most notable (7). In addition, the 300 diagnostic catheterizations per 100,000 population performed in the precapitation reimbursement contract were decreased to 90 catheterizations in the capitated agreement, which is a 70% reduction (7). Such drastic reductions in utilization rates raise serious questions about quality of care under both managed-care and fee-for-service models.

In 1994, Miller and Luft (11) reviewed 167 HMO quality studies and concluded that managed care was equal to or better than fee-for-service care on 14 of 17 measures of quality. Another study refuted the notion that use of primary-care gatekeepers in HMOs results in delayed referral and suboptimal outcomes (12). Vernon et al. (13) studied 330 patients with colorectal cancer to determine quality outcomes in managed-

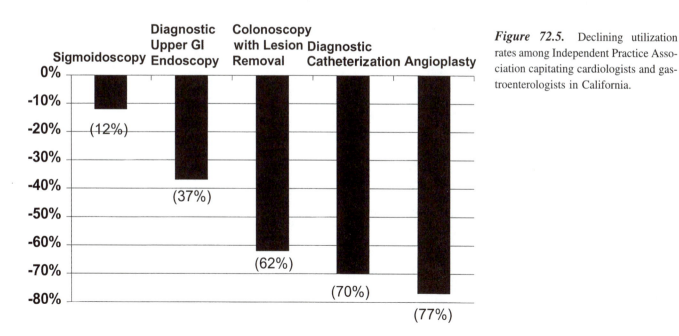

Figure 72.5. Declining utilization rates among Independent Practice Association capitating cardiologists and gastroenterologists in California.

care versus fee-for-service insurance plans. The nature of this study was to determine whether patterns of care that may lead to earlier diagnosis and better prognosis were different depending on the patient's health-care coverage. Their findings suggest no overall differences in the stage of disease at diagnosis or in patient survival. The variable patterns seen at diagnosis, controlling for age, support there being no systematic differences in the care offered to fee-for-service and HMO patients. Overall, findings from these studies are consistent with those from other studies reporting little or no difference in the process and outcome of care for patients with different types of medical coverage. Much more research is needed, however, concerning both short- and long-term outcomes.

Recently, purchasers of health care have begun demanding proof for improved quality of care and cost efficiencies. This has led to greater focus on measurement and reporting of both quality and outcomes through quantifiable, provider-specific data and information. Managed-care organizations have responded by developing disease-management programs for several conditions. In addition, they have begun to examine aggregate patient data to identify indicators of quality. From this, managed-care organizations are developing standards of care that can demonstrate a consistent relationship with improved clinical outcomes. Managed-care organizations then attempt to implement the standards that will control cost as well as ensure quality of care (14).

EFFECTS ON CLINICAL CARE

Managed-care plans have begun focusing on a variety of health-care cost and utilization efforts, particularly those associated with high cost–disease categories. All areas of health-care delivery are being scrutinized, however, to maximize efficiency, quality, and savings.

Health-care delivery under the various managed-care models has—and will—continue to change in several ways. These include:

- The decline in length of stay and reduction in use of technical and professional services will continue.
- The focus on having patients utilize primary-care physicians and obtain referrals to specialists will increase.
- Physicians will need to apply principles of population-based medicine.
- Providers, including physicians, will need to implement patient education and demand-management programs to increase patient satisfaction and lower costs.
- Physicians will need to work with, employ, and provide oversight for allied health-care professionals, who will act as physician extenders.

Physicians need to embrace the changes resulting from an increased focus on managed care, and they must become leaders in facilitating many of these on-going changes. This includes being more flexible and willing to accept new roles,

such as coordinating patient care as well as managing patients through the continuum of care and increased paperwork associated with managed care.

REIMBURSEMENT METHODOLOGIES

Reimbursement to hospitals and physicians has evolved over time, as managed-care plans have introduced new products and risk-bearing arrangements. Before the 1980s, most hospitals and physicians were reimbursed for the actual services performed and billed; this has been known as *fee-for-service*. As managed care evolved, however, discounts from fee-for-service arrangements were introduced.

Hospital per diem methodology is an approach that is designed to shift some of the risk from payors to providers. So-called "per diems" are negotiated, daily payment rates for delivery of all inpatient hospital services that are provided each day, regardless of the actual services provided. Per diem rates differ by the type of care provided (8).

Diagnosis-related groups (DRG) is a methodology that defines the hospital payment rate for Medicare patients. Originally introduced by the HCFA in the 1980s, the DRG system categorizes patients on the basis of demographics, diagnosis, and therapeutic characteristics. A DRG is used to predict medical services, average length of hospitalization, and reimbursement. The system offers hospitals a financial incentive to provide services at a lower cost than the DRG reimbursement. Because of this prospective-payment system, hospitals must be certain their average cost per DRG does not exceed the HCFA rates (15). Since the 1980s, the DRG methodology has been adopted by other payors as well.

In the 1990s, the resource-based relative-value scale (RBRVS) was developed and introduced by the HCFA as a fee schedule for physicians participating in Medicare. The RBRVS assigns a relative value to each current procedural terminology (CPT) code for services on the basis of the provider's practice, malpractice, and work experience, geographic region, and historical trends. Use of the RBRVS has resulted in dramatic changes in physician payment patterns. This system originally increased reimbursement to family- and general-practice physicians by approximately 15%. Payments to ophthalmologists and anesthesiologists decreased by approximately 35%, however, and payments to other procedure-based specialists (e.g., surgeons) decreased as well (15).

With the capitation methodology, physicians, hospitals, or both agree to accept a prepaid amount per person (i.e., member per month [PMPM]) to provide medical services. This amount is determined on the basis of a defined set of services or benefits. Providers must manage patient care within a preset budget or incur a financial loss. Because the monthly capitation amount is fixed for a given period of time (usually 1 year), HMOs or insurance companies can predict and control their medical expenses (16). Table 72.2 shows how capitation rates are calculated and the resultant PMPM reimbursement to hospitals and physicians; Table 72.3 shows

Table 72.2. Calculating Capitation Rates to Determine the Prepaid Amount Available per Member per Month

	Services (per 1000 enrollees/year)	Costs ($)	PMPM ($)
Hospital inpatient			
Medical/surgical/ pediatric, intensive, and cardiac care	182	1401.20	20.36
Neonatal	15	1339.99	1.60
Maternity	32	1216.89	3.11
Hospital outpatient			
Surgery	70	1772.10	9.71
Radiology	173	191.52	2.67
Pathology	212	143.33	2.45
Emergency room	84	260.50	1.59
Professional Services			
Plan office visits	2536	54.90	11.27
Plan surgery	258	365.78	7.64
Plan maternity care	27	838.83	1.83
Plan radiology	551	90.73	4.05
Plan pathology	657	42.25	2.25

the average capitated costs to HMOs for various medical specialty services (16).

MANAGED-CARE CONTRACTING

In today's environment of proliferating managed-care organizations and increasingly complex interrelationships between financing and health-care delivery, physicians must understand managed-care contracting to successfully establish and maintain practices. When developing and evaluating opportunities with an assortment of payors, certain steps can help to improve the success rate:

1. Size up the payor.
2. Evaluate the proposed reimbursement.
3. Analyze and negotiate the contract terms.
4. Assess the payor's requisite procedures and implications of administrative costs and resources.
5. Continually evaluate the compliance and performance of specific contracts, as well as of the entire portfolio.

SIZE UP THE PAYOR

As with other business relationships, certain steps should be taken to assess the business opportunity and any associated liabilities before entering into a managed-care contract. Sizing up the payor often is overlooked, however, especially when

physicians are confronted with a barrage of contracts, too few resources to evaluate them, and a take-it-or-leave-it approach by the payors. Assessment of a contract should include, at minimum, the following basic information:

- Ownership of the health plan
- Number of members (by product and geographic location)
- List of clients (i.e., employers, other payors)
- Years in business
- Other health-plan providers in the same specialty (request a provider directory)
- Advertising and promotion of the network
- Financial position of the health plan
- Administrative procedures

Typically, larger HMOs and PPOs employ provider representatives, who are responsible for directly negotiating and servicing physician contracts. Recently, physician–hospital organizations (PHOs) have emerged as an alternative for pay-

Table 72.3. Average Physician Capitation from a Commercial Population

Specialty	PMPM ($)
Allergy	0.384
Anesthesiology	3.380
Cardiology	1.268
Cardiology (invasive)	0.380
Dermatology	0.552
Endocrinology	0.181
Gastroenterology	0.613
General surgery	1.466
Hematology	0.523
Nephrology	0.230
Neurology	0.450
Neurosurgery	0.373
Obstetrics/gynecology	3.623
Oncology	0.791
Ophthalmology	0.728
Optometry	0.663
Oral Surgery	0.289
Orthopedics	2.074
Otolaryngology	0.656
Podiatry	0.234
Plastic surgery	0.247
Psychiatry/mental health	2.271
Pulmonary	0.179
Radiology	2.654
Rheumatology	0.146
Urology	0.500

Adapted with permission from The HMO salary survey. Rockford, IL: Warren Surveys, 1996. (For further information, call 1-815-877-8794.)

ors who wish to develop physician panels and, therefore, eliminate the more resource-intense individual contracting. Certain payors, however, are philosophically opposed to PHO contracting and the associated loss of control in selecting and establishing the credentials of their physician panel.

EVALUATE THE REIMBURSEMENT (FEE SCHEDULES AND CAPITATION)

Most payors reimburse physicians according to a CPT-specific fee schedule. Generally derived from Medicare's RBRVS fees, these schedules are a percentage of the RBRVS (e.g., 100%, 115%, or 130%). Reimbursement levels vary depending on the penetration or stage of managed care in the market, geographic region, size of payor, and other factors (e.g., negotiating strength, reputation, type of services offered, type of institution).

One common method to evaluate proposed reimbursement is to identify the top 25 or 50 revenue-generating CPT codes for the practice and then request a sample reimbursement for these codes. By adjusting for relative frequencies, an average-weighted impact of the proposed reimbursement then can be projected. Table 72.4 provides an example of a fee-analysis worksheet.

In mature managed-care markets, capitation may be a more prevalent form of reimbursement, particularly for primary care. Capitation places the physician, who typically is paid on a PMPM basis, at risk for the membership base for a defined set of benefits. Capitation rates vary by geographic region, size of the payor, and other factors. A typical commercial (i.e., non-Medicare/Medicaid) capitation rate for primary care can range from $10 to $13 PMPM for the same defined set of benefits or services. When assessing a proposed capitation rate, it is essential to define which services are included as part of the capitation. Such services should be defined by CPT code and included in the contract or contractually binding attachments. The contract must specify how and when the payor will pay the physician, and it should obligate the payor

to provide essential membership and eligibility information on a timely basis to identify and manage both the members and the associated financial risk.

Other payment features that may be somewhat less obvious but are important nonetheless include withheld payments, incentives, penalties for services denied, prompt-pay terms, and terms for payment after termination. These features also should be spelled out clearly in the contract.

ANALYZE/NEGOTIATE THE CONTRACT

All the provisions of a contract should be reviewed thoroughly. At minimum, standard provisions should include:

*   Definitions for covered benefits/services, medical necessity, and emergency services
*   Roles and responsibilities as related to:
    *   Payment
    *   Coordination of benefits (i.e., primary and secondary coverages)
    *   Reporting/data requirements
    *   Membership/eligibility data (for risk contracts)
    *   Patient identification
    *   Benefits and incentives as related to steerage
    *   Marketing
*   Confidentiality
*   Reviewing/establishing credentials
*   Audit rights
*   Insurance requirements
*   Indemnification
*   Use of payor or provider's name, trademark
*   Utilization review and medical-management procedures
*   Grievance and appeals procedures
*   Governing law
*   Severability
*   Term of contract
*   Termination for breach, cure of breach, and without cause
*   Financial terms

		(A) Your Current Price	(B) Network Fee	(C) (6 mo/1 y) Volume	(A) × (C) Unadjusted Revenue	(B) × (C) Adjusted Revenue
Procedure Costs	**Procedure Description**					
99201	Nonpatient level I					
99211	Established patient level I					
81002	Urinalysis					
90703	Tetanus toxoid immunization					
82962	Glucose blood test					
36415	Drawing blood					
				Total	$ _____	_____
					% Discount	_____

Table 72.4.   Managed-Care Fee Analysis Worksheet

Lesser of fee or charge? Then modify accordingly (lesser of (A) or (B) × (C)).

Typically, payors have an administrative manual that may be referenced in the contract, but it often is not provided unless specifically requested. The physician should obtain a copy of this manual and review it thoroughly before signing the contract.

Negotiating strength is a function of the size, location, reputation, and overall demand for a physician's practice. Payors tend to be somewhat inflexible in physician contracting, especially as it relates to solo physicians, but there usually is some latitude for achieving more favorable terms than those in the standard contract. Dealing with a senior manager versus the provider representative can improve the outcome of these negotiations as well.

ASSESS THE PAYOR'S PROCEDURES

Administrative procedures can make or break the effectiveness of the payor/physician relationship, both on a day-to-day and an overall basis. As mentioned, the physician or office manager should request and thoroughly review the payor's administrative manual. Understanding the following procedures are of great importance:

- Eligibility
- Utilization/medical management
  - Precertification requirements/penalties
  - Outpatient authorizations
  - Concurrent review
  - Denial/appeals
  - Emergencies
- Phone numbers related to medical-management activities
- Reviewing/establishing credentials
- Audits
- Data collection/physician profiles
- Utilization reports

EVALUATE CONTRACT COMPLIANCE AND PERFORMANCE

Each physician's office needs to establish procedures and train its staff in how to handle and support the various contract requirements. Monthly or quarterly reports, or both, should be developed to track membership, revenue by payor, capitation details, denials, administrative issues, and other data that may be required for the contract. Developing a system to monitor each payor's compliance with the terms of their contract also is very beneficial in evaluating those contracts.

EMERGING TRENDS IN MANAGED CARE

Both employers and payors have moved from purchasing traditional fee-for-service health benefits to managed-care plans, primarily to control rising health-care costs. Purchasers of health care have become facilitators for value-based, health-system choice. Employers and payors are demanding price stability or premium rollbacks, choice, flexibility in provider networks, provider performance data, a broad range of benefit alternatives, and continuity of primary care–provider relationships for the employee/patients.

Several efforts have been initiated by providers, payors, and employers to better manage their patients. Providers, payors, and employers have begun to work separately and, in many cases, cooperatively on these initiatives.

DISEASE MANAGEMENT

Because of the increased focus on quality of care and cost efficiency, many managed-care organizations, employers, and payors (on behalf of their customers) are developing and implementing disease-management programs for chronic and difficult-to-manage diseases. Diagnosing, properly treating, and monitoring a patient's disease reduces hospitalizations, improves health outcomes, and decreases costs.

MEDICAL MANAGEMENT

The concept of medical management may encompass total care for high-risk patients, including 24-hour care referrals through the case manager, assessing the home environment for healthful living, educating enrollees on the best way to stay healthy, and even providing cellular phones for patients to contact their case manager, primary-care provider, or hospital. In addition, provider groups often will offer and facilitate support groups and workshops for management of specific diseases (e.g., asthma care). Such preventive measures, which are monitored and implemented by the primary-care provider, may increase the quality of both care and life for enrollees. To identify high-risk patients, provider groups also are performing health risk appraisals.

DEMAND MANAGEMENT

A patient-centered approach to reduce consumer demand for medical services, demand management uses decision- and self-management support systems that enable and encourage consumers to make appropriate use of medical care. Demand management can be accomplished through disease prevention, wellness promotion, and nurse triage (17).

OUTCOMES MANAGEMENT

Outcomes management is the use of information and knowledge gained from a patient-outcome assessment to achieve optimal patient outcomes. Outcomes management programs usually target medical conditions in which pharmaceutic and educational interventions can produce clinical as well as cost-effective improvements. The patient-outcome assessments provide a quantitative comparison of treatment programs; this comparison typically maps the course of a chronic disease across the continuum of care or identifies variations in the

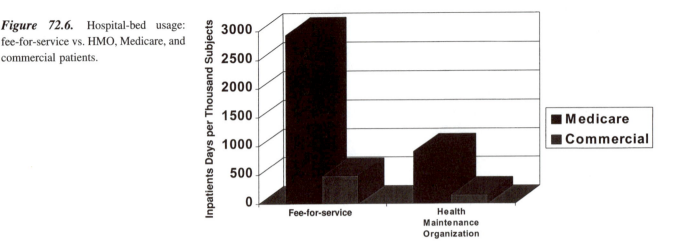

Figure 72.6. Hospital-bed usage: fee-for-service vs. HMO, Medicare, and commercial patients.

outcomes of care to better determine the best process of care management (4).

WIDE GEOGRAPHIC ACCESS NETWORKS

Purchasers of health care (i.e., employers, payors) as well as employees want a broader choice of physicians and hospitals in their managed-care networks. In return for access to larger networks, patients (i.e., employees) may be required to pay higher deductibles, coinsurance, and copayments.

MEETING THE CHALLENGE

The dynamic and changing health-care environment requires physicians to increase their understanding and responsibilities associated with managed care. With decreased bed usage, decreased length of stay, and better case management, the setting for delivery of health care has altered. Figure 72.6, for example, compares hospital-bed usage with fee-for-service coverage to hospital-bed usage with HMO coverage for patients with Medicare or commercial insurance (7). Health-care delivery has moved toward a post-acute and outpatient-dominated system, and allied health professionals have become increasingly important in helping physicians to care for patients. In addition, medical management is driving health-care delivery into less costly settings.

Increased payor contracting, new reimbursement method-

ologies, and a host of emerging trends have changed the role of physicians, and they will continue to do so. These changes also have produced a new level of excitement, anxiety, and challenges for physicians. The prevalence of managed-care contracts and new reimbursement methodologies should give physicians the incentive to learn the basics of managed care and to adapt their practices to maximize reimbursement and meet the needs of their patients.

Managed care alters some of the rules of medical practice, and it introduces medical-management processes for patient care. Good medical management creates an environment in which physicians both participate and understand that how they deliver care will be scrutinized by their peers and managed-care companies. Comprehensive intervention and medical management can improve the quality and clinical outcomes of patient care, and they can reduce the costs associated with providing that care. Both primary- and specialty-care physicians must be aware of how patients access the health-care system, especially because this is critically important in documenting appropriate medical care and assuring financial success.

With increasing pressure to reduce costs, providers are developing PSN and IDS organizations to improve operating efficiencies, better manage patient care, and participate in managed-care contracts. In some cases, there are mergers between providers, such as hospitals, physicians, and sometimes, payors, that enable very large IDS organizations to be created. Such delivery systems are—and will be—the driving force in future health-care delivery.

REFERENCES

1. Bischof RO, Nash DB. Managed care past, present, and future. In: Merli GJ, Brooks RJ, Epstein KR, Reife CM, eds. Med Clin North Am 1996;80(2):225–244.
2. Williams SJ, Torrens PR. Introduction to health services. New York: John Wiley & Sons, 1980.
3. Mayer TR, Mayer GG. HMOs: origins and development. N Engl J Med 1985;312:590–594.
4. Kongstevdt PR. The managed health care handbook. 2nd ed. Gaithersburg, MD: Aspen Publications, 1993.
5. Kongstevdt PR. Ernst & Young LLP. 1995.

6. Managed Care Digest Series: HMO/PPO Digest (corporate publication). Kansas City, MO: Hoechst Marion Roussel & SMG Marketing, 1995.

7. The Grand Alliance II, capitation strategy: the governance committee. Washington, D.C.: The Advisory Board Company, 1994.

8. Friendly Hills Health Care Network. Glossary of managed care terms. La Habra: California Friendly Hills, 1995.

9. Schaller DF: The HMO component model and a managed care dictionary. Phoenix, AZ: Schaller Anderson.

10. Miller R. Health system integration: a means to an end. Health Affairs 1996:Summer;92–106.

11. Miller RH, Luft JS. Managed care plan performance since 1980: a literature analysis. JAMA 1994;271:1512–1519.

12. Paone G, Higgins RS, Spencer T, Silverman NA. Enrollment in the Health Alliance Plan HMO is not an independent risk factor for coronary artery bypass graft surgery. Circulation 1995;92(Suppl 9):1169–1172.

13. Vernon SW, Hughes JT, et al. Quality of care for colorectal cancer in a fee-for-service and health maintenance organization practice. Cancer 1994;69:2418–2425.

14. Phoon J, Corder K, Barter M. Managed care and total quality management: a necessary integration. J Nurs Care Qual 1996;10:25–32

15. Rakich JS, Longest BB Jr, Darr K. Managing health services organizations. 3rd ed. Baltimore, MD: Health Professions Press, 1992.

16. The HMO salary survey. Rockford, IL: Warren Surveys, 1996. (For further information, call 1-815-877-8794).

17. Lester J, Breudigam M. Nurse triage telephone centers: key to demand management strategy. HAHAM Manage J 1996;22(4):13–14.

SUGGESTED READINGS

Boland P. Making managed healthcare work: a practical guide to strategies and solutions. Gaithersburg, MD: Aspen Publications, 1993.

Dacso ST, Dacso CC. Managed care answer book. 2nd ed. New York: Aspen Publications, 1997.

Doyle RL. Healthcare management guidelines. Volume 1: inpatient and surgical care. Millman & Robertson: October 1993.

McCally JF. Capitation for physicians: how to negotiate the contract, maximize reimbursement, and manage financial risk. Chicago, IL: Irwin Professional Publishers (Healthcare Financial Management Association), 1996.

Nash DB, Todd W. Disease management: a systems approach to improving patient outcomes. Chicago, IL: American Hospital Publishers, 1997.

Zablocki, E. Changing physician practice patterns: strategies for success in a capitated health care system. Gaithersburg, MD: Aspen Publications, 1995.

Computers and Medicine

Neil B. Mehta

Personal computers (PCs) have become increasingly common, and since the advent of the World Wide Web in the early 1990s, their use has grown dramatically. By 1995, more than 35% of U.S. homes had PCs.

Most physicians use a computer either at work or at home, but the health-care industry as a whole has been relatively slow getting on the "Information Superhighway." The reasons for this are numerous. They include:

- *Computer applications in health care lack universal standards.* If a patient switches physicians, the electronic record of his or her medical history may be difficult to import into (i.e., to add to) the new physician's database.
- *Computer technology is rapidly and constantly changing.* Faster, more powerful computers as well as newer, more complex software are regularly appearing. New software usually has many desirable features over the older versions, but it often is designed to make use of the power and abilities of the newer computers and, thus, does not function well (if at all) on older machines. Keeping up-do-date requires an on-going investment in new equipment and in training.
- *The health-care industry is changing rapidly.* Numerous health-care plans are evolving today, and both patients and employers are frequently switching between these plans. Because investing in a computerized medical office is a long-term commitment, physicians may hesitate to move forward when the health-care environment itself is unstable.
- *Many physicians are unfamiliar with the information resources available on computers and find it difficult to keep up with the advances in this field.* As it is, physicians, who constantly are urged to see more

patients in less time, are finding that there is less time to keep up even with medical literature.
- *The security of sensitive patient information is uncertain.* This includes information maintained on computer databases as well as that transferred over the Internet.
- *Most hospitals find it difficult to reach a majority of physicians because of resistance from a few.* A majority (i.e., critical mass) of physicians in any organization must use computers on a regular basis for these systems to work and to show both cost- and labor-saving benefits.

Solutions to these formidable problems may lie in the appropriate application of computer technology by the health-care industry.

AN HISTORICAL PERSPECTIVE
A BRIEF HISTORY OF COMPUTERS

For centuries, man has attempted to build devices that could help with repetitive, complex, or mathematic tasks. The first such computational device is attributed to Blaise Pascal, a French scientist, who in 1642 constructed a "computer" box with eight wheels that could add and subtract (1). In 1832, when the British government was trying to eliminate costly mathematic errors from navigation charts, which put lives and cargo in danger, and from accounting, which caused overpayments to pensioners, Charles Babbage developed the prototype of a computer that could address these computational problems (1). Called the "Difference Engine," his device earned him a government grant to develop an even more powerful computer, the "Analytical Engine." In 1842, however, after sizable cost overruns and numerous designs, this project was abandoned (1).

On the other side of the Atlantic, the United States also faced computational challenges. The 1880 U.S. Census took 9 years to complete, and the U.S. government was concerned the 1890 census would not be completed before 1900! Therefore, Hermann Hollerith, who worked on the 1880 census, designed a "Tabulating Machine" that could mechanically compute census results using punch cards. With Hollerith's machine, the 1890 census was completed in 7 years, and by 1924, Hollerith's Tabulating Machine Company had evolved into International Business Machines (IBM).

Early computers were large, often occupying an entire wall of a huge room, and because of their high maintenance needs and enormous costs, they were strictly the domain of the military, universities, and large corporations. After 1970, however, this began to change (2):

- In 1971, Intel released the first microprocessor, which made possible the development of PCs.
- In 1975, the Altair 8800 minicomputer kit was released. Users not only had to assemble the computer but to write the software to operate it, because software was not commercially available. In response, two young computer enthusiasts—Bill Gates and Paul Allen—wrote a program called Beginners' All-purpose Symbolic Instruction Code (BASIC), which could run on the Altair allowing its users to program their computers. (Gates and Allen eventually formed Microsoft.)
- In 1977, Steve Jobs and Steve Wozniak formed Apple Computer Company. In that same year, they also exhibited the first Apple II computer.
- In 1984, Apple released the Macintosh, a new type of computer that incorporated a Graphic User Interface (GUI) and a "mouse." The GUI and mouse helped to create an intuitive, user-friendly, point-and-click interface, which eliminated the need for users to know complex commands. With the Macintosh, even novices could use computers.

Around this time, IBM started working on a PC called the Acorn. In 1981, the Acorn was released under the name of IBM-PC (2). Since then, the personal-computer industry has seen an explosion of progress and change, with faster and more powerful microprocessors being developed almost every year.

A BRIEF HISTORY OF THE INTERNET

Both *Internet* and *World Wide Web* have become buzzwords in the last 4 to 5 years, but their roots can be traced to the 1960s and the Cold War. To understand some of the concepts and components of the Internet today, it is helpful to understand how the Internet developed.

In 1962, Paul Baran and his colleagues at the Rand Corporation wondered how U.S. military databases at different sites could communicate with each other if the network that connected them was destroyed by a nuclear strike (3). In response, they developed a technique called "packet switching," which would be integral to development of the Internet. (In packet switching, data is divided into small "packets" for transmission, with each packet carrying both the source and the destination address. After transmission, the data is reassembled.)

By 1966, several computer sites were communicating with each other using long-distance telephone lines. (The Advanced Research Projects Agency [ARPA] financed the long-distance connections.) There was, however, a problem: a computer at one site could not "talk" to all the other computers without a separate computer terminal and phone line for each of the other sites. To overcome this, ARPA connected all of these sites in 1969 using the packet-switching technology developed by Baran (4). The first four sites to be connected were the University of California at Los Angeles (UCLA), University of California at Santa Barbara (UCSB), University of Utah at Salt Lake City, and Stanford Research Institute in Menlo Park, California. The network connecting these four sites, which was known as the ARPANET, was the first network of the future Internet.

Because access to the ARPANET initially was restricted, several other universities and organizations developed their own networks, which were extremely useful in bringing together people of similar interests into one global community. Nevertheless, even though computers now could talk to others on the same network, they could not communicate with computers on other networks. Thus, to enable broader communication, ARPA commissioned in 1983 implementation of the Transmission Control Protocol/Internet Protocol (TCP/IP), which allowed computers on different networks to communicate. Thus, the Internet—essentially a network of networks connected by the TCP/IP— was born.

The services provided by this young Internet included:

- Terminal user remote login, now known as Telnet
- File-transfer protocol (FTP)
- Electronic mail (e-mail)

Telnet allows individuals to log onto a remote computer; for example, using Telnet, you could work with your office computer even when you are on the road. FTP allows one computer user to exchange files with a remote computer. Many computers on the Internet maintain large collections of files, and by using FTP, one can transfer these files from the remote computer without having an individual account on that computer. Unlike Telnet, however, FTP does not let a user write or modify files on the remote computer. (Telnet, FTP, and e-mail are discussed in greater detail below.)

At this time, the Internet was poised to help build one global community, but several hurdles remained. These included:

- Users had to know commands in the UNIX computer language.

- The Internet did not support the GUI and mouse, which would help novices to get started.
- Only simple text was supported (no pictures, sound, or video).
- Information was hard to find, with no catalogs or ''search engines'' (i.e., computer programs developed to search for data on the World Wide Web).

As a consequence, only academicians, researchers, computer professionals, and certain military personnel regularly used the Internet. Two events in the early 1990s, however, changed this situation dramatically, and traffic on the Internet began to rise exponentially. These events were:

- In 1992, Tim Berners-Lee, a physicist working in the European Laboratory for Particle Physics (CERN) in Geneva, developed the Hypertext Markup Language (HTML). Berners-Lee named his system the World Wide Web (also known as WWW, or simply as the Web). HTML permits users to cross-link different documents or ''pages'' on the Web by embedding links to other pages. HTML also is platform-independent, which means it is compatible with different types of computers (e.g., Macintosh and IBM) as well as with different operating systems (e.g., Windows, UNIX, and so on).
- In 1993, Marc Andreessen and his colleagues at the National Center for Supercomputing Applications developed the Mosaic ''browser,'' which is a software program that lets viewers see Web documents written in HTML. In addition to displaying text, Mosaic also automatically handled graphics, images, and sound. It also was very user-friendly: by using a mouse, a viewer could intuitively click from one document to another without having to know a single UNIX command.

These two developments—HTML and the Mosaic browser—made it possible for almost anyone to navigate the Internet, regardless of their computer type, operating system, or computer skills, and after the introduction of Mosaic, traffic on the Internet grew at an astonishing 350,000% per year (5). Since then, several different browsers have been developed, with Netscape Navigator and Microsoft Internet Explorer being the most popular today. In addition, traffic generated by the Web now exceeds all other forms of Internet traffic, and it is expected to soon surpass telephony as the busiest medium for information transfer. More than 80% of the U.S. population now lives in areas with access to the Internet for approximately $20 or less a month.

MEDICAL INFORMATICS TECHNOLOGY PRODUCTS

Physicians can use computers in their practice in many ways. Because computer technology is advancing rapidly, however, it is wise to obtain the most current information before invest-

ing in any hardware or software. Ironically, one of the best ways to find this information is the Internet. Unlike books and printed catalogs, which can be outdated by the time they are published, Internet sites can be renewed and updated at any time, and they are more likely to contain current information.

Medical informatics technology products can be classified broadly, with some overlap, into the following categories (6):

- Medical-practice management
- Computer-based patient records (CPR)
- Medical-literature management
- Diagnostic-decision and pharmaceutic support
- Patient-education material
- Physician continuing medical education (CME) resources

Another product, the portable computing device, is discussed at the end of this section. (These products also have applications in fields other than medicine.)

MEDICAL-PRACTICE MANAGEMENT

Medical-practice management systems help to automate the business aspects of a medical practice. Uses of such products include:

- Automated billing procedures
- Laboratory interface
- Appointment scheduling
- Reminder notices
- Cost analysis
- Time management

Medical-practice management products currently on the market include:

- Medical Manager, Medical Manager Corporation (7)
- PCN Health Network, Physician Computer Network, Inc. (8)
- Practice Partner, Physician Micro Systems, Inc (9).

Released in 1982, Medical Manager was one of the earliest—and most popular—medical-practice management products in the United States. Medical Manager works with DOS and UNIX, and it also can be run over networks. It does not, however, run on the Windows platform. Standard features include:

- Procedure entry
- Billing
- Payment entry
- Insurance office management
- Clinical history
- Appointment scheduler
- Recall notices
- Encounter-form tracking
- Procedure
- Diagnosis
- Financial history and reports

In addition to these features, several optional modules are available, including:

- Managed care
- Claims adjudication
- Electronic-media claims module
- Electronic remittance system
- Data merge
- Custom report generator
- Electronic data interchange interface
- Automated collections module
- Laboratory interface

The other medical-practice management products have features somewhat similar to these, and all of these products are constantly updated.

Some of the features included in these programs can be very time-saving. For example, some products allow creation of customized "macros," which let users post multiple current procedural terminology (CPT) codes with a single entry. This feature could be useful when ordering a panel of laboratory tests frequently ordered together, such as for a "diabetes follow-up panel" (i.e., glycosylated hemoglobin, urinalysis, serum creatinine, and blood glucose level). The macro would allow a user to order and bill for these tests with a single keystroke.

Continuing with the diabetes follow-up example, a "laboratory interface" would send this request electronically to a laboratory. On completion, the laboratory would send back the results, which then would be downloaded directly into the electronic patient file, thus increasing efficiency and reducing errors. The data also can be imported into word-processing software, allowing the physician to create customized letters and reports, and into a spreadsheet program, allowing the creation of graphs to track trends.

Scheduling software, which helps to plan patient appointments, physician activities, and room as well as resource assignments, allows users to create appointment templates for both individual and groups of physicians. The software also can generate automatic appointment reminder notes for regularly scheduled appointments, such as Pap smears. The patient database can be searched and sorted by various parameters (e.g., number of women older than 50 years who missed their annual mammography appointment). This would allow, among other things, birthday notes, thank-you letters, and other correspondence to be generated automatically.

Billing products help to improve cash flow and give physicians more control over their accounts receivable. The software can store insurance information about individual patients and also track claims sent to insurance companies or health-plan offices. In addition, it can generate the amount of copayment required at the time of the service, thus improving cash collection.

COMPUTER-BASED PATIENT RECORDS

Computer-based patient record systems automatically process a wide range of information. Though we have been hearing about a "paperless" medical office for years, CPR systems are taking a long time to arrive, and significant hurdles still remain. Potential benefits of CPR systems (aside from being environmentally correct) include:

- Decreased storage-space requirements
- Increased security of patient information (if proper precautions are taken)
- Potentially instantaneous access to patient data from local or remote sites
- Ability to search for and sort data by different parameters (e.g., the ability to find all patients with diabetes and hypertension who have proteinuria and are not receiving an angiotensin-converting enzyme inhibitor, which can be very helpful for patient care, research, and quality assurance)
- Unified patient records, even when care is administered at different locations at different times, thus resulting in:
  - Improved patient care
  - Cost savings from nonduplication of tests
  - Time savings from eliminating the transfer of medical records
- Improved patient and provider satisfaction
- Prevention of polypharmacy, adverse drug reactions, and drug interactions by incorporating information on allergies, medication lists, creatinine clearance, and other relevant parameters (formulary information of various plans also can be added to help guide prescription writing)
- Increased legibility and consistency of medical records

In short, CPR systems can result in a general improvement of the quality of care. In turn, this can result in significant cost savings.

Some of the stumbling blocks in development of a comprehensive CPR system include:

- To take advantage of all these features, a patient database must be created, which is a tedious, time-consuming, and expensive undertaking.
- Available commercial CPR products can handle most of the functions described here, but they often lack some of these features.
- Choosing the right CPR system and then adapting it to the needs of an individual practice requires a great deal of labor and planning.
- No product will fit into an individual practice without some staff retraining and workflow modification.
- Software and hardware suffer from the absence of uniform standards and from constant revisions.
- Constant changes in the health-care industry challenge clinicians to keep abreast.
- Once a CPR system is implemented, office personnel must enter all data into the new system for it to be effective. This requires persistence and force of will to use only the newer, less familiar system to enter all

data. Both physicians and their staffs must avoid reverting to older, paper-based systems for any operation covered by the newer CPR system.
- Everyone entering data should use uniform terminology. ''Difficulty breathing'' and ''shortness of breath,'' for example, will appear as different items when sorting data by symptoms. This can lead to problems if the person analyzing data is not aware of it.

To solve some of these vexing issues and bring diverse stakeholders together in a neutral forum to develop common health-care information management solutions, a Computer-based Patient Record Institute was formed in 1992 (10). This followed the recommendations of the Institute of Medicine report on Computer-based Patient Records (11). Today, several CPR products are available, including:

- Logician is a CPR system produced by MedicaLogic (12). A demonstration of this software can be downloaded from their Web site.
- Turbo-Doc is ''Pen''-based software, designed by Dr. Lyle Hunt, to help complete patient-encounter notes in less time. You can see the features of this product and order a demonstration disk from their Web site (13).
- Pathways Smart Medical Record is produced by HBO and Company. A demonstration of the product can be downloaded from their Web site (14).

Another Web site maintains a comprehensive list of such CPR products (15). These allow one to generate a patient-encounter note by clicking on a menu of choices. The note that is generated can be modified or added to before printing. These programs also often include a collection of images, which can be quickly modified by the physician (e.g., the site of a murmur can be drawn on the image showing the chest). In addition, some of these systems allow one to dictate a short sentence or note, which then is transcribed by the computer. Such voice recognition technology is still in its infancy, however. Newer versions of these products can run on Windows, thus making it easy to integrate them with existing software. Some also have a range of electronic data interfaces that enables data sharing with practice-management software, laboratories, transcription services, and other hospital information systems.

Even after the right system is purchased and adapted for a particular practice, however, much work still remains. All the patient data on paper must be entered into the CPR system to create a database. Other information (e.g., addresses and phone numbers of referring physicians, consultants, laboratories, and other members of the group; formulary information; range of available laboratory and radiologic tests, and so on) must be imported into the new system and updated to make use of all the software's features. The better the data interface of the system, the easier this process is. Otherwise, all of these data need to be entered manually.

The CPR system should be compatible with the data system used by your laboratory. This will allow importing or downloading of results directly into the CPR system, thus saving time and reducing errors. It also should be possible to enter data into the patient record at multiple sites (e.g., the nurse should be able to enter the vital signs and medication lists; the physician should be able to enter the patient history, physical examination findings, and the assessment and plan of treatment). On selecting the plan of treatment, most systems automatically will generate the requisitions for investigations and prescriptions, which can be printed or sent electronically to the laboratory or pharmacy.

Despite all efforts, however, there always are some pieces of the patient record, such as external reports, that continue to be on paper. To integrate these into the CPR may require scanning of the document, which produces a facsimile, but this facsimile can be difficult to modify or edit. Optical character recognition is a technology by which text on scanned documents can be captured in a word-processing format. Voice and handwriting recognition technology are two other ways of inputting data without having to type it manually, but neither of these technologies is practical for widespread use as yet.

Digital data require very little storage space. For example, Microsoft Bookshelf 1997, a popular software package on a computer compact disc (CD) measuring 5.25 inches, holds the entire content of the *American Heritage Dictionary, Columbia Dictionary of Quotations, Columbia Encyclopedia, Concise Encarta World Atlas, Internet Directory of Web Sites, Peoples Chronology, Roget's Thesaurus,* and *The 1996 World Almanac.* The advantages of this in terms of saved storage space are obvious.

One concern about digital data is that without proper safeguards, it can be altered without leaving a trace of an alteration having occurred. This problem can be overcome, however, by periodically backing up the data and storing a copy off-site (e.g., at a legal office). This also protects the data from being destroyed by any system breakdown or disaster.

Data security is another issue that always crops up during talk of digital data. The concern is that data, whether on computers connected with networks or otherwise, can be accessed by unauthorized individuals. Compared with paper-based data, digital data is easier to transcribe into different formats and then copy. The small storage size makes it easier to hide and transport as well. On the other hand, data on computers can be protected better than that on paper records. Use of encryption, automatic password generators, and firewalls can make data theft almost impossible. In addition, audit trails, which are mechanisms that make it is possible to track every user who has looked at a digital record, can determine whether the use was unauthorized and record if the data were modified after being created. Use of audit trails and strict company policies about CPRs can be very strong deterrents to unauthorized use.

MEDICAL-LITERATURE MANAGEMENT

Medical-literature management consists of using a PC to access and retrieve relevant medical literature and then maintain that information in a computerized database. Physicians and patients both are switching from anecdotal to evidence-based medicine. Printed textbooks often are somewhat out of date by the time they are published, however, and even if physicians read two or three journal articles each day, they will be years behind in their reading by the end of the first year. Having ready access to a searchable database of medical literature thus is becoming a necessity.

The Medical Literature Analysis and Retrieval System (MEDLARS) is the information retrieval system of the U.S. National Library of Medicine (NLM). It provides access to over 40 online databases, containing roughly 18 million records. MEDLINE (MEDlars onLINE) is NLM's premier bibliographic database covering the fields of medicine, nursing, dentistry, veterinary medicine, and preclinical sciences. Journal articles are indexed for MEDLINE, and their citations are searchable using NLM's controlled vocabulary, the Medical Subject Headings. MEDLINE contains all citations published in *Index Medicus,* and it corresponds in part to the *International Nursing Index* and *Index to Dental Literature.* Citations include the English abstract when published with the article (approximately 75% of the current file). MEDLINE has over 8.5 million citations of articles from over 3700 international biomedical journals published between 1966 and the present. More than 30,000 new citations are added each month. A searchable file of each monthly update is available as the Selective Dissemination of Information Online (SDILINE).

MEDLARS also includes other databases, such as AIDS-LINE, AIDSDRUGS, TOXLIT, and CHEMLINE. Another useful database is Health Services, Technology, Administration, and Research (HealthSTAR), which covers both clinical (i.e., emphasizing evaluation of patient outcomes and effectiveness of procedures, programs, products, services, and processes) and nonclinical (i.e., emphasizing health-care administration and planning) aspects of health-care delivery.

Physicians can access MEDLINE either directly through the NLM or through commercial services. Several Internet sites also provide free access to the MEDLINE database. The search engines used by each of these services differ in their features, however. For direct access through the NLM, you may use either Grateful Med (i.e., NLM's user-friendly interface), PubMed, or direct commands (i.e., command language searching) via Telnet to search the MEDLARS databases:

- Grateful Med is available for Windows and Macintosh platforms as well as in an Internet version. These can be downloaded from the NLM Web site (16). One can use a dial-up modem (i.e., modulator-demodulator) connection to the NLM's computer to search their databases using Grateful Med, or one can use the Internet Grateful Med through the Web.
- PubMed (17) is a Web search tool developed by the National Center for Biotechnology Information at the NLM. It is used to access literature citations and link to full-text journals at Web sites of participating biomedical publishers.

The amount you are charged per search depends on the length of time you are connected to the NLM computer and the amount of information you retrieve. A typical search can cost between $1.25 and $5.00.

As mentioned, several commercial services also provide access to MEDLINE and some of the other databases of MEDLARS. These services include:

- Ovid, Ovid Technologies (18)
- SilverPlatter, SilverPlatter Information (19)
- PaperChase, (20)

These services have their own search engines and interfaces, and they vary in their pricing and the number of databases that can be accessed.

MEDLINE systems are available as CD sets, which are periodically updated databases on CDS, or as on-line databases. The CD sets can be quite expensive for individual physicians, unless they are interested in a limited number of databases covering only a few years. The advantage is that a physician owns the set and does not incur charges for each search and retrieval. In addition, a search done in this manner is quicker, because it does not require connection to a remote computer either over telephone lines or the Internet. These sets can be purchased with a multiuser license by a group of physicians, and they even can be placed on a network. The initial set-up cost can be quite high in such cases, however, and also may require maintenance of the network connections.

The quicker, easier, and often, cheaper option may be to access an on-line database, either over the Internet or by a dial-up modem connection. The current trend is to connect with one of these services via the Internet, either for a fixed fee of approximately $20.00 per month for unlimited searching or in a "pay-as-you-go" format. The advantage here is that Web technology allows access to the service from your home, office, hospital, or anywhere there is a PC or Macintosh, with only a user name and a password required. The only other charge incurred is the Internet access, which many physicians already have. Most services provide full-text articles, which can be mailed or faxed to you for a fee of $10.00 to $20.00. Some even provide a hypertext link to the full-text article, which then can be viewed or printed instantly.

In addition to commercial services, a number of Internet sites provide free access to MEDLINE and some of the other MEDLARS databases (21–24). Quite a few of these do not have as advanced a search capability as the commercial services, however, do not provide full-text articles, or are financed through advertisements.

Physicians' Online is a proprietary service that also provides free MEDLINE searches and other services for physicians, residents in training, and medical students. First, however, one must install the free software provided by the company. This software can be ordered from their Web site (25).

Aside from accessing citations, literature management also involves creating and maintaining a personal, searchable database of articles and citations. This includes—but is not limited to—citations and articles retrieved from MEDLINE searches, copied (or cut out from) journals, personal bibliography and teaching notes, talks, and slide collections. A number of database products are available to help automate these tasks. These products include:

- ProCite, Research Information Systems (26)
- Reference Manager, Research Information Systems (27)
- EndNote Plus, Niles Software, Inc. (28)

The advantages of using such systems are numerous:

- They allow automatic importing of electronically retrieved citations into the database.
- Notes can be added to citations, either by typing or scanning.
- Searching the database is possible by subject, keywords, journal, or author name.
- When writing a research project or book chapter, copying and pasting information from the database into a word processor can automatically create a bibliography.
- The bibliography can be quickly formatted to a particular style (e.g., uniform abbreviations for journal names).
- The same system can be used to file administrative, financial, and other documents that may be needed in the future.

Several of these products also provide a periodic update of the medical literature from certain databases, such as MEDLINE. These updates are mailed as diskettes or e-mail, or they can be retrieved by FTP from the vendors' computers. These updates make it easy to keep up with the literature in one's field. Updates usually work only with the database product sold by the vendor, however. For example, UnCover Reveal is a product designed to work with EndNote, and Reference Update works with Reference Manager. QuickScan Reviews is produced by Educational Reviews, Inc., and it comes with its own database-management software called KeyInfo Manager.

DIAGNOSTIC DECISION SUPPORT SYSTEMS OR COMPUTER-AIDED DIAGNOSTIC SYSTEMS

Diagnostic decision and pharmaceutic support (DDS) provide searchable references to guide test, prescription, and treatment strategies. That computers will be able to diagnose medical conditions has been the subject of many science-fiction movies. Unfortunately, or fortunately as the case may be, this is still just a pipe dream. There are products that generate a list of differential diagnoses in response to some clinical or laboratory finding, but none of these can substitute for the common-sense approach of a competent physician. What they can do—as the name indicates—is support the diagnostic process.

Typical products include:

- Quick Medical Reference, or QMR, University of Pittsburgh and Camdat Corporation (29)
- Iliad—Univ. of Utah and Mosby Consumer Health (30)
- DXplain Massachusetts General Hospital (31)
- Meditel Adult Diagnostic System

These products have received a somewhat unfavorable review for computer-assisted diagnoses (32). Nevertheless, they still can be useful in certain ways:

- They may help to generate a more complete differential diagnosis, which may be useful for patients in whom common or obvious diseases have been ruled out or are considered to be unlikely.
- In cases with seemingly unrelated clinical findings, a DDS system may be able to determine a set of possible, unifying diagnoses.
- They may be used to find out how common a particular symptom, sign, or test result is among patients with a particular disease and, thus, help to rule out (or rule in) a certain condition.
- Some of these products come bundled with simulated cases, which can be used as academic exercises, especially for medical students and residents.
- They may be used in ''browse'' mode as textbooks. Unlike textbooks that describe all findings associated with a particular disease, however, these can be used to list all diseases associated with a particular clinical finding as well as the strength of the association.

The limitations of these systems partly result from their finite database and the logic that they use. Not all diseases and findings can be included in a DDS. System databases include 600 to 2000 diseases and 400 to 4500 clinical findings. In addition, these programs may not be up-to-date with current medical literature.

The inference engine of these programs may use a probabilistic approach (i.e., one based on Bayes' theorem) or a heuristic approach (i.e., one that tries to emulate human reasoning by using weights and strengths of association). There are drawbacks to each approach, the descriptions of which are beyond the scope of this chapter. These programs also depend on the completeness of the data input by the user. For example, in a case of pulmonary embolism, if one enters ''shortness of breath'' and ''chest pain'' as symptoms, the program may rate pneumonia and myocardial infarction as being more likely than the correct diagnosis. If one adds some data about a swollen leg or a duplex ultrasound that is positive for acute thrombophlebitis, however, pulmonary embolism may be included into the top three possible diagnoses listed.

It is easy to be critical of these programs but one should remember that DDS systems were designed to support the clinician and not replace him or her. When this is kept in mind, there are a number of uses that these can be put to as pointed out above.

Pharmaceutic support systems (PSS) are reference materials in an electronic format that can help to guide decisions about use of medications and to screen for drug interactions.

In addition, they may help to educate patients about their medications, automatically maintain and update medication lists, and print prescriptions. Access to such reference sources can be through CDS on a PC, over a network, or through a Web site featuring such material. Pharmaceutical reference products currently available on CDS include:

- AskRx (33) Camdat Corporation
- Clinical Pharmacology (34) Gold Standard Multimedia
- Clinical Reference Library (35) Lexi-Comp Inc.
- PDR (36) Medical Economics Company
- Drugdex (37) Micromedix Inc.
- Mosby's GenRx (38) Mosby Inc.

Some of these products are designed mainly as reference sources with search capabilities. Others have additional features, including:

- Automatic screening for drug interactions
- Printing of prescriptions
- Generating patient education and information material
- Allowing for easy refills by presenting a menu of previous prescriptions for each patient
- Maintaining records of allergies, and alerting physicians about them
- Providing a list of all medications that can be used to treat a particular disease
- Generating lists of all medications that may cause a particular side effect

Other products combine a standard medical reference source with a PSS. These products include:

- Harrison's Plus (39) contains the entire text of *Harrison's Principles of Internal Medicine* plus selected references from the last 10 years of MEDLINE and the USP DI, Volume 1.
- I-MED (40) has the entire text of *Stein's Internal Medicine, Mosby's GenRx,* and selected references from the last 7 years of MEDLINE.
- STAT!-Ref (41) is available in various packages for internal medicine, and it includes *Stein's Internal Medicine, The Merck Manual, Current Diagnosis and Treatment,* and drug information from the USP DI, Volume 1, and the *Medical Letter.* Some packages also include material from additional reference sources.

These products combine the most commonly used reference sources, and they provide cross-links so that one can read about a disease, see what medication is used for treatment, and then read details about the medication. Using such a product on a computer in the examination room can save time, decrease errors, improve the quality of care, and increase both patient and provider satisfaction.

Limitations of such products, however, include:

- They usually are designed for only one or two operating systems.
- The physician must change the CD to access the information on another CD.

- The CDS must be carried home if the physician needs access to them from there.
- The CDS are difficult to share between several physicians in a group.

Some of these problems can be overcome by putting the CDS on an office network. One difficulty with this, however, is that this approach increases overhead and requires maintenance. A solution to this is taking advantage of such reference material on the Web. An increasing number of sites now offer a combination of such products. Some require a subscription; others provide free service to the physicians with a valid Drug Enforcement Administration number. On registering, an account is created that can be accessed by typing in a unique identification code and password. These sites can be accessed by any computer connected to the Web, regardless of its operating system and geographic location. The only other cost is that for Internet access. Representative sites include:

- Clinical Pharmacology Online (42)
- PDRnet (24)
- Medical Economics Interactive (43)
- Mosby's GenRx (38)
- Physicians' Online (25)
- InteliHealth (44)
- Rxlist (45)

PATIENT-EDUCATION MATERIAL

Patient-education software generates customized instructional material. A patient who is better educated is more likely to participate productively in his or her own care. In the present health-care environment, in which physicians are expected to increase their efficiency and productivity, physicians often do not have the time to go over the various aspects of diseases and medications with their patients. On the other hand, patients who know more about their disease and medications may have fewer adverse effects from their treatment, need fewer visits to the emergency room, and have fewer complications from chronic diseases. Thus, patient education may improve patient satisfaction and decrease the cost of health care.

One way to improve patient education without taking precious time away from the physician schedules is an electronic patient-education system. Such a system may include information about diseases, diet and nutrition, medications, and even advice about first aid and self-treatment of nonurgent medical conditions.

Patient education can be in the form of handouts generated by a computer or of interactive, computer-based programs. Programs that allow a physician to generate customized patient handouts include:

- Adult Health Advisor (46), which comes as a DOS- or Windows-based program for patient education about medical conditions, procedures, and so on.
- Patient Instruction Generator (47), which is a Windows-

based program that produces handouts for disease conditions and medications.

- AskAdvice (48), which is linked to AskRx and generates patient-education leaflets regarding medications.
- Patient Ed (49), which is a Windows-based program that generates customized care instructions and documents these in an electronic record.

Interactive, computer-based patient-education programs include:

- The Mayo Clinic Family Health Book (50)
- The Mayo Clinic Family Pharmacist (51)

As with most areas of software development, much progress is being made in using the Web to better educate patients. Increasingly, patients are turning to the Internet to find answers to their health-care questions. There are several Web sites that physicians can recommend, and there are other sites that physicians can use to print out patient-education material. One difficulty with these sites, however, is that it is difficult to customize the material. There also are issues of copyright violation if the material is downloaded into a computer and then modified by the physician. Another issue is that at the time of this writing, most sites were not sufficiently comprehensive; therefore, one might have to search three or four different sites to find the material one wants. Typical Web sites of this nature include:

- Aetna U.S. Healthcare, a managed health-care company, has a site with patient-education leaflets regarding various medical conditions. Aetna U.S. Healthcare also finances a site called InteliHealth, which is a consumer health information site maintained by the Johns Hopkins University and Health System (44).
- The American Association of Family Physicians has its Web site at HealthAnswers (52).
- Healthtouch provides information on various disease conditions. This information is reviewed and approved by national health associations or health agencies (53).
- UCLA Student Health Services, which includes topics of interest to adolescent and young-adult patients (54).

Some potential advantages of such patient-education material are:

- Time saved in the physician's schedule
- Improved patient and provider satisfaction
- Increased patient compliance
- Increased patient involvement in their own health care and, thus, improved outcomes
- Better utilization of health-care resources.

PHYSICIANS' CONTINUING MEDICAL EDUCATION RESOURCES

Continuing medical education software and Internet products help physicians to conveniently and cost-effectively acquire

CME credits. Most physicians in academic settings receive CME credits from attending grand rounds, institutional conferences, and teaching residents. Many other physicians, however, are forced to attend regional or national conferences to meet their CME credit requirements. This often requires traveling to out-of-town sites and leaving a practice for that period of time. This can be difficult for solo practitioners, and even for physicians practicing in small groups. There also may be personal or family reasons to avoid such travel.

For this group of physicians, there are journals and CME programs such as the Medical Knowledge Self-Assessment Program (MKSAP) of the American College of Physicians, which provides CME credits on completion of multiple-choice questions based on material in a journal or book. This process has been made more interesting and interactive with the advent of computer-based CME material and CME programs on the Internet. These programs are feasible for physicians with multimedia-capable computer that, in the latter case, also is connected with the Internet.

Some sources for CD (compact disc) or diskette CME programs include:

- Med-Challenger IM 97 and Med-Challenger FP 97 (55), which contain clinical reference and educational materials on CDs that provide CME credits for internists and family practitioners, respectively. Each CD comes bundled with 50 hours of category 1 CME credits.
- Scientific American Medicine CD (56), which is the CD version of the popular *Scientific American Medicine*. It is updated quarterly and, with the recent inclusion of USP DI, is a complete reference tool. It also includes the DISCOTEST, which are interactive patient modules that offer up to 32 category 1 CME credits from Stanford University.
- PrimePractice (57), which is a CD series for primary-care practitioners. Each CD consists of simulated cases in a particular subspecialty. One can get 10 category 1 CME credits per year from each CD.
- The MKSAP (58) from the American College of Physicians is now available on CD. It is a valuable reference tool, a great way to keep up with current medical practice, and a source for 146 category 1 CME credits.
- Core Curriculum in Primary Care (59), which is available as a series of 18 CD titles, each covering a different area of primary care. Each disc is worth four category 1 CME credits.

In addition to being a source of CME credits, these products are also valuable reference tools.

Recently, a number of Web sites have begun offering CME credits as well. These CME modules usually consist of several questions based on an article or a case presentation. The article may be viewed online or downloaded from the site. Questions generally are answered online. With the improvement in Web technology, an increasing amount of interaction is being included in these modules.

One problem in this area is the lack of uniform standards for multimedia files on the Web. These files can be in various audio, video, animation, three-dimensional, and interactive formats, and depending on the operating system and browser being used, one may need special software called "plug-ins" to view these files. Some of these plug-ins are available for, and supported by, only the two most popular browsers (i.e., Netscape Navigator and Microsoft Internet Explorer). These files are best viewed with the higher-end computers and monitors. The speed at which these files are downloaded depends on the type of connection one has to the Internet, and because these multimedia files can be quite large, the download process sometimes can be quite slow.

Despite these limitations, a number of Web sites provide interesting ways to get CME credits. These include:

- Physicians' Online (25) hosts modules offering CME from the University of Arizona, and the Cleveland Clinic Foundation is starting a series of CME modules in various subspecialties of internal medicine, which will also be at this site. These modules will be based on articles from the *Cleveland Clinic Journal of Medicine.* A sample of one such module already is available on the Web (60). The entire article can be viewed online or printed, and then five to seven multiple choice questions need to be answered. The viewer must get the correct answer to proceed to the next question. An explanation is offered for each choice that the viewer makes, and the entire process, including submission of an application for CME credits, can be completed online. The exercise itself is free, but the if viewer wants CME credits, there is an $8.00 fee for each credit.

- American Health Consultants (61) offer CME modules based on its publications, such as *Internal Medicine Alert.*

- The University of Florida College of Medicine (62) has, at the time of this writing, one internal medicine online module offering one free category 1 credit. The viewer must print out a form containing eight questions based on four cases that can be seen online. The form must be faxed or mailed back to get the CME credit.

- Marshall University School of Medicine (63) has one case called the "Interactive Patient." This module offers one category 1 CME credit for $15.00. The format is extremely user-friendly and allows viewers to ask questions of a simulated patient using a natural language search tool. After going through a patient history and physical examination, the participant is asked to select a diagnosis and a treatment. The correct answer, along with an explanation, is e-mailed to the viewer. To apply for CME credits, a form must be printed and mailed back.

This area is still in its infancy, with most sites offering only one or, at most, few such CME modules. Other specialty sites offer CME over the Web in specialty areas like cardiology, emergency medicine, radiology, and pathology. The number of sites offering online CME surely will increase as the popularity of the Internet does among physicians.

PORTABLE COMPUTING DEVICES

Portable computing devices (also known as Portable Digital Assistants [PDAs]) have been around for many years and, simply stated, were something of a cross between a laptop computer and an electronic organizer. Just a few years ago, they were basically overgrown organizers, cost 10 times as much as they do today, were heavier, could not communicate with a desktop PC, and entailed much difficulty in entering information. Since then, however, a lot has changed. A large number of models and brands now are available, and Microsoft recently entered the market with its own operating system, called Windows CE for PDAs. At the time of this writing, five different PDAs that run on Windows CE are available. These PDAs are called Handheld PCs (HPA) and include:

- Casio Cassiopeia
- Compaq PC Companion
- NEC Mobile Pro
- Philips Velo 1
- HP 300 series

Other PDAs that have been around longer and use proprietary operating systems include:

- Apple Newton Message Pad 2000
- Sharp Zaurus ZR-3000
- U.S. Robotics Pilot
- Psion Series 3c
- HP 200LX (DOS-based)

A full discussion of each individual PDA and HPA is beyond the scope of this chapter. Information can be found on the Web, however, at a site that compares some of these handheld PCs (64). The HP 300 series is the most recent addition, and it boasts a wide screen that displays the entire breadth of the desktop screen, with no need to scroll sideways.

Considering recent advances, much can be accomplished by these palmtop computers:

- They have smaller versions of word-processing, spreadsheet, database, and appointment-and-scheduling software.
- Some have handwriting recognition software, which allows data entry by writing on the screen with a stylus. (The U.S. Robotics Pilot has a system called "Graffiti," which requires modified printing and a little training but, thereafter, seems to work very well.)
- You can receive e-mail and even browse the Web. Unfortunately, however, in most cases the screens are too small, the lighting is too dim, or navigation of the Web hypertext links must be done with arrow keys. Therefore, these devices generally are not ideal for Web browsing.

- Using either built-in modems or PC Memory Card International Association (PCMCIA) cards, one can send and receive faxes.
- They communicate with desktop PCs using either cable, docking stations, or infrared technology. Thus, it is easy to update files on the desktop with work done on the PDA, or to download addresses and schedules to the PDA from the desktop.
- Medical software has been developed for some of these systems by third parties. The HP 200LX, being DOS-based, probably has the most third-party applications available. These can allow you to calculate creatinine clearance or body mass index without remembering formulae, carry a database of patients, print notes instead of writing them by hand, teach medical students and residents from electronic teaching files such as electrocardiograms (ECGs), and so on. With the introduction of a popular operating systems like Windows CE, one can expect much software to be developed for these devices.
- It is possible to attach a pager card to the PDA and, thus, use these devices to receive messages.

Thus, a possible scenario in the not-too-distant future could be:

- A patient calls your office while you are out.
- Your secretary takes down the message and pages you on your PDA.
- The PDA displays the entire text of the message.
- You look up the patient information on your PDA database, maybe use some of its medical software, and make your clinical decision.
- Using wireless communication, you e-mail a message to your secretary, asking her to set up an appointment with a consultant. You also send a copy of this e-mail to the consultant with a copy of the message sent to you by the secretary as an attachment.

This may sound very futuristic, but the technology is already available. The question remaining is agreeing on a uniform technology and deciding whether it is worth the investment for your practice.

TELECOMMUNICATIONS, THE INTERNET, AND MEDICINE

The changes now occurring in the health-care industry have coincided with explosive changes in the telecommunication industry. It has been said that the speed of the microprocessor driving PCS approximately doubles every year. The number of subscribers connected to the Internet also is growing at an exponential rate, with an increase of almost 100% each year. (Compared with this, the worldwide population "explosion" is a paltry 1.6% annual increase.) It is believed that the number of subscribers on the Internet worldwide will surpass 1 billion by the year 2000. If the Internet continues to grow at the present rate, the number of subscribers would theoretically surpass the world population by the year 2004 (65)!

The Internet is the biggest advance in communications since the invention of the printing press. It will change how we do business, and the health-care industry will be no exception. We now look at some features of the Internet, as it exists today, that contribute to its tremendous popularity.

ELECTRONIC MAIL

Electronic mail is an asynchronous mode of communication between two or more people using computers that are connected to each other through a local or a wide area network, or that are on separate networks that are connected to each other (e.g., over the Internet). E-mail was a serendipitous discovery of the original ARPANET, but it has grown to be one of the most powerful and popular features of the Internet. The advantages of e-mail include:

- *Asynchronous mode of communication:* Physicians can communicate with other health-care providers or patients without being interrupted by phone calls and pagers.
- *Ability to save or print the messages:* Unlike voice messages, which are difficult to include in patient records, e-mail messages can be printed and attached to the chart. If the office has a CPR system, the message can be saved on the computer or copied and pasted into the patient record without any typing or manual filing. This leads to more complete, legible, and error-proof medical records.
- *Speed:* Compared to traditional mail service (or "snail mail"), e-mail usually is faster and more reliable. On closed networks, protocols can allow one to find out if a message was received and if it was opened. If the address is incorrect, most systems on the Internet will return the original message, along with an explanation, almost instantly.
- *Ability to send or forward a copy to a number of recipients:* A copy of an e-mail message to a referring physician can be sent to a patient without much additional secretarial labor. In the same way, a copy of an e-mail received from a consultant can be forwarded to a patient.
- *Attachment of files:* Files attached to an e-mail message are delivered in the same way. This allows a physician to send research data, ECGs, radiographs, and other kinds of files. It is, of course, necessary that these files be in a digital format and accessible to the physician, either on the computer or on the network. Otherwise, the material can be scanned into a digital format. Radiologic data generated by computers (e.g., computed tomographic [CT] scans) are already in digital format and can be sent easily in this manner.
- *Automatic filing:* It is possible to set up rules within the e-mail system so that messages from certain people or

containing certain subject matter are filed automatically in the appropriate folders.

- *Cost savings:* Except for the initial set-up cost and the on-going expense of Internet access, the entire process is free, thus saving on stationery and postage expenses. In addition, the features mentioned earlier also increase efficiency and reduce costs.

Concerns and problems with using e-mail in the medical field include:

- *Privacy and security:*
  - This is always a concern, but it is especially so with e-mail. Data transmitted over the Internet are broken up into small bits or packets. These data then pass from node to node, until they reach their final destination. There, the data are reassembled into the complete message. It is possible to intercept this message as it passes through one of the nodes, and certain people have set up programs that search for information streams coding for credit-card numbers as it passes through a given computer on the Internet. This is called "sniffing," and it has led to fear about use of this medium for transmitting sensitive patient information.
  - Techniques have been developed to counter this problem. Encryption of e-mail messages is possible. Paul Zimmerman has developed a program called Pretty Good Privacy (PGP), which is available, along with instruction on using it, as freeware (66). Other commercial programs also are available. RSA Data Security (67) is a pioneer in this field and has developed the RSA public key encryption system, which is utilized by PGP. Verisign (68) is another prominent company in the field. Using their software, Secure/Multipurpose Internet Mail Extensions (S/MIME), it is possible to send encrypted e-mail and also put a personal digital identification on it; therefore, the recipient knows that you, and no one else, sent it and that it has not been altered.
- *Compatibility of various e-mail systems:*
  - Most large group practices with a computer network usually will have the same e-mail client (i.e., software). This permits transmission of attached files in various formats. This may not be quite as easy, however, if files need to be transferred to a separate network over the Internet. Several protocols are available for transmitting these attached files, and if the protocols being used by the sender and receiver are not compatible, the receiver will get a series of mathematic or other symbols instead of, for example, a CT scan.
  - Multipurpose Internet Mail Extensions refers to an official Internet standard that specifies how messages must be formatted so they can be exchanged between different e-mail systems. MIME is a very flexible format, permitting one to include virtually any type of file or document in an e-mail message. Thus, MIME messages may contain text, images, audio, video, and so on. To ensure that e-mail messages containing images or other nontext information will be delivered with maximum protection against corruption, MIME provides a way for nontext information to be encoded as text. This encoding is known as "base64 encoding."
  - Users of e-mail clients that do not support MIME need a program that will decode this text and convert it back into an image (or the original nontext format). Two such programs are "mpack" and "munpack," which are available as freeware from the Carnegie Mellon University FTP site (69). Another such program, which is easier to install, is Wincode; it is available as shareware (70). (After a trial period, shareware must be registered for a small fee). Other encoding standards for transferring nontext files are called UUencode and BinHex.
  - Using decoding programs is not a panacea, however. Sometimes, encoded files get damaged (i.e., corrupted) during transit from one network and server to another. For example, with BinHex encoding, every line in the file is 64 characters long. If this gets changed, then it cannot be properly decoded. Until uniform standards are developed and accepted, some of these problems will persist.
- *Computer or network breakdowns:*
  - If the network or computer system goes down, then a practice or group that depends almost exclusively on e-mail for communication may run into difficulties. (This is true even for the telephone system, however.) To keep such "crashes" to a minimum, it is best to have a temporary back-up system that can provide temporary power to individual computers so that data are not lost.
- *Access to physician's e-mail address:*
  - It is possible to find your e-mail address using search engines on the Internet. Some physicians may find this objectionable, but if you think about it, it is no different from any other database with your address. Also, getting e-mail is no different from the other "junk" mail or other unsolicited mail that you get at your home or office. In fact, it is easier to delete an undesirable e-mail message than to tear up and throw away a piece of paper.

DISCUSSION GROUPS

Discussion groups are "virtual dinner parties" or "cyber cafes," in which like-minded people "meet" and discuss common interests. One such arrangement is called a "listserv," which is a system whereby e-mails are sent to one address and then redistributed to all the subscribers in that group. Thousands of such listservs are in operation on the Internet.

To join a listserv, one sends an e-mail to a specific address. Either in the subject area or the body of the message, a particular phrase is included. This automatically starts the subscription to that listserv. The arrangement to unsubscribe is similar, but the address to which e-mails are sent for discussion usually is different from the one to which the subscription message is sent.

Another arrangement is called a bulletin board. Here, all messages sent to the discussion group are posted at a particular site. This is the system by which Usenet newsgroups operate on the Internet. There are eight major categories of Usenet newsgroups:

1. COMP (computer-related topics),
2. MISC (miscellaneous topics),
3. REC (recreation topics),
4. SCI (science topics),
5. SOC (social-related issues),
6. TALK (anything goes, like talk radio),
7. NEWS (news-related topics), and
8. ALT (alternate topics that do not fit anywhere else).

Thousands of groups can be in each category, and each group is dedicated to a particular subject. For example, "sci.med.informatics" is a newsgroup dedicated to discussing medical informatics on the Internet. Unlike listservs, however, most newsgroups do not need subscriptions.

In addition to listservs and newsgroups, there also are mailing lists, which operate similarly to listservs but do not allow one to send e-mails. Mailing lists are used to distribute electronic newsletters to a group of people over the Internet. The process of subscribing and unsubscribing is very similar to that for listservs. Lists of health-related Usenet newsgroups and health topic–related mailing lists can be found on the Web (71–73). There also are mailing lists that update subscribers about general health news, which may be of interest to health-care professionals or the general public. Health-update mailing lists include:

- Medscape Medpulse (23)
- InteliHealth (44)
- Doctor's Guide to the Internet, E-mail Edition (74)

Discussion groups can be useful in several ways:

- Geographically diverse people can meet and discuss common interests. This helps to break down ethnic and geographic barriers, overcome prejudice, and build a truly global community. It also can help speed multicenter research projects, find answers and compare notes on treatment of worldwide diseases, and so on.
- It is possible to conduct journal clubs or educational courses at a distance. (I recently participated in a journal club on medical education and another course on clinical epidemiology, each of which had participants from many countries.)
- Subscribing to mailing lists is an easy way to keep updated on the medical field. The Centers for Disease Control and Prevention Web site (75) lets one subscribe to an e-mail version of the *Morbidity and Mortality Weekly Report,* which is sent to your computer every week free of charge.
- One can find answers to problems that other people have faced and solved. It is possible to post questions about a difficult case on a discussion group and get a free consult!
- It is often useful to "lurk" on medical-related groups to see what patients are discussing. This can give physicians a new perspective on the disease and also prepare them for questions a patient might ask the next day.
- An ideal use for discussion groups is to continue a conversation after a conference is over and its participants have dispersed.

Some problems and concerns about discussion groups include:

- Because it often is not possible to identify who is posting information, one should be careful before accepting it at face value. One solution is to subscribe to moderated discussion groups, in which someone attempts to monitor the whole process. In addition, some discussion groups are limited to physicians (e.g., the ones on Physicians' Online).
- Certain discussion groups collect messages and then distribute them at periodic intervals. Others send them as soon as they are received. If a group is very large or busy, your e-mail in-box can be flooded with messages. Therefore, it is a good idea to unsubscribe to groups that are not as useful, stimulating, or interesting as expected. Bulletin boards avoid this problem by posting messages at one place rather than e-mailing them to participants. Bulletin board messages also are threaded by topic, which makes it easier to follow the discussion.
- Certain people take advantage of discussion groups by posting advertisements for products related to the subject. Most groups have a moderator who, if informed of this, will remove that person from the discussion list. Such removals may be necessary to prevent the group from degenerating from its original intent.

FILE TRANSFER PROTOCOL

As discussed earlier, FTP allows the transfer of large files in various formats over the Internet. This is different from attaching files to an e-mail. Usually, FTP is used for downloading large files from remote computers that are repositories for many such files. A number of universities and other sites maintain collections of files for downloading. Most of these sites allow anonymous logins (i.e., one does not need a special account to be set up to download the files). Generally, the user ID is "anonymous," as is the password, or it is one's e-mail address. Medical software also sometimes can be downloaded in this manner.

Today, most allow automatic downloading of files by FTP, so there is no need for special FTP software (unless you want to upload files to a remote computer). Unless they are in charge of maintaining a Web site, most physicians will not need to upload such files. If they are in charge of such a site, the Web pages are created on the PC and then uploaded by FTP to the server connected to the Internet. One site with a collection of patient-education material, medical-education software, statistical programs, and so on available for download by FTP is at the University of California, Irvine (76).

TERMINAL EMULATION (TELNET)

Terminal emulation, or Telnet, is a protocol for one computer to talk with another computer over a network. In most situations today, this means the desktop PC is talking with another computer and acting like a display terminal, thus the name ''terminal emulation.'' This protocol allows you to perform tasks using applications on the remote computer.

You need to have an account with the remote computer before you can use Telnet to work on it. Another problem is that Telnet requires some complex UNIX commands, with which most physicians are not familiar. Some interface programs are available that can make this task easier, however, and this often is the case with certain hospital scheduling and results-reporting systems. Here, the computer on the desk acts like a ''dumb'' terminal and relays commands to the mainframe computer over the network. Based on those commands, the desktop screen displays the laboratory results or appointment schedules, but the results being displayed actually are on the mainframe, not the desktop PC. The desktop machine is acting simply as the display screen or dumb terminal; its microprocessor is not involved in the process.

The problem with this type of system is that the capacity of the desktop microprocessor is being wasted. If the data actually were residing on the desktop PC, physicians would be able to work with it in many ways, such as sorting it by name of physician, importing it into a personal database, writing reminder notes next to the laboratory results, and so on.

Telnet has other uses as well. For example, it allows you to login to your computer or network when you are out of town or at home to check your e-mail, work on files, and so on.

THE WEB

Since the introduction of HTML and the browser in 1991 and 1992, the number of people using the Internet has increased exponentially, and new advances are being made at breakneck pace. New browsers also have been developed to view these HTML files over the Internet. In addition, these browsers can send and receive e-mail, let you participate in newsgroups, and retrieve files automatically from sites allowing anony-

mous FTP. Thus, most of the original functions of the Internet can be accomplished by a single application: the browser.

Out of this explosion of activity, two browsers have emerged as leaders in the field. These are Netscape Navigator and Microsoft Internet Explorer.

Many different types of content besides text can be seen on the Web today, including images, audio, animation, video, and interactive content. These multimedia files require special applications (i.e., plug-ins) that work with the browser. Some of these applications come bundled with the browser; others are developed by third parties and need to be downloaded off the Web. In addition, some plug-ins may work only with specific browsers.

Because developing this type of software requires a large investment in both time and money, most plug-ins are first developed for the more popular browsers, such as Netscape Navigator and Microsoft Internet Explorer, for which the returns are likely to be higher. This has set up a cycle that propagates the dominance of these two companies in this field. Both companies, in their bid to outdo the other, keep making new versions of their software with additional capabilities, and new plug-ins are developed to take advantage of these capabilities, thus perpetuating the cycle. A very large amount of money is being funneled into this technology, and consumers are seeing the benefits, with most of plug-ins being available for free. At the same time, it is easy to be overwhelmed by these changes—and frustrated by one's inability to keep up with them.

To develop common protocols for the evolution of the Web, the World Wide Web Consortium (W3C) was founded in 1994. The W3C is an international industry consortium cohosted by the Massachusetts Institute of Technology Laboratory for Computer Science along with centers in Europe and Asia (77). It is directed by Tim Berners-Lee, the father of the Web. The W3C works to develop standards for the Web so that individuals can see the same content regardless of their operating system and browser.

The rapid increase in Web sites has meant that the information one desires is more likely to be on the Web, but that it also is more difficult to find. In fact, the W3C Web site describes the Internet as ''The universe of network-accessible information, the embodiment of human knowledge.'' To find information on the Internet, a number of search engines are available, and certain sites maintain an updated catalog of Web sites of medical interest available for search. These sites include:

- Medical Matrix (78)
- MedWeb (79)
- Doctor's Guide to the Internet (74)
- Health A to Z (80)
- Wellness Interactive Network (81)
- CliniWeb (82)

Browsers also allow you to set up Web sites as ''bookmarks.'' Using bookmarks, one can quickly visit these Web sites to find medically related material. Another option is to set up one of these sites as the start-up page. Then, every time you start your browser, it will load this page first; thus, that page can be your launching pad to the Information Super-highway.

Another time-saving way of using the Web to gather information is an off-line browser service. This allows your computer to do the work of gathering information while you are out of the office (e.g., seeing patients). Periodically, the offline browser will download information from specified sites on the Web, and it will either display this information on your computer screen or let you browse through it quickly. Pointcast maintains one of the most popular off-line browser services (83). Besides providing daily content on hundreds of topics (e.g., national and international news, sports, weather, finance, the computer and Internet-based industry), it also provides health updates through Reuters and InteliHealth. The updates cover articles from the latest issues of major medical journals, and they include commentaries by physicians working at the Johns Hopkins University or at Reuters. Links to related discussion sites are provided as well. Within a few minutes, one can catch up with all the latest news in the health-care industry.

Some Web sites also let you create a personal page by choosing the kinds of information and topics that interest you. The site then stores this information and displays it in a customized format whenever you log on. Most such services are free at the time of this writing, being funded by revenue from advertisements (84).

The potential of the Internet for medical care and communication has increased tremendously with browser support for various types of file formats on the Web. It is easy to see how audio, video, and images can help in medical education, and it now is possible to hear and view such prerecorded information using the browser. An excellent example of this is the Virtual Hospital site at the University of Iowa (85).

With recent advances in technology, live Internet broadcasts of audio and video also are possible. Live-video technology still needs to improve before it can match what is seen on television (TV), but audio quality can be almost perfect with the right equipment. An example of this technology can be heard on a site maintained by a Cleveland FM radio station (86), which plays live classical music on the Internet. Similarly, an example of live video can be seen at a site that constantly shows surf conditions at the Sebastian Inlet State Park in Florida (87). Both these technologies can be used by the health-care industry. Physicians can provide consultations at a distance (i.e., telemedicine), stay updated with events at a conference without leaving their offices, get CME credits, and so on. Many such sites likely will be available in the near future.

Another area now being developed is interactivity. So far, Web pages have done what they are programmed to do. Based on the link that a viewer clicks, the appropriate file is loaded and displayed. Beyond that, however, it has been very difficult to program a Web page to respond to more complex viewer input, such as allowing a user to move an object on the screen and give an appropriate response based on the final location. Today, however, even this is becoming easier. Both Java, developed by Sun Microsystems, and ActiveX, developed by Microsoft, are two tools that can be used to add interactivity to a Web site. Another program is Shockwave, developed by Macromedia, which works with browsers to view interactive content that has been created by other software from Macromedia. A simple example of how animation and interactivity can be used to teach the pathophysiology of Parkinson's disease can be viewed on the San Diego State University Web site (88). Another sample of interactivity is available on the Cleveland Clinic Web Server (89); this site is still under development but demonstrates how patients with high cholesterol levels can be taught how to eat wisely at restaurants. In the near future, using multimedia and interactivity on the Web may become a feasible alternative for patient education, telemedicine, and aspects of health-care administration.

HTML supports the use of forms and user-entry options such as check boxes and radio buttons. These forms can be used to gather data for surveys, and the data can be collected automatically into databases and later imported into statistical programs for analysis. Because these forms look similar and work in the same manner on any computer or operating system, large, multicenter surveys can be conducted easily. Individual sites participating in a multicenter trial can enter data into a common database using the same Web form, and they can share the information on the database without having to transfer files back and forth. One such form, which is used to collect data on demographics and performance of participants in a CME program, can be viewed on the Cleveland Clinic Web site (90).

CONCERNS AND PROBLEMS WITH THE INTERNET

Many exciting changes are occurring with the Internet, but there are some concerns and difficulties that need to be overcome. These include bandwidth; privacy, security, and confidentiality; overflowing mailboxes; and rogue files.

Bandwidth

Bandwidth is a term that originally was used for the transmission capacity of a cable. It is highest for a fiberoptic cable and lowest for a copper telephone wire. Today, however, this term generally is used to describe the total transmission capability of the Internet. Multimedia files are generally much larger than text, and they can take an excessive amount of time to download. This is a particular problem when using a computer connected to the Internet via a telephone line (called the ''plain old telephone service'' [POTS]).

Currently available modems can transfer data at a speed

Table 73.1. Transmission Speeds on the Internet		
Type of Connection	*Transmission Speed*	*Time to Download a 1-Hour Video*
Modem	14.4–56.0 Kbps	Approximately 145 hours at 28.8 Kbps
ISDN	128 Kbps	Approximately 32 hours
T1	1500 Kbps or 1.5 Mbps	Approximately 2.7 hours
T3	45 Mbps	Approximately 6 minutes

of 14.4 to 56.0 Kilobits per second (Kbps), and Table 73.1 compares the transmission speeds of different types of Internet connections. Most of host computers on the Internet are connected by T1 or T3 links. Data can travel extremely fast on such connections. To get to the viewer, however, who is using a computer at his or her home, data must pass through a modem on the POTS, which acts as a bottleneck. Most homes use copper telephone wires to connect with the Internet, and improving transmission speeds over this type of connection is called the "last-mile problem." Must research is being done to address this issue.

One possibility is using cable TV connections to transmit Internet data. Satellite dishes also can be used to download data from the Internet. The problem with both of these solutions, however, is that the communication is asymmetric. In other words, data can be downloaded, but it is not easy to upload data with currently existing cable TV and satellite systems.

Another issue related to bandwidth is the number of users connected to the Internet who are using the same link, or trying to view the same site, at any particular moment. Most people who "surf" the Web regularly will have noticed that the speed at which data can be downloaded varies with the time of day.

These issues are relevant to use of the Internet by the health-care industry. For the advanced Internet medical applications such as telemedicine and interactive teaching to reach their potential, we need a system that is symmetric and can work uniformly well. Until these issues are adequately addressed, one must develop Internet medical applications from the user's perspective. Another possible solution is use of "streaming," in which data (e.g., an audio file) can be seen and heard while they are still downloading. Thus, users do not need to wait for the entire file to download to begin viewing.

Privacy, Security, and Confidentiality

Privacy, security, and confidentiality are some of the main concerns preventing the medical community from embracing the Internet whole-heartedly. We already have seen how it is possible for hackers to "sniff" e-mail and other data as they pass from node to node on the Internet. To counter this threat,

encryption protocols such as PGP, which still has not been broken despite numerous attempts, have been developed. Secure servers that can handle sensitive information (e.g., patient records, credit-card numbers) also have been developed.

On the Web, secure sites are identified by "https" instead of "http" before the Uniform Resource Locator (URL). In addition, Netscape Navigator indicates secure sites by an intact-key icon, and Microsoft Internet Explorer by a lock icon, at the bottom of the browser window. Data collected securely from Web pages can be stored offline to prevent hackers from accessing it. Medical sites on the Web often include disclaimers that data transmission over the Internet is not secure; one such site at the Stanford Medical Group (91) advises patients not to use the Internet for matters related to human immunodeficiency virus, psychiatric records, and work-related injuries. This last point is particularly important for patients using the Internet at work. Employers generally have the right to view electronic data—such as e-mail—that employees receive at work.

Another problem is that even if an e-mail message itself is encrypted, hackers can find out who is sending the message and to whom it is addressed. This information is contained in a separate part of the e-mail, called the "header," which is not encrypted. There is a solution to this issue, however. A number of sites on the Web act as "remailers," removing the part of the header that indicates the sender of the e-mail. Thus, in essence, you are sending an anonymous message. Alternatively, you can put your own name in the encrypted part of the message so that only the recipient, who has the key to the code, can see it (66).

Overflowing Mailboxes

Physicians may be concerned that patients will flood them with e-mails asking for all kinds of medical information. This may, indeed, happen, but these same patients also have access to physicians' phone numbers. So, why the hesitation in giving out e-mail addresses?

Systems such as "nurse-on-call" can be set up to "triage" all e-mail messages sent to a medical group. The nurse handling the e-mail can decide whether to respond herself or to forward the message to a physician (or the physician's secretary). Patients often are more forthright when using e-mail compared with when they are talking to a stranger on the phone. E-mail inquiries also give the nurse or physician enough time to find the appropriate information and to provide a better response. A permanent record of this encounter also can be maintained and added to the patient's electronic medical record.

Physicians should be careful about the discussion groups and mailing lists to which they subscribe as well. Some of these are very prolific, generating a lot of mail for your inbox. "Spamming" is an Internet colloquialism that means using a mailing list or newsgroup to send the same message to many recipients. This often is used for commercial reasons, and it is frowned upon by the Internet community. Moderators

Table 73.2.   Web Sites of Medical Interest

Medical search sites:
Medical Matrix	http://www.medmatrix.org/
MedWeb	http://www.cc.emory.edu/WHSCL/medweb.html
Doctor's guide to the Internet	http://www.pslgroup.com/medres.htm
Health A to Z	http://www.healthatoz.com/
Wellness Interactive Network	http://www.stayhealthy.com/index.html
CliniWeb	http://www.obsu.edu/cliniweb/

Medical Mega-Sites:
Medical Economics Interactive	http://www.medecinteractive.com/
Physicians' Online	http://www.po.com/ (order special software from this site)
InteliHealth	http://www.intelihealth.com/ih/ihtHome
The Virtual Hospital	http://indy.radiology.uiowa.edu/

Pharmaceutic Reference Sites:
Rxlist	http://www.rxlist.com/
Clinical Pharmacology Online	http://www.cponline.gsm.com/
PDRnet	http://www.pdrnet.com/
Mosby's Physicians' GenRx	http://www.mosby.com/Mosby/PhyGenRx/group.html

Sites with Free MEDLINE:
Avicenna	http://www.avicenna.com/
Healthgate	http://www.healthgate.com/
Medscape	http://www.medscape.com/
PDRnet	http://www.pdrnet.com/
PubMed	http://www4.ncbi.nlm.nih.gov/PubMed/

Patient Education Materials:
InteliHealth	http://www.intelihealth.com/ih/ihtHome
HealthAnswers	https://www.healthanswers.com/health_answers/aafp/conditions_frame.htm
Healthtouch	http://www.healthtouch.com/level1/hi_toc.htm
UCLA Student Health Services	http://www.saonet.ucla.edu/health/healthed/handouts/hndhome.htm

Journals:
Annals of Internal Medicine	http://www.acponline.org/journals/journals.htm
New England Journal of Medicine	http://www.nejm.org/
Journal of the American Medical Association	http://www.ama-assn.org/public/journals/jama/jamahome.htm
British Medical Journal	http://www.bmj.com/bmj/
The Lancet	http://www.thelancet.com/
Canadian Medical Association Journal	http://www.cma.ca/journals/cmai/

Organizations:
American College of Physicians	http://www.acponline.org/
American Medical Association	http://www.ama-assn.org/
Society of General Internal Medicine	http://www.sgim.org/
World Health Organization	http://www.who.ch/
Center for Disease Control	http://www.cdc.gov/
National Institutes of Health	http://www.nih.gov/
Bureau of Primary Health Care	http://www.bphc.hrsa.dhhs.gov/
National Library of Medicine	http://www.nlm.nih.gov/
Agency for Health Care Policy Research	http://www.ahcpr.gov/
National Center for Quality Assurance	http://www.ncqa.org/

Daily Health News Updates:
New York Times	http://nytsyn.com/live/Lead/
InteliHealth	http://www.intelihealth.com/ih/ihtHome
ReutersHealth	http://www.reutershealth.com/

Research Funds Information Sites:
Federal Grants at the National Institutes of Health	http://www.nih.gov
Agency for Health Care Policy and Research	http://www.ahcpr.gov
American Cancer Society	http://www.cancer.org
American Heart Association	http://www.amhrt.org
Nonprofit Organization Listing with hot links	http://fdncenter.org
Philanthropy Links	http://philanthropy-journal.org/plhome/plhome.htm

of discussion groups generally will remove such users from the groups.

Rogue Files

Periodically, concerns are raised about the lack of security regarding certain browsers. As new versions are introduced, they increase the number of types of files that can be viewed and downloaded over the Web. Files that have an interactive content are programmed in languages like Java, and these files sometimes contain software that can read the contents of your hard drive—and even modify those contents. As these security problems are recognized, they are fixed as soon as possible, but with new versions of browsers being introduced at a hectic pace, this potential problem will always be a concern.

One should be careful not to download files from sites that are not well known. A number of established software makers have a digital certificate authenticating their sites. One should look for such certificates before downloading files or viewing interactive content on the Web.

THE FUTURE OF THE INTERNET

The early period of the Internet, before the introduction of HTML, browsers, and the Web has been termed *Internet 1.0.* The present Internet, with the Web is called *Internet 2.0.* The future is called *Internet 3.0.*

It is believed that in the next few years, a general unification of technology will occur, and that this will provide information, entertainment, and communication to consumers through a single medium. The computer, TV, and telephone will merge into one tool, which will be connected to the Information Superhighway. Most households will link with the Internet using this new technology, which will use some of the existing cable TV connections with high bandwidth. This network will be symmetric and global, much like the existing telephone system. Most office applications like word processing, spreadsheets, database tools, and graphic as well as slide packages will integrate seamlessly with the browser. The entire content will be based on HTML and be compatible with all computers and operating systems.

Using these tools, hospitals will be able to place physicians' schedules, laboratory results, education material, and so forth on their computer networks, all of which will be based on the Web standards (i.e., Intranets). Physicians will have browsers on their desktops that can access all this information. Personal pagers, organizers, PDAs, and cellular phones will be combined into one portable, miniaturized product that will meet all of the information and communication needs of physicians.

Some of these changes already are underway. For example, Microsoft, the maker of the Microsoft Internet Explorer browser, has invested in WebTV (a device that allows viewers to use a TVs to connect with the Web), Comcast (a large cable TV company), and MSNBC (a provider of informational content). Other mergers and acquisitions similar to this are underway.

The recent and on-going changes in the health-care industry mean that physicians need to be more efficient, different health-care service providers need to be better organized and integrated, and patients need to be better educated to improve their utilization of resources. Both computers and the Internet are tools that can be used for this purpose. The wheels of change are already in motion, and physicians will need to stay abreast of these changes if they want to succeed in the changing worlds of health care and information and communication technology. Table 73.2 contains the Web (URL) addresses of relevant sites at which pertinent information can be obtained.

REFERENCES

1. Mark Brader. Chronology of digital computing machines (URL http://www.best.com/ ~ wilson/faq/chrono.html).
2. Ken Polsson.Timeline of microcomputers (URL http://www.islandnet.com/ ~ kpolsson/comphist.htm).
3. Robert Hobbes Zakon. Hobbes' Internet timeline (URL http://info.isoc.org/guest/zakon/Internet/History/HIT.html).
4. Daniel P. Dern. Internet timeline (URL http://www.discovery.com/area/history/internet/inet1.html).
5. Mehta NB. Medicine and the Internet: why physicians should pay attention. Cleve Clin J Med 1996;63:315–316.
6. Osheroff JA, ed. Computers in clinical practice. Philadelphia: American College of Physicians Information Technology Series, 1995.
7. Medical Manager Corporation. The Medical Manager Home Page (URL http://www.medicalmanager.com/, 6/10/97).
8. Physician Computer Network (URL http://www.pcn.com, 6/10/97).
9. Physician Micro Systems (URL http://www.pmsi.com/).
10. Computer-based Patient Records Institute. CPRI Home Page (URL http://www.cpri.org/).
11. Dick RS, Steen EB, ed. An essential technology for health care. Washington, D.C.: National Academy Press, 1991 (URL http://www.nap.edu/readingroom/enter2.cgi?MS.html).
12. MedicaLogic. Logician (URL http://www.medicalogic.com/about/logician.html).
13. Turbo-Doc. Welcome to Turbo-doc (URL http://www.jayi.com/sbi/turbodoc/index.html).
14. HBO and Company (URL http://www.hboc.com/).
15. Healthcare Information Systems Directory (URL http://www.health-infosys-dir.com/MedRec.html).
16. National Library of Medicine. NLM's databases and elec-

tronic information sources (URL http://www.nlm.nih.gov/databases/databases.html).

17. National Library of Medicine. Welcome to PubMed (URL http://www.ncbi.nlm.nih.gov/PubMed/).

18. Ovid Technologies Home Page (URL http://www.ovid.com).

19. SilverPlatter Information. SilverPlatter worldwide directory (URL http://www.silverplatter.com).

20. PaperChase. The power of MEDLINE and more (URL http://www.paperchase.com/).

21. Avicenna Systems Corp. Avicenna medical information supersite of the WWW (URL http://www.avicenna.com/).

22. HealthGate Data Corp. Home Page (URL http://www.healthgate.com/).

23. Medscape (URL http://www.medscape.com/)

24. Medical Economics Publications. Welcome to PDRnet (URL http://www.pdrnet.com/).

25. Physicians' Online (URL http://www.po.com/).

26. Research Information Systems (URL http://www.risinc.com/procite/procite.html).

27. Research Information Systems. Reference manager product information (URL http://www.risinc.com/rmprod.html).

28. Niles Software, Inc. (URL http://www.niles.com/).

29. BIOSIS, General medical and miscellaneous software reviews (URL http://www.biosis.org/htmls/reviews/gmm.html#06).

30. Mosby Consumer Health. Iliad at ami-med.com (URL http://www.ami-med.com/ILDTEMP.HTM).

31. Laboratory of Computer Science at Massachusetts General Hospital, MGH Laboratory of Computer Science (URL http://www.lcs.mgh.harvard.edu/).

32. Brenner ES, Webster GD, Shugermann AA, et al. Performance of four computer-based diagnostic systems. N Engl J Med 1994;330:1792–1796.

33. First DataBank, Medical Products (URL http://www.firstdatabank.com/medical products.html).

34. Gold Standard Multimedia, Inc. Clinical pharmacology (URL http://www.gsm.com/products/cp/).

35. Lexi-Comp Home Page (URL http://www.lexi.com/).

36. Medical Economics Company Home Page (URL http://www.medec.com/).

37. Drugdex (URL http://www.mdx.com/pd-ddex.htm).

38. Mosby–Year Book, Inc. Physicians GenRx products (URL http://www.mosby.com/Mosby/PhyGenRx/group.html).

39. The McGraw-Hill Companies, Health Professions Division (URL http://www.mghmedical.com/harrison.htm).

40. Mosby–Year Book, Inc. Mosby's internal medicine multimedia catalog (URL http://www.Mosby.COM/Mosby/Catalogs/MultiMedia/InternalMedicine/).

41. Digital Med, STAT!-Ref CD-ROMs (URL http://www.telemedical.com/ ~ drcarr/Telemedical/Products/teton.html).

42. Gold Standard Multimedia, Inc. Clinical pharmacology online (URL http://www.cponline.gsm.com/).

43. Medical Economics Company, Med Ec Interactive (URL http://www.medecinteractive.com/).

44. Aetna U.S. Healthcare and the Johns Hopkins University Health Systems, Johns Hopkins Health Information (URL http://www.intelihealth.com/ih/ihtHome).

45. Sandow N. RxList—the Internet drug index (URL http://www.rxlist.com/).

46. Clinical Reference Systems, Ltd. Clinical reference systems (URL http://www.patienteducation.com/).

47. Mad Scientist Software. PAIGE—the patient instruction generator (URL http://www.madsci.com/paige/index.htm).

48. First DataBank, AskAdvice (URL http://www.firstdatabank.com/askadvice.html).

49. Medifor (URL http://www2.medifor.com/medifor/).

50. Wave Press, Inc. The Mayo Clinic family health book CD-ROM (URL http://www.healthnet.ivi.com/ivi/ivistore/common/htm/mcfhd.htm).

51. IVI Publishing, Inc. The Mayo Clinic family pharmacist (URL http://www.healthnet.ivi.com/ivi/ivistore/common/htm/pharm.htm).

52. Orbis-AHCN, L.L.C. HealthAnswers: AAFP (URL https://www.healthanswers.com/health answers/aafp/conditions frame.htm).

53. Medical Strategies, Inc. HealthTouch Medical Information: table of contents (URL http://www.healthtouch.com/level1/hi toc.htm).

54. UCLA Student Health Services handouts (URL http://www.saonet.ucla.edu/health/healthed/handouts/hndhome.htm).

55. Challenger Corporation (URL http://www.chall.com/1product.htm).

56. Scientific American Scientific American Marketplace CD-ROMs (URL http://www.sciam.com/marketplace/mrktcdrom.html).

57. Continuing Medical Education Associates (URL http://www.cmea.com/cme/159.html).

58. Mosby–Year Book, Inc. Multimedia: MKSAP 10 Electronic (URL http://www.Mosby.COM/Mosby/Catalogs/MultiMedia/InternalMedicine/0-8151-0718-8.html).

59. SilverPlatter Information. Core curriculum in primary care (URL http://php2.silverplatter.com/physicians/products/ccpc.htm).

60. Mehta N. Cleveland Clinic Foundation (URL http://www.ccf.org/pc/gim/cme/opencme.htm).

61. American Health Consultants (URL http://www.cmeweb.com/).

62. University of Florida Health Science Center. UF continuing medical education learning modules (URL http://www.med.ufl.edu/cme/cme.html).

63. Marshall University School of Medicine. Interactive patient: case #1 (URL http://medicus.marshall.edu/mainmenu.htm).

64. CNET reviews. Comparative reviews: the handheld that rocks the cradle (URL http://www.cnet.com/Content/Reviews/Compare/Handheld/).

65. University Video Communications. Mapping the Internet: a virtual presentation by Gordon Bell (URL http://www.uvc.com/gbell/promo.html).

66. Seattle WebWorks. PGP and remailers made simple using Windows (URL http://www.seattle-webworks.com/pgp/).

67. RSA Data Security (URL http://www.rsa.com/).

68. URL http://www.verisign.com/

69. Carnegie Mellon University (URL ftp://ftp.andrew.cmu.edu/pub/mpack/).

70. ComputerLink Online, Inc. Compression utilities for Windows (URL http://tucows.1st.net/tucows/comp.html).

71. Internet Health Resources. Internet health newsgroups and listserver groups (URL http://www.ihr.com/newsgrp.html).

72. Guided Tour Software, Inc. Newsgroups—the good health web (URL http://www.social.com/health/newsgroups.html).

73. Guided Tour Software, Inc. The good health web—mailing lists (URL http://www.social.com/health/mlists.html).

74. P\S\L Consulting Group, Inc. Doctor's guide to the Internet (URL http://www.pslgroup.com/docguide.htm).

75. Centers for Disease Control and Prevention Home Page (URL http://www.cdc.gov).

76. University of California, Irvine. UCI medical education software archive (URL http://sun3.lib.uci.edu/~sclancy/med-ed/).

77. The World Wide Web Consortium (URL http://www.w3.org/).

78. Healthtel Corporation. Medical Matrix (URL http://www.medmatrix.org/).

79. Emory University Health Sciences Center Library. MedWeb: biomedical internet resources (URL http://www.cc.emory.edu/WHSCL/medweb.html).

80. Medical Network, Inc. Healthatoz—the search engine for health and medicine (URL http://www.healthatoz.com/).

81. Interactive Services, Inc. Welcome to the Wellness Interactive Network (URL http://www.stayhealthy.com/index.html).

82. Oregon Health Sciences University. Cliniweb (URL http://www.ohsu.edu/cliniweb/).

83. PointCast Home Page (URL http://www.pointcast.com).

84. URL http://edit.my.yahoo.com/config/login

85. University of Iowa. Virtual hospital home page (URL http://vh.radiology.uiowa.edu/).

86. WCLV. AudioActive on WCLV! (URL http://www.wclv.com/audio/).

87. URL http://www.ronjons.com/ronjon.htm

88. San Diego State University College of Sciences Instructional Technologies. Parkinson's disease tutorial (URL http://www.sci.sdsu.edu/multimedia/basalgang/).

89. Mehta N. Cleveland Clinic Foundation (URL http://www.ccf.org/pc/gim/trial2.htm).

90. Meha N. Cleveland Clinic Foundation (URL http://www.ccf.org/pc/gim/cme/case 1.htm).

91. Stanford University Medical Center (URL http://www-med.stanford.edu/shs/smg/).

Index

Page numbers in *italics* denote figures; those followed by the letter "t" denote tables.

A

effect on serum triglyceride levels, 491, 496
and intracranial hemodynamics, 532
Antimicrobial therapy, (*see also* Antibiotics)
for pneumonia, 147–148, 148t
Antinuclear antibody test, to diagnose systemic lupus
erythematosus, 305–306
Antiparkinsonian drugs, causing delirium, 102
Antiphospholipid antibodies, to diagnose systemic lupus
erythematosus, 305–306
Antiphospholipid antibody syndrome, 307
Antiphospholipid antibody syndrome and deep venous
thrombosis, 357
Antiphospholipid syndrome and adrenal hemorrhage, 467
Antiplatelet drugs, (*see also specific drugs*)
in membranoproliferative glomerulonephritis, 514
in thrombotic thrombocytopenic purpura, 218
Antipsychotic drugs, (*see also specific drugs*)
causing delirium, 102
in delirium, 72
Antiretroviral drugs, (*see also specific drugs*)
for autoimmune thrombocytopenic purpura and HIV
infection, 219
for HIV, 124–126
and Kaposi's sarcoma, 252
Antithrombin III, for disseminated intravascular
coagulation, 218
Antithrombotic therapy, (*see also* Anticoagulants)
recommendations in atrial fibrillation, 710t
α 1-antitrypsin
augmentation therapy, for chronic obstructive lung
disease, 380
deficiency, 576
and arterial blood gas pattern, 420
and chronic obstructive lung disease (COPD), 378–379
and pulmonary function test results, 418–419
Anxiolytics, for panic attacks, 101
Aortic coarctation, 728, 728t, 758
Aortic regurgitation, 695–696, 757
Aortic stenosis, 693–695, 757
Aortitis, 340, *340,* 346
Aphthae, 84
Aphtoid ulcers, in Crohn's disease, 629
Aplastic anemia, 266
and Parvovirus B19, 156
Arimidex, for breast cancer, 242
Arrhythmias, 700–722, (*see also specific arrhythmias*)
in acute myocardial infarction, 736
bradyarrhythmias, 720–722
in acute myocardial infarction, 737
association with torsades de pointes, 719
atrioventricular block, *721*
atrioventricular dissociation, 720
hypersensitive carotid sinus syndrome, 720
indications for pacing, 721
sinus node dysfunction, 720
and electrocardiography, 759

and hyperkalemia, 538
as a result of pulmonary artery catherization, 406
tachyarrhythmias, 700–720, 702t, *703, 704, 705, 706*
diagnosis, 701–707
mechanisms, 700–701
pharmacologic therapy, 719
supraventricular arrhythmias, 707–717 (*see*
Supraventricular arrhythmias)
ventricular tachyarrhythmias, 717–719 (*see* Ventricular
tachyarrhythmias)
Arrhythmogenic right ventricular dysplasia, 718
Arterial blood gases, in interstitial lung disease, 386
Arterial embolization, for hepatocellular carcinoma, 583
Arterial ligation, for hepatocellular carcinoma, 583
Arteriography, pulmonary
compared with spiral computerized tomography, 359t
to diagnose pulmonary embolisms, 359
Arteritis, temporal, 325
Arthritis
acute monoarticular, 277–286
diagnosis, 277–279
etiology, 277, *278*
gouty arthritis, 279–283
history, 277
physical examination, 277–278, *278*
screening tests, 278–279
septic arthritis, 283–286
acute polyarticular, 290–291
and ankylosing spondylitis, 294
chronic non-erosive synovitis, 294–295
crystal negative, 284
crystal-induced, 281
culture negative, 284
and dermatomyositis, 294–295
due to bacterial endocarditis, 299
due to rubella, 292
due to Salmonella, 293
due to Shigella, 293
due to viral hepatitis, 292–293
due to Yersinia, 293
giant-cell arteritis, 300
gonococcal, 336
diagnosis, 284–285, *285*
gouty, 290–291
treatment, 343, 348
and hemochromatosis, 298
and hypothyroidism, 297–298
infectious
differential diagnosis, 156t
and Parvovirus B19, 156
and inflammatory bowel disease, 294, 630
Lyme disease, 293
and malignancies, 296–297
metabolic arthropathies
treatment, 298–299
microcrystalline, 290, 291–292

C